Patient Care Standards

Collaborative Practice Planning Guides

Patient Care Standards

Collaborative Practice Planning Guides

Susan Martin Tucker, RN, MSN, PHN, CNAA
Patient Care Services Director
Kaiser Permanente Medical Center
Walnut Creek, California

Mary M. Canobbio, RN, MN
Cardiovascular Clinical Specialist
University of California, Los Angeles
Los Angeles, California

Eleanor Vargo Paquette, RN, BS, PHN
Nursing Consultant, Raleigh, North Carolina
    formerly Assistant Director of Education and Training
Kaiser Foundation Health Plan of North Carolina
Raleigh, North Carolina

Marjorie Fyfe Wells, RN, BSN, PHN
Director of Illness Prevention Clinic
Senior Citizen's Guild
Ann Arbor, Michigan

Sixth Edition
with 171 illustrations

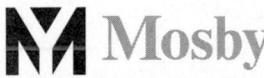 Mosby

St. Louis Baltimore Boston Carlsbad Chicago Naples New York Philadelphia Portland
London Madrid Mexico City Singapore Sydney Tokyo Toronto Wiesbaden

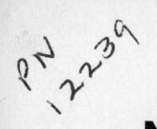 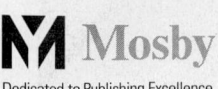

Mosby

Dedicated to Publishing Excellence

A Times Mirror
Company

Vice President and Publisher: Nancy L. Coon
Senior Editor: Susan R. Epstein
Associate Developmental Editor: Laurie K. Muench
Project Manager: Deborah L. Vogel
Production Editor: Jodi Willard
Manuscript Editor: Shepherd, Inc.
Designer: Judi Lang
Manufacturing Supervisor: Betty Richmond

SIXTH EDITION

Copyright © 1996 by Mosby-Year Book, Inc.

Previous editions copyrighted 1975, 1980, 1984, 1988, 1992

Printed in the United States of America
Composition by The Clarinda Company
Printing/binding by Von Hoffmann Press, Inc.

Mosby-Year Book, Inc.
11830 Westline Industrial Drive
St. Louis, Missouri 63146

Library of Congress Cataloging in Publication Data
Patient care standards : collaborative practice planning guides /
 Susan Martin Tucker ... [et al.]. — 6th ed.
 p. cm.
 Includes bibliographical references and index.
 ISBN 0-8151-8856-0 (softbound)
 1. Nursing care plans. 2. Nursing—Standards. I. Tucker, Susan
Martin.
 [DNLM: 1. Nursing Care—standards. 2. Patient Care Planning–
 –standards. WY 100 P297 1996]
 RT49.P38 1996
 610.73'0218—dc20
 DNLM/DLC
 for Library of Congress   95-50439
                                                   CIP

96 97 98 99 00/9 8 7 6 5 4 3 2 1

Contributors

Barbara Boylan-Lewis, RN, BSN, MA

Enterostomal Therapist
St. Joseph Mercy Hospital
Ann Arbor, Michigan

Victor G. Campbell, RN, PhD

Senior Director of Patient
    Care/Director of Education
Columbus Community Hospital
Columbus, Ohio

Donna L. Cramer, RN, BS, BA

Medical-Surgical Nurse Educator
Kaiser Permanente Medical Center
Martinez, California

Roxanna C. Hammer, RN, BA

Staff Nurse-Gynecology
St. Joseph Mercy Hospital
Ann Arbor, Michigan

Cindy Heberlein, RN, ADN

Staff Nurse-Surgical Unit
St. Joseph Mercy Hospital
Ann Arbor, Michigan

Marcia M. Hegstad, RN, MN, CS, CDE

Outpatient Education
St. Joseph Mercy Hospital
Ann Arbor, Michigan

Bonni Horwitz, RNC, MSN

Nursing Coordinator
Hartford Hospital
Hartford, Connecticut

Judy Kaye, RN, MSN, ARNP, CCRN, CS

Clinical Nurse Specialist/Adult Nurse Practitioner
University Hospital
Augusta, Georgia

Teresa Choate Loriaux, RN, MSN

Managing Editor
The Endocrinologist
West Linn, Oregon

John Novak, RPh, BSPh

Cancer Center
St. Joseph Mercy Hospital
Ann Arbor, Michigan

Laura S. Rogers, RN, BSN

Staff Nurse-Gynecology
St. Joseph Mercy Hospital
Ann Arbor, Michigan

Kathleen Rice Simpson, MSN, RNC

Perinatal Clinical Nurse Specialist, St. John's Mercy Medical Center
Adjunct Clinical Professor, Barnes College of Nursing at the University of Missouri
St. Louis, Missouri

Ellen Whalen, RN, BS, MS, CNA, CCRN

Director, Medical Nursing/Home Health Services
USC University Hospital
Los Angeles, California

Reviewers

Judith Albers, RN
Staff Nurse
Deaconess Hospital
  Central-Rehabilitation
St. Louis, Missouri

Lynn W. Andrews, BSN, MSN, RNC
Clinical Assistant Professor
St. Mary's School of Nursing
Huntington, West Virginia

Sarah E. Angermuller, RN, MSN,
  MEd, CCRN, CNRN, CEN, TNCC
Associate Professor
Columbus College
Columbus, Georgia

Jan Treston Aurand, RN, MSN
Infection Control Practitioner
St. Joseph Mercy Hospital
Ann Arbor, Michigan

Patricia L. Baker, RN, MS
Quality Specialist/Nursing
St. Joseph Mercy Hospital
Ann Arbor, Michigan

Patricia Bates, RN, BSN, CURN
Staff Nurse-Urology
Kaiser Permanente Medical Clinic
Portland, Oregon

Patricia Carter, RN, MSN, AOCN
Clinic Manager-Infusion Center
Texas Oncology, PA
El Paso, Texas

Patricia Dettenmeier, MSN(R),
  CCRN
Asst. Clinical Professor of
  Nursing/Instructor in Medicine
St. Louis University-Health
  Sciences Center
St. Louis, Missouri

Susan W. Donckers, RN, EdD, CS,
  FNP
Family Nurse Practitioner, Internal
  Medicine
Lewis Gale Clinic
Salem, Virginia

Emily Drake, MSN, RNC
Clinical Instructor
University of Virginia School of
  Nursing
Charlottesville, Virginia

Ellen Stoetzner Duke, RN, MSN,
  CCRN
Instructor of Nursing
Angelina Community College
Lufkin, Texas

Sheila A. Dunn, RN, MSN, ANP
Clinical Instructor-School of Nursing
St. Louis University
St. Louis, Missouri

Kristen L. Easton, RN, MS, CRRN
Assistant Professor of Nursing
Valparaiso University-College
  of Nursing
Valparaiso, Indiana

Frances C. Gaskin, RN, PhD
President and CEO
Frances Christian Gaskin, Inc.
Albany, New York

Bette B. Hammond, RN, BSN, MSN
Assistant Professor
St. Charles County Community College
St. Peters, Missouri

Judy Kaye, RN, MSN, ARNP, CCRN, CS
Clinical Nurse Specialist/Adult Nurse Practitioner
University Hospital
Augusta, Georgia

Patricia T. Ketcham, RN, BSN, MSN
Adjunct Asst. Professor/Manager, Learning Resource
  Laboratory
Oakland University School of Nursing
Rochester, Michigan

Kathleen J. Lauwers, RN, MSN
Director of Nursing Practice
  Services
St. Joseph Mercy Hospital
Ann Arbor, Michigan

Cheryl L. Pratt, RN, BSN, MA
Nursing Instructor
Rochester Community College
Rochester, Minnesota

Joanne Santangelo, RN, MSN
Family Nurse Practitioner
University of California-San Diego
San Diego, California

June Thompson, RN, DrPH
Epidemiologist, New Mexico Department of Health
Staff Nurse, University of New Mexico Health Sciences
  Center Hospital
Albuquerque, New Mexico

Golden Tradewell, RN, MSN
Assistant Professor
McNeese State University-College of Nursing
Lake Charles, Louisiana

Catherine A. Ultrino, RN, MSN, OCN
Administrative Coordinator-School of Practical Nursing
Youville Hospital and Rehabilitation Center
Cambridge, Massachusetts

Rose Wagner, RN, MSN
Inpatient Psychiatric Services Manager
Kaiser Foundation Hospital
Martinez, California

Pamela Becker Weilitz, RN, MSN(R), CS
Manager, Nursing Care Delivery
Barnes and Jewish Hospitals
St. Louis, Missouri

Laurel A. Wiersema, RN, BA, BSN, MSN, CS
Clinical Nurse Specialist
Barnes Hospital at Washington University Medical
  Center
St. Louis, Missouri

Linda M. Wray, RN, BSN, MSN
Assistant Professor-Department of Baccalaureate
  Nursing
Eastern Kentucky University
Richmond, Kentucky

Preface

When the first edition of *Patient Care Standards* was published some 20 years ago, the hospital was the center of the health care system. That is no longer true. The focus of health care has become a continuum of care that includes the outpatient or ambulatory setting, and inpatient hospitalization is but a blip on that continuum. Improvements in technology, such as the increase in laser techniques, laparoscopic and endoscopic procedures, and an ever-changing payment/reimbursement system have all contributed to the shift in the focus of health care. Patient care has changed. The average length of stay is down and acuity is up on the general medical-surgical units. Conditions such as Adult Respiratory Distress Syndrome went undiagnosed many years ago. Now it is routinely recognized and managed in critical care units across the nation. What was once in the critical care units is now commonplace on the medical-surgical units, and what was on those units in the past is now being successfully managed in the home. There has been a proliferation of short-stay units, same-day surgeries, and an increased reliance on home health agencies and staff for home care needs.

What does all this mean to the practicing nurse? The role of the nurse has changed from a directive to a participative approach, where the patient becomes a partner in the process of care provided by a multidisciplinary health care team. Nurses have become information brokers in sharing knowledge and information with patients. Many years ago it was considered highly inappropriate for nurses to divulge to patients the types of medications that they were receiving. Now it is imperative that patients become knowledgeable about their plan of care so they can be partners in the creation of the plan, develop mutually agreed upon goals with the health care team, understand the nature of their condition or procedures performed, and learn to self-manage after discharge from the inpatient setting. The role of the nurse is directed toward achieving desired patient outcomes including improvements in bio-psychosocial health status, knowledge of self-care management, and engagement in the therapeutic treatment regimen as created by the multidisciplinary health care team in a collaborative manner with the patient as a partner in the entire process.

Patient Care Standards can be used by the bedside nurse for planning and implementing care of the hospitalized patient as well as by the primary nurse, case manager, charge nurse, team leader, and clinical nurse specialist. The nursing administrator, nurse manager, or quality performance improvement staff can use these standards as the basis for evaluating the provision of care and patient outcomes and identifying opportunities for improvement. Student nurses learning the nursing process and patient care planning will find these standards invaluable as a ready reference with instant information and rationales as to the plan of care. These standards will be and have been useful to nurses working within the continuum of care from the physician's office, the multidisciplinary health care provider's office, home health agencies, skilled nursing facilities, public health nurses, and extended care facility staff by building upon the patient teaching and plan of care, especially for patients with chronic conditions. Discharge planners, case managers, utilization managers, quality professionals, patient educators, and ambulatory care professionals will find these standards helpful in evaluating and promoting a seamless approach to patient care based on consistency and continuity of care across all health care settings.

Patient Care Standards has been extensively revised to address the myriad of changes in health care. New sections on **Patient/Family Teaching and Home Care Considerations** have been added. Most nursing interventions are accompanied by rationales which are highlighted in italics. These rationales are designed to help both students and patients understand specific components of the plan of care. **Assessment** is divided into **Subjective** and **Objective** components to facilitate the data collection process. **Collaborative Management** includes **Therapeutic Management,** which addresses non-nursing health care providers, and **Nursing Management,** which discusses interventions appropriate to the **Patient Problem/Nursing Diagnosis.** The interventions presented include independent (within the scope of professional registered nursing practice), interdependent (performed interdependently with other health care disciplines), and dependent nursing actions (based on physician order). New standards include Domestic Violence, which reflects the increasing awareness in today's society of factors that may implicate and/or complicate the patient's status.

Organization

The first chapter of the book provides guidelines for the planning of patient care and demonstrates the use of this book as an as-is, single source of patient care planning guides, or as a tool for the creation of a multidisciplinary time line plan of care known by several names including care paths, care tracks, and critical paths. Examples of these are provided at the end of most chapters to demonstrate the variety of formats in use. The second chapter of the book includes specific North American Nursing Diagnosis Association (NANDA) nursing diagnoses and care for physiologic and psychobehavioral patterns as well as some general care standards that relate to patients with special needs and special equipment. The subsequent chapters are divided into body systems, and the related standards are preceded by an extensive assessment tool, which includes Gerontologic Considerations. The following describes the components of the standards.

● Title

The medical condition, surgical intervention, procedure, or pharmacological agent that is the basis for the standard is identified.

● Definition

A brief description of the condition, surgical procedure, disease, or condition is given.

● Assessment

Subjective

Descriptive terms used by patients are listed and are based on the patient's perception.

Objective

Observable signs and symptoms are listed from the viewpoint of the nurse or health care provider.

Diagnostic tests

Condition-appropriate tests and studies are identified as well as some laboratory values.

Potential complications

Potential condition/procedure-related complications are identified. Nursing interventions are directed toward preventing these complications.

● Collaborative Management

This section includes the *Therapeutic Management* as provided by non-nursing multidisciplinary health care providers and *Nursing Management* with a continuation of the utilization of the nursing process.

● Patient Problems/Nursing Diagnoses

Problems and diagnoses are listed in a priority sequence and are those most commonly associated with the condition. They are related to the etiologies or other factors from the assessment data to assist the nurse in understanding the reason or rationale for performing the intervention. Although the rationale for each of the interventions is directed toward reducing, correcting, or eliminating the patient problem or nursing diagnosis, there are many intervention-specific rationales provided that are italicized. This is important to the student population but also serves to support the practicing nurse in providing explanations to the patient for the purpose of the intervention.

● Expected Outcomes

This section serves three purposes as goals, expectations, and an evaluation. Worded prospectively, these phrases are goals for the patient. They are expected outcomes and, in addition, provide an evaluation upon which the success of the interventions can be measured through quality/performance improvement activities.

● Additional Nursing Diagnoses to Consider

This list includes problems or diagnoses that the nurse should keep in mind as they are possible, but not highly probable.

● Patient/Family Teaching

This section provides the educational component, which is a nurse-sensitive indicator of the success of the patient's outcome. The patient and/or family should be able to articulate the information and understand their role in engaging or complying with the plan for continuing care in the outpatient setting. The reiteration of information learned by the patient and family is important and indicates that they know something about the patient's condition and plan of care. But mere possession of information does not necessarily mean that it will be used appropriately. (Consider the diabetic patient with multisystem deterioration who correctly articulates all there is to know about diabetes but who demonstrates lack of compliance or engagement in care as reflected by the pounds of chocolates consumed daily!) It is critical to determine if the patient and family plan to engage in the plan of care. This can only be determined by dialogue as to intent when the patient is hospitalized. Follow-up may be indicated to determine the patient's engagement in care by post-discharge phone calls or home health visits as necessary.

● Home Care Considerations

These are factors that the nurse should consider to help the patient get ready for going home. These could include things to anticipate at home or potential problems that might be encountered, such as stairs, privacy, a place to store dressings or supplies, security, and telephone access. In addition, community service agencies may be identified for further support.

Patient Care Standards is provided to promote consistency and continuity of quality care by the multidisciplinary health care team across the continuum of care. The key to success is in partnering with the patient and family for quality outcomes by all health care providers as a "team". . . together each achieves more!

Susan Martin Tucker
Mary M. Canobbio
Eleanor Vargo Paquette
Marjorie Fyfe Wells

Contents

Patient
Care
Standards

Collaborative
Practice
Planning Guides

Introduction: A Guide for Collaborative Practice

Patient care standards are guides for collaborative practice representing the predicted care requirements for patients. They are based on an analytical and problem-solving sequence of assessment, planning, intervention, and evaluation. Expected outcomes, patient/family teaching, and home care considerations are delineated. At one time planning for patient care was done exclusively by nurses based on requirements and standards of licensing and accrediting bodies and taught in the curriculum of nursing education programs. The nursing process (assessment, diagnosis, planning, intervention, and evaluation) has been successfully used by nurses to plan patient care for years. Now that patient care is more patient centered or focused, and because patients and their families/significant others are involved as partners in the planning and often the provision of patient care, it has become imperative to provide a more collaborative approach to the planning of care.

The goal of patient care is to provide individualized, planned, and appropriate care in settings that support the patient's care, treatment, rehabilitation goals, and specific needs. The patient's individualized plan of care must be consistent with the medical plan for care, as well as the therapeutic plans of care by other disciplines. Patient care standards focus on the recipient of care, the patient, and provide the framework for effecting multidisciplinary care.

Many healthcare organizations use published references, such as *Patient Care Standards,* on each patient care unit for guiding patient care planning. Others create their own institution-specific plans of care for their patients via preprinted care plans or computer-based online plans of care. The requirements and standards of licensing and accrediting bodies such as the Joint Commission on Accreditation of Healthcare Organizations (JCAHO) accept a variety of means for patient care planning. The JCAHO does not prescribe any particular format for the planning of care but evaluates compliance with the standards of the *Accreditation Manual for Hospitals* based on the scoring guidelines. A clear understanding of the standard, associated intent language and scoring guidelines is all that is necessary to ensure that the patient care planning of the institution is congruent with JCAHO standards.

Many inpatient facilities in the mid-1980s began using a timeline-based care plan. Initially these guidelines were focused on the care provided or directed by physicians and other healthcare providers. These critical paths or maps contained many aspects of nursing care and sometimes replaced nursing care plans. The initial focus of the timeline plan of care was to address variations in the patient's length of stay caused by a new reimbursement methodology from the Health Care Financing Administration (HCFA) for Medicare patients. Essentially a fixed amount of money would be reimbursed to a facility based on a patient's particular Diagnostic Related Category (DRG) and not based on the patient's actual length of stay, which had been a past practice. Facilities quickly learned that there were significant variations in practices in their institutions and they could easily lose revenues if patients were staying longer than the expected DRG time frame. The timeline care paths or plans provided a guide to ensure consistency in practice within the designated time frame allotted per DRG. Significant achievements were made in the controlling of healthcare costs but, interestingly, various disciplines also had learned to cooperate with one another in a more collaborative patient-centered manner. All disciplines could look at one document to track the patient's progression across the timeline care path as opposed to reviewing each provider's notes contained in different places in the medical record. In addition to the document being patient centered, it was multidisciplinary and ensured congruity of all the disciplines' therapies.

Critical paths, care paths, and clinical maps have provided a more consistent timeline methodology to plan for patient care. The timeline is viewed from left to right and divided into days, periods, or hours depending on the condition or diagnosis. Variation exists among institutions in the categories of care that are delineated across the course of time. The content of *Patient Care Standards* can be used to create a timeline care path by denoting the particular assessment, diagnosis, intervention, and expected outcomes in the appropriate category identified by the institution. A variety of timeline care paths are provided as examples to the user of *Patient Care Standards* in this chapter, as well as in most of the other chapters. There is no right or wrong means to the development and use of timeline care paths. Variations in format will and should occur in different institutions in order to meet the particular needs of patients and multidisciplinary providers of care in a particular facility.

It is important for any institution creating timeline care paths to list the items that are important to include, and the examples herein should provide a springboard for discussion of these items. Chart reviews of the past several patients with a particular diagnosis (DRG) may be helpful if there is no consensus as to when an activity should occur. Significant learning can be gleaned from plotting out the activities in a timeline format on the same diagnosis of multiple patients, especially when managed by multiple providers. Physicians and other healthcare providers are often surprised at the differences in managing the same type of condition, and this data-driven approach is more objective than unsupported subjective comments as to the appropriate time frame for the management of patient care.

In summary, the strides being made in providing a multidisciplinary approach to patient-centered care can only enhance the well-being of the population and better use our precious and limited resources. *Patient Care Standards* is a guide for collaborative practice whether used exclusively or as a source for creating a multidisciplinary timeline plan of care.

DIAGNOSIS ___ Glioma

SURGERY ___ CRANIOTOMY FOR RESECTION OF TUMOR

USC UNIVERSITY HOSPITAL
1500 San Pablo
Los Angeles, CA 90033 ©1991

NAME ___
ALLERGIES ___

SIDE 1

MULTIDISCIPLINARY PLAN

ADMIT DATE ___

DRG _001_ ALOS _14.7_

DISCHARGE OUTCOMES

PHYSIOLOGICAL: ADLs will be met by self or c̄ assistance of others(s). Complications/injury will be prevented or minimized, discomfort relieved/controlled, and infectious process(es) resolving/absent.

COGNITIVE: Verbalizes disease process/prognosis and therapeutic regimen. Will be able to explain surgical care, verbalizes precautions to take for medication use, and state s/sx to report to the health care team.

PSYCHOLOGICAL: Verbalizes acceptance of potential lifestyle changes and incorporates them into ADLs. Able to verbalize fears/anxieties and demonstrate effective coping mechanisms. Able to participate in self-care decisions.

DISCIPLINE	PRE-OP/PRE-ADMIT DAY 1 DATE ___	DOS DAY 2 DATE ___	POD #1 DAY 3 DATE ___	POD #2 DAY 4 DATE ___	POD #3 DAY 5 DATE ___	POD #4 DAY 6 DATE ___
LOCATION	MED/SURG	SURGERY/PAR/NSICU	NSICU→DOU	DOU	DOU→MED/SURG	MED/SURG
LABS	Chem 20, CBC, PT, PTT, UA, T & screen 2u PRBCS, Antiepileptic drug levels	Chem 20 ⟩ on arrival to unit, CBC	Lytes, WBC	Lytes, WBC, Antiepileptic drug levels		
CARDIO-PULMONARY	ECG: R/O Arrhythmia	Pulse oximetry, O₂ 40% face mask, I.S. q 1° W/A, A-line	DC A-line, DC face mask & pulse oximetry	Encourage I.S. q 1° W/A		
IMAGING/NUCLEAR MEDICINE	CXR: 2 Views	MRI c̄/s̄ contrast in am pre-op				
SOCIAL SERVICES D/C PLAN REHAB. SERVICES	Social services consult		Assess need for OT/PT/speech evaluation	Assess need for rehab evaluation	Assess need for home health evaluation	Ordered therapies to assess pt D/C needs
PHARMACY	S.L. Corticosteroids, antiepileptics, H₂ Antagonist	Antiepileptics IV/po, IV fluids, Corticosteroids IV/po, H₂ Antagonist IV/po, Antiemetic, Analgesics, Antibiotics x 24°	Convert IV to S.L. if tolerating po's	Taper corticosteroids		DC S.L., DC H₂ antagonist p̄ corticosteroids DC'ed
DIETARY/NUTRITION	Regular diet, NPO p̄ midnight	NPO: ice chips when fully awake	Advance diet as tolerated			Regular diet

Continued.

PATIENT NAME: _____

MULTIDISCIPLINARY PLAN

DISCIPLINE	PRE-OP/PRE-ADMIT	DAY 1 DATE___	DOS DAY 2 DATE___	POD #1 DAY 3 DATE___	POD #2 DAY 4 DATE___	POD #3 DAY 5 DATE___	POD #4 DAY 6 DATE___
PATIENT ACTIVITY	Ad lib		BR c̄ HOB ↑30° Leg squeezers (begun in OR)	OOB to chair	Ambulate c̄ assistance TID	DC leg squeezers Ambulate as much as tolerated	
EDUCATION		I.S. instruction CDB Teach reason for surgery, postop restrictions, & expected LOS Orient to room, unit, & hospital routine	Reorient to present unit Teach monitoring of dressing & drainage Discuss need for foley	DC foley I & O cath q 6° prn	Review disease process, prognosis, and understanding of therapeutic regimen during hospitalization		Teach s/sx to report to the health care team Instruct pt in care of surgical site Pharmacy to educate pt on D/C medications

COLLABORATIVE PROBLEMS

DATE		DATE		DATE INIT
❶ Anxiety/fear R/T surgery, change in health status, & terminal illness.		❼ Knowledge deficit R/T lack of exposure to hospital, misinterpretation of information received, or limitation of cognitive ability; discharge planning.		
❷ Potential for altered cerebral tissue perfusion R/T cerebral edema altering or interrupting cerebral blood flow.		❽ Denial R/T severity of diagnosis; terminal illness.		
❸ Potential for injury R/T seizure activity, weakness, paralysis, paresthesia.				
❹ Potential for impaired physical mobility R/T neuromuscular impairment & strength, perceptual/cognitive impairment, pain, or restriction in activity.				
❺ Potential for infection R/T suppressed inflammatory response, medication induced, or exposure to pathogens.				
❻ Alteration in comfort R/T headache &/or surgical procedure.				

OUTCOMES

❶ Will acknowledge and discuss fears. Reports anxiety reduction to a manageable level.	❷ Maintains usual or improved level of consciousness and motor/sensory function.	❺ Demonstrates timely healing free from infection. Afebrile.	❺ Continues to demonstrate healing free from infectious spread.
	❸ Seizures controlled, free from injury during hospitalization.	❻ Verbalizes pain control c̄ ordered medication. Able to sleep/rest.	❻ Verbalizes pain control c̄ po medication.
		❼ Verbalizes understanding of condition/disease process.	❼ Verbalizes understanding of D/C plans.
		❹ Regains and maintains optimal physical mobility.	❼ Able to correctly perform procedures necessary.	❽ Pt & S/O verbalize understanding of treatment plan and begin to show signs of acceptance.

KEY

❶ To initiate a problem or intervention, document under corresponding date.

❷ Document outcomes under appropriate date for achieving the goal.

❸ To discontinue an intervention or resolve a patient problem highlight, date, and initial.

PLAN OF CARE DISCUSSED WITH	DAY 1 DATE	DOS DAY 2 DATE	POD #1 DAY 3 DATE	POD #2 DAY 4 DATE	POD #3 DAY 5 DATE	POD #4 DAY 6 DATE
INITIAL / S.O. / Pt. / DATE			INTERVENTIONS			
	– Assess pt and/or S/O level of anxiety – Answer questions & explain all procedures before initiation – Clarify misunderstanding of info & involve pt & S/O in decision making, care planning & evaluation – Assess baseline neurological status	– Assess neurological status per MD order, report changes to MD – Strict I & O – Monitor temp per routine – Monitor respiratory status – Reposition frequently & encourage use of I.S. – Evaluate for s/sx of ↑ ICP: • decreased response to stimuli • changes in VS	– Increase activity & participation in ADLs – Encourage S/O to assist c̄ increased activity – Assess for need of stool softener – Assess pt & S/O understanding of disease process, prognosis, & therapeutic regimen – Continue use of I.S. – Temperature elevation may indicate meningitis	– Reassess pt and/or S/O level of anxiety – Support planning of a realistic lifestyle p̄ hospitalization within limitations but fully using capabilities – Explore sources of support: • S/O • Clergy – Social worker – Encourage use of oral pain medications	– DC leg squeezers once pt fully ambulatory – Reassess need for stool softener – Encourage increased activity – Allow pt time to adjust to illness – Solicit help from S/O's, clergy during denial	– Instruct in showering technique – Teach s/sx to report to health care team • changes in vision • elevated temperature • intense headache • drainage from surgical site – Teach pt how to care for surgical site: • avoid scrubbing • dab very dry • keep hair off of wound x 72°
Case Manager:		• restlessness • weakness/paralysis of extremities • changes in vision or pupillary changes • worsening of headache	– Monitor for CSF leakage – Assess for factors that impair physical mobility: • pain/nausea • dislodging tubes • compromising surgical wound	– Assess need for home health evaluation & outpatient therapies		• avoid sun exposure • OK to shampoo hair p̄ staples out x 24°
Consulting MD:		– If pt has headache, reduce bright lights & room noises if possible – Medicate for pain as ordered & assess pain relief – Note location, intensity & duration of pain	– Treat those items present above &/or educate pt prn – Assure pt that activity ordered will enhance rather than compromise healing process	– Continue to monitor for CSF leakage		• keep clean & dry x 72° p̄ staples out – Instruct pt & S/O regarding discharge medications including name, purpose, route, dosage, frequency, time of administration, and side effects
Social Service		– Provide info to pt & S/O in short segments – Discuss expected length of recovery – Assess pt ability to swallow before advancing diet	– Provide praise and encouragement for all efforts to ↑ mobility – Reinforce need for assistance when getting OOB – Provide pt c̄ safe environment; seizure precautions may be indicated – Assess respiratory status, neurological status & VS per unit routine p̄ transfer			
Anointing of The Sick Date: _____						

MULTIDISCIPLINARY PLAN UPDATE

DATE	SIGNATURES	DATE	SIGNATURES	DATE	SIGNATURES

Continued.

DIAGNOSIS ___Glioma___

SURGERY _CRANIOTOMY FOR RESECTION OF TUMOR_

NAME _____

ALLERGIES _____

USC UNIVERSITY HOSPITAL
1500 San Pablo
Los Angeles, CA 90033   ©1991

SIDE 2   **MULTIDISCIPLINARY PLAN**

ADMIT DATE _____

DISCHARGE OUTCOMES	DRG _001_ ALOS _14.7_						
PHYSIOLOGICAL	ADLs will be met by self or c assistance of other(s). Complications/injury will be prevented or minimized, discomfort relieved/controlled, and infectious process(es) resolving/absent.						
COGNITIVE	Verbalizes disease process/prognosis and therapeutic regimen. Will be able to explain surgical care, verbalize precautions to take for medication use, and state s/sx to report to the health care team.						
PSYCHOLOGICAL	Verbalizes acceptance of potential lifestyle changes and incorporates them into ADLs. Able to verbalize fears/anxieties and demonstrate effective coping mechanisms. Able to participate in self-care decisions.						
DISCIPLINE	PRE-OP/ PRE-ADMIT	POD #5 DAY 7 DATE____	POD #6 DAY 8 DATE____	POD #7 DAY 9 DATE____	POD #8 DAY 10 DATE____	POD #9 DAY 11 DATE____	POD #10 DAY 12 DATE____
LOCATION		MED/SURG→HOME					
LABS							
CARDIO-PULMONARY							
IMAGING/ NUCLEAR MEDICINE							
SOCIAL SERVICES D/C PLAN REHAB. SERVICES							
PHARMACY		DC c̄ po pain medications & antiepileptic therapy					
DIETARY/ NUTRITION		Regular diet					

MULTIDISCIPLINARY PLAN

PATIENT NAME:

DISCIPLINE	PRE-OP/ PRE-ADMIT	POD #5 DAY 7 DATE___	POD #6 DAY 8 DATE___	POD #7 DAY 9 DATE___	POD #8 DAY 10 DATE___	POD #9 DAY 11 DATE___	POD #10 DAY 12 DATE___
PATIENT ACTIVITY		Ad lib					
EDUCATION		DC teaching: • staples to be removed 7-10 days post-op • shower instructions • staples may be wet • towel dry thoroughly p̄ showering					

COLLABORATIVE PROBLEMS

DATE		DATE	
	❼ Knowledge deficit R/T lack of exposure to hospital, misinterpretation of information received, or limitation of cognitive ability; discharge planning.		

OUTCOMES

❼ Verbalizes understanding of D/C plans	

KEY _____

❶ To initiate a problem or intervention, document under corresponding date.

❷ Document outcomes under appropriate date for achieving the goal.

❸ To discontinue an intervention or resolve a patient problem highlight, date, and initial.

Continued.

PLAN OF CARE DISCUSSED WITH		POD #5 DAY 7 DATE ___	POD #6 DAY 8 DATE ___	POD #7 DAY 9 DATE ___	POD #8 DAY 10 DATE ___	POD #9 DAY 11 DATE ___	POD #10 DAY 12 DATE ___
DATE	INITIAL S.O. Pt.	INTERVENTIONS					
		– Explain safety precautions to maintain at home: continue to monitor for CSF leak					
		– Reinforce those s/sx that need to be reported to the health care team					
		– Encourage tips for recovery: • return to normal social & physical activity					
		• verbalization of concerns c̄ health care team • emphasize the importance of ongoing outpatient care & follow-up visits					
		– Review those medications pt will take at home					
Case Manager: ___							
Consulting MD: ___							
Social Service ___							
Anointing of The Sick Date: ___							

MULTIDISCIPLINARY PLAN UPDATE

DATE	SIGNATURES	DATE	SIGNATURES	DATE	SIGNATURES

Interdisciplinary Care Path:

UNCOMPLICATED MI CARE PATH

Expected Length of Stay: 4.5

This Plan of Care has been discussed with patient/significant other. Date: _____
Signature: _____, RN
If discussed with someone other than the patient, specify.
Name: _____ Relationship _____
If "NA," explain: _____

Addressograph

Patient Care Problems	Patient Outcomes	INTERVENT					
		Date: Emergency Dept.	Date: Day 1	Date: Day 2	Date: Day 3	Date: Day 4	Date: D/C
1. Alteration in comfort related to anginal pain/myocardial hypoxia.	1. The patient will report pain level of 0 on a scale of 0-10. Date: _____ *If not achieved, a narrative note must be written.*	— BR — O₂ — Cardiac monitor — IV access — RN cardiac assessment — Discuss plan of care	— BR — O₂ — ASA — NTG SL ordered — MS IV ordered — Cardiac monitoring — IV access — RN cardiac assessment — Obtain rhythm strip — Assess CP q4 hrs Scale 0-10	— BR with BRP — O₂ — Cardiac Monitoring — IV access — RN cardiac assessment — Obtain rhythm strip — Assess CP q4 hrs Scale 0-10	— Ambulate — DC O₂ — Telemetry Monitoring — RN cardiac assessment — Obtain rhythm strip — Assess CP q4 hrs Scale 0-10	— Ambulate — DC Telemetry Monitoring — O₂ — RN cardiac assessment — Obtain rhythm strip — Assess CP q4 hrs Scale 0-10	— DC Saline Lock
2. Alteration in tissue perfusion related to cardiac ischemia/damage and dysrhythmia.	2. The patient will be hemodynamically stable with a MAP≥60. Date: _____ *If not achieved, a narrative note must be written.*	— ECG — CXR — CBC — LYTES	— CPK#1 with ISOS on admission — CPK#2 8 hours after admission — CPK#3 16 hours after admission — Continue CPK every 8 hours until CPK is normal	— ECG	— ECG	— ECG	

INSTRUCTIONS FOR USE:
Initial if intervention initiated
Leave blank if intervention not initiated
Write NA if intervention not applicable

If the intervention is not initiated within 24 hours, document a narrative note. A narrative note is not required for NA (not applicable).

Staff assures that the care path is reviewed and variances are documented.

Discharge to: Home □ SNF □ HH □ SOC □
Date: _____
Time: _____
SOC: _____

Used by permission of Kaiser Permanente Medical Center, Kaiser Foundation Hospital, Martinez, California.

Continued.

INTERVENTIONS

Patient Care Problems	Patient Outcomes	Emergency Dept. Date:	Day 1 Date:	Day 2 Date:	Day 3 Date:	Day 4 Date:	D/C Date:
2. continued					— Chest pain ☐ None ☐ Relieved with medication ☐ ECG done with persistent chest pain ETT ☐ Scheduled ☐ Not indicated ☐ Not available	— Chest pain ☐ None ☐ Relieved with medication ☐ ECG done with persistent chest pain ETT ☐ Scheduled ☐ Not indicated ☐ Not available	
			— Chest pain ☐ None ☐ Relieved with medication ☐ ECG done with persistent chest pain	— Chest pain ☐ None ☐ Relieved with medication ☐ ECG done with persistent chest pain			
3. Knowledge deficit related to disease process, prescribed regimen, and diagnostic tests.	3. The patient/ significant other will communicate understanding of diet, activity, and disease process. ___ Date: _____ *If not achieved, a narrative note must be written.* 4. The patient will be provided with referrals, resources, and teaching. ___ Date: _____ *If not achieved, a narrative note must be written.*		— Discuss Plan of care with patient and/or family. — Assessment of discharge needs. — Patient copy of care path given to patient and/ or family.	— Implement cardiac patient learning checklist — Review patient copy of care path with patient and/or family — Give patient An Active Partnership for the Health of Your Heart book	— Continue patient learning checklist with patient and/ or family.	— Continue patient learning checklist with patient and/ or family.	— Complete patient learning checklist — Review discharge instructions — Review discharge medication — Schedule return appointment — Give patient copy of discharge instructions

| | | GRASP: 8 am-4 pm _____ | GRASP: 8 am-4 pm _____ | GRASP: 8 am-4 pm _____ | GRASP: 8 am-4 pm _____ | GRASP: 8 am-4 pm _____ | GRASP: 8 am-4 pm _____ |

Emergency Dept.		Admission Shift		#2 Shift		#3 Shift		DC	
INIT	PRINT NAME	TITLE	INIT	PRINT NAME	TITLE	INIT	PRINT NAME	TITLE	INIT	PRINT NAME	TITLE

All assigned registered nurses are responsible to update/review and sign the patient care path each shift.

* 6/94 This care path is to be used as a guideline only and does not necessarily imply a standard of care.

PATIENT STANDARD OF CARE
Chest Pain

1. We will make a plan of care to meet your basic care needs.
2. It is important that you and your family let us know about any questions or concerns.
3. We will provide a safe and clean environment.
4. We will help you understand your condition and treatments.
5. You will be asked to participate in your care.
6. We will help you plan for your continued care.

PATIENT CARE ISSUES	WHAT WE WILL DO	WHAT YOU CAN DO	EXPECTATIONS
You need information about your condition.	Health care team members will provide you with information about your condition. We will tell you about treatments, medicines you receive, and follow-up care.	Please ask any questions about your treatment and follow-up care. Let us know if you do not understand something we say or if you still have questions.	You will have the information you need and want about your treatment plan.
What will happen to you during your hospitalization?	We will take your temperature, pulse, and blood pressure as needed. We may need to wake you up at night. We may keep track of how much you eat and drink and how much you urinate. You may be on a special diet. It may be difficult for you to rest as a result of lights, noise, and treatments. We will control these as much as we can.	If you are able, help us keep track of what you eat, drink, and urinate. Ask us any questions you have about your diet. Check with the nurse before you eat or drink anything that we have not brought to you. Let us know if there is something we can do to help you rest.	You will understand the treatments and activities you experience in the hospital.

Continued.

PATIENT CARE ISSUES	WHAT WE WILL DO	WHAT YOU CAN DO	EXPECTATIONS
(During your hospitalization, cont.)	You will have tests that have been ordered by your physician such as blood samples, x-rays, and ECGs. You may have tests done while you are uncomfortable to help us diagnose or treat your problem.	Ask us if you have questions or concerns about these tests.	
	We will watch your heart rhythm continuously, through the small sticky patches we put on your chest. The signal from them appears on a special monitor screen at the nurses' station.	Try not to pull on the patches or wires.	
	We will let you know how active you can be while hospitalized and will gradually increase your activity level.	Remain in bed until instructed by staff to get up. Rest between activities.	You will be up and about with no chest discomfort or new shortness of breath.
You may experience discomfort or shortness of breath.	We may give you medicines urder your tongue, on your skin, by pill, or through your IV. Oxygen, if used, will be stopped when you no longer have any discomfort and are up and around.	Tell your nurse if you have any body symptoms that make you uncomfortable or uneasy. Do not wait to see if the sensations go away on their own.	Your discomfort will be controlled or relieved to a level acceptable to you.
Plan for your continued care.	We will ask you about any special needs you have at home. We will give you written instructions about diet, activity, medications, and things you need to tell your physician. We will help you to schedule your follow-up vists with your physician.	Tell us about any concerns or needs you have. Review the instructions we give you; ask about anything that is unclear before you leave. Follow instructions closely. Before discharge, confirm the name of your physician. Arrange for someone to drive you home before 11 AM.	You will be able to care for yourself at home and gradually increase your activity to prehospitalization levels.

NOTES:

_____

_____

PATIENT LEARNING CHECKLIST   page 1 of 2

DIAGNOSIS: **MI, R/O MI, UNSTABLE ANGINA, CAD, ANGINA**
(Circle appropriate diagnosis)

INTERVENTION CODES	PATIENT / SIGNIFICANT OTHER CODES
A. Questions answered **B.** Information provided; list written materials **C.** Task demonstrated **D.** Multidisciplinary referrals; specify **E.** Refer to class	**A.** Needs instruction/reinforcement **B.** Demonstrates verbal understanding **C.** Returns demonstrations **D.** See flow record

TEACH / DEMONSTRATE	INTERVENTION				PATIENT/SIGNIFICANT OTHER RESPONSE				COMMENTS
	CODE	DATE	TIME	INITIAL	CODE	DATE	TIME	INITIAL	
A. Patient has been oriented to plan of care									
• ECG									
• Enzymes									
• Activity restriction									
• Oxygen									
• Reportable symptoms									
• Report chest pain using 0-10 scale									
B. Patient has reviewed *Take Heart* packet									
C. Patient has been referred to *Take Heart* class									
D. Teach/Demonstate									
• Anatomy and Physiology: Video 1									
• Signs and Symptoms: Videos 1, 2, and 7									
• Risk Factors: Videos 1 and 2									
• Sexual Activity: *Sensuous Heart* (Binder)									
• Diet: Video 4									
• Emotional Health: Video 6									
• Activity Programs: Videos 2 and 5									
• Quitting Smoking: Video 3									
• Other_____									

Continued.

TEACH / DEMONSTRATE	INTERVENTION				PATIENT/SIGNIFICANT OTHER RESPONSE				COMMENTS
	CODE	DATE	TIME	INITIAL	CODE	DATE	TIME	INITIAL	
E. Tests									
• Stress tests									
• Cardiac catheterization									
• Other _____									
F. Notify advice nurse of the following									
• Shortness of breath									
• Unrelieved chest pain or pain level/ patterns new to the patient									
• Fainting									
G. Discharge									
• Medications reviewed with patient									
• Instructions reviewed with patient									

INITIAL	SIGNATURE	TITLE	INITIAL	SIGNATURE	TITLE

USC UNIVERSITY HOSPITAL

1500 San Pablo
Los Angeles, CA 90033

MULTIDISCIPLINARY PLAN

DIAGNOSIS HIV with Fever of Unknown Origin	NAME
SURGERY	ALLERGIES
	MR#

ADMIT DATE:

DRG 490   ALOS 8.4

DISCHARGE OUTCOMES	
PHYSIOLOGICAL	Physiological symptoms controlled with treatment of causative organism. Vital signs within normal limits. Adequate nutritional intake as evidenced by maintenance of weight, and laboratory tests within normal limits.
COGNITIVE	Patient/significant other verbalizes medical follow-up plan, signs and symptoms to report to healthcare team. Verbalizes modes of transmission of infection of HIV, universal precautions, high- and low-risk behaviors.
PSYCHOLOGICAL	Anxiety/fear controlled as evidenced by ability to participate in medical decisions/care. Demonstrates methods to manage fear/anxiety. Knowledgeable about available community support.

DISCIPLINE	PRE-OP/ PRE-ADMIT	DOS DATE	DAY 1	PO#1 DATE DAY 2	PO#2 DATE DAY 3	PO#3 DATE DAY 4	PO#4 DATE DAY 5	PO#5 DATE DAY 6
LOCATION			Med/Surg	Med/Surg	Med/Surg	Med/Surg	Med/Surg	Med/Surg
LABS		CBC, Chem 20, U/A If abnormal U/A, urine for C/S Blood culture¹ for conventional bacteria, mycobacteria, viral (CMV). Blood cryptococcal Ag. Histoplasmosis Ag. coccidiomycosis².	If CBC indicates cytopenias, bone marrow bx.	Sputum for AFB. If chest x-ray positive, and cough, LDH abnormal, induce sputum for PCP and AFB.		If blood cryptococcal Ag. positive, lumbar puncture. If abnormal liver function studies, hepatitis serology, liver biopsy.		
CARDIO-PULMONARY								
IMAGING/ NUCLEAR MEDICINE		Chest x-ray. Sinus x-ray if respiratory symptoms.				Absence of focal findings, CT of chest, head, and abdomen.	Abnormal lymph adenopathy, consider biopsy. If skin lesion, biopsy.	
SOCIAL SERVICES D/C PLAN REHAB. SERVICES		Assess home situation and psychological response to illness. Provide support prn.		Assess support system. Discharge planning. Home health as indicated.			Reassess DC plan.	
PHARMACY		PPD and anergy screen. IV fluid replacement. If FUO and clinical findings consistent with pneumonia, PCP, empiric therapy. Suspect bacterial findings, broad spectrum antibiotics.						
DIETARY/ NUTRITION		DAT. Dietary consult prn.	NPO status as indicated for testing; otherwise, advance diet.					

Used by permission of USC University Hospital, Los Angeles, California.

Continued.

PATIENT NAME _____

MULTIDISCIPLINARY PLAN

MEDICAL RECORD # _____

DISCIPLINE	PRE-OP/ PRE-ADMIT	DOS DATE ___ / DAY 1	PO#1 DATE ___ / DAY 2	PO#2 DATE ___ / DAY 3	PO#3 DATE ___ / DAY 4	PO#4 DATE ___ / DAY 5	PO#5 DATE ___ / DAY 6
PATIENT ACTIVITY		Up ad lib, as tolerated.	Up ad lib, as tolerated. Daily weight before breakfast.	Daily weight before breakfast.	Daily weight before breakfast.	Daily weight before breakfast.	Daily weight before breakfast.
EDUCATION	Hospital orientation. Preprocedure instructions. Medical treatment plan.	Preprocedure instructions. Medication education.	Preprocedure instructions.	Preprocedure instructions. Nutritional education.	Side effects of medication.		

COLLABORATIVE PROBLEMS

	DATE	DC DATE ___ INIT ___
1. Hyperthermia.		
2. Fluid/electrolyte imbalance, potential.		
3. Potential/actual for infection, R/T immunodeficiency.		
4. Alteration in comfort, pain.		
5. Anxiety/fear.		
6. Potential for injury R/T drug administration (liver/renal toxicities).		

COLLABORATIVE PROBLEMS

	DATE	DC DATE ___ INIT ___
7. Alteration in coping related to diagnosis/prognosis.		
8. Knowledge deficit related to disease, transmission, medications, and/or follow-up plan.		

KEY

1. To initiate a problem or intervention, document under corresponding date.

2. Document outcomes under appropriate date for achieving the goal.

3. To discontinue an intervention or resolve a patient problem highlight date and initial.

OUTCOMES

1. Patient will maintain/regain near normal body temperature.
2. Fluid/electrolyte balanced throughout hospitalization.
3. No infection throughout hospitalization, or infection managed with no evidence of systemic infection.
4. Pain controlled at a level ≤3 on 1-10 scale.
5. Verbalizes anxiety/fears.
6. No injury related to drug administration

4. Continued pain control less than or equal to 3 on 1-10 scale.
5. Anxiety diminished. Verbalizes understanding of anxiety and demonstrates methods of manage.
2. Fluids, electrolytes within normal limits.
7. Identified appropriate resources to seek prn.
8. Verbalizes signs and symptoms of side effects of meds. Knowledgeable about S/E to report to medical team.

PATIENT NAME _____

MEDICAL RECORD # _____

MULTIDISCIPLINARY PLAN

DISCIPLINE	PRE-OP/ PRE-ADMIT	PO#6 DATE DAY 7	PO#7 DATE DAY 8	PO#8 DATE DAY 9	PO#9 DATE DAY 10	PO#10 DATE DAY 11	PO#11 DATE DAY 12
PATIENT ACTIVITY		Up ad lib.					
EDUCATION		Disease process methods to prevent transmission. Patient risk reduction. Risk factors for infection.					

COLLABORATIVE PROBLEMS

	DATE				DC DATE / INIT	DATE				DC DATE / INIT
3. Infection, actual.										
4. Alteration in comfort.										
8. Knowledge deficit R/T to disease, transmission, medications, &/or follow-up plan.										

KEY

1. To initiate a problem or intervention, document under corresponding date.

2. Document outcomes under appropriate date for achieving the goal.

3. To discontinue an intervention or resolve a patient problem highlight, date, and initial.

OUTCOMES

3. Infection managed throughout hospitalization.						
4. Pain control ≤3 on scale of 1-10.						
8. Pt verbalizes medical follow-up plan, s/sx to report to team, modes of transmission of infection, & preventative interventions.						

Continued.

PLAN OF CARE DISCUSSED WITH	DOS DAY 1 DATE	PO#1 DAY 2 DATE	PO#2 DAY 3 DATE	PO#3 DAY 4 DATE	PO#4 DAY 5 DATE	PO#5 DAY 6 DATE
DATE INIT SO/P	**INTERVENTIONS**					
	Continued assessment/management of elimination, infection, skin integrity, fluid & electrolyte, & pain problems.					
	Confirm fever. Question if temperature log maintained. Thorough med hx to R/O cause.					
	Obtain recent travel hx. Implement cooling measures. Avoid inducing shivering/chills.	Encourage participation as much as possible		Create private/supportive environment for pt family. Explore pt/family perceptions.	Pace care/rest activities to provide for as much independence as possible.	Explain disease process, methods to prevent transmission.
	Provide ↑ nutritional/fluid intake. Strict I & O.	Monitor for s/sx of adverse effects from meds:		Promote strengths & appropriate coping mechanisms providing	Consult P.T./O.T. prn.	Discuss need to follow safe sex guidelines.
CASE MANAGER:	Monitor for signs & symptoms of fluid electrolyte imbalance. Monitor temperature q 4°.	• nausea/vomiting, diarrhea, bone marrow suppression • renal/liver toxicity		support & MSW consult. Assist pt/family to use social network for support assistance in care.	Education regarding support available in the community.	Discuss pt risk reduction. Maintenance of home environment.
CONSULTING MD:	Assess pain level, characteristics. Medicate as ordered.	• anorexia/rash		Discuss possible areas of conflict that may arise.	Teach pt about prescribed meds, indications for use, side effects.	Adequate nutritional intake.
	Monitor for s/sx of septicemia temp >101 or <98 WBC/bacteria in urine & blood cultures.	Assess nutritional status, height, wt, total protein/albumin.		When appropriate, encourage pt to document preferences regarding decision		Avoidance of people with infection.
SOCIAL SERVICE:	Institute measures to prevent exposure to known sources of infection.	Consult dietary prn. Provide small, frequent high-calorie meals as tolerated/desired.		maker/advance directive. Continued nutritional support.		Prevention of injury. Management of activity/rest.
ANOINTING OF THE SICK DATE:	Assess level of anxiety • provide opportunities to express feelings	Allow for adequate rest & assist with ADLs prn. Monitor tolerance to visitors/phones.		Lumbar Puncture • maintain activity as specified • hand carry all specimens to laboratory		Avoidance of high-risk behaviors (i.e., use of ETOH, tobacco, recreational drugs).
	• MSW consult prn	Assess psychological response to illness.				Teach reduction of risk factors for infection:
	Maintain immediate environment to allow for self-control	Bone Marrow Biopsy • monitor site for hematoma, bleeding • maintain activity as specified • hand carry all specimens to laboratory				• malnutrition • exposure to infectious sources or invasive procedures
						Avoidance of frequent venipuncture.

MULTIDISCIPLINARY PLAN UPDATE

SIGNATURES	DATE	SIGNATURES	DATE	SIGNATURES

Basic Nursing Diagnoses, Special Needs, and Equipment

Patient Care Planning Guides Related to Nursing Diagnoses

The planning guides for care in this section are the basic nursing functions required for all patients regardless of their medical or surgical diagnosis. The planning guides are included to assist the nurse in selecting appropriate interventions, on which the nurse may act independently. To list by priority and to combine related diagnoses, they are divided into Functional Health Patterns.* The interventions under each diagnosis are not meant to be inclusive. The nurse must select the appropriate interventions based on the related factors, the risk factors, and the defining characteristics. The nursing diagnoses included here were approved in 1994 by the North American Nursing Diagnosis Association (NANDA). This is a partial list of NANDA-approved nursing diagnoses.

*From Gordon M: *Manual of nursing diagnosis: 1995-1996,* St. Louis, 1995, Mosby.

Functional Health Pattern I: Health Perception and Management

● Risk for Infection

Definition*

The state in which an individual is at increased risk for being invaded by pathogenic organisms

Risk factors

Inadequate primary defenses (e.g., broken skin, traumatized tissue, decrease in ciliary action, stasis of body fluids, change in pH secretions, altered peristalsis)

Inadequate secondary defenses (e.g., decreased hemoglobin, leukopenia, suppressed inflammatory response, immunosuppression)

Inadequate acquired immunity

Tissue destruction and increased environmental exposure to the sun, cold, or rain

Chronic disease

Invasive procedures

Malnutrition

Pharmaceutical agents and trauma

Rupture of amniotic membranes

Insufficient knowledge to avoid exposure to pathogens

Interventions

Assess body systems for type, location, and cause of infections
  Wear gloves, gown, mask, goggles as appropriate to procedure
  Wash hands after patient contact and before self-contact
Monitor vital signs
Monitor laboratory values (e.g., elevated WBC, urinalysis, positive blood culture)
Initiate cooling measures as prescribed
Administer antipyretics and antibiotics as indicated; assess for effectiveness and side effects
Discuss with and teach patient about adequate nutrition and fluid intake

Provide and review immunization requirements to help patient maintain his or her health
Discuss health practices and teach patient about hazards of substance abuse, unsafe sexual behaviors, and smoking
Integumentary system
  Maintain aseptic technique during dressing changes; change dressings prn
  Promote and provide skin care and oral hygiene daily
  Assess pressure points prn; apply lotion and protective covering as needed; massage skin only if it is not reddened
  Monitor intravenous insertion sites and central lines daily
  Maintain IV sites and dressings according to policy
  Discuss with and teach patient about principles of autocontamination and cross-contamination
Respiratory system
  Assess for dyspnea, shortness of breath, and rales
  Assess frequency, color, and consistency of expectorate; culture as indicated
  Encourage coughing and deep breathing at least once q1h to 2h
  Assist patient with respiratory aids (e.g., incentive spirometer) and oxygen therapy
  Encourage ambulation or frequent position changes
  Elevate head of bed to promote more comfortable breathing
  Encourage fluid intake to liquefy sputum
Genitourinary system
  Maintain intake (oral/IV) at 2000 to 2500 ml/day, unless contraindicated
  Encourage fluids and foods high in acid content (e.g., cranberry, plum) to help prevent bacteria from adhering to bladder wall where they can multiply and cause infection
  Maintain closed drainage system for urethral catheters as indicated
  Monitor intake and output
  Provide daily catheter care as indicated
  Culture urine as indicated
Gastrointestinal system
  Instruct patient to ingest only USDA-inspected meats
  Encourage patient to handle and store food properly

Expected outcomes

Patient
  Understands cause of infection
  Expresses knowledge of methods of preventing further or recurring infections
  Demonstrates ability to promote own wellness

---

*Definitions, risk factors, related factors, and defining characteristics in this section for NANDA nursing diagnoses are from Kim MJ et al: *Pocket guide to nursing diagnoses,* ed 6, St Louis, 1995, Mosby.

● Risk for Injury

Definition

The state in which an individual is at risk of injury as a result of environmental conditions interacting with the individual's adaptive and defensive resources

Risk factors

Interactive conditions between individual and environment that impose a risk to defensive and adaptive resources of individual

Internal factors
  Biochemical factors
    Regulatory function
      Sensory dysfunction
      Integrative dysfunction
      Effector dysfunction
    Tissue hypoxia
    Malnutrition
    Immunity-autoimmunity
    Abnormal blood profile
      Leukocytosis or leukopenia
      Altered clotting factors
      Thrombocytopenia
      Sickle cell anemia
      Thalassemia
      Decreased hemoglobin
  Physical factors
    Broken skin
    Altered mobility
  Developmental factors
    Age
      Physiologic
      Psychosocial
  Psychologic factors
    Affective factors
    Orientation
External factors
  Biologic factors
    Immunization level of community
    Microorganisms
  Chemical factors
    Pollutants
    Poisons
    Drugs
      Pharmaceutical agents
      Alcohol
      Caffeine
      Nicotine
    Preservatives
    Cosmetics and dyes
    Nutrients (e.g., vitamins, food types)

Physical factors
  Design, structure, and arrangement of community, building, and/or equipment
  Mode of transport/transportation
  Nosocomial agents
People/provider
  Nosocomial agents
  Staffing patterns
  Cognitive, affective, and psychomotor factors

Interventions

Assess patient's mental, visual, and auditory acuity

Review patient's neuromuscular status, age, medication history (including home remedies), and nutritional status

Assess patient's ability to perform activities of daily living (ADLs), exercise, and ambulate

Maintain safe environment for patient

Orient patient to surroundings

Provide needed equipment and ensure patient's ability to reach it easily; avoid clutter

Maintain side rail, bed position, and use of restraints per policy

Remind patient about no smoking policy

Assist patient with ADLs; teach safe use of mobilizing devices as needed

Explain all treatments, procedures, and care; be aware of any language barriers

Provide adequate lighting

Ensure that electrical and hospital equipment is in good working condition

Practice safe medication administration

Monitor laboratory profiles for signs of impending problems

Administer medications according to policy
  Understand and monitor side effects
  Instruct patient to take medications as prescribed on discharge; explain that any side effects should be reported to physician
  Advise patient to avoid over-the-counter (OTC) medications unless advised by physician

Provide home safety teaching according to maturational age
  Avoid scatter rugs, icy steps or ramps, and wet or waxed floors
  Avoid loose or flowing gowns near stove, use thick pot holders, and keep pan handles toward front of stove
  Install handrails and antislip cover for bathtub or shower
  Avoid heat or cold overexposure
  Maintain adequate lighting for dispensing medications

Separate oral and eye medications from topical medications

Keep all medications out of reach of children

Expected outcomes

Patient

Demonstrates understanding of potential health hazards

Practices injury prevention measures for self

Remains injury free

Functional Health Pattern II: Nutritional and Metabolic

● Altered Nutrition: More Than Body Requirements

Definition

The state in which an individual experiences an intake of nutrients that exceeds metabolic needs

Related factor

Excessive intake in relation to metabolic need

Defining characteristics

Weight 10% to 20% over ideal for height and frame

Triceps skinfold (TSF) greater than 15 mm in men and 25 mm in women

Sedentary activity level

Reported or observed dysfunctional eating patterns

Pairing food with other activities

Concentrating food intake at end of day

Eating in response to external cues (e.g., time of day, social situation)

Eating in response to internal cues other than hunger (e.g., anxiety)

Interventions

Assess patient for signs of fluid retention

Weigh patient daily in same clothes and at same time, using same scale

Assess patient's desire for weight loss and his or her history of dieting

Obtain triceps skinfold measurements

Determine patient's height and ideal body weight (Table 2-1 and Table 2-2)

Assess patient's dietary history, taking heredity, age, culture, religion, and medical problems into consideration; include laxative use

Collaborate with nutritionist or registered dietitian and patient. Help patient set realistic goals for weight loss; reward goals attempted and attained

Table 2-1 Height and Weight Table for Men and Women

	Weight (pounds)	
Height	**Ages 19-34**	**Ages 35 and Older**
5'0"	97-128	108-138
5'1"	101-132	111-143
5'2"	104-137	115-148
5'3"	107-141	119-152
5'4"	111-146	122-157
5'5"	114-150	126-162
5'6"	118-155	130-167
5'7"	121-160	134-172
5'8"	125-164	138-178
5'9"	129-169	142-183
5'10"	132-174	146-188
5'11"	136-179	151-194
6'0"	140-184	155-199
6'1"	144-189	159-205
6'2"	148-195	164-210
6'3"	152-200	168-216
6'4"	156-205	173-222
6'5"	160-211	177-228
6'6"	164-216	182-234

Source: *Nutrition and your health: dietary guidelines for Americans,* Washington, D.C., 1990, USDA.

Table 2-2 Height and Weight Assessment*

Females:	45 kg (100 lbs) for first 150 cm (5ft), plus 2.25 kg (5lbs) for each additional 2.5 cm (1 in)
Males:	47.7 kg (106 lbs) for first 150 cm (5ft), plus 2.4 cm (6 lbs) for each additional 2.5 cm (1 in)

*Yield ideal body weight + 10%

Encourage patient to keep a diary of intake (i.e., what, when, and where food is eaten) and feelings at time of eating

Emphasize importance of a regular exercise program

Provide information on a reputable weight loss program

Refer patient for counseling as needed

Expected outcomes

Patient

Expresses understanding of factors causing weight gain

Demonstrates desire to maintain normal weight for age and height

● Altered Nutrition: Less Than Body Requirements

Definition

The state in which an individual experiences an intake of nutrients insufficient to meet metabolic needs

Related factor

Inability to ingest or digest food or absorb nutrients because of biologic, psychologic, or economic factors

Defining characteristics

Loss of weight with adequate food intake (see Table 2-2)

Body weight 20% or more under ideal for height and frame

Reported inadequate food intake, (i.e., less than the RDA)

Weakness of muscles required for swallowing or mastication

Reported or evidence of lack of food

Lack of interest in food

Perceived inability to ingest food

Aversion to eating

Reported altered taste sensation

Satiety immediately after ingesting food

Abdominal pain with or without pathological conditions

Sore, inflamed buccal cavity

Interventions

Assess patient's nutritional status, past eating patterns, and medications (Table 2-3 and Table 2-4)

Assess causative factors; (e.g., anorexia, bulimia, dysphagia, altered taste, age, unavailability of food)

Assess patient's cultural food preferences (i.e., likes and dislikes)

Monitor patient's intake and output; weigh patient weekly at the same time and in the same clothes, using same scale

Table 2-3 Effect of Drugs on Nutritional Status*

Drug	Effect
Antacids (aluminum)	Malabsorption of medications and some nutrients
Aspirin	Malabsorption of folate
	Excretion of vitamin C
Barbiturates	Malabsorption of thiamin, vitamin B_{12}
Corticosteroids	Malabsorption of calcium, zinc, phosphorus
Hydralazine	Excretion of pyridoxine
Laxatives	Loss of fluid/electrolytes
Methotrexate	Malabsorption of vitamin B_{12}, folate, fat
Mineral oil	Malabsorption of fat-soluble vitamins, calcium, phosphorus
Neomycin	Malabsorption of major nutrients
Oral contraceptives	Possible decreased absorption of vitamin C, B complex vitamins, magnesium, zinc
Penicillin	Loss of potassium
Tetracycline	Malabsorption of calcium, iron, magnesium, pyridoxine
	Excretion of vitamin C, riboflavin, niacin, folic acid
Thiazides	Excretion of potassium, magnesium, zinc, riboflavin

*Updated from Long BC, Phipps WJ: *Medical-surgical nursing: a nursing process approach,* ed 3, St Louis, 1993, Mosby.

Table 2-4 Medications to be Taken With Food*

Aspirin	Nitrofurantoin (Macrodantin)
Aminophylline	
Chlorothiazide (Diuril)	Phenylbutazone (Butazolidin)
Ferrous sulfate	
All nonsteroid antiinflammatory drugs	Phenytoin (Dilantin)
	Prednisolone
Metronidazole (Flagyl)	Reserpine (Serpasil)
	Triamterene (Dyrenium)

*Updated from Long BC, Phipps WJ: *Medical-surgical nursing: a nursing process approach,* ed 3, St Louis, 1993, Mosby.

Monitor laboratory values (e.g., complete blood count, electrolytes)

Maintain calorie count chart

Establish rest/activity pattern

Encourage patient to keep a food intake diary

Encourage a well-balanced diet of 2400 calories every day

Provide four to six meals per day as needed

Encourage patient to establish regular exercise habits

Assess patient's oral cavity and ability to chew and swallow

Provide meals in a quiet environment; encourage patient to eat slowly and chew well

Help patient adjust to a comfortable position for meals

Encourage family or significant other to be involved with meals, eat with patient, and to bring food from home

Maintain clean environment to prevent nausea and anorexia

Collaborate with nutritionist or registered dietitian about cultural food preparation

Discuss and teach patient and significant other about nutritional guidelines, importance of eating regular meals, and appropriate foods to include

Refer patient for nutritional counseling as needed

Expected outcomes

Patient

Expresses understanding of nutritional deficit

Demonstrates knowledge of adequate nutritional intake

Gains weight as needed to meet body needs

● Altered Oral Mucous Membrane

Definition

The state in which an individual experiences disruptions in the tissue layers of the oral cavity

Related factors

Pathologic conditions: oral cavity (radiation to head and/or neck)

Dehydration

Trauma

    Chemical (e.g., acidic foods, drugs, noxious agents, alcohol)

    Mechanical (e.g., ill-fitting dentures, braces, endotracheal tubes, nasogastric tubes, surgery in oral cavity)

NPO instructions for more than 24 hours

Ineffective oral hygiene

Mouth breathing

Malnutrition

Infection

Lack of or decreased salivation

Medication

Defining characteristics

Coated tongue

Xerostomia (dry mouth)

Stomatitis

Oral lesions or ulcers

Lack of or decreased salivation

Leukoplakia

Edema

Hyperemia

Oral plaque

Oral pain or discomfort

Desquamation

Vesicles

Hemorrhagic gingivitis

Carious teeth

Halitosis

Interventions

Assess patient's mucous membranes, tongue, and gums daily

Observe for moisture, cleanliness, integrity, edema, color, bleeding, and odor

Assess patient's teeth for cleanliness, integrity, sensitivity to heat or cold, presence of dentures, and sordes

Brush patient's teeth bid and prn with toothpaste, powder, baking soda, or mouthwash

Promote regular flossing

Advise patient to avoid foods that cause discomfort (e.g., hot, cold, and spicy foods)

Encourage adequate fluid intake

Advise patient to rinse with water or mouthwash after brushing

Apply petroleum jelly, lip balm, or glycerin-lemon mixture to patient's lips to prevent dryness and chapping

Remove patient's dentures (if applicable) and cleanse bid with toothpaste or powder and running water. Protect dentures from breaking by placing them in a marked denture cup when not in use

Cleanse patient's mouth with equal parts of hydrogen peroxide and water prn for crust removal

Perform oral cleaning as needed with toothettes or disposable foam swabs; avoid lemon-glycerine swabs because they can irritate the mucosa

Encourage routine dental checkups

Expected outcomes

Patient

Demonstrates correct technique to promote proper oral care

Has oral cavity that is pink, clean, moist, and odor free

Reports a feeling of oral cleanliness

● Risk for Impaired Skin Integrity

Definition

The state in which an individual's skin is at risk of being adversely altered

Risk factors

External (environmental) factors

Hypothermia or hyperthermia

Chemical substance

Mechanical factors

Shearing forces

Pressure

Restraint

Radiation

Physical immobilization

Excretions and secretions

Humidity

Internal (somatic) factors

Medication

Alterations in nutritional state (e.g., obesity, emaciation)

Altered metabolic state

Altered circulation

Altered sensation

Altered pigmentation

Skeletal prominence

Developmental factors

Alterations in skin turgor (e.g., change in elasticity)

Psychogenic factors

Immunological factors

Interventions

Assess causative factors

Assess patient's bathing needs (e.g., complete or partial bed bath, tub or shower using warm water and mild superfatted soap)

Provide privacy and ensure adequate temperature to avoid chilling

Massage patient's skin gently with mild lanolin-based lotions to increase circulation and maintain integrity; never massage broken areas because it may provoke further ulceration

Dry skin thoroughly

Consider using "bagbath" method of bathing: place four washcloths in plastic baggies; add nonrinsable cleaner, such as Septisoft; and dilute according to directions; heat bag in microwave for 60 to 90 seconds; use one cloth for each part of body; allow patient to air dry, which takes about 30 seconds; discard cloths in laundry hamper

Assess patient's skin for redness, lesions, blisters, swelling, or drainage; notify enterostomal nurse if these conditions occur

Monitor for incontinence; cleanse area with mild soap and water prn

Encourage patient to ambulate; limit chair sitting to 1 hour

Assist with and/or teach range-of-motion (ROM) exercises

Provide nutritious diet and adequate fluid intake

Assess patient's perineal and perianal areas as needed; observe for excoriation, vaginal or penile discharge, and pain; apply lotions or cornstarch to area prn

Assess patient's feet and hands; observe nail beds and look for signs of rash, dryness, or skin breaks; use side lighting to assess rash

Soak patient's feet and hands in warm soap and water, dry well, and apply lotion prn

Cleanse and trim patient's nails as needed

Assess condition of patient's hair; observe for matting, tangles, signs of alopecia, lice, cradle cap scales, and dryness

Comb hair daily and shampoo prn, with patient's permission; start with edges and work toward scalp, holding shaft of hair to prevent discomfort

Apply baby oil and massage it into scalp; leave oil on for 1 hour to remove scales, then gently shampoo and comb

Apply alcohol to release tangles

Style patient's hair for attractiveness, comfort, and easy care

Assess male patient's shaving needs

Apply warm towels to patient's face before shaving

Rinse skin well and apply lotion after shaving

Maintain physical comfort

Change bed linen prn; keep linen neat, dry, wrinkle-free, and clean

Provide adequate warmth

Change patient's position frequently to prevent pressure and fatigue

Expected outcomes

Patient

Maintains skin integrity

Nails and hair are in optimal condition

Impairment is minimal if present

Maintains maximal circulation

Demonstrates optimal nutrition

● Risk for Altered Body Temperature

Definition

The state in which an individual is at risk for failure to maintain body temperature within normal range

Risk factors

Extremes of age

Extremes of weight

Exposure to cold/cool or hot/warm environments

Dehydration

Inactivity or vigorous activity

Medications causing vasoconstriction or vasodilation, altered metabolic rate, sedation

Inappropriate clothing for environmental temperature

Illness or trauma affecting temperature regulation

Interventions

Hyperthermia

Assess causative factors (e.g., heatstroke, lesions of anterior hypothalamus)

Monitor patient's vital signs qlh

Monitor patient's mental acuity

Monitor intake and output; report output less than 30 ml/hr to physician

Monitor electrolytes, CBC, glucose, and liver function

Monitor for tachycardia or tachypnea

Maintain parenteral fluids as indicated

Initiate cooling measures as indicated; cool slowly, and handle body gently

Monitor patient's temperature q10min during procedure and qlh after procedure

Discontinue cooling measures when temperature is 1° F above normal

Dry patient's skin thoroughly (avoid friction) and provide clean, dry linen

Encourage patient to reduce physical activity and to drink plenty of fluids

Administer prescribed antibiotics and antipyretics

Reinstitute cooling measures as needed

Maintain cool room temperature

Hypothermia

Assess causative factors (e.g., accidental hypothermia, lesions of posterior hypothalamus)

Monitor patient's vital signs qlh

Monitor patient's mental acuity

Initiate warming measures as prescribed; warm body slowly, and handle body gently

Monitor for bradycardia or hypotension

Monitor blood gases, electrolytes, and glucose; report any abnormal results to physician

Monitor intake and output qlh. If urine output is less than 30 ml/hr, notify physician

Maintain warm, comfortable environment

Expected outcomes

Patient's

Temperature is normal

Vital signs are normal

Skin is warm and dry

Functional Health Pattern III: Elimination

● Constipation

Definition

The state in which an individual experiences a change in normal bowel habits characterized by a decrease in frequency and/or passage of hard, dry stools

Related factors

Less than adequate intake

Less than adequate dietary intake and bulk

Less than adequate physical activity or immobility

Personal habits

Medications

Chronic use of medication and enemas
Gastrointestinal obstructive lesions
Neuromuscular impairment
Musculoskeletal impairment
Pain on defecation
Diagnostic procedures
Lack of privacy
Weak abdominal musculature
Pregnancy
Emotional status

Defining characteristics

Frequency less than usual pattern
Hard-formed stool
Palpable mass
Reported feeling of rectal fullness
Straining at stool
Decreased bowel sounds
Reported feeling of abdominal fullness or
  pressure
Less than usual amount of stool
Nausea

Other possible defining characteristics

Abdominal pain
Back pain
Headache
Interference with daily living
Laxative use
Decreased appetite
Appetite impairment

Interventions

Assess cause(s) of constipation
Determine patient's normal elimination pattern
Assess patient's daily defecation routine and encourage
  him or her to maintain pattern as much as possible
Provide natural stimulants (e.g., coffee, prune juice) as
  allowed
Provide privacy
Monitor and record patient's daily bowel movements;
  monitor for melena as needed
Initiate diet changes to maintain normal consistency;
  provide high-fiber foods (e.g., fruits, vegetables,
  whole grains)
Initiate high-fiber foods slowly to prevent intestinal distention and gas formation
Avoid excessive use of bran, which can increase gas
  formation
Increase activity, exercise, and fluid intake (6 to 8
  glasses every day)

Provide natural laxatives initially (e.g., lemon juice in a
  glass of warm water, prune juice qAM) before admin-
  istering laxative or enema
Instruct patient to avoid routine use of laxatives
Explain that medications often cause constipation
Explain importance of defecating as soon as urge
  occurs
Instruct patient to set schedule for defecating daily,
  such as after a meal.
Initiate relaxing techniques to assist in defecation
Reduce rectal pain and discomfort from hemorrhoids
  through use of lubricants, cool compresses, stool soft-
  eners, and suppositories
Administer perianal care after each defecation

Expected outcomes

Patient
  Expresses understanding of causative factors of con-
    stipation
  Demonstrates knowledge of the importance of diet,
    fiber, fluids, regularity, and exercise
  Verbalizes need to avoid straining and using laxatives
    to defecate

● Diarrhea

Definition

*The state in which an individual experiences a
change in normal bowel habits, which is characterized
by the frequent passage of loose, fluid, and unformed
stools*

Related factors

Stress and anxiety
Dietary intake
Medications
Inflammation, irritation, or malabsorption of bowel
Toxins
Contaminants
Radiation

Defining characteristics

Abdominal pain
Cramping
Increased frequency of bowel movements
Increased frequency of bowel sounds
Loose, liquid stools
Urgency
Color changes

Interventions

Assess causative factors, including impaction

Maintain NPO and parenteral fluids as indicated

Collaborate with physician; initiate fluids and progress to soft, bland diet as tolerated

Encourage dietary bulk in diet as soon as possible; Psyllium (Metamucil) may be indicated

Avoid irritating foods (e.g., milk, caffeinated products, and raw fruits and vegetables)

Weigh patient daily (same time, clothes, and scale)

Assess usual elimination pattern

Monitor serum electrolytes

Monitor bowel sounds

Encourage patient to verbalize situations that cause stress

Assist and teach stress management techniques

Assess patient's perineal area for excoriation and irritation

Provide perineal skin care after each bowel movement; apply soothing ointments as indicated

Provide bedpan or commode, and place it within easy reach

Maintain uncluttered room for easy access to bathroom; provide a night light

Allow for privacy

Suggest methods of eliminating odors

Expected outcomes

Patient

Verbalizes causative factors of diarrhea

Reports improved frequency and consistency of stools

Presents normal electrolytes and fluid intake

● Altered Urinary Elimination

Definition

The state in which an individual experiences a disturbance in urine elimination

Related factors

Sensory motor impairment

Neuromuscular impairment

Mechanical trauma

Defining characteristics

Dysuria

Frequency

Hesitancy

Incontinence

Nocturia

Retention

Urgency

Interventions

Assess causative factors, including family history of kidney problems and peripheral edema

Determine patient's usual urinary pattern; inquire about any recent alterations in patient's pattern

Measure intake and output

Monitor urine for color, frequency, amount, odor, and consistency

Monitor urine for sugar, acetone, blood, and pH levels

Monitor for residual urine

Monitor for frequency, urgency, dysuria, and distension

Administer and teach female patient about perineal care after urination; explain correct wiping procedure

Provide privacy

Maintain uncluttered room for easy access to bathroom; provide a night light

Increase fluid intake, if allowed, to maintain hydration

Institute voiding measures (e.g., running water, leaning forward, standing position, peppermint in bedpan) as needed

Maintain bedpan within easy reach

Monitor indwelling urethral catheters for patency, correct position of collection unit, and infection; teach self-catheterization as needed

Provide daily urinary meatal care according to policy

Monitor for incontinence

Initiate voiding schedule q2h to 4h

Provide protective padding as needed

Expected outcomes

Patient

Expresses understanding of causative factors of altered urinary pattern

Verbalizes and demonstrates correct posturinating hygiene

Reports urination returning to a normal pattern

Functional Health Pattern IV: Activity and Exercise

● Risk for Activity Intolerance

Definition

The state in which an individual has insufficient physiologic or psychologic energy to endure or complete required or desired daily activities

Related factors

Generalized weakness
Sedentary lifestyle
Imbalance between oxygen supply and demand
Bed rest or immobility

Defining characteristics

Verbal report of fatigue or weakness
Abnormal heart rate or blood pressure in response to activity
Exertional discomfort or dyspnea
Electrocardiographic changes reflecting dysrhythmias or ischemia

Interventions

Physical interventions
  Assess body systems for possible cause of inactivity
    Disturbance in oxygen maintenance
    Fluid or electrolyte imbalance
    Deficiencies in nutrition
    Neuromuscular disorders
  Observe patient for pain and insufficient rest or sleep
  Monitor side effects of all medications and diagnostic studies
  Collaborate with physical and occupational therapists as needed
  Assess patient's tolerance of activity
    Assess past activity pattern
    Explain procedure, activity, or treatment
    Monitor resting vital signs
    Have patient perform activity at his or her own rate
    Monitor vital signs immediately and again in 3 minutes
    Discontinue activity if any of the following occur: chest pain, dyspnea, cyanosis, vertigo, confusion, hypotension, failure of systolic pressure increase, increased diastolic pressure, decreased respiratory rate, continuing tachycardia
    Reduce energy expenditure where possible
  Increase activity slowly to increase patient's tolerance
    Assist as needed
  Coordinate care and medication schedule to allow for rest periods
  Maintain and increase strength with active or passive range-of-motion (ROM) exercises
  Encourage self-care activities when patient is able
  Provide adaptive devices, such as padded eating utensils and long-handled tongs, to assist in activities of daily living (ADLs) as needed
Psychologic interventions
  Assess patient for presence of depression or lack of incentive; assess for maladaptive behaviors
  Explain importance of activity to tolerance
  Involve patient in care plan and short-term goal setting
  Acknowledge and praise patient for attempting or completing tasks
  Discuss and assist patient with identifying possible incentives to increase activity
  Assist patient in identifying successful past coping behaviors
  Involve family or significant other in supporting and participating with patient in daily activities

Expected outcomes

Patient
  Participates in activities that increase ability to perform ADLs and other activities
  Expresses understanding of a balanced rest/activity program
  Seeks support of others to maintain optimal level of activity

● Impaired Physical Mobility

Definition

The state in which an individual experiences a limitation of ability for independent physical movement

Related factors

Intolerance of activity (i.e., decreased strength and endurance)
Pain and discomfort
Perceptual or cognitive impairment
Neuromuscular impairment
Musculoskeletal impairment
Depression or severe anxiety

Defining characteristics

Inability to purposefully move within physical environment, including bed mobility, transfer, and ambulation
Reluctance to attempt movement
Limited range of motion (ROM)
Decreased muscle strength, control, and/or mass
Imposed restrictions of movement, including mechanical and medical protocol
Impaired coordination

Interventions

Assess patient's mobility tolerance and motivation
Maintain circulatory function

Encourage and teach arm and leg exercises to be performed q1h

Apply antiembolic hose

Monitor for thrombophlebitis; symptoms include pain, warmth, and edema of extremity

Assist and teach patient turning techniques

Monitor patient's vital signs after activity at 3 minutes and 15 minutes

Observe for hypertension or hypotension, tachycardia, or bradycardia

Maintain respiratory function

Encourage and teach deep breathing q1h

Assist and teach patient how to use incentive spirometer

Maintain patent airway

Monitor respirations g1 to 2h

Increase fluid intake to liquefy secretions

Monitor vital signs after activity

Observe for dyspnea, cyanosis, shortness of breath, tachypnea, or bradypnea

Maintain normal elimination

Increase fluid intake

Encourage exercise and activity

Provide diet that will promote elimination

Bowel: high fiber, roughage, prunes

Bladder: meat, fish, cereals

Provide privacy

Assist and teach perianal and perineal hygiene

Provide bedpan within easy reach

Maintain musculoskeletal function

Collaborate with physical and occupational therapist for supportive exercises

Perform active exercises or assist with and teach passive ROM exercises q4h; note patient's tolerance and motivation

Maintain bodily alignment while in bed

Provide bed cradle as needed

Prevent footdrop with foot board

Support dependent limbs as needed with pillows or immobilizing devices; avoid placing pillow under knees

Avoid letting patient remain in any one position for long periods; frequent small changes prevent pressure, discomfort, and fatigue

Maintain casts, braces, traction, or prosthetic devices in correct position to avoid discomfort or pressure

Help patient progress toward mobility slowly as tolerated

Assist patient as needed with sitting up, dangling, standing, and ambulation

Initiate and teach use of mobilizing devices (e.g., crutches, walker, wheelchair, sling) as needed

Maintain skin integrity

Assess pressure points for signs of breakdown

Administer gentle massage to pressure areas; apply lotion as needed

Encourage activity as tolerated

Prevent shearing force with use of turn sheet

Provide nutritious diet of proteins and carbohydrates

Increase fluid intake; monitor intake and output

Change patient's position often if he or she is in wheelchair

Maintain psychologic integrity

Encourage patient to express fears and anxieties

Promote support of significant others

Provide diversional activities

Encourage patient to be involved in his or her care

Maintain positive communication

Reinforce positive coping patterns

Provide and teach patient about available support resources; distribute handouts and telephone numbers of rehabilitation and social services

Expected outcomes

Patient's

Ability to interact with others, make own decisions, and use positive coping behaviors is increasing

Vital signs are normal

Elimination is normal

Activity is at optimal level

Skin integrity is maintained

Functional Health Pattern V: Sleep and Rest

● Sleep Pattern Disturbance

Definition

Disruption of sleep time causes discomfort or interferes with desired lifestyle

Related factors

Sensory alterations

Internal factors

Illness

Psychologic stress

External factors

Environmental changes

Social cues

Defining characteristics

Verbal complaints of difficulty in falling asleep

Awakening earlier or later than desired

Interrupted sleep

Verbal complaints of not feeling well rested

Changes in behavior and performance

Increasing irritability

Restlessness
Disorientation
Lethargy
Listlessness
Physical signs
  Mild, fleeting nystagmus
  Slight hand tremor
  Ptosis of eyelid
  Expressionless face
Thick speech with mispronunciation and incorrect
  words
Dark circles under eyes
Frequent yawning
Changes in posture

Interventions

Assess and identify causative factors
Assess patient's normal rest/sleep pattern
Control environmental disturbances, noise, and lighting
Maintain quiet environment; close doors and pull
  drapes and dividers; decrease incoming stimuli
Provide night lights and soft music
Coordinate nursing functions to allow for rest periods
  and fewer interruptions during night
Limit visitors during rest periods
Limit fluid intake where possible after 6 PM
Maintain balance of daytime activity and rest
Increase activity to point of tolerance to promote
  tiredness
Limit sleep during daytime and stimulate wakefulness
  as required
Involve patient in unit and diversional activities
Provide comfort measures
Maintain warm, clean, and comfortable bed
Provide needed equipment within easy reach
Encourage usual sleeping aids
Administer hs care as close to bedtime as possible
Assess any sleep medication for effectiveness
Encourage patient to express fears and anxieties that
  may prevent or disrupt sleep
Monitor for pain or discomfort; administer analgesics if
  needed
Teach patient alternative pain/stress management
  techniques

Expected outcomes

Patient
  Expresses understanding of causative factors of sleep
    disturbance
  Demonstrates optimal balance of rest and activity
  Expresses increased ability to sleep

Functional Health Pattern VI: Cognitive/Perceptual

● Pain

Definition
  The state in which an individual experiences and reports the presence of severe discomfort or an uncomfortable sensation

Related factors

Injuring agents
Biologic factors
Chemical agents
Physical factors
Psychologic factors

Defining characteristics

Subjective data
Communication (verbal or coded) of pain descriptors

Objective data
Guarding behavior (i.e., protective)
Self-focusing behavior
Narrowed focus (altered time perception, withdrawal
  from social contact, impaired thought process)
Distraction behavior (moaning, crying, pacing, seeking
  out other people and/or activities, restlessness)
Facial mask of pain (eyes lack luster, "beaten look,"
  fixed or scattered movement, grimace)
Alteration in muscle tone, which may span from listless
  to rigid
Autonomic responses not seen in chronic, stable pain
  (e.g., diaphoresis, blood pressure and pulse rate
  change, pupillary dilation, increased or decreased respiratory rate)

Interventions

Assess location, type, duration, and frequency of pain
Assess intensity of pain using scale of 0 to 5 (0 being
  absence of pain and 5 being intense pain)
Assess causative factors
Discuss past effective and ineffective pain relief
  measures;
Assess effect of pain on patient
  Altered sleep/activity pattern
  Decreased energy, sexual activity
  Reduced feelings of self-worth

Assess effectiveness of pain-relief measures
Encourage patient to keep a pain diary
Develop trusting relationship
  Encourage patient to talk about himself or herself
  Be a good listener
  Avoid making judgmental statements
  Be truthful and consistent
  Accept patient's view of pain
  Set realistic goals
  Assist patient in describing pain
  Explain relationship of pain to disease process
  Estimate duration of pain when possible
  Explain painful procedures realistically
Involve patient in his or her care; allow some control
  over his or her daily activities when possible
  Encourage pain reduction techniques as appropriate:
    (e.g., rocking movements, external warmth, visual
    focal point with breathing patterns, imagery, relax-
    ation techniques, touch)
  Suggest self-help groups that assist in coping with
    pain
  Collaborate with physician regarding central lines; pe-
    ripherally inserted central catheter (PICC) (see p.
    88); intravenous continuous opioid infusion (ICOI)
    (see p. 89); continuous subcutaneous opioid infusion
    (CSI) (see p. 90); epidural analgesia (see p. 92); and
    patient controlled analgesia (PCA) (see p. 92).
Discuss alternate interventions such as biofeedback,
  transcutaneous electrical nerve stimulation (TENS)
  unit, hypnosis, and self-controlled pain procedure
Encourage support of family and significant others

Expected outcomes

Patient
  Expresses understanding of causative factors of pain
  Demonstrates ability to reduce or control pain using
    learned skills

● Knowledge Deficit

Definition

The state in which specific information is lacking

Related factors

Lack of exposure
Lack of recall
Misinterpretation of information
Cognitive limitation
Lack of interest in learning
Unfamiliarity with information resources
Patient's request for no information

Defining characteristics

Verbalization of the problem
Inaccurate follow-through of instruction
Inadequate performance of test
Inappropriate or exaggerated behaviors (e.g., hysteri-
  cal, hostile, agitated, apathetic behavior)
Statement of misconception
Request for information

Interventions

Establish patient's expected outcomes for learning
Use information obtained in assessment; be aware of
  any language barriers
Set patient's expected outcomes according to priority
  and to patient's needs and readiness to learn
Set small, specific, and realistic expected outcomes to
  provide patient with a sense of accomplishment
Reward goals that are attempted or completed
Write expected outcomes in nursing care plan
Incorporate principles of learning and teaching
  Patient's desire to learn must be present before learn-
    ing can take place
  Each individual learns at his or her own pace
  Environment must be free from stress, discomfort,
    pain, or distractions
  Information is best learned if it is meaningful, orga-
    nized, and relevant
  Individual will learn only if he or she sees value in the
    information
Present information in small segments
Use language that is easily understood
Teach from a well-organized plan
Allow time for questions
Obtain feedback from patient after each segment is pre-
  sented
Continue with teaching plan only when patient under-
  standing is ensured
Maintain eye contact during discussions
Present information step by step and request a return
  demonstration when teaching a procedure
Present information using different techniques based
  on patient's learning preference and/or ability
Involve family and significant others in learning
  process
Use as many audiovisual aids as possible
  Films
  Slides
  Booklets
  Diagrams
  Procedure pictures
  Procedure equipment
Praise patient when learning takes place
Initiate teaching plan as soon as possible after admission,

based on patient's condition, level of perception, and readiness to learn

Expected outcomes

Patient
  Verbalizes understanding of given instructions and information
  Demonstrates learned procedure(s) correctly
  Seeks assistance in clarifying misconceptions or misunderstandings

● Altered Thought Processes

Definition

The state in which an individual experiences a disruption in cognitive operations and activities

Related factors

Physiologic changes
Psychologic conflicts
Loss of memory
Impaired judgment
Sleep deprivation

Defining characteristics

Inaccurate interpretation of environment
  Cognitive dissonance
    Distractibility
    Memory deficit or problems
    Egocentricity
    Hypervigilance/hypovigilance
    Decreased ability to grasp ideas
    Impaired ability to make decisions
    Impaired ability to solve problems
    Impaired ability to reason
    Impaired ability to abstract or conceptualize
    Impaired ability to calculate
    Altered attention span (i.e., distractibility)
    Obsessions, phobias
    Inability to follow commands
    Disorientation to time, place, person, circumstances, and events
    Changes in remote, recent, or immediate memory
    Delusions
    Illusions*
    Ideas of reference
    Paranoid ideation*

Hallucinations
Confabulation
Inappropriate social behavior
Altered sleep patterns
Inappropriate affect

Other possible defining characteristic

Inappropriate or nonreality-based thinking

● Disorientation*

Description

Disorientation is the inability to correctly identify self in relation to time, place, or person

Defining characteristics

Chronic dementia
Acute delirium
Psychomotor agitation
Insomnia
Excessive fear
Visual or auditory hallucinations
Aggressive behavior
Purposeless or repetitive activity
Reversible causes (e.g., alcohol intoxication, altered cerebral blood flow, dehydration, electrolyte imbalance, high fever, infection, metabolic disturbance, sleep pattern disturbance, toxic reactions, head trauma, malnutrition, sensory deprivation or overload, overmedication)
Irreversible causes (e.g., senile dementia [Alzheimer's disease], AIDS dementia, chronic progressive neurological conditions, neoplasms that are present with the following behaviors: psychomotor agitation or retardation, disinterest in personal care, confabulation, "sundowner's" syndrome (extreme nocturnal agitation), short-term memory loss, inability to concentrate, loss of intellectual abilities, delusions, lability of affect and concrete thinking)

Interventions

Assess causative factors and possible etiology of disorientation (acute and reversible delirium versus chronic and irreversible dementia)
Treat acute delirium as a medical emergency

---

*These defining characteristics are not NANDA approved.

*Not a NANDA-approved diagnosis

Protect patient from self-injury with attention to equipment at bedside

Provide soft restraints or restraint jacket to prevent unescorted wandering

Cover patient adequately to avoid unintentional physical exposure

Wear clearly visible name tag

Orient patient to place and time before giving him or her care

Speak in kind tone; use short and simple sentences

Give one direction at a time

Adjust lighting to prevent shadows and distortions

Leave on a night light

Assist patient in self-care activities

Maintain a therapeutic environment; orient patient to room: display familiar items, place personal items in accessible place, display clock and calendar, and keep equipment and possessions in same place

Post list of daily activities in clear view

Label bathroom and other areas with large-lettered signs or use a color code to help patient identify personal items and room

Encourage ambulation when possible

Encourage socialization

Provide radio, television, or newspapers

Address patient by name

Tell patient when you do not understand his or her statements

Do not point out deficits of behavior

Do not laugh at misinformation or misperceptions

Provide repetitive schedules

Encourage independence

Encourage visits from family and significant others

Assess patient's response to visitors

  Assist family with its emotional reactions

  Help family to set realistic goals

Provide patient with tasks that do not require new learning

Give positive reinforcement for participation in activities

Provide same staff when possible

Expected outcomes

Patient

  Demonstrates reality testing

  Dismisses internal voices

  Demonstrates increased cognitive functioning

  Controls inappropriate and impulsive behaviors

  Demonstrates ability to function in a structured setting

  Interacts with environment

● Decisional Conflict

Definition

A state of uncertainty about the course of action to be taken when choice among competing actions involves risk, loss, or challenge to personal life values (specify focus of conflict, [e.g., choices regarding health, family relationships, career, finances, or other life events])

Related factors

Unclear personal values and beliefs

Perceived threat to value system

Lack of experience or interference with decision making

Lack of relevant information

Support system deficit

Defining characteristics

Verbalized feeling of distress related to uncertainty about choices

Verbalization of undesired consequences of alternative actions being considered

Vacillation between alternative choices

Delayed decision making

Self-focusing behavior

Physical signs of distress or tension (e.g., increased heart rate, increased muscle tension, restlessness)

Questioning personal values and beliefs while attempting to make a decision

Interventions

Assess any physical condition that may affect decision-making or cognition

Encourage patient not to make serious decisions while under severe stress

Practice relaxation techniques before decision making to decrease anxiety

Assist patient with clearly identifying a problem

Provide accurate data; be consistent to avoid misconceptions

Decrease anxiety (see anxiety interventions, p. 36)

Assist patient with identifying potential alternatives; encourage patient to write down pros and cons of each alternative

Assist patient with identifying previous successful decisions

Encourage verbalization and recognition of factors that hinder decision making

Reassure patient that it is acceptable to make mistakes

Remind patient that any decision will have negative aspects

Encourage patient to make simple choices first

Allow patient to make choices (e.g., select an item from menu or choose a time for a procedure)

Explain importance of not making decisions based on preference of others

Reinforce patient's verbalization of independent opinions, thoughts, and decisions

Assist and reinforce progression to more complex decision making

Point out available resources to assist in decision making

Teach assertive communication techniques

Assist with appropriate action once decision has been made

Expected outcomes

Patient
  Makes contribution to treatment plan
  Seeks increasing responsibility for own activity and behavior
  Verbalizes alternative solutions to problems
  Involves others in decision-making process

Functional Health Pattern VII: Self-perception and Self-concept

● Anxiety*

Definition

A vague, uneasy feeling, the source of which is often nonspecific or unknown to the individual

Related factors

Unconscious conflict about essential values and goals of life
Threat to self-concept
Threat of death, real or perceived
Threat to or change in health status
Threat to or change in socioeconomic status
Threat to or change in role functioning
Threat to or change in environment
Threat to or change in interaction patterns
Situational and maturational crises
Interpersonal transmission and contagion
Unmet needs

Defining characteristics

Subjective data

Increased tension
Apprehension
Increased helplessness

Uncertainty
Fear
Feelings of being scared
Panic*
Feelings of inadequacy
Shakiness
Fear of unspecific consequences
Regret, obsession, rumination*
Guilt, shame*
Overexcitement
Feelings of being rattled
Distress
Jitters

Objective data

Sympathetic stimulation (e.g., cardiovascular excitation, superficial vasoconstriction, pupil dilation)
Dizziness, hyperventilation*
Restlessness
Insomnia, somnolence, fatigue*
Headaches, GI discomfort*
Muscle tension*
Glancing about
Poor eye contact
Trembling (especially hand tremors)
Extraneous movements (e.g., foot shuffling, hand and arm movements)
Expressed concern regarding changes in life events
Worried behavior
Inability to concentrate*
Crying, irritability*
Anxiety
Facial tension
Voice quivering
Self-behavior focus
Increased wariness
Increased perspiration, sweaty palms, and/or flushing*

● Mild Anxiety

Description

Mild anxiety is normal anxiety that motivates an individual on a daily basis to perform and problem solve

Defining characteristics

Slight discomfort
Restlessness
Mild insomnia
Mild change in appetite

---

*All of the NANDA nursing diagnoses may be associated with anxiety in one of its levels.

*These defining characteristics are not NANDA approved.

Irritability
Repetitively questions
Attention-seeking behaviors
Increased alertness
Increased perception and problem solving
Easily angered
Focus on future problems
Fidgety movements

Interventions

Watch for signs of increasing anxiety
Help patient channel energy constructively
Use prn medication sparingly
Provide supportive listening
Encourage problem solving
Provide accurate and factual information
Be aware of patient's defense mechanisms
Assist in identifying successful coping skills
Maintain a calm, unhurried manner
Teach patient that mild anxiety is a normal part of
  living
Teach relaxation exercises and techniques

Expected outcomes

Patient
  Identifies source of own anxiety
  Employs stress management techniques
  Modifies behavior related to anxiety stressors
  Learns and employs relaxation techniques
  Practices cognitive reframing of negative stressors
  Works to achieve balance in life activities

● Moderate Anxiety

Description

Moderate anxiety is anxiety that interferes with new learning by narrowing the perceptual field so that the individual grasps less but is able to attend with direction by others

Defining characteristics

Progression of mild anxiety
Selective attention to environment
Concentration on individual tasks only
Moderate subjective discomfort
Increase in amount of time spent on problem situation
Voice tremors
Change in voice pitch
Tachypnea
Tachycardia
Tremulousness

Increased muscle tension
Nail biting, finger drumming, toe tapping, or foot swinging
Increased obsessive, ruminating thoughts
Inability to concentrate
Panic, guilt, shame, crying, irritability*

Interventions

Maintain calm, unhurried manner when dealing with patient
Speak in calm, firm, reassuring manner
Use short, simple, and direct sentences
Avoid becoming anxious, angry, or defensive
Listen to patient with respect and interest
Offer physical touch or comfort only if patient desires it
Administer antianxiety medications as ordered
Assist patient with labeling and recognizing anxiety
Assist patient with identifying and describing feelings
  and the source of distress
Do not probe
Allow patient to cry
Allow for verbal expression of anger
Assist patient with correcting events that precipitated
  anxiety
Encourage participation in diversional activities
  Reading
  Watching television
  Listening to the radio
  Writing letters
  Walking and other physical activity
  Visiting with relatives or friends
Assist patient with identifying coping mechanisms that
  will reduce anxiety and with using those that have
  been successful in the past
Teach patient to use relaxation techniques
Encourage patient to engage in activities that use large
  muscle groups
Establish and maintain familiar routines
Teach patient the importance of establishing daily exer-
  cise to control stress level
Continue with mild anxiety care

Expected outcomes

Patient
  Has a decrease in anxiety symptoms
  Is able to work on adaptive behaviors related to anxiety

● Severe Anxiety

Description

During an episode of severe anxiety, an individual's perceptual field is narrowed to the point that he or she is

---

*This defining characteristic is not NANDA approved.

unable to problem solve or learn; the focus is on small or scattered details, and communication patterns are disrupted; the patient may exhibit many aborted attempts to reduce anxiety and usually verbalizes great subjective distress

Defining characteristics

Sense of impending doom
Excessive muscle tension (headache, muscle spasms)
Diaphoresis
Respiratory changes
  Sighing
  Hyperventilation
  Dyspnea
  Dizziness
GI changes
  Nausea, vomiting
  Heartburn
  Belching
  Anorexia
  Diarrhea or constipation
Cardiovascular changes
  Tachycardia
  Palpitations
  Precordial discomfort
Greatly reduced range of perception
Inability to learn
Inability to concentrate
Sense of isolation
Difficult or inappropriate verbalization
Purposeless activity
Hostility

Interventions

Provide quiet and safe environment for patient
Provide frequent-to-constant contact and care
Administer medications as ordered
Assist and/or make decisions for patient; do not ask patient to do this entirely for himself or herself
Observe for signs of increasing agitation
Do not touch patient without his or her permission
Assure patient that he or she will be safe
Assess for safety in immediate environment

Expected outcomes

Patient
  Verbalizes decreased behavioral, affective, physiologic symptoms of anxiety
  Demonstrates ability to concentrate and attends with assistance to immediate environment and care needs
  Uses coping strategies to reduce anxiety
  Identifies thoughts and perceptions that preceded anxiety

● Panic

Description

Anxiety has escalated to the level that the individual is now a danger to self and/or others and may become immobilized or strike out in a random fashion

Defining characteristics

Severe hyperactivity or immobility
Extreme sense of isolation
Loss of identity; personality disintegration
Severe shakiness and muscular tension
Inability to communicate in complete sentences
Distortion of perception and unrealistic appraisal of environment and/or threat
Disorganized behavior in attempting to escape
Assaultive behavior
Avoidant behavior, phobia,* agoraphobia*

Interventions

Remain with patient; call for assistance
Remove as many physical and psychologic stressors from environment as possible
Speak in a calm, reassuring manner, using low voice tones
Tell patient that you (or staff) will not allow him or her to harm self or others
Isolate patient in quiet, safe area
Continue with severe anxiety care

Expected outcomes

Patient
  Does not harm self or others
  Has a decrease in physiologic anxiety or panic symptoms
  Has a decrease in anxiety or panic behaviors
  Has regained some reality-oriented cognitive abilities

● Hopelessness

Definition

The subjective state in which an individual sees limited or no alternatives or personal choices available and is unable to mobilize energy on own behalf

---

*These defining characteristics are not NANDA-approved.

Related factors

Prolonged activity restriction creating isolation
Failing or deteriorating physiologic condition
Long-term stress
Abandonment
Loss of belief in transcendent values/supreme being

Defining characteristics

Passivity, decreased verbalization
Decreased affect
Verbal cues (indicating despondency, "I can't," sighing)
Lack of initiative
Decreased response to stimuli
Turning away from speaker
Closing eyes
Shrugging in response to speaker
Decreased appetite
Increased or decreased sleep
Lack of involvement in care (i.e., passively allows care)

Interventions

Maintain a kind but firm attitude in all patient care activities
Maintain adequate hydration and nutrition
Measure intake and output as ordered or if indicated
Allow patient to wear his or her own clothes when possible
Involve patient in decision-making process when formulating care plan
Help patient set small, realistic goals
Give positive reinforcement for independent functioning
Assess patient with identifying areas over which he or she has control
If patient's appetite is poor and he or she is eating insufficiently, offer soft, nutritious foods that are easily chewed; include high-protein, between-meal snacks and a variety of liquids such as milkshakes, custards, and eggnog
Maintain liquids and food within easy reach
Offer food in frequent small amounts
Discourage intake of nonnutritive items such as coffee and foods high in refined sugar
Encourage water intake
Serve food attractively and at proper temperature
Provide foods that patient prefers; assist with menu selection
Do not give patient choice of not eating by asking, "Do you feel like eating?" Offer foods and say, "I have something for you to eat"
Administer stool softeners or laxatives as needed
Encourage intake of foods rich in fiber
Reinforce and assist grooming efforts and personal hygiene; encourage male patients to shave and female patients to apply makeup and to style their hair

Encourage patient to do things for himself or herself in order to feel better rather than waiting to feel better first before doing things for self
Assist with positioning in bed, sitting, and ambulation
Offer positive recognition for increased activity level
Provide noncompetitive activities (e.g., handicrafts, sewing, simple puzzles) before progressing to competitive activities such as board games
Promote planned rest periods during the day based on patient's physical condition
Discourage patient from sleeping all day or remaining in bed
Decrease environmental and other stimuli at night to promote sleep
Promote bedtime rituals
  Avoid stressful conversation
  Discourage caffeine-containing substances
  Discourage exercise before bedtime
  Offer back rub and warm milk
  Do not encourage dependence on hypnotics, especially those that suppress rapid eye movement (REM) sleep
Continually assess for suicide potential
If patient expresses plan for suicide, ask for details of plan
Support all verbalization of feelings, especially anger
Report suicidal ideation to attending physician
Observe closely for any self-destructive behavior when mood-elevating medications take effect or if patient demonstrates a sudden change in affect or behavior
Plan time to sit with patient; do not act rushed and remain comfortable during silent periods; do not require patient to always talk
Do not discourage patient from crying; remain with and support patient unless he or she requests privacy
Do not belittle patient's statements or offer inappropriately cheerful remarks or platitudes such as "Everything's going to be all right"
Be sure that your reassurances are realistic and are meant for patient, not for yourself
Assess your own feelings of powerlessness and helplessness
Avoid agreement with self-deprecating statements and cast doubt on their validity, but do not argue with patient
Reinforce positive statements about self and others; do not be overcomplimentary
If patient expresses feelings of guilt, assist him or her with exploring its origin and with exploring associated feelings of anger and resentment
Respect denial of illness if patient is unable to accept it; do not force reality on patient
Assist and support gradually increasing amounts of independent self-care
Provide for physical exercise at patient's level of tolerance

Maintain a clean, orderly environment

Ask if visit by religious or spiritual support person is desired

Administer antidepressants as ordered

Be aware of lag time of up to 2 weeks before they take effect

Familiarize yourself with side effects; most common are anticholinergic effects

Be aware of possible "cheeking" of medication or hoarding at bedside; antidepressants are lethal

Expected outcomes

Patient

Identifies cause(s) of hopelessness and depressions

Reaches acceptance stage of death and dying if terminal illness is present

Develops and implements plan of adaptive behaviors for depression

Has reduction in the vegetative signs and symptoms of depression

Verbalizes no self-destructive thoughts

● Body Image Disturbance

Definition

Disruption in the way one perceives one's body image

Related factors

Biophysical factors

Cognitive perceptual factors

Psychosocial factors

Cultural or spiritual factors

Defining characteristics

Either of the following (A or B) must be present to justify the diagnosis of body image disturbance:

A. Verbal response to actual or perceived change in structure and/or function

B. Nonverbal response to actual or perceived change in structure and/or function

The following clinical manifestations may be used to validate the presence of A or B:

Objective data

Missing body part

Actual change in structure and/or function

Not looking at body part

Not touching body part

Hiding or overexposing body part (intentional or unintentional)

Trauma to nonfunctioning part

Change in social involvement

Negative feelings about body

Feelings of helplessness, hopelessness, or powerlessness

Preoccupation with change or loss

Emphasis on remaining strengths, heightened achievement

Extension of body boundary to incorporate environmental objects

Personalization of part or loss by name

Depersonalization of part or loss by impersonal pronouns

Refusal to verify actual change

It may be possible to identify high risk populations such as those with the following conditions:

Missing parts

Dependence on machine

Significance of body part or functioning with regard to age, sex, developmental level, or basic human needs

Physical change caused by biochemical agents (drugs)

Physical trauma or mutilation

Pregnancy and/or maturational changes

Interventions

Determine patient's perception of change in body image and subsequent threat to self

Encourage verbalization of emotions such as anger, fear, frustration, and anxiety about altered functioning or lost body part

Encourage patient to look at and touch changed or lost body part

Assist family or significant other to adapt to change by providing resources, encouraging verbalization, and including them in care of patient

Encourage discussion of physical change in simple, direct, and factual manner

Assess your own attitudes and values related to wholeness and physical appearance

Give realistic feedback about loss or change

Discuss any sexual concerns openly and honestly

Encourage patient to participate in all therapeutic modalities offered in treatment

Give positive feedback for attempts to enhance and integrate new body image

Allow patient to progress at his or her own rate; do not force independent functioning or allow too much dependency

Help patient discriminate between internal stimuli and those that come from environment

Use active listening for nonverbal clues and verbal statements

Assess previous adaptive and maladaptive responses to stressors and illness

Assess for self-destructive behavior

Display empathy rather than sympathy

Provide patient and family/significant other with hospital and community resources

Discuss options available, such as cosmetic procedures, mechanical devices, and rehabilitative services

Teach patient and family/significant other the stages of grief and importance of grief work

Expected outcomes

Patient

Progresses toward completion of grief work

Verbalizes an acceptance of altered body functioning or loss

Plans realistically for future role functioning

Incorporates prosthesis, stoma, or device into changed body image

Verbalizes an interest and willingness to rejoin and resume social interactions and activities

Uses hospital and community support systems

● Self-Esteem Disturbance

Definition

Negative self-evaluation or feelings about self or self-capabilities, which may be directly or indirectly expressed

Related factors*

Loss of significant others

Change in body function or loss of part

Role change

Chronic illness

Aging

Defining characteristics

Self-negating verbalization

Expressions of shame and/or guilt

Evaluation of self as unable to deal with events

Rationalizing away or rejecting positive feedback and exaggerating negative feedback about self

Hesitancy to try new things and situations

Denial of problems obvious to others

Projection of blame and responsibility for problems

Rationalizing personal failures

Hypersensitivity to criticism

Grandiosity

---

*Related factors in this section are not NANDA approved.

Interventions

Provide for success experiences by introducing tasks at patient's level of functioning

Assess for possible alcohol or drug dependency

Communicate acceptance of patient and show genuine concern by spending unstructured, undemanding time

Explore patient's feelings and give validation for their expression

Provide for positive feedback on accomplishments

Explore alternative approach or coping strategies by giving observations; comment on positive attributes; avoid false praise

Explore with patient his or her current strengths

Encourage group interaction and explore possible support groups for aftercare

Assist with grooming and hygiene when necessary; promote attractiveness

Help patient list past success experiences

Teach assertive techniques (e.g., use of "I" statements, ability to say "no," body posture, eye contact, tone of voice, personal space, tactics for negotiation)

Teach difference between assertion and nonassertion, and aggressive and passive behaviors

Practice role playing and self-affirmation

Discuss activities that might increase self-esteem

Expected outcomes

Patient

Verbalizes realistic appreciation of self, including attributes and limitations

Reframes losses or changes into opportunities for personal development

Presents a positive personal appearance that reflects good grooming and hygiene

Initiates approach strategies to potentially threatening events or changes in environment

Demonstrates appropriate assertive behavior in social interactions

Reports a minimal level of interpersonal anxiety

Displays no overt self-destructive behaviors

Communicates needs effectively

● Personal Identity Disturbance

Definition

Inability to distinguish between self and nonself.

Personal identity is the coherent sense of self as a unique and separate identity that develops through successful resolution of developmental issues; identity rests on the ability to distinguish self from nonself, others, and the environment

Defining characteristics*

Disturbance in body image
Sex role disturbance
Gender identity confusion
Pathologic symbiotic relationships
Undifferentiated or fused family
Dissociative states
Developmental crisis such as adolescence
Delirium or dementia
Functional psychotic states (e.g., schizophrenia, bipolar disorder)
Severe anxiety and/or panic
Hypnagogic states

Interventions*

Assist patient with identifying actual threats to himself or herself from misinterpretation of perceived threat
Provide accurate information about threat
Provide calm, structured environment
Encourage self-care activities and taking responsibility for self
Direct activities that are simple and concrete and that support reality issues
Use simple, direct, and concise statements
Assess for altered homeostasis caused by physiologic disequilibrium
Assess developmental issues (e.g., age, crisis, regression)
Encourage verbalization of anxiety concerning sexual identity and sexual preference; be nonjudgmental
Assess for loss of contact with reality (i.e., for hallucinations and/or delusions)
Do not argue with delusions; do not reinforce them; look for needs patient might satisfy and find more appropriate manner of meeting them
Help patient to distinguish what is real and what is hallucination, delusion, or illusion; focus on here and now, decrease stimuli
Use anxiety-reducing interventions
Teach principles of normal growth and development
Refer patient to psychiatric unit or to psychotherapy as necessary

Expected outcomes*

Patient
Distinguishes self from others
Engages in interpersonal relationships without ego-merger or dissociation
Performs age-appropriate developmental tasks

*These sections are not NANDA approved.

Functional Health Pattern VIII: Role and Relationship

● Dysfunctional Grieving

Definition

The state in which actual or perceived object loss (object loss is used in the broadest sense) exists; objects include people, possessions, a job, status, home, ideals, parts and processes of the body, etc.

Related factors

Actual or perceived object loss
Thwarted grieving response to a loss
Absence of anticipatory grieving
Chronic fatal illness
Lack of resolution of previous grieving response
Loss of significant others
Loss of physiopsychosocial well-being
Loss of personal possessions

Defining characteristics

Verbal expression of distress at loss
Denial of loss
Expression of guilt
Expression of unresolved issues
Anger
Sadness
Crying
Difficulty in expressing loss
Alterations in the following:
  Eating habits
  Sleep patterns
  Dream patterns
  Activity level
  Libido
Idealization of lost object
Reliving of past experiences
Interference with life functioning
Developmental regression
Labile effect
Alterations in concentration and/or pursuits of tasks

Interventions

Identify significance of loss or multiple losses
Discuss ambivalence
Assess stage of grief and support patient's expression of grief

Use active listening and permit verbalization of anger

Observe for suicidal ideation

Facilitate discussion of positive and negative aspects of loss

Facilitate exploration of support groups

Provide opportunities for social interaction, especially with those who have coped successfully with similar loss

Teach patient and significant other about grief process

If patient attempts to consistently deny grief, plan to spend time each shift talking about loss, but avoid confrontation during discussion if patient changes subject and shifts reference; take cues from patient; be available to reopen subject when patient initiates conversation; use times of silence to convey support by offering your presence nonverbally.

Assure patient that all feelings are normal, including anger, hatred, and feelings of desertion, guilt, or betrayal

Expect patient to meet responsibilities; give positive reinforcement for resuming role responsibilities

Assist patient with identifying ways of adapting his or her lifestyle to accommodate the loss

Explore ways to assist patient to make new emotional investments

Be aware that it is acceptable to share your feelings with patient as long as these activities serve to support patient through his or her grief and are not expressions of unresolved loss on your part

If you become uncomfortable with your own unresolved feelings of loss, have another nurse who is comfortable talk with patient

Expected outcomes

Patient

Demonstrates engagement in the first steps of the grieving process

Demonstrates ability to express feelings of anger, guilt, sadness, depression

Is able to talk about loss and its impact on own life situation

Resumes some prior-to-loss role functions

Mobilizes network of supportive relationships

For anticipatory grief: patient maintains a constructive and meaningful relationship with the dying significant other without displaying characteristics of dysfunctional grief

● Altered Role Performance

Definition

Disruption in the way one perceives one's role performance

Defining characteristics

Change in self-perception of role

Denial of role

Change in others' perception of role

Conflict in roles

Change in physical capacity to resume role

Lack of knowledge of role

Change in usual patterns of responsibility

Interventions

Assess nature and degree of disturbance in role performance

Assess patient's and significant other's perceptions of role disturbance

Assess cultural and economic factors

Determine number and types of roles within family structure

Assist patient and family with clarifying expected roles and those that must be relinquished or altered

Assist patient with verbalizing realistic expectations of role and concrete behaviors necessary to implement performance

Support grief work if role has been lost

Allow time for expression of fears and anxieties

Be nonjudgmental

Determine if patient is in role that is compatible with his or her sexual orientation, sexual functioning, and self-concept

Provide role model for patient or refer him or her to groups that supply new models

Assist in role rehearsal through role playing

Expected outcomes

Patient

Verbalizes realistic perception and acceptance of new, lost, or altered role

Demonstrates role mastery

Develops with family or significant other specific behavioral strategies for assimilating role-specific changes in existing system

● Risk for Violence: Self-Directed or Directed at Others

Definition

The state in which an individual experiences behaviors that can be physically harmful either to the self or others

Risk factors

Anorexic or bulimic behaviors*
Antisocial character
Assaultive behavior*
Battered women
Catatonic excitement
Child abuse
Command hallucinations*
Drug and alcohol abuse*
Homicidal behavior*
Impulse disorders*
Manic excitement
Organic brain syndrome
Panic states
Rage reactions
Self-destructive behaviors of borderline
  personalities*
Suicidal behavior
Temporal lobe epilepsy
Toxic reactions to medication

● Risk for Violence:
  Self-Directed—Suicide†

Description

Self-directed violence is characterized by any activity that has negative consequences for the individual's physical or mental well-being

Defining characteristics

Low self-esteem
Major loss
Terminal illness or major disability
Lack of future orientation
Lack of impulse control
History of substance abuse
Severe depression
Agitation and increased restlessness
Excessive guilt
Hopelessness (i.e., the person feels like a failure)
Moderate or greater levels of anxiety
Powerlessness
Verbal statements concerning thoughts of death (e.g.,
  "I just can't cope with life anymore" and "My family
  would be better off without me")
Decreased verbal communication with family and/or
  significant others

Giving needed things away
Making a will
Checking on life insurance
Refusing to spend money for new possessions
Diminished ability to care for self
Writing letters saying "goodbye" or asking for forgive-
  ness
Suicidal plan

Interventions

Obtain psychiatric consultation for patient; active suicidal patients need to be seen daily by psychiatric consultant for evaluation and treatment
Administer antidepressant, antianxiety, and/or antipsy-
  chotic medications as ordered
    Administer prns as needed; watch for anticholinergic
    effects and extrapyramidal symptoms
Consider inpatient psychiatric hospitalization for mod-
  erate to severe depression
Refer patient to outpatient psychiatry for aftercare
Assess patient's suicidal ideation or plan each shift that
  patient is awake; note patient's sleep/wake patterns,
  ADLs, and eating behaviors
Assess patient for his or her level of agitation or energy
  to commit suicide
Assess environment for potential suicidal means such
  as sharp objects and remove them
Active suicidal patients require one-on-one
  staffing
Allow patient to talk about his or her depressed/suici-
  dal feelings and respond with active listening
Discuss suicide alternatives and options with
  patient
Discuss past coping strategies that have lifted
  depression and ask why patient may want to go
  on living
Discuss anger management and thought-stopping techniques
Report any increase in suicidal ideation/plan or
  mood changes to physician; evaluate for use of
  medications
Engage patient in adaptive activities (e.g., exercise, expressive therapy [music/art/writing], talk therapy) to
  decrease depression

Expected outcomes

Patient
    Demonstrates ability to manage stressors without re-
    sorting to violence against self
    Expresses satisfaction with current life situation
    Demonstrates increased self-esteem
    Develops discharge plans with staff

---

*These risk factors are not NANDA approved.
†Although this is a NANDA-approved diagnosis, the description,
 defining characteristics, interventions, and expected outcomes are
 not NANDA approved.

● Risk for Violence: Directed at Others—Excessive Hostility or Assaultive Behavior*

Description

A potential for violence directed at others is characterized by the acting out of anger, hostility, or resentment in such a manner that it brings threat or harm to others in a socially unacceptable context. Hostility may be considered different from anger in that it is viewed as destructive, whereas anger can be seen as constructive. Anger is often justified and can be a healthy response to threatening, fearful, or frustrating situations. Expressing anger may enhance self-esteem and give an individual a sense of power in a situation. Expressing anger appropriately involves the creative use of energy. Unexpressed anger tends to pile up and create a negative and resentful individual who often vents anger inappropriately or not at the original source. Aggressive behavior is hostility acted out and may involve significant danger to others. There are important ethical and legal issues involved in managing aggressive behavior. It is the responsibility of the nurse to become familiar with those issues within the institution. Aggression indicates that behavior is out of control, and it is the responsibility of the staff to protect the patient and others from harm, not to punish the patient.

Defining characteristics

Verbal abuse, increased voice volume (shouting, swearing)
Actual threats of harm or death
Rising agitation, pacing
Low self-esteem
Lack of impulse control, actual hitting or throwing things
Panic
Resistance to hospitalization or treatment
Psychosis: loss of contact with reality (delusions and/or hallucinations)
Intoxication by drugs or alcohol; history of substance abuse
Destruction of property

Interventions

Intervene early; prevention is the best strategy
Call patient by name; speak in calm, firm, manner and

tell patient to stop his or her violent or assaultive behavior
Direct patient to calm and control himself or herself
Do not approach an openly hostile, aggressive patient by yourself; obtain assistance from other staff members
Listen to what patient has to say
Do not invade personal space
Do not touch patient
Remove others from immediate area
Do not threaten, argue, or respond with hostility
Do not approach patient who has a weapon by yourself or attempt to disarm him or her; get appropriate assistance
State that you cannot allow patient to harm himself or herself or anyone in environment
Do not leave patient alone
Be aware of your own feelings and behavior
Maintain and communicate control to patient
    Do not become personally insulted or demonstrate anger at patient's behavior
    Do not submit to patient's inappropriate demands
    Have another nurse remain with patient if you become upset or defensive
Decrease environmental stimulation
Give patient as much control over his or her own area as is safely possible
Focus on patient's feelings
Avoid pat reassurances and overgeneralizations
Use the same terms that patient uses (e.g., "upset," "frustrated," "ticked off")
Make every attempt to talk patient out of intended assaultive behavior
Apply mechanical restraints only if absolutely necessary and according to policy; have a plan
Offer medication early in preescalation phase
Administer chemical restraint (medications) according to policy
When incident has passed, complete the following:
    Assist patient with identifying and discussing his or her feelings
    Assist patient with identifying what triggered loss of control
    Assist patient with identifying alternative ways of expressing emotion and relieving tension
Be aware of importance of staff continuing with routine patient care activities
Manage emotional reactions of other patients to the incident
Involve patient in activities to promote release of energy and feelings (e.g., large muscle movement)
Understand that rejection of patient by staff can increase patient's anxiety and perpetuate anger
Teach difference between assertive and aggressive behavior

---

*Although this is a NANDA-approved diagnosis, the description, defining characteristics, interventions, and expected outcomes are not NANDA approved.

Expected outcomes

Patient
Will not direct excessive hostility or assaultive behaviors toward others
Will use alternate ways to manage expression of anger
Displays effective coping strategies in reducing anxiety and in assessing potentially threatening situations
Develops increased self-awareness and increased self-esteem

● Domestic Violence*

Description

The physical or emotional harassment, assault and battery, including rape, between family members, significant others, or acquaintances; nearly 30% of all homicides in the United States occur among family members

Assessment

Subjective data

Pain associated with physical trauma (including rape)
Anxiety, depression, apprehension, or hopelessness
Suicide attempts
Describes typical behaviors of potential or actual batterer
Actual injuries including rape; injuries during pregnancy
Controlling behavior; manages person's schedule, comings/goings, and decisions
Jealousy of person's time with friends, family, and coworkers
Isolation; cuts person off from supportive resources such as talking with friends on phone or socializing with coworkers
Batterer blames others for personal problems; it is always someone else's fault; past history of battering with a list of excuses why someone else caused the battering behavior; disavows responsibility for personal actions
Hypersensitive and easily upset by minor annoyances (e.g., criticism of any kind, request to assist with child care or chores)
Cruelty to children and animals with seeming insensitivity to their pain and suffering; teases and/or hurts children and animals

"Playful" use of force in sex; holding the person down or initiating sex when the person is asleep, sick, or tired
Verbal abuse including degrading, cruel, and humiliating language; prevents person from going to sleep to argue or wakes person up to verbally abuse
Mercurial behavior; sudden mood swings with unpredictability of demeanor
Demonstrates loving remorse/sorrow and vows never to repeat the battering but does so
Breaks or strikes objects narrowly missing or actually hitting person or children; beats on furniture/table
Threatens violence including threats to kill the person, hurt them, break their neck
Uses physical force during an argument by holding person down or against a wall; pushes, hits, slaps, shoves, or kicks; chokes, stabs, or shoots

Objective data

Injuries on face, neck, throat, chest, abdomen, or genitals
Multiple injuries in various stages of healing
History of injuries during pregnancy
Substantial delay between onset of injury and presentation for treatment
Minimization of the seriousness of the situation and the injuries
Flat affect; tearfulness; verbalization of hopelessness, helplessness, and apathy
Extent or type of injury inconsistent with explanation given
Evidence of alcohol or drug abuse
Partner appears to be overly (out of norm) concerned with patient's care; does not leave when requested; intrusive regarding patient's medical care
Evidence of nonspecific physical or psychological complaints such as frequent headaches, nonorganic GI complaints, depression, anxiety, exhaustion, difficulty in concentrating

Diagnostic tests (for rape)

Cultures for gonorrhea and chlamydia
Microscopic examination of vaginal secretions for motile sperm
Baseline serologic tests for hepatitis B virus; human immunodeficiency virus (HIV), and syphilis
Pregnancy test

Diagnostic tests (for battery)

Radiologic examination, including MRI, CT scans, and ultrasound

---

*Not a NANDA-approved diagnosis.

Endoscopic/laparoscopic procedures as indicated
Assessment for compartmental syndrome
CBC and coagulation factors

Potential complications

Noncurable sexually transmitted disease (herpes, AIDS)
Pregnancy
Intracranial bleed
Fractures
Internal bleeding
Hemorrhage, shock, death

Collaborative management

Therapeutic management

Manage evident trauma: hematomas, fractures, lacerations
Photographs of injuries
Prophylaxis for sexually transmitted disease if raped
Postcoital hormonal prophylaxis to prevent pregnancy if raped
Tetanus injection
Psychologic counseling
Notification of police department and/or child protective services
Referral to a "safe house" or shelter
Collection of evidentiary material for authorities, including pubic hair combings, samples of pubic and head hair, vaginal secretions, cultures, results of microscopic evaluation for motile sperm, and collection of patient's bagged clothing in rape cases

Nursing management

PATIENT PROBLEMS/NURSING DIAGNOSES

● **NDX:** Rape-trauma syndrome associated with attempted or actual attack

Provide safe and protected environment
Ensure considerate physical examination
Assist to establish a close relationship with a safe person *to ensure presence of an ongoing support person*
Assist patient and support person to discuss and focus on the subjective experience *to express feelings*
Discuss anger and related feelings *to avoid social withdrawal and isolation*
Assist patient to establish self-control over personal decisions
Counsel patient regarding stress response images, sounds, or sensations that provoke anxiety
Counsel immediate family about rape-trauma syndrome

and how symptoms are manifested in patient and their response to the patient

EXPECTED OUTCOMES

Patient verbalizes that support person has expressed concern and warmth
Patient verbalizes understanding of rape-trauma syndrome or retains document describing anticipated future reactions, signs, and symptoms
Patient verbalizes intent to adhere to decisions made about keeping follow-up appointments (medical, psychological counseling, HIV results counseling, rape-support groups), taking of medications, and following through with legal authorities

● **NDX:** Powerlessness related to victimization by a violent individual

Encourage patient to identify the areas over which she or he has power, such as managing the care and nutrition for children, and reinforce those capabilities *to promote a sense of control and of capability*
Identify areas of perceived powerlessness and assist patient to consider alternatives and other courses of action
Assist patient to identify a resource person while he or she is safe; encourage patient to contact this person before leaving the health care provider's office *to ensure patient safety and security*
Provide opportunities to express feelings *to increase understanding of individual coping styles and mechanisms to provide a more objective perception of the violence/battering*
Encourage expressions of positive thoughts and emotions including the will to live, hope and faith, and a sense of purpose
Assist patient to develop a "safety plan" for self and children in order *to be able to leave the home environment at any time day or night*

EXPECTED OUTCOMES

Patient verbalizes positive feelings and confidence in ability to increase control over life circumstances
Patient demonstrates effective coping strategies based on realistic assessment of personal situation (e.g., seeks protective services for self or children and has a safety plan)
Acknowledges abilities for managing nutrition for self and children

Patient/family teaching and home care considerations

Instruct patient to go to any emergency room if future injuries occur by calling an ambulance, friend, relative, or the police

Contact personal physician or other health care provider immediately if future injuries occur

Learn how to obtain a copy of patient's medical record, which will be needed when the district attorney files charges against the abuser

Develop a safety plan for self and children for leaving the abuser because this may need to occur during, after, or when anticipating a beating

A safety plan might include the following measures:

Pack an extra set of clothes, toilet articles, and necessary medications for self and children; store this with a friend or neighbor; include an extra set of keys to the house and car

Have extra cash, credit cards, checkbook, or savings account book hidden or with a friend; have identification for self and children such as birth certificates, social security cards, voter registration, marriage and/or driver's license and children's immunization records, which may be required to enroll children in a school or to obtain financial assistance

Have a list of important phone numbers in a protected place, including police, attorney or legal aid, relatives, friends, social service agencies, crisis hotlines, or safe houses

Take something special or meaningful, such as a favorite toy, blanket, or book, for each child if possible

Take or have photocopies of important financial records, such as tax returns, grant deed, house payment or rent receipts, insurance, and title to the car, in a protected place

Have a plan and know exactly where to go and how to get there even if the battering should occur in the middle of the night

Explain that a period of loving remorse by the batterer who promises never to beat the victim again is a typical response of batterers who feel ashamed and horrified by their actions

Ensure that patient understands that remorseful batterers *do* typically repeat the battering and rarely discontinue battering without being brought into the legal system and that legal intervention *does* have a positive effect

● Impaired Social Interaction

Definition

The state in which an individual participates in an insufficient or excessive quantity or ineffective quality of social exchange

Related factors

Knowledge/skill deficit about ways to enhance mutuality

Communication barriers
Self-concept or self-esteem disturbance
Absence of available significant others or peers
Limited physical mobility
Therapeutic isolation
Sociocultural dissonance
Environmental barriers
Altered thought processes
Inadequate personality*

Defining characteristics

Verbalized or observed discomfort in social situations

Verbalized or observed inability to receive or communicate a satisfying sense of belonging, caring, interest, or shared history

Observed use of unsuccessful social interaction behaviors

Dysfunctional interaction with peers, family, and/or others

Family report of change in style or pattern of interaction

● Manipulative Behavior†

Description

Manipulative behavior involves two ways of controlling the behavior of others to achieve one's goals: passive behavior gets needs met indirectly through others; aggressive behavior is directed against or toward others in an attempt to get one's own needs met; these two ways of interacting are used when an individual feels powerless to meet his own needs through assertive interaction

Defining characteristics

Lack of insight toward problems and/or denial of problems

Inability to express anger openly
Changing subject of conversation or activity of group
Crying or acting helpless when confronted
Attention-seeking behavior such as monopolizing conversations in both social and therapeutic interactions
Constantly seeking approval and recognition
Being overly solicitous and ingratiating
Attempting to gain special attention or privileges
Demonstrating anger and feeling hurt, deserted, and unworthy when above attempts are denied
Reporting confidential information to others
Attempting to use others' weaknesses against them; playing one person against the other

---

*This related factor is not NANDA approved.
†Not a NANDA-approved diagnosis.

Consistently breaking rules and routines and disrupting procedures
Intellectualizing and rationalizing problems away
Projecting blame onto others
Viewing self as uniquely special and deserving
Attempting to get others to rescue him or her by being helpless and boosting others' self-esteem by relying on them to fix the problem

Interventions

Assess needs that patient is trying to meet through manipulation
Decrease patient's manipulation of staff
Avoid discussing yourself and other staff members with patient
Assign consistent staff when possible
Develop plan of care with other staff members and communicate with everyone involved with patient's care
Communicate often with other staff members to ensure continuity and consistency of approach
Point out manipulative behavior to patient if he or she states:
"You're the only one who understands . . ."
"You're the only one who cares about me"
"You're the only one I can talk to"
Caution staff not to attempt to be liked or to be patient's favorite nurse
Do not accept favors as gifts; this fosters a personal relationship
Be matter of fact in any interactions with patient
Avoid angry, negative, and punitive responses to patient when patient is being manipulative
Offer limited choices (e.g., "Would you like to ambulate now or at 9 o'clock?")
Be direct in your interactions; do not bargain or rationalize
Assist patient in recognizing his or her own patterns of manipulative behavior by providing nonthreatening similar examples
Point out relationship between need to control and inability to achieve self-control
Encourage identification of alternate and appropriate behaviors for meeting needs; use role playing
Give verbal and nonverbal positive reinforcement when patient functions without being manipulative
Encourage and support patient to verbalize his or her feelings, medical conditions, and/or surgery and current treatment; listen nonjudgmentally
Build trust through consistency and keeping promises
Assure patient that if limits are set, it is because you care and that caring and limit setting are neither mutually exclusive nor opposites
Involve patient in his or her own plan of care without allowing patient to dictate aspects of care

Expected outcomes

Patient verbalizes satisfaction with improved social interaction
Demonstrates ability to define and meet needs without manipulative behavior
Participates actively in planning own care

● Demanding Behavior*

Description

Demanding behavior occurs in syndromes involving anxiety, fear, helplessness, inadequacy, inferiority, hostility, manipulation, and dependent behavior; the individual believes he or she is incapable of fulfilling own needs or having his or her needs met by making requests in a direct, matter-of-fact manner; attempts are then made to coerce others to meet these needs by making requests with forceful and manipulative behavior with implied threat

Defining characteristics†

Making frequent requests
Constant attention seeking
Attempting to coerce others to meet needs
Asking others to do what he or she is capable of doing
Displaying helplessness when making requests
Displaying anger when requests are not met immediately
Detaining staff with subsequent requests after initial request has been met
Domineering, sarcastic, or ridiculing behavior
Using threats if requests are not met
Not using proper channels of communication (e.g., goes over nurses' authority by talking to supervisors)

Interventions

Be aware that dynamics between staff and patient can create and maintain the problem situation
Be aware that staff's responses to patient will influence whether or not patient continues to be demanding; avoid displaying annoyance or anger with patient's request; understand that such a display perpetuates patient's demands
Be aware that depersonalization caused by hospitalization promotes anxiety and contributes to patient's perception of lack of control and self-esteem
Assess patient's unfilled needs
Involve patient in deciding how his or her needs will be met

---

*Not a NANDA-approved diagnosis.
†Defining characteristics in this section are not NANDA approved.

Assist patient with identifying demanding behaviors

Relate to patient your own responses to demanding behavior in nonemotional tone of voice

Assist patient with developing alternative behavior by the following actions:

Asking directly for what is wanted

Taking responsibility for behavior by using the personal pronoun "I" before a request

Becoming more aware of responses and associated feelings when requests are not met immediately

Reinforcing independently made direct questions

Do not refuse or ignore patient's request

Give reasons why requests cannot be met

Anticipate realistic requests and meet them rapidly

Allow patient as much control in his or her own care as possible

Spend time with patient when he or she is not demanding; set up a regular schedule of checking in with patient that is independent of call light usage

Give patient your full attention during verbal interactions and recognize positive qualities to promote self-esteem

Demonstrate interest and be attentive to patient as a person

Allow opportunity for appropriate ventilation of feelings regarding annoyances, restrictions, and feeling of powerlessness

If you tell patient that you will return in 20 minutes, be sure that you do

Avoid withdrawing from patient by insensitive mechanistic actions

Expected outcome

Patient demonstrates ability and willingness to learn to meet needs without having to resort to demanding behaviors

● Withdrawn Behavior*

Description

Withdrawn behavior is an attempt to avoid interaction with others and thus avoid relatedness; it is a defense against anxiety that is related to a stressor or threat; the range of behavior can be from disinterest in others to severe withdrawal with an accompanying increase in primary process thinking; this may ultimately lead to autistic behavior or delusions and hallucinations as the individual withdraws more from the environment and attends to internal thoughts and stimuli

---

*Not a NANDA-approved diagnosis.

Defining characteristics

Dull, flat, or inappropriate affect/mood

Apathy

Depression

Absence of spontaneity

Inappropriate response to environmental stimuli

Excessive fear and increasing levels of anxiety

Decreased or absent verbalization

Decreased motor activity or agitation

Lack of awareness of surroundings

Inattention to grooming and personal habits

Inappropriate social behavior, including open masturbation, obscene language, handling of excreta

Regression (the patient may assume the fetal position)

Disturbance in thought content, such as delusions

Disturbance in perception, such as hallucinations

Interventions

Communicate with patient in a positive, accepting manner

Plan time to sit with patient

Make sure that you have patient's attention before speaking or giving directions on care

Avoid attempts to oververbalize with patient

Remain comfortable during silent periods

Ask open-ended questions, not "yes" or "no" questions

Expect patient to respond to conversation

Provide reality-oriented conversation focusing on the here and now; avoid generalizations and abstract concepts

Allow sufficient time for patient to respond

Avoid placing patient in a private room

Administer psychotropic medications and antidepressants as ordered

Measure intake and output if indicated

Assist with meeting patient's basic needs (e.g., eating, drinking, elimination, bathing, and ambulation)

Assist and teach ROM exercises; turn patient q2h if bedridden

Maintain skin integrity

Use television and/or radio in room

Provide newspapers and magazines

Involve patient in his or her plan of care

Assist patient with identifying alternate and appropriate behaviors

Orient patient to time, place, and person; use clock and calendar in room

Provide positive reinforcement for self-care activities

Be aware that logical arguments only increase delusional thought content

Encourage and support verbalization of feelings about concrete issues (e.g., medical condition, menu)

Decrease anxiety level (see anxiety care plan, p. 36)
Provide a regular schedule of activities (routines)
Use empathy (e.g., "That must be frightening.")
Gradually introduce patient to more people in
  environment

Expected outcomes

Patient
  Exhibits a decrease in withdrawn behavior, depres-
    sion, and social isolation
  Demonstrates an increase in social interactions
Patient exhibits an increase in self-care and other func-
  tional task activities

● Dependent Behavior*

Description

*Dependent behavior includes impaired decision mak-
ing; a tendency to lean on others for guidance, direction,
support, protection, and advice; and a compelling need to
relate to a stronger person in coping with stressors*

Defining characteristics

Constant attention seeking
Whining
Helplessness when making a request
Refusing to make decisions
Asking others to do what he or she could do himself or
  herself
Feeling no responsibility for the following:
  Decisions
  Behaviors
  Feelings
  Thoughts
Lack of initiative
Low self-esteem
Procrastination
Passiveness
Low frustration tolerance
Lack of social skills
Few adaptive coping skills
Lack of problem-solving skills
Moderate interpersonal anxiety
Moderate-to-severe depression
Covert expressions of anger

---

*Not a NANDA-approved diagnosis.

Repeated hospitalizations; many physical
  complaints
Substance abuse and/or dependency
Inability to define or express needs appropriately

Interventions

Assess for suicidal thoughts and behaviors
Assess patient's dependence on drugs and/or
  alcohol
Maintain consistent approach
  Set limits for unrealistic and inappropriate
    requests
  Use calm, firm tone of voice when speaking
  Do not display anger or frustration toward patient
  Do not reward attention-seeking behavior
  Meet patient's dependency needs at first, then gradu-
    ally assist patient to become more independent in
    stages: (1) do for patient; (2) do with patient; (3) al-
    low patient to take lead while you provide support;
    (4) provide positive reinforcement for independent
    behaviors
Avoid making simple decisions for patient
Offer alternative choices
Investigate physical symptoms reported by patient,
  but do not encourage "sick role" behavior
Assist patient with verbalizing and identifying
  strengths
Do not be the only person with whom the patient can
  talk; involve other staff with patient
Avoid feelings of sympathy; do not give your phone
  number to patient or allow patient to call you at work
  or home
Assist patient with identifying consequences of behav-
  ior, including indecisiveness
Assist patient with expressing anger in open and direct manner when his or her demands or requests
  are not met
Positively reinforce expression of genuine feelings
Refer patient to self-help groups when appropriate
Teach patient about physical and/or psychologic dependency that occurs with continued use of tranquilizers and/or alcohol

Expected outcomes

Patient
  Assumes responsibility for major areas of life
  Resumes appropriate role functioning
  Reports satisfying social interactions
  Makes decisions independently
  Copes with stressors without using tranquilizers
    and/or alcohol

Functional Health Pattern X: Coping/Stress Tolerance

● Ineffective Individual Coping

Definition

Impairment of adaptive behaviors and problem-solving abilities of a person in meeting life's demands and roles

Related factors

Situational crises
Maturational crises
Personal vulnerability
Multiple life changes
No vacations
Inadequate relaxation
Inadequate support systems
Little or no exercise
Poor nutrition
Unmet expectations
Work overload
Too many deadlines
Unrealistic perceptions
Inadequate coping methods

Defining characteristics

Verbalization of inability to cope or inability to ask for help
Inability to meet role expectations
Inability to meet basic needs
Inability to problem solve
Alteration in societal participation
Destructive behavior toward self or others
Inappropriate use of defense mechanisms
Change in visual communication patterns
Verbal manipulation
High illness rate
High rate of accidents
Overeating
Lack of appetite
Excessive smoking
Excessive drinking
Overuse of prescribed tranquilizers
Alcohol proneness
High blood pressure
Chronic fatigue
Insomnia
Muscular tension
Ulcers
Frequent headaches
Frequent neckaches
Irritable bowel
Chronic worry
General irritability
Poor self-esteem
Chronic anxiety
Emotional tension
Chronic depression

Interventions

Understand that patient may not know what the problem is
Assist patient with clearly identifying precipitating event
Explore major changes that have occurred in previous 2 weeks, past 6 months, or last year
Ask patient how he or she feels and help patient to put a label on emotion
Assist patient with identifying
  How problem affects his or her life and future
  How problem is affecting patient's family or significant other
  If other factors could be influencing the way he or she sees problem
Assist patient with identifying his or her strengths and coping skills
  Ask patient if anything like this has happened to him or her in past
  Ask how past crises were handled
  Inquire as to how patient usually decreases tension and anxiety
  Ascertain whether patient has tried to use any of the same anxiety-reducing methods this time; if not, attempt to explore possible reasons or blocks to using prior coping skills
  If anxiety-reducing methods were tried and were unsuccessful, ask what kept them from working
  Assist patient with exploring and identifying what else he or she thinks might work
Assist patient with identifying nature and strength of situational supports; collect data about current and potential sources of support:
  Persons with whom patient lives
  Persons with whom patient is close
  Friends or best friend
  Persons available to help
  Persons whom patient trusts and feels are understanding
  Community services
Assist patient with planning alternative solutions using patient's own coping skills and situational and environmental supports
Offer suggestions of other adaptive coping strategies
Confront self-defeating and destructive behavior in a

factual and nonjudgmental manner; make observations about amount of alcohol intake, use of tranquilizers, or overindulgence in food or smoking

Acknowledge patient's feelings about crisis

Assist patient with sorting out his or her feelings and validate them as acceptable and normal

Assist patient with exploring alternative coping skills

Assist patient with role playing or rehearsing new approaches to deal with problems

Present yourself as role model for open and direct communication, innovative thinking, flexibility, and self-awareness

Provide positive reinforcement for all adaptive coping skills used in situation

Teach relaxation techniques

Teach patient about psychologic and physiologic effects of chronic stress

Expected outcomes

Patient

Returns to precrisis level of functioning

Develops an adequate response repertoire

Displays no symptoms of excessive anxiety or lasting physiologic responses to stress

Increases self-esteem

Acknowledges increased confidence to solve future problems effectively

Functional Health Pattern XI: Value and Belief

● Spiritual Distress (Distress of the Human Spirit)

Definition

Disruption in the life principle that pervades a person's entire being and that integrates and transcends one's biologic and psychosocial nature

Related factors

Separation from religious and cultural ties

Challenged belief and value system (e.g., result of moral or ethical implications of therapy or result of intense suffering)

Defining characteristics

Concern expressed regarding the meaning of life and death and/or belief systems

Anger toward supreme being (as defined by the person)

Questioning the meaning of suffering

Verbalizing inner conflict about beliefs

Verbalizing concern about relationship with deity/supreme being

Questioning meaning of own existence

Inability to choose or choosing not to participate in usual religious practices

Seeking spiritual assistance

Questioning moral and ethical implications of therapeutic regimen

Displacement of anger toward religious representatives

Description of nightmares or sleep disturbances

Alteration in behavior or mood evidenced by anger, crying, withdrawal, preoccupation, anxiety, hostility, apathy

Regarding illness as punishment

Not experiencing that God is forgiving

Inability to accept self

Engaging in self-blame

Denying responsibility for problems

Describing somatic complaints

Interventions

Assess cause(s) of spiritual distress

Assess patient's belief in divine power, its existence, and credibility

Meaning of religion; description or relationship of divine power

Means of communicating with divine power

Effect of beliefs on personal life

Sense of identity, worth, and purpose

Relationship with others: value, need, changes caused by illness

Meaning of illness or suffering in relation to belief

Important features of religious faith

Assistance with fear, pain

Source of strength, hope, love

Religious practices, symbols, medals, garments

Provide a quiet, private atmosphere for patient's expressions of faith, self, and meaning of life

Listen with attention, understanding, and compassion

Be available and sensitive to patient's needs to express his or her feelings

Talk *with,* not *at,* the patient

Be cognizant of your nonverbal behavior, biases, preconceptions, and judgments

Do not impose your beliefs on patient

Accurately interpret and clarify meanings expressed and behavior observed

Assist patient with facing reality; explore patient's experience with illness and meaning of suffering

Encourage self-awareness and mobilization of internal strengths and resources

Assist patient through uncompleted developmental

stages to attain trust, hope, love, forgiveness, and purpose in life

Assist patient with exploring life situations and discov-
ering practical solutions to problems

Allow and encourage free choice and decision making

Praise physical, emotional, and spiritual successes

Convey to patient that he or she is important and what
he or she does with his or her life matters

Use touch therapeutically (e.g., stroking, holding
hands, and grooming) when providing daily care if patient desires

Provide pleasant view and special pictures

Control odors and smoking as necessary

Provide articles necessary for religious practice (e.g.,
special clothing, rosary, books)

Arrange patient's religious symbols for easy viewing

Arrange for patient's favorite music (i.e., obtain
recordings)

Read favorite, comforting passages from Bible, Koran,
Torah, Book of Mormon, poetry, or other meaningful
works

Share in prayers or special practices when appropriate

Provide uninterrupted time for meditation, silence, and
prayer

Arrange for communion, Holy Eucharist, anointment,
and other practices

Arrange easy access for communication with loved
ones, chaplain, priest, rabbi, or minister

Provide special foods, meals, and periods of fasting as
needed

Consider needs in special situations
 Birth: baptism or circumcision
 Medical procedures: amputation, burial, transfusions
 Schedule for holy days
 Religious observances
 Anointment
 Laying-on of hands
 Healing services
 Confession
 Communion, Holy Eucharist
 Restrictions or needs in diet or appearance
 Not cutting or shaving of hair
 Use of special clothing
Death
 Baptism
 Rite for anointing the sick
 Bathing and placement of body
 Positioning of extremities

Expected outcomes

Patient
 Expresses increase in spiritual wellness
 Expresses increased sense of hope and well-being
 Uses available religious resources

Care of Patient With Special Needs

● General Perioperative Care and Education

Preoperative assessment

Observations/findings

PSYCHOLOGIC STATUS

Understanding of operative, preoperative, and postoperative procedures

Ability to verbalize fears and anxieties

Ability to concentrate

Past successful coping behaviors

Previous experience with pain relief measures

Relationship, response, and behavior of patient and
family

Family's knowledge of operative procedure

PHYSICAL STATUS

Nutritional and hygienic state

Elimination habits

Medication history

Medical background
 Preexisting diseases (e.g., diabetes, hypertension,
 bleeding disorders)
 Prior surgery
 Anesthesia history
 Substance abuse history

Socioeconomic background

Allergies

Physical handicaps and other limitations

Signs of infection

Mental, visual, and auditory acuity

LEGAL STATUS

Informed consent signed for operation

Physician's preoperative orders complete

Identification bands on and correct

Patient's willingness to receive blood documented

Environmental orientation recorded
 Use of equipment in room
 Use of call bell
 Purpose and use of side rails

Interventions

Maintain NPO after midnight or according to policy

Take and record patient's baseline BP, T, P, R, and
weight; report any abnormalities to physician

Check for and record any allergies

Monitor laboratory work; report any abnormalities to physician

Assess surgical preparations for completeness

Monitor for electrocardiogram (ECG) and chest x-ray examinations

Assess patient's skin for baseline color

Assess patient's history, physical, and anesthesia records for completeness

Assess patient's blood type and cross match results; note number of units of blood available

Administer preoperative medications; make sure that side rails are up after you complete injection

Insert nasogastric tube and/or indwelling bladder catheter according to policy

Initiate parenteral fluids

Encourage patient to void before leaving for operating room

Ensure that patient removes dentures, contact lenses, nail polish, makeup, prosthesis, and/or valuables before leaving for operating room; religious medals may be pinned to gown

Preoperative education

PSYCHOLOGIC STATUS

Reinforce physician's explanation of surgical procedure

Answer any questions as honestly as possible

Allow time for and encourage verbalization of fears and anxieties

Avoid standard clichés such as "Don't worry," "Everything is just fine," or "I know how you feel"

Listen to and *hear* patient

Avoid rushing through explanations

Accept patient's behavior unless it is unsafe; avoid judging patient's behavior or trying to change it

Involve family or significant other in patient's care and instructions when possible

Explain pain management plan: using patient controlled analgesia (PCA), determining pain scale, asking for medication before pain becomes severe

PHYSICAL STATUS

Explain all procedures and their reasons and importance

Preoperative
I.V. line, indwelling urethral catheter
Skin preparation
NPO
Laboratory work

Postoperative
Parenteral fluids
Vital signs
Dressings
Pain and availability of medications
Nasogastric and other tubes
Indwelling urethral catheter

Incentive spirometer, oxygen therapy
Not touching the incision

Teach patient, using return demonstration, how to do the following:
Turn, cough, and deep breathe, depending on surgical procedure
Use spirometer
Support incision during coughing
Breathe deeply every hour after surgery
Exercise lower extremities actively
Sit up, get up, and ambulate; Prolonged chair sitting should be avoided

Explain importance of progressive care
Early ambulation
Self-care encouraged as soon as patient is able

Discuss purpose of recovery room with patient and family
Visiting policies
Type of care
Length of stay if applicable
Possibility of placement in intensive care unit (ICU) if indicated

Explain other hospital policies as indicated
Visiting hours
Number of visitors
Location of waiting rooms
How physician will contact them after operation

● Immediate Postoperative Care

Assessment

Observations/findings

GENERAL ANESTHESIA

Level of consciousness
Unconscious state
Absence of cough or gag reflex
Presence of endotracheal tube or airway
Semiconscious state
Absence of endotracheal tube
Presence of oral or nasal airway
Partial return of all reflexes
Conscious state
Return of all reflexes

Respiration: rate, rhythm, depth, quality

Laryngospasm

Endotracheal tube or airway present
Position
Adequate ventilation

Pulse: rate, rhythm, quality

Blood pressure: hypotension, hypertension, normal

Parenteral infusion: flow rate, type of solution, site, patent vein, medications; observe for infiltration

Pain: location, amount, severity, type, tolerance of

Skin
  Color: normal, flushed, cyanotic, pallid
  Condition: dry, moist, hot, cold
Nail beds: color, pink, cyanotic, purple, dark brown
Return of reflexes
Type of surgery performed
Site of incision: dry, bleeding, drainage, drains
Dressing: dry, intact
Drainage tubes: patency and connections
Past and current medical problems

SPINAL ANESTHESIA

Monitor each item under the general anesthesia section and check the patient's legs for the following:
Mobility
Color in dependent and independent position
Temperature, pedal pulses
Return of sensation

Interventions

Maintain patent airway
  Maintain endotracheal tubes; nasal or oral airway
    Suction prn
  For an inadequate airway
    Hyperextend neck
    Bring chin forward
    Turn head to one side
    Insert oral or nasal airway
    Notify anesthesiologist of respiratory impairment
Take initial BP, P, and R and report findings to anesthesiologist
Monitor patient q15min and prn until stable
  BP, R, and apical pulse
  Oxymetry pulse if applicable
  Level of consciousness
  Return of reflexes
  IV site
  Site of incision
  Drainage tubes and equipment
  Movement of extremities
Monitor rectal or axillary temperature q1h to 4h
Auscultate chest for breath sounds q30min
Administer oxygen, or incentive spirometer
Maintain NPO
Maintain parenteral fluids
Measure intake and output; report less than30 ml/hr of output to physician
Reinforce dressing prn; notify physician if drainage is excessive
Administer blood and blood components as indicated
Administer all medications as ordered
Encourage patient to move his or her legs and feet, if not contraindicated

Position patient to maintain optimal ventilation and comfort
Maintain pain management; administer narcotics in one-fourth, one-third, or one-half doses until patient has reacted fully
Monitor patient-controlled analgesia (PCA) or continuous epidural anesthesia (CEA) as warranted
Keep patient warm and dry; cover him or her with warm blankets if necessary
Remain with patient if he or she is restless
Turn patient's head to one side at first sign of vomiting; suction as needed
Administer oral hygiene q1 to 4 hrs; keep patient's mouth and tongue moist
Assist patient to turn, cough, and deep breathe q1h to 2h when reactive; provide support to incision as needed
Monitor traction equipment for accurate placement and weights
Monitor casts for position and body alignment
Maintain quiet environment; avoid discussions over patient's bed
Discharge to unit occurs at the following times:
  Patient is fully reactive
  Patient is moving extremities well
  Patient's vital signs have been stable for 1 hour
  Patient is medicated for pain and vital signs are stable
  Dressings have been checked and no bleeding or excessive drainage is noted
  All drainage tubes are functioning
Notify unit of patient's arrival and any equipment needed.
Accompany patient to unit and give receiving nurse a comprehensive report of his or her condition, including type of surgery, last time he or she was medicated for pain, and his or her latest vital signs

● Care of the Aging Patient

Description

Aging: part of the continuum of life; effects vary widely from one individual to the next; does not progress at a uniform rate, and at any given time the patient may exhibit only a few of the characteristics (disease should not necessarily be equated with aging; however, when one health problem is identified, others must be suspected because multiple disease conditions are a primary characteristic of advancing years); classification of aging has changed in recent years because of increasing longevity— 65 to 75 years: older adult; more than 75 years: elder-older adult

● Normal Variations During the Aging Process

Assessment

Observations/findings

Eyes
  Dry and lusterless
  Discoloration of sclera, conjunctiva
  Arcus senilis (opaque ring near edge of cornea)
  Diminished pupil size, which may be opaque
  Pale brown discoloration in iris
  Diminished peripheral vision
  Decreased lens accomodation, tearing
Ears
  Hearing loss
  Initial loss of high frequency tones
  Suspiciousness and irritability may or may not be
    present
Mouth
  Loss of taste perception; dry mucous membranes
  Recession of gums if not edentulous
  Reduced acuity of taste buds
  Decreased mastication
  Increased difficulty in swallowing
Respiratory system
  Decreased tidal volume
  Decreased peripheral perfusion
  Tracheal deviation if upper dorsal scoliosis present
  Increased rigidity of chest wall
  Decreased pulmonary elasticity
Cardiovascular system
  Decreased resting heart rate and cardiac output
  Easily palpable peripheral pulse
  Decreased arterial circulation
  Increased blood pressure; orthostatic hypotension
Gastrointestinal system
  Diminished salivation and gastric acid secretion
  Reduced gastrointestinal motility
  Decreased esophageal peristalsis
  Weight gain in women; weight loss in men
  Constipation
Renal system
  Decreased renal blood flow
  Frequent nocturnal micturition
  Incontinence
  Difficulty in initiating and ending the stream in male
    (caused by prostatic hypertrophy)
Female reproductive system
  Narrowing and shortening of vagina
  Diminished vaginal lubrication
  Dyspareunia
  Decreased estrogen production

Uterine contractions with orgasm may be uncomfort-
    able
  Pendulous, elongated, and/or flaccid breasts
Male reproductive system
  Decrease in size and firmness of testes
  Enlarged prostate gland
  Decrease in amount and viscosity of seminal fluid
  Increased diameter of penis
  Longer duration of excitement and plateau of orgas-
    mic phases; resolution phase may last 12 to 24 hours
  Libido and sense of satisfaction usually do not
    change
  Decreased testosterone production
Musculoskeletal system
  Decrease in quick voluntary movements
  Decrease in muscle mass (not necessarily associated
    with loss of strength)
  Diminished height, 2.5 to 10 cm
  Osteoarthritic changes in joints
    Heberden's nodes at distal finger joints
    Bouchard's nodes at proximal finger joints
  Dupuytren's contracture of lateral fingers, preventing
    full extension
  Osteoporosis (kyphosis may be an early indication)
  Broad-based stance; flexion of hips and knees
Integumentary system
  Thinning of skin over back of hands
  Decreased activity of sebaceous and sweat glands,
    which may result in "dry skin"
  Thinning and/or loss of scalp, pubic, and axillary
    hair
  Small, scattered scarlet growths (senile telangiectasis)
  Paler skin with increased pigment deposition
    (freckles)
  Local or general skin areas lacking pigmentation
    (vitiligo); increases with age
  Hyperkeratosis, or warts with raised pale, brown, or
    black epidermal overgrowth usually located over
    long axis of skin creases
  Cutaneous skin tags (acrochordons) around lower
    neck, axillary area; usually soft and flesh colored and
    on pedicles
  Ears and nose appear large in relation to face
  Dry, wrinkled, and sagging skin
  Loss of hair and pigmentation
Neurologic system
  Decrease in conduction velocity of some nerves
  Diminished sense of smell
  Diminished sense of position
  Decreased tactile sense
  Deep tendon reflexes may be decreased
  Diminished sensitivity to hot and cold extremes in
    temperature
  Altered sleep patterns
  Decreased range, duration, intensity of voice

Interventions

Assess support systems and recent changes in patient's
life that may have bearing on his or her ability to meet
own needs
Monitor fluid and nutritional intake
  Observe for retention, dehydration, malnutrition, or
    overhydration
  Assess skin turgor
  Provide fluids and food within parameters of disease
    process
  Assess patient's ability to chew and swallow; check for
    the presence of dentures
  Assess patient's food likes and dislikes
  Allow patient time to finish his or her meals
Monitor elimination patterns
  Observe for incontinence, constipation, or diarrhea;
    note frequency
  Provide bedpan or urinal within easy reach
Maintain safe environment
  Adequate lighting
  Clear passage for moving about
  Use of canes, walkers
  Assist with activities as needed
Monitor patient's activity and rest
  Observe patient's ability to perform ADLs and ROM
    exercises
  Provide balance between activity and rest
Monitor communication and social skills
  Provide alternate means of communicating as needed
  Involve patient in his or her care plan
  Encourage family or significant other to support patient
Monitor medications
  Administer medications judiciously
  Absorption, detoxification, and excretion of drugs is
    diminished; lower dosage levels and decreased fre-
    quency of administration may be indicated
  Assess need for analgesia carefully because sensitivity
    to pain is usually decreased
  Monitor side effects carefully
Monitor vital signs to assess cardiopulmonary function
Monitor patient's skin for redness and/or broken areas
  Provide support and frequent position changes to pre-
    vent pressure ulcers
  Encourage and teach good physical hygiene
  Avoid dryness by applying lanolin-based lotions on pa-
    tient's skin

● Care of the Dying Patient

Death

*An unavoidable part of life and the part most difficult
to accept; each person dies uniquely and therefore must be
cared for uniquely; that is, the nurse must develop and*
*maintain a positive needs-perceptive relationship with the
patient and family that will allow the patient to die in
comfort and with dignity*

Nurse self-assessment/interventions

To care for the dying patient, you must:
  Learn about yourself and your own feelings concern-
    ing dying
  Look at your own ethno-cultural background
  Examine your own exposure to death
    Family and friends
    Reactions to these experiences
  Be honest about your own feelings (anxiety, depres-
    sion, avoidance, coping mechanisms)
  Examine how you view your own death
  Share your feelings about death with others; initiate
    open discussion to better understand behavior
  Learn to listen; realize that all of patient's questions do
    not require answers; often patient will answer his or
    her own questions if you do not provide "pat"
    answers
  Explore your feelings about life (respect, discontent)
  Recognize your own power in controlling patient and
    his or her responses to care
    Avoid using this power as threat to patient
    Use it to give respectful, humane care
  Consider effect patient has on you; examine how you
    see patient as an individual human being
Consider the following in caring for the dying patient:
  Be aware of what physician has told patient; avoid con-
    flicting statements
  Realize that decision to tell patient of outcome of dis-
    ease lies with physician, patient, and family
  Be honest in dealing with patient who has not been
    told of impending death; ask patient what he or she
    thinks or feels about his or her question, "Am I go-
    ing to die?"
Communicate situations and conversations with patient
  to others on the staff; provide continuity and avoid dis-
  crepancies in emotional care

Family assessment/interventions

Realize that family or significant other will need sup-
  port during patient's illness
Assess and evaluate patient's and family's feelings
  about death and work within the framework of those
  feelings
Do not judge actions or behavior of family
  Realize that family members may have gone through a
    lot with a long illness and are no longer able to cope
  Understand that a change in family structure is occur-
    ring

Emotional: loss of a loved member

Financial: long illnesses become a burden

Be aware that pre-illness relationships and/or problems will continue

Encourage family to be involved with patient's care

Frequent visits and telephone calls

Staying with patient

Bringing valued objects to patient

Providing home-cooked meals

Bringing children and pets for visits

Assist family in grieving process

Understand that they also will go through the stages of dying

Be aware that timing of stages is very often not the same as the patient's timing

Understand that family very often may not reach stage of acceptance

Work with family members so that they can let patient know the truth, thus permitting open and frank communication with patient past denial stage

Assist family in making both intermediate and long-term plans

Help family see patient's need to live as normally as possible for as long as possible

Assist family in making arrangements for home care when it is possible and desirable for patient

Teach methods of care that will be required

Arrange for help through social service department and community resources

Explore possibility of hospice care

Patient assessment/interventions

Realize that patient needs compassionate, consistent, and realistic care during terminal illness

Be aware that he or she is sensitive to feelings of others

Understand that patient will avoid discussing his or her death and feelings if he or she senses others are unable to talk of dying

Be aware that patient will often discuss feelings with nursing staff rather than with the physician

Provide needed hope, human contact, and caring

Understand that hope must be realistic; patient needs treatment for alleviation of pain rather than getting well

Do not avoid patient during any of the stages of dying

Realize that patient needs continuous caring by all members of staff

Be aware that patient has many fears

Encourage expression of feelings

Provide an accepting environment

Demonstrate warmth and friendliness

Encourage use of spiritual resources

Explore past coping strengths

Explain all procedures and nursing functions

Discuss patient's fears with him or her

Fear of the unknown

Loss of control of body and behavior

Pain: Patient needs explanation of availability of different drugs and therapies, such as radiation or surgery

Helplessness: Patient needs general nutrition, some activity, and deep breathing every day, which usually helps initially

Understand that patient needs to have each day be as comfortable, positive, and productive as possible

Promote self-care and diversional activities

Help patient to maintain a normal lifestyle for as long as possible

Care During the Stages of Dying

● Denial and Shock

Assessment

Observations/findings

Ignoring or distorting reasons given for illness

Refusal to participate in care

Refusal to follow directions of physician or staff

Interventions

Recognize that denial and shock will be used by the patient after he or she is told of his or her impending death

Do not interfere with this mechanism unless it becomes destructive (e.g., patient refuses further treatment and care)

Spend time with patient to show that he or she will not be left alone

Do not support denial; conversations should include reality

Continue to teach and encourage self-care and activities

● Anger

Assessment

Observations/findings

Abusive language

Refusal of care

Refusal of nutrition and self-care
Negative criticism of staff
Striking out
  Not permitting others to be close to him or her
  Throwing objects
  Removing IV needle, leads
  Calling for nurse and then asking why nurse is there

Interventions

Recognize that patient is not angry with you personally
Do not allow physically harmful behavior to continue
  Spend time with patient and discuss his or her
   anger
  Encourage verbalization of anger; be empathetic
Plan patient's care with him or her and encourage mutual problem solving
Question how patient evaluates care being given
Continue to question and discuss patient's anger

● Bargaining

Assessment

Observations/findings

Statements such as "I hope I live until. . .," "If only I could . . ."

Interventions

Realize that patient needs time to accept his or her impending death
Spend time with patient
Discuss importance of valued objects and people
Set small, realistic, attainable goals
Provide praise for goals reached or attempted

● Depression

Assessment

Observations/findings

Apathy
Decreased ability to concentrate
Insomnia
Inability to wake up
Crying
Constant fatigue
Poor appetite
Lack of interest in people or environment
Sitting alone

Interventions

Recognize that patient is beginning to separate himself or herself from life
Do not attempt to cheer patient
Be available to sit quietly and, if appropriate, to hold patient's hand
Accept crying; do not interrupt
Realize that patient may only want his or her most beloved person to be with him or her
Promote positive relationships to maintain patient's dignity
Soothe patient with gentle back care and oral hygiene

● Acceptance

Assessment

Observations/findings

Devoid of feelings
Absence of emotional affect
Peacefulness
Less pain and discomfort (usually)

Interventions

Plan patient's care to allow person with whom patient is comfortable to care for patient
Realize that patient may not want to be alone

Nutritional Problems

● Enteral Nutrition

Provision of nutritional support to meet nutritional requirements via a nasogastric tube, orogastric tube, esophagostomy, gastrostomy, duodenostomy, or jejunostomy; preferred for the patient who has a functional GI tract but is unable to consume an adequate nutritional intake or when oral intake is contraindicated; may be indicated in the following clinical conditions: physical impairments (e.g., obstructive lesions of the esophagus or pharynx, following radical head and neck surgery, following fracture of facial bones); neurologic conditions associated with impaired swallowing and oropharyngeal trauma; increased metabolic needs caused by trauma, burns, or sepsis; or the presence of an endotracheal tube

Assessment

Subjective data

Abdominal cramping, pain, feeling of fullness
Nausea
Dry mucous membranes
Constipation

Objective data

Dietary history
Lactose intolerance
Food allergies, dietary restrictions
Medical history
  Chronic renal disease
  Liver disorders
  Diabetes mellitus
  Heart disease
Cerebrovascular accident (CVA)
  Coma
Respiratory problems
  Respiratory distress
  Aspiration
  Coughing
  Choking
  Cyanosis
  Increased respiratory rate
  Decreased breath sounds
  Rales at lung bases
Skin and mucous membranes
  Skin irritation and/or breakdown, nares, ostomy tube
  Poor skin turgor
  Diaphoresis
Level of consciousness
  Coma
  Change in mental status
Gastrointestinal
  Vomiting
  Diarrhea
  Abdominal distention, delayed gastric emptying
  Decreased or absent bowel sounds
  Esophageal reflux
  Gastric residual
  Tube placement: nasogastric, nasoduodenal, nasojejunal, gastrostomy, jejunostomy, percutaneous endoscopic gastrostomy (PEG)

Diagnostic tests

Serum electrolytes, CBC
Serum osmolality
Serum glucose
Urine glucose
Urine specific gravity
BUN
Serum creatinine
Serum albumin
Serum transferrin

Potential complications

Hypernatremia (see p. 74)
Hyperchloremia
Azotemia
Dehydration
Tube feeding syndrome
Hyperglycemia
Nausea
Vomiting
Pulmonary injury during insertion
Aspiration/pneumonia
Diarrhea
Constipation
Gastric retention
Fluid overload (see p. 82)
Gastric rupture
Dumping syndrome
Weakness
Diaphoresis
Light-headedness
Tachycardia
Cramping
Tube displacement
Tube obstruction
Intraperitoneal leakage and leakage of fluid around catheter (associated with gastrostomy and jejunostomy tubes)

Collaborative management

Therapeutic management

Treatment of underlying disease process
Desired route (e.g., ostomy, percutaneous esophageal gastrostomy [PEG])
Tube selection (small bore tubes generally used)
Type of formula (concentration and rate)
Intermittent or continuous feeding
Antidiarrheal agents
Laxatives
Insulin
Intake and output
Daily weights
Daily laboratory studies
Formula preparation and distribution

Nursing management

PATIENT PROBLEMS/NURSING DIAGNOSES

● **NDX:** Diarrhea related to altered dietary intake, malabsorption, concomitant drug therapy, type of formula, bacterial contamination, stress/anxiety

Record color, odor, amount, and frequency of stool every day

Monitor intake and output q8h

Monitor stool for occult blood

Weigh patient daily at same time and in same clothing, using same scale

Assess for signs and symptoms of dehydration
  Poor skin turgor
  Decreased urine output
  Increased urine specific gravity
  Dry mucous membranes

Monitor laboratory results; report any abnormalities to physician

Review current medications, antibiotics, cimetidine, other H_2 blockers, electrolyte elixirs, and antacids for possible side effects such as diarrhea

Assess for intolerance to feeding solution q4h

Report untoward reactions to physician immediately:
  Abdominal distention, delayed gastric emptying
  Nausea
  Vomiting
  Cramping

Auscultate bowel sounds q4h

Report hyperactive or hypoactive bowel sounds to physician

Assess for gastric residual q4h

If gastric residual is greater than 100 ml, discontinue feeding and notify physician (replace residual)

Avoid rapid rate of infusion
  Initiate tube feeding slowly at half-strength concentration or as ordered by physician
  Increase rate according to patient tolerance
  Regulate flow rate using enteral pump (some IV infusion pumps can be adapted to deliver enteral feedings)
  Place time tape on formula bag or bottle; monitor rate q1h
  Give formula at room temperature
  Administer antidiarrheal agents as ordered

Avoid formula with high osmolality and high fat content
  Contact physician regarding change in formula
  Administer enteral feedings at approximate serum osmolality
  Administer dilute strength and/or decrease volume as ordered by physician

Intervene for lactose intolerance
  Contact physician regarding change to lactose-free formula
  Delete all milk products from patient's diet

Avoid bacterial contamination

Wash hands thoroughly before preparing and handling formula

Use ready-mix formula whenever possible

Allow formula to hang for no longer than 8 to 12 hours; nocturnal feedings are best because they interfere less with daily activities

Refrigerate unused formula

Rinse feeding container and gavage set between feedings

Flush tube with water when feeding tube is disconnected

Change feeding container and gavage set daily

EXPECTED OUTCOMES

Patient
  Tolerates tube feeding volume, concentration, and formula type
  Evacuates soft-formed stool every other day
  Maintains hydration and weight

● **NDX:** Risk for aspiration related to reduced level of consciousness, diminished or absent cough and gag reflexes, incompetent esophageal sphincter, delayed gastric emptying, displaced feeding tube

Use small-bore feeding tubes: less likely to disrupt the esophageal sphincter and cause reflux

Ensure correct placement of tube in stomach q4h; with small-bore tube, a x-ray examination may be necessary to confirm tube's placement

Confirm placement of all intestinal tubes by x-ray examination

Keep head of bed elevated at 30 to 45 degrees during feeding periods and 1 hour after feedings

Clamp feeding tube when patient must be placed flat

Check for gastric residual q4h for continuous feeding and before each intermittent or bolus feeding

Report to physician if gastric residual is 100 ml or more; discontinue feeding

Replace aspirate: prevents loss of gastric juices and electrolytes

Assess patient for cramping, bloating, nausea, and abdominal distension

Auscultate bowel sounds q4h

Monitor vital signs T, P, R, and BP q4h

Inflate cuff for cuffed tracheostomy tube or endotracheal tube; keep it inflated for 1 hour after feeding

Assess for signs and symptoms of aspiration; report any findings to physician
  Shortness of breath
  Fever
  Cough
  Discolored tracheal aspirate
  Increased respiratory rate
  Cyanosis
  Diminished breath sounds
  Rales/rhonchi

Before removal of orogastric or nasogastric tube, irrigate and clamp or pinch tube to minimize risk of aspiration when tube is withdrawn

EXPECTED OUTCOMES

Patient's
  Breath sounds are normal as evidenced by
    No rales or rhonchi
    No cough
  Temperature is within normal limits

● **NDX:** Fluid volume deficit related to insufficient fluid intake and abnormal fluid loss associated with high osmolality of enteral feeding

Assess patient q8h for signs and symptoms of fluid volume deficit
Report the following to physician
  Poor skin turgor
  Decreased urine output
  Dry mucous membranes
  Weight loss greater than 0.5 kg/day
  Decreased blood pressure
  Increased urine specific gravity
Measure intake and output q8h
Weigh patient daily at same time and in same clothing using same scale
Increase free water administration via feeding tube as prescribed; thereafter, flush feeding tube with 30 to 50 ml of water q4h to 6h
Monitor urine specific gravity q8h
Administer hypertonic formulas using a half-strength concentration
Change hypertonic formula to isotonic formula
Document patient's baseline mental status
Assess patient's mental status q4h; report any changes to physician
Monitor continuous feedings qh
Use enteral pump to regulate rate of feedings
Monitor urine or serum glucose levels q6h or as ordered

EXPECTED OUTCOMES

Patient
  Maintains good skin turgor and color
  Maintains moist mucous membranes
  Maintains weight
  Maintains urine specific gravity within normal limits

● **NDX:** Constipation related to formula composition, inadequate water intake, and immobility

Ensure administration of high-residue formula
Increase free water administration via feeding tube as prescribed
Flush feeding tube with 30 to 50 ml of water every 4 to 6 hours
Administer stool softener as prescribed
Administer 4 to 6 oz of prune juice daily through tube, if prescribed
Monitor medications (e.g., narcotics) for their possible side effects
Encourage physical activity within limits
  Assist with ambulation
  Assist patient to chair twice a day
  Change patient's position q2h
Monitor for fecal impaction
Allow patient adequate time in bathroom or with commode or bedpan
Provide privacy
Monitor patient's bowel elimination pattern

EXPECTED OUTCOMES

Patient
  Tolerates tube feeding and maintains weight
  Evacuates soft, formed stool every day

● **NDX:** Impaired tissue integrity related to pressure from feeding tube and/or drainage from ostomy tube insertion site

Use small-bore feeding tube when possible
Position tube to prevent undue pressure on nares
Cleanse and lubricate nares q4h and prn
Provide oral care q4h and prn
Provide skin care at insertion site of ostomy tube
Encourage nasal breathing, rather than oral, to prevent dry mouth
Provide lozenges or hard candy, if allowed
Assess tube insertion site q8h for tenderness, redness, and drainage
Report any abnormalities to physician
Change ostomy/PEG site dressing q2h and prn
Cleanse site with soap and water and allow it to air dry
Apply stoma adhesive around tube at insertion site
Cover site with transparent or similar dressing
Secure ostomy/PEG tube
Report any continuous leakage around tube to physician

EXPECTED OUTCOME

Patient's skin around the tube insertion site is clean and dry

● **NDX:** Body image disturbance related to change in appearance resulting from nasal or ostomy tube

Assess patient's level of anxiety and understanding of need for tube feedings; if feasible, select and/or change to a feeding tube that patient tolerates physically and psychologically

Encourage patient to express his or her feelings about the way he or she feels and looks

Reassure patient that his or her feelings are appropriate

Continue to be sensitive to patient's needs and feelings

Assess for patient's readiness to begin self-care

Instruct patient and/or significant other regarding feeding procedure

Provide emotional support and positive feedback for patient's participation in his or her feeding

Provide opportunity for questions and reinforce instructions as necessary

Continue to support coping efforts

Provide referrals (e.g., social service, nutritionist or registered dietitian, support groups, clergy) as necessary

Encourage ambulation if not contraindicated

Provide small amounts of patient's favorite foods orally, if allowed

EXPECTED OUTCOMES

Patient

Expresses understanding of need for tube feeding

Copes with imposed restrictions

Participates in own care

Shares feelings about how he or she views himself or herself

ADDITIONAL NURSING DIAGNOSES TO CONSIDER

Perceived constipation related to belief that lack of daily bowel movement indicates constipation

Fatigue related to nutritional deficiencies

Patient/family teaching

Purpose and administration of tube feedings

Explain that all necessary nutrients—protein, fats, carbohydrates, vitamins, and minerals—will be supplied by tube feeding

Discuss formula selection and reason for its choice

Instruct patient and/or significant other in formula preparation, storage, feeding schedule, and proper cleaning of equipment

Instruct patient and/or significant other how to administer formula and medications via feeding tube; administer only prescribed medications

Complications

Discuss signs and symptoms of feeding intolerance (e.g., nausea, vomiting, diarrhea, cramping, bloating, flatulence); discuss importance of reporting any signs and symptoms to physician

Explain reasons for administering feeding with patient in a upright position

Demonstrate procedure for checking placement of feeding tube to patient and family or significant other

Discuss signs and symptoms of possible aspiration (e.g., coughing, choking, difficulty in breathing, elevated temperature); discuss importance of reporting any signs and symptoms to physician

Discuss importance of flushing tube with water after each feeding and after administration of medications

Demonstrate urine and/or serum glucose checking procedure; discuss importance of reporting any abnormalities to physician

Discuss measures to prevent constipation

Contact home health nurse if tube is clogged, broken, or dislodged

Nasal, PEG tube, and enterostomy care

Demonstrate proper taping of tube to prevent slipping

Demonstrate cleansing and lubrication of nares; explain that this should be done q4h and prn

Teach importance of maintaining good oral hygiene

Demonstrate ostomy/PEG care

Discuss importance of reporting any redness, drainage, foul odor, or tenderness around stoma to physician

Teach patient how to remove and insert ostomy feeding tube per physician order; (esophagotomy and gastrostomy tubes may be removed after several weeks and inserted only for feedings)

Demonstrate use of flow sheet for record keeping

Activity

Instruct patient to increase activity/exercise as desired and tolerated

Discuss benefits of exercise

Promotes feeling of well-being

Increases gastric motility

Home care considerations

Assess and continue with patient and family education; monitor following:

Caregivers' ability to prepare and administer tube feedings

Purchasing of needed supplies

Use of flow sheet

Ability to care for tube/PEG

Activity tolerance

Rest and exercise
Urine, serum glucose testing
Presence of telephone and numbers of home health team

● Total Parenteral Nutrition

Infusion of necessary nutrients—amino acids, fat, trace elements, carbohydrates, vitamins, and electrolytes— through a peripheral or central vein; peripheral or central venous nutrition may be chosen when the enteral route is not available because of mechanical or functional abnormalities of the GI tract; clinical conditions that may indicate the need for parenteral nutrition are short bowel syndrome, ileus, malabsorption, pancreatitis, hypermetabolic states (trauma, sepsis), altered metabolic states (acute renal failure, hepatic insufficiency), burns, and cancer

Assessment

Subjective data

Pain, discomfort at insertion site

Objective data

Insertion site
  Warmth
  Redness
  Edema
  Drainage at insertion site
  Leakage at insertion site
Fever
Leukocytosis
Glucose intolerance

Diagnostic tests

Potassium
Phosphorus
Magnesium
Blood glucose
Calcium
Sodium
Chloride
Blood urea nitrogen (BUN)
Prothrombin time (PT)
White blood cell (WBC) count, urinalysis
Liver enzymes
Bilirubin
Serum albumin
Transferrin

Potential complications

Mechanical complications
  Pneumothorax (with subclavian vein catheterization)
  Air embolism
  Catheter and venous thrombosis
Septic complications
  Catheter sepsis (bacterial or fungal)
Metabolic complications
  Hyperglycemia
  Hyperosmolar nonketotic coma
  Hypoglycemia
  Fatty acid deficiency
  Electrolyte abnormalities
  Liver dysfunction
  Mineral and trace elements deficiency

Collaborative management

Therapeutic management

Route of administration; peripheral or subclavian
X-ray examination to determine placement of central line
Keeping vein open with isotonic solution until catheter placement is confirmed
Rate of flow
Increase or decrease in rate of solution
Lipid emulsion
Daily weights
Urine glucose
Blood glucose monitoring
Administration of insulin, glucose
Intake and output
Daily laboratory studies (see above)
Preparation, storage, and/or dispensing of formula

Nursing Management

PATIENT PROBLEMS/NURSING DIAGNOSES

● **NDX:** Risk for infection related to invasive procedure and delivery of high concentrations of glucose parenterally

Peripheral venous nutrition
Wash hands thoroughly before inserting IV needle or catheter
Wear gloves per universal precautions
Select distal veins in upper extremities
Clip or shave any hair at site according to policy
Prepare site with povidone-iodine swab and allow site to air dry
Cover site with occlusive dressing
Monitor for signs and symptoms of phlebitis and/or infiltration

Remove catheter or needle if phlebitis or infiltration is present

Rotate catheter site q72h or according to policy

Tape IV tubing securely

Monitor catheter site every hour

Change IV tubing q24h or according to policy

Use strict aseptic technique when assembling and changing administration set

Monitor vital signs T, P, and R q4h; report elevation of temperature to physician

Monitor blood glucose as ordered

Monitor urine for glucose as ordered, usually q6h; glucosuria may indicate impending sepsis

Ensure that final amino acid concentration does not exceed 10% dextrose

Ensure continuous infusion of lipid emulsion when 10% dextrose is infused

Refrigerate total parenteral nutrition (TPN) solution until it is ready to use

Allow solution to hang for no longer than 24 hours

Never piggyback medications other than lipid emulsion via TPN line

Securely tape needle used for piggybacking lipid emulsion

Central venous nutrition

Assist physician with inserting central line catheter

Ensure that catheter insertion is completed under sterile conditions

Ensure proper site preparation

Change central line dressing using sterile technique

Prepare site with povidone-iodine and allow it to air dry

Apply povidone-iodine ointment to catheter site

Cover site with sterile occlusive dressing

Observe site for signs of sepsis (e.g., erythema, swelling, tenderness, drainage at insertion site)

Monitor vital signs T, P, and R q4h; report temperature elevation to physician

Monitor blood glucose

Monitor urine for glucose as ordered, usually q6h; glucosuria may indicate impending sepsis

Monitor catheter site q1h

Tape tubing securely

Do not use stopcocks on TPN line

Change IV tubing q24h or according to policy

Use strict aseptic technique when assembling and changing administration set

Allow solution to hang no longer than 24 hours

Never use line for piggybacking medications, taking central venous pressure (CVP) readings, or aspirating blood for laboratory studies

EXPECTED OUTCOMES

Patient's

Temperature is within normal limits

Catheter insertion site is clean, dry, and intact with no sign of redness, edema, or drainage

Laboratory values are within normal limits

● **NDX:** Altered protection related to inadequate nutrition, age, anorexia, adverse reaction to therapy, surgery

Metabolic abnormalities

Monitor for signs and symptoms of hyperglycemia

Polyuria

Glycosuria: elevated blood sugar

Polydipsia, polyphagia

Dimmed, blurred vision

Monitor for signs and symptoms of hypoglycemia

Tachycardia

Cold sweat

Posterior occipital headache

Irritability, jitteriness

Lethargy

Blood glucose level of less than 60 mg/dl

Perform urine and/or serum testing q6h

Monitor vital signs and electrolytes q4h

Assess patient's neurologic status q8h

Monitor intake and output q8h

Weigh patient daily at same time and in same clothing, using same scale

Initiate TPN solution slowly

Increase rate per patient's tolerance and physician's order

Do not increase rate to "catch up"

Monitor flow rate of solution, using infusion control device

Do not interrupt infusion for more than 1 hour q8h

Ensure patency of line

For hyperglycemia, administer insulin

For hypoglycemia, administer IV 50% dextrose

Taper solution before discontinuing

Review medications that may affect glucose metabolism

Assess for possible sepsis

Monitor for signs and symptoms of fluid overload

Pedal or sacral edema

Rapid weight gain: 1 lb (0.45 kg) or more a day

Pitting edema

Increased blood pressure

Bounding pulse

Monitor for signs and symptoms of fluid deficit

Review all routine laboratory tests for any abnormalities

Assess for signs and symptoms of fatty acid deficiency, alopecia, brittle nails, desquamating dermatitis, decreased immunity, thrombocytopenia, and delayed wound healing

Report any abnormalities to physician

Pneumothorax

Auscultate patient's chest for breath sounds q1hr

Assess patient's respiratory status q1h and report any signs and symptoms to physician

Sudden onset of sharp chest pain

Coughing secondary to pleural irritation

Dyspnea, cyanosis, hypotension

Obtain baseline BP, apical pulse, T, and R

Keep vein open with isotonic solution until chest x-ray examination confirms correct placement of central line

Air embolism

Assess for signs and symptoms of air embolism, dyspnea, tachycardia, cyanosis, and hypotension

Place patient in head-down position during subclavian or jugular vein insertion

Use Luer-Lok connections on all central line tubing

Securely tape all tubing connections

Use air-eliminating filters when possible

Clamp catheter or assist and teach patient to perform Valsalva's maneuver during tubing changes

Reaction to Total Parenteral Nutrition

Assess patient for dyspnea; chest, abdominal, or back pain; fever; flushing; chills; headache; decreased blood pressure; cyanosis; diaphoresis; and/or urticaria

Stop infusion and report any of above reactions to physician

Monitor and report elevated triglyceride levels and/or elevated liver function tests

EXPECTED OUTCOMES

Patient's

Central line is patent

Laboratory results are within normal limits

Weight is stabilized and/or progressing toward his or her ideal

Skin turgor is good

Cardiopulmonary status is within normal limits

ADDITIONAL NURSING DIAGNOSIS
TO CONSIDER

Fatigue related to increased psychological, physical demands and/or discomfort

Patient/family teaching

Provide patient and/or significant other with instructions regarding the following:

Reasons for TPN

Importance of therapy

Expected outcome

Need for protection of IV site

Need for prevention of tension on central venous catheter

Importance of intake and output measurement (provide flow sheet)

Explain signs and symptoms to report to nurse and/or physician, including the following:

Excessive urination

Chills

Elevated temperature

Feeling of warmth

Shortness of breath

Excessive thirst

Leakage of fluid at catheter site

Pain or tenderness at catheter site

Swelling and/or redness at catheter site

Instruct patient about the following:

Amount of physical activity allowed

Need to keep follow-up appointments

Poor skin turgor

Dry mucous membranes

Tachycardia

Hypotension

Weight loss or gain

Ensure that patient and/or significant other understands the following:

Resources for assistance as needed

Importance of avoiding crowds and persons with infections

How to recognize and handle possible complications (e.g., air embolism, blood backup, catheter injury)

Ensure that patient and/or significant other demonstrates the following:

Proper handwashing technique

Preparation and infusion of TPN solution

Use of infusion pump

Clamping catheter

Flushing catheter

Changing injection site cap

Central line dressing change

Care of catheter insertion site

Measuring and recording intake and output

Testing urine for sugar and acetone

Taking and recording temperature

Home care considerations

Assess and continue with patient and family education and monitor the following:

Type of solution

Schedule of infusion

Obtaining the solution
Storage of solution
Inspection of solution
Procedure for changing central line dressing
Frequency of dressing change
Supplies needed
Where to obtain supplies
Cleansing of site
Observation of site
Procedure for flushing catheter
Purpose of flushing
Frequency of flushing
Solution used for flushing
Changing injection site cap
Frequency of change
Clamping of catheter before cap change
Signs and symptoms to report to physician
Elevated temperature
Rapid weight loss or gain
Increased fatigue
Shortness of breath
Tightness in chest
Redness, swelling, or drainage at insertion site
Glucose present in urine
Presence of telephone and emergency phone numbers as well as those of home care team

● Electrolyte, Fluid, and Acid-Base Balance (Table 2-5)

Electrolytes are substances that have been dissolved in the body fluids; they are potassium, sodium, chloride, calcium, soda bicarbonate, magnesium and phosphate; the fluid concentration of these electrolytes must be maintained at a very narrow margin of normal; many diseases, conditions, and/or medications can cause an imbalance

Fluid in the body accounts for about 60% of body weight and is found in two areas: in the cells (intracellular/ ICF) and between the cells and blood vessels (extracellular/ECF); it is also located in the gastrointestinal tract and the cerebrospinal fluid; an increase/decrease of the ECF can cause a fluid imbalance.

Acid-base balance is regulated by the concentration of the hydrogen ion in the body fluids; pH is the term used to represent this concentration; as the concentration increases, the pH decreases, causing acidosis; as the concentration decreases, the pH increases, causing alkalosis; the pH normal range in the plasma is 7.35 to 7.45.

Care of Patient With Special Equipment

● Central Lines

A venous catheter inserted into the superior vena cava through the subclavian, internal, or external jugular vein; can be used for monitoring of venous pressure, infusion of medications and TPN, rapid infusion of fluid and blood products, and blood withdrawal

Insertion of catheter

Auscultate chest for breath sounds
Obtain baseline BP, apical pulse, T, and R
Provide emotional support
  Explain procedure to patient
  Reinforce physician's explanation of procedure
Prepare to assist physician with inserting central venous catheter
  Maintain sterile technique
  Remove any hair from insertion site with razor or depilatory agents
  Prepare skin around insertion site with povidone-iodine solution
  Establish and maintain a sterile field throughout insertion procedure
Place patient in supine or Trendelenburg position if subclavian or jugular vein is chosen as insertion site
Administer isotonic IV solution at a keep-open rate until position of catheter is verified by chest x-ray examination (Table 2-6)
Apply sterile occlusive dressing to catheter insertion site; label dressing with date and time of insertion
Obtain chest x-ray film

Postinsertion assessment

Subjective data

Chest, shoulder, or neck pain

Objective data

Edema in catheterized arm
Neck vein distention
Redness, swelling, or drainage at insertion site
Temperature elevation
Elevated WBC count
Occlusion of central line
Rejection of catheter
Air embolization
Accumulation of serous fluid around site

Text continued on p. 84.

Table 2-5 Observation of Electrolyte, Fluid, and Acid-Base Imbalances

Imbalances	Causes	Neuromuscular System	GI System
ELECTROLYTE IMBALANCES			
Hyperkalemia (potassium excess): normal values, 3.5-5.0 mEq/L; critical values, >6.5 mEq/L	Excessive administration of potassium chloride Decreased renal excretion, as in renal failure, hypovolemia, potassium-sparing diuretics Trauma to tissues such as burns and crash injuries (will release intercellular potassium and result in hyperkalemia) Aldosterone insufficiency Respiratory or metabolic acidosis Banked blood Medications including: aminocaproic acid (Amicar), antibiotics, antineoplastic, Captopril (Capoten), epinephrine, heparin, histamine, isoniazid (INH), lithium, mannitol, potassium-sparing diuretics, succinylcholine (anectine) Hemolysis	Weakness, flaccid paralysis, twitching, hyperreflexia, paresthesia or numbness and tingling sensations, (usually affect the face, tongue, hands, and feet), apathy, confusion	Diarrhea, intestinal colic, nausea
Hypokalemia (potassium deficit): normal values, 3.5-5.0 mEq/L; critical values, < 2.5 mEq/L	Increased renal loss (diuretics; diuresis phase after burns; diabetic acidosis, Cushing's syndrome; nephritis) Hypomagnesium Inadequate intake of potassium	Muscular cramps, paresthesias, muscular weakness to flaccid paralysis, fatigue, mental confusion, hyporeflexia, drowsiness, apathy, irritability, tetany, coma	Anorexia, nausea and vomiting, abdominal distension, paralytic ileus

Respiratory System	Cardiovascular System	Renal System	Skin and Mucous Membranes	Blood Gas Values	Interventions
Respiratory paralysis and involvement of muscles of phonation	Bradycardia, lethal dysrhythmias, and cardiac arrest ECG changes: tall peaked T waves, shortened QT interval, disappearance of P waves, widening of QRS complex, flat-to-absent P wave and asystole				Observe patient for changes in heart rate, rhythm, and ECG pattern Be aware cardiac arrest can occur Restrict potassium-containing foods, fluids, and salt substitutes Monitor serum potassium levels Do not give calcium if patient is on digitalis since calcium potentiates the effect of digitalis Avoid potassium-containing medications such as potassium penicillin Administer IV glucose, insulin, and sodium bicarbonate as ordered (helps shift potassium into the cells) Administer cation-exchange resins as ordered (helps to remove potassium by way of GI tract) Peritoneal or hemodialysis may be ordered if other therapy fails
Respiratory muscle weakness, paralysis of the diaphragm, shallow respirations, apnea, and death may result	Irregular rhythm, ECG: flat or inverted T wave, appearance of U wave, short and depressed ST segment, peaking of P waves, QT interval prolonged, circulatory failure, hypotension and systolic arrest				Monitor serum potassium and report significant changes Observe for signs and symptoms of metabolic alkalosis Watch for signs of toxicity in patients receiving digitalis (blurred vision, nausea, and vomiting)

Continued.

Table 2-5 Observation of Electrolyte, Fluid, and Acid-Base Imbalances—cont'd

Imbalances	Causes	Neuromuscular System	GI System
Hypokalemia (potassium deficit)—cont'd	Acid base imbalance: alkalosis; loss from vomiting, diarrhea, excess use of laxatives, GI suction or fistulas, steroid administration Medications including: acetazolamide (Diamox), aminosalicylic acid (PAS), amphotericin D, carbenicillin, cisplatin (Platinol), diuretics (potassium wasting), glucose infusions, insulin, lithium carbonate, penicillin G sodium (Bicillin), salicylates (aspirin), sodium polystyrene sulfonate (Kayexalate)		
Hypercalcemia (calcium excess): normal values, 9.0-10.5 mg/dL (total), 4.5-5.6 mg/dL (ionized); critical values, >14 mg/dL (total)	Hyperparathyroidism Prolonged immobilization (causes calcium displacement from bone to blood) Hypophosphatemia Metastatic carcinoma Alkalosis Thyrotoxicosis Vitamin D overdose Addison's disease Multiple myeloma Skeletal muscle paralysis Cardiac failure Prolonged thiazide diuretic therapy Excessive calcium intake Parathyroid tumor Sarcoidosis Medications including: hydralazine (Apresoline), lithium, parathyroid hormone	Generalized muscle weakness Depressed or absent deep tendon reflexes (DTRs) Drowsiness Lethargy Headaches Loss of muscle tone Ataxia Mental confusion Impairment of memory Slurred speech Personality or behavior changes Stupor or coma Pathologic fractures may occur Flank or deep bone pain	Anorexia Nausea Vomiting Constipation Epigastric pain Polydipsia

Respiratory System	Cardiovascular System	Renal System	Skin and Mucous Membranes	Blood Gas Values	Interventions
	Effectiveness of digitalis enhanced (to the point of toxicity)				Monitor rate of IV administration of potassium Monitor intake and output (report changes) Encourage intake of food and fluids rich in potassium (orange juice, bananas, bouillon, meat broths, colas, tea, leafy vegetables) Observe for changes in heart rate, rhythm, and ECG pattern Determine source of potassium losses
	Bradycardia Hypertension ECG: QT interval shortened, T waves inverted Ventricular dysrhythmias Enhanced effectiveness of digitalis	Development of renal calculi, kidney stones Polyuria			Assess for causes Administer loop diuretics to increase excretion of calcium Administer corticosteroids and mithramycin as ordered (lowers serum calcium concentration) Administer antacids cautiously: some contain calcium Position and move patient carefully to prevent pathologic fractures Administer isotonic fluids as ordered Encourage fluid intake of 2000 to 3000 ml a day Monitor intake and output Avoid dietary intake of calcium (dairy products and green leafy vegetables)

Continued.

Table 2-5 Observation of Electrolyte, Fluid, and Acid-Base Imbalances—cont'd

Imbalances	Causes	Neuromuscular System	GI System
Hypercalcemia (calcium excess—cont'd			
Hypocalcemia (calcium deficit): critical values < 6 mg/dL (total)	Inadequate intake of calcium Decreased absorption from intestine Hypoparathyroidism Vitamin D deficiency Rapid dilution of the plasma by intravenous calcium free solutions Chronic renal failure Chronic malabsorption syndrome Neoplastic diseases Hypomagnesemia Cushing's syndrome Acute pancreatitis Hyperphosphatemia Extreme stress situations Excessive citrated blood, alkalosis Medications, including: acetazolamide, anticonvulsants (Dilantin), asparaginase, aspirin, calcitonin, cisplatin (Platinol), corticosteroids, heparin, laxatives, oral contraceptives	Muscle tremors, paresthesias, especially numbness or tingling, skeletal muscle cramps, abdominal spasms and cramps Hyperactive reflexes Convulsions Positive Trousseau's sign Positive Chvostek's sign Emotional depression or confusion	Paralytic ileus GI bleeding

Respiratory System	Cardiovascular System	Renal System	Skin and Mucous Membranes	Blood Gas Values	Interventions
					Monitor serum calcium levels
					Observe for changes in heart rate, rhythm, and ECG pattern
					Observe for digitalis toxicity
	Dysrhythmias				Monitor rate, rhythm, and ECG pattern
	Hypotension				Administer calcium gluconate or calcium chloride 10% as ordered
	Prolonged QT interval with normal T wave on ECG				Monitor serum calcium levels every 12 to 24 hr
					Report calcium deficit to physician
					Monitor PT and platelet levels
					Observe for signs and symptoms of tetany
					Provide dietary calcium (e.g., cheese, cream, milk, yogurt)
					Administer vitamin D as ordered
					Monitor prothrombin and platelet levels
					Check for bleeding from any source (calcium aids in blood clotting)
					Monitor use of laxatives and antacids (those containing phosphate affect calcium metabolism)

Continued.

Table 2-5 Observation of Electrolyte, Fluid, and Acid-Base Imbalances—cont'd

Imbalances	Causes	Neuromuscular System	GI System
Hypernatremia (sodium excess): normal values, 136-145 mEq/L; critical value, >160 mEq/L	Primary aldosteronism: excessive steroids (Cushing's disease) Excessive IV administration of large amounts of sodium chloride solution without water replacement Renal failure (with sodium retention) Neurohypophyseal dysfunction (as in diabetes insipidus) High-protein diets with minimal fluid intake Diabetes mellitus Excessive ingestion of sodium chloride Decreased water intake, severe vomiting or diarrhea Inadequate circulation of blood to the kidneys (congestive heart failure [CHF]) Cirrhosis of the liver Recent trauma, surgery, shock Medications including: anabolic steroids, antibiotics, clonidine (Catapres), corticosteroids, cough medicines, laxatives, methyldopa (Aldomet), NSAIDS, oral contraceptives	Sodium ↑, water ↓ CNS depression (lethargy to coma), muscle weakness, muscle rigidity, muscle tremors	
Hyponatremia (sodium deficit): critical values, <120 mEq/L	Inappropriate ADH syndrome Excessive intake of hypotonic fluids Severe malnutrition Vomiting Diarrhea GI drainage from suction or fistulas Severe diaphoresis Trauma such as surgery or burns Small bowel obstruction and peritonitis	Headache Vertigo Anxiety Muscle weakness and cramps Lassitude, apathy, confusion Hyperreflexia	Anorexia, nausea, vomiting, diarhea, cramping

Respiratory System	Cardiovascular System	Renal System	Skin and Mucous Membranes	Blood Gas Values	Interventions
Sodium ↑, water ↑ (increase in extracellular fluid volume) may cause pulmonary edema: shortness of breath, coughing, cyanosis, increased respiratory rate	Sodium ↑, water ↑: postural hypotension Sodium ↑, water ↑: elevated blood pressure; pitting edema		Increased sodium with decrease in fluid intake: observe for signs and symptoms of dehydration (dry mucous membranes, flushed skin, elevated temperature)		Sodium ↑, water ↓: Increase po fluid intake Administer IV fluids as ordered Instill water with or between tube feedings Sodium ↑, water ↑ Administer diuretics as ordered Restrict NA intake Restrict fluid intake Monitor intake and output q8h Weigh daily Monitor vital signs q8h Check urine for specific gravity
Hyperpnea	Hypotension Orthostatic hypotension Tachycardia Thready peripheral pulse or loss of peripheral pulse, collapsed neck veins	Decreased urine output Oliguria to anuria	Flushed, dry, hot skin Fever Loss of skin turgor		Administer IV normal saline solution as ordered (monitor rate carefully) Monitor serum sodium and potassium levels Administer sodium orally as ordered Maintain intake and output q8h Weigh daily

Continued.

Table 2-5 Observation of Electrolyte, Fluid, and Acid-Base Imbalances—cont'd

Imbalances	Causes	Neuromuscular System	GI System
Hyponatremia (sodium deficit)—cont'd	Renal disease Administration of sodium-removing diuretics Water intoxication (IV therapy, tap water enemas) Medications including: carbamazepine (Tegrefol), sulfanylureas, triamterene (hydrochlorothiazide), vasopressin		
Hypermagnesemia (magnesium excess): normal values, 4.4-5.5 mEq/L; critical values, >6.5 mEq/L	Renal failure Adrenal insufficiency Excessive ingestion of magnesium-containing medications Diabetic ketoacidosis (with severe water loss) Hyperparathyroidism	Drowsiness, lethargy, loss of deep tendon reflexes Respiratory depression, coma, and cardiac arrest	Nausea
Hypomagnesemia (magnesium deficit): critical values, <3.0 mEq/L	Acute pancreatitis Malabsorption syndrome (nontropical sprue or steatorrhea) Diarrhea, vomiting Excessive calcium intake Primary hyperparathyroidism and other hypercalcemic states Alcoholism Bowel resection, small bowel bypass, or inherited intestinal defects Gastrointestinal fistulas Excessive renal secretion Nasogastric suctioning Diabetic ketoacidosis Toxemia of pregnancy	Neuromuscular irritability Tremors, tetany, increased reflexes, clonus Convulsions Disorientation Agitation, depression Hallucinations Athetoid or choreiform movements, convulsions, clonus, positive Babinski's sign, positive Chvostek's sign, and positive Trousseau's sign Paresthesias of feet and legs	Anorexia Nausea

Respiratory System	Cardiovascular System	Renal System	Skin and Mucous Membranes	Blood Gas Values	Interventions
					Encourage foods and fluids high in sodium (milk, meat, eggs, fruit juices, bouillon) Use normal saline for all irrigations
Depressed respirations	Hypotension Bradycardia, weak pulse, prolonged QT interval on ECG Heart block				Avoid use of all magnesium-containing medications (Maalox, Mylanta, and Milk of Magnesia) Monitor vital signs and level of consciousness qlh Encourage fluid intake Administer IV calcium gluconate as ordered Monitor serum magnesium levels q6h Observe for flushing of skin and diaphoresis
	Tachycardia Hypotension Atrial or ventricular premature contractions Nonspecific T wave changes				Administer magnesium sulfate as ordered When administering IV magnesium sulfate, observe patient carefully Monitor for signs and symptoms of high serum magnesium Check for loss of patellar reflex q5 min Monitor respiratory rate q5 min Observe for increased thirst, flushing of skin, diaphoresis, anxiety, or drowsiness

Continued.

Potential complications

Infection at site
Venous thrombosis
Catheter migration
Catheter embolus
Occlusion of catheter
Extravasation
Septicemia
Pneumothorax
Hemothorax
Hematoma
Cardiac tamponade
Cardiac dysrhythmias

Postinsertion care

Immediate care

Observe patient for signs of pneumothorax until chest
x-ray film is read
Auscultate chest for breath sounds q15 min ×4 and
then q1h; report diminished or absent breath sounds
to physician
Report any respiratory distress and presence of chest
pain to physician
Prepare to insert chest tubes if pneumothorax is
present

Interventions

Check BP, T, P, and R q4h
Avoid using arm with line for BP
Auscultate chest for breath sounds q8h
Monitor parenteral fluids
Maintain a closed system
Keep system free of air
Have a rubber-tipped hemostat available to clamp
catheter if necessary
Maintain a continuous drip of parenteral solutions at
all times unless obtaining a CVP reading or aspirat-
ing a blood specimen
Change dressing daily
Inspect catheter insertion site for any signs of infec-
tion, redness, tenderness, drainage, and edema
Cleanse skin around insertion site with povidone-
iodine solution
Apply bacteriostatic ointment to catheter insertion
site; avoid antibiotic ointment
Apply sterile occlusive dressing
Secure tubing to patient's skin to prevent tension on
catheter
Measure intake and output every 8 hours
Send tip of catheter to laboratory for culture when
catheter is removed

Table 2-6 Regulation of IV Drip Rates

Amount/ hr (ml)	Amount/8 hr (ml)	Amount/24 hr (ml)	Drops/min
PEDIATRIC MICRODRIP (60 DROPS/ML)			
4	30	90	4
5	40	120	5
6	50	150	6
8	60	180	8
9	70	210	9
10	80	240	10
12	100	300	12
14	110	330	14
18	150	450	18
22	180	540	22
25	200	600	25
30	250	750	30
37	300	900	37
ADULT IV SET (10 DROPS/ML)			
125	1000	3000	21
100	800	2400	16
90	720	2160	15
80	640	1920	13
70	560	1680	11
60	480	1440	10
50	400	1200	8
40	320	960	6
30	240	720	5
ADULT IV SET (15 DROPS/ML)			
125	1000	3000	30
100	800	2400	25
90	720	2160	22
80	640	1920	20
70	560	1680	17
60	480	1440	15
50	400	1200	12
40	320	960	10
30	240	720	7

Patient/family teaching

Ensure that patient and/or significant other describes
and understands the following:
Purpose of central catheter
Importance of not touching catheter and tubing

Importance of reporting any difficulty in breathing, sudden chest pain at insertion site, or fever to nurse

When to flush catheter

When to change dressing

Type and amount of parenteral solutions to be infused daily

Where to purchase solution and supplies needed

Need to keep solution refrigerated (bring to room temperature before administration)

Name of medication, dosage, time of administration, and side effects

Need to avoid crowds and persons with infections

Ensure that patient and/or significant other demonstrates the following:

Proper handwashing technique

Dressing change

    Inspect catheter insertion site for redness, tenderness, drainage, or swelling

    Clean skin around insertion site with povidone-iodine solution

    Apply bacteriostatic ointment to insertion site

    Apply sterile occlusive dressing

Flushing catheter

Administration of parenteral solutions and/or medications as ordered by physician

Use of infusion pump if necessary

● Multilumen Subclavian Catheters

Three separate subclavian catheters contained in one sheath; allows infusion of incompatible drugs simultaneously—the solutions do not mix but exit via separate lumens; the catheters vary in length, gauge, and volume (Figure 2-1)

Postinsertion assessment

Observations/findings

See Central Lines (p. 67)

Potential complications

See Central Lines (p. 67)

Interventions

Postinsertion care

Use large-gauge lumen for administration of blood products or blood withdrawal (e.g., 16-gauge CVP readings can be taken from distal lumen only)

Reserve one lumen for TPN use only

Keep occlusive clamp available at bedside

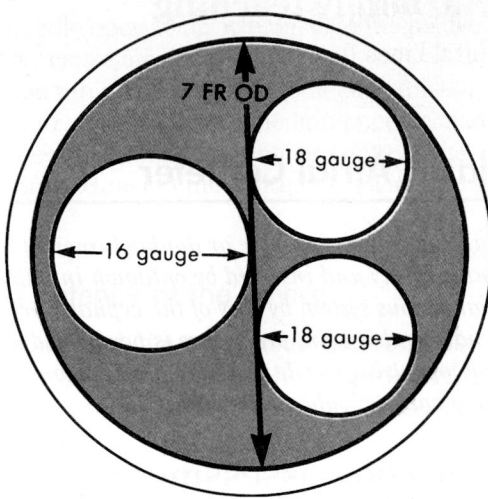

Figure 2-1   Multilumen catheter. French polyurethane catheter featuring three internal lumens: 18-gauge proximal, 18-gauge middle, and 16-gauge distal. (Redrawn from Recker DH, Metzler DJ: *Crit Care Nurse* 4[3]:92, 1984.)

Site care

Observe site qh

Inspect site for redness, pain, drainage, swelling, leakage of fluid, or loose sutures; notify physician if any of these occur

Change dressing daily for gauze dressing and q5d for transparent dressing (or when nonocclusive dressing is used)

Cleanse site with povidone-iodine solution

Apply povidone-iodine ointment to catheter insertion site

Apply occlusive gauze or transparent dressing

Maintaining patency of lumens

Flush each catheter lumen with heparin q12h if catheter lumen is not in use

Flush lumens after each intermittent medication infusion or blood sampling

Change injection site cap q3d or according to policy

Cap change should coincide with heparin flush

Blood withdrawal

Collect blood specimen for laboratory studies as ordered

Stop infusion through other lumens

Perform procedure using sterile technique

Aspirate and discard the first 3 ml of blood

Withdraw amount of blood needed for laboratory studies

Flush lumen with normal saline, then with 3 ml heparin solution

Resume infusion through other lumens

Decreased GF motility
Vomiting
Alterations of endocrine and autonomic nervous
  systems
Desired effects
Analgesia
Alertness
Increased coherence
Decreased anxiety
Improved coping ability
Improved relationships with others
Improved cardiac function
  Decreased tachycardia
  Modulation of BP
Regular respiratory rhythm

Interventions

Choose opioid based on minimum toxicity; drug of
  choice is morphine (Dilaudid) and hydromorphine hydrochloride
Dilute solution based on dosage required for analgesia
  and amount of fluid per hour that is therapeutic for
  patient
Titrate hourly drip rate to level of analgesia desired
  without untoward effects
Regulate drip carefully with controller or pump as indicated (see box on p. 91)
Involve patient in his or her care plan; encourage
  patient to communicate how he or she feels
Monitor BP, P, R, and level of consciousness qh while
  dosage is being adjusted
Monitor BP, P, R, and level of consciousness q2h when
  optimum dosage is achieved
Check arterial blood gases as ordered
Initiate flow sheet and enter patient's vital signs and
  dosage per hour as indicated

Patient/family teaching

Ensure that patient and/or significant other knows and
  understands the following:
  Purpose of central catheter
  Importance of not touching catheter and tubing
  Importance of reporting any difficulty in breathing,
    pain at insertion site, or fever to nurse
  When to change dressing
  Type and amount of solutions to be infused daily
  Need to keep solution refrigerated (bring to room
    temperature before administration)
  Name of medication, dosage, time of administration,
    and side effects
  Need to avoid crowds and persons with infections
Ensure that patient and/or significant other demon-
  strates the following:

Proper handwashing technique
Dressing change
  Inspect catheter insertion site for redness, tender-
    ness, drainage, or swelling
  Clean skin around insertion site with povidone-
    iodine solution
  Apply bacteriostatic ointment to insertion site
  Apply sterile occlusive dressing
Use of infusion pump with alarm if necessary
Knowledge of side effects to report to physician
  Respiratory distress
  Drowsiness
  Decreased mental acuity
  Vomiting

Home care considerations

Assess and continue with patient and family education
  and evaluate for the following:
  Ability of patient and caregiver to perform needed
    tasks
  Correct type and amount of infusion
  Ability to care for insertion site and to change
    dressing
  Knowledge and use of infusion pump
  Use of flow sheet for record-keeping tasks
  Mental acuity and signs of toxicity to opioid
  Amount of rest and exercise
  Intake and output
  Elimination status
  Nutritional status
  Presence of telephone and emergency phone num-
    bers as well as those of home health team

● Continuous Subcutaneous Opioid Infusion

*An alternate method of administering opioids to the
terminally ill who have intractable pain when other
accesses are not desirable*

Indications

Rectal and oral routes contraindicated
Intravenous sites not accessible or desirable
Intramuscular sites painful and/or damaged

Assessment

Subjective data

Injection site pain
Nausea

Objective data

Dosage necessary for maximum pain relief and minimum side effects
Side effects
  Drowsiness
  Mood changes
  Decreased mental acuity
  Respiratory depression
  Increased $Paco_2$—arterial carbon dioxide
  Decreased gastrointestinal motility, constipation
  Nausea/vomiting
Desired effects
  Analgesia
  Alertness
  Decreased anxiety
  Improved interacting/coping ability
  Improved vital signs

Interventions

Choose opioid based on minimum toxicity; drug of choice is morphine or hydromorphine hydrochloride (Dilaudid)
Dilute solution based on analgesic requirement and hourly therapeutic intake
Select subcutaneous site using either abdominal, thigh, or clavicular area
Using sterile technique, insert small-bore (27-gauge) butterfly needle and connect it to a controller or infusion pump
Titrate hourly drip rate to desired level of analgesia
Monitor BP, P, R and mental acuity qh until patient is stable and then monitor them q4h
Monitor infusion site q8h for swelling and pain
Change site at least q6d to 7 d and prn

Electronic Infusion Devices

Nonvolumetric devices	Deliver solution in drops/min	Drop rate–calibrated infusion pumps	Are designed to count drops and are set in terms of gtt/min; move solution through the line by application of positive pressure
Volumetric devices	Deliver a specific volume in a given time as shown in ml/hr		
Drop rate–calibrated infusion controllers	Regulate infusion rate via gravity by electronically counting or measuring drops (controllers that set the rate in drops/min are now considered obsolete)	Volumetric infusion pumps	Have rate setting adjustment calibrated in ml/hr rather than drops/min; pump output pressure limits are established by manufacturer and can range as high as 25 psi
Volumetric infusion controllers	Count the volume in each drop; permit flow rate to be set in ml/hr rather than gtt/min (controllers *do not* add pressure to the line to overcome resistance to flow)	Variable pressure limit volumetric infusion pumps	Are designed to provide only the pressure needed for specific clinical situations; allow nurse to set pressure limit based on clinical considerations
Infusion pumps	Apply positive pressure to the line to overcome flow; most deliver solution to a vein at an average pressure of psi (pounds per square inch) *(pressure can increase if a line is occluded partially or totally)*		

Patient/family teaching

See ICOI (p. 89)

Home care considerations

See ICOI (p. 89)

● Patient-Controlled Analgesia

Patient-controlled analgesia (PCA) enables the patient to self-administer a physician-prescribed dose of analgesia on demand; with PCA acute as well as chronic pain can be managed; more severe pain such as that encountered by a patient with terminal cancer can be controlled through the use of the continuous infusion feature; the continuous infusion rate may also be used in conjunction with PCA to control severe chronic pain

Indications

Acute postoperative pain
  Laminectomy
  Chest surgery
  Major abdominal surgery
  Orthopedic surgery
Acute pain in disease, such as sickle cell crisis
Chronic severe pain

Assessment

Subjective data

Nausea
Constipation

Objective data

Ability of patient, mentally and physically, to operate the device
Dosage adjustment for maximal pain relief with minimal side effects
Ability of patient to participate in his or her care
Side effects
  Respiratory depression
  Drowsiness
  Vomiting
  Mental cloudiness
  Increased $Paco_2$—arterial carbon dioxide
  Anxiety
  Decreased GI motility

Interventions

Ensure completeness of physician's order
  Name of drug
  Concentration of drug
  Loading dose
  Lock-out interval
Program prescribed information into PCA unit
Verify accurate program entry with another RN
Monitor patient's baseline vital signs and level of consciousness
Instruct patient about purpose of PCA and operation of unit
Stay with patient when first dose is administered
Be prepared to place the unit in stop mode if respiratory distress or change in sensorium is noted at any time during the infusion
Have naloxone hydrochloride (Narcan) available at all times
Monitor BP, P, R, and level of consciousness 30 minutes after the first dose and q4h thereafter
Monitor BP, P, R, and level of consciousness whenever a change in PCA dose occurs, when administering a loading dose, or when a change in the lock-out interval occurs
Monitor patient for adequate pain relief; use flow sheet and pain rating scale
Collaborate with physician to determine dosage needed if pain relief is not obtained
Monitor for side effects of the opioid drug

● Permanent Epidural Catheter

The placement of a radiopaque silicone catheter into the epidural space for the administration of a narcotic drug can be used as a method of pain control; the catheter has two segments; the one with the smaller lumen is inserted at L1, and the proximal end is placed between T11 and C3 at the appropriate level to obtain pain relief; the segment with the larger lumen is inserted in the abdomen, tunneled to the lumbar site, and joined to that segment; a Dacron filter cuff is attached to the catheter 2 inches from the abdominal incision; subcutaneous tissue adheres to the cuff, preventing bacterial entry

Indications

Chronic pain such as that in the following
  conditions:
  Cancer
  Degenerative joint disease
  Spinal trauma
Pain not controlled by conventional therapy
Restriction of activity by usual pain therapy

Assessment

Subjective data

Insertion site pain
Nausea

Objective data

Severity of pain (rating scale)
Amount of pain relief (rating scale)
Dosage of opioid that will control pain with minimal
side effects
Side effects
Respiratory depression
Drowsiness
Vomiting
Mental cloudiness
Increased Pa_{CO_2}
Anxiety
Decreased GI motility
Constipation

Potential complications

Infection
Displacement of catheter
Catheter malfunction

Interventions

Immediate postoperative care

Obtain epiduragram to confirm placement and deter-
mine the spread of fluid in the epidural space
Maintain dressings at both lumbar and abdominal inci-
sion sites for the first 24 hours after operation
Assess for bleeding at sites
Reinforce dressings prn
If bleeding is noted, apply ice packs or apply pressure,
using sand bags, to the subcutaneous tunnel
Catheter care
Change dressings at both incision sites daily until su-
tures are removed from lumbar site
Continue to change dressings at abdominal site on a
daily basis
Cleanse site with hydrogen peroxide followed by io-
dine solution
Cover site with sterile occlusive dressing
Administration of drug
Dilute prescribed drug with preservative-free normal
saline solution to a volume of 5 to 10 ml because
epidural space can safely handle only 15 ml/hour
Stay with patient during first few infusions
Monitor BP, P, and R q15min to 30min

Keep injection of naloxone (Narcan) available
Cleanse injection site of the catheter cap with iodine
Inject the drug into the catheter as rapidly as is com-
fortable
Change catheter filter daily for continuous infusion
and q4d for intermittent infusion
Assess for signs and symptoms of infection at exit site
q8h and report presence to physician
Redness and edema
Pain
Seepage of fluid around catheter
Fever of unknown origin
Assess severity of pain and pain relief q4h; use a rating
scale
Monitor for medication side effects and toxicities q4h
to 8h
Assess BP, P, R, and level of consciousness
If you are unable to inject medication into catheter, do
the following:
Change the filter
Change patient position while trying to inject medica-
tion
NOTE: If label on catheter indicates that it is not for
IV access, and if IV is accidently infused, remove fil-
ter, aspirate as much of drug or solution as possible,
attach a new filter, and notify physician *before* injecting any other drugs or solutions
If previously mentioned interventions fail, report
problem to physician

Patient/family teaching

Ensure that the patient and/or significant other de-
scribes and demonstrates the following:
Purpose of epidural catheter
Proper handwashing and sterile technique
Method of dressing change
Name, purpose, dosage, and frequency of medication
Side/toxic effects of medication to report
Need to notify physician if pain relief is not obtained
Preparation of medication
Administration of medication
Method of changing filter and injection cap
Symptoms of infection/inability to inject medication to
report to physician

Home care considerations

Assess and continue with the patient and family educa-
tion and evaluate for the following:
Proper handwashing and sterile technique
Ability of caregiver(s) to perform tasks
Preparation of opioid solution and administration
Dressing change technique
Mental acuity

Response to infusion; decreased pain and discomfort
Signs of side effects, toxicity of opioid infusion
Presence of telephone and emergency phone numbers as well as home care team
Nutritional and elimination status

● Transcutaneous Electrical Nerve Stimulation

Transmission of an electrical impulse to the body from a battery-powered device through electrodes attached to the skin; pain is relieved by production of a pleasant tingling, tapping, or massaging sensation

Indications

Postoperative use
During labor and delivery
Acute injuries
Chronic conditions (Herpes Zoster, osteoarthritis, neuralgia)

Contraindications

Cardiac pacemaker
Significant dysrhythmias
Myocardial infarction (MI)
Cardiac monitoring (creates artifact)
First trimester of pregnancy
Placement over carotid sinus nerve, eyes, laryngeal/pharyngeal muscles

Assessment

Subjective data

Muscle spasm
Increased pain
Nausea
Headache

Objective data

Skin irritation
Sensations produced
  Tingling
  Pleasure
  Itching
  Burning
  Prickling
Unit function
  No stimulation
  Cuts in and out

Unit settings
  Rate: 2 to 200 pulses/min (hertz [Hz])
  Pulse width: 0 to 500 μsec
  Amplitude

Interventions

Assist patient in placing electrodes according to the manufacturer's recommendations
Maintain electrodes in total contact with patient's skin
Change electrode positions prn to prevent skin irritation
Monitor patient for appropriate pain relief
Adjust rate and pulse width settings to prevent unpleasant sensations
Maintain electrodes in place
Activate unit in response to patient's pain
For skin irritation,
  Remove electrodes
  Expose skin to air
  Apply skin cream
  Reposition electrodes away from irritation
  Change type of electrode if necessary
For nausea,
  Reposition electrodes
  Vary rate, pulse width, and amplitude
For headache,
  Turn down pulse width dial
  Turn down amplitude
  Use shorter stimulation period
  Place electrodes farther apart
  Vary rate
If problems are not resolved,
  Try different TENS device
  Discontinue using TENS device
Refer patient for assistance from a TENS specialist, if available
Refer patient to pain clinic

Patient/family teaching

Ensure that patient and/or significant other describes and demonstrates the following:
  Mechanisms of rate, pulse width, and amplitude adjustments
  Appropriate sensations to be achieved
  How to adjust settings to do the following:
    Achieve maximum pain relief
    Avoid unpleasant sensations
    Avoid muscle spasm and pain exacerbation
  Need to do the following:
    Change electrode placement prn
    Maintain skin integrity

Wear TENS all day: on for 2 hours, off for 1 hour (total stimulation of 6 to 8 hours)

Wear TENS all night if sleep is interrupted (turn unit on if awakened by pain)

Maintain a record of settings that achieve desired effect

BIBLIOGRAPHY

Andresen GP: How to assess the older mind, *RN* 55(7):34, 1992.

Beare PG, Myers JL: *Principles and practice of adult health nursing,* ed 2, St Louis, 1994, Mosby.

Bender P: Deceptive distress in the elderly, *Am J Nurs* 92(10):29, 1992.

Bockus S: Troubleshooting your tube feedings, *Am J Nurs* 91(5):24, 1991.

Christopher M, Lajkowicz C: Patient teaching by the book, *RN* 56(7):48, 1993.

Doenges ME et al: *Nursing care plans: guidelines for planning and documenting patient care,* ed 3, Philadelphia, 1993, FA Davis.

Eisenberg PG: A nursing guide to tube feeding, *RN* 57(10):62, 1994.

Greene LM, Gerlach CJ: Central lines have moved out, *RN* 57(5):26, 1994.

Groah L, Howery D: 25 Predictions for perioperative nursing, *Nursing '92* 22(1):48, 1992.

Hamblelton NE: Dealing with complications of epidural analgesia, *Nursing '94* 24(10):55, 1994.

Hogstel MO: Understanding hoarding behaviors in the elderly, *Am J Nurs* 93(7):42, 1993.

Hummer A: Get your patient moving, *RN* 56(6):34, 1993.

Kim MJ et al: *Pocket guide to nursing diagnoses,* ed 6, St Louis, 1995, Mosby.

Marshall M: Postoperative confusion, *Nursing '93* 23(1):44, 1993.

McCance KL, Huether SE: *Pathophysiology, the biological basis for disease in adults and children,* ed 2, St Louis, 1994, Mosby.

McFarland GK, McFarlane EA: *Nursing diagnosis and intervention: planning for patient care,* ed 2, St Louis, 1993, Mosby.

Meares C: P.I.C.C. and M.L.C. lines, *Nursing '92* 22(10):52, 1992.

Pasero C, McCaffery M: Unconventional PCA: making it work for your patient, *Am J Nurs* 93(9):38, 1993.

Skewes SM: No more bed baths! *RN* 57(1):34, 1994.

Smith RM: A nurse's guide to implanted ports, *RN* 56(4):48, 1993.

Stewart KB, Walton RL: Tips on teaching the elderly, *Nursing '92* 22(10):66, 1992.

Tasota FJ, Wesmiller SW: Assessing ABGs, *Nursing '94* 24(5):34, 1994.

Uram MS: A new delivery system makes pain control easier, *RN* 55(5):46, 1992.

Walsh J: Postop effects of OR positioning, *RN* 56(2):50, 1993.

Waltman RE: 5 goals for managing older patients, *Nursing '93* 23(1):62, 1993.

Wild L, Coyne C: Epidural analgesia, *Am J Nurs* 92(4):26, 1992.

Woodin LM: Cutting postop pain, *RN* 56(8):26, 1993.

Young C: Tube feeding at home, *Am J Nurs* 92(4):46, 1992.

	Rex Healthcare Clinical Pathway Prevention of Noscomial Pneumonia for Ventilator ICU Patients	

Admission Date/Time:_____

Clinical Path Date/Time:_____

Discharge Date/Time:_____

Case Manager/Phone:_____

Patient/Family Contact/_____
Phone Number:

Category	Day 1/Placed on Ventilator	Day 2	Day 3	Day 1/Post Extubation	Day 2/Post Extubation	Day 3/Post Extubation
TESTING	M12 (1) ABG ———————— CBC ———————— M6 PT/PTT ———————— EKG (1) CXR ————————	M7—————	—— PRN ———— —— PRN ———— — PRN —— PRN —— — PRN —			■ ■ ■ ■ ■
MEDICATIONS	Sedation per Protocol (on back of path) Reassess to D/C antibiotic (2 ———— Antacid: H2 Blocker until GI track function returns (5)					■
PATIENT CARE/ TREATMENTS	Assess for specialty bed Assess need for CPT Mouth Care Q4 and PRN per protocol (on back of path) Verify NG placement per protocol ——— Verify NT or ET tube place— ment Q shift ———— Suctioning PRN ———— RN/RT document secretion PRN (based on assessment of patient) —— Turning Q2H ———— Skin integrity Q shift ———— I & O ———— Weight ——————Daily Weight— Vent setting ———— Nebulizer meds (2) if ordered/as ordered ——— Tube changing per Protocol Retaping ET tube (per Protocol to be developed) ————	PT assess OOB with RT/PT OOB		Incentive spirometry Swallowing Assessment post extubation or > 5 days intubated ■ ■ Assess for Ambulation ——— ■		■ ■ ■ ■ ■ ■ ■
DIETITIAN		MD assess for enteral parenteral feeding Dietitian Screening				
CONSULTS	As directed: — Anesthesiology — Pulmonology — IM — Surgeon — Nephrology — Infectious Disease — Cardiology	Wound/Ostomy/Skin Care per Clinical Nurse Specialist				
DISCHARGE PLANNING	D/C Plan Consult	D/C Plan Assessment completed		D/C Plan in place or disposition determined		
EDUCATION	Use of Nebulizer Turning, coughing, deep breathing, splinting Trach Care education*			Incentive Spirometry Smoking Cessation (to be developed)		
PROCEDURES	A—Line IV: — CVP* — Swan* NG Dialysis*	MD assess for small bore feeding tube, Gastrostomey, Jejunostomy			MD assess for Small bore feeding tube	

NOTE: CLINICAL PATHWAYS ARE GUIDELINES FOR CONSIDERATION WHICH MAY BE MODIFIED ACCORDING TO INDIVIDUAL PATIENT NEEDS.

* As individual patient's condition indicates appropriateness. (1) Required only if previously done >12 hours prior to intubation. (2) Prophylactic antibiotics discouraged. (3) Bed assessment guidelines/at reisk: (a) weight >250 lbs (b) age >60 (c) Neuro, abdominal and throacic surgery. (4) Recommended mertered dose inhaler as ordered. (5) Best oral antacid is Carafate (R). Best IV antacids are Pepcid (R), Tagamet (R), or Zantac (R).

KEY TO DISCIPLINES PERFORMING SERVICES	
RN — Registered Nurse	MD — Physician
RT — Respiratory Therapist	RP — Registered Pharmacist
RD — Registered Dietitian	Lab — Laboratory
PFS — Patient & Family Services	US— Unit Secretary
CM — Case Manager	PT — Physical Therapist

Form Date: July 5, 1995
Form Revision Date: August 23, 1995

Prevention of Noscomial Pneumonia
for Ventilator ICU Patients

Category	Day 1/Placed on Ventilator	Day 2	Day 3	Day 1/Post Extubation	Day2	Day 3
OUTCOMES	Lab WNL – – – – – – – –					■
	Chest x–ray clear – – – –					■
	Patient is comfortable and cooperative with treatment and tolerating vent status – –			■		
	Patient will be free from signs of GI bleeding – –					■
	Patient bed type is appropriate – – – – –					■
	Patient has breath sounds WNL – – – – –					■
	Patient exhibits mucosal intgrity – – – –					■
				Patient has normal gag reflex (immediatly post extubation) – – – – – – –		■
				Patient understands and independatly performs incentive spirometry (80% of predictated value) – – – – – – –		■
	Patient has clear secretions – – – – – –					■
	Patient's skin integrity is is maintained – – – – –					■
		Patient activity level increasing – – – – – –				■
		Patient is receiving adequate nutrition – –				■
				Patient/Family verbilizes and understands D/C Plan		
				Patient demostrates understanding through performance of turning, coughing, deep breathing and splinting		

Pathway Daily Variance Tracking

Variance Type/Date Occured	Initials	Reason/Comment	Initials	Action Taken/Date Resolved	Initials
1.					
2.					
3.					
4.					
5.					
6.					
7.					
8.					
9.					
10.					

Protocol for Mouth Care and Assessment for Patient's with Endotracheal Tube

NOTE: The following information presents the standard of mouth care for patients who are intubated.

A. Comprehensive Mouth Care Performed q12h by RN and RT:
1. RT loosens ties and manually holds the ET tube.
2. RN brushes teeth using toothpaste and PlaqVac brush or removes dentures and soaks them in cleaning solution.
3. Cleanse mouth by instilling diluted H202 (1 part H202 to 1 part NaC1) while maintaining continuous oral suction.
4. Rinse mouth by instilling NaC1 (remove residual H202) while maintaining continuous oral suction.
5. Apply moisturizer to mucosa (mouthcare kit) and lips.
6. Inspect mouth for lesions, xerostomia, or stomatitis.
7. Reposition ET tube and apply new ties PRN.

B. Routine Mouth Care performed q4h, with each ET suctioning and PRN.
1. Suction mouth of all accumulated saliva.
2. Rinse mouth by instilling diluted H202 while maintaining continuous oral suction.
3. Rinse mouth by instilling NaC1 (remove residual H202) while maintaining continuous oral suction.
4. Apply moisturizer to mucosa and lip balm to lips.

C. Minimize the following conditions by:
1. Xerostomia (dry mouth)
   * Obtaining order for moisturizing spray and use per mouth care protocol and PRN.
   * Swabbing mouth with moist Toothette q4h and PRN.
   * Applying lip balm.
2. Stomatitis:
   * Obraining order for magic mouthwash (MMW).
   * Using MMW with mouthcare q8h.
   * Obtaining Viscous Lidocaine order for placement on lesions PRN pain relief.

D. Post extubation, mouthcare should be performed at least qid by the patient or nurse. An oral assessment is done b.i.d.

E. For patients who are neutropenic and/or thrombocytopenic or on chemotherapy, see Nursing Division Protocol #242.

Form Date: July 5, 1995
Form Revision Date: August 23, 1995

Cardiovascular System

Cardiovascular Assessment

● Subjective Data

Pain
  Onset
  Duration
  Location
  Radiation
  Description
Indigestion
Weakness
Fatigue
Fainting
Dizzy spells, lightheadedness
Shortness of breath with or without activity or on waking at night
Palpitations
Sudden awakening at night with shortness of breath
Fever
Cough, wheezing, hemoptysis
Swelling of extremities
Blue discoloration of lips, fingers
Nausea
Numb, cold extremities
Changes in vision
Headaches

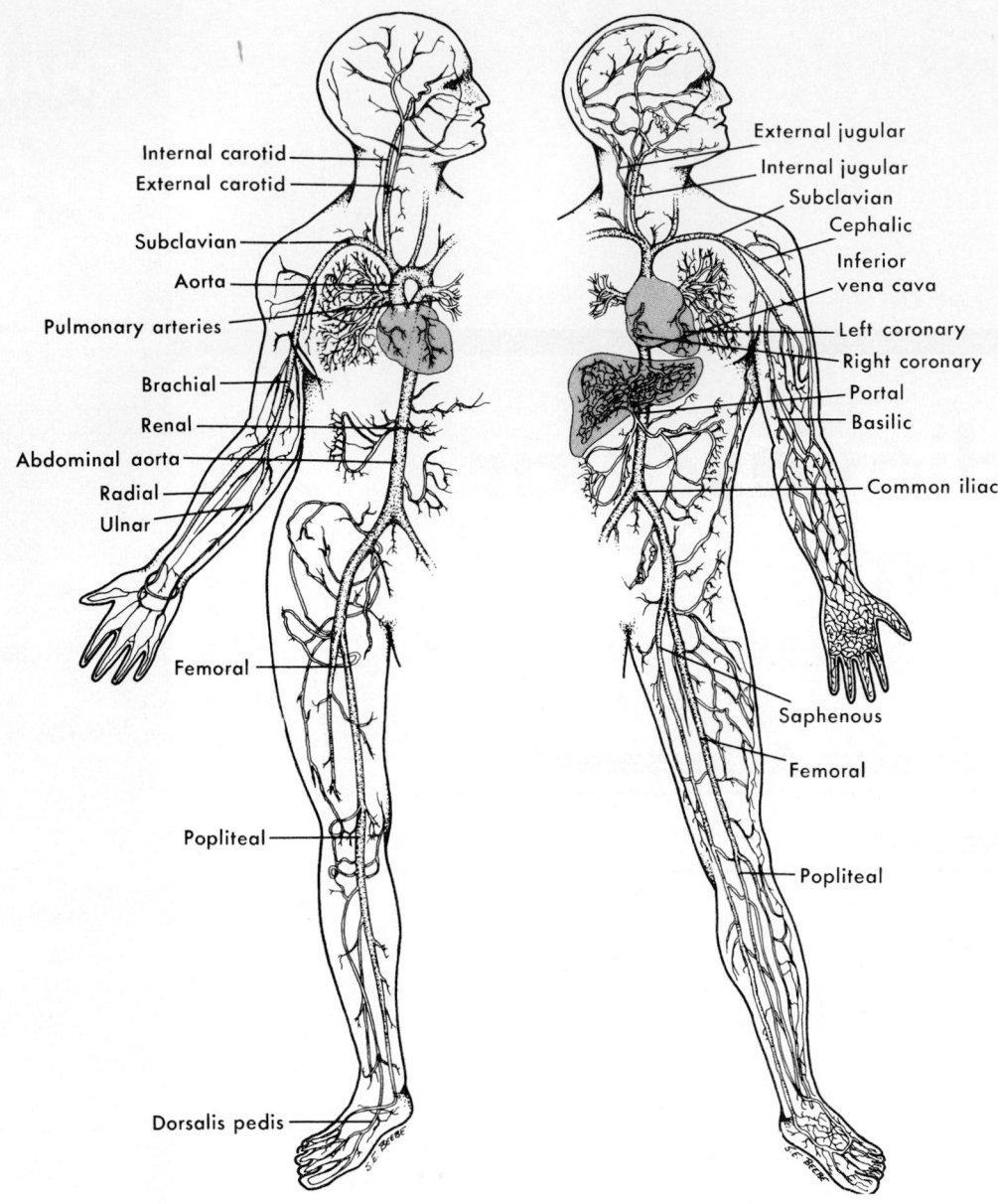

Figure 3-1 Arterial system *(left)* and venous system *(right)*.

● Objective Data

Age
Sex
General appearance
  Color
  Assumed position
Vital signs
  Arterial pulses
    Rate
    Rhythm
    Equality
    Presence

Absence
Respirations
  Rate
  Character
  Type
  Temperature
Neck veins
  Distension
  Venous pressure
  Pulsation
BP
  Position and extremity
  Pulse pressure

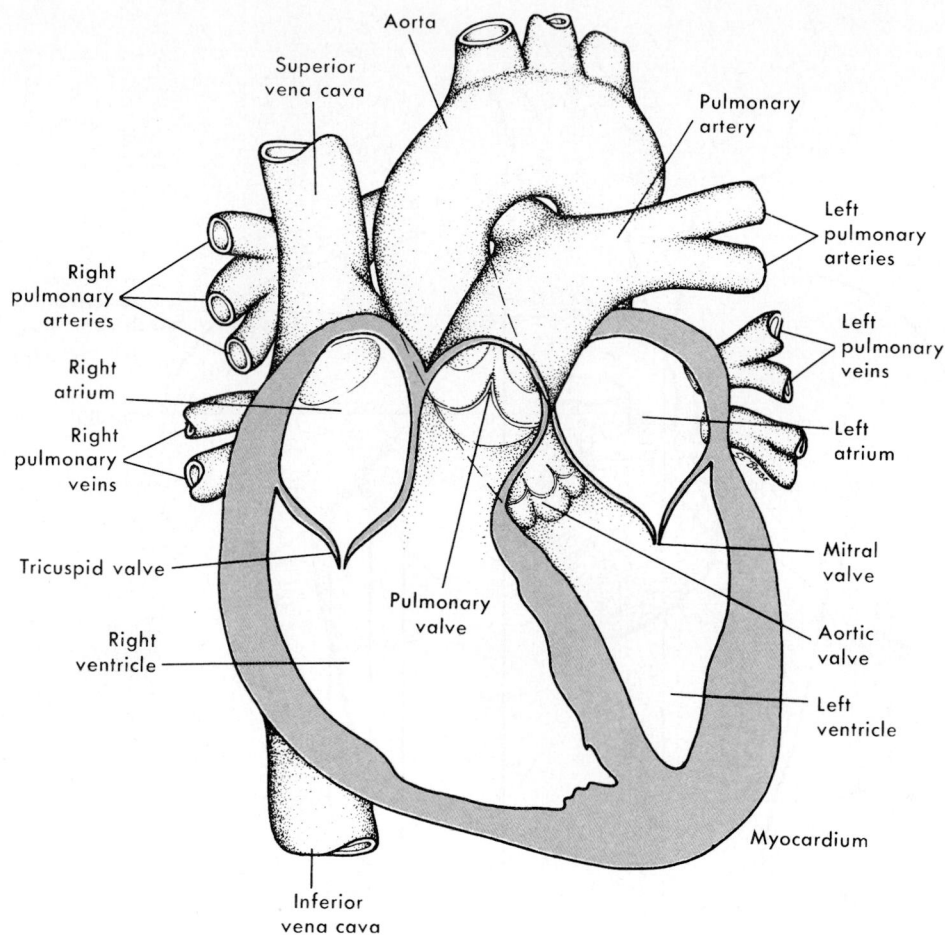

Figure 3-2 Circulatory system (heart).

Pulsus paradoxus
Pulsus alternans
Urinary output
  Amount
  Character
  Color
Precordium (Figure 3-3)
  Point of maximal impulse (PMI)
  Lifts
  Bulges
  Pulsations
  Thrills
  Symmetry
  Cardiac border
Heart sounds (Figure 3-4)
  Intensity
  Pitch
  Duration
  Timbre
  Origin
  S_1, S_2
  Presence of S_3, S_4

Murmurs
Pericardial friction rub
Breath sounds
  Location
  Description
    Normal
    Decreased
    Pleural friction rub
    Adventitious
    Rhonchi
    Crackles
Skin
  Color
  Temperature
  Turgor
  Diaphoresis
  Dryness
Extremities
  Appearance
  Color
  Temperature
  Edema

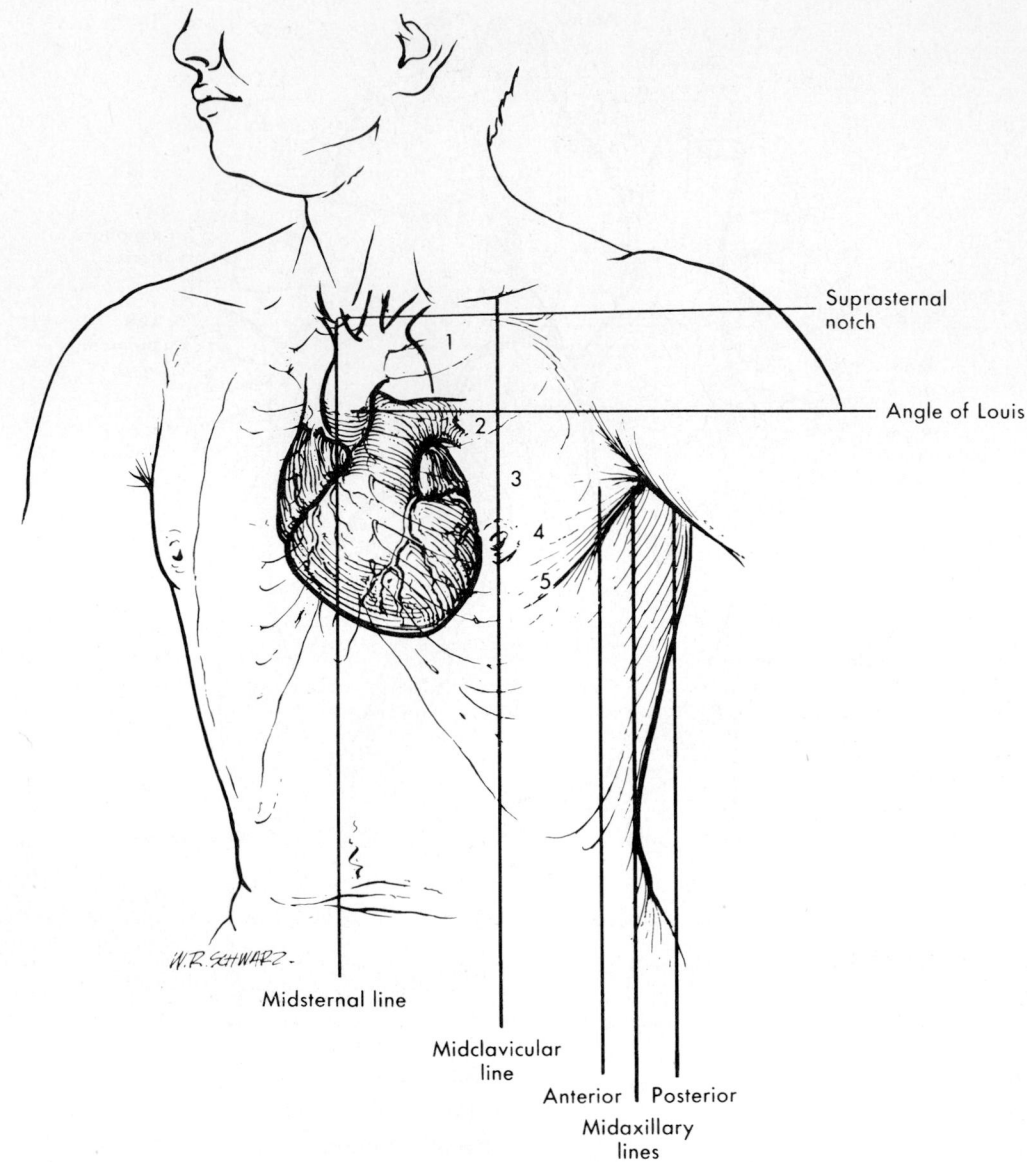

Figure 3-3   Chest wall landmarks. (From Malasanos L et al: *Health assessment,* ed 4, St Louis, 1990, Mosby.)

Capillary filling time
"Clubbing"
Nail shape
Description of lesions
Central nervous system (CNS)
    Level of consciousness
    Neurologic signs
    Reflexes
    Response to pain
Gastrointestinal system
    Ascites
    Hepatomegaly

● Pertinent Background Information

Concurrent diseases or conditions

Atherosclerosis
Hyperlipoproteinemia
Hypertension
Obesity
Diabetes
Pulmonary conditions
    Pneumonia
    Emphysema

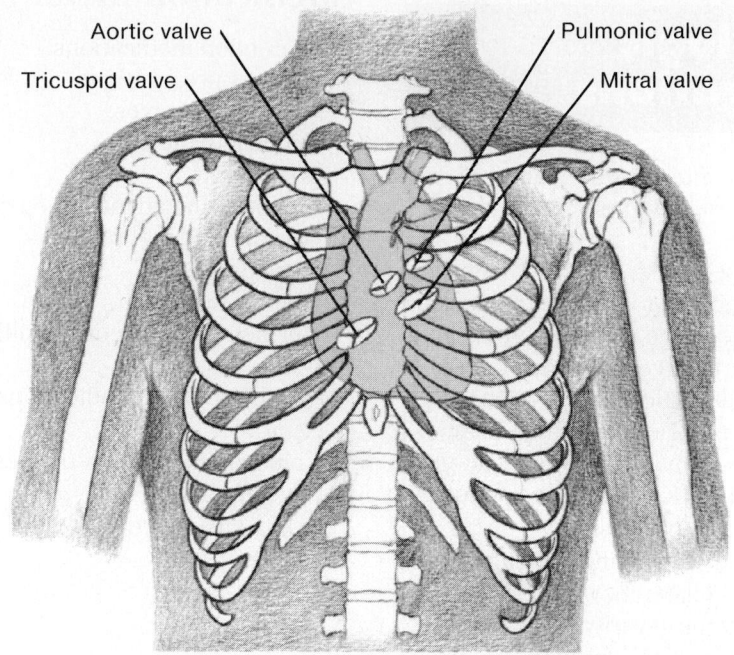

Figure 3-4 Anatomic location of cardiac valves. (From Canobbio MM: *Mosby's clinical nursing series: cardiovascular disorders,* St Louis, 1990, Mosby.)

Cor pulmonale
Renal conditions

Behavioral responses

Response to stress
Methods of coping
Response to pain
Relationships with others
Recent stressful life events

Medical history

Infancy and childhood
  Cyanosis at birth
  Murmurs
Systemic infection
  Rheumatic fever
  Endocarditis
  Kawasaki disease
Coronary artery disease
  Myocardial infarction (MI)
  Angina
  Heart failure
Heart murmur
Congenital heart disease
Cardiovascular surgery
Thromboembolism

Occlusive vascular disease
Pulmonary conditions
Renal conditions

Family history

Heart disease
Hypertension
Diabetes
Obesity
Arterial and venous diseases
Cerebrovascular accident (CVA)
Kidney disease

Social/cultural history

Cultural orientation
Educational level
Smoking
Alcohol use
Exercise and activity levels
Nutritional status
  Height
  Weight
  Less or more than body requirements
Occupation (sedentary or active)
Sleep patterns
Leisure activities

Gerontologic Considerations

- Changes in the cardiac musculature lead to reduced efficiency and strength, resulting in decreased cardiac output.
- Disorientation, syncope, and decreased tissue perfusion to organs and other body tissues can occur as a result of decreased cardiac output.
- Aging causes sclerotic changes in blood vessels and leads to decreased elasticity and narrowing of the lumen. Arterial pathology resulting from the aging process causes hypertension because of the increased cardiac effort needed to pump blood through the circulatory system.
- Progressive coronary artery changes can lead to the development of collateral coronary circulation. This can modify the severity of signs and symptoms seen in myocardial infarction. Angina symptoms may be less pronounced, and dyspnea may replace angina as a key symptom of acute infarction.
- Congestive heart failure can result from rapid intravenous infusion.
- Edema secondary to congestive heart failure may cause tissue impairment in the immobile older adult. Immobility leads to venous stasis and increases the risk of venous thrombosis and embolus formation.
- Older adults with cardiac disease often receive several medications, which are often prescribed at lower doses than for younger adults. Even with lower doses of medications, the older adult should be observed closely for signs of toxicity, since the rate of drug metabolism and excretion decreases with age.
- Independent older adults with cardiac conditions should receive adequate teaching regarding medication, diet, and warning signs of complications. They should be encouraged to maintain regular contact with the physician and to seek care at the first sign of problems.

From Christensen BL, Kockrow EO: *Foundations of nursing,* ed 2, St Louis, 1995, Mosby.

Environmental factors
Economic resources
Insurability status
Social support resources
  Marital status
  Number of siblings, children

Medication history

Prescription medications
  Digitalis preparations
  Antihypertensives
  Anticoagulants
  Beta blockers
  Angiotensin-converting-enzyme (ACE) inhibitors
  Calcium channel blockers
  Vasodilators
  Diuretics
  Hormones: birth control pills, replacement therapy
  Other
Over-the-counter medications
  Aspirin
  Cold and influenza remedies
  Sleeping pills
Street or illicit drugs
  Cocaine
  IV drug use

● Diagnostic Tests

Enzyme profile
  Aspartate aminotransferase (AST)
  Creatine phosphokinase (CPK-MB)
  Lactic acid dehydrogenase (LDH)
Electrolyte profile
Cholesterol value
Lipid levels: high density lipoprotein (HDL) to low density lipoprotein (LDL) ratio
Triglyceride value
Complete blood cell count (CBC)
Erythrocyte sedimentation rate (ESR)
Hemoglobin (Hgb)
Hematocrit (Hct)
Clotting profile
Prothrombin time (PT)
Activated partial thromboplastin time (APTT)
International Normalize Ratio (INR)
Heparin time
BUN, creatinine level
Glucose level
Urinalysis

Electrocardiogram (ECG)

P wave
P-R interval
QRS complex
Q-T interval
ST segment
T wave
U wave
Axis calculation

Rhythm identification
Chamber enlargement

Other procedures

Noninvasive

Radiologic studies
  Chest x-ray examination
  Fluoroscopy
Echocardiography
  M-mode
  Two-dimensional
  Doppler ultrasound
Transesophageal echocardiogram (TEE)
Treadmill (stress test)
Holter monitor
Signal averaging (SA) ECG
Atrial electrogram (AEG)
Nuclear studies
  Thallium uptake
  Computed tomography (CT) scan
  Multigated cardiac blood pool imaging (MUGA)
  Magnetic resonance imaging (MRI)

Invasive

Arterial pressure
Digital subtraction angiography (DSA)
Digital vascular imaging (DVI)
Cardiac catheterization
Coronary angiography
Ventriculography
Electrophysiologic (EP) studies
  His bundle recordings
  Programmed electrical stimulation (PES)
  Mapping (endocardial, epicardial)

Peripheral Vascular Assessment

● Subjective Data

Limb pain
  Initiating factors: onset
    Continuous exercise
    Rest
    Amount of exercise tolerated
  Provoking factor: change in environmental temperature, exercise
  Alleviating factors
    Rest
    Exercise

  Effect of prescribed medication
  Location
    Calf
    Foot
Swelling of extremity
Skin discoloration: pale, red, blue tinged
Numb, cold extremities
Transient ischemic attack (TIA)
Abdominal or back pain

● Pertinent Background Information

Concurrent diseases or conditions

Atherosclerosis
Hyperlipoproteinemia
Hypertension
Diabetes
Obesity
Heart failure
Renal conditions

Medical history

Thrombophlebitis
Cerebrovascular disease
Coronary artery disease
Aneurysm

Family history

Premature or sudden deaths
Cerebrovascular diseases
Atherosclerosis

Medication history

Over-the-counter: aspirin
Prescribed medications
  Antihypertensives
  Anticoagulants
  Antiinflammatories
  Steroids
  Hormone therapy
  Fibrinolytics
  Vasodilators

Social history

Tobacco use
Alcohol and caffeine use
Occupation (sedentary or active)
Environmental factors

Exercise and activity levels: recent changes caused by
  increased symptoms
Leisure activities

● Diagnostic Tests

Noninvasive

Segmental limb systolic pressure (SLP)
  Normal
    Lower extremities
      Midthigh: 16 mm Hg
      Upper third of leg: 3 to 12 mm Hg
      Above ankle: 1 to 18 mm Hg
      Foot: 0.2 to 1 mm Hg
    Upper extremities
      Upper arm: 4 to 16 mm Hg
      Elbow: 3 to 12 mm Hg
      Wrist: 1 to 10 mm Hg
      Hand: 0.2 to 2 mm Hg
Phlebography (venography)
Intermittent claudication determination
Doppler flow velocity tracings
Plethysmography
Radioactive fibrinogen uptake
Infrared thermography (IRT)
Carotid phonoangiogram (CPG)
Stress testing
Allen test
  Radial
  Ulnar
Radionuclide studies

Invasive

Digital subtraction angiography (DSA)
Angiography

OBJECTIVE DATA
General appearance
  Color
  Assumed position
Age
Vital signs: BP, T, P, and R
Pulses
  Rate
  Equality
  Rhythm
  Amplitude
    4+: strong, bounding (normal)
    3+: easily palpable
    2+: difficult to palpate

1+: weak, thready
0: absent
Bruits
  Carotid
  Subclavian
  Femoral
Skin
  Temperature
  Tissue loss
    Ulceration
    Gangrene
  Lesions
Color
  Pale: increased pallor of lower extremities with walk-
    ing, with elevation
  Mottled
  Cyanosis
  Redness (rubor): increased in dependent position
Hair loss
Opacification of nails
Lower extremities
  Cold feet
  Intermittent claudication
    Pain: calves, thighs, buttocks
    Onset with continuous exercise
    Localized or radiates from calf to thigh
    Relieved by rest or stopping activity
  Pain with rest
  Tissue loss
Upper extremities
  Digital ischemia
  Fingertip ulcerations
  Gangrene
  Positive Allen test
Abdomen
  Pulsatile abdominal mass
  Bruits
Capillary filling time
  Normal: <3 sec
  Abnormal: >3 sec

Venous Thrombosis

*An abnormal vascular condition associated with
  thrombus formation within a blood vessel, which
  develops as a result of stasis, hypercoagulability, or
  damage to the internal lining of the vein; can occur in
  superficial or deep veins (Figure 3-5); the following
  are terms used to describe venous disorders that reflect
  thrombus (clot) formation*
phlebitis: *Inflammation of a vein*
phlebothrombosis (venous thrombosis):
  Intraluminal thrombus with minimal or no

inflammatory component; these have a greater tendency to embolize

thromboembolism: *Phenomenon of thrombus dislodgment and migration*

thrombophlebitis: *An acute condition characterized by thrombus and inflammation in deep or superficial veins*

Assessment

Subjective data

Pain: ache, cramping, tenderness, heavy feeling over involved extremity

Objective data

Lower extremity (deep veins)
  Calf pain with dorsiflexion of foot (Homan's sign)
  Redness
  Taut, shiny skin
  Swelling and edema
  Ulcerations

Increased size compared with nonaffected extremity
Increased skin temperature
Peripheral pulses: present, absent
Upper extremity (superficial veins)
  Redness
  Warmth
  Tenderness
Elevated temperature

Diagnostic tests

Phlebography (venography)
Doppler ultrasound
Phlethysmography
125 I fibrinogen uptake test

Potential complications

Venous ulcers
Pulmonary embolism
Chronic venous insufficiency
CVA

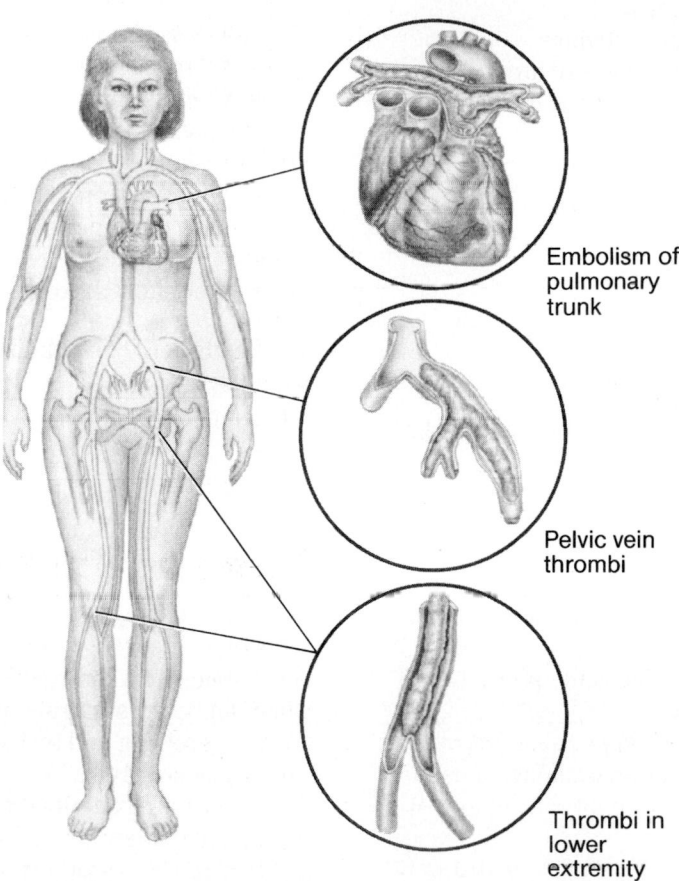

Embolism of pulmonary trunk

Pelvic vein thrombi

Thrombi in lower extremity

Figure 3-5   Venous thrombosis. (From Canobbio MM: *Mosby's clinical nursing series: cardiovascular disorders,* St Louis, 1990, Mosby.)

Collaborative management

Therapeutic management

Medications
   Anticoagulant therapy: heparin, warfarin
   Fibrinolytic agents: streptokinase
   Antiplatelet agents
   Dipridamole (Persantine)
   Analgesics
Surgical management
   Iliofemoral thrombectomy
   Procedures to prevent distal embolization
   Extravascular vena cava interruption
   Intracaval filter (Mobin-Udden umbrella, Kimray-
      Greenfield filter)

Nursing management

PATIENT PROBLEMS/NURSING DIAGNOSES

● **NDX:** Pain: peripheral related to inflammatory
process

Assess quality and location of pain
Maintain bed rest; limit self-care activities
Elevate affected limb above level of right atrium
Apply warm, moist compresses as ordered; avoid burn-
   ing edematous skin
Use bed cradle over affected extremity
Provide support or antiembolic stockings
Administer analgesics as ordered

EXPECTED OUTCOME
Patient verbalizes relief from pain and absence of
   swelling and redness

● **NDX:** Altered tissue perfusion: peripheral related
to interruption of venous flow

Assess circulation of affected extremity q4h; measure
   and record size of affected limb qd *to identify presence
   of deep vein thrombosis*
Assess pulses in all extremities q4h; use Doppler sensor if pulse seems absent
Maintain complete bed rest during acute phase (4 to 7
   days) *to prevent embolization*
Position patient comfortably; avoid *position that restricts
   venous blood flow by venous compression;* avoid use
   of pillows; never gatch knees without raising foot of
   bed
Elevate affected limb above the level of right atrium *to
   lessen venous stasis and improve venous flow*
Do not wash or massage affected extremity
Provide support or antiembolic stockings

Administer anticoagulation and fibrinolytic therapy as
   ordered
Assess laboratory values as indicated *to reduce risk of
   bleeding*
   Activated partial thromboplastin time (APTT): q4h to
      12h to maintain 1½ to 2½ times control for heparin
      therapy
   Prothrombin time (PT): qd to maintain level 1½ to 2½
      times control for warfarin therapy
Instruct patient *to avoid use of tobacco products to pre-
   vent vasoconstriction caused by tobacco*
Implement progressive exercise program as or-
   dered *to improve venous return and avoid venous
   pooling*
   Ambulate as ordered
   Alternate with bed rest
   Never let legs dangle
   Ambulate 10 min qh while awake or as ordered
   Apply support stockings before ambulating
   Avoid having patient stand for long periods
   Have patient alternate position by standing on toes,
      then on heels
   Exercise toes and change weight distribution q10min
      to 15 min
Elevate legs 10 min qh when sitting
   Do not constrict circulation in groin area
   Flex calf muscles and perform quadriceps contrac-
      tions 10 min qh
   Avoid having patient cross legs at the knees
Advise patient to build exercise tolerance by
   increasing walking distance each day; continue
   after discharge, increasing distance to 1 to 2
   miles
Refer to monitored exercise program

EXPECTED OUTCOME
Patient demonstrates adequate tissue perfusion as evidenced by palpable pulses and warm extremities

● **NDX:** Impaired gas exchange related to embolization of thrombus

Assess for signs of pulmonary embolism: chest pain,
   dyspnea, tachypnea, tachycardia, hemoptysis, pallor,
   anxiety
Auscultate chest for breath sounds q4h
Maintain bed rest during acute phase
Avoid exercising and massaging affected extremity
   during acute phase
Administer anticoagulant therapy as ordered
Encourage patient to turn, cough, and breathe deeply
   q2h to 4h
Obtain and monitor Po_2 and Pco_2
Apply elastic support stockings when patient is ambu-
   lating or sitting for prolonged periods

EXPECTED OUTCOME

Patient demonstrates effortless breathing and performs self-care activities without becoming short of breath

● **NDX:** Risk for impaired skin integrity related to venous stasis and fragility of small blood vessels

Assess skin for redness, breakdown, or ulcerations
Administer daily hygiene measures
Use small amount of mild soap
Rinse well
Dry gently but thoroughly; avoid vigorous rubbing
Do not allow skin to remain wet
Use bed cradle for affected extremity
Do not wash or massage affected extremity
Assist and teach patient as appropriate to make small changes in position
Perform active or passive range of motion (ROM) exercises with unaffected extremities

EXPECTED OUTCOMES

Demonstrates no signs of skin breaks or ulceration
Demonstrates management of home care

Patient/family teaching

Assess level of understanding
Discuss importance of not using any tobacco products
Discuss symptoms of recurrence to report to physician (see Objective data, p. 107)
Review medications: name, dosage, time of administration, purpose, and side effects
Explain need to avoid taking over-the-counter medications without checking with physician
Discuss anticoagulant precautions if appropriate (p. 191)
Discuss symptoms of complications to report to physician
Pulmonary emboli
MI
CVA
Explain importance of ongoing outpatient care

Home care considerations

Explain skin care
Avoid use of harsh soaps
Do not rub or massage affected extremity
Keep extremity warm and avoid exposure to temperature extremes
Discuss need to avoid use of constrictive clothing (e.g., garters, girdles, underwear with elastic groin bands, knee-high or ankle stockings with elastic tops)
Teach application of support or antiembolic stockings

Review activity program
Develop a planned exercise program that includes aerobic activities (e.g., swimming, progressive walking)
Never let legs dangle; elevate legs when sitting
Avoid standing for long periods

Vein Ligation and Stripping

Ligation of the saphenous vein and its branches and stripping (removal) from the groin to the ankle to treat varicosities

Assessment

Subjective data

Leg cramps when standing

Objective data

Color, warmth, and sensation of affected extremity
Edema or heaviness of affected extremity
Dilation of leg veins

Potential complications

Thrombophlebitis
Phlebitis
Leg ulcers
Hemorrhage

Collaborative management

Therapeutic management

Medications: analgesics

Nursing management

PATIENT PROBLEMS/NURSING DIAGNOSES

● **NDX:** Altered tissue perfusion: peripheral related to inadequate venous return and/or immobility

Assess color, warmth, and sensation of affected extremity qh for 6 hr to establish a baseline; report any change to physician
Maintain bed rest
Elevate legs as ordered
Do not gatch knees
Do not let legs dangle

Apply elastic bandages from toes to groin to promote venous blood flow and decrease venous stagnation; leave in place for 24 hr; remove elastic bandages or stockings as indicated

Reapply bandages q8h and prn

Avoid constriction

Keep bandages snug and wrinkle free

Assess bandages frequently for slippage, especially after ambulation

Assist patient with ambulation within 24 hr as ordered

Have patient increase activity as ordered; ambulate with assistance

Do not allow chair sitting (patient must be either walking or in bed)

Perform active and/or passive ROM exercises to unaffected extremities q4h and dorsiflexion of foot of affected extremity

EXPECTED OUTCOMES

Patient has improved tissue perfusion

Peripheral pulses are palpable

Extremities are warm with normal color

● **NDX:** Pain of lower extremities related to surgical incision

Assess quality and degree of pain

Determine source of pain

  Incision

  Constrictive dressings

  Bleeding

  Local site infection

Assess bandages for bleeding qh; report excessive bleeding to physician

Assess dressings for signs of wound infection; report to physician

  Low-grade temperature

  Swelling, redness, pain, purulent drainage

Reinforce and/or change dressings

Assess BP, T, P, and R q4h and as indicated

Administer analgesics as indicated

EXPECTED OUTCOME

  Patient verbalizes absence of pain

Patient/family teaching

Assess level of understanding

Discuss need to maintain normal weight for age and height and reduce if overweight

Explain need to check with physician before taking oral contraceptives

Discuss signs and symptoms of wound infection and bleeding to report to physician

Redness, drainage

Edema

Pain

Explain importance of ongoing outpatient care

Discuss possibility of varicosities recurring

Home care considerations

Explain importance of avoiding constriction of venous blood return in extremities

  Do not wear tight garters or girdles

  Avoid crossing legs

  Walk rather than sit or stand

  Wear full-length support hose, elastic stockings, or bandages as ordered

  Elevate legs while sitting

  Sleep with legs elevated

Explain importance of skin care

  Keep legs and feet warm and dry

  Avoid chilling

  Avoid extreme temperatures

  Do not massage affected area

Chronic Arterial Insufficiency

Inadequate blood flow in arteries caused by occlusive atherosclerotic plaques or emboli, damaged or diseased vessels, aneurysms, hypercoagulability states, or heavy use of tobacco

Progressive narrowing of the arterial tree gives rise to collateral vessels to ensure adequate blood supply and prevent peripheral ischemia. Progressive occlusion leads to hypoperfusion and ischemia. The arms and legs are the most vulnerable to ischemia.

Assessment

Subjective data

Pain

  Foot, calf, thigh, or buttocks

  Sharp and viselike

  Cramping

  Tired feeling in legs

  Usually occurs during exercise; decreases when exercise stops (intermittent claudication)

  May occur at rest, especially at night, accompanied by very hot or cold feeling

  Increases with elevation of legs

Objective data

Pulses: diminished-to-absent pedal and popliteal pulses
Extremities
  Numbness
  Hair loss
  Skin: glossy, thin, smooth, cold, discolored,
    atrophied
  Ulcerations, poor wound healing
  Nails thickened: accumulation of cornified material
  Pigmentation, rashes
  Pallor
    Increased with elevation of extremity
    Decreased with extremity below heart level
  Rubor
  Edema
  Delayed venous filling in dependent position

Diagnostic tests

Doppler ultrasonography
Angiography
Arteriography

Potential complications

Peripheral ischemia, necrosis
Cellulitis
Gangrene

Collaborative management

Therapeutic management

Medications
  Thrombolytic enzymes: urokinase, streptokinase, tis-
    sue plasminogen activator
  Antiplatelets: aspirin, dipyridamole
  Pentoxifylline (Trental)
Regular walking program
Diet therapy
  Weight reduction
  Low-saturated-fat, low-cholesterol diet
Percutaneous or peripheral transluminal angioplasty
  (PTA)
Laser thermal angioplasty (LTA)
Surgical management
  Arterial reconstruction and/or revascularization
  Endarterectomy
  Bypass graft surgery
  Femoropopliteal reconstruction: femoropopliteal by-
    pass (Figure 3-6), profundoplasty
  Lumbar sympathectomy
  Amputation of limb

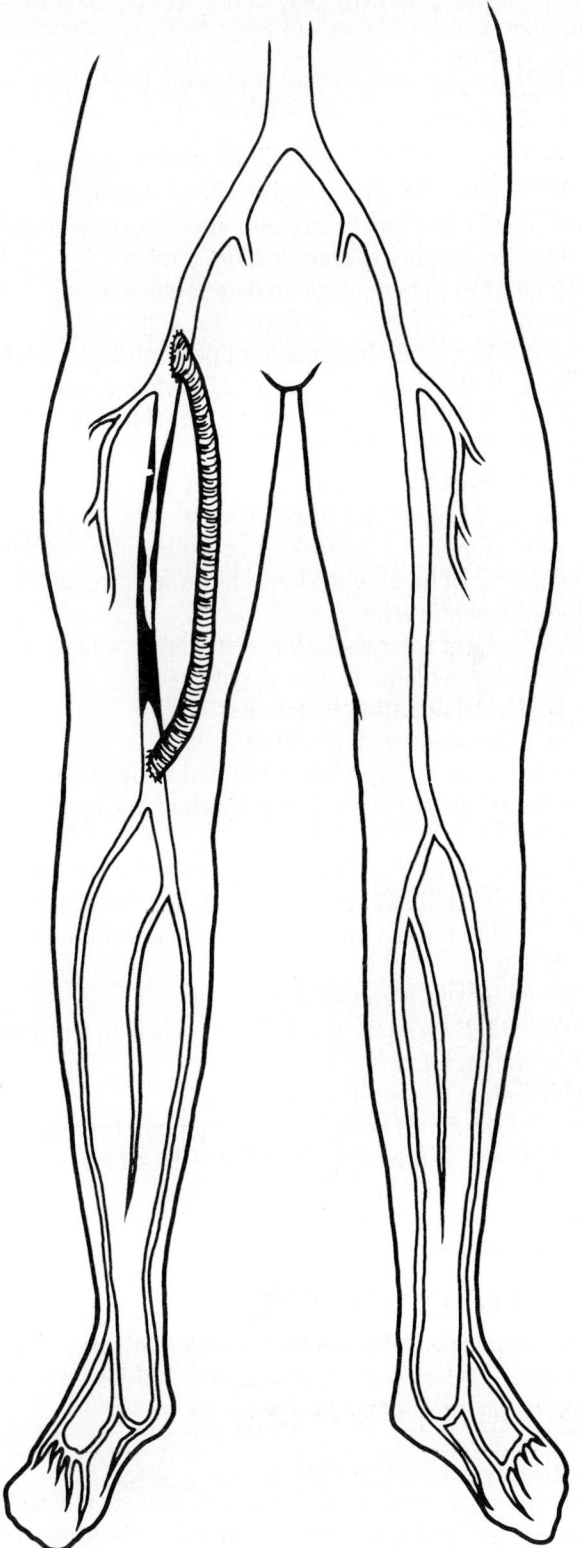

Figure 3-6 Femoropopliteal bypass graft to revascularize right lower limb. (From Guzzetta C, Dossey B: *Cardiovascular nursing: bodymind tapestry,* St Louis, 1985, Mosby.)

Nursing management

PATIENT PROBLEMS/NURSING DIAGNOSES

● **NDX:** Alterated tissue perfusion related to interruption of arterial flow

Assess arterial pulses; determine pulse volume qid *to determine adequacy of peripheral circulation*

Auscultate for bruits before and after exercise; *presence confirms existence of atherosclerotic lesion*

Elevate head of bed; use 4- to 6-inch block as ordered

Maintain extremity in dependent position *to maintain optimal and/or improve arterial blood flow;* avoid use of knee gatch or other positions *that interfere with gravitational flow*

Protect affected extremity

Place bed cradle over affected area

Use heel guards (sheepskin) or white cotton socks

Avoid use of heating devices on lower extremities

Keep patient warm

Have patient wear socks when in bed or walking

Place cotton blankets next to patient

Use flannel or cotton bedclothes

Use extra blankets if required

Assist patient with getting out of bed as ordered; avoid one position, sitting or standing, for long periods

Initiate scheduled walking exercise program *to promote development of collateral flow;* with increased pain, have patient stand until pain eases, then continue walking

Have patient sit with feet dependent

Perform active or passive ROM exercises to all extremities q4h to 6h

Turn patient q2h while on bed rest

Change patient's position slightly q20min to 30min

Avoid raising lower extremity above heart level

Instruct patient to avoid use of nicotine

Administer medications as ordered

EXPECTED OUTCOMES

Patient reports relief of pain (no claudication)

Peripheral pulses are present, equal, and bilateral

Skin is warm with normal color

● **NDX:** Pain related to peripheral ischemia

Assess quality and degree of pain *to determine degree of claudication and exercise tolerance*

Assist patient with identifying activities that precipitate or aggravate pain and understanding nature of pain

Instruct patient to stand or dangle at side of bed *to obtain relief from ischemic pain*

Encourage regular exercise program but instruct patient to stop and rest before claudication occurs

Administer analgesics as indicated

Initiate alternate pain relief measures

Relaxation techniques: meditation, deep breathing

Guided imagery

Biofeedback

Involve patient in decision making regarding measures to reduce pain

Assess effectiveness of pain relief measure(s)

EXPECTED OUTCOMES

Patient reports relief or control of pain

Patient verbalizes and demonstrates a variety of strategies to reduce pain level

● **NDX:** Risk for impaired skin integrity, actual or potential, related to impaired circulation

Assess skin daily for signs of scaling, breaks, or cuts

Administer daily hygiene measures

Use small amount of mild soap

Rinse well

Dry gently but thoroughly; avoid vigorous rubbing

Apply lanolin-based lotions; do not allow skin to remain wet

Assess skin color and temperature in both legs qid

Treat ulcerated areas as they occur

Administer soak, topical, and/or systemic antibiotics and dressings as ordered

Avoid use of adhesive tapes directly on skin

Avoid use of tight, constrictive socks or hose; use cotton socks; avoid use of knee gatch; reposition extremities frequently

EXPECTED OUTCOMES

Patient shows no signs of skin breakdown

Patient demonstrates progressive healing of ulcerations

Patient/family teaching

Provide information regarding disease process and associated risk factors (see the box on p. 117)

Explain need to avoid using tobacco products

Discuss symptoms of recurrence to report to physician (see Subjective data, Objective data, pp. 110 and 111)

Explain importance of maintaining diet (low calorie, low cholesterol, low fat) as ordered

Discuss medications: name, dosage, time of administration, purpose, and side effects

Explain need to avoid taking over-the-counter medications without checking with physician

Explain importance of ongoing outpatient care

Home care considerations

Explain importance of care of legs and feet
  Inspect legs, feet, and toes daily for blisters, skin
    breaks, and discolored areas
  Wash daily with mild soap, dry well, and apply lanolin-
    based lotion; do not leave skin wet
  Clean small cuts or abrasions with soap and water;
    protect from further injury
  Report to physician cuts or skin breaks that do not be-
    gin healing in 2 to 3 days
  Trim toenails straight across; refer older or frail pa-
    tients to podiatry department
  Do not cut, file, or use over-the-counter medications
    on corns or calluses
  Avoid exposing legs to temperature extremes; wear
    warm coverings in cold weather and avoid exposure
    to sunshine
  Do not apply indirect heat to legs (e.g., hot water bot-
    tles or electric pads); wear cotton or woolen socks to
    warm feet
  Avoid injury to legs and feet
  Always wear well-fitting shoes or slippers; never go
    barefoot
  Wear well-fitting, correct size stockings
  Avoid tight-fitting or constrictive clothing (e.g.,
    garters, girdles, underwear with elastic legs,
    and knee-high or ankle stockings with elastic
    tops)
  Avoid crossing legs
  Avoid scratching legs or feet
  Turn on lights when getting up at night to avoid
    bumps
  Sleep with bed level or with head elevated
  Avoid tight-fitting covers over legs and feet
Instruct and help patient plan a daily progressive walk-
  ing program
  Walk to tolerance; increase time each week until able
    to walk without pain for 30 to 60 min (may initially
    experience decreased ability)
  Walk until pain increases, stop and stand still to de-
    crease pain, then continue to walk
  Do not sit or raise legs above heart level to decrease
    pain
  Remember that same distance walked in one direction
    must also be walked on return

Carotid Endarterectomy

*Surgical removal of atherosclerotic plaques or thrombus
  from the inner lining of the carotid artery to increase
  blood flow to the brain. Indicated for patient suffering
  from reversible ischemic neurologic deficit, transient
  ischemic attacks (TIAs), syncope, and dizziness.*

Assessment

Objective data

Respiratory distress
  Bradypnea
  Tachypnea
  Cyanosis
  Tracheal deviation to opposite side
  Laryngeal edema
  Stridor
Neurologic deficit
  Cerebral ischemia, TIAs
    Decreasing BP, increasing P and R
    Dizziness
    Altered level of consciousness
    Confusion
    Disorientation
    Memory loss
  Unequal reaction of pupils to light
  Unequal handgrips
  Inability to protrude tongue
  Muscle weakness of mouth on operative side
  Dysphagia
  Altered speech
    Slurred
    Indistinct
Dysrhythmias

Potential complications

Seizure activity
Hemorrhage
Shock
Embolism
Infection
CVA
Neurologic deficit
Hematoma

Collaborative management

Therapeutic management

Parenteral fluids
Medications
  Antihypertensive
  Vasopressor

Nursing management

  PATIENT PROBLEMS/NURSING DIAGNOSES

● **NDX:** Altered cerebral tissue perfusion related to
    interruption of arterial flow (see Care of pa-
    tient in recovery room, p. 54)

Assess for changes in mental status

Assess and compare temporal pulses q15min for four times, then q2h to 4h

Mark pulse site on skin; note rate and volume

Assess neurologic signs q15 to 30min, increasing to qh

Assess BP, R, and apical pulse q1h to 2h for 24 hours; report increase or decrease to physician immediately

Maintain bed rest in quiet environment; position with head elevated 30 to 45 degrees

Check temperature q2h to 4h for 24 hours

Administer medications as ordered

Inspect incision qh *for bleeding and edema;* report excessive bleeding or edema to physician

Control pain as ordered; apply ice collar to neck as ordered

Provide emotional support

Gentle reassurance

Means of communicating; phrase questions for *yes* or *no* answers

Continue with immediate postoperative care and decrease frequency of nursing functions as patient's condition improves

Ambulate as ordered; check and report any altered gait

Change dressing prn

Continue assessing neurologic signs q8h

EXPECTED OUTCOMES

Patient demonstrates adequate cerebral blood flow as evidenced by the following:

Mental alertness and orientation

Absence of dizziness

Equal and reactive pupils

Normal motor-sensory function

● **NDX:** Risk for injury: respiratory distress

Maintain patent airway

Perform oropharyngeal suctioning only if ordered

Assist and teach patient to turn and breathe deeply q1h to 2h

Avoid having patient cough

Auscultate chest for breath sounds q1h to 2h

Report complaints of severe hoarseness, sore throat, or dysphagia to physician

Monitor oxygen saturation via arterial blood gases or peripheral O_2 saturation as indicated

EXPECTED OUTCOME

Patient demonstrates effortless breathing

Patient/family teaching

Assess level of understanding regarding disease process

Discuss diet restrictions as ordered; encourage low-fat, low-cholesterol diet

Explain importance of ongoing outpatient care

Explain importance of reporting sudden changes in vision, gait, speech or the experience of muscle weakness to physician immediately

Home care considerations

Discuss risks associated with activities

Exercise to tolerance

Avoid bending from waist

Plan rest periods

Avoid lifting or straining

Demonstrate care of incision

Discuss signs of wound infection

Redness

Pain

Drainage

Edema

Aortofemoral Bypass Graft

Surgical resection of an aortic aneurysm and insertion of a graft conduit to deliver blood to the femoral vessels, bypassing diseased segments

Assessment

Subjective data

Pain related to surgical incision versus pain related to development of graft thrombosis

Objective data (Postoperative findings)

Marked increase or decrease in BP, P, and R

Decreased arterial pressure or CVP

Signs of arterial graft occlusion of lower extremities (lower limb ischemia)

Mottled or pale skin

Skin cool to touch

Absence of pulses

Site of incision

Redness

Pain

Swelling

Diagnostic tests

Doppler: systolic ankle pressure
White blood cell count (WBC), chemistries, electrolytes

Potential complications

Embolism to extremities, cerebrum, or heart
Cardiac complications
  Congestive heart failure (CHF)
  Dysrhythmias
  Acute myocardial infarction (AMI)
Hemorrhage
Shock
Renal failure
  Decreased urine output
  Specific gravity <1.030
Bowel ischemia
  Diarrhea with or without blood
  Abdominal tenderness
  Leukocytosis
  Metabolic acidosis
Prosthetic graft infection
  Purulent wound drainage
  Low-grade fever without chills
  Sepsis
  Graft occlusion
  Local hemorrhage
  Septic embolization: cellulitis
  Sinus tract infection
Spinal cord ischemia
  Paraplegia
  Paraparesis

Collaborative management

Therapeutic management

Hemodynamic monitoring: pulmonary artery pressure
  (PAP), arterial pressure
Cardiac monitor
Medications
  Anticoagulation therapy
  Antibiotic therapy
  Vasodilators
Ankle-to-brachial systolic pressure index (0.95 mm Hg
  or more)

Nursing management

PATIENT PROBLEMS/NURSING DIAGNOSES

● **NDX:** Risk for altered tissue perfusion related to interruption of arterial flow secondary to development of graft thromboses

Assess affected extremity *to detect development of graft thromboses*
Compare pedal pulses q15min for four times, then q4h; mark pulse site on skin
Assess lower extremities for color, warmth, and sensation q15min for 4 hr
Assess and compare ankle-to-brachial systolic pressure index (ratio) as ordered; report if <1mm Hg
Maintain bed rest; elevate head 30 to 45 degrees (Figure 3-7)
  Do not gatch knees; avoid sharp hip flexion *to prevent graft pressure*
Provide antiembolic stockings or elastic bandages as ordered; remove, reapply, or rewrap bandages q8h
Do not massage or apply heat to lower extremities
Ambulate as ordered; no chair sitting
Administer daily skin care
  Observe for signs of breaks or drainage
  Avoid use of adhesive tape on sensitive skin of distal lower extremity
  Protect affected extremity
  Place bed cradle over affected area
  Use sheepskins

EXPECTED OUTCOMES

Patient demonstrates improved tissue perfusion
  Graft is patent
  Peripheral pulses are palpable
  Extremities are warm with normal color
  Ankle-to-brachial pressure index is normal or improved

● **NDX:** Risk for infection related to arterial prosthetic graft procedure

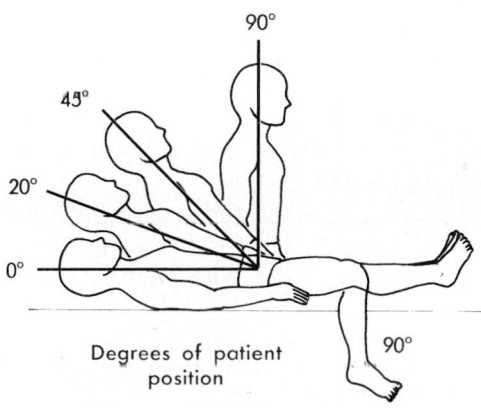

Figure 3-7 Degrees of patient position.

Observe for signs of infection of incision (see Objective data, p. 114)
Check T q4h
Inspect dressing q1h to 2h
  Observe for healing process
  Reinforce dressing prn
  Report excessive drainage to physician
Administer prophylactic antibiotic as ordered
Avoid prolonged use of urinary catheters, nasogastric tubes, or pressure catheter, which may cause transient bacteremia
Use strict aseptic technique in dressing change, venipuncture, or suctioning procedures
If graft infection occurs
  Administer antibiotic therapy as ordered
  Perform irrigation of graft and wound as ordered
  Prepare for surgical intervention as ordered
    Graft removal
    Revascularization
    Amputation

EXPECTED OUTCOMES
Patient demonstrates absence of graft infection
Temperature is normal
Graft is patent
Skin integrity is maintained

● **NDX:** Risk for complications: cardiac, bowel ischemia, renal failure, and hemorrhage*

Cardiac complications
  Monitor ECG, arterial pressures, PAP, CVP qh
  Assess BP, R, and apical pulse q4h for 48 hr
  Auscultate heart and lung sounds q4h to 6h or as indicated
  Record description of chest pain; report increase or significant change to physician
  Obtain ECG rhythm strip during episodes of chest pain
  Obtain isoenzymes (CPK-MB) as indicated
  Monitor potassium levels
Bowel ischemia
  Maintain NPO, usually for first 12 hours or until bowel sounds are present
  Progress diet as tolerated and ordered after nasogastric tube removal
  Connect nasogastric tube to intermittent suction as ordered
  Auscultate abdomen q2h to 4h
  Measure abdominal girth for distension q8h

---

*Not a NANDA-approved nursing diagnosis.

Assess for and report increased distension to physician
Renal failure
  Administer parenteral fluids with electrolytes as ordered
  Measure intake and output
  Use indwelling urethral catheter as ordered
    Measure urine output qh
    Report urine output <30 to 50 ml/hr
Hemorrhage
  Assess for signs of bleeding q4h to 8h
    Hematoma in groin area
    Bleeding of skin incision
    Retroperitoneal bleeding: signs of hypovolemia— low CVP and pulmonary capillary wedge pressure (PCWP), decreased urine output, severe back pain
  Evaluate laboratory studies q4h to 8h

EXPECTED OUTCOME
Patient demonstrates no signs or symptoms of complication

Patient/family teaching

Assess for level of understanding
Explain importance of not using tobacco products
Discuss symptoms of recurrence to report to physician
Explain importance of ongoing outpatient care

Home care considerations

Explain importance of exercise and activity
  Avoid sitting or standing without moving for long periods
  Do not cross legs
  Exercise up to level of tolerance, with caution not to push beyond tolerance
  Discuss importance of maintaining planned rest periods
  Exercise feet and legs as ordered
Demonstrate correct application of antiembolic stockings or elastic bandages
Discuss care of legs and feet
  Do not wear constrictive clothing (e.g., girdles, garters)
  Avoid temperature extremes
  Keep feet warm
Demonstrate care of incision
Discuss signs of wound infection
  Redness
  Pain
  Swelling
  Drainage

Cardiovascular Risk Factor Profile

Family history of heart disease
Sex: Males (35-55)
    Females (>50 or
      after menopause)
Hypertension
Tobacco use
Overweight/obesity
Elevated serum level of lipids and cholesterol
Diabetes mellitus
Physical inactivity; sedentary lifestyle
Stress
For women <40 years: use of estrogen (i.e., birth
   control pills) and smoking

Hypertension

Arterial hypertension is a persistent elevation of systolic blood pressure greater than 140 mm Hg and diastolic pressure equal to or greater than 90 mm Hg. It is a major risk factor for coronary artery, renal cerebral, and peripheral vascular disease. It is classified according to cause, severity, and type.

primary (essential, idiopathic): Most common form constituting 90% to 95% of all cases. No single known cause but familial tendencies, race, and obesity are known risk factors. The disease begins insiduously and may be slow progressing. If uncontrolled or untreated, it may lead to serious complications such as malignant hypertension. Early detection and treatment can lead to good control and improved prognosis.

secondary: Results from other diseases such as renal failure, dysfunction of adrenal medulla or cortex, coarctation of aorta, or other identifiable causes (e.g., estrogen-containing oral contraceptive).

malignant: Sudden severe elevation of BP (systolic greater than 200 mm Hg, diastolic greater than 140 mm Hg) with mean arterial pressure greater than 150 mm Hg. This is a medical emergency necessitating aggressive therapy to prevent severe complications.

Assessment

Subjective data

Symptoms range from no symptoms to the following:
  Morning occipital headaches
  Neck stiffness, soreness
  Dizziness, vertigo
  Nausea, vomiting
  Palpitations (heart pounding)

Objective data

Arterial blood pressure
  Systolic BP >140 mm Hg
           >160 mm Hg over age 65
  Diastolic BP >90 mm Hg
           >96 mm Hg over age 65
  Pulse
    Pulsus alternans
    Tachycardia
    Bounding
    Femoral delays

● Malignant Hypertension

Severe suboccipital headache radiating frontally
Skin: pallor, diaphoresis
Hypertensive encephalopathy
  Confusion
  Irritability
  Stupor
  Somnolence
  Coma
  Eye signs and symptoms
    Diplopia
    Visual loss
    Optic fundi hemorrhage, cotton exudates, arterial-venous nicking papilledema
Cardiac symptoms
  Angina
  Dyspnea on exertion (DOE)
  Paroxysmal nocturnal dyspnea (PND)
  Orthopnea
  S_4 gallop
Renal symptoms
  Hematuria
  Nocturia
  Azotemia

Diagnostic tests

Blood
  Electrolytes, chemistries
  Aldosterone
  Cholesterol, triglycerides
Urine
  Steroids, catecholamines; renin
  Urinalysis: BUN, uric acid levels

24-hour VMA levels
  Aldosterone
Electrocardiogram (ECG)
  Left ventricular hypertrophy (LVH)
  Ischemia
Echocardiogram
  LVH with/without dilation
Chest x-ray examination
  Increased cardiothoracic ratio
CT scan
  Cerebral ischemia, infarct
  Encephalopathy

Potential complications

Cardiac dysrhythmia
MI
Renal failure
Heart failure
CVA

Collaborative management

Therapeutic management

For primary hypertension, a stepped approach to medical treatment is recommended (see the box below)

For malignant hypertension, admission to intensive care

unit (ICU) with continuous arterial pressure and cardiac monitoring.
Medications
  Diuretics: thiazide, Loop, potassium sparing
  Beta blockers (e.g., propanolol, atenolol)
  Vasodilators (e.g., minoxidil, hydralzine)
  Angiotensin-converting-enzyme (ACE) inhibitors
    (e.g., captopril)
  Calcium channel blockers (e.g., nifedipine,
    diltiazem)
  Adrenergic inhibitors (e.g., clonidine HCL)
Diet: sodium restricted, fat reduced
Intake and output

Nursing management

PATIENT PROBLEMS/NURSING DIAGNOSES
(For Patients With **Malignant Hypertension**)

● **NDX:** Pain (headache) related to increased cerebral vascular pressure

Maintain bed rest; provide a quiet, low-lighted environment
Minimize environmental distractions and stimulation
Limit activities
Avoid use of nicotine products
Administer analgesia and sedation as ordered
Administer comfort measures as indicated
Apply ice packs
Give reassurance and frequent, simple explanations

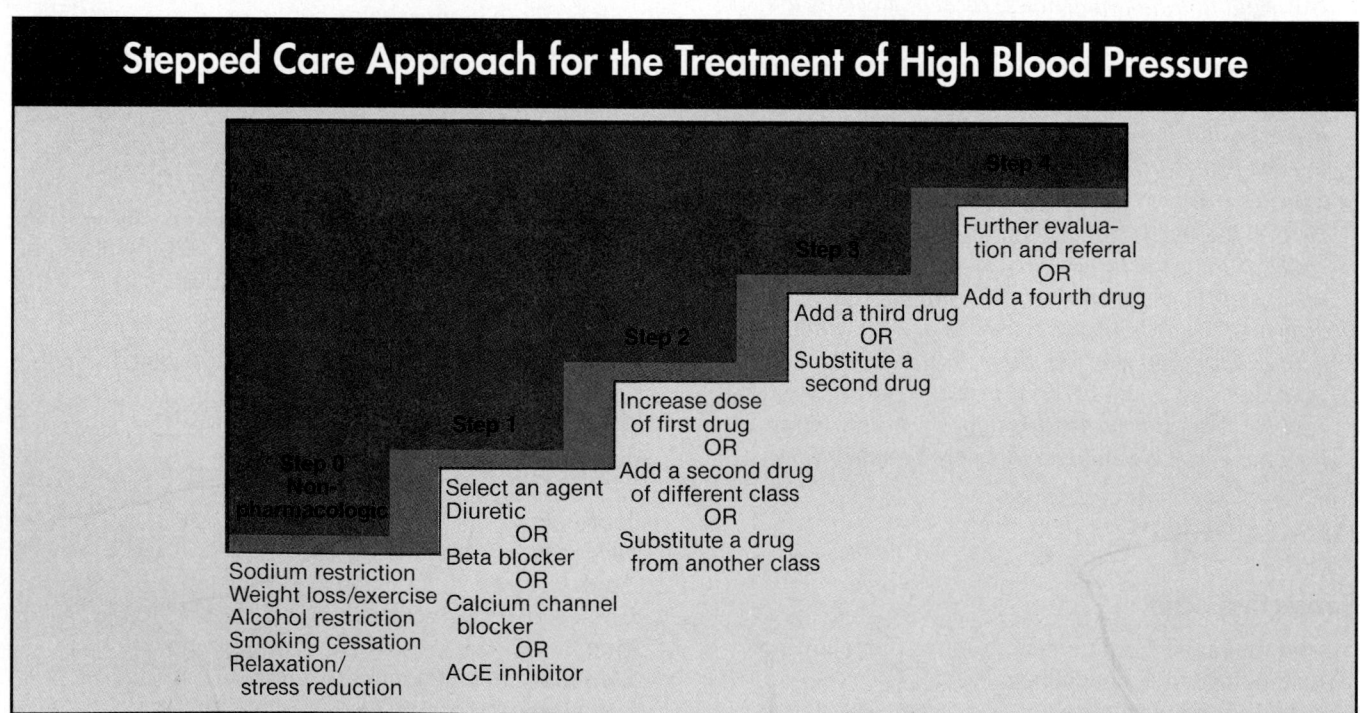

Stepped Care Approach for the Treatment of High Blood Pressure

Step 4
  Further evaluation and referral
  OR
  Add a fourth drug

Step 3
  Add a third drug
  OR
  Substitute a second drug

Step 2
  Increase dose of first drug
  OR
  Add a second drug of different class
  OR
  Substitute a drug from another class

Step 1
  Select an agent
  Diuretic
  OR
  Beta blocker
  OR
  Calcium channel blocker
  OR
  ACE inhibitor

Step 0
  Non-pharmacologic
  Sodium restriction
  Weight loss/exercise
  Alcohol restriction
  Smoking cessation
  Relaxation/stress reduction

From Canobbio MM: *Mosby's clinical nursing series: cardiovascular disorders,* St Louis, 1990, Mosby.

Place patient in comfortable position; assist with turning gently, using pull sheet as indicated

Medications: vasodilators (nitroprusside, nitroglycerin)

Teach relaxation techniques

Suggest guided imagery

Explain need to avoid Valsalva maneuver

Explain need to avoid constipation

EXPECTED OUTCOMES

Patient verbalizes absence of headache

Patient appears comfortable

● **NDX:** Risk for altered tissue perfusion: cerebral, renal, cardiac related to impaired circulation

Acute malignant hypertension

Maintain bed rest; elevate head of bed; shock blocks may be ordered

Assess BP on admission in both arms: lying, sitting, and with arterial pressure monitor if available

Assess BP, R, apical pulse, and neurologic signs q5min to 10min

Use same arm for BP reading each time

Use Doppler sensor if indicated

Monitor arterial pressure as ordered

Maintain parenteral fluids with medications as ordered

Administer medications as ordered

Antihypertensives: IV, IM

Observe for side effects or toxic effects of each medication

Monitor IV medications continuously

Titrate according to prescribed BP parameters as ordered

Observe for sudden hypotension

Place on cardiac monitor; record ECG rhythm strip q4h to 6h and prn

Measure intake and output

Measure output qh; note amount and color of urine

Report urine output <30 ml/hr

Monitor electrolytes, BUN, creatinine levels as ordered

Check specific gravity and perform urinalysis as ordered

Keep NPO if nausea and/or vomiting is present

Restrict fluids as ordered

Do not allow the use of tobacco products

Ongoing care:

Continue with immediate care and decrease frequency of nursing functions as patient's condition improves

Maintain progressive ambulation, observing at all times for orthostatic hypotension

Elevate head of bed slowly in beginning, then take BP reading

Progress to dangling for 10 min as ordered if BP is stable

Take BP reading while patient is sitting up

Take reading while patient is standing at bedside; then have patient take small steps when ordered

Ambulate to tolerance; avoid fatigue

EXPECTED OUTCOMES

Patient demonstrates improved tissue perfusion as evidenced by BP within acceptable limits

No complaints of headache, dizziness

Laboratory values within normal limits

Urine output ≥30 ml/min

Patient's vital signs stable

Patient/family teaching

Explain nature of disease, associated risk factors, and means of reducing risk factors; describe and explain purpose of stepped care treatment for hypertension

Discuss medications: name, dosage, time of administration, purpose, and side effects or toxic effects

Explain need to avoid taking over-the-counter medications without checking with physician

Discuss symptoms of recurrence or progression of disease to report to physician

Headache

Dizziness

Faintness

Nausea, vomiting

Bloody nose

Explain importance of not using tobacco products

Explain need to avoid constipation and straining

Home care considerations

Diet

Sodium restriction, weight reducing (low fat, low calorie)

Discuss importance of decreasing weight or maintaining stable weight

Explain importance of maintaining proper fluid intake; amount allowed, limitations such as caffeinated beverages and alcohol

Activity

Discuss need to avoid fatigue and heavy lifting

Discuss importance of planned daily exercise program and rest periods

Demonstrate taking and recording of BP and P using home monitoring equipment

Angina Pectoris

Chest pain or discomfort caused by myocardial ischemia, which occurs when myocardial oxygen demand exceeds the supply. Myocardial ischemia commonly occurs as a result of coronary atherosclerotic heart disease, although angina pectoris may occur in patients with normal coronary arteries. Classification of angina is found in Table 3-1.

Assessment

Subjective data

Chest pain or pressure: mild to severe aching; sharp, tingling, or burning sensation or pressure described as heavy, squeezing; heartburn or tight chest lasting 5 to 30 min

Table 3-1 Different Patterns of Angina

Observations	Stable Angina Pectoris	Variant (Prinzmetal's) Angina	Unstable Angina Pectoris
CHEST PAIN			
Quality	Aching, sharp, tingling, or burning sensation or pressure	Similar to stable angina pectoris	Similar to stable angina pectoris but may be more severe
Location and radiation	Substernal with radiation to left shoulder, down inner aspect of left arm or both arms; neck, jaw, and scapula may be additional sites of radiation	Similar to stable angina pectoris	Similar to stable angina pectoris
Precipitating factors	Onset classically associated with exercise or activities that increase myocardial oxygen demand (e.g., physical exercise, heavy lifting, emotional stress, cold temperatures)	Onset at rest; pain is cyclic, often occurring during sleep (most common in early morning hours)	Pain may be brought on with less than usual exertion; may occur at rest
Duration and alleviating factors	3-15 min; relieved by rest, stopping pain-inducing activities, taking sublingual nitroglycerin (NTG) tablet	Characteristically, pain intensifies quickly, tends to last longer than angina, and subsides with exercise	Prolonged and not usually as quickly relieved by rest or taking NTG
Associated signs and symptoms	During anginal attack: dyspnea; anxiety; diaphoresis; cool, clammy skin	Similar to stable angina pectoris	Similar to stable angina pectoris but symptoms may be more prominent and may persist; may be associated with nausea
PHYSICAL EXAMINATION			
	Normal during asymptomatic periods; during anginal attacks, increased HR, pulsus alternans, and transient abnormal findings including precordial bulge and atrial and ventricular gallops (S_3, S_4)	Similar to stable angina pectoris	Similar to stable angina pectoris; may also demonstrate irregular pulse, hypotension, or signs of LV dysfunction

From Canobbio MM: *Mosby's clinical nursing series: cardiovascular disorders*, St Louis, 1990, Mosby.

Complains of lightheadedness, palpitations, shortness of breath (SOB)

OBJECTIVE DATA

Precipitating factors
  Physical or emotional stress
  Exposure to temperature extremes
  Eating a heavy meal
Alleviating factors
  Termination of precipitating factors
  Taking nitroglycerin (NTG) tablets
Diaphoresis
Anxiety
Indigestion
Skin: pallor, diaphoresis
Respiration: shortness of breath
Cardiac: tachycardia, pulsus alternans, atrial and/or
  ventricular gallops (S_3, S_4)

Diagnostic tests (Table 3-2)

Cardiac enzymes: CPK-MB, LDH
Lipid profile: LDL, HDL, LDL:HDL ratio, triglyc-
  erides
ECG changes recorded during episodes of pain
Exercise stress test (EST): ECG changes recorded dur-
  ing chest pain
  Protocols: Bruce, Naughton
Echocardiography
Thallium 201 scintigraphy (viable myocardial cells ex-
  tract thallium from blood)
Radionuclide blood pool imaging with technetium
  99 m
Coronary angiography

Potential complications

Myocardial infarction
Heart failure

Collaborative management

Therapeutic management

Medications
  Short- and long-acting nitrates
  Beta-adrenergic blocking agents
  Calcium antagonists
  Analgesics, sedatives
Oxygen therapy
Diet: low saturated fat, low cholesterol, low sodium
Percutaneous transluminal coronary angiogram
  (PTCA)
Direct coronary atherectomy
Surgical management
  Coronary artery bypass graft

Nursing management

PATIENT PROBLEMS/NURSING DIAGNOSES

● **NDX:** Pain, chest related to imbalance of myocardial oxygen supply and demand

Maintain rest during episodes of pain *to reduce
  myocardial oxygen demand*
Assess pain: location, duration, radiation, and onset of
  new symptoms
Administer oxygen as indicated *to increase oxygen supply to myocardium*
Assess and record description of pain *to establish baseline description and/or to detect extension of
  ischemia*
Obtain 12-lead ECG during anginal pain episodes *to
  document ischemic episodes; monitor RV leads*
Monitor for signs of associated symptoms
Monitor BP and apical pulse during episodes of pain
Administer medications as indicated; assess and record
  response
Maintain diet as ordered; if chest pain occurs during
  eating, advise small feedings rather than two or three
  large meals

EXPECTED OUTCOMES

Patient verbalizes relief of pain
Patient appears relaxed and verbalizes a sense of calm

Patient/family teaching

Assess level of understanding *to determine any misconceptions or areas of deficit*
Explain atherosclerotic process and its different clinical
  manifestations
Discuss contributing risk factors and importance of
  modification (see the box on p. 117)
Discuss management and nature of chest pain; assist in
  identifying precipitating factors
Discuss importance of avoiding use of all tobacco products
Explain importance of controlling any coexisting diseases that may aggravate atherosclerotic process: hypertension, diabetes, hyperlipidemia
Explain importance of weight control, avoiding obesity
Explain role that stress plays in aggravating heart disease; need to identify stress-producing factors; methods of stress management using relaxation techniques
Discuss medications: name, dosage, time of administration, purpose, and side effects

Home care considerations

Discuss activity allowances and limitations
  Avoid isometric-type activity: heavy lifting and
  pushing

Table 3-2 Diagnostic Tests

	Findings			
Diagnostic Test	**Variant (Prinzmetal's) Stable Angina Pectoris**	**Angina**	**Unstable Angina Pectoris**	**Myocardial Infarction**
Electrocardiogram (ECG)	Changes usually seen during anginal episodes; 50%-70% of patients have normal ECG during pain-free episodes; ischemia determined by horizontal ST segment or downsloping with depression of >1 mm; T wave inversion represents impaired repolarization caused by ischemia	Ischemia appears as ST elevation during anginal attack but regresses as pain subsides; ECG changes may be seen before patient complains of chest pain or may be recorded in absence of pain; A-V conduction defects may occur, particularly when right coronary artery is involved, and include Mobitz type II and complete A-V block; ventricular irritability such as premature ventricular contractions, ventricular tachycardia, or fibrillation can occur, particularly during ischemic attack	Ischemia determined by horizontal ST segment or downsloping with depression of >1 mm; T wave inversion represents impaired repolarization caused by ischemia; ventricular irritability such as premature ventricular contractions, ventricular tachycardia, or fibrillation	Changes are evolutionary and indicate progression of infarction; in acute stage, ST elevations with subsequent T wave inversion and Q wave formation; Q waves indicate necrosis and are considered pathologic if they are 0.04 sec or greater in duration, 0.4 mm or greater in depth, or present in leads that do not normally have Q waves; ST elevations reflect myocardial injury that interferes with polarization of cells, are seen in leads facing injured area, and return to normal (isoelectric) within days; ST elevations beyond 4-6 wk should raise suspicion of ventricular aneurysm; infarction location determined by identifying leads that demonstrate characteristic ECG changes; such leads are those with positive terminals that face injured site of heart; reciprocal changes, seen in leads that face *opposite* surface of damaged heart, are absence of Q wave, increase in R wave amplitude, depressed ST segment, upright tall T wave *RV infarction*: ST elevation in right precordial leads (V$_1$, V$_3$R-V$_6$R). V$_4$R-V$_6$R may be more sensitive indicators
Laboratory tests Enzymes	No elevation; checked to rule out MI	No elevation; checked to rule out MI	No elevation; checked to rule out MI	

	Onset	Peak	Return to normal
AST	6-12 hr	36 hr	3-4 days
CPK-MB	4-12 hr	24 hr	3-4 days
LDH (iso-enzyme)	24-48 hr	3-6 days	8-14 days
LDH$_1$ to LDH$_2$ ratio >1.0			

Test				
Complete blood count (CBC)	No elevation; checked to rule out anemia-induced angina	No elevation; checked to rule out anemia-induced angina	No elevation; checked to rule out anemia-induced angina	Elevated WBC and ESR reflect tissue necrosis
Glucose	No elevation	No elevation	No elevation	Transiently elevated owing to adrenergic response
Lipid levels (triglycerides, cholesterol, high- and low-density lipids)	Checked to determine any lipoprotein abnormalities	Checked to rule out presence of atherosclerotic process	Checked to determine any lipoprotein abnormalities	Checked to determine any lipoprotein abnormalities; total cholesterol and HDL may drop 48 hr after admission
Chest x-ray examination	Normal	Normal	Normal; may show signs of cardiomegaly or signs of left ventricular failure	Same as unstable angina
Exercise stress test (EST)	Chest pain; horizontal ST segment or downsloping of 1 mm or more; failure of systolic blood pressure to rise or drop; ST elevations	Normal stress test done to differentiate between variant and classic angina; ST elevation with or without associated chest pain occasionally develops	As in stable angina pectoris, should not be done until patient has been stable and pain free for 24 hr	Not done in presence of documented MI, low-level test may be performed before discharge from hospital
Echocardiography	Limited use, but performed after EST may detect wall motion abnormalities	Limited use, but performed after EST may detect wall motion abnormalities	2-dimensional: may show transient abnormalities of ventricular wall motion	Identifies area of abnormal regional wall motion; aids in detecting complications associated with acute MI: papillary dysfunction, septal rupture; visualizes LV thrombus *RV infarction:* dilated RV, abnormal RV wall motion
Thallium 201 scintigraphy	Ischemic areas appear as "cold" areas, reflecting reduced thallium uptake; when ischemia relieved, "cold" areas show normal thallium uptake	Ischemic "cold" areas may be demonstrated once involved coronary artery has been identified	Similar to stable angina pectoris	Similar to stable angina pectoris

Continued.

From Canobbio MM: *Mosby's clinical nursing series: cardiovascular disorders,* St Louis, 1990, Mosby.

Table 3-2 Diagnostic Tests—cont'd

Diagnostic Test	Findings			
	Variant (Prinzmetal's) Stable Angina Pectoris	Angina	Unstable Angina Pectoris	Myocardial Infarction
Radionuclide blood pool imaging with technetium 99 m			Positive findings suggest recent (previous) minor degrees of subendocardial necrosis or infarction	Confirms myocardial damage by localizing and permitting estimation of size of transmural infarction; must be done within 2-6 days after acute infarction; determines wall motion abnormalities; permits estimation of ventricular function by determining ejection fractions
Magnetic resonance imaging (MRI)				Differentiates ischemic, infarcted, and normal myocardial tissue; used in early detection of MI to assess areas of perfusion and detect jeopardized or vulnerable tissue
Cardiac catheterization and coronary angiography	Determines number and location of obstructive lesions, "graftability" of artery distal to obstructive lesion, and ventricular function	Distinguishes spasm in normal coronary arteries from those with severe obstructive lesions; intravenous injection of ergonovine maleate provokes coronary artery spasm in patients with variant angina	As in stable angina pectoris, used in conjunction with PTCA	Generally not performed as diagnostic procedure during acute period unless done in conjunction with intracoronary thrombolysis

Exercise regularly; encourage regular home exercise program

Avoid sexual activities when fatigued; if chest pain occurs during sexual activity, stop and take nitrates if ordered; if pain persists or extreme fatigue occurs, report symptoms to physician

Self-management during episodes of pain
Stop activity and rest
Take nitrates as ordered

Report to physician if pain persists longer than 15 min or diaphoresis and SOB appear

Discuss importance of maintaining diet that is low in saturated fats, cholesterol; avoid caffeine intake; refer to dietitian for counseling

ADDITIONAL NURSING DIAGNOSIS
TO CONSIDER

Anxiety related to perceived biologic threat and pain

Acute Myocardial Infarction

Complete occlusion of the coronary artery and/or its branches, resulting in myocardial ischemia and necrosis (Figure 3-8). It occurs as result of a sudden decrease in coronary perfusion or an increase in myocardial oxygen demand without adequate coronary perfusion. Two types of infarction are the following:

subendocardial infarction (non-Q wave): *Confined to a small area of myocardium, usually within the subendocardial wall of the left ventricle, ventricular septum, and papillary muscle.*

transmural or full thickness (Q-wave): *Infarction is widespread myocardial necrosis, extending from the endocardium to the epicardium.*

Assessment

Subjective data

Severe, crushing chest pain
Precordial
Substernal
Unrelated to exertion or respiration
Dizziness, faintness
Indigestion, nausea

Objective data

Diaphoresis
Skin
Cold
Clammy
Pale

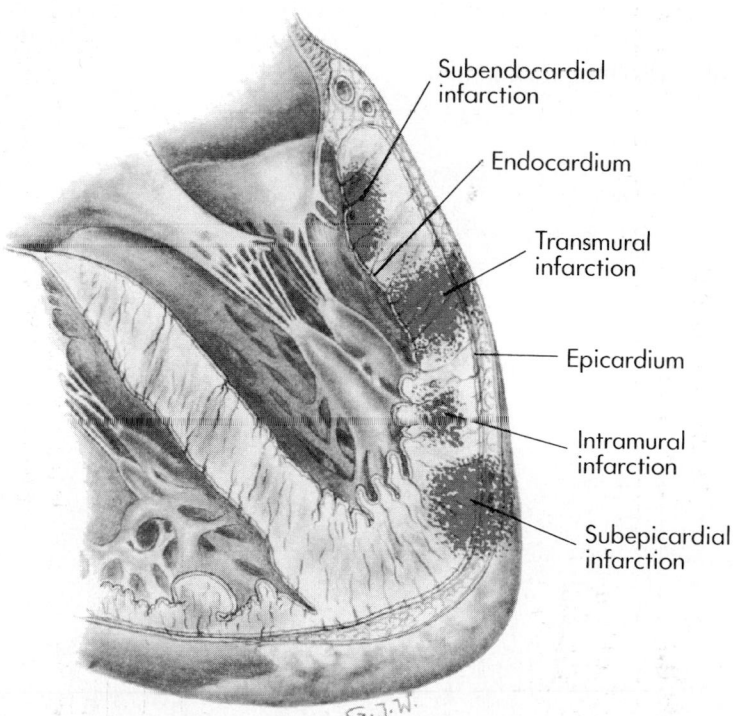

Figure 3-8 Location of infarctions in the ventricular wall. (From Thelan LA et al: *Critical care nursing: diagnosis and management,* ed 2, St Louis, 1994, Mosby.)

SOB
Decreased BP
Tachycardia
Elevated temperature
Anxiety
Restlessness
Behavioral responses
  Denial
  Depression
Heart sounds
  S₃ gallop
  Pericardial friction rub
  Murmurs
Right ventricular infarction
  Increased jugular venous distension
  Peripheral edema
  Liver tenderness

Diagnostic tests (see Table 3-2)

Serum studies
  Elevated enzymes: Creatine phosphokinase (CPK-MB, CPK), LDH, AST
  Elevated ESR
  Elevated WBC
ECG changes (Figure 3-9)
  ST segment elevation
  T wave depression, inversions
  Q waves
  Dysrhythmias
Echocardiography: ventricular wall motion abnormalities
Radionuclide blood pool studies: thallium, technetium

Localization of infarct area
  Ventricular function
Magnetic resonance imaging
Angiography

Potential complications

Dysrhythmias
Heart failure
Cardiogenic shock
Extension of MI
Pulmonary/systemic emboli
Pericarditis
Rupture
  Ventricular
  Papillary muscle
Ventricular septal defect: systolic murmur LLSB
Valvular dysfunction
Ventricular aneurysm
Postmyocardial infarction syndrome (Dressler's syndrome)

Collaborative management

Therapeutic management

Coronary care unit (CCU) admission with continuous cardiac monitoring
Oxygen therapy: 2 to 4 L/min
Thrombolytic therapy: myocardial reperfusion within 4 to 6 hr of onset of pain
Diet: NPO until stable; low fat, low sodium, low cholesterol

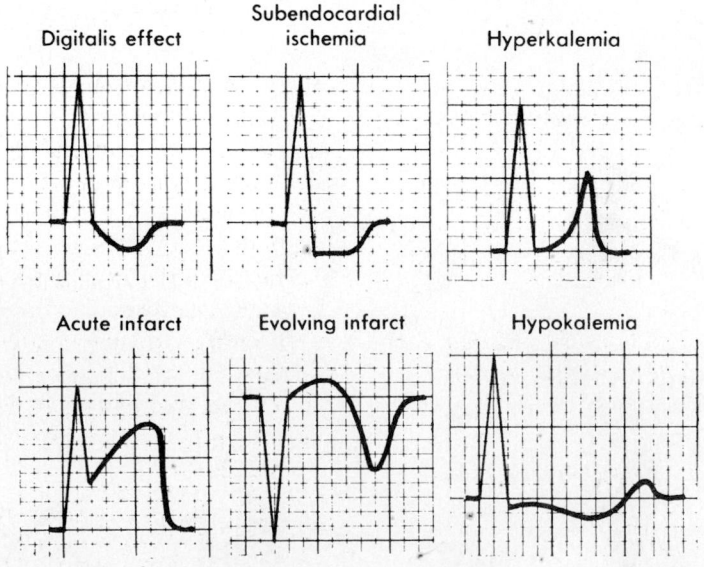

Figure 3-9 ST-T segment changes. (From Goldberger AL, Goldberger E: *Clinical electrocardiography: a simplified approach,* ed 4, St Louis, 1990, Mosby.)

Parenteral fluids
Medications
    Pain management: morphine sulfate
    Sedation
    Antiarrhythmics
    Beta-adrenergic blocking agents
    Vasodilators
    Antiplatelets
    Calcium antagonist
Hemodynamic monitoring; SVO$_2$
Surgical reperfusion: coronary artery bypass graft

Nursing management

PATIENT PROBLEMS/NURSING DIAGNOSES

● **NDX:** Pain, chest related to myocardial ischemia or necrosis

Maintain bed rest for first 24 to 30 hr and as indicated; position patient comfortably *to conserve myocardial oxygen consumption*

Assess and record description of pain and factors that aggravate pain; determine if influenced by respiration or body position

Administer oxygen as ordered

Administer drug therapy as ordered; assess and record response

Obtain BP, P, and R during pain episode to monitor for signs of hypotension, *which may reflect hypoperfusion*

Initiate nonpharmacologic measures *to relieve pain* (e.g., relaxation techniques; guided imagery; quiet, restful environment)

EXPECTED OUTCOME
Patient verbalizes absence of pain and appears relaxed

● **NDX:** Decreased cardiac output related to electrical factors (dysrhythmias), decreased myocardial contractility, and structural defects

Maintain bed rest with head of bed elevated 30 degrees for first 24 to 48 hr *to reduce myocardial oxygen demand*

Assess and report signs of decreased cardiac output; incidence of morbidity and mortality are greatest in first 24 hr

    Decreased BP, increased heart rate
    Decreased urine output
    Fatigue and weakness
    Cool, pale, clammy skin

Assess and monitor BP, T, R, and apical pulse q2h to 4h or as indicated by clinical status

Monitor and record ECG continuously *to assess rate and rhythm* q2h to 4h or as indicated

Obtain and compare 12-lead ECG and/or RV leads as ordered *to confirm and identify location of MI*

Administer oxygen therapy as ordered

Prepare and/or initiate thrombolytic therapy as ordered *to limit size of infarction by reperfusing ischemic heart muscle*

Auscultate breath and heart sounds q1h to 2h or as indicated

Monitor serial serum enzymes

Monitor PAP, PCWP, or CVP as indicated

Monitor intake and output q2h to 4h

Maintain parenteral fluids as ordered

Administer medications as ordered

Provide diet as tolerated; avoid use of caffeine

Avoid straining such as Valsalva's maneuver; use stool softeners or laxatives

EXPECTED OUTCOMES
Cardiac output remains stable or improved
Patient demonstrates hemodynamic stability
Vital signs and urine output are within normal limits
Patient is able to perform activities of daily living (ADLs)

● **NDX:** Anxiety related to perceived or actual threat to biologic integrity

Assess for signs and verbal expressions of anxiety

Initiate comfort measures such as a quiet, restful environment and relaxation techniques (e.g., visual imaging, soft rhythmic music *to decrease unnecessary external stimuli that can stimulate sympathetic response)*

Minimize contact with stressful stimuli such as other anxious patients

Use calm, reassuring voice

Discuss and orient patient to CCU environment and equipment

Administer sedation as indicated

Stay with patient during periods of highest anxiety and offer reassurance

Give simple explanations regarding care and procedures

Encourage expression of feelings; accept crying

Permit family member to assist patient whenever possible

EXPECTED OUTCOMES
Patient's anxiety level is reduced
Patient appears relaxed and verbalizes sense of calm

Patient/family teaching

Assess level of understanding and degree of readiness to learn

Review physician's explanation of heart condition
  Extent of infarction
  Associated complications
    Dysrhythmias
    Angina
    Postmyocardial infarction syndrome
    Heart failure

Describe the nature and course of coronary artery disease including
  Risk factors involved and methods of modification (p. 117)
  Precipitating factors of angina

Discuss importance of controlling any coexisting disease that may aggravate recovery
  Hyperlipidemia
  Hypertension
  Diabetes

Explain importance of weight control

Explain stress management: need to control stress-producing events and activities

Discuss signs and symptoms of an extending MI versus angina
  Extending MI: chest pain, shortness of breath, perspiration, weakness not relieved by medication or rest, pain not always associated with physical exertion
  Angina: chest pain or pressure is usually relieved by rest and/or vasodilators; pain is usually associated with physical or emotional strain

Explain importance of calling physician if chest pain lasts longer than 15 min (if pain is associated with other symptoms, call physician immediately)

Explain names of medications, dosages, times of administration, purposes, and side effects

Explain need to avoid taking over-the-counter medications without checking with physician

Home care considerations

Assist with development of exercise and activity plan
  Review limitations and allowances of activity; check with physician for walking and exercise limitations
  Avoid or modify activity after heavy meals, alcohol consumption, periods of emotional stress, or in temperature extremes
  Explain importance of planned rest periods
  Discuss importance of activity limitations as related to healing process (healing takes approximately 6 to 8 weeks)
  Explain need to exercise at regular intervals; encourage home exercise program

Explain importance of checking with physician with regard to resuming sexual activity, travelling, and driving automobile

Explain need to avoid isometric-type activity (e.g., heavy lifting and pushing)

Explain need to monitor daily activities (space activities with periods of rest; stop when fatigued; avoid rushing)

Discuss importance of encouraging independence in self-care activities

Discuss importance of communication with significant other or family

Explain need to deal with feelings about possible role change and sexual activity

Explain importance of maintaining dietary restrictions including low-sodium, low-cholesterol, low-fat, and low-calorie diet as ordered; refer to dietitian for education; if no specific diet is ordered, instruct to limit intake of eggs, cream, butter, and foods high in animal fat; modify or restrict salt intake

Explain need to rest after meals (avoid exercising up to 2 hours after having meals)

Explain need to avoid use of caffeine products (e.g., coffee, certain teas, and cola drinks)

Explain need to avoid use of tobacco products such as cigarettes, cigars, and chewing tobacco

Explain need to avoid constipation and straining

Explain need to avoid sitting in same position for long periods

Infective Endocarditis

An inflammatory process involving the endothelium of the heart, including the cardiac valves (Figure 3-10). Infective endocarditis begins as an infection that causes bacteremia. It is characterized by vegetations or thrombus composed of fibrin and platelets that form on

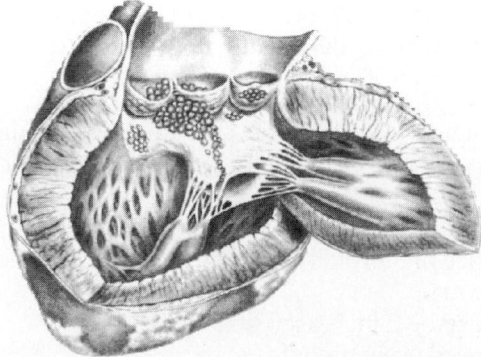

Figure 3-10 Endocarditis. (From Canobbio MM: *Mosby's clinical nursing series: cardiovascular disorders,* St Louis, 1990, Mosby.)

valves and adjacent areas when endocardial tissue is damaged.

Affected structures such as valves eventually become scarred, impeding function. The infection may also burrow into the myocardium, causing conduction defects, abscesses, and rupture of the chordae tendineae or ventricular septum.

Assessment

Subjective data

Complains of flulike symptoms: malaise, weakness, arthralgias

Objective data

Recurrent temperature elevation
  Acute: 102° to 104°F (39° to 40°C)
  Subacute: 102°F (39°C)
Alternating chills and diaphoresis (may occur at night)
Signs of embolization
  Petechia
    Conjunctiva
    Palate, buccal mucosa
    Extremities
Osler's nodes
"Café-au-lait" complexion
Anorexia
Weight loss
Headache
Splenomegaly
Heart sounds
  Early: usually normal
  Late: murmurs

Diagnostic tests

Positive blood cultures
CBC
  Normocytic, normochromic anemia
  Elevated ESR
  Leukocytosis
Rheumatoid factor: positive in patients with infection 6 wk or longer
Echocardiogram: presence of vegetation or abscesses; valve involvement; LV dysfunction
Electrocardiogram: atrial fibrillation or flutter
Radionuclide studies
  Galluim 67 citrate

Potential complications

Cardiac
  Abscesses

Valvular heart disease
Heart failure
Myocarditis
Embolization: cerebral, renal, splenic, coronary
Mycotic aneurysms

Collaborative management

Therapeutic management

Parenteral therapy
Medications
  IV antibiotics
  Antipyretics: salicylates
  Analgesics
  Anticoagulation

Nursing management

PATIENT PROBLEMS/NURSING DIAGNOSES

● **NDX:** Altered nutrition: less than body requirements related to biologic factors (e.g., fever, infection)

Assess for progressive weight loss and signs of malnutrition *because infectious process increases metabolic* needs (chronic illness leads to anorexia)
Monitor daily caloric intake
Weigh daily *to determine amount of weight loss and need to add supplemental feedings*
Offer high-calorie and high-protein supplemental feedings *to ensure adequate intake of nutrients*
Consult with dietitian regarding nutritional requirements
Ensure patient comfort during meals

EXPECTED OUTCOMES
Nutritional status is maintained or improved
Age-appropriate, sex-appropriate body weight is achieved or maintained
Patient verbalizes improved appetite

● **NDX:** Diversional activity deficit related to prolonged antibiotic therapy

Assess for diversional deficit; differentiate from progression of disease process
Encourage patient to explore diversional activities (e.g., reading, puzzles, and out-of-hospital passes) as indicated
Initiate occupational therapy if indicated
Encourage daily structured exercise program *to maintain muscle tone and promote sense of well-being*

EXPECTED OUTCOME

Patient engages in identifiable inpatient diversional activities

● **NDX:** Altered body temperature related to infectious process

Assess for dehydration: diaphoresis, poor skin turgor, dry mucous membrane
Obtain temperature q4h to 8h as indicated *to detect presence of infectious process*
Monitor fluid intake and output q8h, noting water loss resulting from perspiration *to avoid negative fluid balance from dehydration*
Encourage fluid intake as tolerated *to maintain fluid balance*
Administer antibiotics as ordered, ensuring they are given on time *to maintain consistent drug levels in blood*
Administer antipyretics as ordered *to reduce temperature*
Monitor laboratory reports on CBC with differential and blood cultures
Monitor IV sites for redness and swelling; change site q48h *to reduce risk of infiltration and infection*

EXPECTED OUTCOMES

Inflammatory process has cleared
Patient demonstrates normal body temperature
Skin is warm and dry

● **NDX:** Risk for altered cerebral tissue perfusion related to embolization

Assess for signs of embolization each shift and prn; report positive signs to physician immediately
Perform neurologic checks every shift or as indicated by patient's condition
Administer anticoagulant therapy as ordered
Instruct patient about need to continue with anticoagulants, if ordered, to prevent future embolic episodes

EXPECTED OUTCOMES

Cerebral tissue perfusion is maintained
Patient is alert and oriented
No signs of embolization are present

ADDITIONAL NURSING DIAGNOSES
TO CONSIDER

Risk for altered tissue perfusion (renal, pulmonary) related to embolization
Risk for decreased cardiac output related to mechanical factors secondary to heart failure

Patient/family teaching

Discuss symptoms of recurrence to report to physician
Fatigue
Elevated temperature
Chills
Weight loss
Just not feeling well
Discuss need to avoid persons with infections, especially upper respiratory infection (URI), and to report symptoms (e.g., cold, influenza, cough) to physician
Explain importance of avoiding fatigue; need to plan rest periods before and after activity
Discuss importance of reporting to physician any event that may predispose to bacteremia
Dental or gum therapy
Surgical procedures
Invasive medical procedures
Childbirth
Trauma
Furuncles
Explain need to maintain good oral hygiene: daily care and regular visits to dentist
Explain importance of ongoing outpatient care
Discuss name of medication, dosage, times of administration, purpose, and side effects
Explain significance of prophylactic antibiotic therapy before procedures that predispose to bacteremia (Table 3-3)

Valvular Heart Disease

An acquired or congenital disease involving the cardiac valves. The disorders fall into two classifications: insufficient (regurgitation), the inability to close sufficiently to permit blood flow; or stenosis, the inability to open sufficiently to permit blood flow. The most common forms of valvular heart disease (VHD) are aortic or mitral stenosis and aortic or mitral regurgitation (Figure 3-11, Table 3-4).

Assessment

Subjective data

General complaints
Fatigue
Malaise
SOB
DOE
Anorexia
Sleep disorders: PND, orthopnea, nocturnal sweats
Palpitations

Table 3-3 Recommended Antibiotic Coverage for Endocarditis Prophylaxis

Drug	Dosing Regimen[†‡§]
RECOMMENDED STANDARD PROPHYLACTIC REGIMEN FOR DENTAL, ORAL, OR UPPER RESPIRATORY TRACT PROCEDURES IN PATIENTS WHO ARE AT RISK*	
Standard regimen	
Amoxicillin	3.0 g orally 1h before procedure; then 1.5 g 6h after initial dose
Amoxicillin/penicillin-allergic patients	
Erythromycin	Erythromycin ethylsuccinate, 600 mg, or erythromycin stearate, 1.0 g, orally 2h before procedure; then half the dose 6h after initial dose
Clindamycin	300 mg orally 1h before procedure and 150 mg 6h after initial dose
ALTERNATE PROPHYLACTIC REGIMENS FOR DENTAL, ORAL, OR UPPER RESPIRATORY TRACT PROCEDURES IN PATIENTS WHO ARE AT RISK[‡]	
Patients unable to take oral medications	
Ampicillin	IV or IM administration of ampicillin, 2.0 g, 30 min before procedure; then IV or IM administration of ampicillin, 1.0 g, or oral administration of amoxicillin, 1.5 g, 6h after initial dose
Ampicillin/amoxicillin/penicillin-allergic patients unable to take oral medications	
Clindamycin	IV administration of 300 mg 30 min before procedure and an IV or PO administration of 150 mg 6h after initial dose
Patients considered high risk and not candidates for standard regimen	
Ampicillin, gentamicin, and amoxicillin	IV or IM administration of ampicillin, 2.0 g, plus gentamicin, 1.5 mg/kg (not to exceed 80 mg), 30 min before procedure; followed by amoxicillin, 1.5 g, orally 6h after initial dose; alternately, the parenteral regimen may be repeated 8h after initial dose
Ampicillin/amoxicillin/penicillin-allergic patients considered high risk	
Vancomycin	IV administration of 1.0 g over 1h, starting 1h before procedure; no repeated dose necessary
REGIMENS FOR GENITOURINARY/GASTROINTESTINAL PROCEDURES[§]	
Standard regimen	
Ampicillin, gentamicin, and amoxicillin	IV or IM administration of ampicillin, 2.0 g, plus gentamicin, 1.5 mg/kg (not to exceed 80 mg), 30 min before procedure; followed by amoxicillin, 1.5 g, orally 6h after initial dose; alternately, the parenteral regimen may be repeated once 8h after initial dose
Ampicillin/amoxicillin/penicillin-allergic patient regimen	
Vancomycin and gentamicin	IV administration of vancomycin, 1.0 g, over 1h plus IV or IM administration of gentamicin, 1.5 mg/kg (not to exceed 80 mg), 1h before procedure; may be repeated once 8h after initial dose
Alternate low-risk patient regimen	
Amoxicillin	3.0 g orally 1h before procedure; then 1.5 g 6h after initial dose

From *JAMA—The Journal of the American Medical Association,* 264:2919-2922, Copyright 1990, American Medical Association.
*Includes those with prosthetic heart valves and other high risk patients.
†Initial pediatric doses are as follows: amoxicillin, 50 mg/kg; erythromycin ethylsuccinate or erythromycin stearate, 20 mg/kg; and clindamycin, 10 mg/kg. Follow-up doses should be one half the initial dose. *Total pediatric dose should not exceed total adult dose.* The following weight ranges may also be used for the initial pediatric dose of amoxicillin: 15 kg, 750 mg; 15 to 30 kg, 1500 mg; and 30 kg, 3000 mg (full adult dose).
‡Initial pediatric doses are as follows: ampicillin, 50 mg/kg; clindamycin, 10 mg/kg; gentamicin, 2.0 mg/kg; and vancomycin, 20 mg/kg. Follow-up doses should be one half the initial dose. *Total pediatric dose should not exceed total adult dose.* No initial dose is recommended in this table for amoxicillin (25 mg/kg is the follow-up dose).
§Initial pediatric doses are as follows: ampicillin, 50 mg/kg; amoxicillin, 50 mg/kg; gentamicin, 2.0 mg/kg; and vancomycin, 20 mg/kg. Follow-up doses should be half the initial dose. *Total pediatric dose should not exceed total adult dose.*

Cardiac Conditions/Procedures for Which Endocarditis Prophylaxis Is Recommended/Not Recommended*

ENDOCARDITIS PROPHYLAXIS RECOMMENDED

Prosthetic cardiac valves including bioprosthetic and homograft valves

Previous bacterial endocarditis, even in the absence of heart disease

Most congenital cardiac malformations

Rheumatic and other acquired valvular dysfunction, even after valvular surgery

Hypertrophic cardiomyopathy

Mitral valve prolapse with valvular regurgitation†

ENDOCARDITIS PROPHYLAXIS NOT RECOMMENDED

Isolated secundum atrial septal defect

Surgical repair without residua beyond 6 months of secundum atrial septal defect, ventricular septal defect, or patent ductus arteriosus

Previous coronary artery bypass graft surgery

Mitral valve prolapse without valvular regurgitation†

Physiologic, functional, or innocent heart murmurs

Previous Kawasaki disease without valvular dysfunction

Previous rheumatic fever without valvular dysfunction

Cardiac pacemakers and implanted defibrillators

The American Heart Association. Reprinted from *JAMA—The Journal of the American Medical Association:* 264, Dec. 12, 1990. Copyright 1990, American Medical Association.

*Cardiac conditions listed for which endocarditis prophylaxis is recommended/not recommended are not meant to be all-inclusive.

†Individuals who have a mitral valve prolapse associated with thickening and/or redundancy of the valve leaflets may be at increased risk for bacterial endocarditis, particularly men who are 45 years of age or older.

Table 3-4 Common Valvular Disorders: Adult Onset

Aortic Stenosis	Mitral Stenosis	Aortic Regurgitation	Mitral Regurgitation
OBSERVATIONS			
DOE	DOE	Dyspnea	Dyspnea
Syncope	Fatigue	Awareness of strong pulsations of heart	Fatigue
Fatigue	Decreased tolerance to exercise	Excessive sweating	Exercise intolerance
Angina pectoris	Orthopnea	Skin warm, flushed, and damp	Orthopnea
Decreased pulse pressure	PND	Dizziness	Palpitations
Carotid pulse	Cough	Neck pain	
Slow with long upstroke	Hemoptysis	Head bobbing (DeMusset's sign)	
Small quality to pulse		Pulses	
		Visible arterial pulsations in neck	
		Bisferiens pulse	
		Water-hammer (Corrigan's) pulse	
		Widened pulse pressure to >80 mm Hg	

Continued.

Table 3-4 Common Valvular Disorders: Adult Onset—cont'd

Aortic Stenosis	Mitral Stenosis	Aortic Regurgitation	Mitral Regurgitation
OBSERVATIONS—cont'd			
Apical impulse: strong, sustained during systole	Apical impulse: tapping quality	Apical impulse: forceful, sustained, displaced downward and outward	Apical impulse; large, laterally displaced
Systolic thrill			
Heart sounds (Figure 3-12)	Heart sounds (Figure 3-12)	Heart sounds (Figure 3-12)	Heart sounds (Figure 3-12)
Moderate: crescendo-decrescendo, rough, harsh systolic murmur heard over aortic area	Loud first heart sound; low-pitched rumbling diastolic murmur with an opening snap heard at apex	Decrescendo: high-pitched blowing heard at left sternal border	Holosystolic systolic murmur heard at apex
Decreased aortic second sound		Systolic ejection sound	First heart sounds diminished
		Diastolic murmur	Splitting of second heart sound
			Third heart sound
POTENTIAL COMPLICATIONS			
Endocarditis	Endocarditis	Endocarditis	Endocarditis
Systemic emboli	Systemic emboli: brain, extremities, abdomen		Rupture of chordae tendineae; systemic emboli
DIAGNOSTIC FINDINGS			
ECG	ECG	ECG	ECG
Left ventricular hypertrophy (LVH)	P waves notched or peaked in I, II, III, and AVF	Normal	Nonspecific ST segment and T wave abnormalities
Conduction defects	Atrial fibrillation	Septal Q waves V_5, V_6	LVH
Left anterior hemiblock	Right ventricular hypertrophy (RVH)	LVH	P waves abnormalities
Left bundle branch block (LBBB)			Atrial dysrhythmias: premature atrial contractions (PACs), atrial fibrillation
Complete heart block			
Dysrhythmias: atrial fibrillation			
Chest x-ray examination: enlargement of LV; calcification of aortic valve	Chest x-ray examination: enlargement of LA, RV, right atria (RA), and pulmonary trunk; calcification of mitral valve	Chest x-ray examination: enlargement of LV; dilation of aorta	Chest x-ray examination: enlargement of LA, LV
Hemodynamic changes: elevated left atrial (LA) and LV pressures	Hemodynamic changes: elevated pressures—LA, pulmonary artery (PA), and RV	Hemodynamic changes: elevated left ventricular end-diastolic pressure (LVEDP)	Hemodynamic changes: elevated LA and PA pressures and PCWP

Objective data

NOTE: Observations and care listed are for moderate-to-severe forms of valvular heart disease (see Table 3-4 for specific findings for most common forms of valvular heart disease)

Diagnostic tests

ECG
  Atrial, ventricular hypertrophy
  Dysrhythmias: atrial fibrillation, flutter
  Conduction defects: bundle branch blocks

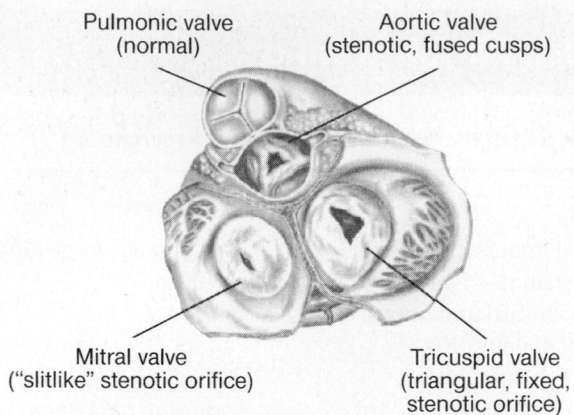

Figure 3-11 Valvular heart disease. (From Canobbio MM: *Mosby's clinical nursing series: cardiovascular disorders,* St Louis, 1990, Mosby.)

Echocardiogram: decreased excursion of leaflets; chamber enlargement; dilation
Chest x-ray examination
  Cardiomegaly
  Pulmonary vascular congestion
  Valve calcification
Cardiac catheterization

Potential complications

Infective endocarditis
Embolism
  Brain
  Lungs
Left ventricular (LV) failure
Right ventricular (RV) failure
Dysrhythmias
Rupture of papillary muscles or chordae tendineae
Pulmonary edema

Collaborative management

Therapeutic management

Medications
  Antibiotics
  Antidysrhythmics
  Diuretics
  Analgesics
  Anticoagulants
Diet: sodium restriction
Cardioversion
Hemodynamic monitoring
Percutaneous balloon catheter dilation (balloon angioplasty)
Surgical management
  Commissurotomy
  Valvotomy
  Valvuloplasty
  Valve replacement

Nursing management

PATIENT PROBLEMS/NURSING DIAGNOSES

● **NDX:** Decreased cardiac output related to mechanical factors (preload, afterload) secondary to valvular dysfunction

Establish baseline assessment of cardiovascular status *to evaluate disease process and development of right or left ventricular failure*
Monitor BP, T, and R with apical pulse q4h or as indicated
Auscultate heart sounds q6h to 8h; record presence or absence of murmurs or gallop sounds *to determine*

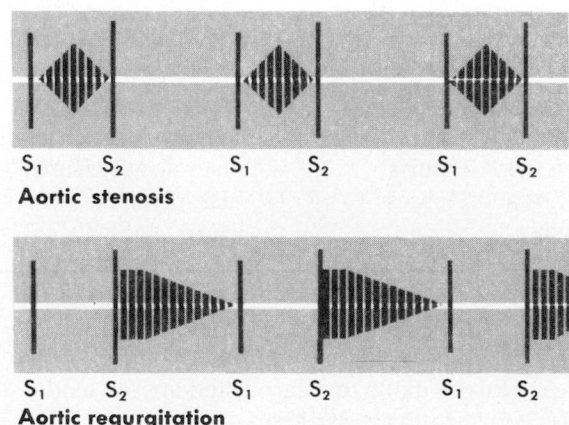

Figure 3-12 Valvular heart disease murmurs. (From Guzzetta C, Dossey B: *Cardiovascular nursing: bodymind tapestry,* St Louis, 1985, Mosby.)

Dental or Surgical Procedures for Which Endocarditis Prophylaxis Is Recommended/Not Recommended*

ENDOCARDITIS PROPHYLAXIS RECOMMENDED

Dental procedures known to induce gingival or mucosal bleeding including professional cleaning

Tonsillectomy and/or adenoidectomy

Surgical operations that involve intestinal or respiratory mucosa

Bronchoscopy with a rigid bronchoscope

Sclerotherapy for esophageal varices

Esophageal dilatation

Gallbladder surgery

Cystoscopy

Urethral dilatation

Urethral catheterization if urinary tract infection is present†

Urinary tract surgery if urinary tract infection is present†

Prostatic surgery

Incision and drainage of infected tissue†

Vaginal hysterectomy

Vaginal delivery in the presence of infection†

ENDOCARDITIS PROPHYLAXIS NOT RECOMMENDED‡

Dental procedures not likely to induce gingival bleeding such as simple adjustment of orthodontic appliances or fillings above the gum line

Injection of local intraoral anesthetic (except intraligamentary injections)

Shedding of primary teeth

Tympanostomy tube insertion

Endotracheal intubation

Bronchoscopy with a flexible bronchoscope, with or without biopsy

Cardiac catheterization

Endoscopy with or without gastrointestinal biopsy

Cesarean birth

In the absence of infection for urethral catheterization, dilatation and curettage, uncomplicated vaginal delivery, therapeutic abortion, sterilization procedures, or insertion or removal of intrauterine devices

The American Heart Association. Reprinted from *JAMA—The Journal of the American Medical Association:* 264, Dec. 12, 1990. Copyright 1990, American Medical Association.

*This table lists selected procedures but is not meant to be all-inclusive.

†In addition to prophylactic regimen for genitourinary procedures, antibiotic therapy should be directed against the most likely bacterial pathogen.

‡In patients who have prosthetic heart valves, a previous history of endocarditis, or surgically constructed systemic-pulmonary shunts or conduits, physicians may choose to administer prophylactic antibiotics even for low-risk procedures that involve the lower respiratory, genitourinary, or gastrointestinal tracts.

progression in valve dysfunction or distention of heart chambers

Monitor cardiac rhythm for changes from baseline; record any dysrhythmia (changes in rhythm *may reflect development of dysrhythmias, which can interfere with ventricular filling*)

Administer medications as ordered

Monitor intake and output

Restrict and monitor dietary intake of sodium *to minimize sodium retention and excrete excess fluid*

Limit and/or modify activity during acute phase *to conserve energy and decrease myocardial oxygen demand*

Avoid fatigue; maintain planned rest periods

Perform active or passive ROM exercises to extremities qid

EXPECTED OUTCOMES

Patient demonstrates stable or improved cardiac output

Reports improvement of symptoms

Lungs are clear

Vital signs and urine output are within normal limits

Patient is able to perform ADLs

● **NDX:** Fluid volume excess related to cardiac decompensation

Assess and monitor intake and output; report output <30 ml/hr or intake greater than output on daily basis

Assess and monitor for signs of fluid retention, increased congestion

Auscultate heart sounds (S_3, S_4) and breath sounds q4h to 8h

Check for increase or decrease in jugular venous pressure

Weigh daily using same amount of clothing and at same time of day

Administer diuretics and vasodilator therapy as ordered
Restrict sodium and fluids as indicated *to control sodium resorption and fluid retention*
Monitor electrolytes, chemistries, Hgb, and Hct

EXPECTED OUTCOMES

Patient's fluid balance is restored
Lung sounds clear
S_3, S_4 absent
Ideal body weight is achieved

● **NDX:** Activity intolerance related to diminished cardiac reserve

Assess and monitor for signs of activity intolerance *as a result of an inability of myocardium to effectively increase stroke volume in response to increased demands*
Check BP, HR, and R before and after activity, report HR >20 bpm above resting HR, marked increase in BP, or complaints of dyspnea, chest pain, diaphoresis, or excessive fatigue
Maintain bed or chair rest as indicated
Identify factors known to cause fatigue *to promote energy conservation*
Space treatments and procedures *to allow for periods of uninterrupted rest to ensure periods of complete rest;* provide periods of rest throughout day and evening
Implement measures that will improve activity tolerance by minimizing fatigue (e.g., toileting via bedside commode rather than bedpan; up in chair with legs elevated rather than complete bed rest)
Increase activity level as indicated by condition; assess activity tolerance and activity progression *to evaluate improved myocardial performance*

EXPECTED OUTCOMES

Activity level improved
Patient reports being able to participate in ADLs
Patient denies having SOB
HR, BP, R within normal limits

ADDITIONAL NURSING DIAGNOSES TO CONSIDER

Risk for injury (cerebral) related to interruption of arterial blood flow secondary to embolization
Risk for infection

Patient/family teaching

Assess level of understanding
Explain nature and cause of disease process
Discuss importance of reporting signs and symptoms of heart failure
  Increased fatigue

Tachypnea
Orthopnea
Cough
Infective endocarditis
  Elevated temperature
  Malaise and anorexia
  Chills alternating with diaphoresis
Discuss importance of reporting to physician any event that may predispose to bacteremia
  Dental or gum manipulation
  Genitourinary procedures
  Drainage of abscesses
  Presence of skin boils
  Gynecologic procedures
    Childbirth
    Dilation and curettage (D & C)
    Therapeutic abortion
    Tubal ligation

Home care considerations

Explain importance of notifying dentist, urologist, and gynecologist of valvular heart disease
For females, provide instruction regarding appropriate choice of contraceptives (i.e., to avoid oral contraceptives and intrauterine devices); explain importance of obtaining counseling regarding pregnancy before conception
Discuss name of medication, dosage, times of administration, purpose, and side effects
Explain need to avoid taking over-the-counter drugs without checking with physician
Explain importance of ongoing outpatient care
Instruct patient about importance of prophylactic antibiotic therapy to prevent endocarditis (see Table 3-3)
Explain need to maintain good oral hygiene, daily care, and regular visits to dentist
Discuss activity allowances and limitations; assist to develop activity plan
  Explain need to avoid fatigue and to plan rest periods before and after activity
  Instruct patient in measures that will minimize fatigue
    Bathing: shower with chair rather than tub bath
    Avoid prolonged periods of standing; use stool to lean against when cooking, ironing

Congenital Heart Disease

Structural or functional abnormalities or defects of the heart or great vessels existing from birth. With the advances in medical and surgical treatment, increasing number of persons are reaching adulthood. However, despite treatment, many of the defects

continue to have residual problems that must continue to be monitored and treated.

Assessment

Subjective data

Dyspnea on exertion
Fatigue
Decreased exercise tolerance
Palpitations
Lightheadedness

Objective data

See Table 3-5

Diagnostic tests

See Table 3-6
ECG
Chest x-ray
Echocardiogram
  Doppler 2D
  Transesophageal
Cardiac catheterization
Serum studies for patient with cyanotic CHD (NOTE:
  HCT is normally elevated more than 45% with a range
  to 60%)
  Hct, Hgb, MCV, platelets
  Uric acid, BUN, creatinine levels

Potential complications

Endocarditis
Dysrhythmias
Heart failure
Eisenmenger reaction

Collaborative management

Therapeutic management

Medical
  Dictated by patient's clinical status
Surgery
  Palliative
    Systemic to pulmonary shunts (e.g., Blalock-
      Taussig, Glenn)
    Pulmonary artery banding
    Atrial septectomy

Corrective
Dictated by specific defect

Nursing management

PATIENT PROBLEMS/NURSING DIAGNOSES

● **NDX:**   Anxiety related to threat to health status

Assess level of anxiety and determine primary cause *to determine patient's appraisal and perception of his or her clinical condition*
Assess usual coping mechanisms *to determine whether appropriate or sufficient to control anxiety and fear*
Provide and/or clarify information relative to condition *because anxiety can be result of misinterpretation of what congenital heart disease means.*
Provide positive reinforcement about prognosis; assist patient in attaining realistic goals and lifestyle *to promote a sense of wellness and optimism about future*

● **NDX:**   Risk for activity intolerance related to immobility, lack of knowledge or progressive decreased cardiac reserve

Assess whether activity level is appropriate for medical condition because *patient may be misinformed about appropriate activity allowances and limitations*
Assess and monitor response to activity noting type, intensity, frequency, and type of symptoms that may develop
Implement measures that will improve activity tolerance if patient has reduced cardiac reserve *to limit myocardial oxygen demand*

ADDITIONAL NURSING DIAGNOSES
TO CONSIDER

Decreased cardiac output related to structural (defect), mechanical (preload, afterload, myocardial contractility), and electrical (dysrhythmias) factors
Ineffective individual and family coping related to incorrect information regarding clinical diagnosis or to progressive lifestyle and role changes imposed by disease process

Patient/family teaching

Ensure patient/family understand primary defect, and what (if any) palliative or corrective surgical interventions have occurred
Explain endocarditis, review preventive measures (see Infective endocarditis, p. 128)

Text continued on p. 143.

Table 3-5 Congenital Heart Disease Objective Findings

Assessment	Patent Ductus Arteriosus	Atrial Septal Defect	Ventricular Septal Defect	Pulmonic Stenosis	Coarctation of Aorta	Ebstein's Anomaly	Tetralogy of Fallot
HISTORY	Small shunt: asymptomatic; large shunt: exertional dyspnea, decreased exercise tolerance	Small shunt: asymptomatic; moderate to large shunt: exertional dyspnea, decreased exercise tolerance, palpitations	Small to moderate shunt: asymptomatic, exertional dyspnea; large shunt	Asymptomatic; if develops symptoms: exertional dyspnea; decreased exercise tolerance	Asymptomatic; symptoms may be related to high BP or increased failure	Clinical symptoms vary from asymptomatic to mild to moderate exertional dyspnea and fatigue; complaints of palpitations and lightheadedness	In adulthood (following palliation): exertional dyspnea, cyanosis with clubbing
PHYSICAL EXAMINATION						Cyanosis: absent to moderate; mean JVP	
PALPATION	Neck vessels dilated and pulsating	Left parasternal lift	Large shunt: left parasternal lift	Left parasternal heave; subxiphoid pulsation	Delayed; diminished femoral pulsations; lag in timing of arterial pulses in lower extremities compared to upper extremities; presence of forceful carotid and suprasternal pulsations; visible collateral arterial pulses over scapula	Normal; RV impulse absent	Precordial prominence; parasternal heave

				Precordium; suprasternal thrill, normal to sustained LV impulse
AUSCULTATION	Systolic pressure normal; diastolic pressure low; wide pulse pressure; harsh, loud, continuous murmur in 1st, 2nd, 3rd ICS at lower LSB; machinerylike murmur best heard when patient is lying, becoming fainter when patient is standing	Small shunt: holosystolic at 3rd, 4th, and 5th ICS, systolic thrill; large shunt: holosystolic murmur at 3rd, 4th, and 5th ICS, splitting of S₂ during expiration, widening during inspiration, systolic ejection sound at 2nd ICS at LSB	Systolic pressure > diastolic, wide pulse pressure, differences in arterial pressure between right and left arms; continuous murmur in interscapular area and/or over upper thorax anteriorly and posteriorly; S₂—normal with loud aortic component; with bicuspid aortic valve—a systolic ejection murmur	S₁ is widely split with a loud, delayed S₂; S₃ may be present because of abnormal filling of RV; early systolic or holosystolic murmur; short mid-diastolic murmur occurs, especially in prolonged P-R interval
	Soft blowing systolic murmur at 2nd ICS at LSB	S₁ normal; early systolic ejection click heard at base; midsystolic murmur at 2nd and 3rd ICS at LSB, radiates to suprasternal notch and to left side of neck; S₂ widely split		Single S₂; systolic ejection murmur at 3rd ICS; may radiate upward to left side of neck

From Canobbio MM: *Mosby's clinical nursing series: cardiovascular disorders*, St Louis, 1990, Mosby.

Table 3-6 Diagnostic Tests

Diagnostic Test	Patent Ductus Arteriosus	Atrial Septal Defect	Ventricular Septal Defect	Pulmonic Stenosis	Coarctation of Aorta	Ebstein's Anomaly	Tetralogy of Fallot
ELECTROCARDIOGRAM (ECG)	Normal (small ductus); LVH; P-R interval may be prolonged; atrial fibrillation	Normal; RVH; RBBB; P-R interval may be prolonged; left axis deviation (ostium primum); normal or right axis (ostium secundum)	Normal if defect is small; if moderate to large, LVH; LVH/RVH in presence of pulmonary hypertension	Normal if stenosis is mild; if moderate to severe, RVH and right axis deviation; if severe, right atrial hypertrophy (RAH)	Normal; LVH (in older patients); T wave inversion, S-T depression ($V_5 V_6$)	Normal; atrial flutter with one-to-one response or atrial fibrillation with rapid ventricular response via a right bypass tract; preexcitation (WPW) occurs in 20%-25% of patients	RVH
CHEST X-RAY	Normal; with moderate to large shunt, enlarged cardiac silhouette with enlarged LA, LV, and pulmonary artery (PA); enlarged aorta; enlarged pulmonary trunk and increased pulmonary flow	Enlarged RA, RV, PA; increased pulmonary vascular markings; LA, LV, and aortic knob may be small	Mild LVH with small shunt; with large shunt, increased LV, dilation of PA, increased pulmonary vascular markings; enlarged LA	Enlarged RV and PA; if severe, decreased peripheral pulmonary vascular markings	Normal; rib-notching caused by dilated intercostal collaterals; prominent ascending aorta; indentation below aortic knob at site of coarctation (3-sign); LV enlargement	Normal or cardiomegaly with enlarged RA; normal or decreased pulmonary vascularity	Small cardiac silhouette; small PA; prominent aorta (may arch to right in 25% of cases)

ECHOCARDIOGRAM	Ductus not visualized; enlarged LA and LV owing to left-to-right shunt	With ostium secundum, enlarged RV, paradoxic movement of septum during systole; with ostium primum, mitral valve displaced inferiorly and anteriorly	Defect not visualized; large shunt; enlarged LA	Normal if stenosis is mild; if moderate to severe, enlarged RA and RV thickness associated with bicuspid aortic valve	Normal; confirms presence of bicuspid aortic valve; increased LV thickness associated with bicuspid aortic valve	12-dimensional: delayed closure and increased amplitude of anterior tricuspid leaflet and displaced septal leaflet; atrialized RV	Overriding aorta visualized; pulmonary stenosis visualized with degree of obstruction; enlarged ventricular septum (septal motion remains normal)
LABORATORY TESTS	No specific findings	No specific findings	No specific findings unless patient is cyanotic, then increased Hct value, decreased Hgb level and arterial oxygen saturation	No specific findings	No specific findings	No specific findings unless patient is cyanotic, then increased Hct	Increased Hct value; degree depends on amount of deoxygenated systemic blood

From Canobbio MM: *Mosby's clinical nursing series: cardiovascular disorders*, St Louis, 1990, Mosby.

Continued.

Table 3-6 Diagnostic Tests—cont'd

Diagnostic Test	Patent Ductus Arteriosus	Atrial Septal Defect	Ventricular Septal Defect	Pulmonic Stenosis	Coarctation of Aorta	Ebstein's Anomaly	Tetralogy of Fallot
CARDIAC CATHETERIZATION	Increased pulmonary blood flow; increased oxygen saturation in PA; intracardiac pressures normal; RV and PA pressures may be slightly elevated	Left-to-right shunt; increased oxygen saturation in RA; RA pressure usually normal; mitral regurgitation	Left-to-right shunt; study determines degree of shunt; increased pulmonary blood flow, oxygen saturation in RV, and systolic pressure	Increased RA pressure, which determines systolic pressure gradient between RV and PA	Aortography confirms obstruction and determines pressure gradient	Done to evaluate degree of tricuspid regurgitation	RV outflow obstruction; increased RV pressure; RV to LV shunt; decreased PA pressure as catheter crosses obstruction

Explain importance of regular or periodic medical
follow-up

Home care considerations

Review activity allowances and limitations as indi-
cated by clinical status including recreational sports,
ADLs
Provide counseling with respect to education, employ-
ment, and insurability
Discuss any dietary limitations
For adolescents and young adults, provide counseling
concerning childbearing, genetics
For women, provide information regarding
Gynecology: report any signs of dysfunctional bleeding (e.g., heavy bleeding, irregular or missed pe-
riods)
Contraception: appropriate forms
Pregnancy and delivery, associated risk with type of
defect, and current clinical status; discuss impor-
tance of obtaining prepregnancy counseling
For cyanotic patient
Describe signs of hyperviscosity: headaches, muscle
aches, visual disturbances, lightedheadness, paresthesia of fingers and toes, and need to report to
physician for laboratory evaluation
Discuss importance of avoiding dehydration and
overexertion, particularly on hot days
Discuss importance of not using tobacco products
Discuss need to avoid aspirin and iron replacement
without checking with physician

Pericarditis

*An inflammatory process involving the parietal and
visceral layers of the pericardium and outer
myocardium. Pericarditis occurs as an acute process;
an exudate of fibrin, white blood cells, and endothelial
cells is released. Chronic pericarditis, referred to as
"constrictive pericarditis," is characterized by dense
fibrous pericardial thickening.*

Assessment

Subjective data

Chest pain
Precordial
May radiate to shoulder or neck
Severe, sharp
Dsypnea
Nausea
Muscle aches

Objective data

Substernal chest pain
Increases with inspiration
Relieved by sitting up and leaning forward
Increased systemic venous pressure
Pericardial friction rub: scratchy sound in time with
heartbeat
Elevated temperature
Chills alternating with diaphoresis
Restlessness
Anxiety
Fatigue
Orthopnea

Diagnostic tests

ECG
Elevated ST segment in LV leads: V_5, V_6, I, II, aV_L and
aV_F
T wave inversion (late stage)
Low-voltage QRS complex in presence of pericardial
effusion
Dysrhythmias
Blood studies
CBC: leukocytosis (increased WBC); increased ESR;
elevated viral titers
Chest x-ray examination: normal or symmetrically en-
larged cardiac silhouette
Echocardiogram: presence of pericardial effusion
Radionuclide blood pool scanning
Technetium label macroaggregated albumin and thal-
lium (confirms presence of pericardial effusion)
Magnetic resonance imaging (MRI): visualizes peri-
cardium

Potential complications

Pericardial effusion
Cardiac tamponade
Heart failure

Collaborative management

Therapeutic management

Medications
Nonsteroidal antiinflammatory agents: indomethacin
Analgesics, antipyretics: aspirin
Corticosteroids
Pericardiocentesis
Surgical procedures
Pericardial window
Pericardiectomy

Nursing management

PATIENT PROBLEMS/NURSING DIAGNOSES

● **NDX:** Pain, chest related to pericardial inflammation

Assess and record quality of chest pain *to distinguish pericardial pain from myocardial ischemia*
Supervise activity
  Maintain bed rest, elevate head 45 degrees, position for comfort, provide padded overbed table *to minimize pain that is aggravated by movements*
Administer pain medications *to provide relief and suppress inflammatory symptoms*

EXPECTED OUTCOME

Chest pain is relieved

● **NDX:** Anxiety related to perceived or actual threat to biologic integrity

Assess level of anxiety and degree of understanding, noting verbal and nonverbal expressions, *to determine source of anxiety and identify any misunderstanding of disease process or treatment*
Provide supportive care *to ensure sense of trust, comfort, and reassurance*
Remain with patient if anxious
Encourage communication with significant other/family
Explain procedures and treatments thoroughly
Ensure quiet environment *to reduce external stimuli*
Use calm, reassuring voice

EXPECTED OUTCOME

Patient's anxiety level is reduced; appears calm

● **NDX:** Risk for decreased cardiac output related to reduced ventricular filling

Assess and monitor for signs of cardiac tamponade, which is a complication
Check for pulsus paradoxus, narrowing pulse pressure, respiratory filling of neck veins *to detect early signs of increasing intrapericardial pressure and development of tamponade*
Monitor BP, T, R, and apical pulse q4h as indicated *to detect pericardial restriction, hypotension, and tachycardia*
Place on cardiac monitor during acute phase, checking rhythm q1h to 2h *to detect nonspecific changes caused by superficial injury to epicardial surface of heart*
Obtain 12-lead ECG as ordered
Auscultate heart sounds for presence of pericardial friction rub, *which may reflect presence of pericardial effusion,* q6h to 8h
Administer medications as ordered
Prepare for pericardiocentesis when ordered

EXPECTED OUTCOMES

Cardiac output and hemodynamic stability maintained
Vital signs within normal limits
Negative for pulsus paradoxus

Patient/family teaching

Discuss symptoms of recurrence to report to physician
  Increasing fatigue
  Elevated temperature
  Difficult respirations
  Chest pain
Explain that symptoms may continue up to 2 wk, but notify physician if symptoms do not diminish or if they increase
Explain need to avoid persons with infections, especially URIs, and to report symptoms (e.g., cold, influenza, cough) to physician
Explain need to avoid overexertion and heavy lifting; alternate periods of activity with rest
Explain importance of ongoing outpatient care
Discuss medications: name, dosage, time of administration, purpose, and side effects
Explain need to avoid taking over-the-counter medications without checking with physician

Cardiac Tamponade

Rapid accumulation of fluid or blood within the pericardial cavity that results in restriction of diastolic filling and causes decrease in the stroke volume and cardiac output

Assessment

Subjective data

Pain or discomfort in chest, abdomen
Dyspnea
Restlessness

Objective data

Distended neck veins with inspiratory rise in venous pressure (Kussmaul's sign)
Decreased systolic BP; narrowing pulse pressure; pulsus paradoxus >10 mm Hg
Decreased and/or distant heart sounds

Pericardial friction rub
Anxiety
Tachypnea
Tachycardia: weak, absent peripheral pulses
Skin
  Cyanotic
  Dusky
  Pale
Posture: Patient sits upright or leans forward
Hemodynamic findings
  Decreased CO
  Elevated RAP
  Elevated CVP
  Lowered left atrial pressure (LAP)

Diagnostic tests

Echocardiogram: pericardial effusion; paradoxic septal
  motion
ECG
  Tachycardia
  Nonspecific ST and T wave changes
  Diminished voltage, altering voltage of both P wave
    and QRS complex
  Dysrhythmias
Chest x-ray examination: enlarged cardiac silhouette
  (globular shape); lung fields clear
Blood pooling scanning
Magnetic resonance imaging (MRI): to show loculated
  effusions
Right heart catheterization: decreased ventricular fill-
  ing pressures, elevated RAP

Potential complications

Heart failure
Cardiogenic shock
Cardiac arrest

Collaborative management

Therapeutic management

NPO
Parenteral fluids: volume expanders
Pericardiocentesis
Medications
  Inotropic, chronotropic
  Corticosteroids
  Antiarrhythmics
12-lead electrocardiogram
Maintain defibrillator and emergency drugs at bedside
Surgery: pericardiectomy

Nursing management

PATIENT PROBLEMS/NURSING DIAGNOSES

● **NDX:** Decreased cardiac output related to restricted ventricular filling

Assess for and estimate degree of pulsus paradoxus
  and increased JVP *to confirm presence of tamponade
  and increased intrapericardial pressure*
Maintain bed rest; elevate head of bed 45 degrees (see
  Figure 3-7)
Place patient on cardiac monitor; check rhythm strip qh
Monitor arterial pressure, pulse pressure, pulse vol-
  ume, ECG, and level of consciousness q5min to 15min
  *to evaluate signs of progressive impairment of ventricu-
  lar filling*
Administer parenteral fluids as ordered
Administer medications as ordered
Assist with pericardiocentesis

EXPECTED OUTCOMES

Patient demonstrates hemodynamic stability
Patient tests negative for pulsus paradoxus
Vital signs within normal limits
Jugular venous distension decreases

● **NDX:** Anxiety (moderate to severe) related to perceived and/or actual threat to biology integrity

Assess level of anxiety, noting both verbal and nonverbal expressions
During this period, remain with patient and offer realistic assurances; use simple explanations *to ensure sense
  of trust and comfort*
Ensure quiet environment *to reduce external stimuli as
  much as possible*

EXPECTED OUTCOME

Patient's anxiety level is reduced (i.e., patient appears
  relaxed)

Pericardiocentesis

*Withdrawal of blood or fluid from the pericardial sac via
  percutaneous needle puncture (Figure 3-13)*

Preparation and patient teaching

Reinforce physician's explanation of procedure
Obtain signed consent
Maintain NPO 4 to 6 hr before procedure when
  possible

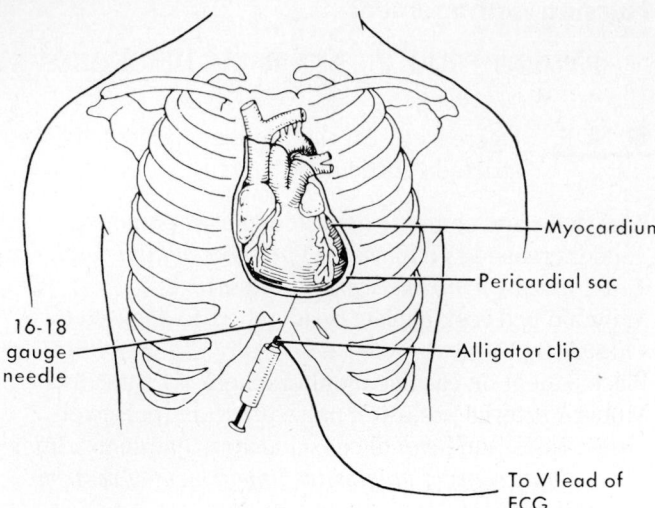

Figure 3-13 Pericardiocentesis. (From Sheehy SA: *Emergency nursing: principles and practice,* ed 3, St Louis, 1992, Mosby.)

Elevate head of bed 20 to 30 degrees as ordered (see Figure 3-7)
Obtain 12-lead ECG and rhythm strip; connect ECG unipolar lead to needle using alligator clip
Obtain laboratory studies as ordered: CBC, PT, PTT, platelets
Administer oxygen by mask or cannula as ordered
Obtain and record baseline arterial pressures, paradoxic pulse, and pulse pressure
Maintain parenteral fluids as ordered
Obtain necessary equipment as ordered
  ECG machine
  Needles: No. 16 spinal
  Syringes: 30 ml and 50 ml
  Three-way stopcock
  Sterile drapes
Administer medications as ordered
  Atropine
  Lidocaine
  Sedatives
Maintain defibrillator and emergency drugs at bedside
Provide emotional support

Assessment during and after procedure

Objective data

Level of consciousness
ECG
  ST elevations
  Increased P-R interval
Arterial pressure
RAP
Pericardial aspirate
  Amount

Color
Turbidity
Presence/absence of blood

Potential complications

Puncture of coronary artery, ventricle, or lung
Dysrhythmias
Ventricular fibrillation
Laceration of lung
Pneumothorax
Recurring cardiac tamponade

Postprocedure care and patient teaching

Maintain bed rest
Assess BP, R, and apical pulse q15min for 1 hr, then q4h as ordered
Monitor arterial pressures; check for decreased pulse pressure or pulsus paradoxus q15min for 1 hr, then q4h as ordered
Maintain NPO as ordered
Auscultate heart sounds q2h to 4h
Observe for recurrence of tamponade; be prepared to repeat pericardiocentesis or surgical intervention
Continue ongoing care for specific disease process

Heart Failure

Inability of the heart to increase cardiac output sufficiently to meet the body's metabolic demand

Assessment

Subjective data

Fatigue
Effort intolerance
Anorexia
Dyspnea
Nocturia

Objective data

  GENERAL
Cachexia
Nausea and/or vomiting
Tachypnea
Tachycardia
Pulsus alternans
Heart sounds: gallop rhythms (S_3, S_4)
Peripheral cyanosis
Anxiety

Restlessness
Lung sounds: crackles, rhonchi
Cheyne-Stokes respiration
Drug toxicity
  Digitalis toxicity
  Hypokalemia
Dysrhythmias

LEFT VENTRICULAR FAILURE

Shortness of breath
Restlessness
Dyspnea, exertional and/or at rest
PND
Orthopnea
Tachypnea
Dry, unproductive cough
Hemoptysis
Elevated BP
Tachycardia
Pulsus alternans
Left ventricular gallop: S_3
Hypoxemia
Crackles, rhonchi
Cyanosis

RIGHT VENTRICULAR FAILURE

Increased venous pressure (rise in "a" and "v" waves)
Distended neck veins
Firm, pitting edema
Peripheral edema
  Sacrum
  Genitalia
  Ascites
Right upper quadrant abdominal tenderness
Hepatosplenomegaly; hepatojugular reflex
Diaphoresis
Weight gain
Right ventricular gallop: S_3
Decreased urine output
Anorexia

Diagnostic tests

GENERAL

Serum
  HcT, HgB
  BUN, creatinine
  Electrolytes
    Hyponatremia
    Hyperkalemia
    Hypokalemia
  Bilirubin: hyperbilirubinemia
  Enzymes: AST, ALT, LDH
  PT/INR

  Albumin
  Glucose
Arterial blood gases
Urine
  Specific gravity
  Protein
  Creatinine
  Sodium
ECG
Chest x-ray examination
Echocardiogram
MUGA
Hemodynamic monitoring
Pulmonary function tests

LEFT VENTRICULAR FAILURE

ECG: left ventricular hypertrophy (LVH), left atrial hypertrophy (LAH), dysrhythmias
Increased PCWP
Decreased CO
Chest x-ray
  Redistribution of pulmonary flow to upper lobes
  Kerley B lines
  Pleural effusion
  Increased cardiac shadow
Pulmonary function test: decreased vital capacity (VC), residual volume, and total lung capacity

RIGHT VENTRICULAR FAILURE

ECG: Right ventricular hypertrophy (RVH), right atrial hypertrophy (RAH)
Elevated RA, RV pressure
Elevated CVP
Chest x-ray examination: generalized enlargement of cardiac shadow

Potential complications

Pulmonary edema
Embolic phenomenon
Pulmonary infarction
Cardiogenic shock

Collaborative management

Therapeutic management

Low-sodium diet
Medications
  Diuretics
  Vasodilators
  Beta-blocking agents
  Inotropic drugs
  Morphine sulfate
Oxygen therapy
Hemodynamic monitoring

SVO_2
Intraaortic balloon pump (IABP)
Ventricular assistive devices (VAD)

Nursing management

PATIENT PROBLEMS/NURSING DIAGNOSES

● **NDX:** Decreased cardiac output related to mechanical factors (preload, afterload, or contractility)

Assess and monitor BP, apical pulse, HR, and R q4h or as indicated *to detect signs of decreased CO*
Maintain bed rest as indicated to conserve energy; elevate head of bed 30 to 60 degrees *to facilitate ventilation;* lean patient forward on padded overbed table as needed
Monitor and record hemodynamic pressures *to evaluate preload and afterload parameters* and *to assess response to therapy*
Administer medications as ordered
Monitor for signs of drug toxicity; monitor drug levels
Restrict activities as indicated by condition
Provide bedside commode
Implement measures that *prevent fatigue*
  Plan rest periods between procedures
  Have patient rest before and after meals
  Maintain planned rest periods
Provide emotional support, offer simple explanations

EXPECTED OUTCOMES
Vital signs within acceptable limits for age
HR, CO, PCWP within acceptable limits
Urine output increased
Activity tolerance is increased

● **NDX:** Fluid volume excess related to compromised regulatory mechanism

Assess and monitor for signs of fluid retention, increased congestion, and/or response to therapy
  Check for increase or decrease in jugular venous pressure
  Auscultate chest for breath and heart sounds (S_3, S_4) q4h to 8h
  Measure intake and output; record output qh; report output <30 ml/hr
  Weigh patient daily (same time, scale, and clothing); report increase of 500 g/day or greater
Maintain parenteral fluids by microdrip when ordered; avoid rapid and excessive hydration; use concentrated IV infusion *to decrease volume administration* when possible

Administer diuretics and vasodilator therapy as ordered; observe for effect and toxicity
Estimate diaphoretic fluid loss
Monitor BUN and electrolytes
Maintain sodium-restricted diet and maintain fluid restrictions *to control sodium resorption and fluid retention;* assist patient with planning distribution of fluids over waking hours

EXPECTED OUTCOMES
Patient exhibits no signs of fluid overload as evidenced by the following:
Absence of edema
Weight loss, return to baseline
Lung sounds clear; heart sounds normal (i.e., no S_3, S_4)
No signs of increased jugular venous pressure

● **NDX:** Impaired gas exchange related to alveolar-capillary membrane changes caused by increased pulmonary capillary pressure

Assess and monitor for changes in respiratory function *to detect signs of impaired ventilation and perfusion*
Monitor serial arterial blood gases *to identify hypoxemia, hypercapnia*
Auscultate lung sounds q4h *to detect increases in congestion*
Monitor chest x-ray examinations for changes
Monitor hemodynamic parameters that are indicators of degree of pulmonary congestion: PAP, PCWP
Elevate head of bed; have patient lean forward on padded overbed table; reposition q2h to 4h as indicated *to enhance ventilation and gas exchange*
Administer oxygen therapy *to increase arterial oxygenation* as ordered; prepare for intubation and assisted mechanical ventilation if required
Provide humidified inspired air *to liquefy secretions as ordered*
Instruct patient to cough and breathe deeply *to facilitate ventilation and remove secretions*
Administer medications as ordered
  Morphine
  Rapid-acting diuretics
Instruct patient to avoid using tobacco products
Provide brief explanations of all treatments and procedures *to prevent hyperventilation resulting from fear or anxiety*

EXPECTED OUTCOMES
Patient demonstrates improved gas exchange as evidenced by the following:
Effortless breathing
Improved respirations
Lungs clear on auscultation
Po_2 and Pco_2 levels within normal limits

● **NDX:** Risk for impaired skin integrity related to impaired circulation and metabolic state

Assess skin integrity and bony prominence daily for signs of redness, scaling, breaks, or ulcerations

Initiate measures *to maintain skin integrity and enhance circulation*

  If patient is on bed rest, turn and reposition q2h

  Provide alternate preventive devices

    Alternating pressure mattress

    Air pressure beds (Clinitron)

  Prevent and eliminate pressure and friction; position pillows or other supports between pressure areas *to avoid two skin areas touching*

Assist patient out of bed frequently or as ordered

Administer skin care q2h

  Keep skin clean and dry

  Massage bony prominence q2h to 4h using lanolin-based lotion

NOTE: To prevent skin excoriations, do not massage reddened area

Initiate decubitus care at first signs of tissue breakdown or ulceration (p. 37)

EXPECTED OUTCOMES

Patient demonstrates maintenance of skin integrity as evidenced by the following:

Skin intact

Warm and dry, normal color

Signs of healing over areas of breakdown

● **NDX:** Altered nutrition: less than body requirements related to impaired absorption of nutrients secondary to decreased cardiac output

Observe daily for signs of malnutrition and cardiac cachexia

  Dry body weight 20% or more under the ideal for age, height, and frame

  Decreased triceps skinfold measurements

  Stomatitis

  Anorexia

  Increasing fatigue and weakness

  Decreased serum albumin, transferrin, iron-binding capacity, BUN

  Lack of interest in food

Determine patient's baseline weight

Weigh patient daily (same time, scale, and clothing) *to determine accurate weight and caloric needs*

Administer oral hygiene q2h to 4h

Administer medications to relieve nausea and/or vomiting; arrange medication schedule so it does not interfere with mealtime

Maintain diet as ordered; consult with dietitian *to evaluate nutritional status and to assist in selection of foods*

Do not force patient to eat

Tempt appetite with food preferences compatible with diet restrictions and cultural values

Remove unsightly and odorous items from room during mealtime

Serve small, frequent meals

Supplement with high-calorie foods *to maintain minimum required caloric intake*

Initiate caloric count if nutritional status fails to improve

Initiate tube feedings or parenteral nutrition as indicated

EXPECTED OUTCOMES

Patient demonstrates adequate nutritional status as evidenced by the following:

Dry body weight that is improved or normal for age and body build

Improved appetite

Good skin turgor, increased muscle mass

● **NDX:** Activity intolerance related to weakness secondary to decreased cardiac output

Assess and monitor for signs of activity intolerance

Check BP, HR, and R before and after activity *to detect orthostatic hypotension,* which can result from prolonged periods of bed rest and inactivity

Maintain patient on bed or chair rest with feet elevated as indicated

Identify factors known to cause fatigue; restrict and/or limit activities as indicated (e.g., number of visitors and their length of stay) *to promote energy conservation*

Space treatments and procedures *to allow for periods of uninterrupted rest;* provide periods of rest throughout day and evening to ensure periods of complete rest

Implement measures that will improve activity tolerance by minimizing fatigue (e.g., bathing in shower with chair rather than self-bathing); using bedside commode rather than bedpan to limit energy expenditure

Increase activity level as indicated; assess activity tolerance and activity progression *to evaluate improved myocardial performance*

EXPECTED OUTCOMES

Patient demonstrates improved activity tolerance

Verbalizes improved energy to perform ADLs

ECG, BP, HR, and R within acceptable limits during and after activity

ADDITIONAL NURSING DIAGNOSES
TO CONSIDER

Fatigue
Ineffective coping; patient, family

Patient/family teaching

Assess level of understanding
Discuss nature and cause of disease process and under-
lying cause
Review symptoms of early heart failure to report to
physician
Decreased exercise tolerance
SOB
DOE
PND
Persistent cough
Swelling of extremities
Sudden weight gain of >3 lb (6.6 kg) in a 24-hr pe-
riod
Nocturia
Discuss need to avoid persons with infections, espe-
cially URIs
Explain importance of not using tobacco
Teach patient/family to monitor and record heart rate
and report any changes
Discuss medications: name, dosage, time of administra-
tion, purpose, and side effects
Explain importance of avoiding extreme temperature
changes
Explain importance of ongoing care

Home care considerations

Discuss importance of daily weighing (same time,
scale, and clothing) and reporting increases of >2
pounds within 24 hr
Refer to home health agency for assistance with ADLs
as necessary
Activities
Discuss importance of pacing activities to avoid
overexertion and fatigue
Alternate exercise and other activities with rest periods
Use energy-saving techniques (e.g., sitting to brush
hair and prepare foods)
Diet
Discuss importance of maintaining prescribed diet
and fluid amounts; need to avoid food high in
sodium
Instruct patient to read labels for sodium content be-
fore buying
Provide information on alternate ways to season
foods
Refer to dietitian for diet planning

Shock

*A clinical syndrome in which blood flow to the tissues is
insufficient to sustain normal cell metabolism,
resulting in a generalized decrease in perfusion to
vital body function (see the box below and
Table 3-7)*
*hypovolemic shock ("cold" shock): Deficient return
of venous blood to the heart caused by external losses of
blood plasma or extracellular fluid or caused by internal sequestration of plasma*
*vasogenic (warm shock): Shock syndrome that results
in massive vasodilation from an increase in total vascular capacity; most common form is sepsis but may occur as a result of other factors including anaphylactic
reactions*
*cardiogenic shock: Shock caused by inadequate tis-
sue perfusion that results from impaired LV function*

Assessment

Subjective data

Restlessness
Anxiety
Irritability

Shock Syndrome: Causes/Etiologies

HYPOVOLEMIC SHOCK

Loss of blood volume (hemorrhage, gastrointestinal bleeding, wounds)
Loss of plasma volume (dehydration, burns, peritonitis)

CARDIOGENIC SHOCK

Acute myocardial infarction
Septal rupture
Other causes (pulmonary emboli, cardiac
surgery, tamponade)

VASOGENIC SHOCK

Sepsis
Immune-mediated reactions (anaphylaxis)
Deep anesthesia effects

Dizziness
Faintness when sitting up

Objective data

HYPOVOLEMIC SHOCK

Decreased or falling BP: determined by patient's base-
line pressure
Narrowed pulse pressure
Hemodynamics
  Interarterial pressure
    Early: normal
    Late: decreased
  Decreased PAP, PCWP
  Decreased CO
  Decreased CVP (<3 cm H_2O pressure)
Low SVO_2
Flat neck veins
Collapsed peripheral veins
Tachycardia: weak, thready pulse
Tachypnea: shallow respirations
Extreme weakness
Altered levels in mental status
  Lethargy
  Semiconsciousness
  Coma
Circumoral pallor
Conjunctival pallor
Lip cyanosis
Skin
  Pale

Cool
Clammy
Cyanotic
  Mottling of extremities
Subnormal temperature
Excessive thirst
Nausea, vomiting
Renal status
  Urinary output below 30 ml/hr
  Elevated serum creatinine
  Elevated serum urea nitrogen
  Low urine sodium (less than 20 mEq/L)
Internal or external circulating blood volume loss
  due to the following:
  Hemorrhage
    Postsurgical
    Gastrointestinal (GI)
    After trauma
  Plasma volume losses
    Burns
    Excessive diarrhea, vomiting

VASOGENIC SHOCK

Early stage
  Normal or slightly decreased BP
  Decreased or normal SVR
  Hemodynamics
    Decreased or normal PCWP
    Greatly increased CO
    Warm skin
    Tachycardia: bounding pulse
Late stage
  Decreased BP
  Increased peripheral vascular resistance
  Decreased CO
  Decreased PCWP
  Increased SVR
  Metabolic acidosis
  Tachycardia
  Low SVO_2
  Excessive thirst
  Nausea, vomiting
  Tachypnea
  Temperature
    Subnormal
    Elevated
  Altered level of consciousness
    Lethargy
    Semiconsciousness
    Coma
  Skin
    Pale
    Cool
    Clammy
    Cyanotic

Table 3-7 Early and Late Signs of Shock Syndrome

Signs	Early	Late
Blood pressure	↓ Pulse pressure ↑ Diastolic pressure	↓ Systolic pressure
Urine output	↓ Urine sodium concentration ↑ Urine osmolality	↓ Urine volume
Acid-base changes	↑ Respiratory alkalosis Metabolic alkalosis	Metabolic acidosis
Tissue perfusion	Occasionally warm, dry skin	Cold, clammy skin
	Slight restlessness	Cloudy sensorium

From *Shock* 1976, The Upjohn Company. Reproduced with permission of The Upjohn Company.

Renal status
  Urinary output below 30 ml/hr
  Elevated serum creatinine
  Elevated serum urea nitrogen
  Wounds
    Swelling, redness
    Abnormal secretions
    Generalized urticaria, pruritus

CARDIOGENIC SHOCK

Decreased or falling BP; determined by patient's baseline pressure
Hypotension: systolic pressures <90 mm Hg
LV pressures
  Increased LVEDP
  Increased LAP
  Increased PCWP
Cardiac output
  2.2 L/min
  Decreased ejection fraction
  Decreased cardiac index
Increased SVR: >1600 dyne/sec/cm^{-5}
Elevated RV filling pressures
  Presence of jugular vein distension
  Increased CVP: above 15 cm H_2O pressure
  Positive hepatojugular reflex
Tachycardia
Thready radial pulse
Diminished or absent peripheral pulses
Presence of S_3, S_4 gallops or murmurs
Increased SVO_2
Respiratory distress
  Tachypnea
  Orthopnea
  Hypoxia
Alteration in level of consciousness
  Apathy
  Lethargy
  Semiconsciousness
  Coma
Skin
  Pale
  Cool
  Clammy
  Cyanosis
Temperature
  Subnormal
  Elevated
Excessive thirst
Nausea, vomiting
Renal status
  Urinary output below 20 ml/hr
  Elevated serum creatinine
  Elevated serum urea nitrogen
ECG changes

Ischemic changes
Dysrhythmias
Ventricular fibrillation
Pain
  Chest
  Abdominal

Diagnostic tests

HYPOVOLEMIC SHOCK

Electrolytes
Chemistries
Arterial blood gases
Specific gravity

VASOGENIC SHOCK

Cultures
Blood
Sputum
Urine
WBC
ESR
Chest x-ray examination
Clotting profile

CARDIOGENIC SHOCK

Serum
Arterial blood gases
Chemistries
Electrolytes
Drug levels
Cardiac enzymes
ECG
Chest x-ray examination
MUGA
Echocardiogram
Radionuclide ventriculography

Potential complications

HYPOVOLEMIC SHOCK

Heart failure

VASOGENIC SHOCK

Adult respiratory distress syndrome
Disseminated intravascular coagulation
Multisystem failure

CARDIOGENIC SHOCK

Metabolic acidosis
  Increased serum lactate levels
  Decreased pH
Electrolyte imbalances
Myocardial ischemia: elevated enzymes
Heart failure

Pulmonary edema
Adult respiratory distress syndrome
  Diminished breath sounds
  Pulmonary congestion

Collaborative management

Therapeutic management

Admission to cardiac intensive care unit
Cardiac monitor
Hemodynamic monitoring
Assisted mechanical ventilation
Oxygen therapy
Medications
  Vasodilator, sodium nitroprusside
  Sympathomimetic: dopamine, dobutamine
  Osmotic diuretics
For vasogenic shock: epinephrine, antihistamine, hydrocortisone
Parenteral therapy
  Blood replacement
  Plasma volume expanders
  Fluid challenges
Ventricular assist devices (VAD)
Intraaortic balloon pump

Nursing management

PATIENT PROBLEMS/NURSING DIAGNOSES

● **NDX:** Altered tissue perfusion (cerebral, cardiopulmonary, peripheral) related to decreased cardiac output

Assess for signs and symptoms of impaired tissue perfusion *to avoid rapid deterioration of vital functions associated with progressive shock*
Maintain complete bed rest; place patient in flat supine position; keep patient warm and position extremities *to minimize metabolic needs and facilitate circulation*
Maintain parenteral therapy as ordered: whole blood, plasamanate, volume expanders *to maintain adequate circulating volume*
Measure intake and output qh to evaluate kidney function and body volume
Connect indwelling urethral catheter to closed gravity drainage system; notify physician if urinary output is <30 ml/hr
Measure all body fluid loss; estimate loss in dressings or perineal pads
Administer medications as ordered
Assess for effects of drug therapy and signs of toxicity
Maintain NPO or only clear liquid diet as ordered

Check R, apical pulse, and femoral pulse q15min and prn *to assess for signs of vasoconstriction and tissue perfusion*
Monitor hemodynamic parameters as ordered *to assess clinical status and/or response to therapy:* cardiac output, PAP, PCWP
Monitor intraarterial pressure (IAP) q1h to 2h, check peripheral arm BP q15min if arterial line is not in place
Apply pressure to wounds *to control bleeding* if necessary
  Pressure dressing
  Direct pressure
  Gastric tube with balloon
Apply shock trousers as ordered; patient may arrive in trousers
Prepare medications to control bleeding if ordered
  Vitamin K
  Protamine sulfate
Prepare for surgery
  Resuturing of the bleeding site
  Removal of ruptured organ or resection of bleeding site
  See General preoperative care/teaching (p. 53)
Avoid routine nursing functions during acute phase

EXPECTED OUTCOMES

Tissue perfusion is maintained
Blood pressure is within normal limits
Urine output is normal
Skin warm and dry
Peripheral pulses more than 2T

● **NDX:** Decreased cardiac output related to mechanical factors (preload, afterload, and myocardial contractility)

Maintain complete bed rest; position *to promote optimal ventilation;* elevate head of bed 30 to 60 degrees and avoid routine nursing functions *to promote energy, increase venous return, and avoid drop in BP*
Initiate IV line: maintain an open vein
Monitor ECG continuously *to detect dysrhythmias that may result from depressed myocardial contractility*
Measure intake and output qh *to assess for signs of decreased CO or presence of hypovolemia*
Maintain parenteral fluids as ordered
Connect indwelling urethral catheter to closed gravity drainage system; notify physician if urinary output is <30 ml/hr
Check BP, R, apical pulse, and femoral pulse q15min and prn
Monitor LAP, PAP, and PCWP q1h to 2h as ordered
Measure and calculate CO, CI *to evaluate cardiac function*

Monitor intraarterial pressure q2h as order

Calculate systemic vascular resistance as ordered *to determine left ventricular afterload*

$$\frac{\text{mean aortic pressure} - \text{mean right atrial pressure (mmHg)}}{\text{cardiac output (L/min)}}$$

Check axillary temperature qh *to assess for elevations,* which can increase myocardial oxygen demand

Administer oxygen as ordered and prn

Administer medications as ordered

  To decrease afterload and O₂ consumption

    Vasodilator

    Corticosteroid

    Adjust flow rate according to BP response

  To increase myocardial contractility and reduce peripheral vascular resistance (PVR)

    Sympathomimetic

    Vasodilator

    Adjust flow rate according to BP response

Administer plasma volume expanders as ordered; adjust flow rate according to PAP and PCWP readings

Keep patient warm and dry

Auscultate heart sounds q2h to 4h

Prepare for and monitor intraaortic balloon counterpulsation as ordered; assess cardiac response

Restrict and plan activities; provide rest periods between procedures

Avoid constipation, straining, or rectal stimulation; give stool softeners or laxatives as ordered

EXPECTED OU.TCOME

Patient demonstrates improved cardiac output as evidenced by the following:

  Vital signs within normal limits

  CO and PCWP within normal limits

  Improved mentation

● **NDX:** Impaired gas exchange related to increased pulmonary capillary permeability

Assess respiratory pattern, noting rate and depth of respirations, *to assess adequacy of blood oxygenation and determine need for intubation*

Auscultate lungs q1h to 2h *to assess for pulmonary congestion*

Monitor serial arterial blood gases *to assess for decreased oxygen lung perfusion*

Monitor SVO₂; report SVO₂ <60% because this reflects decreased tissue perfusion

Administer oxygen as ordered *to ensure oxygen delivery and gas exchange*

Suction as ordered *to ensure patent airway, clear airway, and improve oxygen delivery*

Assist and teach patient to cough and breathe deeply q1h to 2h

EXPECTED OUTCOME

Patient demonstrates improved ventilation as evidenced by the following:

  Effortless breathing

  Clear lungs

  Po₂ and Pco₂ levels within normal limits

● **NDX:** Anxiety/fear related to actual or potential biologic threat

Determine patient's source of fear and anxiety *to understand patient's perception of situation*

Explain all procedures and treatments; offer brief explanations *to minimize feelings of uncertainty*

Remain with patient *to offer reassurance*

Anticipate needs *to minimize expenditure of energy*

Maintain quiet, nonstressful environment

Allow family or significant other to remain with patient as condition permits

Encourage verbalization of needs and fears of dying

Maintain calm and reassuring manner

EXPECTED OUTCOME

  Patient verbalizes decrease in anxiety level

ADDITIONAL NURSING DIAGNOSES TO CONSIDER

Altered nutrition: less than body requirements related to depleted glycogen stores

Risk for infection related to sepsis and impaired immune response

Risk for impaired skin integrity related to mechanical and internal factors

Cardiac Surgery (Open-Heart Procedure)*

Care depends on whether the operation is an open-heart procedure, requiring use of the cardiopulmonary bypass machine, or a closed-heart procedure that does not require use of the bypass machine

---

*The standard for postoperative care of the patient with open-heart surgery can be used in either cases of open-heart or closed-heart procedures. The patient with closed-heart surgery will usually require less specialized equipment with decreased frequency of nursing functions; however, such a patient may have complications that would also be seen with open-heart surgery (e.g., atelectasis and hypertension).

● Classification of Cardiac Surgery

Closed-heart surgery

Coarctation of aorta
Palliative pulmonary shunts
 Blalock-Taussig
 Potts anastomosis
 Glenn's
Closed mitral commissurotomy

Open-heart surgery

Congenital defects

Atrial septal defect (ASD)
Ventricular septal defect (VSD)
Transposition of great vessels
Tetralogy of Fallot
Truncus arteriosus
Tricuspid atresia
Aortic stenosis

Acquired defects, disorders

Coronary artery disease
Valvular heart disease
Aneurysm, ventricular, aortic

Procedures

Coronary artery bypass graft (CABG)
Aneurysm, repair, resection
Valve repair: commissurotomy, reconstruction, annulo-
 plasty
Valve replacement
Procedures for congenital heart defects
Cardiac transplantation

● Preoperative Care

Assessment

Subjective data

Emotions
 Anxiety: adaptive vs. maladaptive
 Euphoria
 Depression
 Denial
 Fear

Objective data

Level of consciousness
BP, T, P, and R
Skin
 Color
 Turgor
 Temperature
Peripheral circulation
Heart sounds
 Murmurs
 Rubs
 Gallops
Breath sounds: abnormal
 Decreased breath sounds
 Rales
 Wheezes
Smoking history
Weight and height
Activity tolerance
Medications being taken
 Cardiac medications
 Anticoagulants/antiplatelets
 Antidysrhythmics
 Birth control pills

Diagnostic tests

ECG: acute changes, increase in dysrhythmias
 12-lead
 Rhythm strip
Chest x-ray examination
 Cardiomegaly
 Pulmonary vascular congestion
Laboratory studies:
 CBC, Hgb, Hct
 Blood type and cross match
 Coagulation studies: PT, INR, APTT, and platelets
 Electrolytes
 BUN
 Creatine
 Urinalysis
 Pulmonary function
  Vital capacity
  Tidal volume
  Minute ventilation

Preoperative teaching

Assess level of understanding
Involve family or significant other in care and instructions
Reinforce physician's explanation regarding
 operative procedure

Location, type, and length of incision(s)
Length of time anticipated for recovery
Explain preoperative procedures
 Skin preparation: shaving, antiseptic bath or shower
 Visits from anesthesiologist and respiratory therapist
Check whether dental clearance was given (dental checks should be done 10 to 14 days before operation)
Explain and review postoperative procedures and routines of CCU or ICU
 How special unit will differ from regular unit
 Types of noises to be experienced
 Visiting privileges
 Usual length of stay in unit
 Pain to be experienced and availability of medications as needed
 Method of communication while intubated
 Disorientation that may occur resulting from medications and/or lack of sleep
Assess patient's awareness, emotional status, and fears regarding
 Surgical procedure
 Heart-lung machine
 Short- and long-term outcomes
 Possible disabilities
 Previous surgical experiences
Report any *acute* changes in emotional status
 Anxiety
 Depression
 Fear of dying
Instruct patient on simple relaxation techniques such as guided imagery
Introduce patient to unit staff who will be providing care postoperatively
When possible, introduce patient and family to CCU or ICU, explaining equipment to be used
 Cardiac monitor
 Hemodynamic monitor
 Drainage tubes
 Pacing wires, pacemaker
 Respirator
 Nebulizer
 Oxygen administration
 IV therapy
  Blood transfusions
  Replacement fluids
Review postoperative medications, particularly those that will be long term such as anticoagulants
Review procedures for and stress importance and purpose of the following:
 Turning
 Coughing
 Deep breathing
 Incentive spirometry
 Foot and leg exercises

Instruct patient to practice these procedures 1 to 2 days before operation
Withhold medications as ordered (e.g., anticoagulants)
Refer to spiritual advisor or social service worker as indicated

● Postoperative Care

Assessment
Observations/findings
 GENERAL
Neurologic: level of consciousness
Pulmonary system
 Respirations
  Quality
  Rate
  Character
 Breath sounds: equal or decreased
  Dullness
  Crackles
  Rhonchi
 Chest drainage
  Amount
  Quality
  Color
Cardiovascular system
 Hemodynamic parameters
  Arterial BP
  HR, rhythms
  SVo_2 LAP, LVEDP, PCWP
  CVP
 Heart sounds
  Rubs
  Murmurs
 Arterial pulses
  Quality
  Rate
  Rhythm
  Equality
Skin
 Color
 Turgor
 Temperature
ECG: check for presence of acute changes or dysrhythmias
Pacemaker: settings
Renal system
 Intake and output
 Urine output
  Amount
  Color
  Specific gravity
  Osmolality

Electrolytes
BUN, creatinine
Gastrointestinal system
Nasogastric tube drainage
Amount
Color
Absence or presence of bowel sounds
Abdominal tone
Flat
Distended
Tenderness
Incision(s), location
Midsternotomy
Submammary
Leg

VALVE REPLACEMENT

Type of valve replaced
Heterograft
Mechanical
Homograft
Valve sounds: normal
Mechanical: opening, closing clicks
Heterograft, homograft: produces no clicks
Valve dysfunction: occurrence of new regurgitant-type
murmur
Obstruction
Perivalvular leak
Rupture

CORONARY ARTERY GRAFT

Graft site
Saphenous vein
Mammary artery

CONGENITAL HEART DISEASE REPAIR

Type of repair: palliative, corrective
Use of conduits, grafts, baffles

Diagnostic tests

CBC, chemistries, electrolytes, platelet function, PT,
INR, APTT
Arterial blood gases
Chest x-ray examination

Potential complications

GENERAL

Cardiovascular system
Dysrhythmias
Premature ventricular contractions (PVCs)
Ventricular tachycardia
Atrial fibrillation

Atrial flutter
Asystole
Complete heart block
Fluid volume excess
Dyspnea, orthopnea
Increased JVD
Lung sounds: crackles
Heart sounds: S_3, S_4
Elevated PAP, LAP, and PCWP
Low CO syndrome
Restlessness, lethargy
Skin: cool, pale, peripheral cyanosis
Tachycardia
Decreased arterial pressure
Decreased urine output
Increased PCWP and LAP
Increased SVR
Hemorrhage
Increased drainage through chest tubes
Presence of bright red drainage
Adults: blood loss >150 ml/hr
Children: blood loss >5 ml/kg/hr
Decreased Hct
Hypotension
Pericarditis
Cardiac tamponade
Shock
Cardiogenic
Hypovolemic
Heart failure
Postpericardiotomy syndrome
Venous thrombosis
Pulmonary system
Atelectasis
Pleural effusion
Diaphragmatic dysfunction
Tension pneumothorax
Respiratory failure
Neurologic system
Altered level of consciousness
Postpump psychosis
Restlessness
Agitation
Confusion
Combativeness
Visual and auditory disturbances
Transient perceptual disorientation
Cerebral embolism; CVA (p. 578)
Renal system
Electrolyte imbalance
Hyponatremia
Hypokalemia
Metabolic
Acidosis
Alkalosis

Acute tubular necrosis (ATN)
Gastrointestinal system
  Stress ulcers
  Paralytic ileus
  Infection
    Sternal wound
    Leg wound

VALVE REPLACEMENT

Disintegration of prosthesis
Vegetations from resected valve
Endocarditis

MITRAL VALVE REPLACEMENT

Brain embolism
Supraventricular tachydisrhythmias
  Atrial tachycardia
  Rapid atrial fibrillation
Low CO syndrome

TRICUSPID VALVE REPLACEMENT/AORTIC VALVE REPLACEMENT

Conduction defects
Subendocardial necrosis

CORONARY ARTERY BYPASS GRAFT

Acute myocardial infarction
Ventricular dysrhythmias
  PVC's
  Ventricular tachycardia
Low CO syndrome
Graft failure
  Angina

CONGENITAL HEART DISEASE REPAIR

Conduction defects
Atrial dysrhythmias
Conduit obstruction
Patch leaks

Collaborative management

Therapeutic management

Admission to cardiac intensive care unit
Oxygen therapy with mechanically assisted ventilation
Cardiac monitor
Hemodynamic monitoring
SVo_2 monitoring
Medications
  Narcotics, analgesics
  Antihypertensives
  Antidysrhythmics

Inotropic agents
  Dopamine
  Dobutamine
  Digoxin
  Vasodilators
  Anticoagulants
  Electrolytes
Parenteral therapy
  Blood replacement
  Plasma expanders
  Colloids
Pacemaker insertion
Intraaortic balloon pump (IABP)
Ventricular assist devices (VAD)

Nursing management

PATIENT PROBLEMS/NURSING DIAGNOSES (ADULTS)

● **NDX:** Impaired gas exchange related to hypoventilation and/or ventilation/perfusion abnormalities

Assess and monitor respiratory function while patient is on ventilator *to detect abnormal ventilation*/perfusion resulting from effects of anesthesia, hypoxia, acid-base abnormalities
Maintain patent airway
Administer oxygen and assisted ventilation as ordered
Elevate head of bed 45 degrees *to promote oxygenation*
Assess quality and rate of R
Monitor FIo_2 tidal volume to yield arterial Po_2 of about 100 mm Hg
Obtain and monitor arterial blood gases as ordered; observe for and report signs of respiratory alkalosis or acidosis
Monitor SVo_2 as indicated
Auscultate lung sounds q1h to 2h *to assess resolving atelectasis and pulmonary congestion*
Suction q1h to 2h; hyperoxygenate 1 to 2 minutes before procedures; monitor and record any dysrhythmias
Assist and teach patient to turn; percuss chest and reposition q2h *to promote removal of secretions*
Encourage patient to turn, cough, and breathe deeply q1h to 2h in absence of endotracheal tube *to loosen secretions*
Have patient use high-humidity face mask after extubation *to avoid hypoxemia*
Obtain serial chest x-rays q4h to 6h as ordered *to detect signs of progressive pulmonary complications*

EXPECTED OUTCOME

Patient demonstrates adequate ventilation as evidenced by the following:
Effortless breathing
Absence of respiratory complications
Clear, equal, and bilateral breath sounds
PO_2 and PCO_2 within normal limits

● **NDX:** Decreased cardiac output related to mechanical factors (altered preload, afterload, contractility, heart rate) or electrical instability

Assess and monitor for signs of decreased CO *to detect early trends and changes*
Assess BP, apical pulse, and peripheral pulses q15min to 30min for 2 hr, then qh as ordered, reporting
Systolic BP: drop of 20 mm Hg
Systolic BP <80 or >180 mm Hg
Diastolic BP >100 mm Hg
Decreased amplitude in pulses
Pulse rate <60 or >100 beats/minute
Monitor PAP, PCWP, arterial pressure, and SVO_2 q15 min during immediate postoperative period, decreasing frequency as clinical status stabilizes
Calculate CO and SVR as ordered
Check temperature on admission once qh × 6, then q4h
Initiate rewarming procedures slowly; monitor for signs of shivering, which can increase metabolic demand
Blankets
Heat lamp
Auscultate heart sounds q2h to 4h
Monitor urine output qh; report outputs <30 ml/h
Administer fluids, blood products *to maintain adequate tissue perfusion*
Perform laboratory studies q4h to 6h as ordered
Cardiac enzymes, CPK-MB, SGOT, LDH *to detect ischemic changes*
Electrolytes and potassium levels (checked more frequently)
Hgb, Hct
Initiate IABP or VAD as ordered *to increase myocardial perfusion*
Avoid Valsalva's maneuver, such as caused by constipation
Bedside commode
Stool softeners
Mild laxative
Monitor and record dysrhythmias *to avoid hemodynamic compromise*
Record ECG rhythm strips qh; measure rate plus P-R, QRS, and Q-T intervals
Initiate temporary pacemaker *to maintain adequate cardiac index;* check rate and milliamperes (MA)
Administer antidysrhythmic agents as ordered

Administer medications to increase myocardial contractility, decrease SVR, control dysrhythmias

EXPECTED OUTCOME

Patient demonstrates improved cardiac output as evidenced by the following:
Vital signs within normal limits
CO, LVEDP, and PCWP within acceptable limits
Increased activity tolerance

● **NDX:** Risk for hemorrhage related to surgically induced fibrinolysis and/or inadequate reversal of heparin*

Assess and monitor for clinical signs of excessive bleeding that may occur as result of the effects heparin given intraoperatively (heparin rebound); platelet function is decreased
Perform blood studies q4h to 6h as ordered
Hgb, Hct
Coagulation: PT, INR, PTT, platelet count
Measure chest drainage qh; report drainage >150 to 200 ml/hr
Administer transfusions, platelets, and plasma expanders as ordered *to control bleeding and/or clotting disorders*
Administer drugs to correct coagulopathy
Protamine sulfate
6-aminocaproic acid (Amicar)
Epsilon aminocaproic acid (EACA)
Vitamin K
Check dressings q1h to 2h
Note drainage: amount, color, and consistency
Change as indicated

EXPECTED OUTCOME

Patient demonstrates stable hemostasis as evidenced by the following:
Progressive decrease in chest tube drainage
Stable or improved Hct, Hgb
Normal bleeding times: PT, INR, PTT, platelet count

● **NDX:** Ineffective breathing pattern related to decreased lung expansion

Assess rate and quality of respiration *to detect signs of decreased lung expansion or splinting*
Observe and maintain patency of chest tubes *to ensure proper drainage;* record drainage amount and color q1h to 2h and prn
Auscultate chest for diminished breath sounds q1h to 2h and later q4h to 6h *to detect and monitor signs of atelectasis*

---

*Not a NANDA-approved nursing diagnosis.

Encourage patient to cough and breathe deeply q1h to 2h *to mobilize secretions*

Assist and encourage patient to use incentive spirometer

Administer oxygen therapy as ordered

EXPECTED OUTCOME

Patient demonstrates fully expanded lung
  Bilateral equal excursion
  Full and clear breath sounds

● **NDX:** Risk for infection related to compromised host defense and environmental exposure

Monitor suture sites for local redness, drainage, and swelling *to detect developing infectious process*

Assess rectal, oral, or axillary temperature q2h as indicated *to detect infectious or inflammatory process*

Change incisional dressings daily

Administer antibiotics as ordered

Change IV and pressure lines and dressings according to protocol *to prevent nosocomial infections and cross contamination*

Remove urethral catheter when patient awakens or as soon as possible *to prevent urinary tract infection*

Obtain laboratory studies as indicated
  CBC with differential
  Blood and urine cultures

EXPECTED OUTCOMES

Patient shows no signs of infection
  Afebrile
  Wounds: no signs of irritation or redness

● **NDX:** Altered thought process related to biophysical changes (cerebral hypoxia, age, metabolic alterations, CNS depressants, sleep deprivation)

Assess level of consciousness and neurologic signs q15min to 30min for 2 hours, then qh or as indicated

Deal with any personality or psychologic changes
  Use reality orientation
  Offer explanations of all procedures
  Administer sedatives as ordered
  Reorient patient to time of day and surroundings
  Use simple, clear sentence structure
  Anticipate needs
  Maintain quiet environment; minimize external stimuli as much as possible
  Remain with patient
Allow family to visit and participate in care when possible

Provide assurance of daily progress

Maintain patient safety; use soft restraints

EXPECTED OUTCOMES

Patient regains baseline level of consciousness
  Arouses easily
  Clear mentation
  Oriented to time, place, situation

ADDITIONAL NURSING DIAGNOSES TO CONSIDER

Fluid volume excess related to expanded extracellular fluid volume

Ineffective family and individual coping: family, individual related to situational disorganization

Patient/family teaching

Assess level of understanding

Review nature and type of operative procedure, emphasizing precautions and complications associated with surgery

Explain importance of wearing medical alert band if patient has (is taking)
  Prosthetic valve
  Pacemaker (p. 182)
  Anticoagulants (p. 191)

Explain need to avoid persons with infections, especially URIs

Discuss symptoms of wound infection to report to physician
  Chest discomfort
  Elevated temperature
  Rapid, irregular pulse
  Chills
  Anorexia
  Redness
  Pain
  Swelling
  Drainage

Explain care of incision

Discuss importance of ongoing care

Discuss importance of contacting spiritual advisor or social worker as necessary

Discuss medications: name, dosage, time of administration, purpose, and side effects

Explain need to avoid taking over-the-counter medications without physician approval

Discuss diet as ordered
  Refer to dietitian for specific diets
  Restrict salt intake

Discuss symptoms to report to physician
  SOB
  Swelling of hands and legs

Home care considerations

Discuss activity limitations and allowances
  Ambulate to tolerance; avoid excessive physical exertion, lifting heavy objects or performing isometric exercises; restrict driving first 4 to 6 wk
  Instruct patient to increase activity gradually to avoid fatigue
  Avoid fatigue and sitting for long periods of time
  Explain that sexual activity may be contraindicated for 2 to 4 wk; need to check with physician for ability to resume

VALVE REPLACEMENT

Provide instruction regarding anticoagulation therapy
  Mechanical valves: life-long therapy
  Heterografts: 3 to 6 months as ordered
Explain importance of reporting to physician signs and symptoms of endocarditis
  Elevated temperature
  Chills, diaphoresis
  Anorexia
Discuss importance of reporting to physician any event that may predispose to bacteremia
  Dental and gum manipulation
  Genitourinary procedures
  Gynecologic procedures (D & C)
  Childbirth
  Skin boils, infective acne
Discuss importance of notifying all physicians, dentists, urologists, and obstetricians of valve replacement before any treatments
Encourage wearing medical alert bracelet or neck chain.
Discuss need to maintain good oral hygiene
  Daily care
  Regular visits to dentist
  NOTE: Patient should wait 6 weeks after surgery before seeing a dentist
Explain significance of prophylactic antibiotic therapy before procedures that predispose to bacteremia

Cardiac Transplantation

Assessment

Observations/findings

Rejection
  Mild to moderate: usually no clinical symptoms
  Severe: weakness, fatigue, malaise, anorexia, nausea and vomiting, decreased urine output, weight gain, peripheral edema, distended neck veins, increased jugular pulsations, decreased perfusion, cool pale skin, diminished pulses, diaphoresis, confusion, restlessness, pulmonary venous congestion, DOE, cough, tachycardia
  S_3, S_4
  Shock state
  Cardiac arrest

Potential complications

Infection: cytomegalovirus (CMV)
  Lymphoma
  Obstructive coronary atheroscleroses

Diagnostic tests

ECG: atrial dysrhythmia (e.g., PAC, atrial fibrillation)
NOTE: With cyclosporine, these ECG changes may not be seen
Chest x-ray examination: increased C-T ratio (cardiomegaly)
Echocardiogram: thickening of LV, decreased LV function, contractility
Endomyocardial biopsy (EMB)
  Lymphocytes (findings vary with degree of rejection)
  Mild, occasional WBCs
  Moderate: myocyte necrosis
  Severe: perivascular infiltration of lymphocytes, interstitial edema, myocyte, necrosis
  Increased CPK-MB, SGOT, LDH

Collaborative management

Therapeutic management

NOTE: Postoperative care is similar to that for any patient who has had cardiac surgery (p. 154)
Strict reverse isolation
EMB: once a week for 1 month, progressing to twice a week for 2 months
Diet: low saturated fat, cholesterol, sodium restriction (2 g)
Medications
  Cyclosporine (Sandimmune)
  Azathioprine (Imuran)
  Antithymocyte globulin (ATG)
  Orthoclone (OKT$_3$, Ortho)
  Corticosteroids
    Prednisone
    Methylprednisone (Medrol, Depo-Medrol, Solu-Medrol)
  Antihistamines
  Acetaminophen

Nursing management

PATIENT PROBLEMS/NURSING DIAGNOSES

● **NDX:** Risk for injury (rejection) related to noncompliance with prescribed medical regimen

Assess and evaluate patient for understanding of prescribed lifelong therapy *to identify potential adherence problems*

Encourage discussion regarding anticipated changes in lifestyle that may have a positive or negative effect

Ensure that patient is aware that skipping cyclosporine will result in rejection

Review prescribed medical treatment and drug therapy

Anticipate and allow questions regarding prescribed therapy

EXPECTED OUTCOME

Patient demonstrates no signs of rejection
  No new change(s) in EMB results
  No clinical signs of rejection

● **NDX:** Risk for infection related to immunosuppressive drug therapies

Assess and monitor for signs of infection *to begin medical therapy*
  Take temperature q4h
  Obtain cultures as indicated: sputum, throat, urine, any suspicious drainage in wounds
  Obtain and evaluate CBC; chest x-ray examination as indicated (NOTE: Laboratory values may be altered if steroids are taken)

Minimize or avoid use of invasive lines and/or procedures *to decrease risk of nosocomial or bacterial infections:* IVs, indwelling catheters

Change IV tubing, bags, and dressings every day using strict aseptic techniques

Do not place patient in room with another patient who is at risk for infection *to avoid potential cross contamination*

Institute reverse isolation for staff and visitors according to institutional protocol *to decrease potential new infections*

Minimize number of visitors; restrict visitors with signs of infections (e.g., colds, herpes simplex)

EXPECTED OUTCOME

Patient demonstrates no signs of infection
  Baseline temperature maintained
  CBC, urinalysis, cultures within normal limits

Patient/family teaching

Discuss and review signs and symptoms of rejection

Emphasize importance of keeping scheduled EMB appointments

Discuss lifelong need to take medications and need to take them exactly as prescribed; caution patient *never to stop* taking cyclosporine and to notify physician if dose is skipped

Review signs and symptoms of infection: elevation of baseline temperature, early signs of sore throat, cold, influenza

Discuss need to reduce risks of infection by avoiding individuals with infections or contagious diseases, avoiding large crowds

Discuss importance of lifelong follow-up: clinic visits, EMB appointments, and periodic stress test

Discuss activity allowances and limitations; instruct patient to check with physician before engaging in strenuous or competitive activities or sports

Discuss importance of daily weighing and reporting >2 lb weight gain in 24 hr

ADDITIONAL NURSING DIAGNOSIS TO CONSIDER

Risk for decreased cardiac output related to severe rejection

Postcardiac Injury Syndrome

A group of signs and symptoms that occur after injury to the myocardium or pericardial cavity, which are thought to be a result of an immune response or hypersensitivity reaction to pericardial injury

postcardiotomy syndrome: *After cardiac surgery (usually 7 to 10 days after surgery)*

postmyocardial infarction syndrome (Dressler's syndrome): *A late-appearing autoimmune response to myocardial necrosis; symptoms usually appear 3 to 6 wk after MI*

Assessment

Subjective data

Chest pain or discomfort
Dyspnea
Anxiety

Objective data

Elevated temperature
Diaphoresis
Pericardial friction rub

Malaise
Arthralgias

Diagnostic tests

Leukocytosis
Increased ESR
Chest x-ray examination: pleural effusions
Echocardiogram: pericardial effusion

Potential complications

Pericarditis
Cardiac tamponade

Collaborative management

Therapeutic management

Medications
  Analgesics
  Antipyretics
  Antiinflammatory agents

Nursing management

PATIENT PROBLEMS/NURSING DIAGNOSES

● **NDX:**   Pain, chest related pericardial irritation

Assess quality of chest pain
Encourage bed rest; position patient for comfort
  Elevate head of bed 45 degrees
  Provide padded overbed table
Auscultate heart sounds q6h to 8h *to detect pericardial rub*
Administer medications as ordered
  Analgesics
  Antiinflammatory agents
  Antipyretics

EXPECTED OUTCOMES
Patient verbalizes absence of chest pain
Activity level returns to normal

ADDITIONAL NURSING/DIAGNOSIS
TO CONSIDER
Anxiety related to perceived threat to health status

Patient/family teaching

Explain that syndrome commonly occurs after trauma
  or injury to heart and pericardial cavity and may clear
  up without specific treatment
Discuss symptoms to report to physician
  Elevated temperature

Chest pain
Chills, diaphoresis
Difficult respirations
Explain need to avoid fatigue, alternate periods of activity with rest
Discuss name of medication, dosage, times of administration, purpose, and side effects

Cardiac Rehabilitation

Physical and psychologic restoration of the patient with heart disease to an enjoyable and productive life as efficiently as possible; suggested for patients with angina, cardiomyopathy, pacemakers, and congenital heart disease and for patients recovering from myocardial infarction, valve surgery, and coronary artery bypass surgery *

● Inpatient Program

Assessment
Observations/findings

CRITERIA FOR TERMINATING EXERCISE
Symptoms during activity and/or 30 min after activity
  or exercise session
  Severe dyspnea
  Chest pain
  Vertigo
  Diaphoresis
  Fatigue
  Leg claudication
  Disorientation or confusion
  Palpitations
Heart rate
  Increase >20 to 25 beats/min during activity or exercise
  Appearance of irregular rhythm
On telemetry: during exercise and rest periods
  ST elevation of 3 mm or more
  ST segment depression of 2 mm
  Multiple premature ventricular contractions (PVCs)

ACTIVITY PROGRESSION PROGRAM
Follow physician's orders for progressive activity program
Initiate program using a predeveloped in-hospital exercise program (Table 3-8)

---

*Definition from *Guidelines for cardiac rehabilitation centers,* June 1985, copyright the American Heart Association Greater Los Angeles Affiliate.

Table 3-8 Cardiac Rehabilitation Program: Inpatient Activity (Myocardial Infarction)*

Level	Self-Care Activities	Position	Exercises	Repetitions	Education
Level I (1 to 1.5 MET†)	1. Absolute bed rest, complete bed bath 2. Begin feeding self while sitting with head of bed elevated to 45 degrees and arms supported 3. Turn self	1. Supine *Advance to:* Supine 2. Supine	a. Passive ROM: all extremities (excluding shoulders in acute MI) b. Active exercises: all extremities except shoulders as tolerated Deep breathing exercises: all levels	5 times 3 times	
Level II (1.5 to 2.5 MET [except bedside commode])	4. Bed rest 5. Feed self, wash face and hands, brush teeth, and shave in bed 6. Bedside commode (3 MET) 7. Up in chair 20-30 min bid 8. Light recreational activity such as reading, writing	3. Supine	Active plantar and dorsiflexion ankle exercises qid		
Level III (1.5 to 3 MET)	9. In bed, patient assists with self-bath (not legs or back) 10. Patient stands and vital signs are taken 11. May walk to bathroom with help 12. Walk to chair and sit 15 to 30 min tid	4. Supine Sitting *Advance to:* 5. Supine Sitting Sitting	a. Advance active exercises to include neck rotation and shoulder flexion to 90 degrees as tolerated b. Active exercises: all limbs including shoulder flexion to 180 degrees c. Knee extension and hip flexion a. Active exercises: all extremities b. Knee extension and hip flexion c. Shoulder flexion to 90 degrees	5 times 5 times 3 times 7 times 7 times 7 times	Begin education a. Energy conservation b. Body mechanics c. Concepts of heart anatomy and physiology
Level IV (3 MET)	13. Same as 9 14. Begin dressing self (gown and pajamas) 15. If vital signs stable, see 10; walk to bathroom for toilet use only 16. Sit in chair 2 to 3 times a day 30 to 60 min with assistance	6. Supine Sitting 7. Supine	a. Exercise 5a b. Exercise 5b Instruct patient to perform independent exercise 3 times a day (patient to take own pulse)	7 times 7 times 5 times	d. Begin instruction in self heart rate measurement e. Discuss inpatient activity: importance of pacing, rest, relaxation

Adapted from *Guidelines for cardiac rehabilitation centers,* June 1985, copyright the American Heart Association Greater Los Angeles Affiliate.
*Recommended levels and times are for average patients and must be individualized.
†MET: metabolic equivalent: the amount of oxygen consumed per kilogram of body weight per minute at rest. Approximately 3.5 cc kg/min.

Table 3-8 Cardiac Rehabilitation Program: Inpatient Activity (Myocardial Infarction)—cont'd

Level	Self-Care Activities	Position	Exercises	Repetitions	Education
Level IV—cont'd					f. Dietary assessment and referral if appropriate g. Begin discussion of: Signs and symptoms Risk factors Medication Warning signs Sexual counseling Activity progress
Level V	17. Sponge bathe self, sitting in bathroom (nurse bathes back) 18. Up in room and chair ad lib 19. Ambulate in hall 5 to 10 min with telemetry bid		Active exercises 5a, b, c; walk slow pace one half length of corridor (50 feet) with telemetry		
Level VI (3 to 4 MET)	10. Sit-down shower 21. Wash hair while seated 22. Shave, apply makeup in sitting position 23. Sit for meals 24. Full bathroom privileges 25. Up and about in room 26. Ambulate in hall 5 to 10 min bid with telemetry	8. Supine 9. Sitting 10. Walk 11. Ascend 12.	Active exercise 5a Active exercise 5b Increase distance walked, as tolerated, using moderate pace Three to six stair steps as tolerated May transport to cardiac rehabilitation center for low-level activity or test	5 to 7 times 7 times	Complete home instruction a. Diet b. Medications c. Activity allowances and limitations
Level VII (4 to 5 MET)	27. Same as level VI with addition of walking in hall 150 feet, advancing as tolerated 28. Evaluate any special requirements for home activities	13.	Continue stairs and ambulation as tolerated		
Level VIII	29. Same as levels VI and VII, advancing in frequency, distance, and time	14.	Establish progressive home activity program		

Assess patient's progress on a daily basis and plan activity levels for the day (done by rehabilitation team and/or charge nurse and physician)

Increase activity levels gradually until discharge date

Avoid exercises
  After meals; allow 1 hr
  In the presence of dysrhythmias
  In the presence of CHF

Begin exercise program while patient is on telemetry

Record and report any signs or symptoms of SOB, fatigue, or nausea if they occur during or up to 24 hr after exercise

Obtain the following baseline information before activity
  On telemetry
    ECG rhythm strip, noting rate and rhythm
    Resting BP, P, and R, noting rate, rhythm, and quality
    Atrioventricular (AV) block
    Paroxysmal atrial tachycardia
  BP
    Drop of 15 to 20 mm Hg when patient stands
    Decrease in pulse pressure
    Increase in systolic-diastolic pressures: >20 mm Hg

Collaborative management

Therapeutic management

Prescription for inclusion to program
Prescription for activity order

Nursing management

MI
  Maintain bed rest for first 3 to 4 days except for use of bedside commode
  Progress to chair rest
  Avoid prolonged bed rest
CABG
  Maintain bed rest for first 1 to 2 days postoperatively or as ordered by physician
  Start activity levels within 24 hr or as ordered by physician
  Off telemetry obtain resting BP, P, and R, noting rate, rhythm, and quality
Assist patient with performing activity
Obtain peak exercise heart rate
Obtain the following information during and 2 min after exercise
  On telemetry
    ECG rhythm strip toward end of activity, noting rate, rhythm, and ST segment changes or arrhythmias
    Postexercise heart rate

Off telemetry
  BP and HR at 1- and 2-minute intervals at end of exercise and at any signs of fatigue, pain, or SOB
Observe and report patient's tolerance

Patient/family teaching

Normal function of the heart
Nature and causes of coronary heart disease
Importance of identifying risk factors and need to modify or eliminate personal risk factors
  Family history of heart disease
  Patient history of heart disease
  Diabetes
  High blood pressure
  Overweight
  High cholesterol and/or triglyceride level
  Smoking
  Sedentary job and/or lifestyle
  Stressful lifestyle
Dietary restrictions and limitations
Importance of controlling weight
Importance of verbalizing any questions and feelings regarding presence of heart disease
Importance of verbalizing any feelings of anxiety and fear regarding sexual impotency, return to work, and death
Warning signs and symptoms of overexercising to report to physician
  Excessive fatigue
  Chest discomfort
  Muscle pain
  Dizziness
  SOB
  Palpitations
Physician's explanation of prescribed exercise program, allowances, and limitations
Need to avoid isometric (static) activities and/or exercises (e.g., pushing heavy objects, doing pushups, or carrying heavy objects)
Importance of taking and recording heart rate before and after exercise, noting rate and rhythm
Importance of reporting heart rate increase >20 to 25 beats/min
Recommended limitations and allowances for first 2 wk after discharge
  Avoid heavy lifting and pushing
  Refrain from extensive housework and gardening
  Avoid sitting in same position for longer than 2 hr
  Plan regular rest periods for at least twice a day
  Avoid vigorous arm and shoulder exercises, especially those that require arms to be held above shoulders (e.g., washing windows or painting house)

Space activities, alternating activity with rest period

Avoid exercising at the following times
  After meals; wait 1 hr
  When feeling very tired
  When suffering from a cold or other illness

Stop activity at onset of warning signs and rest

Importance of avoiding sexual activity for at least 2 wk (check with physician when feasible to resume; once resumed, avoid after eating heavy meals, drinking alcoholic beverages in excess, or becoming emotionally stressed)

Need to avoid travel by car, bus, airplane, or train without first checking with physician

All walking and exercise activities must be preceded by warm-up exercises

● Prescribed Exercise Program

Initial postdischarge activities for cardiovascular reconditioning

Continue predischarge activities; actively exercise all extremities including shoulder flexion and knee extension

Distance walking

Week after discharge	Total distance (mile)	Time (min)
1	0.25	8 to 10
2	0.25	5
3	0.5	15
4	1.0	30

Adjust speed and time to maintain heart rate at <100 beats/min

Record all exercise sessions, noting distance, time, and resting and peak heart rates (see chart below)

Exercise Record: Target Heart Rate: ___ beats/min

Date	Resting Heart Rate	Distance	Time	Peak Heart Rate	Comment
1-3-96	80	¼ mile	5 min	100	No complaints

Follow all exercise sessions with a cooling down period

Cardiovascular reconditioning program

Ordered approximately 6 to 8 wk after discharge (done by physician)

Follow prescription for exercise determined by treadmill stress test before start of program

Electrocardiogram Rhythms

● Rhythms of Sinus Origin

Rhythms originating in the sinus (sinoatrial; SA) node (located in the right atrium near the opening of the superior vena cava, the sinus node functions as the normal pacemaker of the heart)

Assessment

Subjective data

Palpitations
Dizziness
Lightheadedness
Chest pain
Syncope

Objective data

Skin
  Pallor
  Diaphoresis

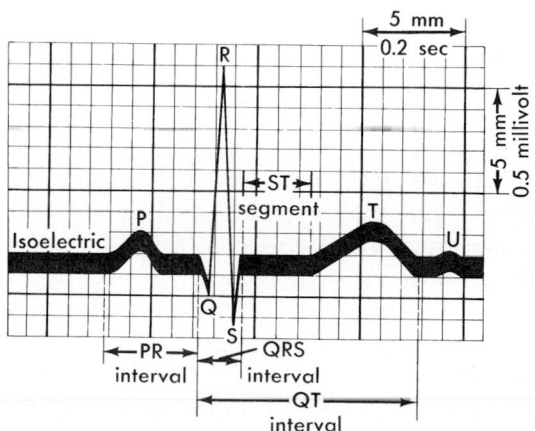

Figure 3-14 Normal electrocardiogram complex.

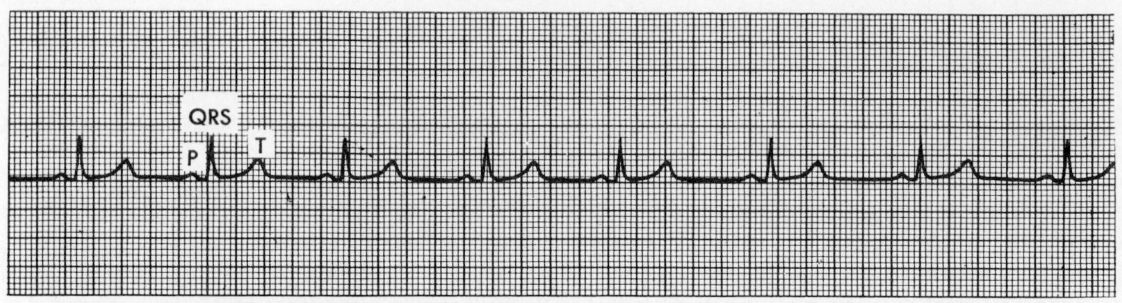

Figure 3-15 Cardiac cycle. Basic cardiac cycle (P = QRS = T). (From Goldberger AL, Goldberger E: *Clinical electrocardiography: a simplified approach,* ed 4, St Louis, 1990, Mosby.)

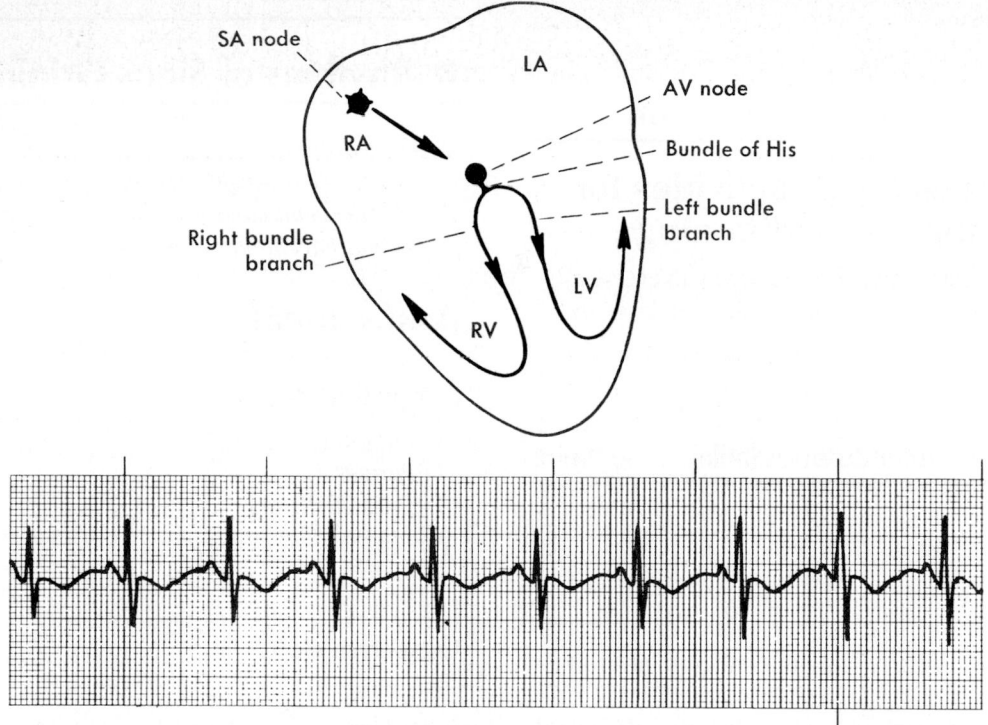

Figure 3-16 Normal sinus rhythm. (From Andreoli KG et al: *Comprehensive cardiac care,* ed 6, St Louis, 1987, Mosby.)

Heart rate
  Normal with ectopy
  Tachycardia
  Bradycardia
Heart rhythm
  Normal or irregular
Hypotension

Diagnostic tests

12-lead ECG
24-hr ambulatory ECG
Electrophysiologic (EP) studies
Signal average ECG

Normal sinus rhythm (Figures 3-14 to 3-16; Table 3-9)

Assessment

OBSERVATIONS/FINDINGS

Rhythm: regular
Rate: 60 to 100 beats/min
P wave: normal configuration, one before each QRS
P-R interval: 0.12 to 0.20 sec
QRS complex: 0.06 to 0.10 sec

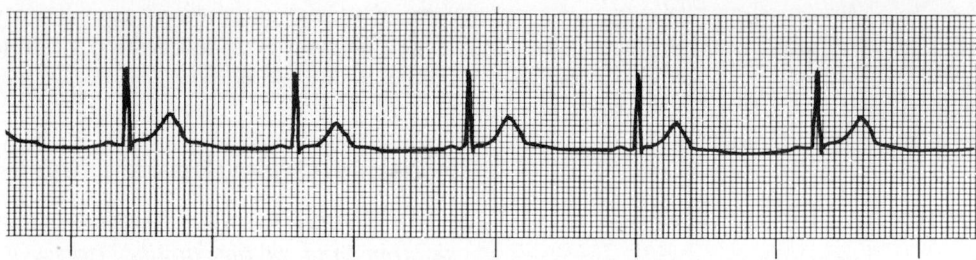

Figure 3-17 Sinus bradycardia. (From Andreoli KG et al: *Comprehensive cardiac care,* ed 6, St Louis, 1987, Mosby.)

Table 3-9 Meaning and Significance of ECG Intervals*

Description	Duration	Significance of disturbance
P-R interval: from beginning of P wave to beginning of QRS complex; represents time taken for impulse to spread through the atria, AV node, His bundle, bundle branches, and Purkinje fibers, to a point immediately preceding ventricular activation	0.12 to .20 sec	Disturbance in conduction, usually in AV node His bundle or bundle branches, but can be in atria as well
QRS interval: from beginning to end of QRS complex; represents time taken for a depolarization of both ventricles	0.06 to 0.10 sec	Disturbance in conduction in bundle branches and/or in ventricles
Q-T interval: from beginning of QRS to end of T wave; represents time taken for entire electrical depolarization and repolarization of the ventricles	0.36 to 0.44 sec	Disturbances usually affecting repolarization more than depolarization such as drug effects, electrolyte disturbances, and rate changes.

From Andreoli K et al: *Comprehensive cardiac care,* ed 6, St Louis, 1987, Mosby.
*Heart rate influences the duration of these intervals, especially that of PR and QT.

Collaborative management

None indicated

Sinus bradycardia (Figure 3-17)

A sinus rhythm <60 beats/min; etiology—may be normal or occur in response to drugs or increased vagal tone

Assessment

OBSERVATIONS/FINDINGS

Faintness
Dizziness
Syncope
Rhythm: regular
Rate: below 60 beats/min

P wave: normal configuration, one before each QRS
P-R interval: 0.12 to 0.20 sec
QRS complex: 0.06 to 0.10 sec

Collaborative management

None indicated unless patient is symptomatic
Medications
  Atropine
  Isoproterenol
Pacing: atrial, ventricular

Interventions

Check BP and apical pulse q4h and prn
Monitor cardiac activity; check rhythm strips q6h to 8h and prn
Administer oxygen therapy as ordered

Patient/family teaching

Ensure that patient and/or significant other knows and understands
  How to take radial pulse
  Pacemaker insertion (p. 182), if indicated

Sinus tachycardia (Figure 3-18)

A sinus rhythm >100 beats/min; causes—drugs, exercise, emotions, fever, increased sympathetic stimulation

Assessment

OBSERVATIONS/FINDINGS
Fatigue
SOB
Rhythm: regular
Rate: 100 to 160 beats/min
P wave: normal configuration, one before each QRS
P-R interval: 0.12 to 0.20 sec
QRS complex: 0.06 to 0.10 sec

Collaborative management

Treatment of underlying factors
Carotid sinus massage

Interventions

Administer medications as ordered
Check BP, R, and apical pulse q4h to 6h and prn

Administer oxygen therapy as ordered
Initiate measures to decrease work of heart: rest, avoidance of caffeine intake

Sinus dysrhythmia (Figure 3-19)

An irregular sinus rhythm; is normally found in children and young adults; causes—respiratory variation

Assessment

OBSERVATIONS/FINDINGS
Rhythm: irregular
Rate: 60 to 90 beats/min; may increase with inspiration and decrease with expiration
P wave: normal configuration, one before each QRS complex
PR interval: 0.12 to 0.20 sec
QRS complex: 0.06 to 0.10 sec

Collaborative management

None indicated

Sinus arrest (Figure 3-20)

A rhythm in which a sinus impulse is not generated; causes—drugs, coronary artery disease, increased vagal tone, sinoatrial node disease

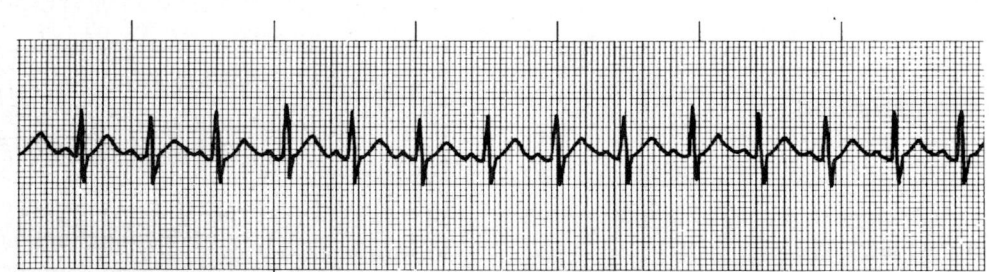

Figure 3-18   Sinus tachycardia. (From Andreoli KG et al: *Comprehensive cardiac care,* ed 6, St Louis, 1987, Mosby.)

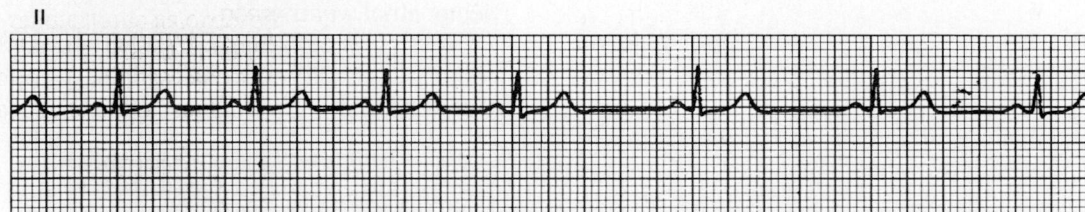

Figure 3-19   Sinus dysrhythmia. (From Conover MB: *Exercises in diagnosing ECG tracings,* ed 3, St Louis, 1984, Mosby.)

Assessment

OBSERVATIONS/FINDINGS

Dizziness
Syncope
Rhythm: irregular during periods of arrest
Rate: variable
P wave: absent during periods of arrest
P-R interval: absent during periods of arrest
QRS complex: absent during periods of arrest

POTENTIAL COMPLICATION

Ventricular standstill

Collaborative management

Medications: atropine
Cardiac pacing
Parenteral fluids
Cardiopulmonary resuscitation (CPR)

Interventions

Monitor cardiac activity; check rhythm strips q4h to 6h
  and prn
Maintain bed rest as indicated
Check BP, R, and apical pulse q4h to 6h and prn
Administer oxygen therapy as indicated

● Rhythms of Atrial Origin

*Supraventricular or atrial rhythms that originate outside
the sinoatrial node and above the bundle of His*

Premature atrial contractions (PACs, APCs) (Figures 3-21 and 3-22)

*premature atrial contractions: Ectopic beats gener-
ated outside the sinoatrial node; causes—anxiety,
ingestion of tobacco or caffeine, electrolyte imbalance,
hypoxia, drug toxicity*

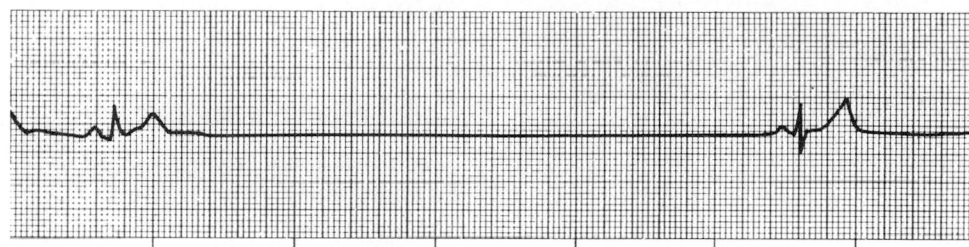

Figure 3-20 Sinus arrest. (From Andreoli KG et al: *Comprehensive cardiac care,* ed 6, St Louis, 1987,
Mosby.)

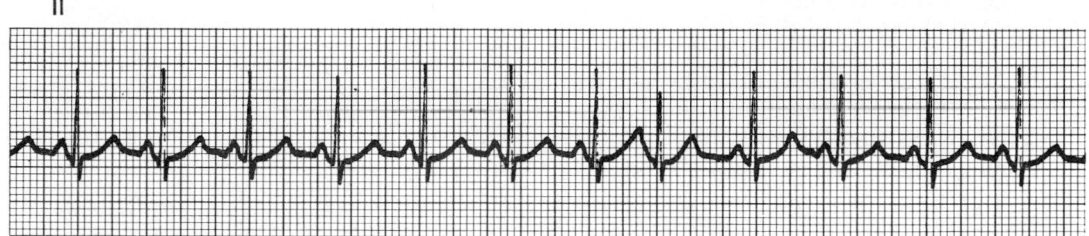

Figure 3-21 Premature atrial contraction. (From Conover MB: *Exercises in diagnosing ECG tracings,*
ed 3, St Louis, 1984, Mosby.)

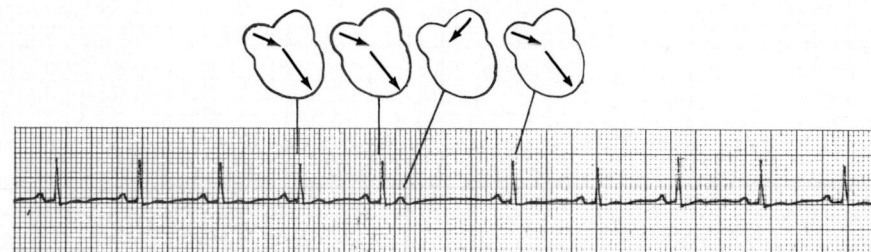

Figure 3-22 Nonconducted premature atrial contraction (PAC). (From Conover MB: *Understanding
electrocardiography: arrhythmias and the 12-lead ECG,* ed 4, St Louis, 1984, Mosby.)

Assessment

OBSERVATIONS/FINDINGS

Palpitations: skipped beats
Anxiety
Dizziness
Rhythm: irregular in presence of PACs
Rate: variable, may be normal or irregular in presence of ectopic beats
P wave: premature P wave is distorted; may be inverted or fused on preceding T wave
P-R interval: may be prolonged
QRS complex: may be normal or may show abnormal conduction in ectopic beat; no QRS will follow if P wave is blocked

POTENTIAL COMPLICATION

Atrial fibrillation

DIAGNOSTIC TEST

Holter monitor examination

Collaborative management

Treatment of underlying disease; none indicated for occasional PACs
Medications: antidisrhythmics

Interventions

Monitor cardiac activity; check rhythm strips q4h to 6h and prn
Check BP, R, and apical pulse q6h to 8h
Restrict caffeine and nicotine as ordered

Atrial flutter (Figure 3-23)

A rapid, regular ectopic atrial rhythm with characteristic "flutter" waves; causes—most forms of cardiac disease

Assessment

OBSERVATIONS/FINDINGS

Tachycardia
Tachypnea
Palpitations
SOB
Rhythm
  Atrial: regular
  Ventricular: may be regular or irregular
  Emboli
Rate
  Atrial: 250 to 350 beats/min
  Ventricular: 100 to 150 beats/min
  P-R interval: unmeasurable
  P wave: absent; rhythm shows F waves in sawtooth shape
  QRS complex: usually normal

POTENTIAL COMPLICATIONS

Emboli
CHF
Shock

Collaborative management

Treatment of underlying disease
Cardioversion
Carotid massage
Medications
  Antidysrhythmics
  Digitalis preparations
Atrial pacing
12-lead ECG

Interventions

Monitor cardiac activity; check rhythm strips q4h to 6h and prn
Check BP, R, and apical pulse q2h to 4h

II

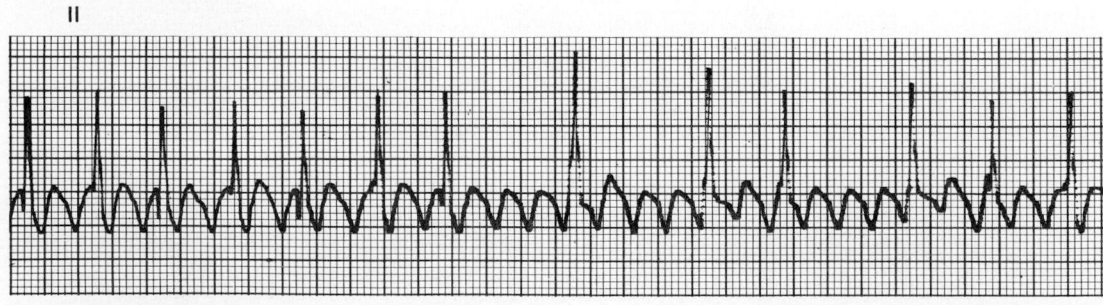

Figure 3-23   Atrial flutter. (From Conover MB: *Exercises in diagnosing ECG tracings,* ed 3, St Louis, 1984, Mosby.)

Maintain bed rest as indicated
Administer oxygen therapy as ordered

Atrial fibrillation (Figure 3-24)

A rapid, irregular, ectopic atrial rhythm with characteristic "fibrillatory" activity; causes—coronary artery disease (CAD), valvular heart disease, hypertension, increased left atrial size in the elderly

Assessment

OBSERVATIONS/FINDINGS

Palpitations
Faintness
Tachycardia
Irregular pulse
Pulse deficit (apical and radial pulses)
Chest discomfort
Nausea
Rhythm: irregular
Rate
 Atrial: 350 beats/min
 Ventricular: 90 to 100 beats/min
P-R interval: immeasurable
P wave: absent; rhythm shows "f" waves that are seen
 as undulations
QRS complex: usually normal

POTENTIAL COMPLICATIONS

Mural thrombi
CHF
Shock

Collaborative management

Medications: antidysrhythmics
Cardioversion
12-lead ECG

Interventions

Monitor cardiac activity; check rhythm strips q4h to 8h
 and prn
Check BP, R, and apical pulse q4h to 6h and prn
Administer oxygen therapy as ordered

Supraventricular tachycardia (SVT)
(Figure 3-25)

An ectopic atrial rhythm that is regular and may start and stop abruptly, originating above AV node; causes—precipitated by sympathetic stimulation (e.g., emotion, caffeine, tobacco, fatigue, excessive alcohol intake); may also be associated with Wolff-Parkinson White (WPW) syndrome

V₁

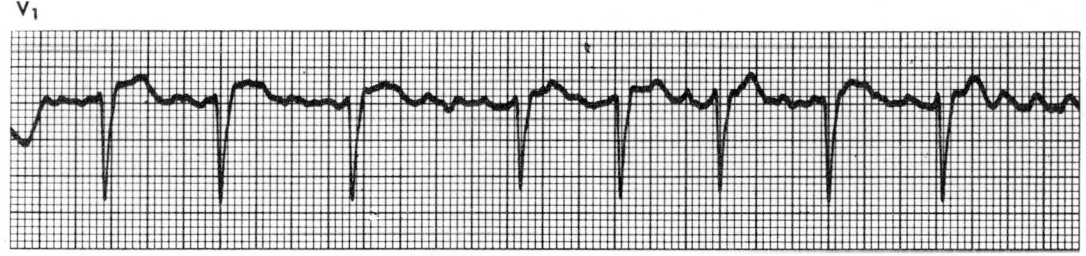

Figure 3-24 Atrial fibrillation. (From Conover MB: *Exercises in diagnosing ECG tracings,* ed 3, St Louis, 1984, Mosby.)

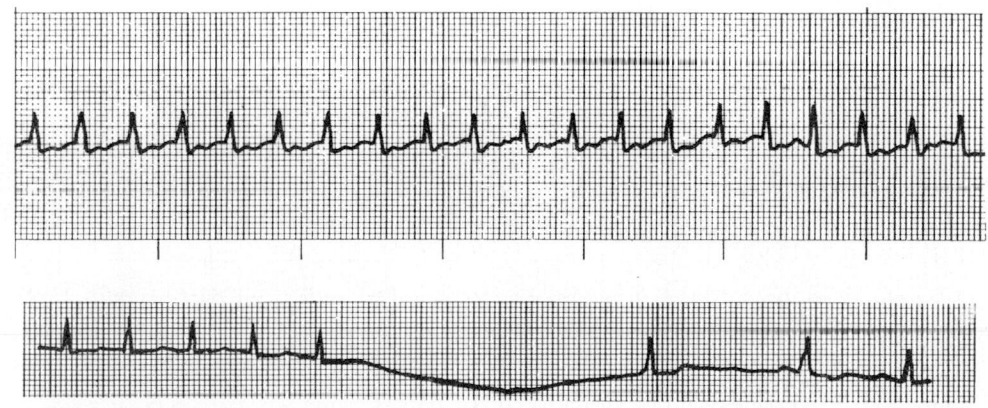

Figure 3-25 Supraventricular tachycardia (SVT). (From Andreoli KG et al: *Comprehensive cardiac care,* ed 6, St Louis, 1987, Mosby.)

Assessment

OBSERVATIONS/FINDINGS

Palpitations
SOB
Lightheadedness
"Frog sign"—rapid, regular venous pulsations in jugular veins during PSVT.
Hypokalemia
Chest pain or discomfort
Abdominal discomfort
Tachycardia of short or prolonged duration
Rhythm: usually regular
Rate: 150 to 250 beats/min
P wave: normal or buried in QRS or T wave; may not be visible
P-R interval: usually normal
QRS complex: usually normal

DIAGNOSTIC TEST

Holter monitor examination

POTENTIAL COMPLICATIONS

CHF
Shock

Collaborative management

Carotid massage (vagal stimulation)
Medications
  Antidysrhythmics
  Vagotonic preparations
Potassium replacement as indicated
Cardioversion
Atrial or ventricular pacing
12-lead ECG
Treat underlying etiology
Radiofrequency catheter ablation for symptomatic dysrhythmias

Interventions

Monitor cardiac activity; check rhythm strips q4h to 6h and prn
Administer oxygen therapy as ordered
Check BP, R, and apical pulse q2h to 4h
Maintain bed rest as indicated
Check serum potassium level if patient is taking digitalis preparations
Maintain quiet environment

● Rhythms of Ventricular Origin

Rhythms that occur as either escape or reentry (overdrive) rhythms arising within the ventricles

Premature ventricular contractions (PVCs) (Figures 3-26 and 3-27)

Premature beats arising in the ventricles below the bundle of His; may be a forerunner of ventricular tachycardia and ventricular fibrillation; causes—increased sympathetic stimulation (e.g., caffeine, tobacco, emotion), most forms of heart disease, electrolyte imbalance

Assessment

OBSERVATIONS/FINDINGS

Palpitations
Precordial pain
Dizziness
Faintness
Momentary loss of consciousness
Rhythm: irregular
Rate
  Atrial: normal
  Ventricular: may be normal or rapid
P wave: does not precede premature beat; premature

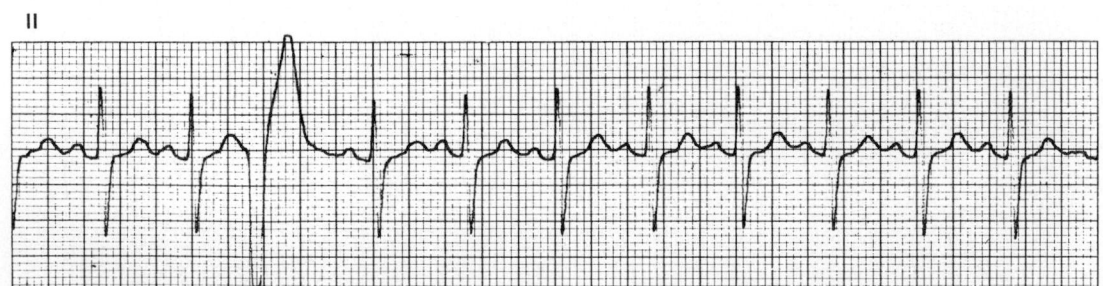

Figure 3-26   Premature ventricular contraction (PVC). (From Conover MB: *Exercises in diagnosing ECG tracings*, ed 3, St Louis, 1984, Mosby.)

beat is usually followed by complete compensatory pause

P-R interval: immeasurable

QRS complex: premature beat is wide and bizarre in appearance, lasting longer than 0.12 sec

DIAGNOSTIC TESTS

12-lead ECG

Holter monitor examination

POTENTIAL COMPLICATIONS

Ventricular tachycardia

Ventricular fibrillation

Collaborative management

Treatment of underlying disease

Medications: antidysrhythmics

12-lead ECGs for

  Multifocal PVCs

R on T phenomenon

Coupling or paired PVCs

Six or more PVCs/min

Radiofrequency catheter ablation

Interventions

Monitor cardiac activity; check rhythm strips q4h to 6h and prn; report if more than 6 PVC/min or if they occur close to preceding T waves

Monitor BP, R, and apical pulse q4h to 6h and prn

Administer oxygen therapy

Restrict caffeine, nicotine, and hot and cold fluids

Ventricular tachycardia (Figure 3-28)

Three or more consecutive PVCs; causes—ischemic heart disease, significant chronic heart disease, drug toxicity

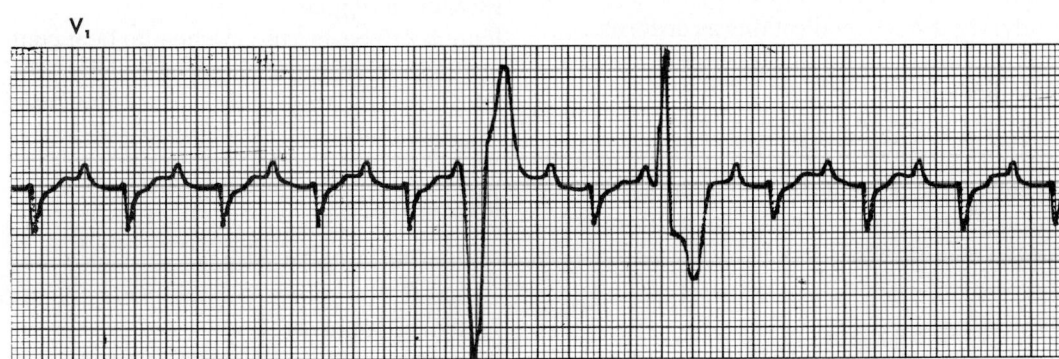

Figure 3-27 Multifocal premature ventricular contractions (PVCs). (From Conover MB: *Exercises in diagnosing ECG tracings,* ed 3, St Louis, 1984, Mosby.)

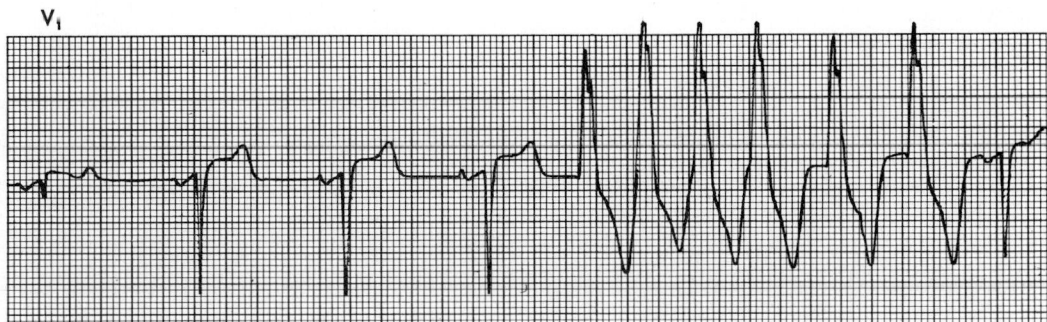

Figure 3-28 Ventricular tachycardia. (From Conover MB: *Exercises in diagnosing ECG tracings,* ed 3, St Louis, 1984, Mosby.)

Assessment

OBSERVATIONS/FINDINGS

Anxiety
Palpitations
Dizziness
Precordial discomfort
Cyanosis
Confusion
Syncope
Altered level of consciousness
Rhythm: usually regular
Rate: ventricular; 150 to 200 beats/min
P wave: absent; may be retrograde to atria
P-R interval: immeasurable
QRS complex: wide and bizarre in configuration, lasting
  >0.12 sec

POTENTIAL COMPLICATIONS

Heart failure
Ventricular fibrillation

Interventions

IMMEDIATE CARE

Apply direct current (DC) countershock
Administer antidysrhythmics medications as ordered:
  lidocaine bolus and drip
Initiate CPR as indicated
Initiate parenteral fluids as ordered
Take 12-lead ECG as ordered
Monitor BP, R, and apical pulse q15min to 30min as in-
  dicated
Administer oxygen as indicated

ONGOING CARE

Monitor cardiac activity; check rhythm strips q4h to 6h
  and prn

Monitor BP, R, and apical pulse q2h to 4h and prn, de-
  creasing frequency as condition stabilizes
Administer medications as ordered
  Antidysrhythmics
  Sedatives
Maintain bed rest as indicated

Ventricular fibrillation (Figure 3-29)

*Disorganized electrical activity of ventricles, which
leads to abrupt cessation of effective blood flow; causes—
severe heart disease, drug toxicity*

Assessment

OBSERVATIONS/FINDINGS

Anxiety
Palpitations
Dizziness
Cyanosis
Precordial pain
Nausea, vomiting
SOB
Syncope
Absence of pulse
Rhythm: irregular
Rate: >210 beats/min; no beat-to-beat count
P wave: not seen; absent atrial activity
QRS complex: wide undulations; wandering, irregular
  baseline

Interventions

IMMEDIATE CARE

Cough CPR if patient is awake and able to cough
Apply DC countershock
Administer CPR; usually indicated
Administer medications as ordered

II

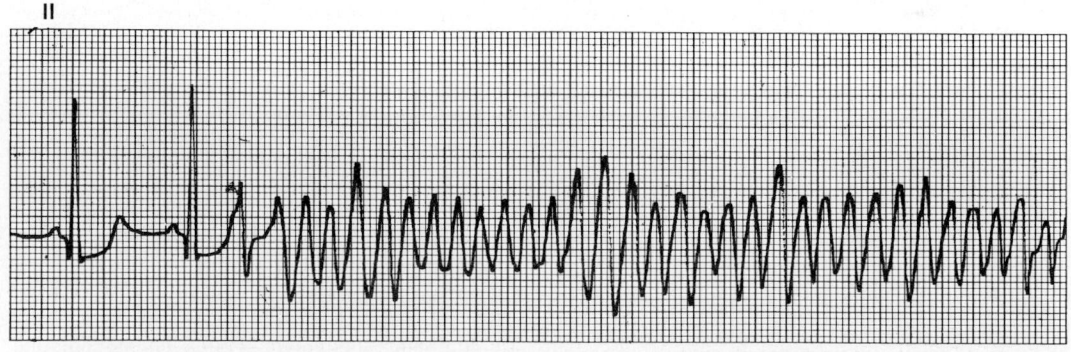

Figure 3-29   Ventricular fibrillation. (From Conover MB: *Exercises in diagnosing ECG tracings,* ed 3,
St Louis, 1984, Mosby.)

Initiate parenteral fluids as ordered
Take 12-lead ECG as ordered
Administer oxygen with assisted ventilation as ordered
Monitor BP, R, and apical pulse q15min to 30min

ONGOING CARE

Monitor cardiac activity; check rhythm strips q1h to 2h, decreasing frequency as condition stabilizes
Monitor BP, R, and apical pulse q1h to 2h and prn
Maintain bed rest as indicated
Keep defibrillator and emergency cart at bedside until condition stabilizes

Torsades de pointes (polymorphous ventricular tachycardia) (Figure 3-30)

Atypical ventricular tachycardia occurring in the setting of delayed repolarization (prolonged Q-T interval); causes—drug toxicity such as quinidine; electrolyte imbalance

Assessment

OBSERVATIONS/FINDINGS

Palpitations
Faintness
Syncope
Rhythm: regular or irregular
Rate: ventricular, 150 to 300 beats/min
P-R interval: not measurable
QRS complex: wide and bizarre in configuration, lasting >0.12 sec; amplitude and direction of QRS complex will vary

Q-T interval during baseline rhythm: >0.46 sec or >33% of baseline
T wave during baseline: very broad and flat

POTENTIAL COMPLICATIONS

Ventricular fibrillation
Sudden death

Collaborative management

Correction of underlying cause if identifiable (e.g., drug toxicity; quinidine, procainamide, amiodarone)
Correction of electrolyte imbalance: hypokalemia, hypomagnesemia
Medications (avoid drugs that prolong Q-T intervals, e.g., quinidine, Norpace)
Overdrive pacing: rate set at 80 to 120 beats/min
Cardioversion
Left stellate ganglionectomy

Interventions

Monitor cardiac activity; check rhythm strips q2h to 4h and prn, decreasing frequency as condition stabilizes
Monitor BP, P, and apical pulse q4h to 6h and prn

● Atrioventricular Block

A conduction disturbance involving the AV junction, which normally functions as a bridge between the atria and ventricles

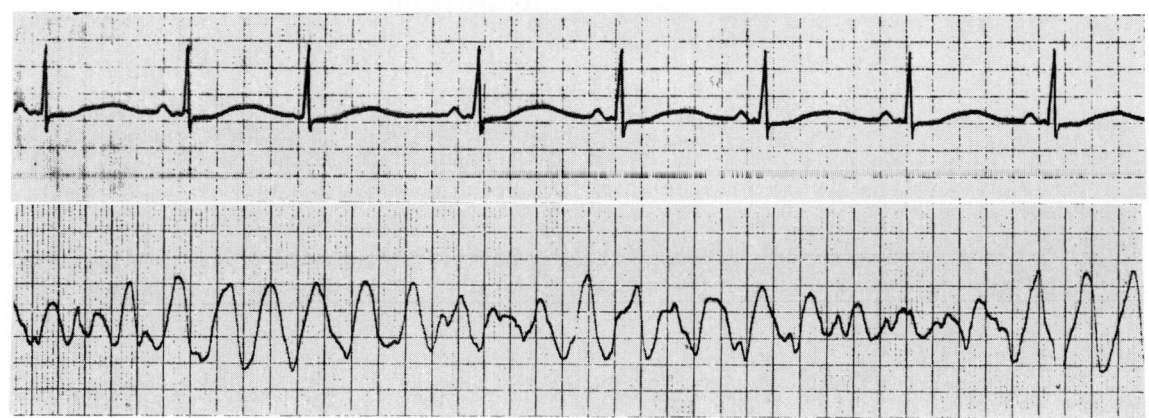

Figure 3-30 Torsades de pointes. Sinus rhythm. T waves are flat and Q-T interval is prolonged. (Courtesy Dr. Daniel H. Schwartz. From Goldberger E: *Textbook of clinical cardiology,* St Louis, 1982, Mosby.)

First-degree atrioventricular block
(Figure 3-31)

A consistent delay in impulse conduction throughout the AV node; causes—digoxin toxicity, ischemic heart disease, hyperkalemia

Assessment

OBSERVATIONS/FINDINGS

Rhythm: regular
Rate: 60 to 90 beats/min
P wave: normal configuration; one before each QRS
P-R interval: prolonged, >0.20 sec
QRS complex: 0.06 to 0.10 sec

Collaborative management

Medications
 Atropine
 Isoproterenol

Interventions

Monitor cardiac activity; check rhythm strips q4h to 6h and prn
Check BP, R, and apical pulse q4h to 6h and prn
Discontinue use of digitalis preparation or quinidine as ordered
Check serum levels of digitalis preparation and potassium as indicated
Observe for changes in P-R interval and measure

Second-degree atrioventricular block

An AV conduction disturbance characterized by nonconducted P waves and classified as type I or type II; causes—digoxin toxicity, ischemic heart disease

Assessment

OBSERVATIONS/FINDINGS

Rhythm: regular
Rate

Atrial: regular
Ventricular: irregular
P wave: may show one or more nonconducted P waves
P-R interval: progressive prolongation of P-R interval until one impulse is completely blocked
QRS complex: 0.06 to 0.10 sec

DIAGNOSTIC TESTS

Serum drug levels
His bundle recording

POTENTIAL COMPLICATIONS

Angina
Heart failure
Complete AV block
Asystole

Collaborative management

Medications
 Atropine
 Isoproterenol
Temporary cardiac pacing

Interventions

Monitor cardiac activity; check rhythm strips q2h to 4h
Monitor BP, R, and apical pulse q4h to 6h and prn

Mobitz type I (Wenckebach phenomenon) (Figure 3-32)

Causes—digoxin toxicity, inferior wall myocardial infarction (MI), rheumatic fever

Assessment

OBSERVATIONS/FINDINGS

Rhythm
 Atrial: regular
 Ventricular: irregular
Rate: atrial > ventricular

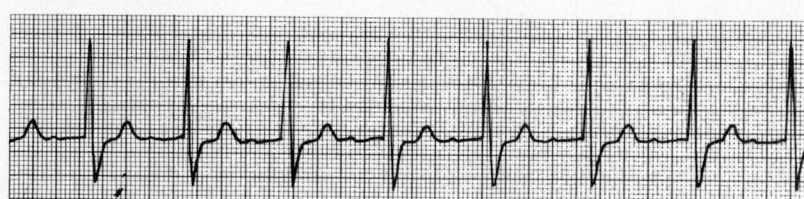

Figure 3-31   First-degree AV block. (From Conover MB: *Understanding electrocardiography: arrhythmias and the 12-lead ECG,* ed 4, St Louis, 1984, Mosby.)

P wave: may have multiple P waves before each QRS
P-R interval: becomes progressively prolonged (>0.28 sec) until one P wave is blocked; cycle will then be repeated
QRS complex: 0.06 to 0.10 sec; RR interval will shorten until QRS complex is dropped

Collaborative management

Medications
  Atropine
  Isoproterenol

Interventions

Withdraw use of digitalis preparation as ordered
Check serum levels of digitalis preparation and potassium as indicated

Mobitz type II (Figure 3-33)

Causes—digitalis toxicity, anterior MI

Assessment

OBSERVATIONS/FINDINGS
Dizziness
Weakness
Rhythm
  Atrial: regular
  Ventricular: irregular
Rate
  Atrial: 60 to 90 beats/min
  Ventricular: will vary according to degree of block

P wave: may have multiple P waves before each QRS
P-R interval: remains constant and may be greater than 0.20 sec
QRS interval: usually normal or slightly prolonged

POTENTIAL COMPLICATIONS
Complete AV block
Asystole

Collaborative management

Cardiac monitor
Medications
  Atropine
  Isoproterenol
Temporary or permanent cardiac pacing

Third-degree heart block (complete) (Figure 3-34)

Atria and ventricles are controlled by independent pacemakers

Causes—chronic conduction defect disease, digoxin toxicity, ischemic heart disease, congenital heart disease

Assessment

OBSERVATIONS/FINDINGS
Bradycardia
Syncope
Altered level of consciousness
Angina
Seizure activity

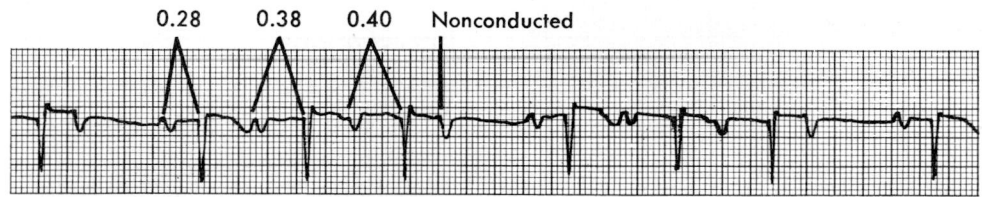

Figure 3-32 Second-degree AV block: Mobitz type I (Wenckebach phenomenon) with narrow QRS complex. (From Conover MB: *Understanding electrocardiography: arrhythmias and the 12-lead ECG,* ed 4, St Louis, 1984, Mosby.)

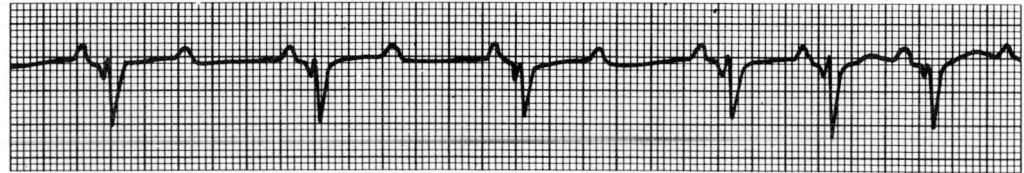

Figure 3-33 Second-degree AV block: Mobitz type II. (From Conover MB: *Exercises in diagnosing ECG tracings,* ed 3, St Louis, 1984, Mosby.)

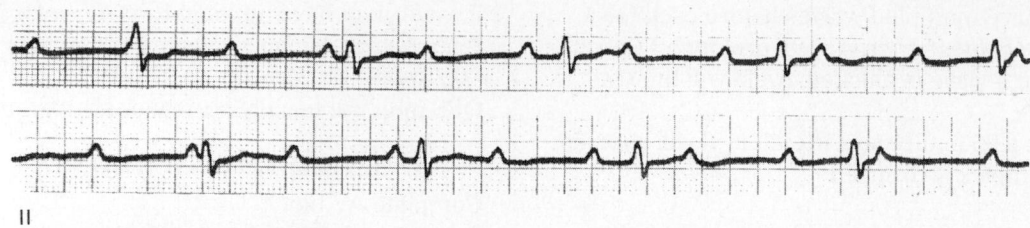

Figure 3-34 Third-degree (complete) AV block. (From Andreoli KG et al: *Comprehensive cardiac care,* ed 6, St Louis, 1987, Mosby.)

Seizure activity
Rhythm: regular; atrial and ventricular rhythms act independently of each other
Rate
  Atrial: 60 to 90 beats/min
  Ventricular: 25 to 45 beats/min
P wave: multiple P waves that occur independently of QRS
P-R interval: immeasurable
QRS complex
  Normal if impulse originates above bifurcation of bundle of His (rate = 40 to 60 beats/min)
  Greater than 0.12 sec of impulse originates below bifurcation (rate = 15 to 40 beats/min)

  POTENTIAL COMPLICATIONS
Heart failure
Shock
Ventricular fibrillation
Asystole

Collaborative management

Transvenous cardiac pacing
Medications
  Atropine
  Isoproterenol
12-lead ECG

Interventions

Monitor cardiac activity; check rhythm strips q2h to 4h or prn
Monitor BP, R, and apical pulse q2h to 4h and prn
Administer oxygen therapy as ordered
Maintain bed rest as indicated

● Atrioventricular Junctional Rhythms

Dysrhythmias that originate at the AV junction; may include premature, escape, and accelerated junctional rhythm; causes—digitalis toxicity, MI, hypoxia, hyperkalemia, tricuspid valve surgery, rheumatic fever, SA node pathology

Atrioventricular junctional escape
(Figure 3-35)

Assessment

  OBSERVATIONS/FINDINGS
Dizziness
Faintness
Heart block
Rhythm: regular
Rate: 40 to 60 beats/min
P wave: may precede or follow QRS; inverted in lead II
P-R interval: not measurable
QRS complex: 0.06 to 0.10 sec; may be slightly abnormal

Collaborative management

Treatment of underlying disease
Medications
  Atropine
  Isoproterenol
Ventricular pacing
12-lead ECG as ordered

Interventions

Monitor cardiac activity; check rhythm strips q4h to 6h
Check serum levels of digitalis preparation and potassium as indicated

● Wolff-Parkinson-White Syndrome (Ventricular Preexcitation)
(Figure 3-36)

Preexcitation of the ventricles over an accessory AV pathway: cause—congenital heart disease

Assessment

  OBSERVATIONS/FINDINGS
Rhythm: regular
Rate: regular

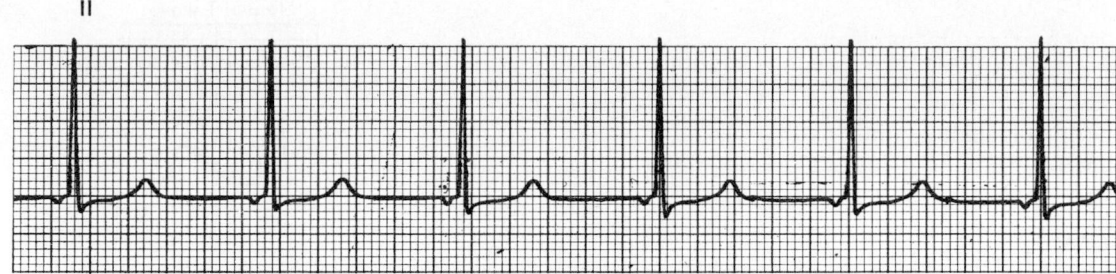

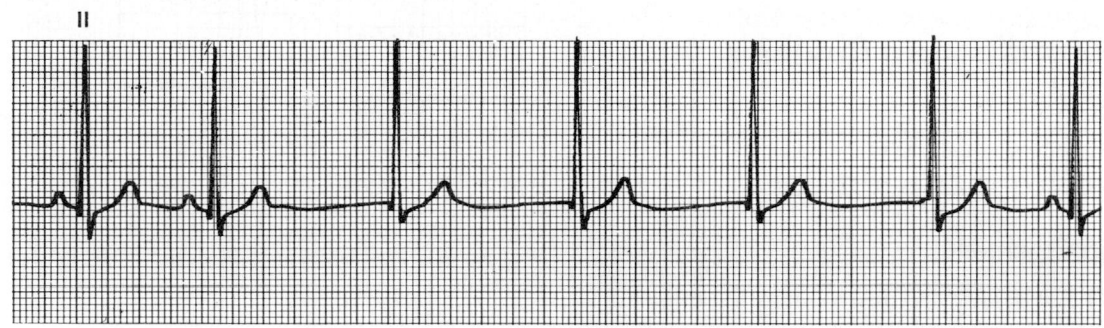

Figure 3-35 Junctional escape rhythms. (From Conover MB: *Exercises in diagnosing ECG tracings,* ed 3, St Louis, 1984, Mosby.)

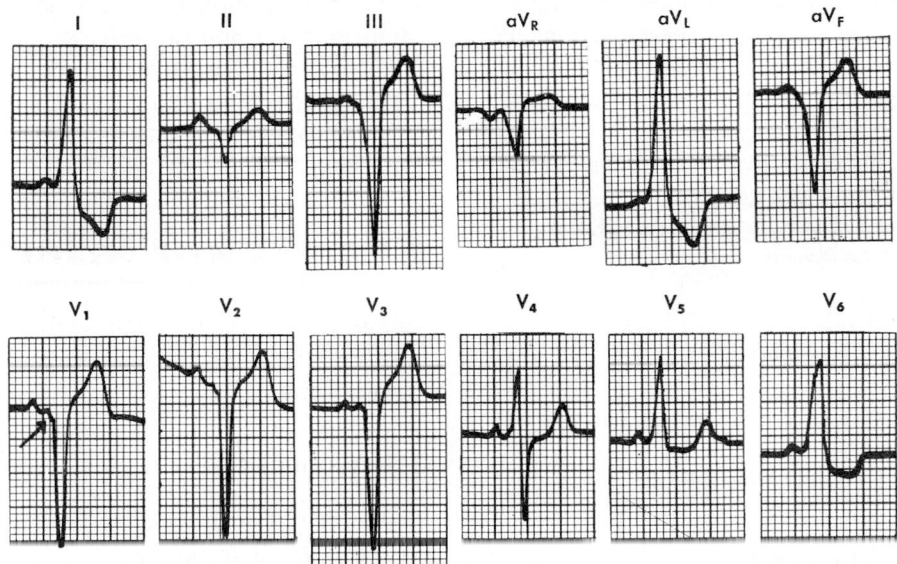

Figure 3-36 Characteristic triad of Wolff-Parkinson-White (WPW) pattern: wide QRS complex, short P-R interval, and delta wave (arrow in lead V_1). (From Goldberger AL, Goldberger E: *Clinical electrocardiography: a simplified approach,* ed 4, St Louis, 1990, Mosby.)

P wave: normal configuration; one before each QRS
P-R interval: <0.12 sec
QRS complex: when following shortened P-R interval, complex is widened and distorted, exhibiting delta waves

DIAGNOSTIC TESTS

Holter monitor examination
Electrophysiologic studies

POTENTIAL COMPLICATIONS

Atrial tachycardia
Atrial fibrillation

Collaborative management

Valsalva's maneuver; eyeball pressure
Medications as ordered
  Calcium channel blocking agents
  Beta-adrenergic blocking agents
Cardioversion

Interventions

Monitor cardiac activity as indicated; check rhythm strips q4h to 6h; report any changes in rhythm to physician

● Electrocardiogram Rhythms

(Figure 3-37)

Collaborative management

Nursing management

PATIENT PROBLEM/NURSING DIAGNOSIS (GENERAL)

● NDX: Anxiety related to altered heart action

Assess level of anxiety and degree of understanding *to identify source of anxiety and clarify any misconceptions*
Provide continuous explanation for various monitoring devices in use and procedures; *information alleviates anxiety*
Remain with patient during periods of heightened anxiety *to provide reassurance and comfort*
Promote physical rest *to decrease cardiac workload*
Administer sedation as ordered

  EXPECTED OUTCOMES
Patient's anxiety level is reduced
Patient appears calm
Verbalizes fears and concerns, asks questions

  ADDITIONAL NURSING DIAGNOSIS
  TO CONSIDER
Risk for decreased cardiac output related to electrical instability

Patient/family teaching

Assess level of understanding
Explain purpose of treatment and equipment
Reinforce physician's explanation of rhythm disturbance and associated symptoms to report
Discuss need to exercise to tolerance and/or as ordered
Explain purpose and demonstrate method of taking pulse

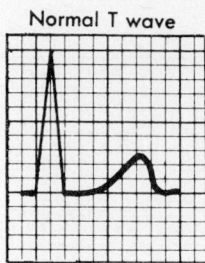

Normal T wave

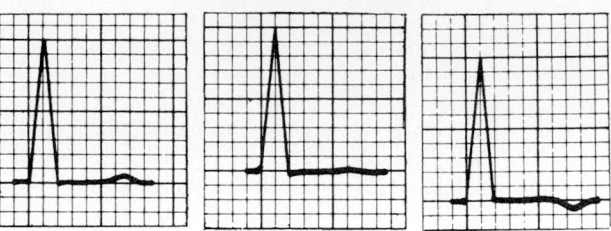

Nonspecific ST-T changes

Figure 3-37 Miscellaneous ECG changes. (Flattening of T wave or slight T wave inversion is abnormal but relatively nonspecific changes.) (From Goldberger AL, Goldberger E: *Clinical electrocardiography: a simplified approach,* ed 4, St Louis, 1990, Mosby.)

Describe dietary restrictions as ordered; need to avoid caffeine and nicotine
Discuss medication: name, dosage, time of administration, purpose, and side effects
Need to avoid taking over-the-counter medications without checking with physician
Importance of ongoing patient care
Pacemaker care when indicated

Pacemaker Insertion

pacemaker: An electronic device used to electronically stimulate the myocardium to control or maintain the heart rate

Preprocedure teaching

Reinforce physician's explanation of procedure
  How pacemaker functions
    To optimize cardiac function
    To restore and/or maintain AV synchronization
  Indications
    To control bradydysrhythmias
    To control tachydysrhythmias
    To control ventricular fibrillation
  Type or mode to be used
    Temporary
    Permanent
  Method insertion
    Transvenous

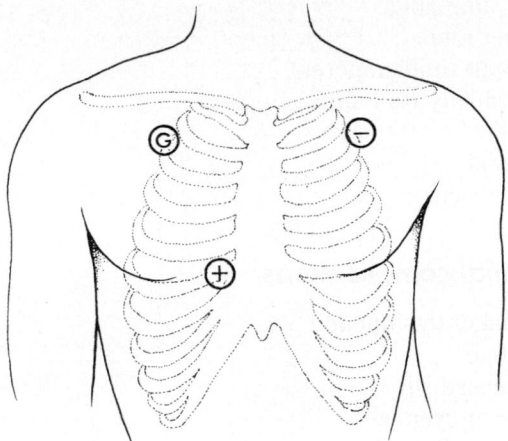

Figure 3-38 MCL. Modified V_1 monitoring lead.

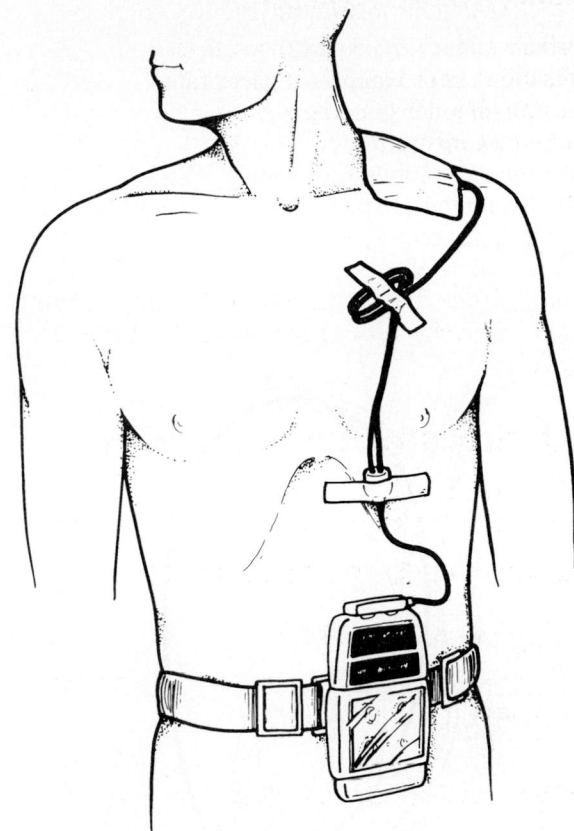

Figure 3-39 Temporary external pacemaker.

Transthoracic
Epicardial
Ensure that patient and/or significant other knows and
understands
Procedure, duration of procedure, where it will be per-
formed (operating room vs. procedure room), equip-
ment that will be used (e.g., fluoroscopy), and type
of anesthesia
Importance of restricting activities for 4 to 6 hr to avoid
lead dislodgment
Importance of performing passive ROM exercises to
extremities postoperatively
Importance of being closely monitored postoperatively
Signs and symptoms of pacemaker malfunction
Faintness
Dizziness
Dyspnea
Twitching
Pectoral muscles
Abdominal muscles
Hiccups
Chest pain

Postprocedure assessment

Observations/findings

TEMPORARY PACEMAKER (Figure 3-39)
Heart rate based on preset pacemaker setting
Pacemaker unit (Figure 3-40)
Firing at preset rate
Output threshold (milliamperes)
Sensing needle
Terminal connections
Electrical grounding
ECG pattern (Figure 3-41)
Pacemaker artifact

Permanent Pacemaker Mode

CHAMBER SENSED

A—atrium
V—ventricle
D—dual
0—none

MODE OF RESPONSE

I—Inhibited
T—Triggered
D—Dual
R—Reserve
0—None

Capturing
Patient's underlying rhythm
Battery failure
Loss of capture
Failure to sense
Sensing needle: not moving

PERMANENT PACEMAKER

Pacemaker unit (Figure 3-42)
  Heart rate: based on preset pacer rate
  Location of pulse generator
  Mode (see box p. 183)
    Ventricular inhibited (demand): VVI
    AV sequential: DVI
    Atrial triggered: VDD
    Universal: DDD

Programmable
  Pacer rate
  Output (milliamperes)
  Sensitivity (to PQRS complex)
  Mode
    Atrial
    Ventricular

Potential complications

Pacemaker dysfunction
  Syncope
  Decreased BP
  Pallor or cyanosis
  Bradycardia
  Fatigue
  Shortness of breath
  ECG pattern changes
  Absent pacemaker artifact
  No ventricular response, absence of QRS complex af-
    ter pacemaker artifact
  Competition; presence of pacemaker response com-
    plex and patient's own complex
  Runaway pacemaker; pacemaker artifact appears at
    several hundred per minute
Catheter dislodgment
  Change in QRS configuration
  Loss of artifact on ECG
  Failure to sense
  Hiccups
  Muscle twitching: chest, abdomen
Stokes-Adams syndrome
  Hypotension
  Vertigo
  Fainting
  Convulsions
  Coma
Cardiac dysrhythmias
  PVCs
  Ventricular tachycardia
Site of insertion
  Discoloration

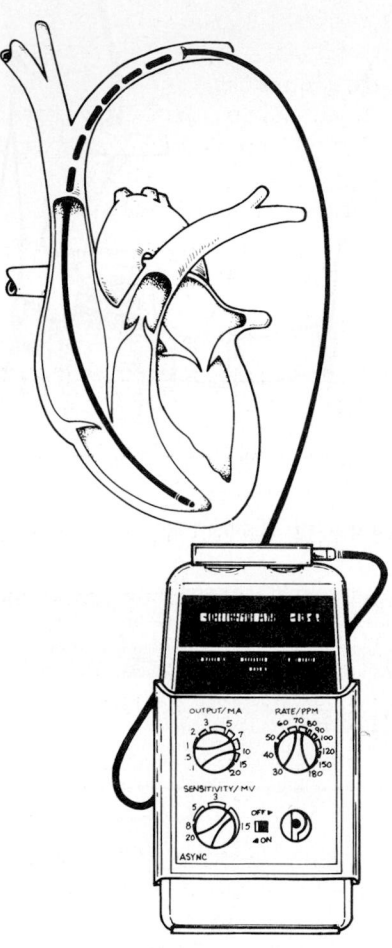

Figure 3-40   Temporary pacemaker unit: transvenous approach.

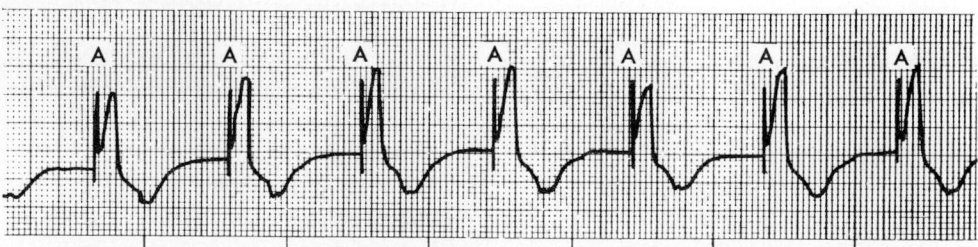

Figure 3-41   Ventricular pacemaker. **A,** Pacemaker spikes. (From Andreoli K et al: *Comprehensive cardiac care,* ed 6, St Louis, 1987, Mosby.)

Pain
 Swelling
 Bleeding
Perforation
 Hiccough
Infection of incisional site
 Elevated temperature
 Redness
 Discoloration
 Pain, swelling
 Fluid collection, drainage
Cardiac tamponade

Collaborative management

Therapeutic management

Cardiac monitor
Pacemaker
 Heart rate setting
 Threshold (milliamperes)
Medications
 Analgesics

Nursing management

PATIENT PROBLEM/NURSING DIAGNOSIS

● **NDX:** Risk for decreased cardiac output related to pacemaker dysfunction secondary to displacement or breakage of pacing catheter, infection, or bleeding

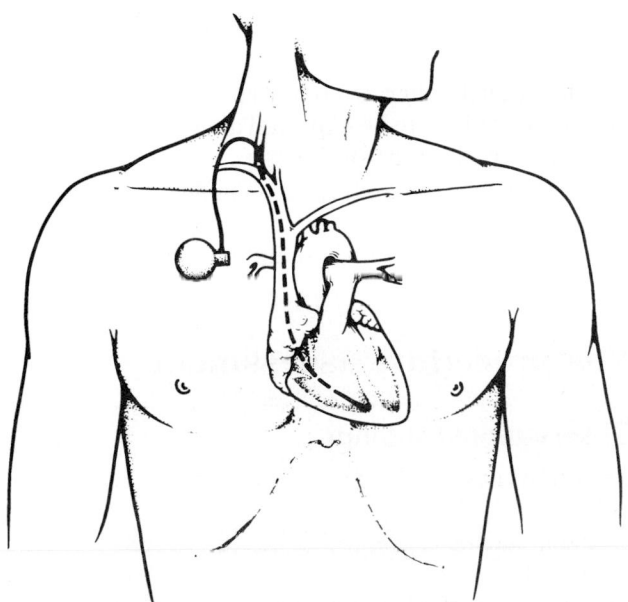

Figure 3-42 Permanent pacemaker.

Assess patient and pacemaker unit *to detect signs of pacemaker failure*
Place patient on cardiac monitor *to evaluate pacemaker function*
Monitor BP, T, and R q4h; check apical pulse q1h to 2h for 7 hr, then q4h *to detect signs of compromised cardiac function*
For temporary pacemaker
 Check settings: output, sensing, and rates
 Immobilize and secure extremity
Check rhythm strips on return to unit q4h and prn noting pacemaker function and rate
Examine site of insertion q2h to 4h; report any excessive bleeding to physician
Continue with immediate postoperative care and decrease frequency of nursing functions as patient's condition improves
Increase activity as tolerated and ordered
Change dressing daily as ordered, using aseptic technique *to prevent infection*

EXPECTED OUTCOME

Patient demonstrates stable cardiac output; pacemaker unit functioning as programmed

ADDITIONAL NURSING DIAGNOSES
TO CONSIDER

Anxiety related to perceived and/or actual changes in health status
Pain related to incision and/or physical immobility of affected arm

Patient/family teaching

PERMANENT PACEMAKER

Assess level of understanding and degree of readiness to learn
Ensure that patient and/or significant other knows pacemaker model, date of insertion, location of pacer generator, and pacer rate
Demonstrate method of caring for pacemaker
Demonstrate changing of dressing
Demonstrate taking of pulse for 1 min; give patient range of normal rates and instruct to report to physician if pulse is less than set range (i.e., <5 beats/min below set rate)
Deal with behavioral changes such as denial
Discuss living with pacemaker, assist patient to adjust to any limitations, and explain that pacemaker will eliminate feelings of faintness and fatigue
Discuss signs of pacemaker failure
 Pulse <60 beats/min or <5 beats/min below set rate
 Dizziness
 Faintness
 Palpitations

Management of Pacemaker Equipment

TEMPORARY PACEMAKER

Ground all equipment
Secure all terminal connections
Avoid use of electrical equipment such as shavers
Insulate exposed pacemaker wires by enclosing
    pacemaker and connections with rubber glove
Avoid wetting pacemaker
Apply soft restraints as indicated

PERMANENT PACEMAKER

Avoid exposure to electrical equipment that
    causes electromagnetic interference (EMI)
    such as diathermy and ungrounded equipment
Ground all equipment
Apply soft restraints as indicated

Hiccups
Chest pain
Discuss method of reporting pacemaker failure
    Telephone monitoring
    Notifying physician
Discuss signs of infection around pacemaker generator
    Fever
    Heat
    Pain
    Swelling
Discuss medications: name, dosage, time of administration, purpose, and side effects
Explain need to avoid taking over-the-counter medications without checking with physician
Review prescribed diet

Home care considerations

Explain importance of ongoing outpatient care: pacemaker clinic, use of transtelephonic system
Describe activity allowances and limitations
    Avoid traveling for at least 3 months after insertion
    Discuss type of employment and make adjustments in
        work accordingly
    Resume sexual activity as tolerated
    Avoid engaging in body contact sports such as baseball, football, and basketball
Discuss need to wear nonrestrictive clothing over site
    of pacemaker

Discuss electrical safety
    Avoid working with radar or electrical equipment
        such as diathermy motors that may cause electromagnetic interference
    Ground home appliances so that they have little or no
        effect on permanent pacemakers
    Wear medical alert band
    Carry pacemaker card with information regarding
        type of pacemaker, set rate, date of implantation, and
        name of physician
    Inform dentist of pacemaker before any extensive
        dental work

Cardiac Catheterization

*An invasive cardiac procedure; assists in detection and
    localization of intracardiac problems, determines
    intracardiac measurements, and shows visualization
    of the cardiac chambers; performed with patient under
    local anesthesia*

Preprocedure teaching

Involve family or significant other in care and instruction
Assess level of understanding
Reinforce physician's explanation of purpose of procedure
Review routine preparation for procedure
    Arm or leg shave and preparation
    Medication for sedation may be ordered
    No food or water 6 to 12 hr before procedure
Review sensations to be experienced during procedure
    Palpitations
    Warm, flushed feeling during injection of dye
    Desire to cough
    Feeling of falling if rotated from side to side
Review sensations to be expected after procedure
    Soreness at insertion site
    Possible backache from lying on table for 1 to 3 hr
    Fatigue
Stress importance of bed rest and immobility of extremity after procedure

Postprocedure assessment

Observations/findings

Hematoma at site of insertion
    Neck
    Antecubital fossa
    Inguinal
Vasospasm of affected extremity
    Numbness

Tingling
Cyanosis
Loss of pulse

Potential complications

Ventricular dysrhythmias
Syncope
Allergic reaction to dye
Nausea, vomiting
Decrease or fall in BP
Thrombus
  Pain at incision site
Thrombophlebitis
Cardiac perforation
Myocardial ischemia
Local infection
Cardiac tamponade

Postprocedure care

Assess BP, T, R, apical pulse, and peripheral pulses, noting quality q15min for four times, then qh for 4 hr, then as ordered
Maintain bed rest for 6 to 8 hr after procedure or as ordered
  Elevate head of bed 20 to 30 degrees
  Keep extremity immobile for 2 to 4 hr after procedure as ordered
  Maintain sandbag over puncture site as ordered
Obtain 12-lead ECG as ordered
Monitor cardiac activity as ordered; check rhythm strips q4h and prn
Examine dressing at site of insertion q2h to 4h, noting amount and color of drainage; change daily and prn
Reinforce dressing as necessary
Inspect surrounding skin
  Redness or discoloration
  Swelling
  Irritation
Control pain as ordered
Ambulate as tolerated
Instruct patient to report any signs of pain, swelling, or discoloration of puncture site
Continue ongoing care for underlying disease process

Percutaneous Transluminal Coronary Angioplasty

An invasive nonsurgical procedure using a balloon-tipped catheter to restore patency of coronary artery by compressing atheromatous plaques within the artery

directional coronary atherectomy (DCA): *Atherectomy is selective excision and removal of atheroma deposits from coronary vessel walls. Catheter introduction and procedure are similar to PTCA.*

Preprocedure teaching

Assess level of understanding and emotional status: fears of procedure and possible necessity of cardiac surgery
Involve family or significant other in care and instruction
Reinforce physician's explanation of purpose of procedure, desired outcome, and associated risks
Explain need to follow directions regarding administration and withholding of medications
Encourage verbalization and questions
Explain that procedure is similar to cardiac catheterization, identifying any previous negative experiences; procedure may last 45 min to 1½ hr
Review routine preparation for procedure
  Skin prepared for coronary bypass surgery
  Medication for sedation may be ordered
  No food or water for at least 8 hr before procedure
Explain sensations to be expected
  During procedure
    Palpitations
    Warm, flushed feeling during injection of dye
    Possible chest discomfort during balloon inflation
  After procedure
    Soreness at insertion site
    Possible backache from lying on table for 3 to 5 hr
    Fatigue
Stress importance of bed rest and immobility of extremity after procedure
Stress importance of drinking fluids for first 6 to 8 hr to wash out contrast material
Explain and review postprocedure activities
  Need to be admitted to CCU for 24 hr for observation
  Routines of CCU
  Visiting privileges
  Equipment to be used
    Temporary pacing electrode
    Cardiac monitor
    Oxygen administration
    IV therapy
NOTE: Cardiac surgical team must be on standby during procedure; see Cardiac surgery on p. 154 for brief explanation of differences in patient care after cardiac surgery
During procedure intraaortic balloon pump must be available on standby

Preparation

Obtain informed consent
Maintain NPO 8 hr before procedure
Withhold anticoagulation therapy 1 to 2 days before
  procedure
Administer medications as ordered
  Salicylates and dipyridamole may be ordered 2 days
    before procedure
  Nitrates
  Beta-blocking agents may be decreased
  Calcium antagonists
  Sedation
Obtain baseline data
  CBC
  Electrolytes
  BUN, creatinine
  Blood type and crossmatch
  Coagulation studies
  ECG
  Chest x-ray

Postprocedure assessment

Subjective data

Chest pain, pressure
SOB
Dizziness, lightheadedness
Anxiety

Objective data

ECG changes
  ST elevations, depressions
  Ventricular dysrhythmias
Skin
  Pale
  Diaphoretic
Hypotension (systolic blood pressure <90 mm Hg)
Hematoma at site of insertion
Vasospasm of affected extremity
  Numbness
  Tingling
  Cyanosis
  Loss of pulse
Dysrhythmias

Diagnostic tests

CBC
Coagulation studies: APTT
Serum potassium and sodium
Cardiac enzymes: CPK
BUN, creatinine
12-lead ECG

Potential complications

Failure to dilate coronary artery
Abrupt coronary occlusion
MI
Bleeding
Rupture or dissection of coronary artery
  Cardiac tamponade
  MI
  Shock
  Cardiac arrest
Cannulated extremity
  Ischemia
  Thrombosis formation
Renal hypersensitivity to contrast material

Collaborative management

Therapeutic management

Admission to CCU for 24 to 48 hr
Bed rest
Cardiac monitor
Parenteral fluids
Medications
  Heparin infusion
  Nitrates
  Calcium channel blockers
  Aspirin
  Dipyridamole

Nursing management

PATIENT PROBLEMS/NURSING DIAGNOSES

● **NDX:** Risk for altered tissue perfusion (peripheral) related to hematoma, thrombus formation, secondary to arterial cannulation

Assess pulses distal to site, noting quality, q15 min for four times, decreasing frequency as ordered; note skin color, temperature
Observe for diminished pulses in extremity distal to cannulation site; report decreased or absent pulses immediately to physician
Maintain bed rest for 6 to 8 hr in supine position until arterial and venous sheaths are removed; when sheaths are removed maintain 5 to 10 lb sandbag over cannulation site
Inspect cannulation site for swelling, tenderness, discoloration, warmth, and drainage
Keep extremity immobile for 2 to 4 hr after procedure; log roll pt side to side; raise head of bed 15 degrees
Inspect dressing at site of insertion q2h to 4h, noting amount and color of drainage
Reinforce dressing as necessary
Inspect surrounding skin

Redness or discoloration
Swelling
Irritation
Administer antiplatelets as ordered
Monitor coagulation studies, reporting prolonged PTT
to physician

EXPECTED OUTCOMES
Patient maintains adequate peripheral tissue perfusion
Pulse is full and bounding
Cannulation site: color is good, there are no signs of
tenderness or swelling

● **NDX:** Risk for decreased cardiac output related to
myocardial ischemia or dysrhythmias

Assess for signs of diminished CO
Monitor BP, R, and apical pulse q15min for 1 hr,
then q30min for 1 hr, then qh for 6 hr, then as
ordered
Monitor cardiac activity, check rhythm strips q4h
and prn, observing for signs of ischemia or dysrhythmias
Obtain 12-lead ECG during episodes of chest pain; observe for and report any signs of ischemic change or
dysrhythmias
Auscultate chest for heart and lung sounds q4h for 24
hr
Monitor intake and output; report output <30 ml/hr or
inability to void within first 4 hr
Administer medications as ordered

EXPECTED OUTCOMES
Patient maintains good cardiac output
Vital signs are stable
Urine output is good
Mentation is clear

Patient/family teaching

NOTE: Refer to p. 120 for education for patients with
angina pectoris
Assess level of understanding
Reinforce physician's explanation of postprocedure results
Review allowances and limitations of activity
Avoid heavy lifting and pushing
Ambulate at regular intervals
Explain importance of calling physician if chest pain occurs lasting longer than 20 min
Discuss medications: name, dosage, time of administration, purpose, and side effects
Explain importance of taking antiplatelet medications
as ordered
Explain importance of ongoing outpatient care

Refer to standard for angina pectoris for patient teaching regarding
Chest pain
Risk factors
Exercise, activities

ADDITIONAL NURSING DIAGNOSIS
TO CONSIDER
Anxiety related to perceived biologic threat

Thrombolytic Therapy

*Infusion of thrombolytic agents to promote clot lysis,
restore coronary blood flow, and limit myocardial
ischemia*

Preprocedure teaching

Assess level of understanding and anxiety level
Involve family or significant other in care and instruction
Reinforce physician's explanation of purpose of procedure, desired outcome, and associated risks
Describe procedure to be performed
Intracoronary: similar to cardiac catheterization, may
last 1 to 2 hr; sensations that may occur: pressure
during insertion of catheter but no discomfort with
infusion
Intravenous: usually in emergency department or in
CCU; infusion administered over 3-hr period
Explain and review intraprocedure and postprocedure
routines
Monitoring in CCU
Visiting privileges
Equipment to be used
Cardiac monitor
Oxygen administration
IV therapy
Explain need for bed rest during and after administration and need for frequent blood sampling to monitor
clotting times
Instruct patient to inform nurse if chest pain develops

Preparation

Obtain informed consents as required: thrombolytic
therapy, cardiac catheterization, PTCA, and CABG
surgery
Obtain baseline laboratory data
To determine hemostatic status: CBC with platelets,
PT, fibrinogen, fibrin split-product labels
To determine degree of myocardial injury:
CPK-MB
Blood type and cross match, electrolytes, BUN
creatinine

Obtain diagnostic data
  12-lead ECG/18-lead ECG
  Chest x-ray examination
Establish two to three patent IV lines
Administer medications as ordered

Postprocedure assessment

Observations/findings

Successful myocardial reperfusion
  Abrupt cessation of chest pain
  ECG changes: return of ST elevations to baseline
  Dysrhythmias: sinus bradycardia, AV block with hypotension, ventricular tachycardia
  Isoenzyme: early peaking of CPK-MB (within 12 hr of onset of symptoms)
Bleeding/hemorrhage:
  Surface bleeding: oozing from puncture or catheter insertion site, gingival bleeding, ecchymoses
  GI: hematemesis, tarry stools, positive occult blood
Coronary artery reocclusion
  Chest pain
  ECG: ST-T wave changes
  Dysrhythmias
Skin
  Pale
  Diaphoretic
  Clammy
Hypotension
Tachycardia
Anxiety

Diagnostic tests

CBC
Serum fibrinogen levels
APTT
CPK-MB

Potential complications

Bleeding
Hemorrhage: GI, intracranial
Myocardial ischemia or infarction

Collaborative management

Therapeutic management

Admission to CCU
Bed rest
Cardiac monitoring

Hemodynamic monitoring
Arterial pressure, PA, PWCP
PTCA
Medications
  During procedure
    Thrombolytic agents
      Streptokinase (SK)
      Urokinase (UK)
      Tissue plasminogen activator (t-PA)
      Anisoylated plasminogen-SK activator complex (APSAC)
    Diphenhydramine
    Heparin
  After procedure
    Heparin

Nursing management

PATIENT PROBLEMS/NURSING DIAGNOSES

● **NDX:** Risk for fluid volume deficit related to bleeding/hemorrhage secondary to thrombolysis-induced coagulopathy

Assess for signs and symptoms of surface or internal bleeding
Monitor BP and HR according to unit protocol during first hr, decreasing frequency as condition stabilizes
Inspect puncture sites every 15 min; apply manual pressure when removing IV catheters
Initiate measures that prevent disruption of vascular integrity and/or keep venous or arterial puncture and injections to a minimum
Instruct patient to avoid vigorous toothbrushing
Avoid removing IV or arterial lines during first 24 to 48 hr or as indicated by specific agents
Use heparin lock for IV access or blood sampling
Monitor PTT valves

EXPECTED OUTCOMES

Patient demonstrates no signs of bleeding
Hemostasis is reestablished
  Coagulation studies are within acceptable limits
  No signs of surface or internal bleeding
  Vital signs are WNL

● **NDX:** Risk for decreased cardiac output related to reperfusion dysrhythmias

Assess and record ECG changes during and after thrombolytic therapy
Assess and monitor BP, HR, R, and hemodynamic response to reperfusion dysrhythmias as they appear
Administer antidysrhythmic medications as ordered; keep medications and defibrillator at bedside

EXPECTED OUTCOMES

Patient maintains good cardiac output
  ECG remains in stable or normal rhythm
  Reperfusion dysrhythmias are controlled or absent
  Vital signs remain stable

● **NDX:** Risk for chest pain related to decreased myocardial tissue perfusion secondary to reocclusion of coronary artery

Assess and monitor complaints of chest pain, noting patient's nonverbal expressions; compare with preprocedural chest pain complaints
Obtain 12-lead ECG during episode of chest pain, comparing with baseline ECG taken after thrombolysis; report any changes
Maintain on bed rest
Monitor BP, HR, R
Administer analgesia: morphine sulfate
Prepare for possible catheterization, repeat thrombolysis, PTCA

EXPECTED OUTCOME

Patient verbalizes absence of chest pain

Anticoagulant Therapy

anticoagulant: Medication administered to prevent or treat arterial or venous thrombosis; used in treatment of pulmonary embolism, cerebral embolism, and valvular heart disease, and with a heart valve prosthesis

Assessment

Observations/findings

Therapeutic serum levels
  Warfarin: protime—1.5 to 2½ × control
  INR—2 to 3
  Heparin: PTT—
    2 to 3 × control
Hematuria
Pain
  Abdominal
  Flank
Tarry stools
Hematemesis
Epistaxis
Bleeding gums
Hemoptysis
Subcutaneous bleeding
Ecchymosis
Hematoma

Joints
  Pain
  Immobility
Site of incision
  Bleeding
  Immobility
Neurologic changes
Increased menstrual flow
Medications
  Potentiate anticoagulation
  Retard anticoagulation

Interventions

Administer parenteral heparin as ordered
  Use heparin lock if ordered
  Give heparin at exact time ordered
  Give dosage over a period of 1 min
  Never skip doses
  Do not remove heparin lock for 2 hr after last dose
  Maintain continuous heparin infusion if ordered
  Never hang more than 4 hr dose at one time; observe rate q30min
  Administer subcutaneous heparin as ordered, rotating sites
  Coordinate all laboratory work; avoid multiple punctures
  Maintain manual pressure for at least 3 min after venous punctures
  Check puncture sites qh
  Monitor BP and P q4h to 8h
Avoid taking rectal temperature
Administer IM medications cautiously; apply manual pressure to injection sites until bleeding stops
Have protamine sulfate or phytonadione (Aqua-Mephyton) available
Administer routine medications cautiously; may potentiate or retard anticoagulation

● Warfarin

Patient/family teaching

Ensure that patient and/or significant other knows and understands
  Name of medication, dosage, time of administration, purpose, and side effects
  Need to avoid taking over-the-counter medications without checking with physician; to read labels of all medications
    Cold prescriptions with aspirin
    Laxatives
    Vitamins

Need to avoid aspirin (acetylsalicylic acid) without
physician's order
Importance of having laboratory work done as or-
dered and of contacting physician for possible
dosage change
General side effects: anorexia, nausea, vomiting, ab-
dominal cramps, dermatitis, and urticaria
Signs of bleeding to report to physician
Hematuria
Vomiting
Elevated temperature
Pain in joints, swelling
Epistaxis
Bleeding gums
Easy bruisability
Increased menstrual flow
Abdominal pain
Diet—moderate- to low-fat content without abundance
of dark, leafy green vegetables; avoid excessive use
of alcohol

Home care considerations

Safety precautions to prevent injury
Avoid vigorous nose-blowing and toothbrushing
Avoid use of sharp-edge instruments such as razors
Refrain from water-jet tooth cleaners; use soft-
bristled toothbrush
Refrain from engaging in dangerous hobbies or con-
tact sports
Wear shoes and slippers at all times
Importance of avoiding pregnancy while on medica-
tion; need to report to physician if pregnancy is sus-
pected
Need to avoid use of intrauterine device (IUD) for
birth control
Importance of ongoing outpatient care
Need to carry medical alert or identification card with
name of medication
Need to inform physician when planning to travel in
order to do the following:
Obtain extra medications
Arrange laboratory test

● Subcutaneous Heparin Injection

Assessment

Observations/findings

Subcutaneous bleeding
Hematoma
Bruises
Intraabdominal bleeding

Pain
Rigid, tender abdomen
Tarry stools
Bleeding gums
Epistaxis
Hematemesis
Hemoptysis
Hematuria
Injection sites
Inflammation
Bruises
Tenderness
Increased menstrual flow
Allergic reactions
Itching
Urticaria
Redness
Joints
Pain
Immobility
Pain
Flank
Abdominal

Patient/family teaching

General guidelines

Ensure that patient and/or significant other knows and
understands
Name of medication, dosage, time of administration,
purpose, and side effects
Importance of giving heparin injections at exact time
designated
Importance of not skipping any doses; keep record of
all missed doses
Need to avoid taking over-the-counter medications
without checking with physician
Aspirin
Salicylates
Need to avoid drinking alcoholic beverages while on
heparin therapy
Importance of having laboratory work done as or-
dered
Signs of bleeding to report to physician
Bleeding gums
Joint pain
Epistaxis
Hematuria
Tarry stools
Increased menstrual flow
Easy bruisability
Safety precautions to prevent injury
Avoid vigorous nose-blowing
Avoid vigorous toothbrushing

Avoid use of sharp-edged instruments such as razors

Refrain from engaging in dangerous hobbies or contact sports

Importance of preventing pregnancy while on medication; need to report to physician if pregnancy is suspected

Need to avoid use of IUD for birth control

Importance of taking correct dosage at correct time

Demonstrate and explain purpose of each step of heparin therapy

Preparation for injection

Rotation of injection sites

Action of heparin

Care of equipment

Have patient repeat steps verbally and then perform procedure

Positively reinforce proper performance of procedure and correct errors

Leave equipment at bedside for practice: syringe (1 to 2 ml with needle (25-gauge, ½ to ⅝ inch), vial of sterile water, alcohol swabs, and flat sponge or orange

Arrange to have equipment that will be used at home available

Have patient continue procedure with supervision while in hospital

Preparation of injection

Ensure that patient and/or significant other demonstrates

Handwashing technique

Preparation of syringe and needle using sterile technique

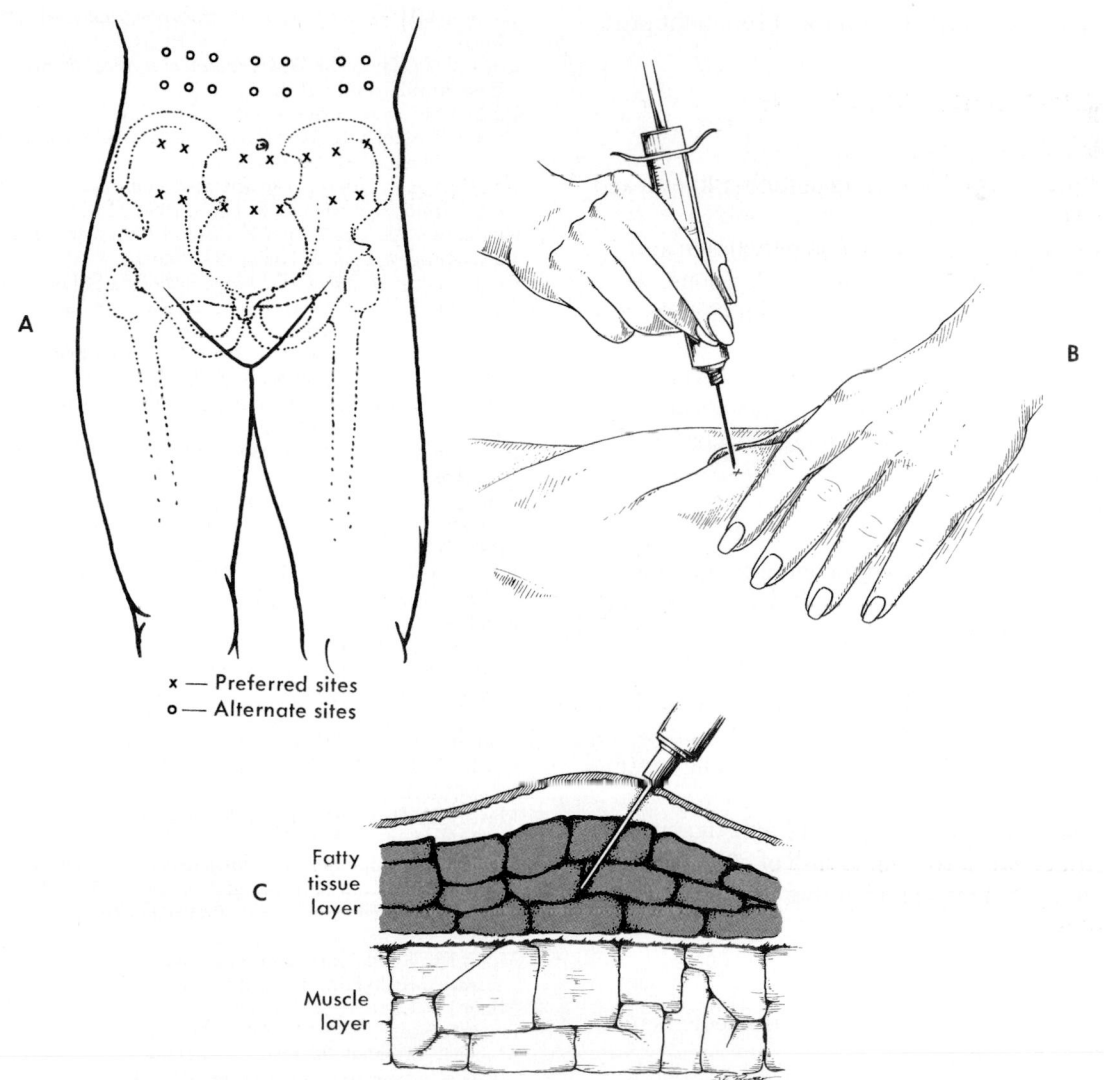

x — Preferred sites
o — Alternate sites

Fatty tissue layer

Muscle layer

Figure 3-43 Subcutaneous heparin injection. **A,** Sites to be used. **B,** Pinching skin to form a flat roll between fingers. **C,** Injection into fatty tissue layer.

Heparin Home Record*

Date	Time	Site	Dosage
1/22/96	6:30 AM	Right upper side	5000 U
	2:30 PM	Left upper side	5000 U
	10:30 PM	Right lower side	5000 U
1/23/96			
1/24/96			

*Physician's order—5000 U heparin injected every 8 hr.

Withdrawal of exact heparin dosage
Ability to maintain sterile technique throughout procedure

Site of injection

Ensure that patient and/or significant other knows and understands
  Importance of using subcutaneous fatty tissue and avoiding bruised areas, hematomas, incisions, or scarred tissue and the area within 5 cm (2 inches) of umbilicus
  Importance of rotating site of injection with every dose of heparin to prevent bleeding or tissue damage
  Importance of recording site of each injection

Injection

Ensure that patient and/or significant other demonstrates injection technique
  Select injection site (Figure 3-43, *A*)
  Prepare skin by cleaning with alcohol
  Hold syringe filled with correct heparin dosage like a pencil or a dart
  Pinch up skin, forming a flat roll between fingers (Figure 3-43, *B*)
  Insert needle at 45-degree angle and quickly push it into subcutaneous tissue up to hub of syringe; may need to guide patient's hand at this point (Figure 3-43, *C*)
NOTE: Do not pull back on plunger
Inject medication slowly
Withdraw needle; gently release skin as needle is removed
Press area gently; avoid rubbing or massaging area
Record date, time, site, and dosage of each injection on home record (see following care paths)

BIBLIOGRAPHY

Abels LF: *Mosby's manual of critical care,* St Louis, 1979, Mosby.
Allen JA, Throm L: Percutaneous transluminal coronary angioplasty: a new alternative for ischemic heart disease, *Crit Care Nurse* 2(1):24, 1982.
American Heart Association: *Guidelines for cardiac rehabilitation,* ed 2, Los Angeles, 1982, American Heart Association, Greater Los Angeles Affiliation.
Braunwald E, ed: *Heart disease: a textbook of cardiovascular medicine,* Philadelphia, 1988, WB Saunders.
Canobbio MM: *Cardiovascular disorders,* ed 3, St Louis, 1990, Mosby.
Canobbio MM: Cardiovascular system. In Thompson JM et al, eds: *Mosby's manual of clinical nursing,* ed 3, St Louis, 1993, Mosby.
Canobbio MM: Congenital heart disease in adults. In Clochesy JM et al, eds: *Critical care nursing,* ed 2, Philadelphia, 1995, WB Saunders.
Cobey JC, Covey JH: Chronic leg ulcers, *Am J Nurs,* 74:258, 1974.
Conn VS, Taylor SG, Casey B: Cardiac rehabilitation program participation and outcomes after myocardial infarction, *Rehabil Nurs* 17(2):58-62, 1992.
Conover MH: *Exercises in diagnosing ECG tracings,* ed 3, St Louis, 1984, Mosby.
Conover MH: *Pocket guide to electrocardiography,* ed 3, St Louis, 1994, Mosby.
Costrini NV, Thomson WM: *Manual of medical therapeutics,* ed 22, Boston, 1977, Little, Brown.
Dasling MC et al: Surgery of the aorta, *CCQ* 8:25, 1985.
Ernst CB, Stanley JC, eds: *Current therapy in vascular surgery,* Philadelphia, 1991, BC Decker.
Fardy PA et al: *Cardiac rehabilitation: implication for the nurse and other health professionals,* St Louis, 1980, Mosby.
Goldberger AL, Goldberger E: *Clinical electrocardiography: a simplified approach,* ed 4, St Louis, 1990, Mosby.
Goldberger E: *Textbook of clinical cardiology,* St Louis, 1982, Mosby.
Guzzetta EE, Dossey DM: *Cardiovascular nursing: holistic practice,* St Louis, 1992, Mosby.
Harris L et al: The cardiovascular effects of caffeine post-myocardial infarction, *Circulation* 72(Suppl III):116, 1985.
Herman JA: Nursing assessment and nursing diagnosis in patients with peripheral vascular disease, *Nurs Clin North Am* 21:219, 1986.
Johanson BC et al: *Standards for critical care,* ed 3, St Louis, 1988, Mosby.
Joint National Committee: The 1984 Report of the National Committee on detection, evaluation, and treatment of high blood pressure, *Arch Intern Med* 144:1045, 1989.
Kayser SR: Drug interaction with coumarin anticoagulants, *Prog Cardiovas Nurs* 8(1):40-45, 1993.
Kim HS, Chung EK: Torsades de pointes: polymorphous ventricular tachycardia, *Heart Lung* 12(3):296, 1983.
Kinney M et al: *Comprehensive cardiac care,* ed 8, St Louis, 1995, Mosby.
Kinney MR, Packa DR, Dunbar SB: *AACN's clinical reference for critical care nursing,* ed 3, St Louis, 1993, Mosby.
Lasater MG: Torsades de pointes: etiology and treatment, *Focus Crit Care* 13(5):17, 1986.
Massey JA: Diagnostic testing for peripheral vascular disease, *Nurs Clin North Am* 21:207, 1986.
McCance KL, Huether SE: *Pathophysiology: the biological basis for disease in adults and children,* ed 2, St Louis, 1994, Mosby.
McCarthy JJ, Williams LR: Femoral artery reconstruction, *CCQ* 8:39, 1985.
Miller DC, Roon AJ: *Diagnosis and management of peripheral vascular disease,* Menlo Park, Calif, 1982, Addison-Wesley Publishing.
Miner PD, Canobbio MM: Care of adult and cyanotic congenital heart disease, *Nurs Clin North Am* 29:249, 1994.
Moore K, Maschak BJ: How patient education can reduce the hazards of anticoagulation, *Nursing '77* 7:24, 1977.
Mosby's Patient teaching guides, St Louis, 1994, Mosby.
Pagana KD, Pagana TJ: *Mosby's diagnostic and laboratory test reference,* ed 2, St Louis, 1994, Mosby.

Painain GA et al: Cardiac transplantation: indications, procurement, operation and management, *Heart Lung* 14:484, 1985.

Parsonnet V et al: A revised code for pacemaker identification: pacemaker study group, *Circulation* 64:60A, 1981.

Ryan TJ, Skolnick AE: Indications for coronary angioplasty, *Heart Dis Stroke* 3(1):29-36, 1994.

Sadler D: *Nursing for cardiovascular health,* East Norwalk, Conn, 1984, Appleton-Century-Crofts.

Sheehy Budassi SA: *Emergency nursing: principles and practice,* ed 3, St Louis, 1992, Mosby.

Skidmore-Roth L: *Mosby's 1996 nursing drug reference,* St Louis, 1996, Mosby.

Smith S: *AACN Tissue and organ transplantation: implications for professional nursing practice,* St Louis, 1990, Mosby.

Spillall JA: Office diagnosis of occlusive arterial disease, *J Cardiovasc Med:* 107, 1984.

Swearingen PL et al: *Manual of critical care: applying nursing diagnosis to adult critical illness,* ed 3, St Louis, 1995, Mosby.

Thelan L et al: *Critical care nursing: diagnosis and management,* ed 2, St Louis, 1994, Mosby.

Underhill S et al: *Cardiac nursing,* ed 3, Philadelphia, 1994, JB Lippincott.

Wang WWT, Engler MM: Hypertension update: highlights from 1993 national report, *Prog Cardiovasc Nurs* 8(1):13-23, 1993.

Whitman G, Hicks LE: Major nursing diagnosis, following cardiac transplantation, *J Cardiovasc Nurs* 2:1, 1988.

Wright JM: Pharmacologic management of congestive heart failure, *CCQ* 18(1):1995.

Zelkovic M, Nichols GG: Carotid endardirectomy in symptomatic patients, *Heart Dis Stroke* 2(4):313-316, 1993.

USC UNIVERSITY HOSPITAL
1500 San Pablo
Los Angeles, CA 90033 ©1991

SIDE 1 **MULTIDISCIPLINARY PLAN**

NAME _____
ALLERGIES _____
ADMIT DATE _____

DIAGNOSIS _____

SURGERY AORTIC PROCEDURES / AORTO-FEMORAL BYPASS/ANEURYSMS

DRG 111   ALOS 8.4

DISCHARGE OUTCOMES

PHYSIOLOGICAL	Patient will maintain patent graft site(s) post-operatively. Patient will be hemodynamically stable, adequate nutrition maintained, and free from complications/infection.
COGNITIVE	Patient will verbalize acceptance of diagnosis and ask pertinent questions regarding future management of health care.
PSYCHOLOGICAL	Patient will verbalize acceptance of potential lifestyle changes, express concerns, and ask questions. Patient will exhibit appropriate coping mechanisms.

DISCIPLINE	PRE-OP/ PRE-ADMIT DAY 1 — MED/SURG	DOS DAY 2 SURGERY/PAR/SICU	POD#1 DAY 3 SICU	POD#2 DAY 4 SICU → DOU	POD#3 DAY 5 DOU	POD#4 DAY 6 DOU → MED/SURG
LOCATION / DATE	MED/SURG	SURGERY/PAR/SICU	SICU	SICU → DOU	DOU	DOU → MED/SURG
LABS	Cell Saver T&C 6 units CBC Chem 20 UA PT PTT	Stat Hct on arrival to unit Spun Hct q 6° x 24° CBC Chem 7	CBC Chem 7	CBC Chem 7	DC daily labs p̄ eating Chem 7 qod	
CARDIO-PULMONARY	ECG Preop non-invasive vascular lab doppler study Pulse oximetry	Intubated → ventilator ABG Invasive monitoring Swan-ganz to monitor	Extubate ECG I.S. post-extubation	DC Swan Ganz & PA-line prior to transfer I.S. q1°	I.S. q1° W/A	I.S. q1° W/A
IMAGING/ NUCLEAR MEDICINE	CXR	Non-invasive intra-operative graft monitoring prior to closure.	CXR if pt remains intubated			
SOCIAL SERVICES D/C PLAN REHAB. SERVICES		Social worker consult Assess for potential home needs				
PHARMACY	Pre-op antibiotics Bowel prep c̄ phospha soda Ancef 1 gm IV	IV antibiotics x 24° Cardiac medication Pain medications Nipride drip for SBP>160 IV-D5LR 100-125cc/hr	If diabetic-pt will require Accu✓ c̄ insulin coverage	DC Nipride if not already done		Convert IV to S.L.
DIETARY/ NUTRITION	Clear liquids NPO p̄ midnight	NPO NG tube to LCS x 24°	DC NG tube Strict NPO		Clear liquids	Advance diet

Used by permission of USC University Hospital, Los Angeles, California.

PATIENT NAME: _____

MULTIDISCIPLINARY PLAN

DISCIPLINE	PRE-OP/ PRE-ADMIT	DAY 1	DOS DAY 2	POD#1 DAY 3	POD#2 DAY 4	POD#3 DAY 5	POD#4 DAY 6
		DATE	DATE	DATE	DATE	DATE	DATE
PATIENT ACTIVITY		Up as tolerated Betadine scrub to abdomen & lower extremities	Bedrest Turn q2° Compression boots	Dangle	OOB to chair Stand at bedside prior to transfer	Ambulate c̄ walker & assistance	Progressive ambulation DC compression boots when fully ambulatory
EDUCATION		Orientation to hospital Pre-op leg exercises I.S. C & DB Foley				Emphasize risk factors associated c̄ vascular disease including diet, smoking & pulse checks DC Foley	Pt to return demonstrate pulse checks Home expectations: • avoid heavy physical activity

COLLABORATIVE PROBLEMS

❶ Tissue perfusion, altered R/T graft, & hemodynamics.

❷ Alteration in comfort; pain R/T incisional site.

❸ Anxiety, fear R/T illness & hospitalization.

❹ Alteration in gas exchange/airway maintenance R/T intubation, mechanical ventilation, & general anesthesia.

❺ Potential for infection R/T surgical procedure & acute care stay.

❻ Knowledge deficit R/T discharge expectations, activity levels & follow-up care.

OUTCOMES

❶ Pt will be free of tissue ischemia c̄ patent graft, adequate arterial blood flow; absence of thrombophlebitis.

❷ Pt will have absence or reduction of pain/discomfort.

❸ Pt will verbalize a reduction in anxiety c̄ provision of information & encouragement

❹ Pt will demonstrate effective use of I.S. q1°

❹ Pt will display adequate respiratory function c̄ sats > 93%.

❺ Pt will remain infection free & afebrile.

❶ Pt will be weaned off vasoactive drips & restarted on pre-op medications.

❷ Pt will exhibit a decreased requirement for pain medications; pain controlled on po medications.

❻ Pt will verbalize understanding of disease processes & risk factors. Able to verbalize expectations for follow-up care & ambulating independently.

KEY

❶ To initiate a problem or intervention, document under corresponding date.

❷ Document outcomes under appropriate date for achieving the goal.

❸ To discontinue an intervention or resolve a patient problem highlight, date, and initial.

KEY _____

Continued.

PLAN OF CARE DISCUSSED WITH			DAY 1	DOS DAY 2	POD#1 DAY 3	POD#2 DAY 4	POD#3 DAY 5	POD#4 DAY 6
DATE	INITIAL	S.O.	Pt.	DATE _____	DATE _____	DATE _____	DATE _____	DATE _____	DATE _____

INTERVENTIONS

DAY 1	DOS DAY 2	POD#1 DAY 3	POD#2 DAY 4	POD#3 DAY 5	POD#4 DAY 6
—Explain disease process, expected outcomes, & provide information as needed	—Monitor all circulatory parameters distal to graft (designated by surgeon): • pulses • color • sensation • numbness • temperature • level of discomfort • immobility —Check pulses by palpation or doppler q1° x 24°	—Check pulses by palpation or doppler q2° x 48°	—Check pulses by palpation or doppler q4°	—Check pulses by palpation or doppler q4° —Assist c̄ ambulation —Begin teaching in reference to risk factors associated c̄ disease —Continue I & O —Assess pt ability to tolerate ordered diet	—Assess ambulation
—Encourage pt to verbalize fears		—Begin weaning off Nipride	—Nipride discontinued prior to transfer		
			—D/C O₂ sats if not on transfer orders		
	—Maintain hemodynamic lines; closely monitor hemodynamic profile & I & O				
	—Turn pt maintaining straight legs; support legs c̄ pillows				
	—Monitor for chest pain & ECG changes —Avoid restriction of affected extremity				
	—Assess pt for nature of pain; note quality, site, & severity of pain —Medicate c̄ analgesics as ordered. Assess for effectiveness				
	—Monitor for ↑ temperature, redness or drainage from surgical site, tachycardia & elevated WBC				
	—Maintain ventilator settings as ordered —Monitor O₂ sats, assess breath sounds q4°: Nipride to keep SBP < 180 (or ordered parameter)				

Case Manager: _____

Consulting MD: _____

Social Service _____

Anointing of The Sick Date: _____

DATE	SIGNATURES	DATE	SIGNATURES	DATE	SIGNATURES

MULTIDISCIPLINARY PLAN UPDATE

DATE	SIGNATURES

USC UNIVERSITY HOSPITAL
1500 San Pablo   Los Angeles, CA 90033 ©1991

SIDE 2

MULTIDISCIPLINARY PLAN

NAME _____
ALLERGIES _____

DIAGNOSIS _____

SURGERY   AORTIC PROCEDURES
AORTO-FEMORAL BYPASS/ANEURYSMS

DRG _____ ALOS _____   ADMIT DATE _____

DISCHARGE OUTCOMES

PHYSIOLOGICAL	Patient will maintain adequate nutrition. Graft site will remain patent postoperatively. Patient will be hemodynamically stable & free from complications/infection.
COGNITIVE	Patient will verbalize acceptance of diagnosis & ask pertinent questions regarding future management of health care.
PSYCHOLOGICAL	Patient will verbalize acceptance of potential lifestyle changes, express concerns and ask questions. Patient will exhibit appropriate coping mechanisms.

DISCIPLINE	PRE-OP/ PRE-ADMIT	POD#5 DAY 7 DATE	POD#6 DAY 8 DATE	POD#7 DAY 9 DATE	POD#8 DAY 10 DATE	POD#9 DAY 11 DATE	POD#10 DAY 12 DATE
LOCATION		MED/SURG	MED/SURG→HOME				
LABS		Chem 7 CBC					
CARDIO-PULMONARY		I.S. q1°	Lower extremity ankle-brachial index prior to discharge				
IMAGING/ NUCLEAR MEDICINE							
SOCIAL SERVICES D/C PLAN REHAB. SERVICES		Discharge planner to re-evaluate home needs prior to discharge					
PHARMACY		DC S.L.	Discharge home c̄ po analgesics for pain control Patient will continue c̄ all pre-op prescribed medications				
DIETARY/ NUTRITION		Diet as tolerated					

Used by permission of USC University Hospital, Los Angeles, California.

Continued.

PATIENT NAME: _____

MULTIDISCIPLINARY PLAN

DISCIPLINE	PRE-OP/ PRE-ADMIT	POD#5 DAY 7	POD#6 DAY 8	POD#7 DAY 9	POD#8 DAY 10	POD#9 DAY 11	POD#10 DAY 12
		DATE ___	DATE ___	DATE ___	DATE ___	DATE ___	DATE ___
PATIENT ACTIVITY		Progressive ambulation					
EDUCATION		Discharge teaching to include: • meds • s/sx to report to health care team	Review discharge teaching Discuss need to return to physician 10 days - 2 weeks post-discharge				

COLLABORATIVE PROBLEMS

DATE	DOC DATE/INIT		COLLABORATIVE PROBLEMS	DATE	DOC DATE/INIT	
		❶	Tissue perfusion, altered R/T graft, & hemodynamics.			
		❷	Alteration in comfort; pain R/T incisional site.			
		❺	Potenial for infection R/T surgical procedure & acute care stay.			
		❻	Knowledge deficit R/T discharge expectations, activity levels, & follow-up care.			

OUTCOMES

❶ Pt will have consistent quality of pulses by palpation or doppler. ❺ Pt will remain free from s/sx of infection.	❻ Pt will verbalize understanding of teaching provided, along c̄ understanding of required follow-up appointments. ❷ Pt will demonstrate pain control c̄ prescribed po medications

KEY

❶ To initiate a problem or intervention, document under corresponding date.

❷ Document outcomes under appropriate date for achieving the goal.

❸ To discontinue an intervention or resolve a patient problem highlight, date, and initial.

		POD#5 DAY 7	POD# 6 DAY 8	POD#7 DAY 9	POD#8 DAY 10	POD#9 DAY 11	POD#10 DAY 12

PLAN OF CARE DISCUSSED WITH

DATE	INITIAL	S.O.	Pt.	DATE ____	DATE ____	DATE ____	DATE ____	DATE ____	DATE ____

INTERVENTIONS

—Review discharge teaching; assess p understanding, & clarify any mis-understandings
—Assess ambulation & ability to perform ADLs
—Re-assess pt tolerance for prescribed diet

—Re-assess pt under-standing of follow-up expectations

Case Manager: _____

Consulting MD: _____

Social Service _____

Anointing of
The Sick
Date: _____

MULTIDISCIPLINARY PLAN UPDATE

DATE	SIGNATURES	DATE	SIGNATURES	DATE	SIGNATURES	DATE	SIGNATURES

BARNES

CARE PATH® 207
23 HR.
CARDIAC CATHETERIZATION

SERVICE		PHYSICIAN	
PRIMARY NURSE		PRIMARY NURSE	
DC DATE	ADM DATE	DATE OF SURGERY	A-8

Problem Number	PATIENT PROBLEMS/NURSING DIAGNOSES
#1	LACK OF KNOWLEDGE R/T POSSIBLE NEW DISEASE OR UNFAMILIARITY WITH PROCEDURE
#2	ACTIVITY INTOLERANCE R/T BEDREST IN SUPINE POSITION FOR 24 HRS.
#3	POTENTIAL ALTERATION IN NUTRITION R/T DECREASED INTAKE, NAUSEA, VOMITING
#4	POTENTIAL ALTERATION IN URINARY ELIMINATION R/T INABILITY TO VOID IN SUPINE POSITION
#5	POTENTIAL FOR INJURY R/T PROCEDURE
#6	ANXIETY R/T PROCEDURE AND COPING MECHANISM * IF APPROPRIATE

Problem Number		PRE-ADMISSION	PRE-CATH
#1 #2	ASSESSMENT / MONITORING	Clinical Coordinator calls pt. to evaluate: – hx of heart disease / symptoms – hx of CABG / PTCA – medication hx – allergy hx – previous CXR / ECG completion – advanced directive	Record height and weight in chart Complete pre-cath orders Complete pre-cath checklist for pts. coming to cath lab from floor **All labs and diagnostic data within acceptable parameters for cath completion** IV site condition, type Nutritional status Pedal pulses prior **VS WNL** and recorded
	CONSULTS	Social Work if Clinical Coordinator identifies need for emotional support, community resources, financial resources, advanced directive Dietary if risk factors identified Pastoral Care	
	PROCEDURE / TEST	Pre-cath labs completed SMA 6 SMA 12 PT / PTT CBC ECG CXR (PA-lateral) within past 6 months	**Pre-cath labs WNL** SMA 6 SMA 12 PT / PTT CBC ECG CXR (PA and lateral) completed within past 6 months
	TREATMENT		
#1 #2	ACTIVITY		Determine past pt. tolerance to maintaining bedrest and initiate plans to reduce discomfort post-cath

Used by permission of Barnes Hospital, St Louis, Missouri.

BARNES

CARE PATH® 207
23 HR.
CARDIAC CATHETERIZATION

CNS	DIETARY	RT
HOME HEALTH	OT	OTHER
PT	SW	OTHER

A-8

Problem Number	PATIENT PROBLEMS/NURSING DIAGNOSES
#7	POTENTIAL ALTERATION IN COMFORT R/T IMMOBILITY, INTERRUPTED SLEEP
#8	POTENTIAL ALTERATION IN BOWEL ELIMINATION R/T IMMOBILITY
#9	POTENTIAL ALTERATION IN SKIN R/T IMMOBILITY

POST-CATH	DC OUTCOMES	RESOURCE INFORMATION
1) VS with pulse check & groin check q 15 mins. x q 1 hr. x 4 and then q 4 hrs. if stable 2) Report the following to House Officer / Cath team / ASM MD immediately: Significant change in VS, diminution or loss of pulse, chest pain / angina equivalent hematoma, back pain, bleeding at groin 3) Notify House Officer / ASM MD if unable to void 4 hrs, post-cath **Pt. will be free of complications post-cardiac cath** I / O Pain / comfort Nutritional status	**Pt. will have no s/sx of impaired circulation R/T cardiac cath** **Groin site without hematoma** **Pedal pulse - normal** **Affected leg - color, temp sensation - normal**	**Cardiac Catheterization DC Instructions** The following information is intended to serve as a guide to assist with your care after DC following cardiac catheterization. 1. Resume your normal diet immediately, unless directed otherwise by your physician. 2. It is important to limit activity of the limb site used for the catheterization for 3 days. This includes, but is not limited to, activities such as aerobics, swimming, jogging, running, bicycling, bowling dancing, rowing, or stair-stepping. If you are involved in activities not listed above, please ask your nurse or physician for specific instructions.
Contact intern / resident / ASM STAT on return of pt. from cath lab for immediate evaluation. Consult Cardiology Fellow or cath lab for significant changes in pt. condition. After hours contact **362-3796** for a cath lab team member. Pastoral Care	**Social Work consult completed** **Dietary completed or** **follow-up appointment arranged**	3. Avoid lifting for 2 days. 4. Gentle walking is permissible but only on level ground.
If hematoma occurs: - Consider Duplex scan and CBC VS **Cardiac cath completed**	**Pt. / signifcant other will verbalize understanding of diagnostic findings**	5. No driving for 2 days. 6. Restrict stair-climbing for 2 days, if possible. If stair-climbing is essential, climb with your non-catheterized leg, then bring the catheterized led up to the same step.
Keep 5 lb. sandbag to _____ groin for _____ hrs. post-cath		7. Customary sexual activity may be resumed after 2 days. Use postures that do not place a strain on the catheterized leg.
Maintain strict bedrest for _____ hrs. after cath. May raise HOB 30° at _____ if VS stable Use electric bed raiser Use orthopedic bedpan for female pts. Place bed in reverse Trendelenberg position to assist males in voiding Utilize appropriate comfort measures to relieve discomfort of bedrest: - pillow under knee of non-affected leg - rolled blanket under back	**Pt. will verbalize understanding of activity restriction the first 3 days post-cath**	8. Avoid straining for bowel movements for 7 days. If you tend to be constipated and/or regularly strain to pass stool, please inform your nurse of this so that a stool softening medication can be ordered. 9. It is common to have some bruising or purple discoloration of the skin near the puncture site.

Continued.

		PRE-ADMISSION	**PRE-CATH**
#1 #2	MEDS / IV	Clinical Coordinator will notify private MD of potential dye allergies to initiate pre-treatment med of Cimetidine, Prednisone and Benadryl	Administer pt. usual PO medications, unless otherwise ordered. Cardiac meds to be taken with sip of water If IDDM, evaluate need for AM insulin requirements and IV hydration. If Cr elevated, consider Mannitol Initiate and monitor IV fluid
#1	NUTRITION	NPO after midnight (except for medications). Limited water intake if specified in pre-cath orders	NPO except meds
#1	PATIENT / FAMILY EDUCATION	**Pt. / family verbalizes understanding of Care Path. Plan of care has been mutually set with pt. / family.** Clinical Coordinator completes pre-cath pt. teaching including: – Remind pt. to bring all current medications with them to hospital – Reminder to bring med records from private MD – NPO after midnight – Remain on bedrest after cath till following morning – No driving for 2 days after cath **Pt. / significant other verbalizes understanding of pre-cath preparation**	Instruct pt. they should wear dentures and may bring glasses to procedure. Remove jewelry and watches, tape rings. Ask pt. to empty bladder and bowel prior to procedure Instruct families that they may not accompany pt. to procedure. **Pt. followed pre-admission instructions** **Pt. / significant other verbalizes understanding of procedure**
#1	DISCHARGE PLANNING		
	PSYCHOSOCIAL / EMOTIONAL / SPIRITUAL NEEDS		Ensure pt. has transportation / accommodation arrangements completed for day of DC Provide opportunity to discuss implications / issues relating to procedure Pt. / significant other exhibits positive coping skills relating to procedure
	SIGNATURES		

POST-CATH	DC OUTCOMES	
4 IV fluids per orders. Resume previous medications when VS stable or as ordered by House Officer / ASM MD	d/c IV if to be DC	However, if any of the following occur, immediately contact your own physician. A. Bleeding from the catheterization puncture site, apply gentle pressure with a clean gauze or cloth (and call your physician or the Barnes Hospital Emergency Department immediately).
Encourage oral fluids, unless nausea / vomiting Withhold solid foods for _____ hrs. Resume previous diet after _____ . **Pt. will not have nausea or vomiting**	**If indicated, pt. verbalizes method to contact outpatient nutritional counseling office for follow-up appointment**	B. If a knot or lump under the skin increases in size, or C. If bruising appears to be worsening or tracking/moving down the leg rather than disappearing. D. If the leg used for catheterization appears pale in color and/or feels cooler to touch compared to the opposite leg.
Pt. will demonstrate compliance with post-procedural instructions	Complete post-cath teaching and provide pt. with instruction sheet **Pt. will verbalize understanding of medication regime** **Pt. / significant other will verbalize understanding of invasive procedure, DC instructions and follow-up** **Pt. / significant other will verbalize s/sx to report to MD when at home**	E. If the leg used for the catheterization appears reddened, swollen and/or feels warmer to touch compared to the opposite leg. 10. You may bathe or shower the day following the catheterization. Be careful to avoid slipping as your leg may feel stiff.
	For delays in DC contact cardiology nurse coordinator 24972	11. Resume the same medication you were taking before the catheterization unless otherwise ordered by your physician. 12. If you have any questions or concerns contact your private physician or call Barnes Hospital Emergency Department at **314 (362-9123).**
Provide opportunity to discuss implications / issues relating to procedure Pt. / significant other exhibits positive coping skills relating to procedure	**Pt. will have adequate transportation and accommodation arrangements for DC** **Pt. / significant other exhibits positive coping skills relating to procedure implications**	

Continued.

BARNES

NURSE ADMISSION NOTE
C-2

Date _____ Time _____ Informant _____ *Age _____

T _____ P _____ R _____ B/P _____ Ht. _____ Wt. _____

Chief Complaint and History of Present Illness _____

_____

_____

_____

ADDRESSOGRAPH

Medical / Surgical History	Date	Medical / Surgical History	Date	Medical / Surgical History	Date

Has received blood products in the past: ☐ Yes   ☐ No   If yes, list dates _____   Reactions: ☐ Yes   ☐ No

Allergies: _____   Advanced Directives: ☐ Yes   ☐ No

Medication / Dose / Freq.	Time of Last Dose	Patient Knows Med Rx	Medication / Dose / Freq.	Time of Last Dose	Patient Knows Med Rx	Medication / Dose / Freq.	Time of Last Dose	Patient Knows Med Rx

Patient Provided: ☐ Admission Kit   ☐ ID Band   ☐ Sensitivity / Allergy Band   ☐ Sensitivity / Allergy Sticker on Chart

Patient Instructed: ☐ Valuables Inventory ☐ Waiver Signed ☐ Smoking / Visitor Policy ☐ Nurse Call / Emergency / TV / Phone

☐ Patient's Rights / Responsibilities   SIGNATURE: _____

Check if infusion device in use _____

Amt.	Types of Fluid	Product # or Medication added	Date/Hr. Start	INT.	Date/Hr. Start	Int.	Amt. Rec'd	IV Site	IV Appearance	✓	IV Site Care Date/Hr.	Tubing Change Date/Hr.	Int.

GRAPHIC SHEET

TEMPERATURE

	DATE:						DATE:					
Centigrade	HOSP DAY#		O.R. DAY#				HOSP DAY#		O.R. DAY#			
TIME:	02 04	06 08	10 12	14 16	18 20	22 24	02 04	06 08	10 12	14 16	18 20	22 24

41°
40°
39°
38°
37°
36°
↓ 35.5°

• = Oral ⓡ = Rectal Ⓐ = Axilliary

BLOOD PRESSURE CHART

PULSE   X = Pulse a = Apical

	DATE:						DATE:					
TIME:	02 04	06 08	10 12	14 16	18 20	22 24	02 04	06 08	10 12	14 16	18 20	22 24

140
130
120
110
100
90
80
70
↓ 50
RESP
WEIGHT
B/P

BARNES

C-10b

NURSING ASSESSMENT FLOWSHEET

DATE

INSTRUCTIONS: CIRCLE IF PRESENT.
WRITE IN ASSESSMENT.
INDICATE N/A NOT APPLICABLE OR NOT ASSESSED.

CODE: S - SELF, A - ASSIST, T - TOTAL, I - INSTRUCTED, C - COLLECTED

ADDRESSOGRAPH

NEURO / CEREBRAL	**NEURO / CEREBRAL**	ALERT CONFUSED MEMORY LOSS AGITATED ORIENTED X _____ _____	ALERT CONFUSED MEMORY LOSS AGITATED ORIENTED X _____ _____
COMFORT / SLEEP	**DISCOMFORT** INTERVENTION	_____ _____ _____	_____ _____ _____
	SLEEP STATUS	AWAKE SLEEP AT INTERVALS SLEPT	AWAKE SLEEP AT INTERVALS SLEPT
ACTIVITY / EXERCISE	**MOBILITY** LIMITATIONS / DEVICES **ACTIVITY**	INDEPENDENT ASSIST DEPENDENT _____ _____ _____	INDEPENDENT ASSIST DEPENDENT _____ _____ _____

SKIN / MUCOSA	**APPEARANCE**
	
	MATTRESS /
	EQUIPMENT
		WARM DRY TURGOR _____
		_____
		_____
		             HEEL AQUA K
		FOAM AIR PROTECTORS PAD TEDS
			WARM DRY TURGOR _____
			_____
			_____
			             HEEL AQUA K
			FOAM AIR PROTECTORS PAD TEDS

WOUND	**LOCATION** APPEARANCE **DRSG. CHANGE**	_____ _____ _____ X _____	_____ _____ _____ X _____
NUTRITION	**MEALS** TUBE-FEEDING INFUSION DEVICE	_____ CONTINUOUS BOLUS FLUSH X _____	% EATEN B: SATL: SAT CONTINUOUS BOLUS FLUSH X _____
ELIMINATION	**URINE** **BOWEL** BOWEL SOUNDS	CONTINENT INCONTINENT FOLEY _____ CONTINENT INCONTINENT GUAIAC _____ FREQ X: ABSENT PRESENT _____ ABDOMEN _____	CONTINENT INCONTINENT FOLEY _____ CONTINENT INCONTINENT GUAIAC _____ FREQ X: ABSENT PRESENT _____ ABDOMEN _____
RESPIRATORY	**AUSCULTATION**	_____ _____ O₂ _____ COUGH / SECRETION _____	_____ _____ O₂ _____ COUGH / SECRETION _____
CIRC	**CIRCULATION**	_____	_____
OTHER	**SPECIMEN**	I C TEST _____ _____	I C TEST _____ _____
	SIGNATURE / STATUS		SIGNATURE / STATUS
	HYGIENE: S A T BATH TUB SHOWER SHAVE HAIR NAILS ORAL	**SAFETY** ID BAND ON _____ SIDERAILS IN USE _____	**HYGIENE:** S A T BATH TUB SHOWER SHAVE HAIR NAILS ORAL **SAFETY** ID BAND ON _____ SIDERAILS IN USE _____

Used by permission of Barnes Hospital, St Louis, Missouri.

USC UNIVERSITY HOSPITAL
1500 San Pablo
Los Angeles, CA 90033 ©1991

NAME _____
ALLERGIES _____

DIAGNOSIS __CAROTID ARTERY STENOSIS__   SIDE 1

MULTIDISCIPLINARY PLAN

SURGERY __CAROTID ENDARTERECTOMY__

ADMIT DATE _____

DISCHARGE OUTCOMES	DRG 005 ALOS 6.5
PHYSIOLOGICAL	Patient will have improved carotid blood flow, be afebrile, healing incision, & VS stable. Patient will maintain baseline neurological status.
COGNITIVE	Patient will verbalize knowledge of risk factors & prevention of disease process as well as expected follow-up regimen.
PSYCHOLOGICAL	Patient will verbalize acceptance of potential lifestyle changes, express concerns, ask questions, & exhibit effective coping mechanisms.

DISCIPLINE	PRE-OP/ PRE-ADMIT	DOS DAY 1	POD#1 DAY 2	POD#2 DAY 3	POD#3 DAY 4	POD#4 DAY 5	POD#5 DAY 6
LOCATION	DATE	SURGERY/PAR/SICU	SICU → DOU	DOU → MED/SURG	MED/SURG	MED/SURG → HOME	DATE
LABS	CBC Chem 20 PT PTT UA Type & screen 4u	Hct stat post-op (Check Blood bank for autologous directed blood ↑ or ↑↑ units)	CBC Chem 7				
CARDIO-PULMONARY	ECG	I.S. Pulse oximetry	D/C pulse oximetry on transfer				
IMAGING/ NUCLEAR MEDICINE	CXR Carotid duplex scan	Arteriogram during surgery Carotid duplex scan intra-op					
SOCIAL SERVICES D/C PLAN REHAB. SERVICES		Social worker support as needed Assess for potential home needs & discharge planning		Re-evaluate needs prior to discharge			
PHARMACY	ASA ↑ prior to OR	Vasoactive drips for BP control (Nipride) Pain medication Start ASA post-op ↑ qd	DC vasoactive drips Change IV to S.L. Change to po anti-hypertensives & pain medications	DC S.L.	Discharge medications: • po analgesics • ASA ↑ tab qd • Continue pre-op prescribed medications		
DIETARY/ NUTRITION		NPO May have clear liquids when fully awake	Advance diet as tolerated				

Used by permission of USC University Hospital Los Angeles, California.

Continued.

MULTIDISCIPLINARY PLAN

PATIENT NAME:

DISCIPLINE	PRE-OP/ PRE-ADMIT	DOS DAY 1	POD# 1 DAY 2	POD#2 DAY 3	POD#3 DAY 4	POD#4 DAY 5	POD#5 DAY 6
		DATE	DATE	DATE	DATE	DATE	DATE
PATIENT ACTIVITY		HOB ↑ 30° Leg exercises compression boots	OOB to chair Ambulate c̄ assistance	Independent ambulation DC compression boots when fully ambulatory			
EDUCATION		Orient to environment Teach purpose/use of I.S., cough & deep breathe, foley, JP Acquaint pt c̄ equipment used for monitoring	Reinforce teaching Observe pt perform I.S. D/C foley	Discuss risk factors associated c̄ vascular diseases. Include diet, smoking, & pulse checks	Discuss home & follow-up expectations: • No driving x 1 week • Avoid heavy, physical activity • May resume usual ADLs • Walking is good exercise	Discuss need for surgeon's office appointment 10 days- 2 wks post-discharge Call office at any time for questions	

COLLABORATIVE PROBLEMS

DATE					DATE		DC DATE/INIT
❶ Potential alteration in LOC, R/T stroke, nerve palsy, & swallowing difficulty.							
❷ Alteration in tissue perfusion R/T hypertension (which may disrupt integrity of graft, sutures, newly manipulated vessel).							
❸ Potential for alteration in gas exchange/airway clearance R/T airway occlusion from hematoma, bleeding, & post-anesthesia complications.							
❹ Alteration in comfort, pain R/T incision site.							
❺ Knowledge deficit R/T discharge expectations, activity levels, & follow-up care.							

OUTCOMES

❶ Any S/SX of neurological damage postop will have immediate intervention & documentation.	❶ Pt will be able to swallow c̄ s difficulty & is awake, alert, & oriented.		❷ Pt will be weaned off vasoactive drips & restarted on pre-op medications.		❺ Pt will verbalize understanding of disease process, risk factors, expectations for follow-up care, & ambulating independently.		
❷ Pt will be hemodynamically stable, including VS which are controlled on prescribed vasoactive medications.			❹ Pt will demonstrate a decreased need for pain medications; po pain medications adequate for pain relief.				
❸ Pt will maintain patent airway c̄ respiratory distress & adequate gas exchange (refer to baseline ABG).							
❹ Pt will have pain controlled/ relieved c̄ prescribed medications.							

❶ To initiate a problem or intervention, document under corresponding date.

❷ Document outcomes under appropriate date for achieving the goal.

❸ To discontinue an intervention or resolve a patient problem highlight, date, and initial.

KEY
△ = Change

PLAN OF CARE DISCUSSED WITH		
DATE	INITIAL	S.O.	Pt.

INTERVENTIONS

	DOS DAY 1	POD#1 DAY 2	POD#2 DAY 3	POD#3 DAY 4	POD#4 DAY 5	POD#5 DAY 6
DATE						
	—Neuro ✓'s q1° x 4, then q4°	—DC PA line p̄ Nipride no longer necessary	—Begin teaching R/T risk factors associated c̄ disease	—Review teaching previously done; —Assess pt understanding & clarify as needed	—Re-assess pt understanding of follow-up expectations	
	—Monitor for s/sx c̄ bleeding: • hematoma • neck swelling • airway occlusion • stridor	—Assist OOB to chair —Assess activity tolerance	—Assist c̄ ambulation —DC compression boots when fully ambulatory	—Explain discharge instructions —Assess ambulation		
	—Maintain JP drain to bulb suction —Assess amount & consistency of drainage	—Assess breath sounds, respiratory status & airway q4° after transfer	—Neuro ✓'s q8° p̄ transfer	—Expect DC of JP drain		
	—Sequential compression boots until fully ambulatory	—I & O qsh				
	—Titrate Nipride to keep systolic BP within prescribed parameters					
	—Monitor ECG for △'s consist c̄ ischemia					
	—Assess breath sounds, respiratory status & airway q1° x 4, then q2°					
	—I & O q2° —Maintain integrity of hemodynamic lines					
	—Assess & document effectiveness of pain medications					
	—Assess for hoarseress; notify MD if this develops					

Case Manager:

Consulting MD:

Social Service

Anointing of The Sick Date:

MULTIDISCIPLINARY PLAN UPDATE

DATE	SIGNATURES	DATE	SIGNATURES	DATE	SIGNATURES

Admission Date/Time: _____ Clinical Path Date/Time: _____ Discharge Date/Time: _____ Case Manager/Phone# _____	Rex Healthcare Congestive Heart Failure (CHF) Clinical Pathway DRG 127 Expected LOS 5.0 Days	Addressograph

NOTE: DID YOU CONTACT YOUR M.D. PRIOR TO COMING TO THE ED? YES____ NO____
Advanced Directive? YES   NO
PATIENT/FAMILY TO CONTACT FOR FOLLOW-UP: PHONE: DATE:

Category	Preadmit/ED_____	Day 1/ Unit _____	Day 2 _____	Day 3 _____	Day 4 _____	Day 5 _____
DIAGNOSTIC TESTING	EKG, CXR, CBC, M7, M12, Magnesium, Blood Gas or Pulse Ox, Coags*, Cardiac Enzymes*, Dig and other appropriate drug levels	Thyroid Profile (3) UA Echo [2] All admission lab and x-ray results on chart Copy of previous Echo report on chart	M7		M7* Dig and other appropriate drug levels*	
PATIENT CARE and TREATMENTS	Obtain previous Echo (US) Pulse Ox (RT) - - - - - - - Monitor Oxygen (RT) I&O (RN) - - - - - - - - - Baseline Weight (RN) Foley* (RN) Hep Lock - - - - - - - - - Cardiac Monitor - - - - - Assessment: Neuro (RN) - - - - - - - - VS (RN) - - - - - - - - - - Breath Sounds (RN) - - - Cardiac (RN) - - - - - - - Home Meds list (RN) - - -	- - - - - - - - - - - - - - - Re-eval O2 (RT) - - - - - Daily Weight (RN) - - - - D/C Foley (RN) F/H Assessment (RN) Complete Survey–(RN) Nutrition/Medications/ Learning Needs Assessment (on back of path)	- - - - - - - - - - - - - -➔ Re-Eval Cardiac Monitor	Spot Check (RT) - - -		▪ ▪ ▪ ▪ ▪ ▪ ▪ ▪ ▪ Repeat Learning Needs Assessment (on back of path)(RN)
MEDICATIONS	IV Diuretics (1) K supplements Nitrates or other Vasodilator Digoxin ACE Inhibitors · - - - - - - Aerosolized Albuterol* Antianxiety medications Laxative of choice - - - - - Morphine - - - - - - - - - ▪		Change to Oral Medications (MD with RN or RP prompt) - - - - - - - - - - - - - - Titrate ACE Inhibitors (MD) - - -			▪ ▪ ▪
DIET	Ice chips until respiratory status is stabilized (RN)	No added salt diet (RD, MD) - - - - - - - - - - - ____ml fluid restriction* (RD, MD) - - - - - -				▪ ▪
ACTIVITY	Fowler's Positioning (RN) Bed rest (RN) Safety & Fall Precautions (RN)	BR with BRP/BR/BSC (RN) Safety & Fall Precautions (RN)	Advanced activity as tolerated (RN, PT) - - -			▪
CONSULTS	Primary Care MD if D/C from Ed	PT, Cardiologist, Clinical Nurse Spec.	RT (4) Nutrition Screening (RD)			
DISCHARGE PLANNING	Preadmission Screening System (PFS or CM) Patient/Family Services or Case Management referral* (PFS or CM) - - - - - - ◀ - - - - -	PFS/Case Management consult (PFS,CM)	PSF/Case Management assessment completed (PFS, CM) Confirm and communicate disposition with patient/family/MD [Rehab, SNF, HH](PFS) Discharge Planning Rounds (all disciplines) - - -			▪ ▪
EDUCATION	Explain testing to patient (RN) Status report to patient/ family (RN) Explain safety measures to patient/family (RN) Discharge instructions if to home (RN) ◀ - - - - -	Orientation to floor, safety measures to patient/family (RN) - - - - - Address specific learning needs (RN, RP, MD) - - - - -	CHF video and pamphlet (RN)			▪ Patient/Family education complete (RN) Patient/Family demonstrates knowledge of disease (RN) Medic-Alert bracelet, (RN, MD) wallet medication card, (RN) information given (RN, MD) Risk factor reduction (RN) Self-care (RN)

NOTE: * If individual patient's condition indicates appropriateness.

(1) Patient's potassium level to be monitored.
(2) If first time with CHF diagnosis or previous test is > one year. (3) If patient has atrial fibrillation or other evidence of thyroid disease, or if >65 and no obvious etiology for heart failure. (5) If inhaler is used.

KEY TO DISCIPLINES PERFORMING SERVICES

RN – Registered Nurse	MD – Physician
RT – Respiratory Therapist	RP – Registered Pharmacist
RD – Registered Dietitian	Lab – Laboratory
PFS – Patient & Family Services	US – Unit Secretary
CM – Case Manager	PT – Physical Therapist

Form Date: June 27,1995
Form Revision Date: August 25, 1995

CHF Clinical Pathway						
Patient's NAME:						

Category	Preadmit/ED	Day 1	Day 2	Day 3	Day 4	Day 5
OUTCOMES		LV function defined within 24 hours O_2 Sat > 92% on oxygen therapy Negative fluid balance defined by: Output > Intake Weight loss				
			Electrolytes/lab values normalizing – – – – – –	– – – – – – – –	– – – – – – –	– – – – – – ■
	Actual weight obtained in ED		Weight loss – – – – – –	– – – – – – – –	– – – – – – –	– – – – – – ■
			No dyspnea at rest – – – –	– – – – – – – –	– – – – – – –	– – – – – – ■
			Patient voiding – – – – –	– – – – – – – –	– – – – – – –	– – – – – – ■
			No symptomatic hypotension – – – – –	– – – – – – – –	– – – – – – –	– – – – – – ■
		Home meds list is obtained				
		VS stable with increased activity – – – –	– – – – – – – –	– – – – – – – ■		
	Primary Care M.D. notified if patient D/C from ED Patient admitted to appropriate level of care Patient/Family demonstrates awareness of path Appropriate test/ treatments initiated based on patient severity of illness at presentation to ED					
			Patient/Family aware of confirmed D/C Plan			
				Patient/Family aware of need for med/ precautions – – – –	– – – – – – –	– – – – – – ■
				Compliance issues identified		

Nutrition – Medication Survey on Admission/Learning Needs Assessment

Nutrition

1. I am supposed to be on a special diet, but I am having trouble following it. yes no

2. I have gained or lost 10 lbs. or more without trying in the past 6 months. yes no

3. My appetite is poor and food does not taste good to me. yes no

4. I do not always have enough money to buy the food I need. yes no

5. (if over 65 years old) I eat alone most of the time. yes no

6. If "yes" to any question 1 – 5; go to # 15.

Medications

7. I do not know why I take each of my medications. yes no

8. I get my medications at different places. yes no

9. I do not always have enough of my medications. yes no

10. I have stopped taking my medicine. yes no

11. If "yes" to any question 7 – 10; go to # 15.

Learning Needs Assessment

(ASK QUESTIONS 12 – 13 – 14 AGAIN UPON DISCHARGE)

12. What is your understanding of your heart condition?

Admission response:_____

Discharge response:_____

13. Name some behaviors that will improve your health.

Admission response:_____

Discharge response:_____

14. Describe the importance of an accurate daily weight in assessing your heart condition and how you would do it.

Admission response:_____

Discharge response:_____

15. If any question(s) has a "yes" response, the nurse will order appropriate dietitian or pharmacist consult.

Pathway Daily Variance Tracking

Variance Type/Date Occurred	Initials	Reason/Comment	Initials	Action Taken/Date Resolved	Initials
1.					
2.					
3.					
4.					
5.					
6.					
7.					
8.					
9.					
10.					

Form Date: June 27, 1995
Form Revision Date: August 25, 1995

Hematologic System

Hematologic Assessment*

● General Observations/Findings

Age
Sex
Ethnic background
Cultural background
Appearance
  Stated age equals appearance
  Pallor
  Facial flushing
  Profuse perspiration
  Signs of pain
  Dehydration
  Abnormal body posture, movements, or gait
  Activity level
  Cachexia
Vital signs
  T, P, R, or BP changes
  Height and weight changes
  Functional health patterns

● Integumentary System

Skin and mucous membranes
  Complaints of
    Pruritus

*See Table 4-1 on p. 216 for possible assessment conclusions.

Bruising and bleeding easily
  Lesions, cuts, infections that do not heal
Pallor
Cyanosis
Plethora
Erythema
Jaundice
Petechiae
Ecchymosis
Purpuric lesions
White patches
Telangiectasis
Rashes
Subcutaneous nodules
Infiltrates
Vesicles
Increased skin temperature
Drainage
Ulcers
Diaphoresis
Turgor
Note distribution of abnormalities
Vascularity
Scars

Pigmentary changes
Nails
  Color
  Brittle
  Ridges
  Flattened dorsal curvature
  Spoon shaped
  Clubbed
  Loosened
  Thickened
Hair
  Texture
  Growth patterns,
    loss or thinning
Eyes
  Edema
  Redness
  Inflammation
  Infection
  Enlarged/engorged vessels
  Vessel tortuosity
  Infiltration
  Hemorrhage
  Cataracts

Table 4-1 Approach to Hematologic Disorders; Various Clues That May Be Found*

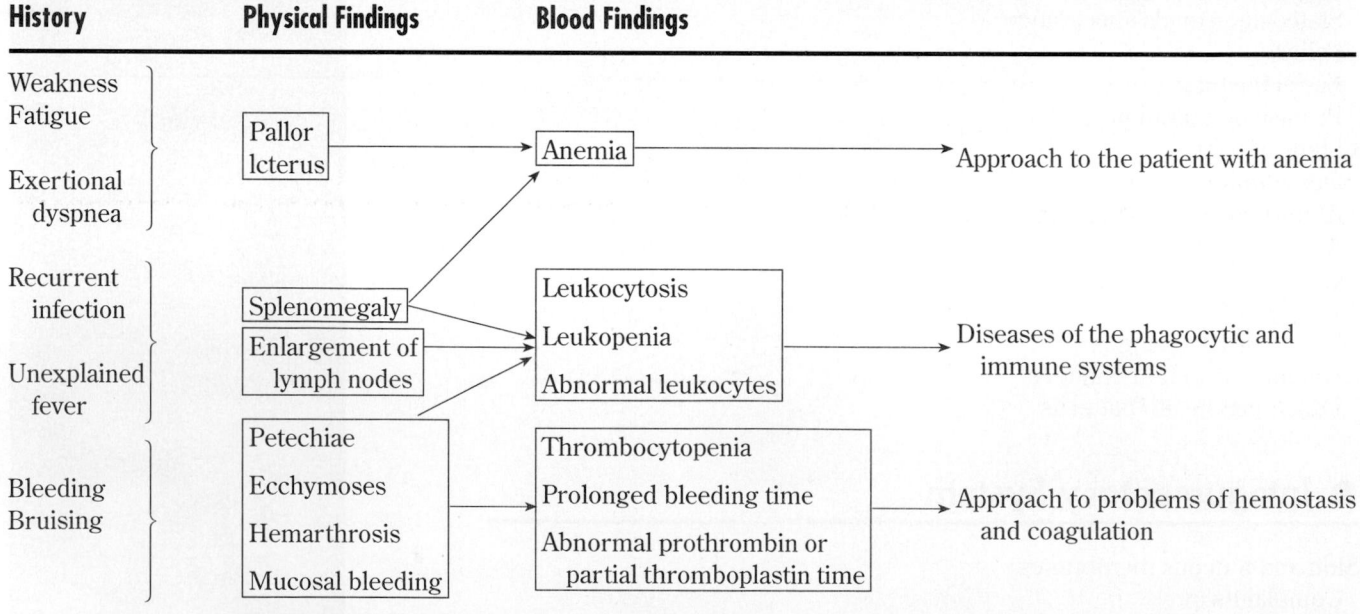

History	Physical Findings	Blood Findings	
Weakness Fatigue / Exertional dyspnea	Pallor Icterus	Anemia	Approach to the patient with anemia
Recurrent infection / Unexplained fever	Splenomegaly / Enlargement of lymph nodes	Leukocytosis Leukopenia Abnormal leukocytes	Diseases of the phagocytic and immune systems
Bleeding Bruising	Petechiae Ecchymoses Hemarthrosis Mucosal bleeding	Thrombocytopenia Prolonged bleeding time Abnormal prothrombin or partial thromboplastin time	Approach to problems of hemostasis and coagulation

From Wintrobe MM et al: *Clinical hematology,* Philadelphia, 1981, Lea & Febiger.
*Features in the history, physical examination, or preliminary blood examination that can guide the examiner toward the solution of a clinical problem.

Position
Alignment

● Lymphatic System

Prominent lymph nodes
  Location
  Size
  Surface characteristics
  Symmetry
  Consistency
  Fixation/mobility
  Tenderness/pain
  Heat
  Vascularity
Erythema
Red streaks

● Gastrointestinal System

Complaints of the following:
  Nausea
  Vomiting
  Dysphagia
  Anorexia
  Weight loss
Mouth
  Red mucous membranes
  Bleeding of gums and mucosa
  Stomatitis
  Purpura
  Telangiectasis
  Tonsillar hypertrophy
  Gingival hypertrophy
  Ulcers
Tongue
  Complaints of pain
  Beefy or swollen appearance
  Texture
    Absence of papillae
    Furrows
  Color: red
Abdomen
  Splenomegaly
  Hepatomegaly
Frank, occult bleeding in stool
  Hemorrhoids, anal/rectal fissures
Bowel habits
Abdomen
  Surface characteristics
    Contour
    Symmetry
    Masses

Pulsations
Bowel sounds
Tenderness
Decreased tympany
Increased dullness
Rigidity
Spasm

● Cardiovascular System

Complaints of the following:
  Palpitations
  SOB
  Fatigue
    After exertion
    All the time
  Angina
Murmurs
Dysrhythmias
Tachycardia
Extremities
  Color
  Response to temperature changes
  Edema

● Respiratory System

Orthopnea
Tachypnea
Dyspnea
Rhythm
Excursion
Breath sounds change
Hemoptysis

● Musculoskeletal System

Range of motion (ROM)
Joints/bones
  Swelling
  Pain
  Stiffness
Romberg's sign
Soft tissue
  Edema
  Hematoma
  Abscess
Muscle loss/weakness
Posture
Flaccidity
Spasticity
Babinski sign

● Genitourinary System

Hematuria
Incontinence
Impotence
Heavy menses
Retention
Difficult urination
Sexual maturity congruent with chronological age
Scrotal masses

● Neurologic System

Complaints of the following:
  Headache
  Numb, tingling extremities
  Paresthesia
  Weakness
  Frequent napping
  Sleeplessness
Behavior/mood changes
Changes in attention span and responses
Convulsions
Visual changes
Syncope
Vertigo
Tinnitus

● Pertinent Background Information

Concurrent diseases or conditions

Frequent illness
Infectious processes
Blood transfusion/component therapy
Multiple allergies
Asthma
Bleeding tendency
Hemorrhage
Renal, cardiovascular, or liver disorders
Cancer
Gastric or duodenal ulcer

Previous surgery or illness

Gastric or duodenal ulcers
Gastric surgery
Hepatic surgery
Cardiac surgery
Renal surgery
Radioactive exposure and irradiation
Exposure to chemical agents
Recurrent infectious processes (e.g., frequent sore
  throats)
Splenectomy

Gerontologic Considerations

- The subjective symptoms of hematological disorders (e.g., fatigue, weakness, dizziness, and dyspnea) may be mistaken for normal changes of aging or attributed to other disease processes commonly seen in the older adult.
- The most common blood disorders are forms of anemia.
- Decreased production of intrinsic factor in the aging gastric mucosa results in an increased incidence of pernicious anemia.
- Many older adults suffer from conditions, such as colonic diverticuli, hiatal hernia, or ulcerations, that can cause occult bleeding. Older adults with these conditions should be observed for iron deficiency anemia.
- Age-related problems such as altered dentition, limited financial resources, difficulty in food preparation, and poor appetite resulting from emotional upset or depression can cause an increased incidence of iron deficiency anemia.

- Severe or persistent anemia can place additional stress on the aging or diseased heart.
- Administration of blood products should be done with caution, since the older adult is at increased risk of developing congestive heart failure. Careful assessment of cardiopulmonary function and intake and output is essential.
- Oral administration of iron preparations increases the risk of GI irritation and constipation in the older adult.
- Ingestion of large amounts of aspirin and other antiinflammatory medications commonly taken by the older adult increases the risk of gastrointestinal bleeding and can lead to alteration in clotting.
- Chronic lymphocytic leukemia is the most common form seen with aging. This form of leukemia usually progresses slowly in the older adult and is rarely treated.

From Christensen BL, Kochrow EO: *Foundations of nursing*, ed 2, St Louis, 1995, Mosby.

Family history

Cancer
Blood dyscrasias, anemias
Immune disorders
Allergies
Rh incompatibility
Cause of death of deceased family members

Social history

Education level
Smoking
Alcohol use
Increased stress
Occupation; exposure to toxic substances
Radiation exposure
Environmental factors
Diet
  Recent changes
  Cultural or religious restrictions
  Decreased protein intake
  Fad diets
  Caffeine intake
  Low iron intake

Medication history

Immunizations
Prescription medications
  Present medications
  Previously taken medications (e.g., chloramphenicol)
Over-the-counter medications
Home remedies
Use of other drugs (particularly quinidines and
  silvadene)

● Diagnostic Tests

Laboratory studies (Figures 4-1 and 4-2)

Complete blood cell count (CBC)
White blood cell count (WBC)/differential
Hematocrit (Hct)
Hemoglobin (Hgb)
Reticulocyte count
Platelet count
Mean corpuscular volume (MCV)
Mean corpuscular hemoglobin concentration (MCHC)
Mean corpuscular hemoglobin (MCH)
Haptoglobin
Methemalbumin
Bleeding time
Prothrombin time/INR (PT)
Thrombin time

Activated partial thromboplastin time
Sedimentation rate
Electrophoresis of serum proteins
Immunoelectrophoresis of serum proteins
Total protein
Fibrinogen
Electrolyte values
Bilirubin level
Direct/indirect Coombs' test
Factor assay
Total iron-binding capacity
Fibrin degradation products
Hemoccult/guaiac tests
Serum iron level
Ferritin titers
Sideroblasts
Gastric analysis
Schilling test
Human lymphocyte antigens (HLA)
Sickle cell test

Other procedures

Biopsies
  Bone marrow
  Lymph nodes
  Spleen
  Liver
Chest and abdominal x-ray examinations
Magnetic resonance imaging (MRI)
Computed tomography (CT) scans
  Bone
  Liver
  Spleen
Intravenous pyelogram (IVP)
Uric acid
Urinary bilirubin
Urine culture
Lymphangiography
Renal ultrasound
Bence Jones protein

PERNICIOUS ANEMIA (CHRONIC, PROGRESSIVE, MACROCYTIC [MEGALOBLASTIC] ANEMIA)

Defective red blood cell production caused by lack of the intrinsic factor essential for absorption of vitamin B_{12} (deficiency of vitamin B_{12} causes gastric, intestinal, and neurologic abnormalities)

Assessment

Subjective data

Central nervous system (CNS)
  Complaints of the following:
    Weakness
    Fatigue
    Numbness of fingers and feet
    Disturbances in taste, vision, hearing
    Poor memory
    Irritability
    Depression
    Mood swings
Cardiovascular system
  Complaints of the following:
    Shortness of breath (SOB)
    Difficulty breathing
    Palpitations
    Rapid heart beat
Gastrointestinal system
  Complaints of the following:
    Loss of appetite
    Abdominal pain
    Nausea
    Indigestion
    Sore mouth
Integumentary system
  Complaints of the following:
    Itching
    Bruising easily
General
  Reports family history of disease

Objective data

Central nervous system
  Impaired judgment
  Impaired fine finger movement
  Paresthesia of hands and feet
  Ataxia
  Disturbed coordination
  Positive Romberg's and Babinski signs
Cardiovascular system
  Tachycardia

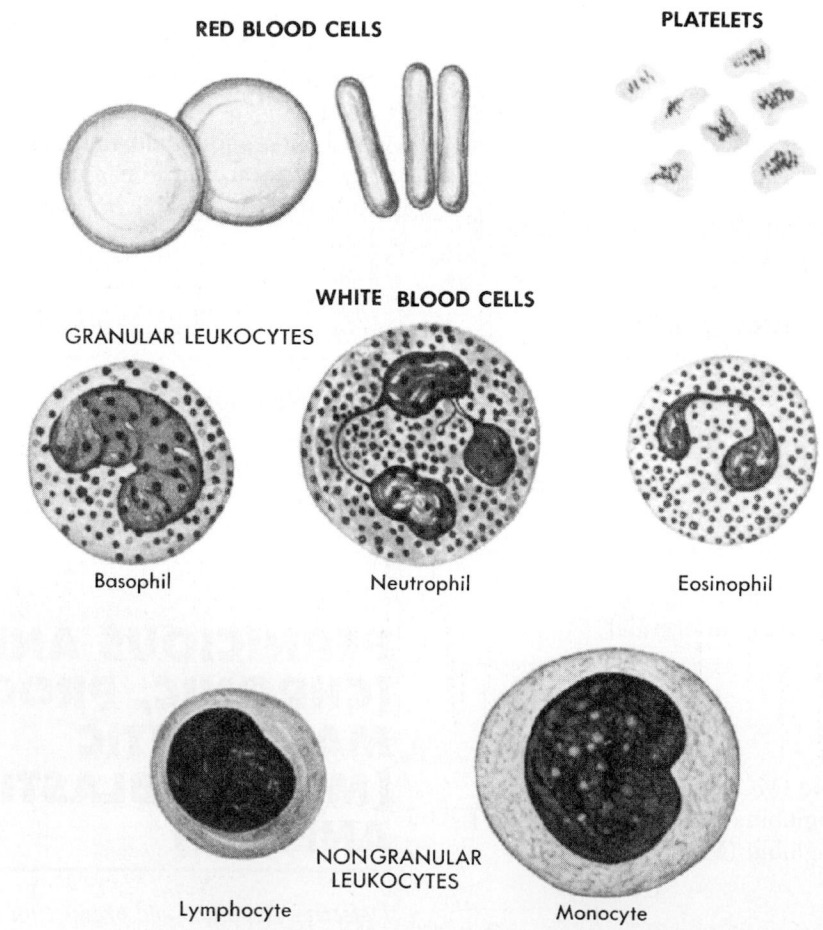

RED BLOOD CELLS

PLATELETS

WHITE BLOOD CELLS

GRANULAR LEUKOCYTES

Basophil   Neutrophil   Eosinophil

NONGRANULAR
LEUKOCYTES

Lymphocyte   Monocyte

Figure 4-1   Human blood cells. (From Anthony CP, Kolthoff NJ: *Textbook of anatomy and physiology,* ed 2, St Louis, 1987, Mosby.)

Wide pulse pressure
Palpitations
Orthopnea
Gastrointestinal system
  Beefy, red, smooth, painful tongue
  Vomiting
  Flatulence
  Constipation or diarrhea
  Weight loss
Integumentary system
  Waxy pallor to lemon-yellow color
  Petechiae
  Purpura
  Jaundiced sclera
  Pale lips/gums
General
  Repeated infections
  Primarily Northern European background

Usually between 50 to 60 years of age
Previous history of gastrectomy

Diagnostic tests

Schilling test ($<3\%$ of radioactive B_{12} excreted in the first 24 hr after injection)
Erythrocyte count <3 million/dl
Hemoglobin reduced to 4 to 5g/100ml
Red blood cells (RBCs) decreased
MCH decreased
MCHC, MCV increased
Bone marrow biopsy: increased megaloblasts
Bilirubin elevated; unconjugated forms
Serum vitamin B low
Serum folate normal or low
Gastric analysis: absence of free hydrochloric acid, decreased secretions, elevated pH

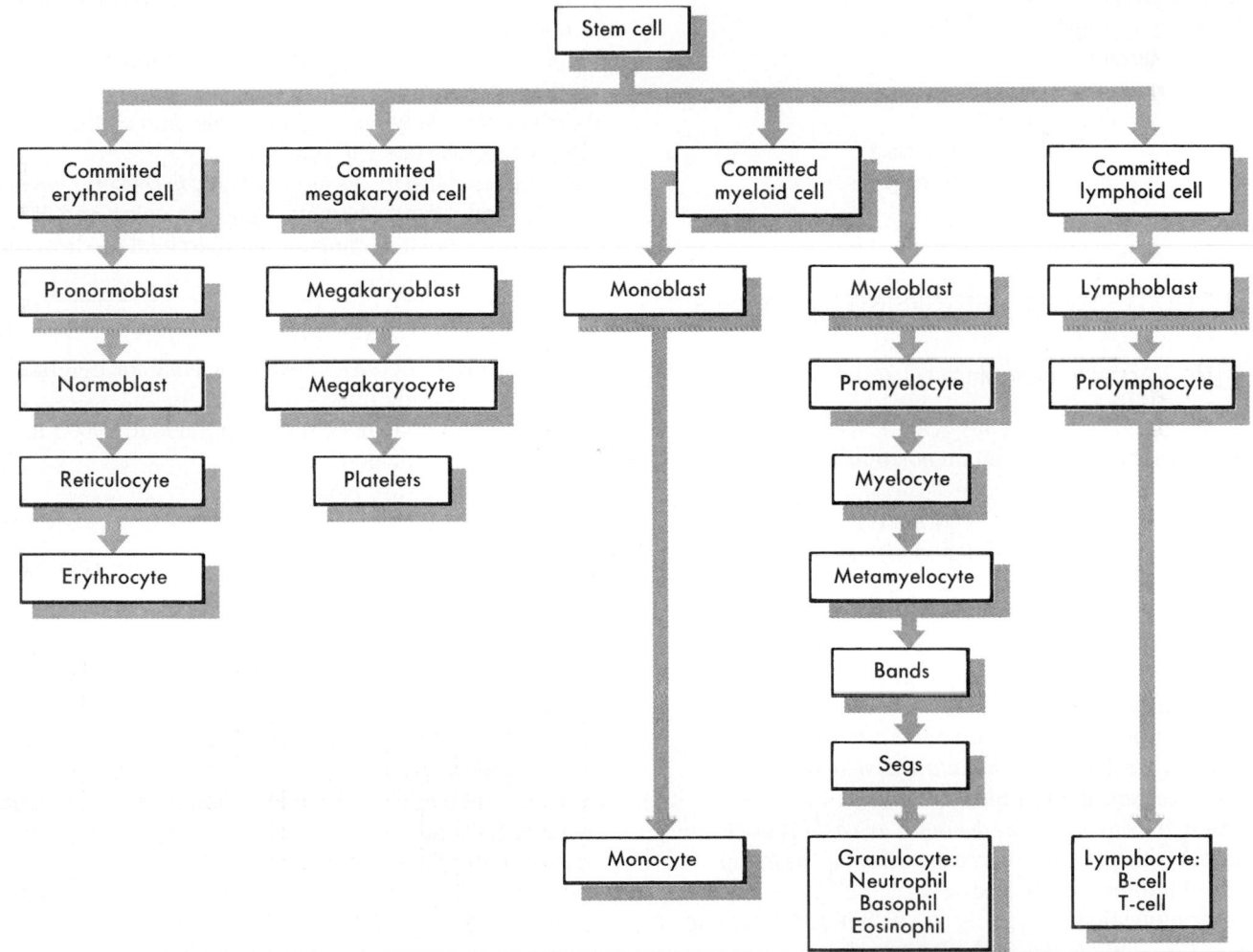

Figure 4-2 Formation and maturation of blood cells. All circulating blood cells originate from a common stem cell. (From Beare PG, Myers JL: *Principles and practice of adult health nursing,* ed 2, St Louis, 1994, Mosby.)

Therapeutic trial with parenteral vitamin B produces a
large number of reticulocytes in the blood 4-5 days after injection

Upper GI Series: atrophy of gastric mucosa

Potential complications

Cardiomegaly
Congestive heart failure (CHF)
Gastritis
Paralysis
Paranoia
Hallucinations, delusions
Infection, usually genitourinary

Collaborative management

Therapeutic management

Blood transfusions
Physical therapy
Respiratory therapy
Hematinic agents
Vitamin supplements
Antifungal, analgesic mouth rinse
Vital sign, pulse pressure monitoring
Diet high in vitamins, iron, and protein

Nursing management

PATIENT PROBLEMS/NURSING DIAGNOSES

● **NDX:**   Activity intolerance related to weakness and
fatigue

If patient on bed rest, maintain position of comfort *to
promote ease of respiration*
Perform active or passive ROM exercises
Assist with ADLs and ambulation *to conserve energy*
Assist patient to identify causes of increased/decreased
activity tolerance *to facilitate development of individu-
alized, safe activity plan*
Develop individualized activity regimen *to maintain
cardiac performance and prevent muscle wasting*
Plan and prioritize ADLs with patient *to reduce fatigue*
Pace activity tolerance *to facilitate development of indi-
vidualized, safe activity plan*
Pace activities *to minimize demands on cardiac workload*
Set goals with patient to increase activities as symptoms of intolerance decrease
Monitor physiologic responses to activities *to evaluate
patient response to the ADL plan*
Assess adverse responses to ADLs (e.g., tachycardia,
dysrhythmias, dyspnea); refer to physician as needed
Encourage use of coping strategies *to reduce fear and
anxiety that may enhance activity intolerance*

EXPECTED OUTCOMES

Patient participates in an activity plan within physiologic limitations without evidence of exertional dyspnea or tachycardia
Patient's activity level progresses to preillness state

● **NDX:**   Altered nutrition: less than body requirements related to inadequate intake of iron
and folic acid

Assess nutritional status and food preferences including cultural, religious, or medical restrictions
Consult dietitian *for further assessment and nutritional
support*
Provide small, frequent feedings *to avoid fatiguing pa-
tient with three large meals*
Provide dietary supplement as ordered *to ensure appro-
priate daily caloric intake*
Encourage family to bring patient's favorite foods from
home if appropriate
Avoid foods that are irritants, spicy, flatus-forming, or
high in caffeine
Monitor intake and output every shift *to aid in early de-
tection of inadequate intake*
Weigh patient daily (same time, scale, and clothing)
Report 2% decrease in weight
Assist patient with meals as necessary *to conserve energy*
Monitor and record character, amount, color, and fre-
quency of stools; administer antidiarrheal medications
as indicated

EXPECTED OUTCOMES

Patient's weight increases toward normal for height,
age, sex, and body build
Patient is taking balanced diet with fluids to 2000 ml,
unless contraindicated
Intake and output are balanced

● **NDX:**   Altered oral mucous membrane related to
nutritional imbalance

Assess oral cavity every shift *to ensure early intervention and treatment*
Assist patient to perform oral hygiene every 2 hr when
awake and before and after meals *to prevent buildup of
plaque and bacteria*
Perform oral hygiene with dilute mouthwash or normal
saline rinse and soft brush or sponge *to avoid irritation of mucous membranes*
Apply topical protective agents (water-based jelly, kaolin
preparations) to lesions as ordered *to promote healing*
Apply topical analgesics 15 to 20 min before meals as
ordered *to facilitate nutritional intake facilitate nutritional intake*
Instruct patient to "swish and swallow" or "swish
and spit"

Apply lubricating, water-based ointment to lips as ordered
Serve foods and fluids lukewarm or cold *to soothe inflamed oral mucosa*
Encourage patient to eat soft, easy-to-chew foods *to
avoid tissue trauma and pain*
Encourage fluids, unless contraindicated; iced liquids
or popsicles may be soothing
Avoid spicy/irritant foods *to decrease mucosal irritation*

EXPECTED OUTCOMES
Patient has pink, moist, intact oral mucosa, tongue, and
lips
Patient verbalizes comfort in chewing, swallowing, and
talking

● **NDX:** Risk for injury related to abnormal blood
profile and hypoxemia

Provide safety measures when needed: side rails up,
bed in low position when patient on bedrest, assist
with ambulation as needed *to prevent falls*
Assess degree of cognitive impairment; monitor emotional state
Identify environmental risk factors *to promote safety*
Apply heat with caution; use extra blankets or layers of
clothing instead of heating devices *to avoid burning
the skin*
Assess skin bid for integrity, color, warmth, texture,
and moisture *to detect peripheral and systemic changes*
Avoid use of restrictive clothing and shoes *to avoid impairment of skin integrity*
Have patient use support-type slippers or shoes and as-
sistive devices as needed *to ensure safe ambulation*
Remind patient to call for assistance when needed

EXPECTED OUTCOME
Patient avoids injury caused by cognitive impairment or
abnormal blood profile

● **NDX:** Risk for infection related to compromised
primary defenses: impaired skin integrity, inflamed mucosa; and compromised secondary defenses: impaired immune system,
abnormal blood profile

Follow Universal Precautions *to minimize risk of nosocomial infection*
Assess for signs and symptoms of infection q8h to 12h
Administer antiinfective agents as ordered
Instruct patient/significant others in proper handwashing technique, including when to perform, *to reduce
exposure to pathogens*
Assist patient to turn, cough, and deep breathe every
4 hr *to prevent stasis of secretions in lungs and
airway*

Encourage fluid intake to 2500 ml per day, unless contraindicated, *to prevent stasis of urine, promote flushing
of kidneys and bladder, and prevent urinary tract infection*
Encourage ambulation as tolerated *to prevent stasis of
body fluids*
Provide for undisturbed rest and sleep periods *to promote healing*
Use soft toothbrush and stool softeners as ordered *to
prevent injury to mucous membranes*

EXPECTED OUTCOMES
Patient remains free of infection
Signs and symptoms of infection are recognized early
and treated promptly

● **NDX:** Impaired gas exchange related to altered
oxygen supply, altered blood flow, and altered oxygen-carrying capacity of blood

Maintain oxygen delivery as ordered *to prevent desaturation*
Monitor pulse oximetry *to assess changes in saturation*
Assess respirations for quality, rate, pattern, depth,
dyspnea on exertion, guarding, use of accessory
muscles
Assess changes in mental status and behavior
Assist patient to maintain position of comfort for optimal respiratory effort *to promote lung expansion and
increase air exchange*
Maintain bed rest with siderails up *to decrease cardiac
workload*
Monitor P, BP, and R *to assess cardiac and respiratory
function*
Assist patient with ADLs as needed to conserve
energy
Increase patient's activity level as tolerated *to maintain
cardiopulmonary fitness*
Change patient's position every 2 hr *to prevent stasis of
secretions and body fluids*
Provide reassurance as needed to reduce patient's anxiety *that may contribute to increased cardiopulmonary
workload*
Instruct patient to report dyspnea and palpitations

EXPECTED OUTCOMES
Patient's vital signs are stable
Patient denies dyspnea
Patient demonstrates increasing activity tolerance

ADDITIONAL NURSING DIAGNOSES
TO CONSIDER
Altered family processes
Ineffective management of therapeutic regimen
Noncompliance

Altered protection
Altered role performance

Patient/family teaching

Medication

Emphasize need to take medications as directed
Instruct patient in name of medication, dosage, time of administration, purpose, side effects, route of administration, and interactions
Instruct patient to avoid over-the-counter medications without checking with physician

Disease process

Discuss signs and symptoms of infection
Instruct patient/significant other in skin integrity maintenance
Instruct patient/significant other in oral hygiene techniques
Instruct patient to observe and report symptoms of recurrence to physician; explain that symptoms will recede with continuing therapy (check with physician for symptoms that may be irreversible)
Explain need to maintain planned rest periods and avoid fatigue
Arrange for visits by home health nurse as needed
Instruct patient to continue follow-up care with physician

Nutrition

Explain need to maintain balanced diet and fluid intake
Review foods high in vitamin B_{12}, folic acid

Activity

Assist patient to practice physical therapy activities and general strengthening exercises
Explain need to increase activities gradually to desired level as tolerated
Instruct patient in measurement of pulse rate and rhythm during activity/exercise; instruct patient to stop if dysrhythmia is noted

Home care considerations

Review history for presence of care giver
Assess knowledge level of patient and care giver about cause and correction of B_{12}/folic acid deficiency
Assess ability of patient/care giver to learn home management techniques including daily weight, maintenance of nutrition log, selection of appropriate foods, oral hygiene, skin care

Iron Deficiency Anemia (Hypochromic, Microcytic Anemia)

Defective red blood cell production resulting from depletion of iron stores in the body needed to synthesize hemoglobin

Assessment

Subjective data

Central nervous system
  Complaints of the following:
    Weakness
    Fatigue
    Numb, tingling extremities
    Headache
    Irritability
    Inability to concentrate
Gastrointestinal system
  Complaints of the following:
    Loss of appetite
    Indigestion
    Vague abdominal pains
    Sore mouth
    Difficulty swallowing
Cardiovascular system
  Complaints of the following:
    Palpitations
    Dizziness
    Rapid heart beat
    SOB with exertion
    Sensitivity to cold
General
  Reports history of taking anticoagulants, aspirin, steroids, or nonsteroidal antiinflammatory agents
  Mother reports history of unsupplemented breast-feeding, bottle-feeding of infant

Objective data

Central nervous system
  Weakness
  Vertigo
  Paresthesia of extremities
  Listlessness
Gastrointestinal system
  Anorexia
  Pica
  Glossitis
  Angular stomatitis
  Dysphagia
  Weight loss

Chronic diarrhea
Flatulence
Cachexia
Cardiovascular system
  Palpitations
  Tachycardia
  Tachypnea
  DOE
  Ankle edema
Integumentary system
  Pale ear lobes, palms, and conjunctivae
  Blue or pearl-white sclera
  Thin, brittle, spoon-shaped fingernails
  Brittle hair
General
  Chronic blood loss: GI bleeding, heavy menses
  Pregnancy
  Premenopausal woman
  Premature, low–birth-weight infant
Malabsorption syndrome: chronic diarrhea, partial or
  total gastrectomy, celiac disease

Diagnostic tests

Hgb reduced as low as 3.6 g/dl
Erythrocyte count rarely below 3 million/dl
MCH decreased
MCHC decreased
Hct reduced
Serum iron low with high binding capacity
Iron-binding capacity increased
Serum ferritin decreased
RBCs decreased with microcytic and hypochromic cells
Bone marrow studies: depleted or absent iron store;
  normoblastic hyperplasia

Potential complications

Chest pain
Cardiomegaly
Hemoglobinuria

Collaborative management

Therapeutic management

Iron therapy, orally or parenterally (see box on p. 226)
Diet high in iron-rich foods to correct nutritional defi-
  ciency
Antifungal, anesthetic mouth rinse
VS monitoring
Hematinic agents
Stool softeners, laxatives
Ascorbic acid

Physical therapy
Respiratory therapy

Nursing management

PATIENT PROBLEMS/NURSING DIAGNOSES

● **NDX:** Altered nutrition: less than body requirements related to inadequate dietary iron intake, inability to absorb iron, and excessive
chronic blood loss

Assess nutritional status and food preferences including cultural, religious, or medical restrictions
Consult dietitian *for further assessment and nutritional
  support*
Provide small, frequent feedings *to avoid fatiguing patient with three large meals*
Provide dietary supplement as ordered *to ensure appro-
  priate daily caloric intake*
Administer iron therapy as ordered *to supplement di-
  etary intake*
Administer ascorbic acid as ordered *to supplement dietary intake*
Weigh patient daily (same time, scale, and clothing) *to
  monitor response to nutritional support*
Encourage family to bring patient's favorite foods from
  home if appropriate
  Avoid foods that are GI irritants, spicy, flatus-forming,
  or high in caffeine
Assist patient with meals as necessary *to conserve energy*
Monitor intake and output every shift *to aid in early detection of inadequate intake*
Review laboratory data *to monitor effectiveness of medication and nutritional support*

EXPECTED OUTCOMES

Patient's weight increases toward normal for height,
  age, sex, and body build
Patient is taking balanced diet with fluids to 2000 ml,
  unless contraindicated
Patient consumes 100% RDA of iron and folic acid daily

● **NDX:** Altered oral mucous membrane related to
nutritional imbalance

Assess oral cavity every shift to ensure early intervention and treatment and monitor response to
  therapy
Assist patient to perform oral hygiene q2h when awake
  and before and after meals *to prevent buildup of plaque
  and bacteria*
Perform oral hygiene with dilute mouthwash or normal
  saline rinse and soft brush or sponge *to avoid irritation of mucous membranes*

Precautions in Iron Therapy Administration

ORAL ADMINISTRATION

Use straw to prevent staining teeth with liquid preparations

INTRAMUSCULAR (IM) ADMINISTRATION

Use second needle after withdrawing solution from ampule to avoid staining tissue
Use Z-tract method of injection
Inject 0.5 ml of air before removing needle from tissue

INTRAVENOUS (IV) ADMINISTRATION

Administer test dose
Remain with patient to assess for symptoms of shock
Use small-gauge needle
Cover solution with dark plastic

Apply topical protective agents (water-based jelly, kaolin preparations) to lesions as ordered *to promote healing*
Apply topical analgesics 15 to 20 min before meals as ordered *to facilitate nutritional intake*
Instruct patient to "swish and swallow" or "swish and spit"
Apply lubricating, water-based ointment to lips as ordered
Serve foods and fluids lukewarm or cold *to soothe inflamed oral mucosa*
Encourage patient to eat soft, easy-to-chew foods *to avoid tissue trauma and pain*

EXPECTED OUTCOMES

Patient has pink, moist, intact oral mucosa, tongue, and lips
Patient verbalizes comfort in chewing, swallowing, and talking

● **NDX:** Risk for injury related to cognitive impairment, alteration in mental status, and abnormal blood profile

Provide a safe environment free of obstacles *to prevent injury to extremities*

Assess degree of cognitive impairment; monitor emotional state
Identify environmental risk factors *to promote safety*
Apply heat with caution; use extra blankets or layers of clothing instead of heating devices *to avoid burning the skin*
Assess skin bid for integrity, color, warmth, texture, and moisture *to detect peripheral and systemic changes*
Avoid use of restrictive clothing and shoes *to avoid impairment of skin integrity*
Have patient use support-type slippers or shoes and assistive devices as needed *to ensure safe ambulation*
Instruct patient to sit at side of bed and stand before walking *to prevent injury as a result of dizziness*
Remind patient to call for assistance when needed

EXPECTED OUTCOMES

Patient avoids injury resulting from cognitive impairment or abnormal blood profile
Patient verbalizes precautions to prevent injury

● **NDX:** Impaired skin integrity related to decreased tissue perfusion

Wash hair gently with conditioning shampoo *to prevent breakage and loss*
Assist patient with nail care as needed *to prevent damage*

EXPECTED OUTCOMES

Patient's hair is strong and shiny
Patient's nails are strong and firm

● **NDX:** Sensory/perceptual alterations related to tissue hypoxia of the nervous system

Assess cognitive functioning every shift
Plan care with patient participation *to promote consistency and sense of calmness*
Maintain a warm environment
Maintain a safe environment *to prevent injury to extremities*
Assist patient with ambulation and positioning *to prevent injury resulting from a fall and increased dizziness*
Administer medications as prescribed *to manage headaches*
Anticipate patient needs, provide instructions and information, allow patient to verbalize concerns *to reduce irritability and manage altered concentration*
Assure patient that altered concentration will improve with therapy

EXPECTED OUTCOMES

Patient exhibits increased concentration when performing ADLs and other activities

Signs of irritability decrease
Patient can change position and ambulate without dizziness or injury to limbs
Patient denies sensitivity to cold, headache

● **NDX:** Activity intolerance related to generalized weakness, fatigue, and imbalance between oxygen supply and demand

Maintain position of comfort
Perform active or passive ROM exercises
Assist with ADLs and ambulation *to conserve energy*
Assist patient to identify causes of increased/decreased activity tolerance *to facilitate development of individualized, safe activity plan*
Develop individualized activity regimen *to maintain cardiac performance and prevent muscle wasting*
Plan and prioritize ADLs with patient *to reduce fatigue*
Pace activities *to minimize demands on cardiac workload*
Set goals with patient to increase activities as symptoms of intolerance decrease
Monitor physiologic responses to activities *to evaluate patient response to ADL plan*
Assess adverse responses to ADLs (e.g., tachycardia, dysrhythmias, dypnea); refer to physician as needed
Provide uninterrupted rest periods *to maintain energy level*
Increase patient activity in small increments until tolerance level is reached

EXPECTED OUTCOMES
Patient participates in an activity plan within physiologic limitations without evidence of exertional dyspnea or tachycardia
Activity level progresses to preillness state

ADDITIONAL NURSING DIAGNOSES
TO CONSIDER
Self-care deficit
Altered parenting
Impaired adjustment

Patient/family teaching

Medications

Instruct patient in names of medications, dosage, time of administration, purpose, side effects, route of administration, and interactions
Inform patient that coffee, tea, eggs, and milk inhibit iron absorption; antacids decrease iron absorption; chloramphenicol delays erythropoiesis
Demonstrate method for parenteral administration of iron
Increase vitamin C/ascorbic acid intake to enhance iron absorption

Instruct patient to avoid over-the-counter medications without checking with health care provider
Explain need to continue iron therapy even when feeling better
Discuss color of stools expected and explain need and methods to avoid constipation
Emphasize need to take medications as directed

Nutrition

Explain need to maintain balanced diet and fluid intake
Review dietary sources of iron
Explain importance of monitoring weight as instructed

Disease process

Discuss signs and symptoms of recurrence to report to health care provider (check with physician for symptoms that may be irreversible)
Instruct patient/significant other in maintenance of skin integrity
Instruct patient/significant other in oral hygiene techniques
Arrange for visits by home health nurse as needed
Instruct patient to continue follow-up care with physician and laboratory
Explain need to increase activities gradually to desired level as tolerated
Explain need to maintain planned rest periods and avoid fatigue

Home care considerations

Review history for presence of care giver
Assess patient's ability to provide balanced diet at home; initiate social services referral as needed
Assess knowledge level of patient and care giver about cause and correction of iron deficiency
Assess ability of patient/care giver to learn home management techniques including daily weight, maintenance of nutrition log, selection of appropriate foods, oral hygiene, ADL plan, medication administration
Assist patient/significant other to assess home environment for environmental safety hazards

HEMOLYTIC ANEMIA

Premature and accelerated destruction of erythrocytes in the presence of normal erythropoiesis; may be acquired or hereditary

Assessment

Subjective data

Central nervous system
  Complaints of the following:
    Weakness
    Fatigue
    Headache
Gastrointestinal system
  Complaints of the following:
    Abdominal pain
    Loss of appetite
    Nausea
Genitourinary system
  Complaints of urinary changes
Cardiovascular system
  Complaints of SOB
Integumentary system
  Complaints of itching
General
  Reports family history of disease
  Reports history of trauma, infection, systemic disease,
    exposure to drugs or toxins

Objective data

Central nervous system
  Weakness
  Irritability
Gastrointestinal system
  Vomiting
  Abdominal tenderness
  Splenomegaly
  Diarrhea
Genitourinary system
  Nocturnal hemoglobinuria
  Urine changes
  Decreased urinary output
Cardiovascular system
  Chills
  Fever
  Venous thrombosis
Integumentary system
  Jaundice
Musculoskeletal system
  Bone deformities

Diagnostic tests

Erythrocyte count low
Hgb low
Hct low
Reticulocyte count high
Erythrocyte fragility increased
Serum bilirubin increased
Urinary urobilinogen increased
Normocytic anemia
Bone marrow biopsy reveals erythroid hyperplasia

Potential complications

Renal failure
Hemoglobinuria

Collaborative management

Therapeutic management

Eliminate causative factors; treat underlying disorder
Management of primary condition
Maintenance of fluid and electrolyte balance
Transfusions as needed
Corticosteroids
Osmotic diuretics
Antidiarrheal medications
Antiemetic medications
Splenectomy

Nursing management

PATIENT PROBLEMS/NURSING DIAGNOSES

● **NDX:** Fluid volume deficit related to active fluid
         loss and blood cell hemolysis

Monitor intake and output every shift *to assess fluid
  needs and prevent overload;* report imbalances
Weigh patient daily (same time, scale, clothing), report
  changes of 2% to 3% of original weight
Monitor vital signs and mental status every 4 hr
Assess skin turgor and peripheral pulses every shift *to
  determine adequacy of hydration*
Monitor character, amount, color, frequency of emesis,
  stools *to assess source, quality of active fluid loss*
Observe color, specific gravity, pH of urine *to ensure
  early detection of renal failure*
Provide oral fluid intake as tolerated *to maintain in-
  travascular fluid volume*
Provide clear liquid diet *to reduce nausea;* progress to
  balanced diet as symptoms abate
Provide oral fluids in small, frequent amounts *to prevent
  abdominal distention*
Administer blood transfusions as ordered *to alleviate
  fluid deficit*
Force fluids to 2500 ml/day unless contraindicated
Administer intravenous fluids as ordered *to correct fluid
  deficit*
Administer urine alkalizers as ordered *to enhance renal
  function*

Chest pai
Fatigue
Difficulty
Rapid hea
Palpitatio
Musculoskel
Complaints
General
Reports fan

Objective

Central nerv
Elevated te
Irritability
Lethargy
Sleepiness
Coma
Gastrointesti
Vomiting
Anorexia
Hepatomeg
Splenomeg
Abdominal
Pale tongue
Musculoskel
Joint swelli
Integumenta
Pallor
Leg ulcers
Jaundice
Pale lips, p
Genitourinar
Polyuria
Hematuria
Enuresis
Dark urine
General
African des
Increased s
Infants and
paired gr
Painful cris
Severe pa
muscles
Increased
Dark urin
Low-grad
Aplastic cri
Associate
Temperat
Pallor
Lethargy
Sleepines

Arrange for quiet rest periods before and after meals *to alleviate nausea, vomiting, gastric distress*

EXPECTED OUTCOMES

Patient's skin turgor and color are normal
Intake and output are balanced
Renal function is adequate
Peripheral pulses are present
Extremities are warm with good color

● **NDX:** Activity intolerance related to generalized weakness, fatigue, and imbalance between oxygen supply and demand

Develop an individualized activity regimen *to maintain cardiac performance and prevent muscle wasting*
Pace activities *to minimize demands on cardiac workload*
Assist patient with ADLs *to conserve energy*
Provide uninterrupted rest periods *to maintain energy level*
Set goals with patient to increase activities as symptoms of intolerance decrease
Monitor physiologic responses to activities *to evaluate patient response to the ADL plan*
Assess adverse responses to ADLs (e.g., tachycardia, dysrhythmias, dyspnea); refer to physician as needed

EXPECTED OUTCOMES

Patient participates in an activity plan within physiologic limitations without evidence of exertional dyspnea or tachycardia
Patient's activity level progresses to preillness state

● **NDX:** Abdominal, back pain related to liver/splenic distention

Maintain position of comfort *to relieve pressure from enlarged liver/spleen*
Administer analgesics as ordered; provide pain-relief measures as needed *to relieve discomfort*
Administer antipyretics as ordered
Provide external sources of warmth *to warm when chilling occurs*
Offer antiemetics, oral care, other measures *to alleviate nausea and vomiting*
Encourage use of coping strategies *to reduce fear and anxiety that may exacerbate pain*
Assess pain for predisposing factors, intensity, frequency, duration, and effective methods of control *to facilitate development of a collaborative pain management program*

EXPECTED OUTCOMES

Patient verbalizes feelings of increased comfort on pain rating scale

---

Temperature is within normal limits

● **NDX:** Impaired skin integrity related to increased serum bilirubin, jaundice, or pruritis

Assess skin condition every shift
Monitor laboratory data daily *to assess liver function*
Provide frequent skin care *to promote comfort and decrease itching* (e.g., soothing baths: sodium bicarbonate, oatmeal)
Avoid skin dryness; apply lotions to slightly moist skin; cool sponge baths or tub soaks may be beneficial
Provide cool ambient temperature with adequate humidity
Avoid constrictive clothing *to prevent friction and impairment of skin integrity*
Elevate bedclothes with bed cradle; keep bed wrinkle-free *to prevent skin irritation*
Launder linen in nondetergents *to prevent skin irritation*
Advise patient to avoid scratching *to prevent irritation and injury*
Instruct patient to apply pressure or cool applications *to alleviate itching*

EXPECTED OUTCOMES

Patient's skin remains intact and moist without evidence of scratching
Patient's skin is warm and dry with good turgor

● **NDX:** Altered nutrition: less than body requirements related to liver dysfunction

Assess nutritional status and food preferences including cultural, religious, or medical restrictions
Consult dietitian *for further assessment and nutritional support*
Provide small, frequent feedings *to avoid abdominal distention*
Provide balanced diet high in iron and protein *to promote erythropoiesis*
Provide dietary supplement as ordered *to ensure appropriate daily caloric intake*
Encourage family to bring patient's favorite foods from home if appropriate
Avoid high-fat foods *to minimize discomfort caused by stress on gallbladder*
Monitor intake and output every shift *to assess patient's appetite*
Weigh patient daily (same time, scale, and clothing) *to assess patient's response to nutritional therapy*
Assist patient as needed with meals *to conserve energy*
Review laboratory data, especially bilirubin, *to assess liver function*

Supportive care; social services

Rest

Hydration with IV fluids and electrolytes

Oxygen therapy

Analgesics

Sedation

Antipyretics

Blood fraction transfusion

Exchange transfusions for aplastic, hyperhemolytic, and sequestration crises

Experimental use of antisickling agents: urea, cyanate, carbamoyl phosphate

Oral maintenance therapy with folic acid and/or iron

Nursing management

PATIENT PROBLEMS/NURSING DIAGNOSES

● **NDX:** Altered cardiopulmonary, cardiovascular, cerebral, renal, peripheral tissue perfusion related to increased blood viscosity, hypoxia, impairment of microcirculation, and hypovolemia

Cardiopulmonary/cardiovascular system

Monitor blood pressure q2h *to assess cardiac function and peripheral resistance to blood flow;* report changes immediately

Monitor respirations and auscultate chest for heart and breath sounds q2h *to assess pulmonary function and detect onset of respiratory failure;* report changes immediately

Maintain patient in semi-Fowler's position when in bed *to promote maximal respiratory excursion*

Encourage frequent rest periods and avoidance of strenuous activity *to decrease cardiac workload and minimize risk of sickling*

Maintain a stress-free environment *to minimize risk of sickling*

Assist with ADLs *to reduce oxygen demand*

Monitor administration of packed RBCs *to prevent circulatory overload and reaction*

Instruct patient to avoid caffeine, tobacco, and other stimulants *to prevent vasoconstriction*

Notify physician for complaints of chest pain, increased dyspnea, cyanosis, restlessness *to facilitate early intervention*

Administer oxygen therapy as ordered *to promote adequate tissue perfusion*

Administer anticoagulants as ordered *to promote tissue perfusion*

Initiate continuous pulse oximetry *to monitor oxygen saturation*

Administer sublingual nitroglycerin as ordered for angina

Review blood studies *to assess adequacy of tissue perfusion and blood flow;* report changes to health care provider

Cerebral system

Assess neurologic signs q2h *to detect increasing intracranial pressure*

Maintain patient on complete bed rest with head of bed elevated *to conserve energy and lower intracranial pressure*

Provide quiet environment *to promote rest and reduce stress*

Instruct patient to avoid stimulants (caffeine, tobacco) *to prevent vasoconstriction*

Renal system

Provide oral/IV intake to 2500 ml/day unless contraindicated *to maintain fluid balance and promote renal perfusion*

Monitor intake and output every shift *to ensure balance is maintained*

Test urine for protein *to detect renal dysfunction*

Weigh patient daily (same time, scale, and clothes) *to monitor fluid retention*

Observe for presence of facial, extremity edema *to detect renal dysfunction, fluid retention*

Monitor vital signs q4h *to ensure adequacy of blood flow*

EXPECTED OUTCOMES

Patient has normal vital signs, pupillary responses, and reflexes

Patient is alert and oriented

Patient denies having headaches

Intake and output are balanced

Skin is warm and dry with good turgor and color

Patient's weight is stable

● **NDX:** Pain related to joint swelling, tissue hypoxia, stasis of RBCs, and sickling

Assess pain location, duration, intensity using pain rating scale *to facilitate development of pain management plan*

Collaborate with patient to develop pain management plan designed to prevent severe pain

Support affected joints with pillows in position of comfort *to minimize pain and discomfort*

Apply warm soaks to joints as ordered *to promote comfort*

Maintain anatomical alignment *to prevent deformity*

Perform back and pressure point care q2h *to prevent skin breakdown*

Move patient with slow, gentle movements *to minimize discomfort of repositioning*

Administer analgesics as ordered *to achieve goal of pain management plan*

Avoid restrictive clothing *to relieve pressure and promote comfort*

Position patient in semi-Fowler's position when in bed *to decrease abdominal pressure and increase intra-abdominal space*

Provide small, frequent feedings *to prevent abdominal distention*

Auscultate bowel sounds *to detect obstruction*

Encourage use of alternate pain management techniques

EXPECTED OUTCOMES

Patient demonstrates relaxed facial expression and posture

Patient verbalizes pain relief using pain scale

● **NDX:** Risk for impaired skin integrity related to altered tissue perfusion, tissue hypoxemia, and immobility

Inspect skin for redness, lesions, swelling, drainage q8h *to detect impairment of skin integrity*

Keep skin warm and dry *to prevent breakdown caused by environmental moisture*

Avoid use of constrictive clothing; maintain ambient and body warmth *to promote circulation and prevent possible sickling*

Assist patient with active and passive ROM exercises as tolerated *to maintain circulation*

Palpate peripheral pulses *to assess status of arterial circulation*

Review blood studies *to evaluate oxygen saturation, blood viscosity, and pH*

If ulceration occurs, maintain patient on bed rest in semi-Fowler's position *to prevent further injury and decrease peripheral vascular resistance*

Elevate affected limb *to promote venous return*

If ulceration occurs, implement wound care procedures as ordered *to remove drainage and necrosis, prevent infection, and promote healing*

Observe reponse of wound, lesions to therapy *to assess effectiveness of interventions*

Cleanse skin with mild soap, rinse well, dry thoroughly *to maintain integrity*

Apply protective cream after bathing and position change

Ensure that bed linens are wrinkle free and nonconstrictive *to prevent mechanical injury*

Reposition patient q2h when on bed rest *to promote circulation and prevent stasis*

EXPECTED OUTCOMES

Patient's skin is warm and dry with good color

Patient's skin is free of ulceration

● **NDX:** Risk for infection related to inadequate primary defenses, inadequate secondary defenses, and chronic disease

Follow Universal precautions/body substance isolation *to prevent transmissions of pathogens*

Maintain aseptic technique for wound care

Limit visitors *to reduce exposure to pathogens*

Encourage high-calorie, high-protein diet as appropriate *to maintain optimal nutritional status*

Encourage fluid intake to 2500 ml/day, unless contraindicated, *to promote dilute urine and frequent emptying of bladder*

Encourage patient to turn, cough, deep breathe *to prevent stasis of secretions*

Administer antibiotics as ordered

Monitor VS and breath sounds q4h *to detect signs/symptoms of infection*

Administer antipyretics as ordered

Obtain cultures of infected areas as ordered *to determine causative agent*

EXPECTED OUTCOMES

Patient remains free of infection

Patient's vital signs are stable and within normal limits for patient

Infection is recognized and treated early

● **NDX:** Risk for injury related to alteration in mental status, abnormal blood profile, bone fragility, and joint swelling

Provide safety measures when needed: siderails up, bed in low position when patient on bed rest; assist with ambulation as needed *to prevent falls*

Assess degree of cognitive impairment; monitor emotional state

Identify environmental risk factors *to promote safety*

Have patient use support-type slippers or shoes and assistive devices as needed *to ensure safe ambulation*

Remind patient to call for assistance when needed

Reposition the patient frequently with joint support *to prevent trauma and injury*

Assist patient with active and passive ROM exercises *to promote circulation, joint movement, and maintenance of muscle strength*

Encourage consumption of diet high in calcium, protein, vitamins, as appropriate, *to prevent bone, tissue injury*

EXPECTED OUTCOMES

Patient ambulates without assistance

Patient avoids injury

Patient denies joint or bone pain

ADDITIONAL NURSING DIAGNOSES
TO CONSIDER

Self-esteem disturbance related to physical, lifestyle, or
role losses
Social isolation related to disease process
Sexual dysfunction related to disease process
Other self-perceptual, role, or coping diagnoses

Patient/family teaching

Discuss need to avoid conditions that precipitate crisis
Infections
Dehydration
Activities that may cause an increase in oxygen re-
quirement: flying in unpressurized planes, high alti-
tudes, cold weather, vasoconstrictive drugs
Explain nutrition requirements and importance of eat-
ing a well-balanced diet with fluids to 2000 ml/day;
avoid iced drinks and foods
Avoid consumption of caffeine and other stimulants
Discuss importance of maintaining relationships with
others and participating in meaningful activity and
work
Teach that balancing exercise/activity with adequate
rest is important
Use stress reduction methods daily
Instruct patient to maintain good hygiene
Teach signs and symptoms of infection to report to
physician or nurse; need to avoid exposure to infec-
tious persons, treat early symptoms, and have early
childhood and yearly immunizations
Instruct about signs and symptoms of recurrence to re-
port to physician
Pain
Persistent low-grade temperature
Decreased fluid intake
Decreased appetite
Increased lethargy or sleeping
Teach name of medication, purpose, side or toxic ef-
fects, time and frequency of administration
Explain that it is necessary to tell all health care
providers about disease
Wear medical alert bracelet and keep follow-up
appointments
Explain that childbearing may cause some risks to fe-
males and refer for gynecologic consultation
Refer family for genetic counseling and psychological
counseling when appropriate

Home care considerations

Review history for presence of care giver
Assess patient/significant other's knowledge level of
disease process

Assess home environment for potential environmental
hazards
Assess ability of patient/significant other to comply
with instructions

Aplastic Anemia

*Anemia, aplastic or hypoplastic, resulting from
destruction of or injury to the bone marrow stem
cells or bone marrow matrix; exposure to toxins,
specifically large doses of radiation, benzene,
metabolites, alkylating agents, chloramphenicol, or
sulfonamides, may cause pancytopenia (bone marrow
failure with granulocytopenia, thrombocytopenia, and
anemia)*

Assessment

Subjective data

Central nervous system
Complaints of the following:
Fatigue
Weakness
Headache
Dizziness
Confusion
Gastrointestinal system
Complaints of the following:
Nausea
Indigestion
Cardiovascular system
Complaints of the following:
Nose bleeds
Bleeding gums
Heavy menses
Bruising easily
Respiratory system
Complaints of the following:
Difficulty breathing
Cold symptoms
Cough
General
Reports exposure to chemical toxin, radiation, or spe-
cific medications
History of frequent infection

Objective data

Central nervous system
Irritability
Slowed thought process
Weakness
Confusion

Gastrointestinal system
  Vomiting
  Bleeding gums
  Flulike symptoms
  Oral ulcers
  Rectal ulcers
  GI disturbances
  GI bleeding
Cardiovascular system
  Tachycardia
  DOE
Integumentary system
  Waxy pallor
  Ecchymosis
  Petechiae
General
  Elevated temperature
  Signs/symptoms of infection
  Cough
  Nonhealing cuts, lesions
  Burning on urination
Documented history of exposure to chemical toxin,
  radiation, or specific medications

Diagnostic tests

RBCs usually normochromic, normocytic potential
  macrocytosis, anisocytosis
Erythrocyte count usually <1 million/mm³
Reticulocytes low
Serum iron elevated
Total iron-binding capacity normal or slightly reduced
WBC count decreased
Platelet count decreased
Coagulation tests abnormal
Bone marrow biopsy demonstrates fatty marrow,
  hypocellular or aplastic

Potential complications

Hemorrhage
Cirrhosis
Diabetes
Heart failure
Blood reactions
Overwhelming infections

Collaborative management

Therapeutic management

Removal of causative agent
Blood transfusion
Packed RBCs
Platelets

HLA-matched leukocyte
Bone marrow transplant
Respiratory support
Antibiotics in the presence of infection
Corticosteroids to stimulate erythroid production
Marrow-stimulating agents
Physical therapy
Nutritional support

Nursing management

PATIENT PROBLEMS/NURSING DIAGNOSES

● **NDX:** Activity intolerance related to imbalance
between oxygen supply and demand, re-
duced number of RBCs, and generalized
weakness/fatigue

Maintain position of comfort *to promote ease of respira-
tion*
Perform active or passive ROM exercises
Assist patient with ADLs and ambulation *to conserve
energy*
Assist patient to identify causes of increased/decreased
  activity tolerance *to facilitate development of individualized, safe activity plan*
Develop individualized activity regimen *to maintain
cardiac performance and prevent muscle wasting*
Plan and prioritize ADLs with patient *to reduce fatigue*
Pace activities *to minimize demands on cardiac work-
load*
Set goals with patient *to increase activities as symptoms
of intolerance decrease*
Monitor physiologic responses to activities *to evaluate
patient response to the ADL plan*
Assess adverse responses to ADLs (e.g., tachycardia,
  dysrhythmias, dyspnea); refer to physician as
  needed
Encourage use of coping strategies *to reduce fear and
anxiety that may enhance activity intolerance*
Provide uninterrupted rest periods *to conserve energy*
Administer oxygen as ordered *to reduce dyspnea*

EXPECTED OUTCOMES

Patient participates in an activity plan within physiologic limitations without evidence of exertional
  dyspnea or tachycardia
Patient's activity level progresses to preillness state

● **NDX:** Risk for injury, bleeding related to bone
marrow malfunction and low platelet count

Avoid IM injections
Apply pressure to injection, venipuncture sites *to prevent extravasation*

Instruct patient to use an electric razor for shaving

Perform oral care with a soft toothbrush or foam stick *to prevent injury to oral mucosa*

Humidify oxygen *to minimize drying of mucous membranes*

Administer stool softener *to prevent constipation and prevent injury to intestinal mucosa*

Monitor VS/q4h *to ensure early detection of signs of hemorrhage;* report changes immediately

Check urine and stool for occult, frank blood

Assess skin for petechiae and ecchymosis

Monitor laboratory results *to ensure early detection of internal bleeding*

Administer blood fractions as ordered

Instruct patient to avoid scratching

Assist with ambulation and ADLs *to prevent injury*

EXPECTED OUTCOMES

Patient's vital signs are stable

Patient exhibits no signs/symptoms of bleeding

Patient's skin and mucous membranes are warm, moist, with good turgor

Patient's laboratory values are within normal limits

● **NDX:** Altered nutrition: less than body requirements related to gastrointestinal disturbances

Assess nutritional status and food preferences including cultural, religious, or medical restrictions

Consult dietitian *for further assessment and nutritional support*

Provide balanced diet high in proteins and vitamins unless contraindicated

Provide small, frequent feedings *to prevent abdominal distention*

Provide dietary supplement as ordered *to ensure appropriate daily caloric intake*

Encourage family to bring patient's favorite foods from home if appropriate

Monitor intake and output every shift *to assess patient's appetite*

Weigh patient daily (same time, scale, and clothing) *to assess patient's response to nutritional therapy;* notify physician for decreases of 2% to 3%

Assist patient as needed with meals *to conserve energy*

EXPECTED OUTCOMES

Patient eats a balanced diet with adequate fluid intake

Patient's weight increases toward normal for height, age, sex, and body build

● **NDX:** Altered oral mucous membrane, related to nutritional imbalance, bleeding, and infection

---

Bone Marrow Study

Bone marrow is obtained by aspiration or biopsy to examine types and numbers of cells, maturation level, and composition of supporting tissue; used for diagnosis and treatment response

INDICATIONS

Evaluation of the hematolymphatic systems for differential diagnosis of various anemias, neutropenia, leukemia, thrombocytopenia, immunoglobulin disorders, lymphoma, or granulomatous disease

CARE

Inform patient that pressure will be felt with insertion of needle and some pain with aspiration; position for good visualization; apply pressure and dressing at site; check BP, P, and R q30 min × 2; maintain bed rest for 1 hr; assess site for bleeding, hematoma, infection

---

Teach and assist patient with routine oral care

Inspect and palpate lips, gums, and buccal mucosa gently q8h

Clean teeth and rinse mouth each morning, after meals, and at bedtime

Increase frequency of oral care to q2h if lesions are present

Choice of dental equipment will depend on state of oral cavity

Soft-bristled toothbrush if there are no breaks or lesions

Gauze or sponge-covered cleaners if there are breaks in skin or gums are bleeding

Assess patient's denture fit

Avoid gumlike grips

Keep dentures scrupulously clean

Remove and clean dentures before using mouth rinse

Keep patient's mouth moist

Provide appealing, tepid liquids for sipping

Flavored ice pops may be soothing

Keep lips moist; use water-soluble gel

EXPECTED OUTCOME

Patient exhibits no oral lesions, or healing of lesions is progressing

● **NDX:** Risk for anxiety related to changes in health, poor prognosis, and uncertainty about tests and treatments

Assess patient/significant other's understanding of disease process, tests, and treatments *to collaboratively identify areas of knowledge deficit*

With patient/significant other, identify available support systems

Assess patient/significant other's coping strategies *to assist in development of effective stress-reducing and anxiety-reducing activities*

Engage patient/significant other in development of the plan of care *to ensure patient needs are met*

Provide care in a consistent and timely manner as agreed upon by staff and patient *to meet expectations and allay anxiety*

Provide instructions and information in a manner consistent with the patient's age, developmental level, and culture

Assess the patient/significant other's understanding of instructions and information

Provide referrals to social worker, clergy, other disciplines as indicated or requested *to assist with development of coping strategies*

Plan care to allow time for the patient/significant other to express fear, anxiety or ask questions

EXPECTED OUTCOMES

Patient and significant other demonstrate knowledge of disease process, tests, and treatments

Patient expresses and discusses fears and anxiety about diagnosis

● **NDX:** Risk for infection related to suppressed immune system, bone marrow malfunction, replacement with factor, and altered blood profile

Observe Universal Precautions/Body Substance isolation *to minimize exposure to pathogens*

Place patient in a private room for absolute neutrophil count <500 mm³ *to minimize exposure to pathogens*

Monitor T, P, and R q4h *to ensure early detection of signs of infection;* report elevations to physician

Monitor breath sounds daily; instruct patient to report sore throat, perirectal discomfort, vaginal itching, or burning on urination *to detect atypical signs of infection*

Observe body fluids for changes in color, odor, and consistency

Administer antibiotics, antifungals, and antivirals as ordered *to treat secondary or opportunistic infection*

Assist patient with daily hygiene and oral care

Assist patient with ambulation, turning, coughing, and deep breathing *to prevent stasis of body fluids*

Ensure fluid intake to 2500 ml/day, unless contraindicated, *to dilute urine and decrease risk of UTI by promoting frequent emptying of the bladder*

Avoid invasive procedures; use strict aseptic technique when invasive procedures must be performed

EXPECTED OUTCOME

Patient is free of respiratory, urinary, GI, or other opportunistic infection

ADDITIONAL NURSING DIAGNOSES TO CONSIDER

Ineffective coping

Ineffective thermoregulation

Self-care deficit

Altered parenting

Social isolation

Patient/family teaching

Nutrition

Explain need to maintain balanced diet of preference and as tolerated; to use frequent, small feedings if preferred; and to avoid foods that irritate oral mucous membranes

Explain need to take fluids of preference—at least 2500 ml/day unless contraindicated

Explain need to perform mouth care routinely before and after meals and prn, to report early signs of mouth lesions or those that do not heal, and to use special mouth rinses as ordered

Demonstrate method of checking for and explain need to report signs and symptoms of mucositis

Explain need to weigh weekly (same time, scale, and clothing)

Activity

Instruct patient to alternate activities with rest periods to conserve energy

Explain need to increase activity gradually and not to become nonfunctional

Instruct patient on placing personal items at hand and furniture to prevent accidents

Demonstrate use of equipment to assist with ambulation when needed

Explain need to monitor activity tolerance (check pulse rate; if elevated or patient is feeling exhausted, rest, then continue)

Instruct patient to report symptoms to physician if no relief occurs with rest

Demonstrate oxygen therapy administration Liters/minute ordered

Use of equipment: changing tank, cleansing or replacement of cannula

Bleeding

Discuss signs and symptoms of bleeding to be reported to physician in any of the following areas
Skin
Oral
Nasal
Rectal
Stomach
Cerebral
Urinary tract
Discuss emergency plan to follow if spontaneous hemorrhage occurs
Have emergency numbers available
Call paramedics
Go to nearest emergency facility
Explain importance of telling dentist and other medical personnel about disease process and low platelet count
Explain importance of maintaining safe, clutter-free environment
Explain importance of avoiding over-the-counter medications, especially those containing acetylsalicylic acid (i.e., aspirin) without checking with physician
Instruct patient to avoid use of sharp objects whenever possible
Instruct patient to avoid harsh coughing and blowing of nose
If cough persists, notify physician
Take cough medication as ordered
Explain need to avoid activities and sports that may cause injury
Explain need to avoid constipation through diet, fluids, and stool softeners
Explain importance of ongoing outpatient care
Routine laboratory appointments
Return physician and nurse appointments
Ensure that patient and/or significant other demonstrates
Method for applying pressure to bleeding site
Apply dressing or clean material directly over site
Apply pressure for 5 min
Apply ice in covered plastic bag over site once bleeding stops
Check site for further bleeding q15 min for 1 hr
Method for testing stool and urine for occult blood

Infection

Discuss signs and symptoms of infection to report to physician or nurse
Explain importance of avoiding persons who may be infectious or who have potentially contagious conditions, as well as persons who have been recently vaccinated and crowds
Explain need to avoid multiple sexual partners
Explain need to wash hands after using bathroom before eating, or before performing any care procedures or food preparation
Discuss importance of preventing injury to skin
Use electric razor
Handle knives and sharp objects carefully
Wear protective gloves when gardening and when using strong household cleaning solutions
Wear broad-brimmed hat and sun screen when in sun
Avoid going barefoot
Wear warm clothing and boots in cold weather
Avoid cutting cuticles, corns, or calluses
Wear padded gloves when using oven
Explain need to perform oral hygiene periodically throughout day and importance of daily hygiene, including perineal and rectal care
Explain importance of drinking up to 2500 ml of fluid each day unless contraindicated; need to avoid using common drinking fountain
Explain need to maintain clean home environment and handle food properly
Explain need to avoid contact with pets or other animals
Demonstrate method for taking and recording temperature
Demonstrate procedure for caring for very small cuts or breaks in skin

Home care considerations

Review history for presence of care giver
Assess patient/significant other's knowledge level of disease process
Assess home environment for potential environmental hazards
Assess ability of patient/significant other to comply with instructions

Polycythemia

An increase in the number of circulating erythrocytes
polycythemia vera: *A chronic disorder in which overproduction of myelocytes and thrombocytes, as well as erythrocytes, occurs with a resulting increase in blood viscosity, blood volume, and Hgb concentration.*
secondary polycythemia: *A compensatory response to hypoxemia, which may result from chronic obstructive pulmonary disease (COPD), congenital heart disease, or prolonged exposure to low oxygen content (high altitude)*

relative polycythemia: A result of decreased plasma volume; erythrocyte level is normal or decreased

Assessment

Subjective data

Central nervous system
  Complaints of the following:
    Headache
    Fullness in the head
    Dizziness
    Visual disturbances
    Fatigue
    Numbness of the fingers
    Double vision
Cardiovascular system
  Complaints of the following:
    Chest pain
    Calf pain with walking
    SOB with exercise
GI system
  Complaints of the following:
    Feeling full
    Constipation
    Weight loss
    Thirst
Integumentary system
  Complaints of the following:
    Itching
    Night sweats
Musculoskeletal system
  Complaints of joint pain

Objective data

Central nervous system
  Paresthesia
  Engorged veins in the fundus and retina
  Congestion of the conjunctiva
  Altered mentation
Cardiovascular system
  Hypertension
  Intermittent claudication
  Thrombus
  Emboli
  Angina
  Hemorrhage
Gastrointestinal system
  Flatulence
  Constipation
  Hepatosplenomegaly in polycythemia vera
  GI bleeding
  Weight loss
  Gingival bleeding

Integumentary system
  Pruritis after hot bath
  Urticaria
  Ruddy cyanosis
  Ecchymosis

Diagnostic tests

Erythrocyte count up to 8 to 12 million per mm^3
Hgb 8 to 25 g/100 ml
Hct > 60%
Mean corpuscular hemoglobin concentration (MCHC) decreased
Leukocytes increased
Thrombocytosis
Granulocytosis
Basophilia
Hyperuricemia
Total blood volume increased
Abnormal coagulation studies

Potential complications

Hypervolemia
Thrombocytosis
MI
CVA
Gangrene of the digits
Hemorrhage
Splenic infarction
Renal calculi
Hypertension
CHF
Peptic ulcers
Leukemia (iatrogenic)

Collaborative management

Therapeutic management

Phlebotomy
Pheresis transfusion
Myelosuppressive therapy (for control of symptoms related to myelocytosis, thrombocytosis, and hyperuricemia)
  Radioactive phosporus po or IV
  Antineoplastic agents
Smoking cessation
Rehydration
Stress management
Respiratory support
Physical therapy
Nutritional support
Treatment of underlying disease, elimination of environmental causes (secondary polycythemia)

Nursing management

PATIENT PROBLEMS/NURSING DIAGNOSES

● **NDX:** Altered cardiopulmonary tissue perfusion related to increased arterial pressure, increased total blood volume, and increased blood viscosity

Monitor BP *to assess cardiac function, peripheral resistance to blood flow, and effectiveness of therapy*

Monitor respirations and auscultate chest for heart and breath sounds *to assess pulmonary function and detect onset of congestive heart failure;* report changes immediately

Encourage frequent rest periods and avoidance of strenuous activity *to decrease cardiac workload*

Assist with ADLs *to reduce oxygen demand*

Apply antiembolic stockings *to enhance peripheral venous return*

Instruct patient to avoid caffeine, tobacco, and other stimulants *to prevent vasoconstriction*

Notify health care provider of complaints of chest pain, increased dyspnea, cyanosis, or restlessness *to facilitate early intervention*

Maintain a stress-free environment *to minimize risk of hypertension and maintain adequate cardiac output*

Administer oxygen therapy as ordered *to promote adequate tissue perfusion*

Initiate continuous pulse oximetry *to monitor oxygen saturation*

Administer sublingual nitroglycerin as ordered for angina

Administer medications as ordered *to promote vasodilatation, diuresis, anticoagulation, pain relief, or treatment of other signs/symptoms and underlying causes*

Instruct the patient to avoid foods high in sodium *to reduce fluid retention*

Maintain the patient in semi-Fowler's position when in bed *to promote maximal respiratory excursion*

Assist the patient to turn, cough, and deep breathe *to ensure an open airway and prevent stasis of body fluids*

Assist the patient to ambulate as tolerated *to prevent stasis of body fluids, maintain cardiac function, and prevent injury caused by falls*

If phlebotomy is required, explain the procedure *to assure the patient that it will relieve distressing symptoms*

Monitor pulse, respirations, and blood pressure *to assess patient response to the procedure*

Have the patient lie down during the procedure *to prevent vertigo and syncope*

Monitor the patient for tachycardia, clamminess, or complaints of vertigo; discontinue the procedure in the event these side effects occur

Check blood pressure and pulse immediately after procedure

Instruct the patient to remain sitting for 5 min before ambulation *to prevent vasovagal attack or orthostatic hypotension*

EXPECTED OUTCOMES

Patient's vital signs are stable

Patient denies complaints of dyspnea, orthopnea, angina, dizziness, headache

● **NDX:** Altered cerebrovascular tissue perfusion related to increased intercranial pressure, intracranial bleeding, cerebral edema, and impairment of microcirculation

Assess neurologic signs *to detect increasing intracranial pressure*

Maintain the patient on complete bed rest with head of bed elevated *to conserve energy and lower intracranial pressure*

Promote a quiet environment *to promote rest and reduce stress*

Instruct the patient to avoid stimulants (caffeine, tobacco) *to prevent vasoconstriction*

Monitor vital signs and blood pressure *to detect the presence of intracranial bleeding*

Assist the patient with ADLs and ambulation *to prevent injury*

Administer medications as ordered for vasodilation and anticoagulation

EXPECTED OUTCOMES

Patient is alert with normal and equal pupillary responses and reflexes

Patient denies visual disturbances, weakness in the extremities, or headache

● **NDX:** Altered peripheral tissue perfusion related to increased blood viscosity and vasconstriction or microcirculation impairment

Observe color of the extremities, face, and mucous membranes *to assess disease status*

Perform passive, active ROM exercises *to prevent venous stasis*

Avoid excessive venipuncture; insert peripherally inserted central catheter (PICC), midline or Aquavene (Menlocare, Inc.) catheter for venous access, consolidate laboratory procedures

Monitor the patient's skin and mucous membranes *to detect lesions and impairment of skin integrity*

EXPECTED OUTCOMES

Patient's peripheral pulses are strong and equal

Patient's skin is intact, warm, and dry

● **NDX:** Altered protection related to abnormal blood profile, drug therapies, and treatments

Assess patient for and report signs and symptoms of
thrombus formation
 Changes in mental status
 Chest pain
 Sudden onset or increase in respiratory distress
 Abdominal pain
 Mottling or coolness of the extremities
Maintain position of comfort *to provide maximal respiratory excursion*
Avoid use of the knee gatch *to prevent venous compromise*
Apply antiembolic stockings as ordered
Perform active/passive ROM exercises *to prevent venous stasis*
Avoid restrictive clothing and bed linens *to prevent injury to skin*
Keep the patient warm and dry *to prevent vasoconstriction*
Avoid sitting for long periods; instruct patient to
avoid crossing legs when sitting *to prevent vasoconstriction*
Assist with ambulation *to prevent injury caused by falls*
Ensure that the environment is free of obstacles *to avoid injury caused by bumps and falls*
Instruct patient to call for assistance
Instruct patient to notify nurse for sudden onset of pain
in the chest, head, extremities, or upon urination

EXPECTED OUTCOMES
Patient verbalizes understanding of instructions to request assistance and notify nursing personnel of onset of pain
Patient exhibits no signs or symptoms of pulmonary, GI, GU, or neurologic involvement
Patient's extremities are warm and dry with good color

● **NDX:** Altered nutrition: less than body requirements related to inadequate intake of iron and folic acid

Assess nutritional status and food preferences including cultural, religious, or medical restrictions
Consult dietitian *for further assessment and nutritional support*
Provide small, frequent feedings *to avoid fatiguing patient with three large meals*
Provide dietary supplement as ordered *to ensure appropriate daily caloric intake*
Encourage family to bring patient's favorite foods from home if appropriate
 Avoid foods that are GI irritants, spicy, flatus-forming, or high in caffeine

Monitor intake and output every shift *to aid in early detection of inadequate intake*
Weigh patient daily (same time, scale, and clothing)
 Report 2% decrease in weight
Assist patient with meals as necessary *to conserve energy*
Monitor and record character, amount, color, and frequency of stools; administer antidiarrheal medications as indicated

EXPECTED OUTCOMES
Patient's weight increases toward normal for height, age, sex, and body build
Patient is taking balanced diet with fluids to 2000 ml/day, unless contraindicated
Intake and output are balanced

● **NDX:** Risk for impaired skin integrity related to altered tissue perfusion, immobility, inadequate nutrition, mechanical forces, and itching

Inspect skin for redness, lesions, swelling, drainage q8h *to detect impairment of skin integrity*
Keep skin warm and dry *to prevent breakdown caused by environmental moisture*
Avoid use of constrictive clothing; maintain ambient and body warmth *to promote circulation*
Assist the patient with active and passive ROM exercises as tolerated *to maintain circulation*
Palpate peripheral pulses *to assess status of arterial circulation*
Review blood studies *to evaluate oxygen saturation and blood viscosity*
If skin impairment occurs, maintain patient on bed rest in semi-Fowler's position *to prevent further injury and decrease peripheral vascular resistance*
Cleanse skin with mild soap, rinse well, dry thoroughly *to maintain integrity*
Apply protective cream after bathing and position change
Ensure that bed linens are wrinkle free and nonconstrictive *to prevent mechanical injury*
Reposition patient q2h when on bed rest *to promote circulation and prevent stasis*
Inspect patient's feet frequently *to ensure early detection of gangrene*
Instruct patient to avoid scratching

EXPECTED OUTCOMES
Patient's skin is warm, moist, with normal color
Patient performs skin hygiene and does not scratch
Patient exhibits no signs or symptoms of gangrene

● **NDX:** Pain related to musculoskeletal problems, impairment of microcirculation, disease process, abdominal distention, ulceration, and headache

Assess patient's pain for location, duration, intensity using a pain rating scale *to facilitate development of a pain management plan*

Collaborate with patient, physician, and other health care team members to develop a pain management plan designed to prevent severe pain

Support painful joints with pillows in position of comfort *to minimize pain and discomfort*

Apply warmth to joints as ordered *to promote comfort*

Administer analgesics as ordered *to achieve goal of the pain management plan*

Use alternate pain management techniques *to achieve the goal of the pain management plan*

Auscultate bowel sounds *to determine presence of obstruction*

Monitor stool and emesis for presence of frank or occult blood *to detect GI bleeding*

Position the patient in semi-Fowler's position *to decrease abdominal pressure and increase intraabdominal space*

Administer antacids as ordered *to relieve epigastric distress*

Provide small, frequent feedings *to prevent abdominal distention*

Palpate the liver *to monitor size and location*

Maintain a quiet environment

Provide uninterrupted rest periods

EXPECTED OUTCOMES

Patient verbalizes relief of pain using the pain management scale

Patient demonstrates a relaxed facial expression and posture

Patient denies headache, joint pain

Patient exhibits normal bowel sounds

ADDITIONAL NURSING DIAGNOSES TO CONSIDER

Altered health maintenance

Altered parenting

Impaired adjustment

Activity intolerance related to immobility caused by joint pain or generalized weakness caused by anemia

Potential for injury related to risk of sensory dysfunction

Patient/family teaching

Disease process

Discuss symptoms of recurrence or progression of disease and complications to report to physician

Demonstrate how to check skin and peripheral pulses

Explain importance of regular follow-up care

Complications

Discuss trauma prevention

Avoid restrictive clothing

Wear well-fitting shoes

Keep home and work area free of clutter

Use assistive devices when needed

Use caution when performing oral hygiene

Avoid sports and hobbies that may cause injury

Handle equipment and sharp objects carefully

Avoid extremes in environmental temperature

Activity

Instruct patient to balance rest and activity periods

Instruct patient not to cross legs when sitting or lock knees when standing; explain need to change position and exercise extremities q30 min

Explain need to plan regular exercise program

Nutrition

Explain importance of well-balanced diet; low-sodium or low-purine diet may be ordered

Instruct patient to take at least 2500 ml of fluid daily unless contraindicated

Discuss foods to avoid: gas-forming, acidic foods

Medication

Teach name of medication, dosage, time of administration, purpose, and side effects

Instruct patient to avoid taking over-the-counter medications without checking with physician

Myelosuppressive treatment

Explain procedure to patient/significant other

Inform patient that risk of infection is increased

Instruct patient to avoid crowds

Instruct patient to notify physician for occurrence of signs and symptoms of infection

Inform patient of potential reactions to alkylating agents (nausea, vomiting, risk of infection); instruct patient to notify physician of side effects

Radioactive phosphorus

Explain procedure to patient/significant other

Inform patient that he or she may require repeated phlebotomies until the treatment takes effect

Instruct patient to lie down during IV administration to prevent extravasation and for 15 to 20 min after injection

Home care considerations

Review history for presence of care giver
Assess patient/significant other's knowledge level of
  disease process
Assess home environment for potential environmental
  hazards
Assess ability of patient/significant other to comply
  with instructions

Thrombocytopenia

*Idiopathic thrombocytopenic purpura (ITP) results from
immunologic platelet destruction and is either acute
(postviral) or chronic. Acute ITP generally occurs in
children ages 2 to 6 years; chronic ITP affects adults
under age 50.*

Assessment

Subjective data

Central nervous system
  Complaints of the following:
    Headache
    Confusion
    Weakness
    Fatigue
Gastrointestinal system
  Complaints of the following:
    Nausea
    Rectal pain
    Abdominal fullness
    Bleeding gums
    Vomiting blood
Cardiovascular system
  Complaints of the following:
    Rapid heart beat
    SOB
    Nose bleeds
    Bleeding gums
Genitourinary system
  Complaints of the following:
    Flank pain
    Blood in the urine
    Frequent, heavy menstrual periods
Integumentary system
  Complaints of the following:
    Bruising easily
    Nasal stuffiness
    Sore mouth
General
  Reports family history of disease or recent exposure

to nonsteroidal antiinflammatory agents, sulfonamides, histamine blockers, alkylating agents, or antibiotic chemotherapeutic agents
Report of recent viral infection
Report of recent excessive bleeding

Objective data

Central nervous system
  Altered pupillary response
  Increased P, R, and BP
  Decreased level of consciousness
  Sluggish reflexes
  Paresthesias of extremities
Gastrointestinal system
  Hematemesis
  Melena
  Guaiac-positive stool
  Abdominal distention
Cardiovascular system
  Tachycardia
  Tachypnea
  Epistaxis
  Oral blood-filled bullae
  Dyspnea
Genitourinary system
  Heavy menstrual flow
  Hematuria
Integumentary system
  Petechiae, purpura
  Ecchymosis
General
  Documented family history
  Documented recent use of specific medications
  Recent infection with Epstein-Barr virus or infectious
    mononucleosis

Diagnostic tests

Platelets <100,000/mm^3
Bleeding time prolonged
Normal coagulation time
Normal prothrombin INR (International Normalize Ra-
  tio) and activated partial thromboplastin times
Increased capillary fragility
Bone marrow biopsy: increased megakaryocytes in the
  presence of increased platelet destruction

Potential complications

Hemorrhage
Transfusion reaction
Death

Collaborative management

Therapeutic management

Treatment of underlying cause, removal of causative
agent
Plasmapheresis
Plasma transfusion
Platelet/blood component transfusion
Splenectomy
Corticosteroids
Respiratory support
Physical therapy
Nutritional support
Analgesics
Stress reduction

Nursing management

PATIENT PROBLEMS/NURSING DIAGNOSES

● **NDX:** Altered protection related to abnormal blood
profile

Maintain patient in a comfortable position; provide support with pillows
Avoid pressure to any area of body; use foam or gel
pads, air mattress, and heel and elbow protection as
needed *to prevent impairment of skin integrity*
Assist with hygiene *to maintain integrity of skin and
mucous membranes*
Monitor vital signs and blood pressure qid *to detect
infection*
Assess skin and mucous membranes for bleeding q4h
to 8h
Check the stool and urine daily for presence of frank or
occult blood
Monitor laboratory studies *to assess status of blood profile*
Avoid frequent venipuncture, IM injections *to maintain
skin integrity and prevent bleeding*
  Consolidate necessary laboratory work
  Use fingersticks when possible
  Apply pressure at injection site for 5 to 10 min or until
    bleeding stops
  Observe injection sites for bleeding or hematoma
    every 15 min for four times after injection
  Observe injection sites every shift for redness, pain,
    swelling, or infiltration
  Clean injection/venipuncture sites with povidone be-
    fore procedure
Use sterile technique for dressing changes
Instruct the patient/significant other in the use of
safety measures *to prevent trauma and bleeding*
Assist the patient with ADLs and ambulation *to prevent
injury from falls*

Provide an environment free from obstructions *to pre-
vent injury from bumps and falls*
Avoid use of constrictive clothing and linens *to prevent
abrasion and impairment of skin integrity*
Pad siderails as needed
Use soft towels and cloths for hygiene; avoid vigorous
skin care
Instruct patient to avoid straining at stool *to prevent in-
creasing intracranial pressure and subsequent bleeding*
Administer stool softeners or laxatives as ordered
Assist patient to perform oral hygiene with soft tooth-
brush or foam stick *to prevent injury to oral mucosa*
Instruct patient to use an electric razor for shaving
Administer platelet transfusion as ordered *to treat com-
plications of severe hemorrhage*
  Administer platelets quickly *to prevent cell destruction*
  Do not administer platelets in the presence of fever *to
    prevent cell destruction*
  Monitor patient for signs and symptoms of febrile
    reaction during administration
  Premedicate as ordered with acetaminophen and
    diphenhydramine
Administer corticosteroid and immunosuppressive
therapy as ordered
Avoid use of antihistamines, phenothiazines, aspirin,
and nonsteroidal antiinflammatory agents in patients
with ITP *to avoid exposure to causative agents*
Instruct patient to avoid use of aspirin *to minimize risk
of bleeding*
Prepare patient for splenectomy as ordered

EXPECTED OUTCOMES
Patient's vital signs are stable
Patient exhibits no signs or symptoms of bleeding

● **NDX:** Altered oral mucous membrane related to altered blood profile

Assess oral cavity q8h to 12h *to ensure early intervention and treatment*
Assist patient to perform oral hygiene q2h when awake
and before and after meals *to prevent buildup of plaque
and bacteria*
Perform oral hygiene with dilute mouthwash or normal
saline rinse and a soft brush or sponge *to avoid irritation of mucous membranes and disruption of bullae*
Apply topical protective agents (water-based jelly,
kaolin preparations) to lesions as ordered *to promote
healing*
Apply topical analgesics 15 to 20 min before meals as
ordered *to facilitate nutritional intake*
Serve foods and fluids lukewarm or cold *to soothe inflamed oral mucosa*
Maintain diet of preference as ordered; avoid spicy/
irritant food *to decrease pain from irritation of mucosa*

Encourage soft, easy-to-chew foods *to avoid tissue trauma and pain*

Encourage fluids, unless contraindicated; iced liquids or popsicles may be soothing

Measure intake and output every shift *to ensure adequacy of dietary intake*

Weigh the patient daily (same time, scale, and clothing) *to assess nutritional status*

EXPECTED OUTCOMES

Patient has pink, moist, intact oral mucosa, tongue, and lips with no bullae

Patient verbalizes comfort in chewing, swallowing, and talking

● **NDX:** Pain related to altered sensations, paresthesias in joints and extremities caused by bleeding

Assess pain location, duration, intensity using a pain rating scale *to facilitate development of pain management plan*

Collaborate with patient, physician, and other health care team members to develop pain management plan designed to prevent severe pain

Support affected joints and extremities with pillows in position of comfort *to minimize pain and discomfort*

Administer analgesics as ordered *to achieve the goal of pain management plan*

Move patient with slow, gentle movements *to minimize discomfort of repositioning and promote relaxation*

Avoid restrictive clothing and linens *to relieve pressure on joints and extremities*

Encourage use of alternate pain management techniques *to enhance effects of analgesics*

EXPECTED OUTCOMES

Patient demonstrates relaxed facial expression and posture

Patient verbalizes pain relief using a pain scale

● **NDX:** Risk for impaired skin integrity related to altered tissue perfusion, mechanical forces, intradermal bleeding, immobility, and altered blood profile

Inspect skin for redness, lesions, swelling, drainage, petechiae, ecchymosis, hematomas every 8 hours *to detect impairment of skin integrity and evaluate need for further intervention;* notify physician of alterations

Keep skin warm and dry *to prevent breakdown due to environmental moisture*

Avoid use of constrictive clothing and maintain ambient and body warmth *to prevent trauma*

Assist the patient with active and passive ROM exer-

cises as tolerated *to avoid injury and maintain circulation*

Avoid excessive venipuncture

Apply ice bag or manual pressure to any puncture site *to control local bleeding*

Gently assist patient with ambulation and repositioning *to avoid injury and tissue trauma*

Cleanse skin with mild soap, rinse well, dry thoroughly *to maintain integrity and avoid trauma*

Apply protective cream after bathing and position change

Ensure that bed linens are wrinkle-free and nonconstrictive *to prevent mechanical injury*

Reposition patient every 2 hours when on bedrest *to avoid pressure injury*

Avoid invasive procedures

EXPECTED OUTCOME

Patient's skin is intact with no discoloration

● **NDX:** Altered cerebral tissue perfusion related to impairment of microcirculation and intracranial bleeding

Assess neurologic signs q2h *to detect increasing intracranial pressure*

Maintain patient on complete bed rest with the head of bed elevated *to conserve energy and lower intracranial pressure*

Instruct patient to avoid coughing, straining at stool, or other Valsalva-type maneuvers *to minimize the risk of bleeding*

Provide a quiet environment *to promote rest and reduce stress*

Instruct patient to avoid stimulants (caffeine, tobacco)

EXPECTED OUTCOME

Patient is alert and oriented with normal reflexes

ADDITIONAL NURSING DIAGNOSES TO CONSIDER

Ineffective coping
Self-care deficit
Altered parenting
Social isolation

Patient/family teaching

Disease process

Demonstrate method to assess for bleeding

Discuss signs and symptoms of recurrence to report to physician: continuous headache, coughing red-streaked sputum, persistent abdominal pain, vomiting frank blood or "coffee ground" material, increased areas of petechiae or ecchymosis, blood-filled bullae in oral cavity, blood in urine or stools

Demonstrate methods of checking for blood in stool and urine

Instruct patient to notify physician when contemplating pregnancy or when pregnancy is first suspected

Caution patient never to donate blood

Explain need to prevent trauma by

Avoiding constipation through diet, fluids, and use of stool softeners or laxatives if needed; avoiding vigorous nose-blowing or coughing; avoiding contact sports or other hazardous hobbies

Careful movements and careful handling of objects that may cause bleeding

Use of nonabrasive skin and mouth care products

Explain importance of notifying all health care providers of diagnosis and keeping follow-up appointments

Nutrition

Explain importance of regular oral hygiene; discuss products to use or avoid; demonstrate method for daily inspection

Explain need to maintain balanced diet with adequate hydration; discuss foods to avoid to prevent trauma

Activity

Explain need to balance rest and activity periods; to increase activity as comfort increases; to use assistance when needed to prevent injury

Medication

Teach name of medication, dosage, time of administration, purpose, and side effects

Teach how to read contents of over-the-counter medications, avoiding those that contain acetylsalicylic acid (antihistamines, phenothiazines, or nonsteroidal antiinflammatory agents in ITP)

Home care considerations

Review history for presence of a care giver

Assess the patient's ability to function independently

Assess the knowledge level of the patient and care giver about the disease process, prevention of trauma, sign and symptoms of bleeding

Assess the patient/significant other's ability to perform necessary procedures and treatments

Disseminated Intravascular Coagulation

Overstimulation of the normal coagulation process associated with underlying conditions such as snakebite, septicemia, severe hypotension, neoplasms, hemolysis, obstetric emergencies, acidosis, cancer chemotherapy, transplant rejection, and extensive burns, trauma, or surgery; the initial accelerated clotting process consumes large amounts of coagulation factors in the formation of fibrin clots; the fibrinolytic system is then activated to lyse fibrin clots into fibrin degradation products; the activity of these products and the depletion of plasma coagulation factors result in hemorrhage

Assessment

Subjective data

Central nervous system
  Complaints of the following:
    Confusion
    Restlessness
    Visual changes
Cardiovascular system
  Complaints of the following:
    Chest pain
    Increasing heart rate
Gastrointestinal system
  Complaints of the following:
    Nausea
    Abdominal pain
Respiratory system
  Complaints of the following:
    Difficulty breathing
    Coughing up blood
Genitourinary system
  Complaints of the following:
    Vaginal bleeding
    Blood in the urine
Integumentary system
  Complaints of the following:
    Oozing of blood from the skin
    Slight blue discoloration of the hands and feet

Objective data

Central nervous system
  Seizures
  Coma

Altered level of consciousness
Restlessness
Vasomotor instability
Cardiovascular system
Increasing hypotension
Postural hypotension
Tachycardia
Epistaxis
Shock
Acrocyanosis
Gastrointestinal system
Nausea/vomiting
Melena
Hematemesis
Increasing abdominal girth
Respiratory system
Hemoptysis
Dyspnea
Tachypnea
Genitourinary system
Hematuria
Oligouria
Integumentary system
Petechiae
Eccymosis
Hematoma
Hemorrhagic bullae
Diffuse oozing of blood or plasma
Palpable purpura, initially on the chest and abdomen
General
Presence of abnormal bleeding in the absence of history of a hemorrhagic disorder
Severe muscle, joint, back pain
Bleeding from surgical incisions, injection sites, IV insertion sites, around chest and nasogastric tubes
Postpartum bleeding
Bleeding into the fundus of the eye

Diagnostic tests

PT, prolonged >15 sec
PTT, prolonged > 60 to 80 sec
Platelet count <100,000/mm³
Fibrinogen level, decreased <150 mg/dl
Antithrombin III level decreased
Thrombin time prolonged
Fibrin degradation products elevated, >100 mcg/ml
Plasminogen levels decreased
Levels of factors V and VIII decreased
Fragmentation of RBCs
Hgb decreased
Urine output, decreased <30 ml per hour
BUN elevated, >25 mg/100 ml
Serum creatinine elevated, >1.3 mg/100 ml

Potential complications

Shock
Acute tubular necrosis
Focal gangrene
Pulmonary edema
CHF
Convulsions
Coma
Failure of major organ systems

Collaborative management

Therapeutic management

Elimination of causative agent
Correction of hypovolemia, hypotension, hypoxia, acidosis
Correction of homeostatic deficiencies
Management of septic shock
Administration of depleted blood fractions
Heparin (early stages and as a last resort for hemorrhage)
Antineoplastic agents
Antibiotics
Respiratory support

Nursing management

PATIENT PROBLEMS/NURSING DIAGNOSES

● **NDX:** Fluid volume deficit related to active fluid loss and bleeding (Table 4-2)

Monitor intake and output q8h to 12h *to assess fluid needs and prevent overload;* report imbalances
Weigh patient daily (same time, scale, and clothing); report changes of 2% to 3% of original weight
Monitor vital signs and mental status q4h
Assess skin turgor and peripheral pulses every shift *to determine adequacy of hydration*
Monitor character, amount, color, frequency of emesis, stools *to detect internal bleeding*
Observe color, specific gravity, pH of urine *to ensure early detection of renal failure*
Provide oral fluid intake as tolerated *to maintain intravascular fluid volume*
Force fluids to 2500 ml/day unless contraindicated
Administer blood fractions as ordered *to alleviate fluid deficit*
Administer heparin as ordered *to control bleeding*
Review laboratory results *to assess degree of blood loss and patient response to therapy*
Apply ice packs and pressure to site of bleeding *to control blood loss*

Table 4-2 Signs and Symptoms of Blood Loss

Volume Lost		Clinical Signs
ml	% TBV*	
500	10	None; occasionally vasovagal syncope in blood donors
1000	20	At rest there may be no clinical evidence of volume loss; a slight postural drop in blood pressure may be seen; tachycardia with exercise
1500	30	Resting supine blood pressure and pulse may be normal; neck veins flat when supine; postural hypotension; exercise tachycardia
2000	40	Central venous pressure, cardiac output, and arterial blood pressure below normal even when supine and at rest; air hunger, rapid thready pulse, cold clammy skin
2500	50	Lactic acidosis, severe shock, death

From Wintrobe MM et al: *Clinical hematology,* Philadelphia, 1981, Lea & Febiger.
*Total blood volume.

Avoid injections, use of straight razors *to minimize risk of injury and bleeding*
Assist the patient with ADLs and ambulation *to minimize the risk of injury*
Use soft towels and cloths for hygiene; do not perform aggressive skin care *to prevent injury*

EXPECTED OUTCOMES

Patient's skin turgor and color are normal
Intake and output are balanced
Renal function is adequate
Peripheral pulses are present
Extremities are warm with good color

● **NDX:** Pain related to tissue hypoxia

Assess location, quality, and intensity of pain; use pain rating scale
Place patient in position of comfort; provide support with pillows to prevent stress on body parts
Assist with care when patient is actively bleeding or experiencing discomfort
Maintain quiet environment

Provide adequate periods of rest; cluster activities and diagnostic studies, when possible, according to patient's tolerance
Assist patient with alternate comfort measures such as music therapy, imagery, or other distractions
Administer analgesics as ordered; assess effectiveness

EXPECTED OUTCOMES

Patient verbalizes no discomfort
Patient's body posture and face are relaxed

● **NDX:** Anxiety related to threat of death and changes in health status

Assess level of patient's fear and current understanding of disease process, treatments, and interventions *to assist in development of an education plan*
Reassure patient as needed; remain with patient *to offer security during periods of anxiety*
Maintain a calm, tolerant attitude during interactions with patient
Provide continuity of care *to facilitate communication of anxieties and fears*
Orientate or reorientate patient to environment as needed *to promote a feeling of control and decrease anxiety, fear of the unknown*
Explain procedures simply and briefly; inform patient of what to expect and when to expect it
Maintain a quiet environment *to reduce stress-inducing stimuli*
Encourage patient to talk about anxiety and fear
Instruct patient to notify staff when he or she feels anxious or fearful *to promote a feeling of security*
Assist patient to develop coping strategies *to promote feeling of control*

EXPECTED OUTCOMES

Patient appears calm and is able to verbalize fears and anxieties
Patient is able to use coping measures independently

● **NDX:** Impaired gas exchange related to altered oxygen supply, altered blood flow, and arterial hypotension

Maintain patient in semi-Fowler's position *to decrease diaphragmatic pressure and promote full respiratory excursion*
Encourage deep breathing *to prevent hyperventilation*
Maintain oxygen delivery as ordered *to prevent desaturation*
Monitor pulse oximetry *to assess changes in saturation*
Assess respirations for quality, rate, pattern, depth, dyspnea on exertion (DOE), guarding, use of accessory muscles

Assess changes in mental status and behavior *to evaluate patient's response to disease state and therapy*

Maintain bed rest with siderails up *to decrease cardiac workload*

Monitor pulse, blood pressure, and respirations *to assess cardiac and respiratory function*

Assist patient with ADLs as needed *to conserve energy*

Increase patient's activity level as tolerated *to maintain cardiopulmonary fitness*

Provide reassurance as needed to reduce patient's anxiety, *which may contribute to increased cardiopulmonary workload*

Instruct patient to report dyspnea and palpitations

Assess skin color and temperature *to determine status of tissue oxygenation*

EXPECTED OUTCOMES

Patient's vital signs are stable

Patient denies dyspnea

Patient demonstrates increasing activity tolerance

Peripheral pulses are strong and regular

● **NDX:** Decreased cardiac output related to decreased oxygenation

Maintain patient in semi-Fowler's to high-Fowler's position *to facilitate cardiac output and venous return*

Administer medications as ordered *to correct dysrhythmias*

Administer cardiotonic and vasoconstrictor medications as ordered *to increase cardiac tone*

Provide quiet, restful environment *to reduce stress that may increase cardiac workload*

Encourage patient to use relaxation techniques

Administer oxygen as ordered

Assess skin color and temperature *to determine status of tissue perfusion*

Monitor laboratory tests *to detect acidosis*

Monitor apical and all peripheral pulses *to determine status of tissue perfusion*

EXPECTED OUTCOMES

Patient's vital signs are within normal limits

Laboratory values are within normal limits

Patient is able to participate in ADLs

Peripheral pulses are strong and regular

Patient's skin is warm, dry, with good color

● **NDX:** Sensory/perceptual alterations (kinesthetic) related to altered sensory reception, hypotension, and hypoxia

Monitor vital signs and blood pressure *to assess cerebral and peripheral bloodflow*

Monitor neurologic signs *to assess cerebral blood flow*

Administer oxygen as ordered *to enhance cerebral blood flow*

Provide quiet, restful environment *to decrease stress on the CNS*

Instruct patient to avoid use of stimulants (caffeine, tobacco) *to minimize vasoconstriction leading to cerebral hypoxia*

Assist patient with ADLs and ambulation *to prevent injury resulting from falls*

Monitor arterial blood gases *to detect impaired cerebral oxygenation*

EXPECTED OUTCOME

Patient participates in ADLs and ambulates without difficulty

Patient/family teaching

Discuss signs and symptoms of DIC that should be reported immediately to physician

Instruct patient/significant other in heparin administration if ordered

Discuss medications prescribed including name, dose, route, time of administration, and side effects

Provide additional teaching applicable to underlying cause of DIC

Instruct patient in ways to prevent trauma and injury

Perform oral care with a soft toothbrush or foam stick

Perform skin care gently with a soft towel

Home care considerations

Review history for presence of care giver

Assess patient/significant other's knowledge level of disease process

Assess home environment for potential environmental hazards

Assess ability of patient/significant other to comply with instructions

Splenectomy

Surgical removal of the spleen to treat traumatic injuries or blood dyscrasias in which hypersplenism occurs (the spleen produces leukocytes, lymphocytes, monocytes, and plasma cells; it also destroys nonfunctional red blood cells and platelets, stores blood, and assists in maintaining hemopoiesis; the spleen indiscriminantly sequesters normal red blood cells and platelets, thereby removing them from the circulation when hypersplenism occurs)

Postoperative assessment

Subjective data

Central nervous system
 Complaints of the following:
  Pain
  Fatigue
Cardiovascular system
 Complaints of rapid heart beat
Respiratory system
 Complaints of inability to take a deep breath
Gastrointestinal system
 Complaints of the following:
  Nausea
  Abdominal pain

Objective data

Central nervous system
 Fatigue
 Weakness
Cardiovascular system
 Bleeding
 Tachycardia
 Thrombosis
Respiratory system
 Splinting with respiration, coughing
 Decreased breath sounds
 Tachypnea
 Atelectasis
 Subdiaphragmatic abscess
Gastrointestinal system
 Nausea/vomiting
 Dehydration
 Abdominal distension
General
 Signs and symptom of infection
 Dehiscence

Diagnostic tests

Thrombocyte level elevated
Normal bleeding, clotting times
Electrolytes
Hgb
Hct

Potential complications

Hemorrhage
Infection
Paralytic ileus
Shock
Thrombophlebitis
Pulmonary embolus

Collaborative management

Therapeutic management

Incentive spirometer
Nasogastric tube
Parenteral therapy
Pain management
Management of complications

Nursing management

PATIENT PROBLEMS/NURSING DIAGNOSES

● **NDX:** Ineffective breathing pattern related to pain, anxiety, decreased energy, and decreased lung expansion

Assess respiratory effort, breath sounds, and rate q4h for 48 hr, then q8h
Position patient to decrease respiratory effort
Assist and teach patient to turn, cough, and breathe deeply q2h to 4h; support incision
Teach patient to use incentive spirometer q4h
Assist with ambulation as soon as possible

EXPECTED OUTCOME
Patient's lungs are clear; respiratory excursion is adequate

● **NDX:** Pain related to abdominal incision, drains, and tubes

Assess pain location, frequency, intensity, and duration; use pain rating scale
Assist patient with assuming position of comfort; support as necessary
Collaborate with physician to establish analgesic schedule and dosage to obtain maximum effectiveness; increased frequency usually required during immediate postoperative period
Teach alternate methods of pain relief (e.g., relaxation, imagery, music)
Administer pain medication before performing activities, thereby increasing compliance with the following:
Coughing and deep breathing
ROM exercises
Early periods of ambulation and self-care activities
If pain increases, assess for other factors (e.g., complications, exacerbation of primary condition)

EXPECTED OUTCOMES
Patient verbalizes feelings of increased comfort
Patient performs activities without limitation
Patient's body posture and face are relaxed

● **NDX:** Risk for fluid volume deficit related to naso-gastric tube, wound drains, blood loss in surgery, NPO status, and vomiting

Maintain NPO as ordered
Connect nasogastric sump tube to low, intermittent suc-tion apparatus as ordered
 Do not change position of tube
 Maintain tube patency
 Check drainage q2h to 4h; report excessive bleeding
Assess skin turgor q8h
Measure intake and output q8h; report imbalance
Weigh patient daily (same time, clothing, and scale)

EXPECTED OUTCOMES
Patient's intake equals output
Mucous membranes are moist
Skin turgor is good

● **NDX:** Altered urinary elimination related to anes-thesia, sensory motor impairment, neuro-muscular impairment, and mechanical trauma

Observe voiding: frequency, amount, color, odor, dis-comfort, distension, q4h to 8h
Insert catheter when ordered for retention or overflow voiding; perform daily catheter care
Institute voiding measures as needed; when catheter is removed; obtain midstream culture

EXPECTED OUTCOME
Patient voids without difficulty and has no signs of in-fection

● **NDX:** Constipation related to less than adequate di-etary intake and bulk, medications, neuro-muscular impairment, musculoskeletal im-pairment, pain on defecation, and emotional status

Auscultate abdomen for bowel sounds q8h; report return of bowel sounds
Begin oral liquids, progressing to regular diet when ordered after return of bowel sounds; note toler-ance
Encourage fluids to 2500 ml/day unless contraindicated
Administer Harris flush q6h or prn for distension if ordered

Monitor for first bowel movement after surgery; give stool softeners or enemas as ordered

EXPECTED OUTCOMES
Patient takes regular diet and fluids to 2500 ml/day
Patient has had soft-formed bowel movement

● **NDX:** Altered gastrointestinal and/or peripheral tissue perfusion related to interruption of flow, venous/arterial, hypovolemia, and hypervolemia

Monitor BP, P, R, CVP, and T q4h for 48 hr, then q8h
Assess for signs of bleeding or thrombosis q4h to 8h
Check dressing for bleeding q2h to 4h for 48 hr
 Reinforce as necessary
 Report excessive bleeding to physician
Change dressing daily and prn; observe healing process; report early signs of infection when present
Position patient comfortably; assist with turning q2h; avoid knee gatch or pillows under knees
Assist with and teach active or perform passive ROM exercises q4h
Provide correct-size antiembolic stockings when or-dered
Plan uninterrupted rest and sleep periods *to prevent fatigue*
Assist with ambulation as necessary
 Avoid sitting for long periods
 Walk in place when standing

EXPECTED OUTCOMES
Patient's vital signs are within normal limits
Peripheral pulses are palpable
Color and temperature of extremities are normal
Incision is healing

Patient/family teaching

Self-care

Instruct patient to shower daily, dry incision well
Teach patient to observe for and report increased pain, swelling, redness, or drainage
Emphasize importance of not applying creams, lotions, or powders to incision
Instruct patient to support incision, if needed, when deep breathing and coughing
Emphasize need for follow-up care

Activities

Explain need to increase ambulation and activities each day and plan regular, uninterrupted rest periods

Explain need to exercise extremities routinely; demonstrate ROM and breathing exercises

Instruct patient to avoid sitting for long periods; explain importance of not crossing legs

Instruct patient to avoid heavy lifting and contact sports for 6 to 8 wk or as directed by physician

Nutrition

Instruct patient to maintain well-balanced diet, taking 2500 ml of liquids daily

Instruct patient to report inability to tolerate food or liquids, nausea, any vomiting, diarrhea, or constipation

Apheresis Therapy

Selective removal of blood or blood components for therapeutic goals; types of apheresis—procedures are named depending on the blood component to be removed (Table 4-3).

Assessment

Assess for appearance of complications during procedure (see Table 4-3)

Continue required assessment for primary condition

Preapheresis care

Reinforce physician's explanation of procedure; include significant other

Obtain written consent after physician has explained procedure

Assess patient's existing condition and note routine and special nursing care requirements for primary condition

Check preapheresis laboratory values

Take and record vital signs and standing and lying BP

Assess patient's heart and lung sounds

Administer medications and fluids as ordered

NOTE: Wear protective gloves and gowns when handling blood components, needles, and centrifuge equipment

Interventions

NOTE: Procedure is performed by a specifically qualified operator

During procedure

Assess vital signs, heart and breath sounds qh

Measure intake and output

Monitor infusions and rates qh

Administer routine medications

Continue care for primary condition

Postapheresis care

If antecubital veins are used for access
  Never use for other venipunctures
  Apply warm soaks qid
  Teach arm-strengthening exercises
If arteriovenous fistula is used for access
  Check patency daily
  Never use for venipunctures
  Never take BP in that extremity; no IM injections in same extremity
  See standard of care for primary condition

Patient/family teaching

Ensure that patient and/or significant other demonstrates
  Care of venous or arteriovenous fistula
  Extremity exercises to perform daily
Ensure that patient and/or significant other knows and understands
  Signs and symptoms of bleeding and infection to report to physician
  To avoid exposure to persons with infections, especially URIs
See standard of care for primary condition

Blood Transfusions

Assessment

Observations/findings

Venipuncture site
  Pain
  Warmth
  Redness
  Swelling
  Leakage at insertion site
Position of extremity
Blood
  Type and Rh factor (Table 4-4)
  Flow rate
  Amount

Potential reactions (Table 4-5)

Hemolysis
  Elevated temperature
  Decreased BP
  Hemoglobinuria

Text continued on p. 260.

Table 4-3 Therapeutic Apheresis Procedures

Considerations	Plasmapheresis	Plateletpheresis	Leukapheresis	Erythrocytapheresis
Indications	Hemolytic anemia (AIHA) acute ITP, nonrelapsing TTP, Guillain-Barré syndrome, myasthenia gravis, renal transplant rejection syndrome, Goodpasture's syndrome, systemic lupus erythematosus, rheumatoid arthritis, multiple myeloma, biliary cirrhosis, hyperlipidemia, hypercholesterolemia, cancer conditions in which plasma substances interfere with immune system	Thrombocytosis	Chronic lymphatic leukemia, rheumatoid arthritis, multiple sclerosis	Acute, severe sickle cell disease, polycythemia vera
Preapheresis laboratory/ diagnostic studies	Total albumin and protein, K, Mg, Ca, CBC, Hgb, Hct, platelet count, PT, activated PTT, hepatitis-associated antigen/VDRL, cold agglutinins, liver/renal function tests, HBSAg if history of hepatitis	Platelet count, CBC, Hgb, PT, activated PTT, cold agglutinins, liver and renal function tests, HBSAg if history of hepatitis	CBC, differential, Hgb, Hct, platelet count, PT, activated PTT, cold agglutinins, liver/renal function tests, HBSAg if history of hepatitis	CBC, Hgb, platelet count, PT, in activated PTT, cold agglutinins, liver/renal function tests, HBSAg if history of hepatitis
Complications	Electrolyte imbalance (hypocalcemia, hypokalemia), hypothermia, hypovolemia, fluid overload, vasovagal reaction, thrombus or air embolus, oliguria or anuria, shock	Air embolus, reaction from anticoagulation: (citrate) tingling chills, seizures, hypotension, hemolysis, bleeding, fluid overload	Air embolus, reaction from anticoagulation: (citrate) tingling chills, seizures, hypotension, hemolysis, bleeding, fluid overload	Hypovolemia, hemolytic transfusion reaction
Usual volume removed	2-4 L	1000 ml, depending on platelet count		
Replacement therapy	Volume removed replaced with normal saline and albumin or fresh frozen plasma (replaces Ig and coagulation factors but increases risk of hypersensitivity and hepatitis)	Albumin 5% add 0.9% NS or plasmanate	Albumin 5% add 0.9% NS or plasmanate	Amount removed replaced with washed, frozen, or WBC-poor RBCs
Usual length of each treatment	2-3 hr usually, dependent on volume to be removed	2-4 hr	3-4 hr	Varies with condition being treated

Continued.

Table 4-3 Therapeutic Apheresis Procedures—cont'd

Considerations	Plasmapheresis	Plateletpheresis	Leukapheresis	Erythrocytapheresis
Usual length of therapy	Six treatments	Varies with primary condition	18-20 treatments, depending on rate of cell proliferation	Varies with primary condition
Usual schedule of treatments	Every other day or every day to total required dependent on antigen/complement levels	Varies with condition, continued until platelet count is at desired level	Three times week 1, two times week 2, then one time a week thereafter to total required	Varies with primary condition

Table 4-4 Blood and Blood Components

Product	Description	Indication(s)	Action	Administration
Red blood cells, packed (PRC)	Concentrated red blood cells that remain after plasma is separated	To improve oxygen-carrying capacity of the blood (hemolytic anemia in aplastic crisis, chronic hypoplastic anemia, leukemia, lymphoma, and other malignant diseases with bone marrow failure); exchange transfusions; surgery; shock; conditions in which sudden changes in blood volume are not tolerated	Increases oxygen-carrying capacity; elevates Hct (3% if unit of PRC has Hct of 70%-80%)	See blood administration standard; administer through a filter; regulate flow to 25 ml/hr for 15 min; remain with patient; observe for reaction; if no reaction, regulate flow to 100-200 ml/hr in adult with no cardiac failure or elevated CVP and in infants and children regulate flow to 2-6 ml/kg/hr; add sodium chloride to PRC before administration when ordered; *no other solution or medication may be added to red cells*
Red blood cells, leukocyte poor	Concentrated red cells with leukocytes removed, usually by continuous flow centrifuge or washing	See PRC; severe febrile transfusion reactions caused by antileukocyte or antiplatelet antibodies; candidates for transplantation	See PRC	See PRC

Table 4-4   Blood and Blood Components—cont'd

Product	Description	Indication(s)	Action	Administration
Red blood cells, frozen	Glycerol added to red cells to protect cell from hemolysis while suspended in hypertonic solution when frozen; glycerol is removed before administration	See PRC; hypersensitivity reactions to plasma components such as IgA	See PRC	See PRC
Whole blood	Plasma and red blood cells; may or may not contain other cells and factors; dependent on length of time transpired after collection; unit usually contains 520 ± 45 ml of anticoagulated blood with Hct of about 40%	Restoration of decreased blood volume caused by hemorrhage or trauma in which more than 25% of volume is lost	Restores blood volume and increases oxygen-carrying capacity	Administer through a filter; remain with patient until 25-50 ml transfused, usually 15-30 min; observe for transfusion reactions; if no reaction, adjust flow rate to administer complete unit within 4 hr; warm unit no higher than 37°C using special coils when refrigerated blood needs to be administered quickly
Whole blood, modified		Hypovolemic shock	Increases oxygen-carrying capacity and provides volume without adding platelets, which release serotonin (a vasoconstrictor)	See whole blood
Whole blood with antihemophilic factor (factor VIII) removed	Prepared by removing factor VIII, using heparin in initial collection, or converting a previously collected unit of blood containing a citrate anticoagulant	Exchange transfusion in the adult	Provides volume without contributing to coagulation ability	See whole blood
Plasma	Plasma prepared from single donor unit of fresh blood	Burns; traumatic shock; replacement of certain coagulation factors	Provides plasma coagulation factors	Administer unit in less than 1 hr in hypovolemic patient; in normovolemic patient, administer at rate of 5-20 ml/kg

Continued.

Table 4-4 Blood and Blood Components—cont'd

Product	Description	Indication(s)	Action	Administration
Plasma, fresh-frozen	Plasma prepared from single donor unit of fresh blood; it is frozen within 6 hr of collection	Source of fibrinogen and factors V and VIII	See plasma; 1 U usually contains approximately 400 mg fibrinogen, 200 U factors VIII and IX, and other stable and labile coagulation factors	Thaw frozen plasma in 37°C water bath with gentle agitation; *do not warm;* administer through a filter; *never add* medications or fluids
Plasma, liquid	Plasma prepared from single donor unit within 5 days after collection; stored frozen	Factor VII, IX, X, XI, and XIII deficiencies or abnormalities	Replacement of factors VII, IX, X, XI, or XIII	See plasma, fresh-frozen
Cryoprecipitated antihemophilic factor (factor VIII)	Preparation containing factor VIII is obtained from a single unit of blood; contains approximately 80 U factor VIII, and 200 mg fibrinogen in 15 ml of plasma	Hemophilia A; von Willebrand's disease (factor VIII deficiency)	Provides high concentrations of factor VIII and fibrinogen	Thaw in warm water bath at 37°C with gentle agitation; administer through filter rapidly within 6 hr after thawing if container not entered; 2 hr after thawing if container entered
Leukocyte concentrate	Leukocytes, platelets, and erythrocytes in varying amounts in 200-500 ml of plasma collected by apheresis; a compatible HLA donor is usually preferred (not identical donor whose use as a tissue donor is anticipated)	Bacterial sepsis not responsive to antibiotic therapy in presence of neutropenia; chronic granulomatous disease when bone marrow recovery is foreseen and temperature elevated for 24-48 hours	Provides granulocytes to more effectively control infection	Administer irradiated leukocytes to prevent engraphment and possible GVHD; regulate rate of flow to give 250-850 granulocytes/µl/M², usually 1 U/day is ordered; slow rate of transfusion at appearance of elevated T wave, chills, and urticaria; stop transfusion when symptoms of transient pulmonary infiltrate appear
Platelet concentrate (random or single donor)	Platelets separated from whole blood suspended in plasma; collection from single donor preferred	Hemorrhage caused by thrombocytopenia; prevention of potential hemorrhage in bone marrow suppression caused by chemotherapy; abnormalities in platelet function	Corrects hemostatic deficit in thrombocytopenia and abnormally functioning platelets; 1 U usually increases platelet count 5000/ml in 70 kg adult	Administer through a filter (*never* a microaggregate filter); regulate flow rate to assure administration of total unit in less than 20 min

Table 4-4 Blood and Blood Components—cont'd

Product	Description	Indication(s)	Action	Administration
Normal serum albumin, USP 25% solution hyperoncotic (NOTE: 5% solution is osmotically equal to plasma)	Derived from pooled venous plasma; contains 25 g normal serum albumin/100 ml	Hypoproteinemia; burns; shock caused by trauma, hemorrhage	Increases oncotic pressure; increases circulating volume by drawing five times the infused volume of albumin into circulation unless patient is dehydrated; reduces hemoconcentration and blood viscosity	Administer at flow rate <2-3 ml/min to prevent rapid rise in BP, circulatory overload, or pulmonary edema
Hespan, Hetastarch	A synthetic colloid derived from a waxy starch composed of amylopectin; it has a molecular weight suitable for use as a plasma expander; Hespan is 6% Hetastarch in 0.9% sodium chloride injection	An adjunct in treatment of hemorrhagic shock, burns, and septic shock	Volume expansion resulting from albuminlike properties Increases ESR when added to whole blood, thereby improving efficacy of granulocyte collection	For hemorrhagic shock, administer at 20 ml/kg/hr, slower rate usually ordered for other indications; contraindications; severe bleeding disorders, severe CHF, renal failure, increased PT or PTT times

Table 4-5 Reactions to Transfusion of Blood and Blood Components

Product	Type of Reaction	Onset	Observations	Nursing Actions
Red blood cells (RBCs), all preparations	Febrile nonhemolytic	Initiation of transfusion to 24 hr post-transfusion	Chills, elevated temperature, headache, nausea, vomiting	Check and record baseline T, P, R, and BP; slow infusion; notify physician; administer antipyretic or antihistamines as ordered; check and record T, P, and R q15min; saline-washed RBCs: frozen, thawed, washed RBCs or leukocyte filter may be ordered to decrease reaction
	Febrile hemolytic	Immediately to 30 min after initiation of transfusion or when 25-50 ml infused	Restlessness, anxiety, precordial oppression, elevated T to 105°F (40.6°C), tachycardia, tachypnea, flushed face, back and thigh pain, generalized	Stop transfusion immediately; change IV tubing; initiate normal saline at 4-6 ml/hr; cap blood tubing with sterile needle or cap; report symptoms to physician and blood bank; recheck identifying blood numbers with patient's numbers; monitor and record T, R, and cardiac rate

Continued.

Table 4-5   Reactions to Transfusion of Blood and Blood Components —cont'd

Product	Type of Reaction	Onset	Observations	Nursing Actions
			tingling, chills, nausea, vomiting, shock, disseminated intravascular coagulation (DIC), renal failure, oliguria, hematuria, anuria	and rhythm q10-15min; measure and record urine output with each voiding or q½ hr; send first specimen to lab for testing; report output <15 ml/30 min or presence of bleeding; ensure that blood samples are drawn for testing; the following are usually ordered: Hgb, haptoglobin level, methemalbumin, bilirubin, differential agglutination, serologic studies, renal function tests, and aerobic and anaerobic cultures; complete transfusion record; send discontinued blood, tubing, and record to laboratory for testing; administer medications and fluids IV as ordered; diuretics, oxygen, electrolytes, and heparin may be ordered; prepare for dialysis
Whole blood	Allergic reaction to plasma proteins	Within 30 min after initiating transfusion	Mild reaction: chills, elevated temperature, backache, pain in legs	Check and record baseline T, P, R, and BP; stop infusion; initiate slow (4-6 ml/hr) infusion of saline using new sterile IV tubing; notify physician and blood bank; monitor T, P, R, and BP q10-15min; ensure that blood specimen is drawn for testing; return remainder of blood product, tubing, and transfusion record to blood bank; indicate observations on transfusion record; usually red cells without IgA will be ordered for administration; oxygen, steroids, vasopressors, or epinephrine may be ordered for anaphylactic shock; prepare for resuscitation
		Immediately to 30 min after initiation of transfusion	Moderate-to-severe reaction: erythematous rash, urticaria, dyspnea, wheezing, hypotension, intestinal hyperperistalsis, anaphylactic shock	
		During transfusion to several days after	Urticaria, swelling of lymph nodes, sore throat	Slow transfusion rate; report observations to physician; administer antihistamines as ordered; blood obtained from a fasting donor may be ordered if reaction is severe
	Circulatory overload	During transfusion to 24	Sharp cough, precordial pain, back pain, dyspnea, cyanosis, increased venous pressure,	Slow transfusion rate; report observations to physician; continue rate of flow as ordered; usually 2ml/kg/hr; monitor, T, P, R, BP, and CVP q15-30min; see CHF (p 835)

Table 4-5 Reactions to Transfusion of Blood and Blood Components —cont'd

Product	Type of Reaction	Onset	Observations	Nursing Actions
			distended neck veins, productive cough, frothy sputum, pleural rales	
	Febrile (hemolytic)	See RBC	See RBC	See RBC
	Febrile (WBC and/ or platelet antibodies)	See Leukocyte concentrate	See Leukocyte concentrate	See Leukocyte concentrate
Massive transfusions of RBCs or whole blood	Metabolic hyperkalemia and citrate toxicity with acid citrate dextrose (ACD) anticoagulant	Citric acid elevations of 100 mg/100 ml	Tremors, prolonged Q-T segment on ECG, hypocalcemia, acidosis then alkalosis, cardiac arrest if citric acid levels higher	When massive transfusions required, transfusion products with citrate-phosphate dextrose (CPD) anticoagulant usually ordered; monitor and record T, R, and cardiac function q10-15min; ensure that blood samples are drawn for electrolytes, calcium, pH, CO_2, bicarbonate levels; administer calcium gluconate IV as ordered; administer oral or rectal cation exchange resins as ordered for hyperkalemia
	Pulmonary infiltrates	During transfusion	Chills, elevated temperature, tachycardia, nonproductive cough, dyspnea, respiratory distress syndrome (p. 225)	Stop blood immediately; change tubing; institute normal saline IV at 4-6 ml/hr; monitor and record T, P, R, and BP; auscultate chest for breath and heart sounds; report observations to physician; see Respiratory distress syndrome (p. 225)
	Bleeding tendency caused by dilutional effect	Transfusion volume equal to blood volume of patient	Bleeding in any body system, thrombocytopenia, coagulation abnormalities	Report observations to physician immediately; check and record T, P, R, and BP q10-15min; monitor cardiac function continuously; auscultate chest for heart and breath sounds q15-30min; administer platelet concentrate, fluids, and medications as ordered; manage hemorrhage as indicated and ordered
	Pulmonary air embolus	During transfusion	SOB, chest pain, cyanosis, syncope, hypotension, shock	Stop transfusion immediately; place patient on left side; administer oxygen as ordered; monitor vital signs, CVP q15min; see Pulmonary embolus (p. 211)
Leukocyte concentrate	Acute reaction Transient pulmonary infiltrate	Immediately	Elevated temperature, chills Retrosternal constriction, pallor, cyano-	Slow transfusion; monitor and record T, P, R, and BP q15-30min; auscultate chest for breath and heart sounds q15-30min; report observa-

Continued.

Table 4-5 Reactions to Transfusion of Blood and Blood Components —cont'd

Product	Type of Reaction	Onset	Observations	Nursing Actions
	GVHD		sis, tachycardia, cough	tions to physician; see Respiratory distress syndrome (p. 225); medicate with Demerol when ordered Usually only irradiated leukocytes are administered for prevention of GVHD
Platelets	Febrile; usually caused by infusion of incompatible leukocytes contaminating platelet preparations	Immediately to 12-24 hr posttransfusion	Chills, hives, flushing	Check and record T, P, R, and BP q15-30min; administer medications when ordered; reaction usually self-limiting; patient may develop antibodies and destroy platelets in subsequent transfusions; check platelet count 1 hr after transfusion
Plasma	Similar to whole blood	Similar to whole blood	Similar to whole blood	Similar to whole blood
Whole blood with factor VIII removed	Bleeding caused by heparin used as anticoagulant; reactions as in whole blood	During and after transfusion when large volumes administered; see whole blood	Bleeding in any body system See Whole blood	Report observations to physician immediately, check and record T, P, R, and BP; monitor cardiac status continuously; administer protamine sulfate as ordered; measure and record urinary output See Whole blood
Normal serum albumin	Reactions are rare	During administration	Chills, elevated temperature, nausea	Slow transfusion rate; report observations to physician; check and record T, P, R, and BP q15-30min
	Circulatory overload/ bleeding during rapid infusion	During transfusion	Rising or elevated, BP circulatory overload, pulmonary edema; new areas of bleeding appear in hemorrhagic shock	Monitor rate of infusion carefully; slow rate of transfusion; report observations to physician; check and record T, P, R, and BP q10-15min; monitor cardiac status continuously; auscultate chest for heart and breath sounds q15-30min; observe closely for new sites of bleeding

Hematuria
Chills
Pain
Circulatory overload
SOB
Lung congestion: rales, rhonchi
Frothy sputum
Pyogenic reaction

Sudden chilling
Elevated temperature
Headache
Allergic reaction
Urticaria
Laryngeal edema
Asthmatic wheezing
Blood-borne infections (e.g., hepatitis, CMV, AIDS)

Pretransfusion care

Select equipment needed for venipuncture according to
  hospital policy, procedure, and physician's order
Prepare equipment and normal saline solution
Obtain blood no more than 30 min before administra-
  tion; check blood according to hospital policy, ensur-
  ing that correct patient receives type-specific blood
Obtain baseline T, P, R, and BP
Prepare venipuncture site

Care during transfusion

Flush blood tubing with normal saline solution before
  starting transfusion
Remain with patient for at least 15 min (or 50 ml) after
  starting blood; check vital signs and compare to
  baseline
Discontinue blood immediately if transfusion reaction
  occurs, call physician, change blood tubing, maintain
  patent IV line, and follow hospital procedure

Posttransfusion care

Apply pressure to venipuncture site
Apply adhesive bandage and/or dressing as indicated
Change blood tubing after transfusion
Observe for reaction 1 hr after infusion of blood
Record whether a reaction occurred

Patient/family teaching

Ensure that patient and/or significant other knows and
  understands the following:
  Importance of maintaining position of extremity
  Importance of reporting symptoms of reaction
  Rash
  Flushed feeling
  Chills
  SOB
  Chest pain
Importance of not regulating flow rate

BIBLIOGRAPHY

American Association of Blood Banks: Blood transfusions outside the
  hospital, *Am J Nurs* 486, 1989.
Belcher, A: *Blood disorders,* St Louis, 1993, Mosby.
Birdsall C, Carpenter K, Considine R: How is autotransfusion done?
  Am J Nurs 108, 1988.
Daeffler RJ: Potential for bleeding. In Daeffler RJ, Petrosino BM:
  Manual of oncology nursing practice: nursing diagnosis and care,
  Rockville, Md, 1990, Aspen Publishers.
Doenges ME, Jeffries MF, Moorhouse MF: *Nursing care plans: nurs-
  ing diagnosis in planning and documenting patient care,* ed 3,
  Philadelphia, 1990, FA Davis.
Griffin JP: The bleeding patient, *Nurs, '86* 34, 1986.
Gulanick M et al: *Nursing care plans: nursing diagnosis and treatment,*
  ed 3, St Louis, 1994, Mosby.
Guyton AC: *Textbook of medical physiology,* ed 8, Philadelphia, 1990,
  WB Saunders.
Huntoon MB: The hematologic system. In Armstrong ME et al, eds:
  McGraw-Hill handbook of clinical nursing, New York, 1979,
  McGraw-Hill.
Ihde JK, Jacobsen WK, Briggs BA: *Principles of critical care,* Philadel-
  phia, 1987, WB Saunders.
Jaffe M, Skidmore-Roth L: *Home health nursing care plans,* ed 2, St
  Louis, 1993, Mosby.
Kaiser Foundation Hospital/Health Plan, Northern California Region:
  *Nursing standards of practice manual, 1994: Blood transfusion stan-
  dard.*
Kim MJ, McFarland GK, McFarlane AM: *Pocket guide to nursing diag-
  noses,* ed 6, St Louis, 1995, Mosby.
Kinney MR et al, eds: *AACN clinical reference for critical care nursing,*
  ed 3, New York, 1993, McGraw-Hill.
Loeb S et al: *Professional guide to diseases,* ed 4, Springhouse, Penn,
  1992, Springhouse.
Pagana KD, Pagana TJ: *Diagnostic testing and nursing implications: a
  case study approach,* ed 4, St Louis, 1994, Mosby.
Phillips L: *Manual of IV therapeutics,* Philadelphia, 1993, FA Davis.
Schechter N, Berrien FB, Katz S: PCA for adolescents in sickle cell
  crisis, *Am J Nurs* 719, 1988.
Simmonson GM: Caring for patients with acute myelocytic leukemia,
  Am J Nurs 304, 1988.
Thompson JM et al: *Mosby's clinical nursing,* ed 3, St Louis, 1993,
  Mosby.
Ulrich C, Canale S, Wendell S: *Nursing care planning guides: a nurs-
  ing diagnosis approach,* ed 2, Philadelphia, 1990, WB Saunders.
Weintrobe MM et al: *Clinical hematology,* ed 8, Philadelphia, 1981,
  Lea & Febiger.
Westphal RG, Kasprisim DO: *Current status of hemapheresis: indica-
  tions, technology and complications,* Arlington, Va, 1987, American
  Association of Blood Banks.

Respiratory System

Respiratory Assessment

● Subjective Data

Cough
Pain
  Chest
  Abdomen
Wheeze
SOB
How many pillows used
Amount of exercise tolerated
Fever
Chills
Rapid breathing
Tiring easily
Change in voice
Dizziness
Sweating
Swelling of feet and hands

● Objective Data

Anxious facies
Dyspnea
Dyspnea on exertion (DOE)
Flaring nostrils
Red, swollen nose
Nasal discharge
Color
  Cyanosis

Lips
 Circumoral area
 Nail beds
 Gums
 Earlobes
 Soles of feet
 Palms of hands
Pallor
Ashen
Gray
Cherry red
Red
Reddish blue
Confusion, restlessness
Hallucinations
Cough
 Onset and duration

Characteristics
 Dry hacking, barking, congested
 Severity
 Nonproductive
 Productive
 Sputum
  When produced
   Upon awakening (morning)
   Afternoon
   Continuously
  Characteristics: color, odor, consistency, amount
Hemoptysis
Stridor
Wheeze
Assuming upright position: orthopnea
Clubbing of extremities: nail beds
Use of accessory muscles of respiration

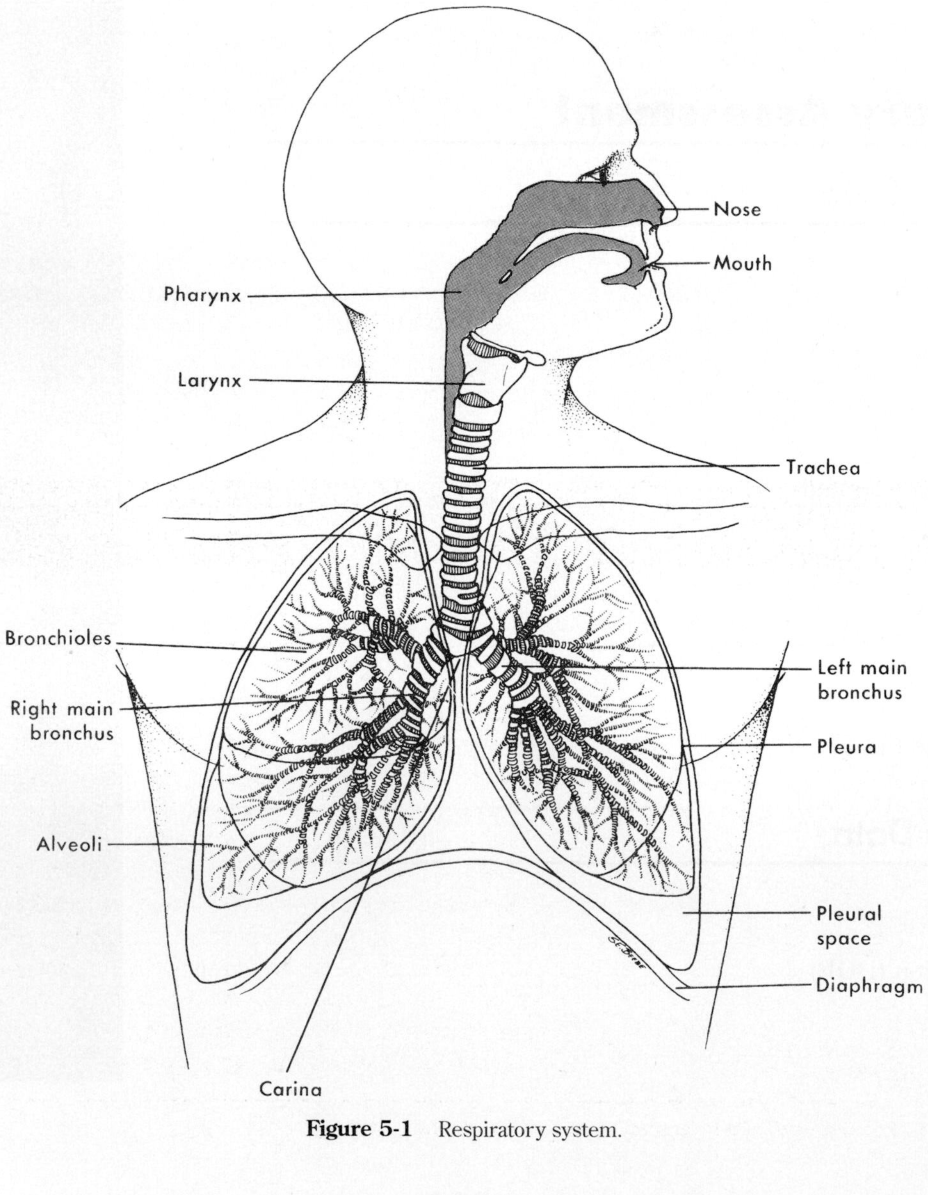

Figure 5-1   Respiratory system.

Telegraphic speech pattern: short, choppy sentences
Eyes
  Engorged veins
  Papilledema
Elevated temperature
Diaphoresis
Anorexia
Weight
  Obese
  Underweight
  Gain
  Loss
Ascites
Rash
Respirations (Tables 5-1 and 5-2)
  Bradypnea
  Tachypnea
  Long expiratory phase
  Irregular
  Asymmetric
  Periods of apnea
  Cheyne-Stokes
  Shallow
  Pursed-lip breathing
  Biot's
  Kussmaul's
  Apneustic
  Hyperventilation
Retractions
  Suprasternal
  Supraclavicular
  Substernal
  Intercostal

Cardiac status
  Elevated BP
  Tachycardia
  Bradycardia
  Sinus dysrhythmia
  Congestive heart failure (CHF)
    Crackles
    Rhonchi
    Jugular venous distention
    Edema
    Abdominal distention and pain
    Hepatosplenomegaly
Thoracic examination
  Scoliosis
  Kyphosis
  Kyphoscoliosis
  Pectus excavatum (funnel chest)
  Pectus carinatum (pigeon chest)
  Barrel chest
  Unequal shoulder height
Palpation
  Thoracic expansion
  Fremitus (vocal/tactile)
  Tracheal deviation
  Crepitus
Percussion
  Resonance
  Hyperresonance
  Tympany
  Dullness
  Flatness
Auscultation (Table 5-3)
  Decreased or absent breath sounds

Table 5-1   Patterns of Respiration

Type		Characteristics
Normal respiration		Rate
		Rhythm, regular
Cheyne-Stokes respiration		Periods of apnea alternating with series of respiratory cycles
		Rate and amplitude of successive respiratory cycles increase to a maximum and then decrease until terminated by period of apnea in a crescendo-decrescendo pattern
Biot's respiration		Variation of Cheyne-Stokes respiration in which periods of apnea alternate irregularly with periods of breaths of equal depth
Sighing respiration		Deep, audible sighs that interrupt normal respiratory rhythm
Painful respiration		Interruption of normal respiratory rhythm caused by pain; breathing frequently becomes shallow during interruption
Ataxic respiration		Gross irregularity in rate, rhythm, and depth of respiration; also referred to as meningitic respirations

Modified from Abels LF: *Mosby's manual of critical care,* St Louis, 1979, Mosby.

Table 5-2 Normal Respiratory Findings

Area of Concern	Normal Adult Findings	Variations in Older Adult
General appearance	Appears relaxed Breathing is quiet and easy without apparent effort Facial expressions and limb movements are relaxed	
Breathing pattern	Diaphragmatic-thoracic pattern is smooth and regular May have occasional sighing respirations Breathing is quiet, and exhalation is passive	Pattern is same as for adults, but calcification at rib articulation points may decrease chest expansion
Respiratory rate	12-20 resp/min Ratio of pulse to respirations is 4:1	
Skin	Appears well oxygenated; no cyanosis or pallor present Palpation of skin and chest wall reveals smooth skin and a stable chest wall; there are no crepitations, bulging, or painful spots	
Nail bed, nail configuration	Minimal angulation between base of nail and finger No thickening of distal finger width	
Chest wall configuration	Symmetrical, bilateral muscle development A:P to transverse ratio is 1:2 to 5:7; larger than these ratios is considered to be barrel chest Straight spinal processes Downward and equal slope of ribs; costal angle 90 degrees or less	Kyphosis is a common finding in older adults; there is dorsal scoliosis with slight tracheal deviation; this may also cause a slight increase in A:P to transverse ratio
Tracheal position	Midline and straight directly above the suprasternal notch	May be slightly deviated if kyphosis is present

Modified from Thompson JM et al: *Mosby's clinical nursing,* ed 3, St Louis, 1993, Mosby.

Crackles
Rhonchi
Wheezing
Friction rubs
Pectoriloquy
Bronchophony
Egophony

Liver disease
Ascites
Polycythemia
Obesity
Hypertension
Guillain-Barré syndrome
Myasthenia gravis or other neurologic disease affecting respiratory function

● Pertinent Background Information

Concurrent diseases or conditions

Cancer
Heart disease
Renal disease

Psychologic responses

Response to stress
Methods of coping
Response to pain
Relationships with others

Table 5-3   Breath and Voice Sounds: Normal and Abnormal

Breath and Voice Sounds	Characteristics	Findings
NORMAL		
Vesicular	Heard over most of lung fields; low pitch; soft and short expirations	Low-pitch, soft expirations
Bronchovesicular	Heard over main bronchus area and over upper right posterior lung field; medium pitch; expiration equals inspiration	Medium-pitch, medium expirations
Bronchial	Heard only over trachea; high pitch; loud and long expirations	High-pitch, loud expirations
ABNORMAL		
Bronchial when heard over peripheral lung fields	High pitch; loud and long expirations	
Bronchovesicular sounds when heard over peripheral lung fields	Medium pitch with inspirations equal to expirations	
Adventitious	Crackles: discrete, noncontinuous sounds *Fine crackles:* high-pitched, discrete, noncontinuous crackling sounds heard during the end of inspiration (indicates inflammation or congestion)	
	Medium crackles: lower, more moist sound heard during the midstage of inspiration; not cleared by a cough	
	Coarse crackles: loud, bubbly noise heard during inspiration; not cleared by a cough	
	Wheezes: continuous musical sounds; if low pitched, may be called rhonchi *Sibilant wheeze:* musical noise sounding like a squeak; may be heard during inspiration or expiration; usually louder during expiration	
	Sonorous wheeze (rhonchi): loud, low, coarse sound like a snore heard at any point of inspiration or expiration; coughing may clear sound (usually means mucus accumulation in trachea or large bronchi)	
	Pleural friction rub: dry, rubbing, or grating sound, usually caused by the inflammation of pleural surfaces; heard during inspiration or expiration; loudest over lower lateral anterior surface	

Modified from Thompson JM et al: *Mosby's clinical nursing,* ed 3, St Louis, 1993, Mosby.

Continued.

Table 5-3 Breath and Voice Sounds: Normal and Abnormal—cont'd

Breath and Voice Sounds	Characteristics	Findings
RESONANCE OF SPOKEN VOICE		
	Bronchophony: using diaphragm of stethoscope, listen to posterior chest as patient says "ninety-nine"	Negative response: muffled "nin-nin" sound heard Positive response: clear, loud "ninety-nine" response heard because the lung tissue is consolidated
	Whispered pectoriloquy: listen to posterior chest as patient whispers "one, two, three"	Negative response: muffled sounds heard Positive response: clear "one, two, three" is heard because of lung consolidation
	Egophony: listen to posterior chest as the patient says "e-e-e"	Negative response: muffled "e-e-e" sound heard Positive response: sound of sound *e* changes to an *a-a-a* because of consolidation

Previous respiratory condition/medical history

Asthma
Bronchitis
Cystic fibrosis
Emphysema
Tuberculosis
Fibrocystic disease
Premature birth
Previous operations

Family history

Heart disease
Hypertension
Diabetes
Cancers
Obesity
Pulmonary disorders

Social history

Smoking (past and present): packs per day × how many years
Alcohol use
Exercise and activity levels
Occupation: current and previous
Sleep patterns

Environmental factors: exposure to dust, fumes, asbestos, or chemicals
Recent exposure to infections
Travel out of country
Available family support

Medication history

Prescription medications
Over-the-counter medications

● Diagnostic Tests

Chest x-ray examination
Complete blood cell count (CBC)
Arterial blood gases (ABGs)
Serum electrolytes
Electrocardiogram (ECG)
Sputum evaluation
  Amount
  Color, odor, viscosity
  Gram stain
  Culture and sensitivity
Throat or nasopharyngeal culture
Pulse oximeter
Pulmonary function tests
  Tidal volume (V_T)

Gerontologic Considerations

- Signs and symptoms of pneumonia are often atypical in older adults. Fever, cough, and purulent sputum may be absent. Generalized signs and symptoms such as lethargy, disorientation, dyspnea, tachypnea, chills, chest pain, and vomiting, as well as an unexpected exacerbation of coexisting conditions, should be viewed with suspicion, because they may indicate pneumonia in the older adult.
- Adequate hydration is very important for the older person with pneumonia. It helps liquefy secretions and promotes expectoration.
- Many older adults have difficulty expectorating, which slows resolution of congestions and increases the difficulty of obtaining sputum specimens. Because deep breathing and coughing are difficult, the older person may require suctioning to remove respiratory secretions. This should be done with discretion, because too-frequent suctioning can stimulate increased production of secretions.
- Older adults, particularly those living in institutions, should have routine skin tests for tuberculosis. Many older adults were exposed to tuberculosis during their childhood and have positive results on skin tests. These individuals should receive routine chest x-ray studies. Older adults who have histories of inactive tuberculosis should be watched for recurrence of active tuberculosis. Signs and symptoms are often vague and include loss of appetite and weight loss.
- Older immigrants and immunosuppressed older adults should be watched closely for drug-resistant strains of tuberculosis.
- Provided that there is no serious disease of the respiratory tract, the older person is generally able to maintain adequate ventilation and oxygenation.

- However, changes of aging do have an impact on respiratory function:
  - Drier mucous membranes and decreased number of cilia affect the older individual's ability to humidify inhaled air and trap debris. These, in turn, increase the risk for inflammation and irritation of the upper respiratory tract.
  - Kyphosis and calcification of costal cartilage are common changes. These restrict expansion of the thoracic cavity and lead to a barrel-chested appearance.
  - Intercostal muscles and the diaphragm lose elasticity, resulting in a decreased ability to breathe deeply and cough.
  - The elasticity of airways and alveoli decreases, alveoli thicken, and pulmonary blood flow decreases, resulting in increased risk for impaired gas exchange.
- Years of exposure to air pollution, smoke, and mechanical irritants increase the risk for respiratory disease in older adults, particularly those who have emphysema and chronic bronchitis.
- Inactivity and immobility increase the risk of stasis pooling of respiratory secretions, which then increases the risk of pneumonia.
- Neurologic damage as a result of cerebrovascular accidents, Parkinson's disease, and other conditions is increasingly common in the older adult. Any neurologic disorder that decreases the gag or swallow reflexes increases the risk of aspiration of fluids and food, with resultant trauma to the respiratory tract.
- Cor pulmonale with right-sided congestive heart failure, as well as left-sided congestive heart failure with pulmonary congestion, are common complications of chronic obstructive pulmonary disease in the older adult.

Modified from Christensen BL, Kockrow EO: *Foundations of nursing*, ed 2, St Louis, 1995, Mosby.

Minute volume (V_E)
Vital capacity (VC)
Forced vital capacity (FVC)
Forced expiratory volume (FEV); in 1 sec (FEV_1)
Inspiratory reserve volume (IRV)
Maximal midexpiratory flow (MMEF)
Peak expiratory flow rate (PEFR)
Residual volume (RV)
Inspiratory capacity (IC)
Expiratory reserve volume (ERV)

Diffuse capacity carbon monoxide (DL_{CO})
 Total lung capacity (TLC)
Gastric lavage
Skin tests
Sweat test
Bronchoscopy
Bronchograms
Lung biopsy
Lung scans
Ventilation/perfusion

Scalene node biopsy
Aortography
Pulmonary angiography
Tomography
Fluoroscopy
Barium swallow
Computed tomography (CT) scan
Pulmonary echograms
Body plethysmography
Thoracentesis

Therapeutic Bronchoscopy

*Direct visual examination of the trachea and tracheo-
bronchial tree by means of a bronchoscope; the flexible
fiberoptic bronchoscope is commonly used because it is
better tolerated by the patient and allows better visualization of distal airways; rigid bronchoscope used to
remove foreign bodies, evaluate tracheal lesions, and
control hemoptysis*

Purpose/indications

Collect secretions for laboratory examinations
Obtain tissue for biopsies
Locate and perform biopsy on tumors
Diagnose hemoptysis, lesions, or masses
Remove foreign bodies or mucous plug secretions
Treat lung abscesses, pneumonia, or aspiration

Preparation

Explain procedure to patient and the need to not talk
  during procedure; procedure may be done under local
  or general anesthetic
Maintain NPO for 6 hr before procedure
Manage pain with sedation as indicated; assess effec-
  tiveness of pain relief measures
Provide emotional support (patient may be fearful of
  discomfort and/or possible findings)
Remove dentures
Place patient in sitting or supine position as directed
Instruct patient to breathe in and out through nose with
  mouth open during procedure
  Fiberoptic bronchoscope is inserted through nose or
  mouth
  Rigid bronchoscope is inserted through mouth

Postbronchoscopic assessment

Observations/findings

Difficulty in breathing
Stridor
Nasal flaring
Suprasternal and/or supraclavicular retractions
Hemoptysis
Hypotension
Tachycardia
Tachypnea
Hyperresonance
Wheezing
Cyanosis
Nausea, vomiting
Absence of gag and cough reflexes
Dysphagia
Hoarseness
Coughing
Throat or nasal pain
Chest pain

Potential complications

Crepitus and/or subcutaneous emphysema
Absence of breath sounds
Decreased S_aO_2
Pneumothorax
Hemoptysis

Immediate postbronchoscopic care

Check BP, P, and R q15min for 1 hr, then q2h to 4h and
  prn
Assist and teach patient to
  Not eat or drink until gag reflex returns, usually 3 to
    4 hr
  Maintain bed rest; elevate head of bed 45 degrees
  Dispose of tissue after coughing
  Understand importance of not using tobacco
  Report signs of crepitus to physician
  Manage pain as indicated; assess effectiveness of pain
    relief measure(s)
  Establish means of communication
    Call bell within reach
    Pad and pencil or Magic Slate*
Auscultate chest for breath sounds q2h to 4h and prn
Report absent or diminished breath sounds to physician
Perform postural drainage as ordered
Perform oropharyngeal suctioning prn
Administer oxygen as ordered

Convalescent care

Check BP, T, P, and R q8h and prn
Assist and teach patient to
  Gargle with warm saline solution q2h to 4h as indi-
    cated

*Registered trademark of Western Publishing Co., Inc., Racine, Wis.

Maintain position of comfort

Progress from liquids to diet as tolerated; avoid extremely hot foods

Patient/family teaching

Ensure that patient and significant other(s) know and understand

Importance of not driving self home if procedure is done as outpatient

Importance of maintaining liquid or soft diet as ordered until throat pain disappears

Importance of forcing fluids to 3000 ml daily unless contraindicated by patient's condition

Need to avoid extremely hot foods and liquids

Need to avoid tobacco use

Symptoms to report to physician

Chest pain

Difficulty in breathing

Inability to swallow

Increased hemoptysis

Change in color and amount of sputum

Importance of ongoing outpatient care

Name of medication, dosage, time of administration, purpose, and side effects

Need to avoid taking over-the-counter medications without checking with physician

Importance of avoiding persons with upper respiratory infections (URIs)

Thoracentesis

Puncture of the chest wall with a large-gauge needle to remove air or fluid from the pleural space

Preparation

Auscultate chest for breath sounds

Obtain chest x-ray examination as ordered by physician

Obtain baseline BP, T, P, and R

Administer sedation as ordered

Prepare local anesthetic as ordered

Position patient on edge of bed with feet supported; head and arms should be resting on overbed table; if patient is unable to sit on edge of bed, have patient lie on unaffected side with head of bed elevated and arm raised over head

Provide emotional support

Obtain signed informed consent

Preprocedure teaching

Ensure that patient and significant other(s) know and understand

Procedure to be performed

Importance of remaining immobile during procedure

Importance of not coughing during procedure; patient may be asked to exhale completely and hold or breathe shallowly during procedure *to decrease risk of puncture*

That sensations of pain and pressure are to be expected

Assessment during and after thoracentesis

Observations/findings

DURING PROCEDURE

Chest tightness

Difficulty in breathing

Tachypnea

Tachycardia

Vertigo

Hypotension

Cyanosis

Diaphoresis

Pallor

Anxiety

POSTPROCEDURE

Difficulty in breathing

Chest pain

Uncontrollable cough

Hemoptysis

Decreased BP

Tachycardia

Tachypnea

Absent or diminished breath sounds

Crepitus

Hyperresonance

Diminished chest wall movement on affected side

Distended neck veins

Cyanosis

Elevated temperature

Deviation of larynx and trachea

Potential complications

Mediastinal shift

Pneumothorax

Pulmonary edema

Immediate postprocedure care

Check BP, P, and R q15min for 1 hr, then q2h to 4h and prn

Check temperature q4h for 24 hr

Apply adhesive bandage or dressing to site of puncture

Check dressing q15min to 30 min

Turn patient on unaffected side for 1 hr, then to position of comfort

Manage pain as indicated; assess effectiveness of pain relief measure(s)

Administer oxygen as ordered

Measure and record total amount of fluid removed; note color and character

Auscultate breath sounds q2h for two times; then q4h for 24hr; report diminished or absent breath sounds and audible crackles to physician

Obtain chest x-ray examination as ordered by physician

Ongoing care

Continue with immediate postprocedure care and decrease frequency of nursing functions as patient's condition improves

Change dressing prn

Assist and teach patient to
Turn and deep breathe q2h to 4h
Ambulate as tolerated
Maintain diet as ordered

Patient/family teaching

Ensure that patient and significant other(s) know and understand
Importance of deep breathing q2h to 4h
Importance of maintaining a well-balanced diet
Importance of forcing fluids to limit allotted for patient's condition
Importance of avoiding tobacco use
Importance of avoiding persons with URIs
Name of medication, dosage, time of administration, purpose, and side effects
Need to avoid taking over-the-counter medications without checking with physician
Symptoms to report to physician
Difficulty in breathing
Chest pain
Vertigo
Elevated temperature
Diaphoresis
Uncontrollable cough
Continued drainage of fluid from puncture site
Hemoptysis
Importance of ongoing outpatient care

Aspiration of Secretions (Suctioning)

Preprocedure assessment

Observations/findings

Restlessness
Wheezing
Inability to expectorate
Difficulty in breathing
Tachycardia
Diaphoresis
Crackles
Rhonchi over large airways
Decreased breath sounds
Cyanosis
Pulse oximetry saturation reading if indicated (use for ventilated patients)

Preprocedure teaching

Explain procedure to patient
Discuss what is expected of patient during procedure
Demonstrate suction equipment
Assist and teach patient to cough and deep breathe before and after procedure

Assessment during procedure

Observations/findings

Tachycardia
Hypoxemia
Trauma to airway; bloody aspirate
Bronchospasm
Aspirate
  Color
  Consistency
  Amount
Cyanosis
Tachypnea
Dyspnea
Nausea

Potential complications

Hypotension
Sudden hypertension
Hypoxemia
Bradycardia
Cardiac dysrhythmias
Atrioventricular (AV) heart block
Premature ventricular contractions (PVCs)
Cardiac arrest

Care during procedure

Auscultate breath sounds
Maintain sterile technique
Use closed ventilation suction system for ventilated patients or use vented catheter
Lubricate sterile catheter
Choose correct catheter to prevent airway occlusion and/or trauma; should be half diameter of airway (general guide)
Adult: 12 to 18 French
Infant: 5 to 6 French
Hyperoxygenate and hyperinflate lungs for four to five breaths × 1 min
Avoid use of force when inserting catheter
Apply suction only while removing catheter; do not exceed 10 sec
Rotate catheter while removing; avoid moving catheter up and down while suctioning
Suction pressure must not exceed
Adult: 80 to 120 mm Hg
Ventilate patient for four or five breaths or longer if necessary as soon as suction has been released
Use closed ventilation suction catheter for tracheal suctioning
Use Yankeur suction tip catheter for oral suctioning
Assess patient for the following:
Adequate chest expansion
Cyanosis: lips, earlobes, fingertips
Increased restlessness
Increased pulse rate
Cardiac dysrhythmias
Bronchospasm
Decrease in O_2 saturation
If bronchospasm, bradycardia, PVCs, or AV block occurs, stop suctioning immediately and ventilate and hyperoxygenate patient
Observe aspirate: if purulent or colored, obtain specimen for culture

● Nasotracheal Suction

Avoid nasotracheal suction if patient has a spinal fluid leak or epistaxis
Elevate head of bed 60 to 90 degrees
Hyperoxygenate and hyperinflate patient's lungs for four to five breaths before suctioning
Lubricate 6 to 8 centimeters of distal end of catheter with water-soluble lubricant or water and insert through nostril to pharynx
Have patient cough or deep breathe and advance catheter into trachea during inspiration
Suction no more than 10 sec at a time

Hyperoxygenate and hyperinflate patient's lungs for four or five breaths after suctioning

● Endotracheal or Tracheostomy Suction

Be aware that a coudé (curved-tip) catheter may be used in an attempt to suction left mainstem bronchus in certain disease states
Hyperoxygenate and hyperinflate patient's lungs for four or five breaths before suctioning
Suction oropharynx and discard catheter after each use
Suction endotracheal tube or tracheostomy tube with a sterile catheter
Suction no more than 10 sec at a time
Hyperoxygenate and hyperinflate patient's lungs for four or five breaths after suctioning

Postprocedure assessment

Observations/findings

Breath sounds
Crackles
Decreased
Increased
Rhonchi over large airways
Decreased
Increased
Arterial blood gases: decreased Pao_2, Sao_2
Elevated temperature
Bronchospasm
Tachycardia
Cyanosis

Immediate postprocedure care

General

Auscultate breath sounds; prepare to repeat suctioning procedure as indicated
Return oxygen concentration to setting ordered by physician
Check apical pulse and/or record ECG rhythm strip
Assist and teach patient to deep breathe after suctioning procedure
Monitor O_2 saturation via pulse oximetry as ordered

Oxygen Therapy

Use of oxygen to relieve hypoxemia and avoid hypoxia; oxygen flow rate and concentration should be regulated to maintain Pao_2 between 60 mm Hg and 100 mm Hg

Preprocedure assessment

Observations/findings

Hypoxemia
  Pao_2 <60 mm Hg
  Sao_2 <85%
Respiratory system
  Cyanosis
  Tachypnea
  Dyspnea
  Shallow respiration
Neurologic system
  Drowsiness
  Disorientation/confusion
  Restlessness
  Decreased attention span
  Impaired judgment
  Delirium
  Decreased long-term and short-term memory
Nausea
Nasal flaring
Muscle weakness
Retractions
Cardiovascular system
  Hypotension
  Sudden hypertension
  Bradycardia
  Tachycardia
  Cardiac dysrhythmias

Preprocedure teaching

Explain procedure to patient
Demonstrate equipment to be used

Assessment during procedure

Observations/findings

Substernal pain with deep inspiration
Somnolence
Respiratory depression
Arterial blood gases
  Pao_2
  $Paco_2$
  pH
  HCO_3
  Sao_2
Tidal volume (V_T)
Vital capacity (VC)
Elevated temperature
Tachycardia
Psychosocial problems
  Anxiety
  Depression
  Dependence

Potential complications

Oxygen toxicity: time and dose related
  Decreased lung compliance
  Reduced VC
  Sore throat
  Nasal drying, bleeding
  Cough
  Diminished breath sounds
  Crackles
CNS toxicity
  Nausea
  Anxiety
  Numbness
  Muscular twitching
Substernal pain with deep inspiration
Circulatory depression: falling central venous pressure
  (CVP)
Visual impairment
  Tearing eyes
  Papilledema

Care during procedure

General

Assess patient for signs of hypoxemia
Maintain patent airway
Assist and teach patient to maintain position best suited for optimal lung expansion; head of bed usually elevated 45 to 90 degrees
Initiate and maintain oxygen flow rate and concentration with humidification as ordered; have portable oxygen tank or extension tubing available if oxygen is to be used continuously and patient is ambulatory or needs to be transported
Monitor BP, T, R, and apical pulse q15min for 1 hr, then q2h to 4h if stable
Assess level of consciousness q15min for 1 hr, then q2h to 4h if no change
Auscultate breath sounds q2h to 4h; report diminished or absent breath sounds or audible crackles and rhonchi to physician
Administer oral and nasal hygiene q2h to 4h
Assist and teach patient to turn, cough, and deep breathe q2h to 4h
Provide emotional support; remain with patient if acutely anxious
Continue other nursing functions required for primary disease process
Avoid high concentrations of oxygen for patients who require some degree of hypoxemia to maintain respirations
Monitor arterial blood gases as ordered
NOTE: Oxygen toxicity can occur with oxygen concentrations of 50% or higher administered for 24 to 48 hr; symptoms include tachypnea, substernal pain, and

dizziness; physiologic effects include atelectasis, ciliary dysfunction, and nitrogen washout; in carbon dioxide retainers, hypoventilation, somnolence, and apnea may occur with minimal elevations in Pao_2

General precautions

Provide humidification with oxygen administration especially for flow rate >2 L/min

Always use sterile equipment when administering oxygen; change connecting tubing, humidification equipment, masks, and nasal cannulas every 24 to 48 hr

Do not allow tobacco use while oxygen is in use

Do not permit oil, grease, or other combustible material to come in contact with cylinders, regulators, gauges, valves, or fittings

Administer oxygen only with a safely functioning and properly fitting regulating device

Cylinders

Secure safely to prevent falling

Transport only in proper carrier

Maintain valve in closed position when not in use

Open valve slowly to full open position when using

Care with use of various devices

NASAL CATHETER

Check catheter patency before insertion

Lubricate catheter with water-soluble lubricant

Avoid kinking or twisting tubing

Position catheter so it cannot be seen when patient's tongue is depressed

Tape securely to nose

Remove catheter q6h to 8h

Reinsert new catheter in opposite nostril if possible

Assess patient for abdominal distention

NASAL CANNULA (PRONGS)

Useful for providing approximately 24% to 44% oxygen at flow rates of 1 to 6 L/min (flow >6 L/min does not deliver more oxygen)

Approximate FIo$_2$ with nasal cannula

1L 24%	4L 36%
2L 28%	5L 40%
3L 32%	6L 44%

Ensure proper positioning; avoid kinking or twisting, which impedes oxygen flow

Apply water-soluble lubricant to nares

Evaluate patient for pressure sores or nasopharyngeal irritation

Reposition q2h

Clean equipment daily

SIMPLE OXYGEN MASK

Can deliver 40% to 60% oxygen at flow rates of 8 to 10 L/min (rate <5 L/min with face mask can lead to carbon dioxide retention in dead space of mask)

Choose correct size for patient

Remove mask q2h to 3h for a few seconds to do the following:

Dry patient's face

Observe for pressure areas

Permit patient communication

Use face mask only with artificial airway in unconscious patient

Have nasal cannula available for patient to use while eating

FACE TENT

Can deliver approximately 40% oxygen at flow rates of 8 to 10 L/min

Useful for patients who cannot tolerate a face mask

Remove periodically for a few seconds

Dry patient's face

Observe chin for pressure areas

Have nasal cannula available for patient to use while eating

PARTIAL REBREATHING MASK WITH RESERVOIR BAG

Used for higher oxygen concentrations (40% to 60%) at flow rates of 8 to 12 L/min

Increases of 1 L/min increased FIo$_2$ by approximately 10%

Select correct size for patient

Ensure proper position of mask

Apply mask as patient exhales

Avoid twisting or kinking bag

Avoid letting bag totally deflate when patient is inhaling; increase oxygen flow rate if necessary

Remove mask periodically for a few seconds

Dry patient's face

Observe for pressure areas

Apply water-soluble lubricant to lips

Provide means of communication

Have nasal cannula available for patient to use while eating

Monitor arterial blood gases

Observe for signs of oxygen toxicity

NONREBREATHING MASK WITH RESERVOIR BAG

Provides 60% to 90% oxygen at flow rates of 6 to 15 L/min

Select correct size for patient

Ensure proper positioning of mask

Avoid letting bag totally deflate

Avoid twisting bag

Ensure that all rubber flaps stay in place
Remove mask periodically for a few seconds
  Dry patient's face
  Observe for pressure areas
  Apply water-soluble lubricant to lips
Observe patient for signs of oxygen toxicity; monitor arterial blood gases as ordered
Have a nasal cannula available for patient to use while eating

VENTURI MASK

Provides 24% to 50% oxygen at 4 to 8 L/min flow rate
Select correct size for patient
Ensure proper positioning; avoid kinking of tubing and blockage of oxygen intake parts, which alter FIO_2
Maintain oxygen flow rate as ordered by physician
Monitor arterial blood gases
Remove mask periodically for a few seconds
  Dry patient's face
  Observe for pressure areas
  Apply water-soluble lubricant to lips
Rid tubing of excessive moisture as necessary
Have nasal cannula available for patient to use while eating

Patient/family teaching

Explain importance of not using tobacco or any open flames in the room with oxygen administration to avoid combustion and fire or explosion
Explain the necessity of checking all electrical equipment used in the same room with oxygen administration for frayed cords or potential for sparking to avoid combustion and fire or explosion
Instruct on proper removal and repositioning of the oxygen equipment because the patient may need to wipe off and dry his or her face, blow his or her nose, or eat
Teach the patient the proper oxygen concentration delivery ordered and the importance of maintaining the appropriate flow rate because high flow rates in CO_2 retainers can suppress the respiratory drive
Explain importance of humidification and adequate hydration because oxygen dries the mucous membranes

Home care considerations

Explain that home oxygen is provided in one of three ways: compressed gas in a cylinder tank, liquid oxygen in a reservoir, or an oxygen concentrator
Provide referral

  To a durable medical equipment company to obtain necessary equipment
  To a home health agency for follow-up care at home
  For patient and family support groups in the area
Demonstrate use, care, and cleaning of all equipment
Teach use of oxygen source, oxygen delivery device, and humidification source
Describe different home oxygen systems
  Liquid oxygen: a portable, relatively lightweight system that is easy to read but costly for continuous use or high flow rates
  Oxygen cylinders: small tanks that need to be changed frequently; least expensive if oxygen delivery is needed for ≤12 hr/day
  Oxygen concentrators: nonportable unit that delivers concentrated oxygen drawn out of room air; indicated for patient requiring oxygen 12 to 24 hr/day and only inside home
Explain the importance of avoiding tobacco use, open flames, and frayed electrical equipment in area of oxygen equipment to prevent combustion, fires, or explosions
Encourage walking and activities with portable oxygen as tolerated because continuous oxygen therapy can limit mobility
Demonstrate care of skin and mucous membrane because oxygen devices can cause skin irritation and breakdown with prolonged wear and provide additional route for microorganisms
Assess body image changes, self-esteem, and sexuality and plan appropriate interventions because alterations may occur

Humidity and Aerosol Therapy

Valuable in loosening thick secretions and in the delivery of medications; aerosol and humidity devices used to provide humidity when artificial airways are being used are as follows

jet nebulizers: *Hand-held nebulizers commonly used to provide medicated aerosol treatment; these are large-reservoir nebulizers for continuous aerosol treatment with or without supplemental oxygen. Cool: delivers 40% to 50% humidity; heated: delivers 100% humidity*

ultrasonic nebulizers: *Can be given to patients breathing on their own or installed into ventilator circuits; treatments generally last 20 to 30 min; deliver 100% humidity*

humidifiers: *Used to prevent humidity deficit when artificial airways are in use; the most commonly used are the bubble humidifiers in conjunction with low-flow oxygen devices, cascade on ventilators*

Assessment

Observations/findings

PATIENT

Respirations
  Quality
  Rate
  Depth
Breath sounds
  Crackles
  Diminished or absent
Secretions
  Amount
  Color
  Character
Fluid overload

EQUIPMENT

Oxygen concentration ordered
Oxygen concentration delivered
Heat control
Connecting tubing is patent, free from excess moisture

Ongoing care

Patient

Maintain patent airway
Monitor patient as frequently as indicated by disease or
  patient's condition during treatment
Suction as indicated
Auscultate breath sounds q2h to 4h; report absent or
  diminished breath sounds to physician

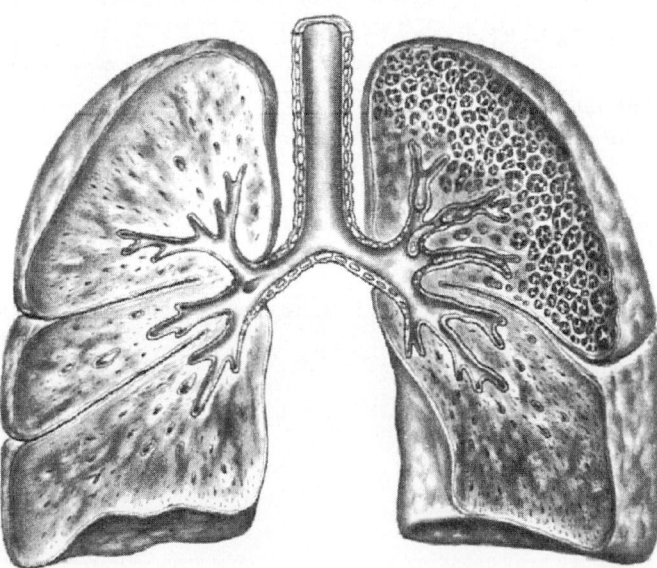

Figure 5-2 Lobar emphysema. (From Wilson SF, Thompson JM: *Mosby's clinical nursing series: respiratory disorders,* St Louis, 1990, Mosby.)

Position patient comfortably
Dry face of moisture as indicated
Assist and teach patient to turn, cough, and deep
  breathe q2h to 4h

Equipment

Use sterile distilled water in nebulizer; check water
  level in reservoir q4h—when adding water, empty
  reservoir, then refill to correct level
Free tubing of excess moisture q2h to 3h and prn
Check heat control q2h to 4h
Maintain temperature between 95° and 97.8°F (35° and
  36.6°C) unless cool mist ordered
Change mask, adaptors, and tubing q24h
Secure and allow sufficient tubing for turning

Patient/family teaching

Teach the patient the importance of humidification and
  nebulization
Demonstrate use of equipment, how to fill humidifiers
  and nebulizers, and proper cleaning and disinfecting
Demonstrate administration of medication via hand-
  held nebulizers
Teach use of medications, dosage, time of administration, purpose, and side effects

Home care considerations

Teach use, care, and cleaning of equipment
Teach to inspect equipment for growth of mold and
  other organisms because water is a medium for
  growth of microorganisms
Check water in humidifiers and nebulizer q8h to maintain adequate level and refill as needed
Explain importance of maintaining temperature of humidifiers between 95° and 97.8°F
Ensure that humidifiers are placed in the room with the
  steam directed into room and set on a table at least 2
  feet from walls and furniture

Chronic Obstructive Pulmonary Disease, Chronic Obstructive Lung Disease

*Chronic condition associated with a history of emphysema
  (Figure 5-2), asthma, chronic bronchitis (see the box
  on p. 278), bronchiectasis, cigarette smoking, or
  exposure to air pollution; there is persistent airway
  obstruction that progressively increases*

Diseases Contributing to Development of COPD

CHRONIC BRONCHITIS

Mucosal swelling and inflammation of the bronchial mucous membrane with excessive mucous secretion in bronchial tree

ASSESSMENT

Observations/Findings
SOB
Cough
  Persistent
  Productive
Sputum (usually morning)
  Thick, tenacious, copious
  Mucopurulent
Breath sounds
  Scattered
  Moist crackles
  Rhonchi
Wheezing respirations
Bronchospasm
Cyanosis

Diagnostic Tests
Arterial blood gases
  Decreased Pao_2
  Increased $Paco_2$
  Increased HCO_3
  Respiratory acidosis
Sputum secretions
  Increased polymorphonuclear
    neutrophil leukocytes
Chest x-ray examination
  Increased peribronchial mark-
    ings at both bases
  Increased cardiac size
Pulmonary function tests
  Decreased FEV_1/FVC ratio
  Increased residual volume
  FRC: may be normal in pure
    bronchitis
  FEV: decreased
  PEFR: decreased

EMPHYSEMA

Destruction of elastic tissues of the alveolar walls, causing a reduced expiratory flow rate and overinflated alveoli; a progressive disease that is irreversible

ASSESSMENT

Observations/Findings
SOB
Difficulty in breathing
Respirations
  Tachypnea
  Shallow
  Prolonged expiratory phase
Use of accessory muscles
  Intercostals
  Neck
  Shoulder
Cough: may be productive
Pursed-lip breathing
Orthopnea
Thoracic changes
  Barrel chest
  Unequal chest expansion
  Increased AP chest diameter
  Skin color: usually normal
Cachexia
Anorexia
Weight loss
Breath sounds
  Distant
  Expiratory wheezes
Hyperresonance
Weakness
Fatigue

Diagnostic Tests
Arterial blood gases
  Decreased Pao_2; normal or in-
    creased $Paco_2$
  pH within normal limits if com-
    pensation has occurred
Chest x-ray examination
  Hyperlucent lung fields; small,
    narrow heart; increased AP
    diameter; low, flat diaphragm;
    widened intercostals
  Apical bullae are common
  Decreased vascular markings
Pulmonary function tests
  Increased total lung capacity
  Increased residual volume,
    FRC
  Decreased PEFR, MMEF,
    FEV_1/FVC
Blood chemistry: α_1-antitrypsin

BRONCHIECTASIS

Chronic dilation of a bronchus or bronchi, secreting large amounts of purulent sputum

ASSESSMENT

Observations/Findings
Cough: paroxysms in early morn-
  ing
Sputum
  Profuse (up to 200-300 ml/day)
  Purulent
  Foul odor
Wheezes
SOB
Prolonged expiration
Hemoptysis
Nasal stuffiness
Breath sounds
  Crackles
  Rhonchi
Recurrent infection, pneumonia
Elevated temperature
Chronic sinusitis

Diagnostic Tests
Chest x-ray examination
  Usually normal
  Air fluid levels and infiltrates
    may be seen in advanced dif-
    fuse disease
Bronchography
Sputum examination: staphylo-
  cocci, streptococci, and
  pseudomonas commonly seen
  on sputum smears and cul-
  tures
Pulmonary function tests
  Normal or slightly decreased
    lung volumes
  Decreased flow rates
Arterial blood gases: mild de-
  crease in Pao_2 and $Paco_2$ are
  common

Assessment

Subjective data

Anxiety
Fear: suffocation, death
Fatigue
Malaise
SOB during exertions; ADLs
Decreased exercise tolerance

Objective data

Audible expiratory wheeze
Prolonged expirations with considerable effort
Pursed-lip breathing
Use of accessory muscles of respiration
Increased AP diameter of chest (barrel chest)
Breath sounds
  Diminished breath sounds
  Crackles
  Rhonchi
Bronchospasm
Restlessness
Anorexia
Weight loss
Cough
  Productive/unproductive
  Hacking, ineffective
Amount and character of sputum
Cardiac
  Hypotension
  Tachycardia
  Dysrhythmia
Pulsus paradoxus
Hypoxemia
Carbon dioxide retention
  Restlessness
  Confusion
  Somnolence
  Loss of memory

Diagnostic tests

ABG studies
  Alveolar-arterial (A-a) oxygen gradient: widened
  Decreased PaO_2, pH
  Increased PCO_2
Chest x-ray examination
  Flattened diaphragm
  Increased AP diameter
  Hyperinflation of lungs
Pulmonary function studies; decreased FEV, FVC, FEV_1/FVC ratio, MMEF, PEFR
Sputum specimen analysis
CBC: polycythemia if chronically hypoxic

Serum electrolytes
ECG: atrial dysrhythmia low voltage, right axis deviation in advanced disease

Potential complications

Dysrhythmias
Acute respiratory failure
Cardiac failure
Cor pulmonale
  Peripheral edema
  Hepatomegaly
  Cyanosis
  Distended neck veins
  Loud P_2
  Murmur of tricuspid regurgitation
Pulmonary hypertension
Blood gas abnormalities
Polycythemia
Peptic and esophageal reflux

Collaborative management

Therapeutic management

Oxygen therapy
Artificial airway/mechanical ventilation as required
Chest physiotherapy
Pulse oximetry
Serial ABG assessment
Medications
  Bronchodilators
  Antibiotics
  Corticosteroids
  Diuretics
  Influenza vaccinations
  Pneumovax
  Cardiotonics
Diet
  High-protein, low-carbohydrate foods and fluids
  Parenteral fluids
  Restriction of tobacco use

Nursing management

PATIENT PROBLEMS/NURSING DIAGNOSES

● **NDX:** Ineffective airway clearance related to tracheobronchial obstruction or secretions

Auscultate lungs q1h to 2h and prn rhonchi, crackles, or wheezing *to determine progression of disease*
Assess secretions noting quantity, color, consistency, and odor *to identify symptoms of infection*

Assess hydration status: skin turgor, mucous membrane, q2h I and O to identify alterations in fluid status

Increase fluid intake to 2000 ml/day unless contraindicated to liquefy secretions

Encourage incentive breathing with large tidal volumes *to open alveoli maximally*

Assist and teach patient to turn and cough q2h; position for optimal coughing: upright and flexed forward *to ensure maximum airway available*

Assist with and monitor chest physiotherapy: postural drainage, percussion *to assist with removal of secretions*

Provide periods of rest between treatments *to prevent fatigue*

Teach controlled cough techniques (see box at right)

Instruct patient in breathing retraining techniques: pursed-lip, diaphragmatic breathing (see the box on p. 281)

Provide humidification via mask, vaporizer

Suction nasopharyngeal airway or artificial airway as indicated *to remove secretions*

Administer medications as ordered
Bronchodilators: observe for therapeutic response; monitor theophylline level as appropriate
Antibiotics

EXPECTED OUTCOME

Patient maintains a patent airway as evidenced by the following:
Improved breath sounds
Cough-produced thinned secretions
Normal rate and depth of respirations
Absence of dyspnea and cyanosis
Blood gases within acceptable levels

● **NDX:** Impaired gas exchange related to alveolar capillary membrane changes

Assess respirations qh; note quality, rate, and use of accessory muscles: changes may indicate altered blood gas state

Auscultate breath sounds q1h to 2h; note area of abnormal sounds

Assess level of consciousness, somnolence, and confusion reporting any changes that *may indicate increase in impaired gas exchange*

Observe color, odor, and amount of secretions: changes may indicate infective process

Maintain bed rest in quiet environment during exacerbation of symptoms *to maximize energy*

Elevate head of bed 45 to 90 degrees
Allow patient to assume position of comfort *to ease work of breathing*
Padded overbed table may be helpful for patient's comfort and breathing

---

Controlled Cough Technique

1. *Maximal inhalation*—an effective cough is contingent on filling the lungs and airways distal to the mucus so that the succeeding forced exhalation will propel the mucus up to the airways. Maximal inhalation also increases airway caliber; as a result, it is more likely that the air will pass distal to partially obstructing mucus or foreign matter.
2. *Hold breath 2 sec*—this step permits the patient to prepare for exhalation and allows distribution of the inhaled air to the lung's periphery.
3. *Cough twice*—the first cough will loosen mucus; the second will propel the mucus. Further coughing may use excessive oxygen and energy at a time when the lung volume has already been expelled with the first two coughs, and the effort is thus wasted.
4. *Pause*—just long enough to regain control.
5. *Inhale by sniffing*—sniffing is recommended, because a deep inhalation through the mouth may drive loose mucus back down into the airways.
6. *Rest.*

Modified from Thelan LA et al: *Critical care nursing: diagnosis and management,* ed 2, St Louis, 1994, Mosby.

Administer humidified oxygen per nasal catheter or cannula at low flow as ordered *to maintain* PaO_2 *of no less than 55 mm Hg*

Observe for signs of cyanosis, which i*ndicates deoxygenation*

Monitor BP, T, and apical pulse q2h to 4h and prn *to assess for hemodynamic stability*

Monitor ABGs: report increase or decreases in $PaCO_2$ and PaO_2 of >10 mm Hg

Assist and teach patient to turn, cough, and deep breathe q2h; note type of cough and color and character of sputum *to maintain airway patency and detect infection*

Collect sputum for culture as ordered

Teach importance of absolutely no tobacco use

Monitor renal function, which may be altered secondary to chronic tissue hypoxia and alterations in metabolism

Administer medications as ordered
Bronchodilators: observe for therapeutic response; monitor theophylline level as appropriate
Antibiotics

Breathing Retraining Techniques

PURSED-LIP BREATHING

- With mouth closed, inhale through nose.
- Exhale through mouth with lips "pursed" (lips in a whistling or kissing position).
- Make exhalation at least twice as long as inhalation (2 seconds in, 4 seconds out).

RATIONALE

Explain to the patient that this maneuver keeps airways open longer during exhalation and evacuates trapped air. The procedure for pursed-lip breathing can be used, along with diaphragmatic breathing, during episodes of SOB.

DIAPHRAGMATIC BREATHING

Have the patient place two fingers just below the xiphoid process and push in with his or her fingers while sniffing gently. Explain that the movement felt at the fingertips is the diaphragm moving as he or she sniffs and that this muscle requires exercise so that it can increase the efficiency of breathing.

TECHNIQUE

- Place one hand on chest, one hand on abdomen.
- Inhale, pushing abdominal hand outward.
- Exhale slowly (through pursed lips), allowing abdominal hand to fall inward.
- Chest hand should remain still.

RATIONALE

Explain that this maneuver saves energy because the diaphragm uses oxygen more efficiently than the accessory muscles and that this technique retrains the diaphragm to assume the work of breathing. Diaphragmatic breathing is useful in terminating episodes of acute SOB but should also be incorporated into a regular routine of muscle retraining.

From Thelan LA, Davie JK, Urden LD: *Critical care nursing: diagnosis and management*, ed 2, St Louis, 1994, Mosby.

EXPECTED OUTCOME

Patient maintains adequate gas exchange as evidenced by the following:
Improved mental status, skin color
Blood gases within acceptable levels for patient
Clear breath sounds

● **NDX:** Altered nutrition: less than body requirements related to decreased oral intake and increased metabolic demand associated with dyspnea, anorexia, and fatigue

Assess nutritional status: weigh daily, monitor dietary intake *to detect signs and symptoms of malnutrition*
Record oral intake using calorie counts *to meet hypermetabolic requirements*
Monitor albumin and lymphocyte levels for indications of adequate protein
Place in high-Fowler's position at meals *to reduce dyspnea*
Encourage rest periods before meals *to reduce fatigue*
Provide liquid-to-soft, high-protein (which supports immune system), low-carbohydrate diet; avoid gas-producing foods, which can limit movement of diaphragm
Administer supplementary feedings
Provide attractive meals
Provide small, frequent meals *to decrease abdominal pressure on diaphragm*
Encourage significant other(s) to bring patient's favorite foods
Administer oral hygiene before meals *to enhance taste and appetite*
Weigh patient daily: same time, clothing, and scale *to assess fluid status and nutritional status*
Administer medications *to relieve constipation* as indicated

EXPECTED OUTCOMES

Patient's nutritional status is maintained or improved as evidenced by weight remaining stable and within or moving toward normal range for patient's height, age, and build

Patient's food intake is increased
Albumin and lymphocytes are within normal limits
  (WNL)

● **NDX:**   Anxiety related to change in health status

Assess level of anxiety (mild, moderate, severe); iden-
  tify any misperceptions of illness or treatment
Assess usual coping skills, which are previously used
  successful methods
Provide quiet, nonstressful environment *to increase re-
  laxation*
Provide emotional support
  Remain with patient during anxious periods
  Encourage significant other(s) to participate in care
  Be aware of patient's subjective statements
  Encourage patient to ask questions and verbalize fears
    and concerns
  Assess whether visitors are helpful during periods of
    heightened anxiety and limit visitation as indicated
  Plan care to provide frequent rest periods
  Avoid blaming attitude
  Explain all procedures and treatment *to reduce fear*
  Introduce support groups available to patient and fam-
    ily: Better Breathing Clubs of American Lung Asso-
    ciation
  Instruct on relaxation techniques such as guided im-
    agery and use of autogenic techniques during peri-
    ods of dyspnea

  EXPECTED OUTCOME

Patient experiences a decrease in fear and anxiety as
  evidenced by the following:
  Relaxed facial expression
  Verbalization of feeling less anxious
  Verbalization of understanding hospital routines, pro-
    cedures, and disease process

● **NDX:**   Activity intolerance related to imbalance be-
    tween oxygen supply and demand

Assess level of response to activities; monitor HR and R
  during and after activity
Plan care to provide optimal rest *to maximize energy*
Instruct patient on energy conservation measures: perform activities such as bathing, shaving in sitting position; rest between activities
Encourage use of pursed-lip breathing during activities
  to decrease the work of breathing
Provide O_2 therapy as indicated; use portable O_2 to facilitate activities
Monitor for signs of extreme fatigue, chest pain, or diaphoresis during and after activity
Assist and teach patient progressive exercise conditioning to increase strength and maintain muscle tone:
  ROM exercises

Encourage participation in Pulmonary rehabilitation
  program (see p. 286)
Determine methods of conserving energy while performing ADLs: stool in bathroom for shower

  EXPECTED OUTCOME

Patient demonstrates an increased tolerance for activity
  as evidenced by ability to resume ADLs without extremes of fatigue or dyspnea

  ADDITIONAL NURSING DIAGNOSES
  TO CONSIDER

Sleep pattern disturbance related to frequent coughing
  and difficulty breathing
Risk for infection related to ineffective airway clearance
  and increased risk factors such as chronic disease,
  steroid therapy
Sexual dysfunction related to activity intolerance secondary to chronic illness

Patient/family teaching

Disease process
  Assess patient level of understanding regarding
    disease process and prescribed home health
    management
  Encourage questions and discussion
  Explain importance of maintaining optimal respiratory
    function by taking medications, eliminating tobacco
    use, and avoiding those who smoke
  Explain need to avoid **respiratory irritants:** dust,
    fumes, smoke, perfume, aerosol sprays, cold
    temperatures
  Explain need to avoid persons with infections,
    especially URIs
  Explain importance of ongoing outpatient care
  Discuss symptoms to report to physician immediately
    Elevated temperature
    Sore throat
    Increase in sputum production
    Change in color and consistency of sputum
    URI
    Increased difficulty in breathing
    Night sweats, chills
    Decreased activity tolerance
    Decreased appetite
    Increased use of IPPB and oxygen
    Change in pulse or feelings of heart fluttering
  Explain need to keep warm and prevent chilling
  Explain importance of influenza immunization and
    pneumovax if ordered
Medications
  Discuss name, dosage, time of administration, pur-
    pose, and side effects

Explain need to avoid taking over-the-counter medications without physician approval

Demonstrate use of bronchodilator nebulizers if ordered

Use tid or qid

Take one or two deep inhalations

Release medication only one or two times with each use

Watch for side effects such as tachycardia

Avoid overuse

Explain need to wear medical alert band identifying COLD

Discuss importance of avoiding emotional stress; teach stress reduction techniques

Diet

Explain need to maintain high-calorie diet as indicated; force fluids to 2000 to 3000 ml/day unless contraindicated

Explain need to avoid constipation and straining

Ensure that patient and significant other(s) demonstrate

Deep-breathing exercises, pursed-lip breathing

Positions for postural drainage if needed

Use of ventilator if applicable

Use of oxygen equipment if applicable

Home care considerations

Initiate contact with Visiting Nurses Association (VNA); determine need for home health care

Instruct patient and family on cleaning of all home respiratory equipment; refer to respiratory therapy as indicated

Assess home for presence of respiratory irritants (see list on p. 282); maintain environment free of irritants

Explain importance of environmental control, maintaining warm house 75° to 80°F (23.8° to 26.6°C)

Teach that some patients tolerate high humidity poorly and may need to have dehumidifier in the home

Provide detailed instruction on use of any oxygen or respiratory equipment to be used at home

Activity level: explain importance of alternating activity and rest periods

Exercise to tolerance

Need to limit activity on days of high air pollution

Plan rest periods during day

Rest before and after meals if SOB increases at mealtimes

Breathe deeply and slowly during periods of activity

Understand own lifestyle and avoid waste of energy

Need to space activities throughout day

Assess economic status and ability to purchase medications and supplies; refer to social services as indicated

Asthma

A reversible obstructive disease characterized by increased reactivity of the trachea and bronchi to stimuli, manifested by wheezing and dyspnea; narrowing is due to a combination of bronchospasm, mucosal swelling, and increased secretions

Assessment

Subjective data

Dyspnea, labored breathing

Chest tightness, pain

Anxiety

Fear of suffocation; death

Decreased activity tolerance

History of allergies

Objective data

Sudden onset of respiratory distress

Prolonged expiratory wheeze

Short inspiratory period

Intercostal and sternal retraction

Use of accessory muscles of respiration

Air hunger

Crackles

Breath sounds

Wheezes

Decreased

Absent

Assumes upright sitting position; leans forward

Diaphoresis

Tachycardia

Distended neck veins

Cyanosis

Circumoral area

Nail beds

Hard, dry cough; productive cough is difficult

Altered level of consciousness

Hypoxemia

Hypotension

Pulsus paradoxus >10 mm

Dehydration

Diagnostic tests

Arterial blood gases

Mild decrease in PaO_2 and $PaCO_2$: normal ABGs common between attacks

Decreased PaO_2, increased $PaCO_2$ with severe attacks

Chest x-ray examination

Normal between attacks

Hyperinflation with allergic attacks

Skin testing (extrinsic asthma)
Pulmonary function tests
  Normal or increased lung volumes
  Decreased FEV, PEFR, MMEF
  Decreased flow rates; improvement with bronchodila-
    tors
WBC and sputum examination
  Sputum and blood eosinophilia are common
  Serum IgE levels are elevated in extrinsic asthma

Potential complications

Pulmonary edema
Respiratory failure
Status asthmaticus
Pneumonia

Collaborative management

Therapeutic management

Oxygen therapy with humidification
Fluid and electrolyte management
Artificial airway and ventilatory support if necessary
Chest physiotherapy: percussion and vibration
Medications
  Bronchodilators (Table 5-4): parenteral, aerosols,
    oral
    Sympathomimetics
    Theophylline
  Steroids
  Antibiotics
Bronchoscopy
Saline lavage
Metered dose inhalers

Nursing management

PATIENT PROBLEMS/NURSING DIAGNOSES

● **NDX:**   Anxiety related to difficulty in breathing, fear
             of suffocation, and/or fear of recurrent at-
             tacks

Assess level of anxiety (mild, moderate, severe)
Assess usual coping skills, which are previously used
  successful methods
Provide emotional support *to increase relaxation and
  coping*
  Remain with patient during acute attack
  Anticipate patient's needs
  Provide quiet reassurance
  Maintain quiet environment
  Encourage significant other(s) to participate in care
    for support

Implement relaxation techniques: guided imagery,
  muscle relaxation *to relieve muscle tension*
Explain procedures; encourage questions *to reduce fear*
Maintain planned rest periods *to conserve energy and
  prevent recurrent attacks*
  Pace and plan ADLs
  Discourage talking if extremely dyspneic
  Limit visitors as necessary
  Encourage frequent rest periods

EXPECTED OUTCOME
Patient demonstrates a reduction in fear and anxiety as
  evidenced by the following:
  Relaxed facial expression
  Verbalization of feeling less anxious
  Vital signs within normal parameters
  Verbalization of understanding procedures

● **NDX:**   Ineffective airway clearance related to ex-
             cessive tenacious secretions and bron-
             chospasm

Assess sputum for color, tenacity, and amount
Auscultate breath sounds q1h to 2h for wheezes, crack-
  les, or rhonchi
Assess respirations noting depth, ease, and rate *to de-
  termine adequate oxygenation*
Observe skin color and temperature q2h
Monitor arterial blood gases
Monitor level of consciousness; report changes to
  physician
Position to level of comfort *to optimize breathing*
  Elevate head of bed 60 to 90 degrees *to facilitate maxi-
    mal air exchange*
  Support back with pillows for comfort
  Provide well-padded overbed table to lean over
  Place siderails up for safety and support
  Place humidifier or steam vaporizer at bedside as or-
    dered *to aid in liquefying secretions*
  Administer low flow of oxygen by nasal catheter as or-
    dered (avoid oxygen mask, which increases sensa-
    tion of suffocation)
  Administer IPPB as ordered
  Encourage patient to cough effectively at frequent in-
    tervals *to clear secretion*
Initiate or assist with chest physiotherapy
Administer medications as ordered
  Sympathomimetic preparations
  Xanthine derivatives: aminophylline—monitor levels
  Antihistamines
  Expectorants
  Adrenal corticosteroids
  Isoproterenol or cromolyn nebulization; avoid using
    isoproterenol and aminophylline together (can cause
    arrest)

Table 5-4 Bronchodilators

Generic Name	Brand Names	Availability	Adult Dosage Range
SYMPATHOMIMETICS			
Albuterol	Proventil, Ventolin	Tablets: 2, 4 mg Aerosol: 90 µg Nebulizer: 0.5%-1%	PO: 2-4 mg 3-4 times daily Inhale: 2 inhalations every 4-6 hours
Ephedrine	Ephedrine	Tablets: 25 mg Capsules: 25, 50 mg Syrup: 11, 20 mg/5 ml Injection: 25, 50 mg/ml	PO: 25-50 mg every 3-4 hr SC, IM, IV: 25-50 mg
Epinephrine	Primatene, Vaponefrin, Bronkaid Mist	Nebulization: 1:100 Aerosol: 0.2, 0.25, 0.3 mg Injection: 1:200, 1:100	See manufacturer's recommendations
Ethylnorepinephrine	Bronkephrine	2 mg/ml	SC or IM: 0.5 ml
Isoetharine	Bronkosol, Beta-2, Bronkometer	Nebulization: 0.125, 0.2, 0.5, 1% Aerosol: 0.61%	See manufacturer's recommendations
Isoproterenol	Isuprel, Aerolone, Norisodrine	Nebulization: 0.25, 0.5, 1% Aerosol: 0.2, 0.25% Injection: 0.2 mg/ml SL: 10, 15 mg tabs	See manufacturer's recommendations
Metaproterenol	Alupent, Metaprel	Tablets: 10, 20 mg Syrup: 10 mg/5 ml Aerosol: 225 mg Nebulization: 5%	See manufacturer's recommendations
Terbutaline	Brethine, Bricanyl	Tablets: 2.5, 5 mg Injection: 1 mg/ml	PO: 5 mg q6h SC: 0.25 mg; repeat, if needed, in 30 min
XANTHINE DERIVATIVES			
Aminophylline		Tablets: 100, 200 mg Elixir: 250 mg/15 ml Liquid: 105 mg/5 ml Suppositories: 250, 500 mg Injection: 250, 500 ml Others	See manufacturer's recommendations
Dyphylline	Dilor, Dyflex, Lufyllin	Tablets: 200, 400 mg Liquid: 100 mg/5 ml Elixir: 100, 160 mg/15 ml Injection: 250 mg/ml	PO: 15 mg/kg, 5 times daily IM: 250-500 mg slowly
Oxtriphylline	Choledyl	Tablets: 100, 200 mg Elixir: 100 mg/5 ml Syrup: 50 mg/5 ml	200 mg 4 times daily
Theophylline	Bronkodyl, Elixophyllin, Theolair, others	Tablets: 125, 200, 225, 300 mg Capsules: 50, 100, 200, 250 mg Elixir: 80 mg/15 ml Liquid: 80 mg/15 ml Syrup: 80 mg/15 ml Suspension: 300 mg/15 ml Others	9-20 mg/kg/24 hr in 4 divided doses

Modified from Clayton BD, Stock YN: *Basic pharmacology for nurses,* ed 10, St Louis, 1993, Mosby.

Force fluids as ordered to keep secretions thin
Collect sputum for culture as ordered
Suction prn: keep suction at bedside

EXPECTED OUTCOME

Patient maintains a patent airway as evidenced by the
following:
Improved breath sounds
Normal rate and depth of respirations
Absence of dyspnea
Absence of cyanosis
Blood gases within normal range

ADDITIONAL NURSING DIAGNOSES TO CONSIDER

Ineffective breathing pattern related to decreased lung
expansion during acute attack
Risk for infection

Patient/family teaching

Assess level of understanding regarding disease
process and self-care management during severe at-
tacks
Explain importance of preventing future attacks
Avoid known irritants and allergens
Avoid stressful situations
Express anxieties and fears
Encourage communication with significant other
and/or family
Provide adequate humidity
Nonflowering plants can increase humidity 5% to
10%
Humidifiers are helpful (provide instructions on use
of humidifiers and need to keep clean)
Avoid persons with infections, especially URIs
Do not use tobacco; avoid persons who smoke
Explain importance of breathing exercises such as
pursed-lip breathing
Explain how to avoid air trapping by slow, extended ex-
halation through pursed lips
Avoid gaining weight
Explain importance of ongoing outpatient care
Discuss symptoms to report to physician
URI
Influenza
Elevated temperature
Discuss medications: name, dosage, time of administra-
tion, purpose, and side effects
Demonstrate proper use of inhalers, peak flow meters
and maintenance of containers
Explain need to wear medical alert band identifying
asthma
Discuss importance of taking medications as
ordered

Home care considerations

Provide detailed instruction on any equipment to be
used at home
Assess home for presence of respiratory irritants that
may trigger asthma attacks
Instruct patient and family on cleaning of all home res-
piratory equipment
Determine need for home care and initiate contact with
home health or visiting nurses
Assess economic status and ability to purchase medica-
tions and equipment; refer to social services or appro-
priate agencies
Activity level: discuss importance of exercising to
tolerance
Avoid fatigue
Plan rest periods
Limit activities during temperature extremes
(hot/cold) and on smoggy days
Diet: explain importance of diet and fluids
Eat balanced, nutritious meals
Force fluids to 2000 to 3000 ml/day unless contraindi-
cated
Develop transportation plan to local health care facil-
ity if symptomatic and if peak flow meter approaches
"red zone" as determined by physician

Pulmonary Rehabilitation

*An inpatient or outpatient program designed to increase
exercise tolerance in patients with lung diseases while
educating them to understand and assist in the
management of their disease; components generally
include physical therapy, respiratory therapy, exercise
conditioning, medications, and education*

Admission criteria

Symptomatic pulmonary disease (Table 5-5)
Dyspnea
Cough
Wheezing
Sputum production
Chest pain
Patient motivation
Restricted ADLs
No underlying condition that would interfere with the
program (psychosis, alcoholism, drug abuse)
Medically stable: no signs of CHF, uncontrolled dys-
rhythmias, or myocardial infarction (MI) in previous 6
months
Adequate financial/insurance status
Family support system

Table 5-5   COPD Disability Scale

Class	Observations/Findings
Class I	No significant restriction of normal activities, but dyspnea on strenuous exertion
Class II	No dyspnea with essential activities of daily living; dyspnea on climbing stairs and in other climbs but not on level walking; employability limited to sedentary occupations
Class III	Dyspnea with some activities of daily living (e.g., showering, dressing), but can perform all such activities without assistance; able to walk at own pace for a city block, but cannot keep up while walking with normal others of the same age
Class IV	Dependent on others in some activities of daily living; not dyspneic at rest, but dyspneic with minimal exertion
Class V	Dyspneic at rest; dependent on assistance from others for most activities of daily living

From Hodgkin J, Zorn E, Connors G, eds: *Pulmonary rehabilitation: guidelines to success,* Stoneham, Mass, 1984, Butterworth. Adapted from Moser KM et al: Results of a comprehensive rehabilitation program, *Arch Intern Med* 140:1596, 1980.

Exclusion criteria

Terminal cancer
Heart failure
Stroke
Alcoholism, active
Drug abuse
Psychiatric disorder, active/uncontrolled
Organic brain disease
End-stage COPD

● Inpatient Program (see box above, right)

Assessment

Observations/findings

Heart rate
  Increase of 30 beats per minute more than resting rate with activity
  HR <50 during activity

Pulmonary Rehabilitation Program: Suggested Class Content

Orientation to rehabilitation program
Anatomy and physiology of pulmonary system
Nutrition
Effects of stress and emotions on lung disease
Coping with chronic lung disease
COPD, specific diseases
Medications
Effect of COPD on family and friends
Oxygen, IPPB treatments
Principles of exercise
Relaxation techniques
Breathing exercises: pursed-lip breathing and diaphragmatic breathing
Energy conservation techniques
Postural drainage
Prevention of infection
Stop-smoking sessions
Discussions on sexuality

Consistent drop in HR of >10 beats per minute during activity
ECG rhythm: presence of irregular rhythm
Blood pressure
  Increase of 20 mm Hg above normal
  Diastolic increase of >10 to 15 mm Hg
  Systolic drop to <90 at rest; diastolic <40

Symptoms during activity

Dyspnea
Dizziness
Fatigue
Pain
Palpitations
Diaphoresis

Indicators of energy expenditure during activity

Arterial oxygen saturation values
Pao_2
Oxygen consumption rate

Indicators of ventilatory response during activity

Minute ventilation
Respiratory rate
Carbon dioxide production

Ongoing care

Activity progression program
  Follow physician's activity prescription
  Initiate exercise program
Evaluate daily progress and plan activity levels
Maintain progressive increase in activities until discharge
Monitor ECG and respiratory parameters
Record and report any signs or symptoms of SOB, fatigue, or nausea during or after exercise
Assist patient in performing ADLs and monitor HR, R, and BP 1 and 4 min after activity (response to activity should return to preactivity level within 5 min; if it does not, monitor every 2 min until pretest levels are reached)
Observe, record, and report patient's tolerance

Discharge evaluation

Self-care/ADL skills
Equipment needs for the home
Weekly schedule of exercise and rest
Assessment of level of knowledge
Knowledge of agency referral sources

● Benefits of Pulmonary Rehabilitation Program

Reduced symptoms
Decreased anxiety and depression
Improved ability to perform ADLs
Increased exercise tolerance
Reduced hospital admissions/days/cost of care
Improved quality of life

Pneumonia/Pneumonitis

Inflammation of the lung parenchyma caused by bacteria, viruses (Table 5-6), chemicals, smoke inhalation, dust, allergens, and aspiration of gastric contents; lung tissue is consolidated as alveoli fill with exudate (Figure 5-3)

Assessment (see box on p. 290)

Subjective data

Dyspnea, malaise, anorexia, and cough
Anxiety or fear of death

Objective data

Difficult and painful respirations
  Pleuritic pain

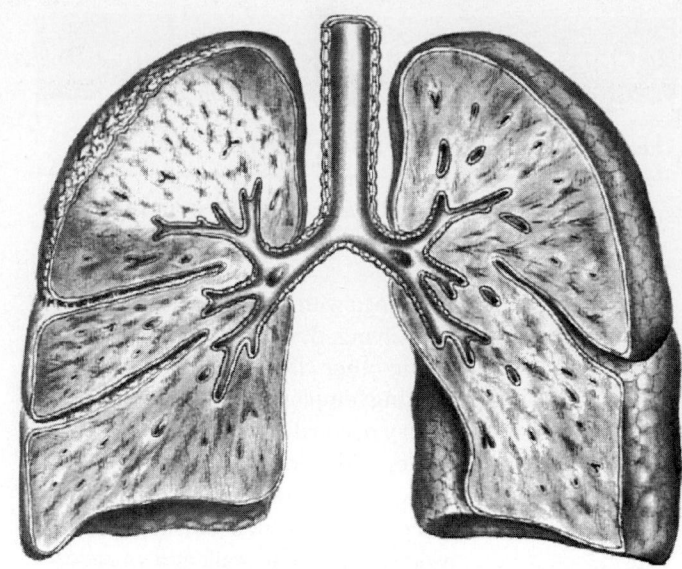

Figure 5-3   Pneumococcal pneumonia. Lobar pneumonia (right upper lobe). (From Wilson SF, Thompson JM: *Mosby's clinical nursing series: respiratory disorders,* St Louis, 1990, Mosby.)

SOB and grunting
Tachypnea
Breath sounds over area of consolidation
  Diminished, progressing to absent
  Crackles
  Rhonchi
  Egophony
Asymmetrical chest movements
Chills and fever (102° to 106°F [38.8° to 41.1°C]); delirium
Diaphoresis
Productive, tenacious cough; may be dry and hacking
  Incessant, painful
  Copious amounts of green-yellow sputum progressing to pink or rusty color
Restlessness
Cyanosis
  Circumoral area
  Nail beds
Tachycardia
Psychosocial problems: disorientation

Diagnostic tests

Chest x-ray examination: patchy or diffuse infiltrates
  Pleural effusion
Sputum examination: Gram stain and culture
WBC count: leukocytosis; neutrophilia
Blood culture
Serological studies: titers, cold agglutinins
Arterial blood gases: PaO_2 <80 mm Hg
Transtracheal aspiration
Bronchoscopy

Table 5-6 Bacterial and Nonbacterial Causes of Pneumonia/Pneumonitis

Pathogen	Persons at Risk	Complications
BACTERIAL		
Streptococcus pneumoniae (pneumonococcus) Gram-positive coccus Accounts for 80% to 90% of community acquired cases	Infants Older adults Alcoholics People with debilitating diseases (diabetes mellitus, sickle cell anemia)	Bacteremia meningitis Emphysema Pericarditis Impaired liver function Pleural effusions Higher mortality if more than one lobe involved
Klebsiella pneumoniae Gram-negative bacillus	Alcoholics Patients with diabetes mellitus or COPD	Lung abscess Emphysema Necrotizing pneumonitis Respiratory failure 25% to 50% mortality
Staphylococcus aureus Gram-positive diplococcus Accounts for 10% of cases in hospitalized patients and 1% of cases in unhospitalized patients	Infants Older adults As complication of influenza As secondary infection after surgery	Necrotizing infections Lung abscess Pleural effusion 15% to 50% mortality Slow response to antibiotics Adult respiratory distress syndrome
Haemophilus influenzae (Type B) Gram-negative bacillus Accounts for 1% of cases	Children under 10 years of age Persons with COPD or immune disease	Bronchiolitis
Legionella pneumophila (Legionnaires' disease) Gram negative	Older adults Smokers Persons with lung diseases	Hypotension Respiratory failure Acute renal failure Shock 15% mortality
Pseudomonas aeruginosa Gram-negative bacillus	Hospitalized patients: endotracheal intubation, respiratory inhalation therapy Burns	70% mortality Rarely occurs in previously healthy adults
NONBACTERIAL		
Mycoplasma (Mycoplasma pneumoniae) Atypical ("walking pneumonia")	School age children Young adults Spreads within family	Interstitial infections Pulse-temperature dissociation
Pneumocystis (Pneumocystis carinii pneumonia) Protozoan organism Viral influenza A	Patients with AIDS, immunosuppressed patients Elderly Symptoms may begin 1 wk after viral infection	Respiratory failure Secondary bacterial infection Respiratory failure
Aspiration pneumonia	Patients with LOC, impaired gag or cough reflex	With aspirated material Atelectasis Pulmonary edema Hemorrhage Necrosis

Observations/Findings of Viral and Bacterial Pneumonia

VIRAL

Symptoms
Usually mild at onset
Headache

Sudden onset of chills followed by fever
Cough (early, nonproductive)
Sputum (late)
 Mucopurulent
 Blood tinged
Myalgia

Photophobia
Anorexia
Nausea

Diagnostic Tests
Sputum examination: Gram stain and culture; influenza A, BC, varicella cytomegalovirus, adenovirus

Blood cultures
WBC normal or low; elevated lymphocytes
Elevated antibody titers
Arterial blood gases: hypoxemia
Chest x-ray examination
 Bronchopneumonic infiltrates

BACTERIAL

Symptoms
Sudden onset of high fever and shaking chills
Streptococcal pneumonia: afternoon, evening temperature; diaphoresis
Pleuritic chest pain
Cough
Sputum
 Rust colored, greenish, or yellow
 Purulent
Breath sounds
 Crackles
 Friction rub
Cyanosis

Diagnostic Tests
Sputum examination: Gram stain and culture streptococcal, pneumococcal, staphylococcal, *Haemophilus influenzae*

Blood cultures
WBC leukocytes with shift to left
Arterial blood gases: hypoxemia

Chest x-ray examination
 Patchy areas of consolidation and infiltrates
 Pleural effusion

Potential complications

Atelectasis
Empyema
ARDS
Pleurosy
Pulmonary edema
Meningitis
Superinfection pericarditis
Lung abscess

Collaborative management

Therapeutic management

Fluid management
Parenteral therapy
Oxygen therapy
Chest physiotherapy
Artificial airway or mechanical ventilation support
Medications

Antipyretics
Analgesics
Antibiotics
Antimicrobials
Expectorants

Nursing management

PATIENT PROBLEMS/NURSING DIAGNOSES

● **NDX:** Impaired gas exchange related to lung consolidation with decrease in surface area available for gas exchange

Auscultate breath sounds q2h to 4h *for adventitious sounds or decreased breath sounds*
Assess respiratory pattern, noting quality and rate
Monitor mental status and LOC *to assess for hypoxia/hypercapnia*
Observe color, odor, and amount of secretions *to assess for signs of infection*

Provide humidified oxygen by mask or nasal catheter as ordered *to avoid drying of upper airway;* maintain continuous vaporizer at bedside

Position patient *to optimize breathing*

Administer oxygen therapy as ordered *to prevent hypoxia*

Assist and teach patient to turn, cough, and deep breathe q2h to 4h *to remove secretions*

Initiate or assist with chest physiotherapy *to mobilize secretions*

Assist with use of incentive spirometer *to open alveoli maximally*

Administer medications as ordered
 Antibiotics
 Expectorants

Pace activities to patient's tolerance *to decrease oxygen demand*

Monitor ABGs, CBC, and serum osmolality

Encourage fluid intake as tolerated *to liquefy secretions*

Assist with administration of mechanical ventilation as indicated

 EXPECTED OUTCOME

Patient maintains adequate gas exchange as evidenced by the following:
 Usual mental status
 Usual skin color
 Blood gases within acceptable range

● **NDX:** Ineffective airway clearance related to increased tracheobronchial secretions secondary to inflammatory process

Assess secretions noting quantity, color, and consistency *to detect signs of infection or need to clear secretions*

Assess hydration status: skin turgor, mucous membranes, 24 hr intake

Auscultate breath sounds for crackles, rhonchi, and friction rubs q2h to 4h

Assist patient with use of incentive spirometer *to open alveoli maximally*

Perform nasopharyngeal or nasotracheal suctioning as needed

Force fluids as ordered *to help liquefy secretions*

Assist and teach patient to turn, cough, and deep breathe q2h to 4h *to maintain patent airway*

Monitor laboratory reports and serial chest x-ray examinations

Position patient *to optimize breathing and coughing*

Provide humidification as indicated

 EXPECTED OUTCOME

Patient maintains an effective breathing pattern as evidenced by the following:

Normal rate, rhythm, and depth of respirations
Clear lungs
Decreased dyspnea
Blood gases within normal range
Cough that has subsided

● **NDX:** Altered body temperature related to infectious process

Assess body temperature: measure temperature and pulse q4h; increase frequency during periods of chilling

Monitor skin color and temperature

Collect blood cultures and sputum cultures as ordered; monitor reports daily

Administer prescribed antipyretics as indicated

Encourage oral fluids as ordered *to ensure adequate hydration*

Administer cooling procedures as indicated: tepid sponge bath

 EXPECTED OUTCOME

Patient demonstrates no signs of elevated temperature as evidenced by the following:
 Temperature within normal limits (35.8° to 37.3°C)
 No signs of shivering, flushing
 Pulse within normal limits

● **NDX:** Pain in chest related to inflammation of lung parenchyma

Assess and monitor quality of pain, noting any changes; ask patients to rate on scale 1-10

Assist patient in chest splinting techniques during coughing episode *to reduce pain*

Administer medications *to suppress cough*

Administer analgesics as ordered
 Be aware of potential for depression of respiratory function
 Evaluate effectiveness

Provide additional comfort measures *to ease pain*

Plan rest periods
 Bed rest
 Quiet environment; soft or low light
 Avoid unnecessary talking if necessary
 Limit visitors as necessary

 EXPECTED OUTCOME

Patient experiences decreased pain as evidenced by the following:
 Verbalization of pain relief
 Relaxed facial expression and body movements
 Improved breathing pattern
 Effective cough

● **NDX:** Altered nutrition: less than body requirements related to decreased oral intake secondary to increased metabolic needs associated with fever and infectious process

Assess and monitor daily food intake *to assess intake of nutrients and need for supplemental feedings*

Identify factors contributing to anorexia: nausea/vomiting, fever, pain

Initiate measures to correct aggravating factors; administer antiemetics, antipyretics, analgesics

Weigh daily and compare to admission weight *to determine weight loss*

Remove sputum containers during mealtimes

Provide small, frequent meals

Have family members bring patient's favorite foods

Schedule respiratory treatments 1 hr before mealtimes

Administer oral hygiene every 2 to 4 hr and after any enemas

EXPECTED OUTCOME

Patient maintains balanced nutritional status as evidenced by the following:

Baseline weight maintained or reestablished

Daily caloric intake equaling nutritional requirement

Patient/family teaching

Disease process

Assess level of understanding regarding disease process

Explain importance of avoiding transmission of disease

Turn head away when coughing and cover mouth with tissue

Use tissue once only

Dispose of tissue in waste container

Explain importance of gradual convalescence

Limit exercise and activity to tolerance

Plan two or three rest periods during day

Avoid fatigue

Explain importance of postural drainage and deep breathing exercises; continue deep-breathing exercises qid for 6 to 8 wk

Diet: explain importance of maintaining diet as tolerated

Avoid high-calorie diet if overweight

Force liquids to 3000 ml/day unless contraindicated

Explain need to prevent recurrence of disease

Keep warm

Avoid chilling

Avoid persons with infections, especially URIs

Receive influenza vaccine and pneumovax as ordered

Discuss symptoms to report to physician

Elevated temperature

Chill

Diaphoresis; night sweats

Difficulty in breathing

Persistent cough

Cold or influenza

Medications

Discuss medications: name, dosage, time of administration, purpose, and side effects

Explain need to avoid taking over-the-counter medications without physician approval

Ensure that patient and significant other(s) demonstrate methods of postural drainage

Home care considerations

Explain need and use of vaporizer or humidifier at home

Explain importance of ongoing outpatient care

Assess home environment for any factors that would contribute to recurrence: adequate heat/cooling, absence of persons with infections

Assess economic status for ability to purchase medications and equipment; refer to social services or appropriate agency as indicated

Pulmonary Edema

Abnormal accumulation of fluid in the alveoli; causes an increase in pulmonary hydrostatic pressure, usually a result of cardiac disorders including AMI, mitral stenosis; noncardiogenic causes resulting from decreased colloid osmotic pressure

Assessment

Subjective data

SOB, dyspnea

Anxiety, fear of suffocation

Objective data

Respiratory distress

Labored, noisy breathing

Orthopnea

Nasal flaring

Tachypnea: shallow, moist respirations

Breath sounds—crackles: in dependent parts of lung initially, extending progressively upward

Cough: pink, frothy sputum
Bounding pulse
Hoarseness
Anxiety
Confusion
Restlessness, thrashing movement
Tachycardia: thready pulse
Diaphoresis
Pallor
Cyanosis
Heart failure (see p. 146)

Diagnostic tests

ABGs: variable
  Early: respiratory alkalosis
  Late: respiratory acidosis and hypoxemia
Chest x-ray examination
  Bilateral interstitial (Kerley B lines are common) and
    alveolar infiltrates
ECG
  Tachycardia
  Dysrhythmias
Pulmonary capillary wedge pressure (PCWP)
  14 to 20 mm Hg: mild
  25 to 30 mm Hg: moderate to severe
Protein concentration of edema fluid

Potential complications

Respiratory failure
Respiratory/cardiac arrest

Collaborative management

Therapeutic management

O_2 therapy: high flow by Venturi mask
Parenteral therapy
Intake and output
Hemodynamic monitoring
Cardiac monitor
Rotating tourniquets
Diet: low sodium
Medications
  Morphine
  Diuretics
  Cardiotonics
  Bronchodilators
  Vasodilators: nitroglycerine, nitroprusside
Mechanical ventilatory support
IABP

Nursing management

PATIENT PROBLEMS/NURSING DIAGNOSES

● **NDX:** Impaired gas exchange related to alveolar
capillary membrane changes

Assess respirations noting rate, depth, and use of acces-
  sory muscles
Assess LOC and mental status *to assess for hypoxia or
  hypercapnia*
Auscultate breath sounds qh
  Decreased breath sounds
  Crackles
Elevate head of bed 60 to 90 degrees with lower
  extremities dependent *to decrease venous
  return*
Monitor ABGs; intraarterial line may be required be-
  cause of frequent need of samples
Monitor serial chest x-rays *to detect signs of improve-
  ment or exacerbation*
Administer bronchodilators *to relieve bronchospasm and
  respiratory effort;* vasodilators *to reduce systemic and
  venous pressure*
Administer oxygen therapy as ordered
Administer IPPB as ordered (p. 326)
Check BP, R, and apical pulse qh and prn
Assist and teach patient to cough and deep breathe qh
  and prn *to maximize air exchange*
Maintain bed rest during acute phase

EXPECTED OUTCOMES

Patient has adequate gas exchange as evidenced by
  demonstrated effortless breathing
Lungs clear to auscultation
Hemodynamic stability
Blood gases within normal range

● **NDX:** Anxiety related to perceived biologic threat
(fear of suffocation)

Assess degree of anxiety (mild, moderate, severe)
Provide emotional support
  Remain with patient
  Reassure that treatments will relieve symptoms
  Reduce environmental stimuli
  Explain procedures and treatments thoroughly
  Use short, simple sentences
  Use calm, reassuring voice
  Assess whether significant family member present
    would reduce anxiety
Position to level of comfort: high-Fowler's position with
  padded overbed table
Plan rest periods *to maximize relaxation and decrease
  oxygen demand*
Encourage patient to verbalize fears and concerns

Administer morphine sulfate or antianxiety medication
to calm patient

EXPECTED OUTCOME

Patient demonstrates decreased anxiety as evidenced
by the following:
Verbalization of reduced anxiety
Demonstration that treatment is understood
Decreased use of tranquilizers and pain medica-
tion

ADDITIONAL NURSING DIAGNOSES
TO CONSIDER

Fluid volume excess related to left ventricular dysfunction (see Heart failure, p. 146)
Ineffective breathing pattern related to tracheobronchial secretions and fluid overload
Activity intolerance related to imbalance between oxygen supply and demand

Patient/family teaching

Disease process
  Assess level of understanding regarding disease
    process and contributing factors
  Provide instruction regarding disease process
Explain need to exercise to tolerance
  Avoid strenuous exercise
  Plan frequent rest periods
Explain need to maintain a low-sodium diet as
  ordered
Explain importance of avoiding tobacco use
Discuss symptoms to report to physician
  Sudden weight increase of >3 to 5 lb/wk
  Decreased urinary output
  Swollen feet and ankles
  Chest pain
  Difficulty in breathing
  Persistent cough
  Decreased activity intolerance
Discuss medications: name, dosage, time of administra-
  tion, purpose, and side effects

Home care considerations

Provide instruction regarding home management including respiratory therapy
Provide instruction on oxygen or respiratory equipment used at home
Teach the patient adaptive breathing techniques
Explain the importance of ongoing outpatient
  care
Explain the importance of avoiding contact with persons who have URIs

Assess economic status for ability to purchase medications and equipment; refer to social services or
agency as indicated

Pulmonary Embolism

*Occurs when the pulmonary artery or one of its branches
is partially or completely occluded; damage to the lung
depends on the number of clots and the extent of
obstruction to pulmonary circulation; most commonly
associated with dislodged clot from systemic circulation
such as deep veins of legs or pelvis, or atrial fibrillation*

Assessment

Subjective data

Dyspnea
Sudden severe substernal pain
SOB
Restlessness
Anxiety and feelings of impending doom
Fear of suffocation/apprehension

Objective data

Diaphoresis
Cyanosis, pallor
Tachypnea
Tachycardia
Hypotension
Hemoptysis (rare)
Cough
Breath sounds
  Decreased
  Crackles
  Pleural friction rub

Diagnostic tests

Chest x-ray examination
  Unilateral elevated diaphragms
  Atelectasis
  Hyperlucent lung fields
  Unilateral pleural effusion
  Area of consolidation (occasional)
ABG
  Decreased Pao_2 (<80 mm Hg)
  Decreased $Paco_2$ (<40 mm Hg)
  Elevated pH (>7.45g)
ECG
  Right ventricular strain
  Right axis deviation

Incomplete right bundle branch block (RBBB)
Atrial fibrillation
Lung (ventilation/perfusion) scan
Pulmonary angiogram
Serum assays
  Elevated LDH, elevated bilirubin
  Fibrin split products (FSP)/fibrin degradation tests
Prothrombin time (PT), partial thromboplastin time (PTT)
International normalized ratio (INR)
Pattern of abnormal perfusion in area of ventilation
  Intraarterial filling defects
  Pulmonary artery obstruction(s)

Potential complications

Extended/recurrent pulmonary embolism
Pulmonary infarction
Atelectasis
Pulmonary hypertension
RV failure
Cor pulmonale
Decreased cardiac output
Shock
Cardiopulmonary arrest

Collaborative management

Therapeutic management

Bed rest
Oxygen therapy
Cardiac monitor
Medication
  Anticoagulants
    Heparin
    Warfarin
  Fibrinolytic enzymes
    Streptokinase
    Urokinase
  Vasopressors
  Analgesics/sedatives
Parenteral fluids
Surgical therapy
  Insertion of umbrella filter for multiple emboli
  Embolectomy

Nursing management

PATIENT PROBLEMS/NURSING DIAGNOSES

● **NDX:** Impaired gas exchange related to ventilation/perfusion abnormalities

Assess, monitor for, and report signs of restlessness, confusion, and irritability, which *may indicate hypoxia or respiratory distress*
Assess quality and respiratory rate q2h to 4h and prn
Administer oxygen as ordered; intubation and assisted ventilation may be indicated
Monitor BP, R, and apical pulse q1h to 2h and prn
Auscultate breath sounds q2h to 4h
Maintain bed rest during acute phase; instruct to turn and deep breathe q2h to 4h; avoid positions that bend knees, which *decreases venous return and can increase risk of PE*
Elevate head of bed *to promote optimal breathing*
Monitor ABGs as ordered: report changes in Pao_2 or Pco_2 >10 mm Hg
Monitor ECG and cardiac status for dysrhythmias secondary to blood gas levels
Monitor for pulmonary hypertension, jugular venous distention, blood gas abnormalities, hepatomegaly, and cardiac compromise, which may indicate cor pulmonale

EXPECTED OUTCOME
Patient experiences adequate O_2/CO_2 exchange as evidenced by the following:
ABGs within normal range
Reports exhibiting no signs of respiratory distress
Normal breath sounds

● **NDX:** Risk for injury related to increased bleeding from anticoagulant therapy

Observe for signs and symptoms of bleeding: stools—occult and frank bleeding, hematuria, sputum, bleeding gums, bruising skin
Monitor PT or INR and clotting functions or coagulation factors daily as ordered
Administer anticoagulants as ordered
Do not administer aspirin-containing products
Provide antiembolic stockings as ordered *to prevent venous status*
Avoid constipation and straining; use stool softeners or mild laxatives

EXPECTED OUTCOME
Patient experiences no bleeding or extension of embolism as evidenced by absence of blood in stool, urine, sputum, or other sites

● **NDX:** Anxiety related to fear of perceived threat (suffocation) or actual threat to biologic integrity

Assess verbal and nonverbal signs and symptoms of anxiety/fear; encourage questions

Provide emotional support; maintain quiet environment

Remain with patient during periods of heightened anxiety

Explain procedures and treatments; use simple explanations

Assess whether significant family members present decrease anxiety: assist them to provide care

Administer antianxiety medications as ordered

EXPECTED OUTCOME

Patient experiences a reduction in anxiety as evidenced by the following:

Relaxed facial expression

Verbalization of feeling less anxious

Decreased use of sedatives and/or tranquilizers

Verbalization of an understanding of routines and treatments

ADDITIONAL NURSING DIAGNOSIS TO CONSIDER

Altered tissue perfusion related to interruption of arterial blood flow secondary to pulmonary embolism

Patient/family teaching

Discuss disease process
  Assess level of understanding regarding disease process
  Provide information on prevention for patients at risk for pulmonary embolism
Discuss symptoms to report to physician
  Sudden, sharp chest pain
  Bloody sputum
  Difficulty breathing
  Blood in stool
Medications
  Discuss medications: name, dosage, time of administration, purpose, and side effects
  Explain need to avoid taking over-the-counter medications without physician approval
  Explain need to check for bleeding in urine, stools, and sputum if sent home on anticoagulants (see Anticoagulant therapy, p. 191)
Activity
  Explain need to exercise to tolerance with planned rest periods
  Review strategies to prevent venous pooling
    Avoid sitting or standing for long periods
    Elevate legs while sitting
    Do not cross legs
    Use antiembolic stockings if ordered
    Perform regular exercise such as walking
Explain need to avoid constipation and straining

Explain importance of avoiding tobacco use

Explain need to wear medical alert band identifying use of anticoagulants

Home care considerations

Discuss any home management issues

Explain importance of ongoing outpatient care

Monitor exercise program

Assess economic status for ability to purchase medications and equipment; refer to social services and appropriate agency as indicated

Pulmonary Hypertension

*An elevation of mean pulmonary artery pressure (MPAP) >20 mm Hg. Pulmonary hypertension may occur as a **primary** disorder or **secondary** to preexisting diseases such as congenital heart disease or other pulmonary disease.*

Assessment

Subjective data

DOE and at rest
Fatigue
Syncope
Chest pain

Objective data

Tachypnea
Breath sounds
  Distant
  Decreased at periphery
  Crackles
Cyanosis
RV failure (Figure 5-4)
  Distended jugular veins
  RV heave
  Loud, accentuated P_2
  RV diastolic gallop
  Murmur of tricuspid insufficiency
  Peripheral edema
Chest pain

Diagnostic tests

Chest x-ray examination
  Enlarged pulmonary artery
  RV dilation or hypertrophy
ECG
  Right axis deviation
  RBBB

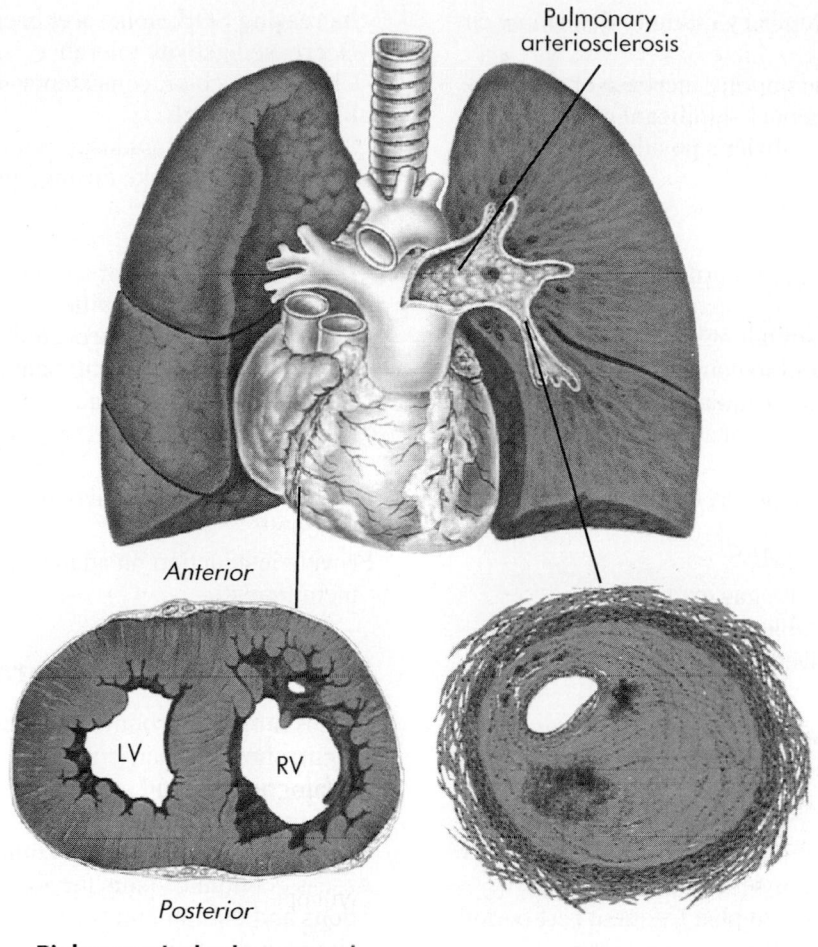

Figure 5-4 Right ventricular hypertrophy. (From Wilson SF, Thompson JM: *Mosby's clinical nursing series: respiratory disorders,* St Louis, 1990, Mosby.)

Echocardiogram
  Enlarged RA, RV
  Diminished wall motion
  PV malfunction
Cardiac catheterization
  Elevated PA systolic and diastolic pressure with
    normal PCWP
  Decreased CO
ABGs
  PaO_2 40 to 60 mm Hg
  $PaCO_2$ will vary depending on cause (40 to 70 mm Hg)

Collaborative management

Therapeutic management

Oxygen therapy
Hemodynamic monitoring
Cardiac monitoring
Medications

Vasodilators
  Prostacyclin
  Hydralazine
Calcium channel blockers
Ace inhibitors
Diuretics
Digitalis (used for biventricular failure)
Lung transplantation (unilateral or bilateral)
Heart/lung transplantation

Nursing management

PATIENT PROBLEMS/NURSING DIAGNOSES

● **NDX:** Impaired gas exchange related to alveolar-capillary membrane changes

Assess and monitor rate and depth of respirations, use of accessory muscles, air hunger, tachycardia

Assess skin color and capillary filling to determine circulatory adequacy

Auscultate breath sounds noting increase or decrease of rhonchi, crackles; report significant changes

Position patient in semi-Fowler's position *to optimize lung expansion*

Monitor serial ABGs and for signs of progressive hypoxemia and acidosis

Administer oxygen therapy as ordered *to optimize gas exchange*

Monitor chest x-ray examinations

Assist and instruct patient to cough and deep breathe; assess need to suction at regular intervals

Monitor for increasing signs of activity intolerance

Plan regular rest periods

Administer vasodilator as ordered

EXPECTED OUTCOMES

Patient maintains adequate gas exchange

ABGs are within acceptable limits

Lung sounds are improved

● **NDX:** Activity intolerance related to fatigue and dyspnea secondary to hypoxemia and decreased LV function

Assess degree of reported activity intolerance; observe respiratory rate in response to activities

Assist and instruct patient to plan frequent rest periods, especially between activities

Monitor signs of progressive deterioration in performing ADLs; report to physician

Provide oxygen therapy as indicated *to prevent hypoxia*: report changes in Pao_2 and $Paco_2$ >10 mm Hg

Assist patient to identify energy-saving methods while performing ADLs: shower chair, sitting while shaving

Instruct and encourage patient to use adaptive breathing techniques

EXPECTED OUTCOME

Patient reports ability to perform ADLs and verbalizes a decrease in fatigue

ADDITIONAL NURSING DIAGNOSIS TO CONSIDER

Fluid volume excess related to RV failure (see p. 147)

Patient/family teaching

Disease process

Assess level of understanding regarding pulmonary hypertension, identifying any misconceptions

Provide patient and significant other(s) with information regarding disease process, signs and symptoms to report

Increasing SOB; noisy, wet breathing

Decreased activity tolerance

Changes in color, consistency of sputum

Increased cough

Swelling of legs, ankles, or abdomen

Discuss action to take during episodes of fatigue or dyspnea

Activity

Discuss importance of spacing heavy workloads and resting between activities

Teach energy-saving procedures: shower chair; sitting while shaving, combing hair, dressing, cooking

Discuss importance of taking prescribed medications: name, dosage, purpose, time of administration, and side effects

Discuss importance of avoiding tobacco or nicotine products

Provide instruction on adaptive breathing techniques

Home care considerations

Assess home environment for energy saving equipment: shower chair, grab bars

Monitor activity and exercise program: walking with rest periods

Teach use of home oxygen equipment

Assess economic status for ability to purchase medications and equipment; refer to social services and agencies as indicated

Pulmonary Tuberculosis

A chronic acute or subacute infectious disease caused by the tubercle bacillus, mycobacterium tuberculosis, most commonly affecting the alveolar structure of the lung; clinical presentation varies from asymptomatic with only a positive skin test to extensive pulmonary and systemic involvement

Assessment

Subjective data

Fatigue, malaise

Headache

Anorexia

Chest pain

Objective data

Low-grade fever, night sweats

Tachycardia

Weight loss

Cough: nonproductive at first
  Blood-streaked sputum
  Mucoid or mucopurulent sputum
Lymph nodes
  Inflamed
  Painful
Crackles over apex of lung
Pleuritic chest pain
Irregular menses

Diagnostic tests

Skin testing
  PPD: 5 units of purified protein derivative
  Mantoux test: PPD or OT—old tuberculin, injected intradermally with pressure gun
  Tine test: OT pressed into skin with tine unit
Gastric washings
Sputum cultures: positive for *M. tuberculosis* within 2 to 3 weeks if active; positive acid-fast bacilli (AFB)
Chest x-ray examination
  Calcification at original site, enlarged hilar lymph nodes, and infiltrates if extension of original site has occurred
  Pleural effusion or cavitation
  CAUTION: Other lung abnormalities (pneumonia, tumors) can look like tuberculosis
Fiberoptic bronchoscopy
Needle biopsy of pleura
WBC: leukocytosis

Potential complications

Atelectasis
Hemoptysis
Pneumothorax
Recurrence
Miliary tuberculosis
Tuberculosis pericarditis, peritonitis, meningitis, lymphadenitis

Collaborative management

Therapeutic management

Antiinfective agents
  Primary drugs
    Isoniazid (INH)
    Ethambutol
    Rifampin
    Streptomycin
  Secondary drugs
    Paraaminosalicylic acid (PAS)
    Pyrazinamide
    Ethambutol

Analgesics
AFB isolation until medication therapy initiated
High-protein, high-carbohydrate diet
Respiratory isolation as necessary
Report to board of health for follow-up on family and contacts
Surgical therapy
  Drainage of lung abscess
  Lung resection

Nursing management

PATIENT PROBLEMS/NURSING DIAGNOSES

● **NDX:** Ineffective breathing pattern related to mucopurulent secretions and poor cough effort

Assess quality and depth of respirations, use of accessory muscles; record any changes
Assess quality of sputum: color, odor, consistency
Auscultate breath sounds q4h for adventitious or decreased breath sounds
Position patient *to optimize breathing:* semi-Fowler's or high-Fowler's position
Assist and teach patient to turn, cough, and deep breathe q2h to 4h *to mobilize secretions and maximize lung expansion*
Instruct patient to splint chest *for more effective and productive cough*
Provide frequent rest periods, avoid fatigue, and exercise to tolerance
Monitor T, P, and R q4h
Administer medications as ordered
Encourage fluid intake *to liquefy secretions*

EXPECTED OUTCOME
Patient maintains an effective breathing pattern
  Normal rate, rhythm, and depth of respirations
  Decreased dyspnea

● **NDX:** Risk for infection, transmission related to insufficient knowledge of pathogen

Discuss importance of maintaining respiratory isolation; avoid direct contact with sputum until antibiotic therapy is initiated and necessary levels obtained
Teach patient to cough into tissues
  Turn head with coughing
  Dispose of tissues properly
  Use mask if unable to follow directions
Instruct patient how to collect and care for sputum cultures and use good handwashing techniques *to reduce risk of spreading infection*
Teach patient importance of not stopping antituberculosis medications until directed by physician

EXPECTED OUTCOME

Patient has decreased potential for transmission of disease as evidenced by failure of patient contacts to convert to positive skin test

● **NDX:** Altered nutrition: less than body requirements related to fatigue, anorexia, or dyspnea

Obtain admission weight and monitor daily for changes

Assess nutritional status on a regular basis; consult with dietitian

Monitor percentage of meals eaten

Maintain high-protein, high-carbohydrate diet with small, frequent feedings

Assess for additional causes of malnutrition such as depression

Monitor albumin, prealbumin, and lymphocytes as *guide to nutritional status*

Place in high-Fowler's position at meals *to reduce dyspnea*

Encourage rest periods before meals *to reduce fatigue*

Encourage oral care before meals

Encourage significant other(s) to bring patient's favorite foods

EXPECTED OUTCOME

Patient maintains an adequate nutritional status; weight remains stable and within normal range for patient's height, age, and build

Patient/family teaching

Disease process
  Assess level of understanding regarding disease process; identify any fears or misconceptions
  Explain nature of disease and purpose of treatment and procedures
Explain importance of good hygiene and handwashing (coughing into tissues, use of mask if unable to follow directions, how to dispose of tissues, to turn head if coughing, and to avoid direct contact with sputum)
Teach importance of maintaining respiratory isolation until necessary medication levels are obtained
Explain importance of exercise, frequent rest periods, and avoiding fatigue
Instruct on importance of avoiding close contact with others until advised by physician
Explain need to avoid crowds and persons with URIs
Discuss symptoms to report to physician
  Hemoptysis
  Chest pain
  Difficulty in breathing
  Hearing loss
  Vertigo

Diet: explain importance of maintaining high-protein, high-carbohydrate diet; need to force fluids to 2000 to 3000 ml/day unless contraindicated

Discuss medications: name, dosage, time of administration, purpose, and side effects

Explain need to avoid taking over-the-counter medications without physician approval

Discuss importance of stopping medication only with physician approval

Home care considerations

Assess patient's ability to maintain isolation in home until necessary medication levels are obtained

Assess home for sanitary equipment for maintaining good hygiene: disposable trash bags, covered waste can for soiled tissues

Assess home for sleeping conditions, crowding, and persons with URIs; also children and others susceptible to infection

Evaluate economic status for ability to purchase medications and supplies; refer to social services and other agencies as indicated

Explain importance of ongoing outpatient care

Encourage PPD testing of family and contacts

Pneumothorax and Hemothorax

Collection of air or gas in the pleural space, causing the lung to collapse; may be partial or total collapse; open or communicating pneumothorax (sucking wound) occurs as result of an open chest wound that permits entry of air; spontaneous pneumothorax (closed) results from rupture of a bleb or bullae on the surface of the lung; may occur as a result of pulmonary disease (COPD, TB); or may be iatrogenically induced (thoracentesis)

tension pneumothorax: *An opening through the pleura that allows air to pass into the pleura on inspiration; however, the air cannot exit on expiration; this produces a shift in the affected lung and mediastinum toward the unaffected side (tension pneumothorax is a medical emergency) (see box on p. 302 and Figure 5-5)*

hemothorax: *Blood in the pleural space, causing the lung to partially or totally collapse; often appears as a complication of chest trauma and after chest surgery (see box on p. 302 and Figure 5-6)*

NOTE: *Symptoms and treatment depend on size of pneumothorax:*
  <15%: small
  15% to 60%: moderate
  >60%: large

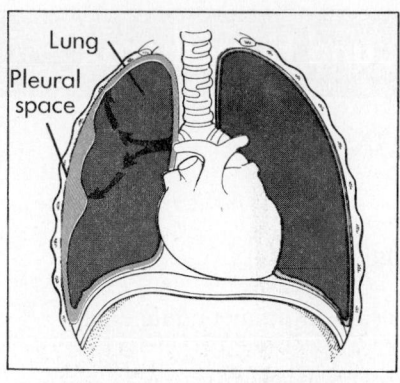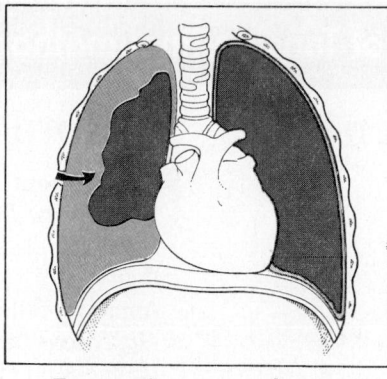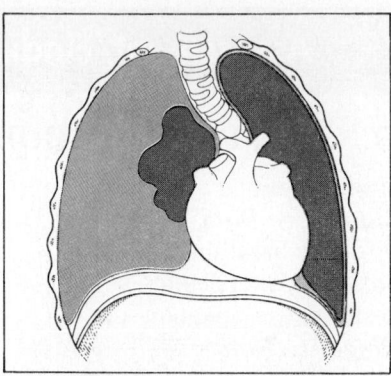

Spontaneous pneumothorax   **Traumatic pneumothorax**   **Tension pneumothorax**

Figure 5-5   Spontaneous, traumatic, and tension pneumothorax. (From Wilson SF, Thompson JM: *Mosby's clinical nursing series: respiratory disorders,* St Louis, 1990, Mosby.)

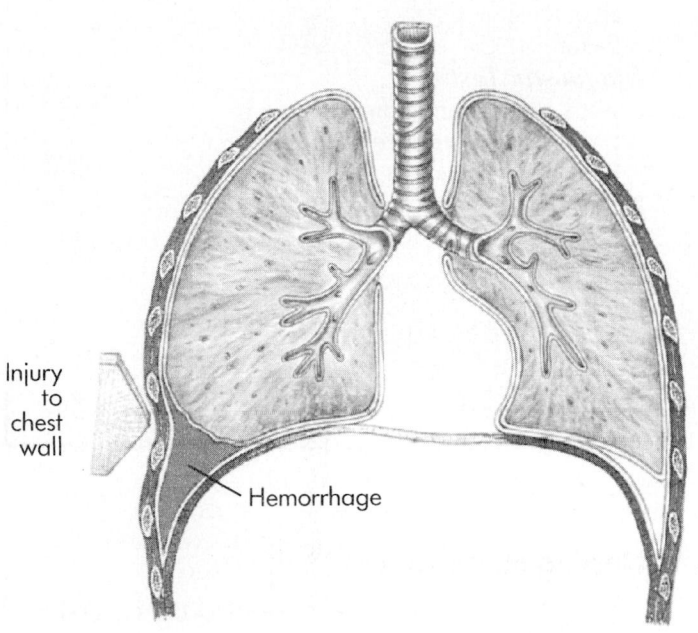

Figure 5-6   Hemothorax. (From Wilson SF, Thompson JM: *Mosby's clinical nursing series: respiratory disorders,* St Louis, 1990, Mosby.)

Assessment

Subjective data

Pain: pleural type, sudden, sharp pain radiating to shoulder or arm of affected side
Anxiety
Dyspnea or SOB

Objective data

Diaphoresis
Tachycardia
Cyanosis
Tachypnea

Absent or decreased breath sounds on affected side
Hyperresonance to percussion over affected thoracic space

Diagnostic tests

Chest x-ray examination
  Unequal lung expansion
  Air in pleural cavity
  Mediastinal shift to unaffected side
Arterial blood gases
  Decreased Pao_2
  Decreased pH
  Increased $Paco_2$

Assessment/Finding of Tension Pneumothorax and Hemothorax

TENSION PNEUMOTHORAX DATA

Assessment
Subjective Data
Difficulty breathing
Anxiety, fear of death
Restlessness, agitation
Objective Data
Respiratory distress: sudden, severe
Use of accessory muscles of respiration
Tachycardia
Cyanosis
Tachypnea
Hypotension
Paradoxic chest movement
Hyperresonance over affected area on percussion
Tracheal and mediastinal shift: toward unaffected
    side
Breath sounds
  Absent (affected side)
  Diminished (unaffected side)
Distant heart sounds
Subcutaneous emphysema
Diagnostic Tests
Chest x-ray examination: complete lung collapse of
    affected side, mediastinal or tracheal shift to unaf-
    fected side

HEMOTHORAX

Assessment
Subjective Data
Difficulty breathing
Pain
Anxiety, restlessness, fear of impending doom
Objective Data
Dullness on chest percussion
Distant to absent breath sounds on affected side
Asymmetric chest movements
Hypovolemic shock if blood loss is severe
  Tachypnea
  Tachycardia
  Hypotension
  Pallor
Diagnostic Tests
Chest x-ray examination
  Blunting of costophrenic angles
  Hazy appearance over lower chest
Hct/Hgb

Potential complications

Decreased cardiac output
Respiratory failure
ARDS
Infection
Cardiac arrest

Collaborative management

Therapeutic management

Chest tube insertion (closed-tube thoracostomy)
Oxygen therapy
Parenteral therapy
Thoracentesis
Blood transfusion (hemothorax)
Mechanical ventilation with PEEP

Nursing management

PATIENT PROBLEMS/NURSING DIAGNOSES

● **NDX:** Ineffective breathing pattern related to inadequate chest expansion caused by air/fluid accumulation

Assess quality, rate, and depth of respirations, nasal flaring, retractions; report any changes
Note chest wall movement and position of trachea *to differentiate tension pneumothorax*
Auscultate breath sounds q2h to 4h *to detect absence of breath sounds*
Reassure and try to calm patient
Place patient in a position *to ensure optimal respiration:* sitting position with head of bed elevated 60 to 90 degrees
Administer oxygen per nasal cannula at 2 to 6 L/min as ordered unless contraindicated *to treat hypoxia*

Assist with insertion of chest tube and provide chest tube care (see Chest tubes, p. 315)

Administer oxygen and IPPB as ordered

Monitor BP, T, R, and apical pulse q2h to 4h: *to detect changes in cardiac output, infective process, or oxygenation*

Assist and encourage patient to

Turn and deep breathe q2h to 4h: diaphragmatic, segmental breathing; instruct patient to suppress cough

Avoid stretching, reaching, or sudden movements

Provide emotional support; remain with patient during periods of heightened anxiety

Continue with acute care and decrease frequency of nursing functions as patient's condition improves

Assess for tiring in relation to breathing attempts

Space activities *to provide periods of rest*

EXPECTED OUTCOME

Patient maintains an effective breathing pattern as evidenced by the following:

Normal rate, rhythm, and depth of respirations

Chest x-ray examinations show full expansion

Breath sounds are clear with full aeration

● **NDX:** Impaired gas exchange related to decreased oxygen supply

Assess for signs and symptoms of hypoxemia: restlessness, confusion, irritability

Monitor ABG results: report changes in $Paco_2$ or Po_2 of >10 mm Hg

Observe for signs of respiratory distress: increased work of breathing, unequal lung expansion, complaints of increased dyspnea

Administer supplemental oxygen as ordered; assist with endotracheal intubation and mechanical ventilation as indicated

Monitor function and patency of chest tube

Provide periods of rest *to decrease oxygen demand*

EXPECTED OUTCOME

Patient maintains adequate gas exchange as evidenced by the following:

Usual mental status

Usual skin color

Blood gases within normal range

● **NDX:** Pain, chest related to biologic factors (tissue trauma) and physical factors (chest tube insertion)

Assess for presence of pain (verbal and nonverbal): rate pain on scale 1-10

Administer analgesic as prescribed (30 min before initiating movement)

Assess effectiveness of pain relief measures

Medicate patient before breathing/coughing exercises

Instruct patient on splinting techniques; move as a unit *to enhance stability and comfort*

Secure chest tubes *to limit movement and resulting irritation*

EXPECTED OUTCOME

Patient experiences decreased pain as evidenced by the following:

Verbalizes pain relief

Relaxed facial expression and body positioning

Improved breathing pattern

Increased activity

Patient/family teaching

Disease process

Assess level of understanding regarding disease process and contributing factors

Explain importance of not smoking

Explain need to avoid persons with infections, especially URIs

Discuss symptoms to report to physician: cold; sore throat; influenza; elevated temperature; cough; sudden, sharp chest pain; difficulty in breathing; any redness, pain, swelling, or tenderness of puncture wound

Diet

Explain importance of maintaining diet as ordered; need to force fluids to 2000 to 3000 ml/day unless contraindicated to liquefy secretions and maintain hydration

Activity

Explain need to exercise to tolerance, avoid fatigue, and plan rest periods

Explain importance of avoiding strenuous activity or exercise, especially contact sports

Discuss medications: name, dosage, time of administration, purpose, and side effects

Home care considerations

Explain importance of ongoing outpatient care for extended period following pneumothorax

Ensure that patient and significant other(s) demonstrate care of chest puncture wound (see Chest tubes p. 315)

Evaluate economic status for ability to purchase medications and supplies and refer to social services or agency as indicated

Teach patient adaptive breathing techniques to maximize lung reexpansion and prevent complications

Teach importance of avoiding persons with URIs and flu

Thoracic Empyema

Pus in the pleural cavity caused by underlying infections of the lung, such as pneumonia or lung abscess, occurring after thoracic surgery or resulting from penetrating chest wounds

Assessment

Subjective data

Difficulty in breathing
Localized chest pain
  Constant
  Only during inspiration
Malaise
Fatigue
History of thoracic surgery, penetrating chest wound, persistent fever despite antibiotic administration

Objective data

Nasal flaring
Asymmetric chest expansion
Decreased or absent breath sounds over affected area
Productive cough
Elevated temperature
Tachycardia
Tachypnea

Diagnostic tests

Chest x-ray examination: unilateral/bilateral pleural effusions
Thoracentesis
Examination of pleural exudate
  Gram stain
  Culture and sensitivity
Examination of pleural fluid
  Fluid cell count/differential
    Specific gravity
    pH <7.2 mm Hg
  Cytologic examination
ABGs: Pao_2 <70 mm Hg; $Paco_2$ and pH within normal limits

Potential complications

Pneumothorax
Pneumonia
Bronchopleural fistula

Collaborative management

Therapeutic management

Chest tube insertion: irrigation of pleural cavity to flush out purulent and necrotic material
Thoracentesis to drain small, localized area
Thoracic drainage to drain large quantities of pus
Intrapleural aspiration and instillation of medications
Thoracotomy if necessary
High-protein, high-carbohydrate diet; force fluids during febrile state
O_2 therapy as necessary
Medications: antibiotics, antipyretics, analgesics
Fluid management

Nursing management

PATIENT PROBLEMS/NURSING DIAGNOSES

● **NDX:** Ineffective breathing pattern related to decreased lung expansion secondary to pus in the pleural space

Assess respirations, noting changes in rate, depth, quality, nasal flaring, or prolonged expiration cycle
Assess chest movement, noting signs of asymmetry
Auscultate breath sounds q2h to 4h for adventitious or decreased sounds
Place patient in a sitting position with head of bed elevated 60 to 90 degrees *to maximize breathing*
Administer oxygen per nasal cannula at 2 to 6 L/min as ordered unless contraindicated *to treat hypoxia*
Assist with insertion of chest tube (see p. 315)
Administer oxygen and IPPB as ordered
Monitor BP, T, R, and apical pulse q2h to 4h *to assess for infective process*
Administer medications as ordered
Review serial chest x-ray and ABGs as ordered
Assist and teach patient to
  Deep breathe q2h to 4h; position onto affected side; use diaphragmatic, segmental breathing
  Encourage use of incentive spirometer (see p. 327)
  Perform passive and active ROM exercises to extremities q4h
Encourage coughing: assist patient to splint affected side when coughing *to mobilize secretions and enhance lung expansion*
Avoid stretching, reaching, or sudden movements

EXPECTED OUTCOME

Patient maintains an effective breathing pattern as evidenced by the following:
Normal rate, rhythm, and depth of respirations

Decreased dyspnea
Blood gases within normal range

● **NDX:** Pain, chest related to biologic factors (tissue trauma) and physical factors (chest tube insertion)

Assess for presence of pain (verbal and nonverbal): rate pain on scale 1-10
Administer analgesic as prescribed (30 min before initiating movement)
Assess effectiveness of pain relief measures
Medicate patient before breathing/coughing exercises
Instruct patient on splinting techniques; move as a unit *to enhance stability and comfort*
Secure chest tubes to limit movement and resulting irritation

EXPECTED OUTCOME
Patient experiences decreased pain
Verbalizes pain relief
Relaxed facial expression and body positioning
Improved breathing pattern
Increased activity

ADDITIONAL NURSING DIAGNOSES
TO CONSIDER
Impaired gas exchange related to alveolar-capillary membrane changes
Self-care deficit related to chest tube placement and fatigue
Risk for fluid volume deficit related to febrile state

Patient/family teaching

Disease process
Assess level of understanding of disease process; identify
Discuss symptoms to report to physician
Difficulty in breathing
Chest pain on inspiration
Elevated temperature
Persistent cough
Coughing up foul-smelling sputum
Explain importance of avoiding persons with URIs
Discuss symptoms of a cold or flu to report to physician
Explain need to exercise to tolerance
Plan rest periods
Avoid fatigue
Medications
Discuss medications: name, dosage, time of administration, purpose, and side effects
Explain need to avoid taking over-the-counter medications without checking with physician

Home care considerations

Explain importance of ongoing outpatient care
Assess for need for influenza vaccination in patient and significant family members
Instruct on home hygiene and handling of tissues using disposable trash bags, covered waste, and good handwashing techniques of patient and all family members
Evaluate economic status for ability to purchase medication and supplies; refer to social services and other agencies as indicated
Assess home for crowding, sleeping conditions, and persons with URI or influenza
Teach and review use of equipment for home use

Atelectasis

Collapse of alveoli or airless condition of the lung caused by mucous plugs, excessive secretions, compression of lung tissue by tumors, effusions, or pneumothorax, shallow breathing, or incomplete lung expansion at birth.

Assessment

Subjective data

Difficulty breathing
SOB
Localized chest pain
Fatigue
Anxiety
Fear of air hunger

Objective data

Elevated temperature
Breath sounds
Absent or decreased over affected area
Crackles
Egophony and bronchophony
Tachypnea
Tachycardia
Labored breathing
Nasal flaring
Restlessness
Asymmetrical chest movement on inspiration

Diagnostic tests

Arterial blood gases
Decreased PaO_2: <80 mm Hg initially
Normal or decreased $PaCO_2$
Significant atelectasis: increased $PaCO_2$

Chest x-ray examination
  Elevated diaphragm on affected side
  Shift of trachea mediastinum toward affected side if
    large area is atelectic
  Narrow rib spaces

Potential complications

Pneumonia
Bronchiectasis

Collaborative management

Therapeutic management

Oxygen therapy as needed
Chest physiotherapy
IPPB/incentive spirometer
High tidal volume and/or PEEP for intubated patient
Bronchoscopy
Nutritional support
Fluid management
Medications
  Antipyretics
  Bronchodilators
  Antibiotics

Nursing management

PATIENT PROBLEM/NURSING DIAGNOSIS

● **NDX:** Impaired gas exchange related to compressed lung tissue

Assess for signs of hypoxemia: labored breathing,
  tachypnea, restlessness, pallor
Assess LOC for signs of hypoxia or hypercapnia
Auscultate breath sounds q2h to 4h
  Check quality and rate of respirations
  Note area of lung without breath sounds
Assist and instruct patient to turn, cough, and deep
  breathe q1h to 2h and prn *to enhance lung expansion
  and mobilize secretions*
Assist and instruct patient to perform postural drainage qid
  and prn; clapping may be ordered *to mobilize secretions*
Assist or initiate chest physiotherapy
Perform nasotracheal suction as indicated *to maintain
  patent airway*
Administer nebulization as ordered *to liquefy secretions*
Administer oxygen and IPPB as ordered
Instruct and encourage patient to use incentive spirom-
  eter as ordered
Encourage early ambulation as soon as possible *to facil-
  itate lung expansion*

Monitor BP, T, and apical pulse q4h *to assess hemody-
  namics and infectious process*
Monitor arterial blood gases as ordered
Administer medication as ordered: antipyretics

EXPECTED OUTCOME
Patient's gas exchange is improved
  ABGs within acceptable limits
  Lungs clear to auscultation
  Normal rate and rhythm of respiration

Patient/family teaching

Assess level of understanding regarding disease
  process: identify fears and misconceptions
Instruct patient in coughing and deep breathing tech-
  niques; teach patient to splint chest when coughing
Instruct patient in use of incentive spirometer and how
  frequently to use if continued at home
Explain need to avoid persons with infections, espe-
  cially URIs
Explain importance of avoiding tobacco use
Discuss symptoms to report to physician
  URI
  Influenza
  Difficulty in breathing
  Persistent cough
  Elevated temperature
Explain importance of exercising to tolerance; need to
  avoid fatigue and plan rest periods
Discuss medications: name, dosage, time of administra-
  tion, purpose, and side effects
Explain need to avoid taking over-the-counter medica-
  tions without physician approval

Home care considerations

Explain importance of ongoing outpatient care
Teach use of home oxygen therapy to patient and significant other(s)
Evaluate economic status for ability to purchase medications and supplies; refer to social services and
  other agencies as indicated

Pleural Effusion

*Excessive amount of nonpurulent fluid in the pleural
  space between the visceral and parietal layers;
  associated with primary diseases in which capillary
  fluid, lymphatic drainage membrane hydrostatic, and
  colloidal pressures of plurae are disturbed. Pleural
  effusion is rarely a primary disease*

Assessment

Subjective data

SOB
Localized chest pain
Fatigue
Fear of suffocation

Objective data

Related to underlying disease and may be asympto-
  matic if effusion is small
Respiratory difficulty
Breath sounds
  Diminished or absent over affected area
  Egophony over effusion area
  Pleural friction rub
Asymmetric chest expansion
Elevated temperature
Cough

Diagnostic tests

Chest x-ray examination
  Blunting of costophrenic angle
  Partially obscured diaphragm
  Complete "white out" (opaque densities) of involved
    area in large effusions
Thoracentesis
Pleural biopsy
Cytologic examination of fluid
Gram stain, culture, and sensitivity of pleural fluid

Potential complications

Pneumothorax
Pneumonia
Empyema

Collaborative management

Therapeutic management

Bed rest
Chest tube insertion (see p. 315)
Thoracentesis
Medications: antibiotics
Fluid management
Chest physiotherapy
Nitrogen mustard instillation or tetracycline via chest
  tube
Treatment of underlying disease process

Nursing management

PATIENT PROBLEM/NURSING DIAGNOSIS

● **NDX:** Ineffective breathing pattern related to decreased lung expansion secondary to fluid
accumulation in the pleural space

Assess rate, depth, and quality of respirations
Auscultate chest q2h to 4h for changes in breath sounds
Maintain bed rest; assist patient to assume position of
  comfort *to maximize breathing*
See Thoracentesis (p. 271) and Chest tubes (p. 315) if
  ordered
Monitor BP, T, P, and R q4h and prn to assess hemody-
  namics and infective process
Administer medications as ordered
Assist and teach patient to
  Turn, cough, and deep breathe q2h to 4h
  Use incentive breathing *to maximize lung expansion*
  Splint chest when coughing
  Perform active ROM exercises to all extremities q2h
    to 4h
Use blow bottles or incentive spirometer *to maximize
lung expansion*
Increase activity as tolerated

EXPECTED OUTCOME

Patient maintains an effective breathing pattern
  Normal rate, rhythm, and depth of respirations
  Decreased dyspnea
  Chest x-ray examination clear

ADDITIONAL NURSING DIAGNOSES
TO CONSIDER

Impaired gas exchange related to alveolar-capillary
  membrane changes
Fear related to suffocation and dying

Patient/family teaching

Disease process
Assess level of understanding regarding disease
  process and allay fears and misconceptions
Discuss symptoms to report to physician: difficulty in
  breathing, chest pain, elevated temperature, persis-
  tent cough
Instruct and encourage patient to cough, deep breathe
  to keep lungs well aerated
Explain importance of avoiding persons with URIs
Discuss symptoms of a cold or influenza to report to
  physician
Explain importance of influenza vaccination as ordered
Medications
  Discuss medications: name, dosage, time of adminis-
    tration, purpose, and side effects

Explain need to avoid taking over-the-counter medications without physician approval
Activity: explain need to exercise to tolerance
  Plan rest periods
  Avoid fatigue

Home care considerations

Explain importance of ongoing outpatient care
Assess members living at home for possible URI or influenza; explain need for influenza vaccination
Evaluate economic status for ability to purchase medications and supplies and refer to social services or appropriate agency as indicated

Flail Chest

Chest cage abnormality usually resulting from crushing chest injury where multiple fractures of ribs have occurred

Assessment

Subjective data

Difficulty breathing
Pain: rib cage
Fear

Objective data

Sharp chest pain
Respirations
  Shallow
  Paradoxical chest wall movement
  Splinting
Tachypnea
Tachycardia
Cyanosis
Decreased breath sounds
Mediastinal and tracheal shift
Sputum
Copious
Blood tinged

Diagnostic tests

Chest x-ray examination
  Atelectasis
  Pneumothorax
  Evidence of fractured ribs
Arterial blood gases
  Decreased PaO_2
  Increased $PaCO_2$
Pulmonary function tests: decreased lung volumes

Potential complications

Tension pneumothorax
Hemothorax
Pulmonary edema
Cardiac tamponade
Respiratory arrest
Shock

Collaborative management

Therapeutic management

O_2 therapy
Chest tube insertion
Intubation and mechanical ventilation with PEEP
Medications
  Neuromuscular blockers
  Sedatives
  Antibiotics
  Bronchodilators
  Analgesics

Nursing management

  PATIENT PROBLEMS/NURSING DIAGNOSES

● **NDX:**   Ineffective breathing pattern related to unstable chest wall movement

Maintain bed rest; assist patient in assuming position of comfort; do not turn patient onto flailed side
Understand that endotracheal tube (p. 317) or tracheostomy (p. 319) may be ordered
Place on continuous mechanical ventilation (p. 323) as ordered
  Positive-pressure ventilator
  Volume-cycled ventilator
  Respirations may be controlled by ventilator
Understand that chest tubes may be ordered (p. 315)
Monitor BP, P, and R q1h to 2h and prn for hemodynamic and respiratory changes
Auscultate breath sounds q1h to 2h and prn for adventitious or decreased sounds
Report decreased or absent breath sounds to physician
Perform oropharyngeal suctioning prn *to maintain patent airway and maximize lung expansion*
Monitor arterial blood gases as ordered; report changes in PCO_2 and PaO_2 of >10 mm Hg
Turn and reposition patient q2h to 4h and prn to provide comfort and skin care
Maintain body alignment
Assist and teach patient to deep breathe q2h to 4h and prn in absence of tracheostomy or endotracheal tube

Continue acute care management but decrease frequency of nursing functions as patient's condition improves

Administer IPPB with humidification as ordered

Assist and teach patient to use incentive spirometer as ordered

EXPECTED OUTCOME

Patient maintains an effective breathing pattern
Normal rate, rhythm, and depth of respirations
Decreased dyspnea
Blood gases within normal range
Breath sounds clear

● **NDX:** Pain, chest related to trauma

Assess for verbal and nonverbal signs of pain: rate pain on 1-10 scale

Manage pain as indicated; assess effectiveness of pain relief measure(s)

Prepare for possible intercostal nerve block

Establish means of communication of pain
Call bell within reach
Pad and pencil or Magic Slate

Explain all procedures thoroughly, using calm, reassuring voice

EXPECTED OUTCOME

Patient experiences decreased pain as evidenced by the following:
Verbalization of pain relief
Relaxed facial expression and body positioning
Improved breathing pattern
Increased activity

Patient/family teaching

Disease process
Assess level of understanding regarding disorder, causes, treatment, and procedures; identify fears and misconceptions

Discuss symptoms to report to physician
URI
SOB
Persistent cough
Persistent chest pain

Activity: explain importance of exercising to tolerance; avoid overexertion, excessive sports and activities, and heavy lifting

Medication
Discuss medications: name, dosage, time of administration, purpose, and side effects
Explain need to avoid taking over-the-counter medications without physician approval

Home care considerations

Explain importance of ongoing outpatient care
Monitor exercise and rest periods to increase strength

Respiratory Failure

Inability of the respiratory system to maintain normal oxygenation of blood (hypoxia: PaO_2 <60 mm Hg) or elimination of carbon dioxide ($PaCO_2$ >45 mm Hg) resulting from problems with ventilation, diffusion, or perfusion

Type I Hypoxemia without hypercapnia
Type II Hypoxemia and hypercapnia
Type III Hypoventilation causing hypercapnia

Assessment

Subjective data

Difficulty breathing
Headache
Fear of suffocation, anxiety
Fatigue

Objective data

Respiratory distress
Nasal flaring
Tachypnea or bradypnea
Retractions
Use of accessory muscles of respiration
Labored breathing
Air hunger
Diaphoresis
Cyanosis
Breath sounds
Crackles
Rhonchi
Wheeze
Increased respiratory secretions
Altered LOC
Restlessness
Confusion
Drowsiness
Impaired motor function; asterixis
Papilledema
Cardiovascular
Tachycardia
Hypertension
Dysrhythmias
Atrial
Ventricular
Decreased cardiac output
Restlessness

Lethargy
Somulena
Tachycardia
Decreased urinary output

Diagnostic tests

ABGs
  Hypoxia
    Mild: Pao_2 <80 mm Hg
    Moderate: Pao_2 <60 mm Hg
    Severe: Pao_2 <40 mm Hg
  Increased or decreased $Paco_2$, depending on stage of failure
Chest x-ray examination: documents underlying pathology or progressive disease process
Hemodynamic findings: type I—increased PCWP
Chest x-ray examination: depends on underlying cause of failure
ECG
  May show evidence of right-sided heart strain
  Dysrhythmias

Potential complications

ARDS
Deterioration from type I to type II
Cardiac failure
Barotrauma

Collaborative management

Therapeutic management

Oxygen therapy
  Low-flow oxygen delivery: nasal cannula, catheter, face mask, partial rebreathing mask with reservoir bag
  Mechanical ventilatory support with constant positive airway pressure (CPAP) or PEEP
  Nebulized inhalation
  Chest physiotherapy
  Hemodynamic/cardiac monitoring
  Parenteral therapy
  Medications
    Bronchodilators
    Steroids
  Nutritional support as needed

Nursing Management

PATIENT PROBLEMS/NURSING DIAGNOSES

● **NDX:** Ineffective breathing pattern related to decreased lung expansion

Assess rate, depth, and quality of respirations, breathing pattern, and use of accessory muscles
Assess vital signs and LOC qh and prn: changes in LOC is one of first signs of ARF
Be aware that endotracheal tube may be inserted or tracheostomy done (see p. 319) if $Paco_2$ is >50 mm Hg or Pao_2 is <60 mm Hg
Administer oxygen with assisted ventilation and humidification as ordered *to correct hypoxia and liquefy secretions*
Monitor and record ABGs as indicated: assess for downward trend in Pao_2 or upward trend in $Paco_2$
Be aware that continuous mechanical ventilation (see p. 323) is indicated if $Paco_2$ is >60 mm Hg, $Paco_2$ increases at a rate of 5 mm Hg or more per hour, Pao_2 cannot be maintained at 60 mm Hg or higher, patient manifests increased fatigue or mental depression, or secretions become difficult to control
Auscultate breath sounds qh for adventitious or decreased sounds
Maintain bed rest with head of bed elevated 30 to 45 degrees *to optimize breathing*
Encourage coughing and deep breathing; assist patient to splint chest during coughing *to optimize breathing and removal of secretions*
Instruct patient to use pursed-lip and diaphragmatic breathing *to reduce work of breathing*

  EXPECTED OUTCOME
Patient maintains an effective breathing pattern
  Normal rate, rhythm, and depth of respirations
  Decreased dyspnea
  Blood gases within normal range

● **NDX:** Ineffective airway clearance related to obstructed airway and poor ventilation secondary to retention of secretions

Assess rate and quality of respirations and use of accessory muscles
Auscultate breath sounds q2h for adventitious or decreased sounds
Assess, monitor, and record amount, consistency, and color of secretions: report changes to physician
Assist and teach patient to turn, cough, and deep breathe *to maximize breathing*
Encourage use of incentive spirometry (see p. 327)
Instruct patient in controlled coughing techniques
Position patient *to maximize breathing*
Assist and teach patient to perform postural drainage as ordered *to mobilize secretions*
Administer oxygen therapy as indicated *to correct hypoxia*
Provide airway humidification *to liquefy secretions*
Maintain adequate fluid intake *to liquefy secretions and prevent dehydration*

Suction secretions if necessary
  Use sterile technique
  Hyperoxygenate and/or hyperinflate patient's lungs
    for four or five breaths before and after procedure
Observe cardiac monitors for dysrhythmias during
  procedure
Administer medications as ordered
  Bronchodilators
  Mucolytic agents

EXPECTED OUTCOME

Patient maintains a patent airway as evidenced by the
following:
  Improved breath sounds
  Normal rate and depth of respirations
  Ability to expectorate secretions
  Blood gases within normal range

● **NDX:** Impaired gas exchange related to ventilation-
  perfusion abnormalities secondary to hypoventilation

Assess for signs and symptoms of hypoxia and hypercapnia
Assess BP, P, apical pulse, and LOC qh and prn; report
  changes in LOC to physician
Monitor and record serial ABGs, *assessing for upward
  trend in $Paco_2$ or downward trend in Pao_2*
Assist with administration of mechanical ventilation as
  indicated; assess need for CPAP or PEEP
Auscultate for diminished breath sounds qh *for adventi-
  tious or decreased sounds*
Review serial chest x-ray examination, noting improve-
  ment or deterioration
Monitor cardiac rhythm for dysrhythmias
Administer parenteral fluids as ordered *to maintain
  hydration*
Administer drugs as ordered
  Bronchodilators
  Antibiotics
  Steroids
Evaluate ADLs in relation to decreased oxygen demands

EXPECTED OUTCOME

Patient maintains adequate gas exchange
  Lungs clear
  Usual skin color
  Blood gases within normal range for predicted age

● **NDX:** Anxiety/fear related to perceived and actual
  biologic threat (inability to breathe)

Assess level of anxiety (mild, moderate, severe)
Encourage patient and family to verbalize fears and
  concerns and ask questions regarding procedures
  and condition

Explain procedures and treatments using simple sen-
  tences
Instruct patient on energy conservation techniques
  Pursed-lip breathing
  Diaphragmatic breathing
Use calm, reassuring manner
Monitor vital signs
Assess to determine whether significant other's partici-
  pation in care relieves anxiety
Reassure patient that he or she will not be left alone
Describe and point out alarms to patient and significant
  other(s) and explain that these alarms will alert staff
  to any problems
Answer any alarms immediately

EXPECTED OUTCOME

Anxiety level is reduced
  Appears calm and relaxed
  Able to verbalize fear

ADDITIONAL NURSING DIAGNOSES
TO CONSIDER

Risk for infection related to invasive procedures, inadequate primary defenses, chronic disease
Sleep pattern disturbance related to sensory alteration:
  illness, disrupted circadian rhythms

Adult Respiratory Distress Syndrome

*Nonspecific result of acute injury to the lung,
  characterized by a group of symptoms that include
  decreased compliance of the lung, noncardiac
  pulmonary edema, and refractory hypoxemia (Figure
  5-7); etiology is diverse and includes shock, chest
  trauma, aspiration, fat embolism, and massive viral
  pneumonia; end result is a uniform hyaline membrane
  development that leads to gas exchange abnormalities;
  mortality is 50% to 60%*

Assessment

Subjective data

Difficulty breathing
Fear of suffocation or death
Anxiety

Objective data

Early phase
  Dyspnea
  Tachypnea

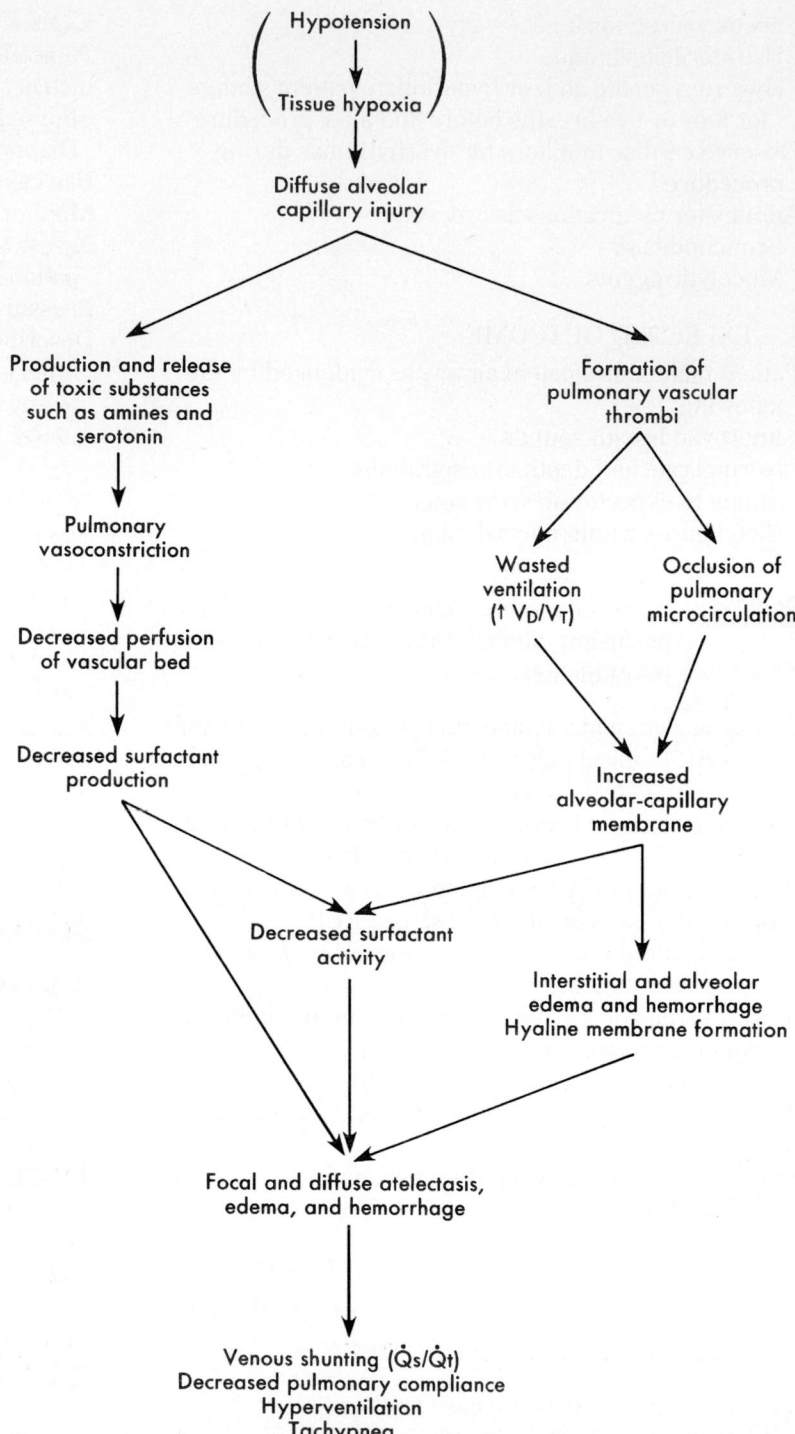

Figure 5-7 Proposed pathogenesis for ARDS. (From Thompson JM et al: *Clinical nursing,* ed 3, St Louis, 1993, Mosby.)

Restlessness
Cough
Clear breath sounds
Late phase
  Grunting respirations
  Use of accessory muscles of respiration

Color
  Pallor
  Cyanosis
  Diaphoresis
Breath sounds
  Crackles

Rhonchi
Tachycardia
Confusion

Diagnostic tests

Arterial blood gases
  Decreased PaO_2 that is unresponsive to increasing
    FIO_2
  Decreased $PaCO_2$ initially; then elevated $PaCO_2$ in later
    stages
  pH initially >7.45 mm Hg; as ARDS worsens, pH
    <7.35 mm Hg
CBC
Chest x-ray examination
  Early: normal
  Late
    Diffuse bilateral pulmonary infiltrates
    "White out" on x-ray film, giving ground-glass ap-
      pearance
Pulmonary artery pressures (PAP, PCWP)
  Early: normal
  Late: elevated
Pulmonary function tests
  Decreased VC, MV, FRC
  Decreased pulmonary compliance of >50 m/cm
    H_2O
Increased shunt fraction ($\dot{Q}s$-Qt) >15% to 20% (normal
  3% to 4%)
Increased lactic acid levels

Potential complications

Dysrhythmias
Low cardiac output
Renal failure
Infection/sepsis
Barotrauma
Disseminated intravascular coagulation (DIC)

Collaborative management

Therapeutic management

Oxygen therapy
Intubation with ventilator support; use of CPAP,
  PEEP
Parenteral therapy
Nutritional support
Medications
  Sedation
  Steroids
  Heparin
  Diuretics

Cardiac monitor
Hemodynamic monitoring

Nursing management

PATIENT PROBLEMS/NURSING DIAGNOSES

● **NDX:** Impaired gas exchange related to ventila-
tion/perfusion abnormalities

See Respiratory failure (see p. 309)
See standard of care for primary condition
Assess and monitor rate, quality, and depth of respira-
  tions
Assess for signs of respiratory distress
Auscultate breath sounds for crackles and wheezes
Place patient on volume-cycled ventilator with PEEP or
  CPAP as ordered; PEEP is contraindicated in patients
  with COPD
Administer oxygen therapy, monitoring FIO_2
Assess ABGs; monitor for increases or decreases of
  PaO_2 and $PaCO_2$
Monitor lactic acid levels
Administer parenteral fluids and electrolytes as or-
  dered by physician
Monitor BP, P, and R qh; assess LOC qh and prn
Suction secretions if crackles or rhonchi are present
Administer corticosteroids and diuretics as ordered by
  physician
Assess PAP and PCWP qh
Measure and record urinary output qh
Maintain bed rest with head of bed elevated 30 to 45 de-
  grees *to maximize breathing*
Reposition from side to side q1h to 2h

EXPECTED OUTCOME
Patient maintains adequate gas exchange as evidenced
  by the following:
  Return to baseline: LOC, skin color, respirations
  Blood gases within acceptable range

● **NDX:** Ineffective airway clearance related to excessive secretions secondary to interstitial edema

Assess and monitor rate and quality of respirations and
  use of accessory muscles
Assess characteristics of secretions; report changes to
  physician
Auscultate for breath sounds qh *to determine presence
  of adventitious or decreased sounds*
Review serial chest x-ray examinations to assess improvement
Assist and teach patient to turn, cough, and deep
  breathe if crackles or rhonchi are auscultated
Suction secretions as indicated to maintain patent airway

If patient is intubated, hyperoxygenate and hyperinflate patient's lung for four or five breaths before and
after procedure
Observe cardiac monitor during suctioning procedure
for dysrhythmias caused by hypoxia
Assist and teach patient to perform postural drainage
as ordered *to mobilize secretions*
Administer bronchodilators and expectorants as ordered

EXPECTED OUTCOME

Patient's airway is patent
Normal rate, rhythm, and depth of respirations
Breath sounds clear
Secretions are diminished/absent

ADDITIONAL NURSING DIAGNOSES
TO CONSIDER

Altered nutrition: less than body requirements related to
insufficient intake verses increased metabolic demand
Activity intolerance related to fatigue of breathing
See standard of care for primary condition
See Volume-cycled positive pressure ventilators
(p. 325)

Home care considerations

Assess for lung damage as a sequela of ARDS to determine need for respiratory equipment including oxygen for home use

Thoracotomy, Lobectomy, Pneumonectomy

thoracotomy: Surgical incision of the chest wall
lobectomy: Removal of one or more lobes of the lung
pneumonectomy: Removal of an entire lung

Preoperative care

See general preoperative care/teaching

Postoperative assessment

Subjective data

Difficulty breathing
Chest pain
Tenderness at chest tube insertion site

Objective data

Patent airway
Respiratory distress
Labored breathing
Use of accessory muscles of respiration
Tachypnea
Shallow respirations
Dyspnea
Tachycardia
Breath sounds
  Present/absent
  Crackles, rhonchi
Elevated temperature
Hemoptysis
Crepitus
Cyanosis
Mediastinal shift
Incision
  Redness
  Pain
  Swelling
  Drainage
Arm contracture: operative side

Diagnostic tests

Chest x-ray examination
ABGs
ECG

Potential complications

Pulmonary embolism
Pulmonary edema
Hemorrhage
Atelectasis
Tension pneumothorax
Infection
Bronchopleural fistula

Collaborative management

Therapeutic management

O_2 therapy
Intubation and ventilator support
NPO until stable
Fluid and electrolyte therapy
Medications: analgesics
Chest tube insertion

Nursing management

PATIENT PROBLEMS/NURSING DIAGNOSES

● **NDX:**   Ineffective breathing pattern related to pain
secondary to surgical incision

Assess and monitor respiratory rate; note use of accessory muscles

Assess chest symmetry for mediastinal shift, paradoxic respirations, or splinting caused by pain

Assess severity and quality of pain: rate on a pain scale 1-10

Administer oxygen as ordered *to treat hypoxia*

Elevate head of bed 60 to 90 degrees *to facilitate maximal breathing*

Assist and teach patient to turn, cough, and deep breathe qh *to promote full lung expansion and promote drainage*

Do not turn to unaffected side when pneumonectomy is done

Pad area around chest tube when turned to operative side

Splint chest to assist with coughing

Administer IPPB as ordered

Assist and teach patient to use incentive spirometer

Provide emotional support

Auscultate breath sounds q2h; report diminished or absent breath sounds on unaffected side to physician

Monitor ABGs

Check function of chest tube: note tidaling in the water seal chamber, prevent dependent loops in tubing

Administer pain medications as indicated

Monitor for signs of gastric distension that may occur secondary to anesthesia or swallowing

EXPECTED OUTCOME

Patient maintains an effective breathing pattern: normal rate, rhythm, and depth of respirations

Decreased dyspnea

Blood gases within acceptable range

Clear breath sounds

● **NDX:** Impaired physical mobility (arm on affected side) related to incisional pain and edema

Consult with physical therapy department to obtain ROM exercises *to prevent stiffness and ankylosis of shoulder on side of chest tube*

Assist and teach patient to exercise to tolerance

Ambulate as ordered *to prevent thrombosis*

Plan rest periods q1h to 2h

Begin ROM exercises, starting with passive and progressing to active

Encourage patient to rotate arm 360 degrees as ordered

Document progress

Medicate for pain as needed

EXPECTED OUTCOME

Patient has full range of motion of affected side by discharge date; able to rotate arm in full 360-degree circles

Patient/family teaching

Disease process

Assess level of understanding regarding surgical procedure

Explain need to avoid tobacco use

Explain that some numbness, pain, or heaviness in operative area is expected; it is caused by interruption of intercostal nerves and is usually temporary

Explain need to avoid persons with URIs

Discuss symptoms to report to physician: persistent dyspnea, cough, elevated temperature, URI, redness, pain, swelling, drainage from incision

Activity

Explain importance of exercising to tolerance

Increase amount of exercise gradually

Adjust activities according to degree of fatigue experienced

Plan rest periods

Medications

Discuss medications: name, dosage, time of administration, purpose, and side effects

Explain need to avoid taking over-the-counter medications without physician approval

Home care considerations

Explain need to continue coughing and deep breathing qid at home

Monitor gradual increase of exercise program and rest periods

Assess for URI or influenza in family members; encourage vaccinations

Explain importance of ongoing outpatient care

Ensure that patient and significant other(s) demonstrate care of incision

Chest Tubes

*Drainage tubes placed in the pleural space and attached to a water seal drainage system and/or suction to remove air and/or fluid to allow expansion of the affected lung and reestablish negative pressure
Indications: pneumothorax/hemothorax, pleural effusion, empyema, postoperative thoracotomy*

Assessment

Observations/findings

PATIENT

Chest drainage

Amount

Color

Character

Dyspnea
Labored breathing
Tachypnea
Tachycardia
Nonsymmetric chest expansion
Breath sounds on affected side
  Diminished
  Absent
  Crackles
  Rhonchi
Crepitus

EQUIPMENT

Patency of tube(s) and water seal drainage system
Continuous fluctuation of water or "tidaling" in water
  seal drainage system
Water level in water seal drainage system
Stability and security of water seal drainage system
Amount of added suction applied to water seal drainage
  system
Assure all tubing connections are securely attached
  and taped

Ongoing care

PATIENT

Position patient on affected side with head of bed
  elevated 45 to 60 degrees after insertion of chest
  tube
Explain purpose of chest tube(s) to alleviate anxiety
Monitor and record BP, T, P, and R q4h and prn
Monitor and record amount, color, and character of
  drainage q2h to 4h; report drainage in excess of 100
  ml/hr to physician
Manage pain as indicated; assess effectiveness of pain
  control measure(s)
Check chest tube site(s) and surrounding area q2h to
  4h for crepitus and air leaks
Assist and teach patient to turn, cough, and deep
  breathe q2h *to facilitate lung reexpansion*
  Splint chest when coughing
  Pad area around chest tube(s) when patient is turned
    to operative side
Assist and teach patient to perform active or passive
  ROM exercises to extremities q2h to 4h *to prevent
  thrombus*
Ambulate patient as indicated
Auscultate breath sounds q2h to 4h; report diminished
  breath sounds in unaffected lung to physician
Change dressing as ordered

EQUIPMENT

Tape connecting tubing and secure chest tube to thorax
  securely
Maintain pressure if patient is on added suction as ordered

Inspect tubing for kinking and obstruction
Keep water seal drainage system lower than patient's
  chest at all times
Secure connecting tubing and chest tube(s) to avoid
  tension and allow freedom of movement
Observe fluctuation of water in water seal drainage system; if patient is breathing spontaneously, fluid level
  rises during inhalation and falls during exhalation
Change water seal drainage system as indicated; never
  allow drainage to fill collection unit
Have petroleum jelly gauze at bedside for emergency use
Do not clamp the chest tube unless closed water seal
  drainage system breaks and the lung is nearly expanded; it can result in a tension pneumothorax
If the system is broken, submerge the end of the tube
  in a cup of sterile water until another system is set up

Patient/family teaching

See standard of care for primary condition
Ensure that patient and significant other(s) know and
  understand
  Purpose of chest tube(s), function, and care
  Importance of turning, coughing, and deep breathing
  Importance of keeping closed water seal drainage sys-
    tem below level of patient's chest when sitting or am-
    bulating
  Importance of not placing tension on chest tube(s)
  Need to report difficulty in breathing and chest pain
    to nurse and/or physician
Ensure that patient understands importance of and
  demonstrates coughing and deep breathing

● Removal of Chest Tube

Interventions

Place patient in a sitting position
Instruct patient to take a deep breath and hold it until
  chest tube is removed
Place pressure dressing with antibiotic ointment or pe-
  troleum jelly gauge over chest wall wound
Instruct patient to breathe normally
Auscultate chest for breath sounds for 24 q4h; report
  diminished or absent breath sounds to physician
Monitor respirations and drainage from pressure dressing

Patient/family teaching

See standard of care for primary condition
Ensure that patient and significant other(s) know and
  understand
  Importance of reporting any sudden chest pain, diffi-
    culty breathing, redness, pain, swelling of puncture site

Importance of coughing and deep breathing
Importance of exercising to tolerance; avoiding strenuous activity or exercise; checking with physician when to resume
Need to avoid contact with any persons with URI
Need to avoid crowds
Importance of not using tobacco

Artificial Airways

● Oral (Oropharyngeal) Airway

An artificial airway that extends from the lips to the pharynx, displacing the tongue anteriorly; oral airway is usually temporary, removed once patient regains consciousness or when more permanent airway is required for ventilation

● Nasal (Nasopharyngeal) Airway

An artificial airway that extends from the nares to the pharynx (Figure 5-8)

Assessment

Subjective data

Difficulty in breathing
Anxiety

Objective data

LOC
Airway obstruction
  Restlessness
  Stridor

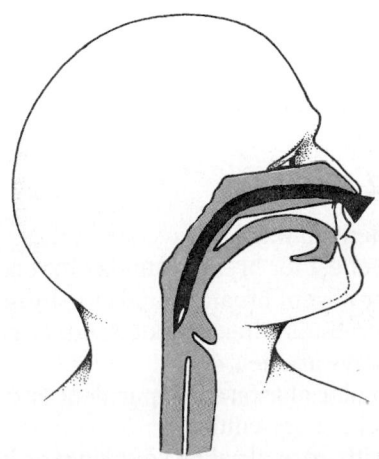

Figure 5-8   Nasopharyngeal airway.

Labored breathing
Retractions
  Intercostal
  Suprasternal
  Supraclavicular
  Nasal flaring
Cyanosis or pallor
Tachycardia
Breath sounds
  Crackles
  Rhonchi
  Decreased
Secretion incrustations
Airway ports: patent or occluded
Oral airway
  Gagging
  Mouth infections
  Oral lacerations or pressure sores
  Position of tongue
  Position of head and neck
Nasal airway
  Mouth breathing
  Pressure sores on nares
  Position of head and neck
Complications: oral airways—airway obstruction, aspiration

Ongoing care

General

Assess airway for patency and proper size of airway
Auscultate chest for breath sounds q2h and prn
Suction oropharynx or nasopharynx as indicated
Administer oxygen as ordered
Tape airway to prevent slippage or dislodgment
Monitor P and R q4h and prn; note quality of respirations
Administer oral hygiene q4h to 8h and prn

Oral airway

Assess LOC
Ensure that tongue is not between teeth and airway
Maintain patient on side to decrease possibility of aspiration; if in supine position and gagging or vomiting occurs, turn head to side
Change airway daily
Reposition airway q1h to 2h if flange of airway contacts lip
Apply cream, petroleum, or water-soluble jelly to lips *to prevent mucosal drying and cracking*

Nasal airway

Change airway q8h, alternating nares if possible *to prevent necrosis*

Clean nares q8h and prn
  Use cotton-tipped applicator with saline solution
  Apply water-soluble lubricant to nares
Assess need for humidification via face mask in long-term use
Use soft restraints if indicated
Establish means of communication when necessary
  Call light within reach
  Pad and pencil, Magic Slate, or communication board at bedside

Removal of airway

Assess LOC
Suction before removal
Remain with patient for 15 min after removal
Assess for any signs of respiratory distress
Monitor vital signs, noting any changes in rate and quality of respirations
Auscultate chest for breath sounds q15 min to 30 min for three times, then q2h to 4h as ordered

Patient/family teaching

Explain purpose of airway as indicated
Explain need to avoid mouth breathing

● Endotracheal Tube

An artificial airway that extends from the nose or mouth into the trachea (Figure 5-9)

Indications
  Upper airway obstruction
  To protect airway from aspiration

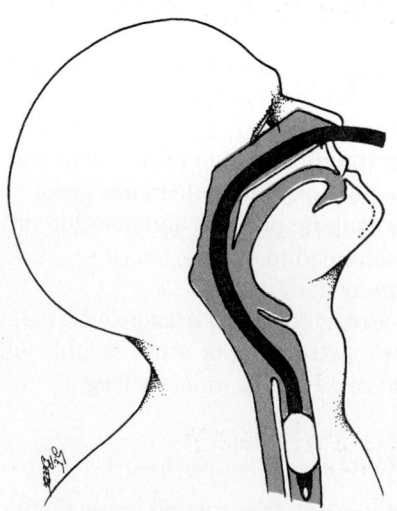

Figure 5-9   Endotracheal tube.

To remove secretions from central airways
To provide mechanical ventilation

Assessment

Observations/findings

  PATIENT
After insertion
Correct position of tube: bilateral breath sounds
Incorrect placement
  Right mainstem bronchus: unilateral (right) breath sounds; decreased breath sounds on left
  Carina: persistent coughing
  Esophagus: absent breath sounds
  Respiratory distress: cyanosis, tachypnea, restlessness, tachycardia, decreased PaO_2, increased $PaCO_2$
Crackles
Rhonchi over large airways
LOC
Pressure sores/infection on nares, ears, lips
Anxiety

Equipment
  Tube and cuff size (average adult is 7.5 to 9.0 mm)
  Hard versus soft cuff
  Inflation pressure
  Inflated cuff
  Minimal leak technique (MLT) pressure
  Minimal occlusion volume (MOV) technique pressure not >20 mm Hg or 5 to 25 cm H_2O
  Deflated cuff
Tube placement should be assessed by chest x-ray examination: tube tip should be 2 to 3 cm above carina
Humidification with room air or oxygen

Complications
  Tracheal injury
    Tracheal ulceration
    Tracheal bronchial fistula
  Aspiration
  Dysrhythmias
  Gag reflex
  Pressure sores on nares, ears, lips

Ongoing care

Maintain patent airway
  Auscultate chest for breath sounds qh; report decreased or absent breath sounds to physician
  Suction secretions when crackles and/or rhonchi over large airways are heard
    Observe color of aspirate: if purulent or colored, obtain specimen for culture
    Irrigate with normal saline solution if ordered *to liquify secretions*

Check position of tube q½h to 1h *to prevent slippage into right or left mainstem bronchus;* average adult tube is placed at 25-26 cm mark at lips

Obtain chest x-ray examination after insertion *to ascertain position of tube*

Keep hand-held resuscitator with adaptor at bedside

Assess respirations for quality and rate qh

Be aware that respirations are usually maintained on a continuous mechanical ventilator

Use air or oxygen blow-by if indicated

Be certain cuff is inflated while patient is on ventilator

Maintain inflated cuff with either a minimal leak or minimal occlusion volume technique

Check cuff pressure: it should not exceed 20 mm Hg

Deflate cuff when patient is off ventilator for long periods of time; suction mouth and trachea before deflating cuff

Monitor ABGs as indicated

Assess LOC qh; establish means of communication if patient is conscious

Call bell within reach

Pad and pencil, Magic Slate, or communication board at bedside

Provide emotional support; explain all procedures

Administer oral hygiene q1h to 2h

Clean nares gently around endotracheal tube q8h and prn; use cotton-tipped applicator with saline solution; apply water-soluble lubricant to nares

Provide oropharyngeal airway or bite-block if patient bites on endotracheal tube

Apply soft restraints as necessary if patient is restless

Provide humidification to endotracheal tube when patient is off ventilator

● Care During/After Extubation

Assessment

Observations/findings

LOC
Gag reflex
Respiratory distress
Laryngeal spasm
  Dyspnea
  Noisy breathing
  Use of abdominal or accessory muscles

Ongoing care

Assess whether patient is able to maintain spontaneous respirations at a rate sufficient to maintain normal ABGs

Auscultate chest for breath sounds: note adventitious or diminished sounds

Assess LOC: change in LOC is early sign of hypoxia

Elevate head of bed 45 to 90 degrees *to maximize breathing*

Preoxygenate and hyperinflate patient's lungs for four or five breaths

Suction oropharynx and/or nasopharynx *to maintain patency and remove secretions*

Suction endotracheal tube *to maintain patency and remove secretions*

Instruct patient to take a deep breath

Deflate cuff at peak of deep breath

Remove tube quickly as patient exhales, using a smooth, slightly downward motion

Administer humidified oxygen

Instruct patient to cough and deep breathe

Auscultate chest for breath sounds q15min for four times, then q1h to 2h; report absent or diminished breath sounds to physician

Monitor BP, R, and apical pulse q15min for four times, then q1h to 2h

Monitor ABGs as ordered

Assess for signs of stridor and/or laryngospasm

Prepare for reinsertion of endotracheal tube if laryngospasm occurs or if patient is unable to maintain adequate respiratory rate

Administer oral hygiene

Provide emotional support

Remain with patient as much as possible

Explain that sore throat, hoarseness, and dysphagia are common after extubation and will resolve in a few days

Encourage patient to minimize talking for a few hours

Provide a pad and pencil, Magic Slate, or communication board

Have call light within reach

Patient/family teaching

Explain all procedures whether patient appears conscious or not; orient patient to date, time, and place

Explain why patient is unable to talk and that it is only a temporary condition

Establish means of communication

Call bell within reach

Pad and pencil, Magic Slate, or communication board at bedside

Emphasize importance of turning and coughing up secretions

Tracheostomy

Insertion of a tube into the trachea through a surgical incision (tracheotomy) (Figure 5-10)

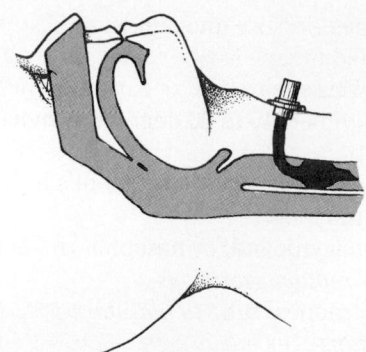

Figure 5-10   Tracheostomy tube with cuff.

Preoperative care

See General preoperative care/teaching (p. 53)
Include as much of the following as possible
Provide emotional support
Explain purpose of tracheostomy
Remain with patient as much as possible
Speak calmly and act unhurried
Involve family or significant other(s) in care and
  instructions
Demonstrate: tracheostomy tube
  Cleaning equipment
  Suctioning equipment; explain suctioning procedure
Determine whether patient can read and write English
  or another language
Determine whether patient can hear
Explain that patient will not be able to talk postoperatively
  Have pad and pencil, Magic Slate, or communication
    board at bedside
  Have picture cards available if patient is unable to write
Explain that patient may be in critical care area after op-
  eration; tour critical care area with patient and family
Review means of contacting nurse
  Call light
  Tap bell

Postoperative assessment

Observations/findings

PATIENT
Position of tracheostomy
Cuff
  Present
  Inflated
  Deflated
Bilateral expansion of chest
Sputum
  Amount
  Character

Stoma
  Pain
  Swelling
  Drainage
Anxiety
Fear of suffocation
Helplessness
Hemorrhage
Airway obstruction
  Restlessness
  Tachycardia
  Tachypnea
  Noisy respirations
  Wheezing
  Stridor
  Pallor
  Cyanosis
Subcutaneous or mediastinal emphysema
Pneumothorax
Injury to thyroid, laryngeal nerve
Complications of tracheostomy
  Stomal infection
  Stomal hemorrhage
  Excessive cuff pressure
Infection
  Elevated temperature
  Purulent aspirate

EQUIPMENT
Tracheostomy tube
  Size
  Type: cuffed versus uncuffed
  Tubes used for weaning from mechanical ventilation
    Fenestrate tube
    Tracheostomy buttons

Immediate postoperative care

See Immediate Postoperative Care (p. 54)
Maintain patent airway
  Administer humidification to tracheostomy *to liquefy
    secretions and prevent drying of trachea*
  Suction prn; need for suctioning is determined by
    auscultation of chest for breath sounds qh
    Suction when crackles and rhonchi over large air-
      ways are heard
    Use sterile technique when suctioning secretions
    Hyperoxygenate and hyperinflate patient's lungs for
      four or five breaths before suctioning *to prevent
      hypoxia*
  Clean inner cannula (if present) q2h to 4h and prn
  Avoid occluding airway with bed linen or when turn-
    ing patient
  Tape tracheostomy obturator to head of bed

Have standby tracheostomy tube available: same size and type

Have hand-held resuscitator with adaptor at bedside

Elevate head of bed 45 to 60 degrees; prevent forward flexion of neck

Remove pillow if necessary

Place small towel under shoulder area

Administer oxygen or mechanical ventilation as ordered; see appropriate standard

If a cuffed tracheostomy tube is used

Maintain inflated cuff with either MLT or MOV technique; test pressure in inflated cuff q8h as indicated; cuff pressure should remain <20 mm Hg

Use a low-pressure, cuffed tube

Auscultate chest for breath sounds q2h to 4h; report diminished or absent breath sounds to physician

Monitor BP, P, R, and rectal T q4h for 48 hr, then qid

Maintain NPO

Assess stoma and neck q2h to 4h as indicated; report a constant ooze, subcutaneous emphysema, pulsation of tracheostomy tube

Assist and teach patient to turn, cough, and deep breathe q2h

Ongoing care

Continue with immediate postoperative care and decrease frequency of nursing functions as patient's condition improves

Maintain diet as ordered

Assess swallowing ability

NOTE: Feedings may begin with nasogastric tube until swallowing ability returns

Begin feedings with semisolid foods (e.g., gelatin)

Inflate cuff before feedings and leave inflated for 30 min after each feeding

Test swallowing reflex with gelatin; have suctioning equipment available

Observe for signs of aspiration and tracheo-esophageal fistula

Cleanse skin around stoma q4h and prn

Wash with hydrogen peroxide

Rinse with saline solution

Pat dry

Change and secure tracheostomy ties prn

Place 4 × 4 inch gauze under tracheostomy tube

Perform tracheostomy care

Postintubation: q4h for 2 days

Routine care: q8h and prn

Be aware that physician may change tracheostomy tube daily using progressively smaller sizes

If tracheostomy is permanent, begin to demonstrate tracheostomy care while patient watches in mirror

Establish means of communication

Have pad and pencil, Magic Slate, or communication board available

Avoid asking questions that require *yes* or *no* answers

Wait for patient to write answer; do not anticipate end of sentence

Read statements aloud

Encourage patient to communicate feelings

Provide emotional support

Encourage communication with significant other; help visitors and staff not to exclude patient from conversation or talk exclusively to one another

Remain with patient as much as possible

Answer call light promptly

Deal with fear of suffocation and helplessness

Decannulate tracheostomy as ordered

Be aware that a fenestrated tube may be used for decannulation process

Partially plug tracheostomy tube

Make sure cuff is deflated throughout procedure

Observe patient for respiratory obstruction

Progressively increase size of cork until tracheostomy is completely occluded; notify physician when patient is able to tolerate complete occlusion of tracheostomy for 24 hr

If tracheostomy is long term or permanent, provide means of communication

Pad and pencil

Magic Slate or communication board

Call light within reach

Tap bell

Initiate instruction on the following:

Care of tracheostomy and stoma; discuss and demonstrate; provide mirror

Handwashing procedure

Suctioning procedure before tracheostomy care: clean procedure, not sterile

Care of inner cannula: clean procedure, not sterile

Changing of tracheostomy ties

Cleansing skin around stoma bid

Use hydrogen peroxide

Rinse with water

Pat dry

Understand that patient may not be motivated to participate initially

Have patient shower daily

Direct spray below neck

Cover tracheostomy with waterproof material

Patient/family teaching

Ensure the patient and significant other(s) know and understand

Purpose of tracheostomy

Care of tracheostomy tube and stoma

Importance of clean not sterile technique; need to wash hands before handling equipment: gloves not necessary unless another person is cleaning tracheostomy

Changing tracheostomy ties

Tracheostomy dressings are not recommended unless excessive secretion occurs

Importance of reporting signs and symptoms of skin irritation, infection, or changes in secretions

Humidification and infection control measures

Safety measures such as having an extra tracheostomy tube and suction equipment available

Home care considerations

Provide referral as necessary to the following:

Home health agency for follow-up care

Durable medical equipment company for required equipment for home therapy: suction equipment, humidifier, tracheostomy supplies

Diet

Maintain as ordered

Explain that tracheostomy tubes at home do not usually have cuffs that need inflating during eating

Encourage patient to force fluids to 3000 ml/day unless contraindicated *to help liquefy secretions*

ADLs

Explain need for daily shower; when showering use a shower hose and direct spray below neck; avoid getting soap into stoma

Instruct male patients to shave with electric razor or safety razor; avoid getting lather into stoma

Encourage to exercise to tolerance; continue work, hobbies, and activities except swimming; plan regular rest periods as needed

Keep stoma covered at all times; wear clothing with high necklines and scarves to protect against foreign materials and warm air

Avoid areas with excessive dust, fumes, aerosols, smoke, and powder

Avoid extremes in temperatures, which can irritate tracheal mucosa

Wear medical alert identification indicating neck breather for emergency situations

Avoid persons with URIs

Explain importance of ongoing outpatient care and physician visits

Explain importance of covering stoma when coughing and need to report persistent cough or change in color of sputum to physician

Teach how to perform a *glottal stop* for secretion removal: take a deep breath then momentarily occlude tracheostomy tube opening; simultaneously cough and move the finger from the opening; this substitutes for the usual way intrathoracic pressure is increased to move secretions into the trachea

Report any respiratory distress to physician

Discuss need to use commercial humidifier or pan of water on stove to add comfort and prevent encrustation; explain importance of changing water daily to prevent growth of microorganisms

Explain the importance of not using tobacco and refer to stop smoking groups as indicated

Teach name of medications, dosage, time of administration, purpose, and side effects

Discuss the need to avoid taking over-the-counter medications without physician approval

Demonstrate clean technique for tracheostomy care

Clean around stoma with mild soap and water as part of hygiene

A pipe cleaner can be used to clean the inner cannula; rinse with running tap water

For plastic tubes: use a clean bowl with half-strength solution of hydrogen peroxide and tap water to clean the tracheostomy tube

Demonstrate suctioning technique

Spontaneously breathing patient: three or four deep breaths before and after suctioning is usually sufficient for hyperoxygenation

Patients not immunocompromised may use clean technique for suctioning

Describe care and cleaning of suction equipment

Rinse suction catheter and allow to dry thoroughly between uses

Store in clean, self-sealing plastic bag

Catheters may be cleaned with hydrogen peroxide and water and used for multiple days

After rinsing thoroughly in running water, soak in hydrogen peroxide 5 min, then rinse thoroughly

Place in boiling water 10 to 15 min and allow to air dry on clean towel

Discard catheters when secretions cannot be completely removed

Assess body image, self-esteem, and sexuality and plan interventions as tolerated

Pulse Oximetry Monitoring

A noninvasive monitor used to measure oxygen saturation of functional hemoglobin (Figure 5-11)

Indications: borderline oxygenation especially: FIO_2 delivery of >50%, PEEP on ventilator >10 cm H_2O; unstable or uncertain pulmonary status; diseases commonly associated with hypoxemia; rehabilitation of patients with increased activity levels following respiratory failure

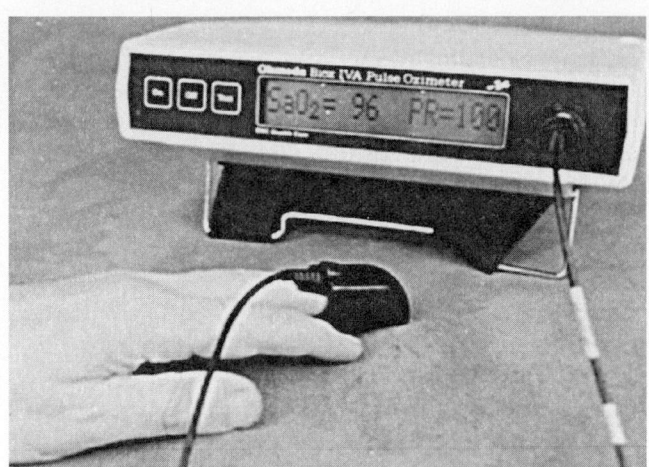

Figure 5-11 Portable pulse oximeter displays oxygen saturation and pulse rate. (Courtesy Ohmeda, Boulder, Colo.)

Assessment

Objective data

Saturation of hemoglobin (SpO_2): normal 96% to 100%, however 95% is usually acceptable; an SaO_2 <70% is life threatening

P, BP

Routine respiratory assessment (see Respiratory failure p. 309)

Activities that may positively or negatively affect oxygenation: suctioning, repositioning, changes in FIO_2, PEEP, medication, and clinical condition)

Ongoing care

Identify type of probe/sensors (see Figure 5-11) and select site by assessing area for warmth, capillary refill, and confirmation of arterial pulse

Place the window for the light source and the photodector directly opposite each other on each side of the arterial bed to ensure accuracy

Assess tissue at sensor site and rotate site q8h and prn to prevent tissue necrosis in hypoxemic patient

Set alarm limits and trouble shoot according to specific patient needs

Shield the sensor from extreme light: heat lamps, procedure lights

Remove nail polish or choose another site because it may interfere with light transmission

Patient/family teaching

Teach the pulse oximetry indications, use of equipment, and SpO_2 values expected

Explain alarms and problems that can cause false alarming

Continuous Mechanical Ventilation

A method of providing ventilatory support for those patients who are unable to spontaneously maintain adequate oxygenation of the blood, with or without carbon dioxide retention; two categories of ventilators are positive pressure (volume-cycled or pressure-cycled) and negative pressure (iron lung, cuirass), which is not commonly used; examples of time, volume-cycled, positive-pressure ventilators are Siemann's Servo 300, Puritan-Bennett 7200, Siemann's Servo 900C, Bear 1000, and Bird 8400ST. Volume-cycled ventilators include Bennett MA3 and the Bourns Bear 1 and 2. Pressure-cycled ventilators include the Bird Mark 7 and 8 and the Bennett PR2.

● Care of Patient on Continuous Mechanical Ventilation

Assessment

Subjective data

Apprehension
Anxiety
Dependence on ventilator
Difficulty in breathing

Objective data

Position of airway
  Endotracheal tube
  Tracheostomy
Patency of airway
Respiratory distress
  Tachypnea
  Tachycardia
  Restlessness
  Anxiety (an early sign of hypoxemia)
  Diaphoresis
  Pallor
  Cyanosis
Breath sounds
  Diminished
  Absent
  Crackles
  Rhonchi
Respiratory acidosis (acidemia)
  Decreased pH: <7.4 mm Hg
  Elevated $PaCO_2$: >45 mm Hg
Respiratory alkalosis (alkalemia)
  Increased pH: >7.4 mm Hg
  Decreased $PaCO_2$: <35 mm Hg

Pulse oximetry saturation ≤90%
Hypoxemia
Sputum
  Amount
  Color
  Consistency
Atelectasis

Potential complications

Disconnection from ventilator
Acid-base imbalance
Respiratory infection
Oxygen toxicity (time and dose related)
  Diminished breath sounds
  Crackles
  Decreased lung compliance
  Decreased VC
  Decreased $Paco_2$ while using same oxygen concentration
  Changes on chest x-ray examination
  Visual impairment
  Papilledema
Fluid and electrolyte imbalance
  Dehydration
  Positive water balance
Decreased cardiac output
Pneumothorax
Barotrauma
GI bleeding

Acute care

Assess quality and rate of respirations
Assess for bilateral chest movement
Ensure that respirations are in phase with the ventilator
Maintain patent airway
  Suction prn; determine need for suctioning by auscultating chest for breath sounds qh—
    suction when crackles or rhonchi are present
    Hyperoxygenate and hyperinflate lungs for four or
    five breaths before suctioning secretions
  Suction patient with closed ventilation suction system
  Monitor pulse oximetry saturation
Keep hand-held resuscitator with adaptor and mask at
  bedside
See Tracheostomy (p. 319)
See Endotracheal tube (p. 317)
Administer medications as ordered
  Sedatives
  Morphine sulfate
  Neuromuscular blocking agents
Monitor ABGs as indicated
Assess BP, R, and apical pulse q1h to 2h
Check rectal T q4h

Auscultate breath sounds q1h to 2h, reporting any
  changes indicating progressive disease
Maintain position of optimal ventilation; elevate head
  of bed 45 to 90 degrees; turn q1h to 2h
  and prn, alternating postural drainage positions
Document ventilator settings q4h to 8h or as indicated;
  readjust as indicated
  FIo_2; measure after suctioning
  Tidal volume (V_T)
  Airway pressure
  Maintain temperature in inspiratory tubing between
    89.6° and 95°F (32° and 35°C)
  Check ventilatory alarms
Administer parenteral fluids as ordered
Provide nutritional support
  Assess nutritional status daily
  Administer tube feedings, total parenteral nutrition as
    ordered
Provide emotional support
  Answer call light promptly
  Establish means of communication: pad and pencil,
    Magic Slate, or communication board
  Allow patient sufficient time to communicate thoughts
    and feelings
  Maintain nonstressful environment
  Be calm, confident, and unhurried when caring for
    patient
  Encourage communication with significant
    other(s)

Ongoing care: subacute

Continue with acute care and decrease frequency of
  nursing functions as patient's condition improves
Wean patient off respirator as ordered
  Obtain baseline respiratory rate, VC, and V_T
  Explain weaning process thoroughly
  Remain with patient during weaning process
  Monitor R and apical pulse q5min to 15min after removal from ventilator
  Place on ventilator immediately if respiratory distress
    occurs
  Be prepared to repeat weaning process several times
    if necessary

Convalescent care

See standard of care for primary condition

Patient/family teaching

Ensure that patient and significant other(s) know and
  understand
  Purpose of ventilator
  Importance of breathing with ventilator

Importance of coughing up secretions
Importance of artificial airway
Need to avoid placing any tension on airway; to never touch airway with hands
Need to communicate in writing
Technique for suctioning
Ventilator alarms and their implications
Use of manual resuscitator bag

Home care considerations

Explain to patient/family that home ventilators are portable, easy to use, and small; home ventilation requires a great deal of commitment on the part of the family or significant other; refer to durable medical equipment company for equipment
Teach care of tracheostomy and suctioning; see Tracheostomy (p. 319)
Demonstrate ventilator connections, alarms, trouble shooting, care, and cleaning
Teach how to drain and change tubing
  Drain tubing to prevent fluid from entering lungs and partial obstruction of system
  Properly draining and changing tubing is an infection-control measure
  Demonstrate manual resuscitator bag and keep one at home in case of power failure
Activity
  Teach and discuss importance of ROM exercises and chest mobility exercises if patient is unable to ambulate
  Encourage patient to sit up in a chair as much as tolerated
  Ambulation with assistance is possible with small, battery-powered ventilators placed on a small cart
Diet
  Diet as ordered
  Patient may be able to eat: check with physician for diet allowances; see Tracheostomy (p. 319)
  If unable to eat, enteral or parenteral feedings are required
Assess body image, self-esteem, and sexuality and plan appropriate interventions
Refer to VNA or other home health agency for follow-up care
Refer family to support group for emotional support

● Pressure-Limited, Positive-Pressure Ventilator

Delivers a volume of air until a preset pressure is reached; used primarily for IPPB treatments in the adult population

Assessment and care of equipment/home care considerations

Attached to gas source
Connecting tubing
  Patent
  Free of excessive moisture
Air leaks
  Cuff of endotracheal tube
  Cuff of tracheostomy
Patent airway
Adequate humidification
  Nebulizer
  Heated humidification
Temperature of inspired gas
Settings as ordered
  Respiratory rate: should not be <12/min
  Oxygen concentration: air-mix control
  Inspiratory pressure control
  Apnea control
  Sensitivity control

Ongoing care

Maintain inspiratory rate and respiratory pressure as ordered
  Patent airway
  System free of leaks
  Connective tubing patent and free of excessive moisture
Be aware that inspiratory, positive-pressure ventilators may not have alarm systems
Remain with patient as much as possible
Determine respiratory rate, oxygen concentration, and inspiratory pressure setting by ABGs
Establish flow sheet
  Record ventilator settings
  Record laboratory values
Maintain oxygen concentration as ordered; measure FIO_2 q8h and prn
Maintain respiratory rate as ordered
  Measure Tidal volume q8h and prn
  Auscultate chest for breath sounds qh
Provide humidification
Make sure that equipment continues to cycle when cuff is deflated
Have patient sigh q15min or as ordered; use hand-held resuscitator
Change connecting tubing, nebulizer, and humidification system q24h; replace with sterile equipment

● Volume-Cycled, Positive-Pressure Ventilator

Delivers breathing gas at a predetermined volume; once the desired volume has been delivered; the ventilator will cycle and patient will passively exhale

Assessment and care of equipment

Electrical system
  Plugged in
  Alarms on
Connecting tubing
  Patent
  Free of excessive moisture
Air leaks
  Cuff of endotracheal tube
  Cuff of tracheostomy
Patent airway
Adequate humidification
  Heated humidification
  Nebulizer
Temperature of inspired gas
Settings as ordered
  Alarms
  Flow rate
  Inspiratory pressure
  Tidal volume (10 to 15 ml/kg body weight)
  PEEP
  CPAP
  Pressure support
  Ventilator rate: 10 to 16 breaths/min
  Oxygen concentration
  Sigh pressure
  Sigh volume
  Number of sighs per hr
  Ventilatory mode
    Control
    Assist
    Assist-controlled
    Synchronized intermittent mandatory ventilation
      (SIMV or IMV)
    Sensitivity
    Peak airway pressure (<40 cm H_2O)
    I:E ratio

Ongoing care

Maintain tidal volume as ordered
  Patent airway
  System free of leaks
  Connective tubing patent and free of excessive moisture
Determine ventilator settings by ABGs

Establish flow sheet
  Record ventilator settings
  Record laboratory values
Maintain oxygen concentration as ordered (determined by PaO_2); measure FIO_2 q8h and prn
Maintain respiratory rate as ordered
Provide heated humidification
Remove excessive water in tubing
Have patient sigh q15min or as ordered; sigh pressure and volume as ordered
Avoid turning alarm system off
Measure V_T q8h and prn
Test alarm system q8h
Change connecting tubing, nebulizer, and humidification q24h; replace with sterile equipment

Intermittent Positive-Pressure Breathing

intermittent positive-pressure ventilator: A ventilator that delivers breathing gas until equilibrium is established between the patient's lungs and the ventilator; depends on pressure buildup in the patient's lungs rather than on time or volume; a valve mechanism shuts off the gas flow when the pressure has been reached and patient exhales passively; should be used only after less expensive modalities have been tried

Pretreatment assessment

Observations/findings

BP
Pulse
Color
Respiratory effort
Breath sounds

Preparation

Observe BP and apical pulse before treatment
Auscultate chest for breath sounds
Place patient in sitting position
Prepare machine
  Secure all tubing connections
  Place medication or saline solution in nebulizer
  Set pressure and oxygen concentration as ordered
  Control nebulizer to produce fine mist

Preprocedure teaching

Explain procedure and what is expected of patient
  Concentrate on using diaphragm

Breathe at normal rate through mouth
Allow machine to fill lungs to desired volume
Prolong expiration
Purse lips around mouthpiece

Assessment during treatment

Subjective data

Fatigue
Restlessness, nervousness
Chest pain

Objective data

Respiratory rate
Chest expansion
Sudden respiratory distress
Hyperventilation
  Circumoral numbness
  Tingling of fingers
  Dizziness
Tachycardia
Function of equipment

Ongoing care

Take pulse one or two times during treatment
Remain with patient during initial treatment
Stop treatment if sudden respiratory distress or chest
  pain occurs
Have patient deep breathe slowly one or two times dur-
  ing treatment
Have patient cough one or two times during and after
  treatment
Check pressure gauge and adjust flow to avoid negative
  inspiratory pressure
Administer oral hygiene after treatment

Patient/family teaching

Ensure that patient and significant other know and un-
  derstand
  Need to follow physician's instructions regarding use
    of IPPB
  Need to cough during and immediately after treat-
    ment
  Importance of using saline solution or medication in
    nebulizer
  Symptoms of respiratory distress to report to physi-
    cian
  Need to stop treatment if dizziness, nervousness,
    chest pain, rapid pulse, or sudden respiratory dis-
    tress occurs during treatment

Symptoms of URI to report to physician
Name of medication, dosage, time of administration,
  purpose, and side effects
Need to avoid taking over-the-counter medications
  without physician approval

Home care considerations

Ensure that patient and significant other(s) demon-
  strate
  Understanding of importance and purpose of treatments
  Preparation of machine for treatment
  Use of machine during treatment
  How to adjust pressure gauge and flow to avoid nega-
    tive inspiratory pressure
  IPPB procedure
    Take pulse one or two times during treatment
    Deep breathing slowly one or two times during treat-
      ment
    Coughing techniques
    Stop treatment if sudden respiratory distress or
      chest pain occurs and contact physician
    Administer oral hygiene after treatment
    Care and cleaning of equipment
Explain importance of ongoing outpatient care and
  physician visits
Teach importance of avoiding persons with URIs
Refer to home health agency for follow-up care

Incentive Spirometer

*A mechanical device that assists patient in maintaining
  maximal inspiratory effort; effective when used by
  postoperative patients to prevent development of
  atelectasis and pneumonia; more physiologic and less
  hazardous than IPPB because it depends only on the
  patient's inspiratory effort (not on electricity, batteries,
  or gas)*

Assessment

Observations/findings

  PATIENT
Presence or absence of pain
Motivation
Weakness
Hyperventilation
  Dizziness
  Lightheadedness
  Numbness around mouth and nose
  Tingling in fingers and toes
Cough
  Productive

Nonproductive
Breath sounds
  Diminished
  Absent
  Crackles
  Rhonchi over large airways

    EQUIPMENT
Type of device
Tidal volume

Ongoing care/home care considerations

Patient must be alert and cooperative
Assess degree of pain present
  Administer analgesics as ordered
  Assess effectiveness of pain relief measure(s)
Elevate head of bed 60 to 90 degrees or have patient sit in chair
Assist and teach patient to use incentive spirometer
  Exhale slowly
  Place mouthpiece in mouth between teeth
  Close lips tightly around mouthpiece
  Inhale through mouth only, taking a slow, deep breath
  Hold breath for 3 to 5 seconds
  Remove mouthpiece from mouth
  Exhale slowly
Repeat procedure 10 to 20 times qh
Caution patient not to breathe too rapidly
Observe for signs of hyperventilation; stop use of incentive spirometer if dizziness or lightheadedness occurs
Assist and teach patient to cough after using incentive spirometer
Auscultate chest for breath sounds q4h
  Assist and teach patient to cough if crackles or rhonchi are heard
  Report diminished or absent breath sounds to physician
Monitor patient's progress q4h
Increase V_T as patient tolerates it

Patient/family teaching

Ensure that patient and significant other(s) know and understand
  Purpose of incentive spirometer
  Importance of using it 10 to 20 times qh
  Importance of holding breath for 3 to 5 sec
  Need to inhale through mouth
  Importance of not exhaling into apparatus
  Importance of reaching desired V_T
  Importance of coughing after using apparatus

Ensure that patient demonstrates
  Use of incentive spirometer
  Coughing productively

BIBLIOGRAPHY

Abels L: *Critical care nursing: a physiologic approach,* St Louis, 1986, Mosby.

Ahrens TS, Rutherford K: *Essentials of oxygenation,* Boston, 1993, Jones & Bartlett.

Alspach JG: *Core curriculum for critical care nursing,* Philadelphia, 1991, WB Saunders.

Bates DV: *Respiratory function in disease,* Philadelphia, 1989, WB Saunders.

Boggs RL, Wooldridge-King M: *AACN procedure manual for critical care,* ed 3, Philadelphia, 1993, WB Saunders.

Burrell LO: *Adult nursing in hospital and community settings,* Norwalk, Conn, 1992, Appleton & Lange.

Carpenito LJ: *Handbook of nursing diagnosis,* ed 5, Philadelphia, 1993, JB Lippincott.

Clayton DB, Stock YN: *Basic pharmacology for nurses,* ed 10, St Louis, 1993, Mosby.

Corbett JV: *Laboratory tests and diagnostic procedure with nursing diagnoses,* Norwalk, Conn, 1992, Appleton & Lange.

Fischback F: *A manual of laboratory and diagnostic tests,* Philadelphia, 1992, WB Saunders.

Guzzetta CE et al: *Critical care nursing: body-mind-spirit,* ed 3, Boston, 1991, Little, Brown.

Hopp L: Ineffective breathing related to decreased lung expansion, *Nurs Clin North Am* 22:193, 1987.

Hudak CM, Gallo BM: *Critical care nursing: a holistic approach,* ed 6, Philadelphia, 1994, JB Lippincott.

Kidd PS, Wagner KD: *High acuity nursing: preparing for practice in today's health care setting,* Norwalk, Conn, 1992, Appleton & Lange.

Kim MJ, McFarland GK, McLane AM: *Pocket guide to nursing diagnoses,* ed 6, St Louis, 1995, Mosby.

Kinney MR, Packa DR, Dunbar SB: *AACN's clinical reference for critical-care nursing,* ed 3, New York, 1993, McGraw-Hill.

Kozier B et al: *Techniques in clinical nursing,* ed 4, Redwood City, Ga, 1993, Addison Wesley.

Laguatra I, Gerlach MO: *Nutrition in clinical nursing,* Albany, NY, 1990, Delmar.

Lehrer S: *Understanding lung sounds,* ed 2, Philadelphia, 1993, WB Saunders.

Luckmann J, Sorensen K: *Medical-surgical nursing,* ed 4, Philadelphia, 1993, WB Saunders.

McCance KL, Huether SE: *Pathophysiology: the biological basis for disease in adults and children,* ed 2, St Louis, 1994, Mosby.

Schlichtig R, Ayers SM: *Nutritional support of critically ill,* Chicago, 1988, Yearbook Medical Publishers.

Swearingen PL: *Manual of critical care: applying nursing diagnosis to adult critical illness,* ed 3, St Louis, 1995, Mosby.

Sweetwood H: *Nursing in the intensive respiratory care unit,* New York, 1979, Springer Publishing.

Thelan LA et al: *Critical care nursing: diagnosis and management,* ed 2, St Louis, 1994, Mosby.

Thompson JM et al: *Mosby's clinical nursing,* St Louis, 1993, Mosby.

Tierney LM et al: *Current medical diagnosis and treatment,* Norwalk, Conn, 1994, Appleton & Lange.

Weilitz PB: *Pocket guide to respiratory care,* St Louis, 1991, Mosby.

Wilkins R, Shelden R, Krider S: *Clinical assessment in respiratory care,* ed 2, St Louis, 1990, Mosby.

Wilkins RL, Dexler JR: *Respiratory disease: principles of patient care,* Philadelphia, 1993, F.A. Davis & Co.

Wilson S, Thompson JM: *Respiratory disorders,* St Louis, 1990, Mosby.

Wright JE, Shelton BK: *Desk reference for critical care nursing,* Boston, 1993, Jones & Bartlett.

ADULT PNEUMONIA CARE PATH

PATIENT PROBLEM

1. Impaired gas exchange related to disease process.
2. Alteration in body temperature (hyperthermia) related to disease process.
3. Fluid volume deficit related to hyperthermia, excess insensible loss, and poor intake.
4. Knowledge deficit related to disease process

ADDRESSOGRAPH

PATIENT OUTCOMES

1. Oxygen saturation > 94% and lung sounds clear before discharge.
2. Temperature will be 100° or below for 24 hours day before discharge.
3. Patient will be hydrated upon discharge as shown by intake and output within 100 cc and have a PO fluid intake of at least 2000 cc per day.
4. Patient will communicate discharge instruction.

DAY	DAY 1 DATE	DAY 2 DATE	DAY 3 DATE	DAY 4 DATE	DISCHARGE DAY 5 DATE
	Emergency Department	Inpatient			
History Physical		Prior history pneumonia, COPD, asthma, TB Wheeze, rales, respiratory distress, shortness of breath, effusion			
Tests	☐ Chest x-ray, if significant effusion consider thoracentesis ☐ CBC, Lytes, Creat, Sputum gram stain STAT, Sputum C + S, Induce PRN ☐ Blood Cult x 2 if temp >101 ☐ Oxygen saturation-oximetry, ABG if indicated	☐ Pulse oximetry if on oxygen ☐ PPD, cocci, controls if indicated	☐ Pulse oximetry if on oxygen	☐ If oxygen saturation greater than or equal to 95% do room air oxygen saturation	☐ If oxygen saturation greater than or equal to 95% do room air oxygen saturation	None
Treatment	☐ Suction if unable to cough	Assessment for following: ☐ Chest PT ☐ Cough, deep breath, q2h ☐ Incentive Spirometry q2h ☐ Deep suction PRN	Assessment for following: ☐ Chest PT ☐ Cough, deep breath, q2h ☐ Incentive Spirometry q2h ☐ Deep suction PRN	☐ Continue treatments if indicated	☐ Continue treatments if indicated	None
Meds	☐ IVs ☐ Parenteral antibiotics oxygen if saturation <94% ☐ Nebulizer/metered dose inhaler with spacer (MDI) if indicated	☐ IVs ☐ Parenteral Antibiotics adjusted for gram stain ☐ Tylenol for temp >101 ☐ Med for pain ☐ Nebulizer/MDI	☐ DC IVs if PO intake tolerated ☐ Heparin lock ☐ Parenteral antibiotics ☐ Tylenol for temp >101 ☐ Med for pain ☐ Nebulizer/MDI	☐ DC Tylenol and pain meds ☐ Heparin lock ☐ Parenteral antibiotics ☐ DC oxygen if indicated ☐ Antibiotics adjusted for sputum/blood cultures if indicated	☐ Heparin lock ☐ Parenteral antibiotics	☐ DC Heparin lock ☐ DC parenteral antibiotics ☐ Discharge on PO antibiotics
Diet	☐ Diet & fluids as tolerated	☐ Regular diet ☐ Encourage fluids	☐ Regular diet ☐ Encourage fluids	☐ Regular diet ☐ Encourage fluids	☐ Regular diet ☐ Encourage fluids	☐ Regular diet

DAY	DATE — DAY 1		DATE — DAY 2	DATE — DAY 3	DATE — DAY 4	DATE — DISCHARGE DAY 5
	Emergency Department	Inpatient				
Activity or Treatment	☐ Bed rest	☐ BRP with assist and ad lib if tolerated	☐ OOB in chair for 20 min. BID ☐ BRP ☐ Ambulate with assists × 1 or ad lib if tolerated	☐ Ambulate × 3 in hall or ad lib if tolerated	☐ Ambulate × 5 in hall or ad lib if tolerated	☐ Ambulate ad lib
Assessment and Evaluation	☐ Collect culture specimens ☐ Induce sputum if needed ☐ If sputum collection attempts are unsuccessful, notify physician ☐ Start antibiotics	☐ Assess lung sounds ☐ Monitor temp. q4h ☐ I&O ☐ Assist with care due to shortness of breath ☐ Document sputum production and color ☐ Pulse oximetry daily if on oxygen	☐ I&O ☐ Encourage fluids at least 2000 cc/day ☐ Assess lung sounds ☐ Monitor temp q shift ☐ Assist with care ☐ Document sputum production and color ☐ Pulse oximetry daily if on oxygen	☐ Assess lung sounds ☐ Document sputum production & color ☐ Monitor temp q shift ☐ D/C I&O ☐ Encourage increased self-care ☐ Pulse oximetry daily if on oxygen	☐ Monitor incentive spirometry ☐ Assess lung sounds ☐ Document any sputum ☐ Temp routine ☐ Increased self-care ☐ Ask patient to arrange transportation in preparation for discharge	☐ Discharge instructions: Include incentive spirometry, fluid intake, MDI if needed ☐ Medication instructions
Teaching	☐ Discuss initial plan of care with patient	☐ Discuss plan of care with patient ☐ Inspirometer, cough, deep breathe	☐ Discuss plan of care with patient ☐ Teaching continues from Day 1	☐ Discuss plan of care with patient ☐ Patient demonstrates appropriate MDI, deep breathing and coughing technique	☐ Discuss plan of care with patient ☐ Patient demonstrates appropriate MDI, deep breathing and coughing technique	☐ Discuss plan of care with patient ☐ Discharge instructions ☐ Vaccinations ☐ Smoking cessation
Discharge Planning			☐ Patient/family assessment	☐ Post-hospital plans documented if needed. Discuss tentative discharge date with physician.		☐ Arrangements made

DATE	SHIFT	SIGNATURE/TITLE	DATE	SHIFT	SIGNATURE/TITLE

Admission Date: _____

Discharge Date and Time: _____

Actual LOS: _____

Date Care Path Discontinued: _____

Implement Compromised Respiratory Status Standard

VARIANCE REPORT

DATE	VARIATION	CAUSE	KEY	ACTION TAKEN	SIGNATURE	DATE RESOLVED	SIGNATURE

CHECK IF PATIENT OUTCOME WAS ATTAINED BEFORE DISCHARGE:

☐ Oxygen Saturation is above 94% and lung sounds are clear

☐ Temperature is 100° F or below during the last 24 hours

☐ The patient has taken oral fluids of 2000 ml/day. I and O is within 500 ml.

☐ The patient is able to communicate discharge instructions.

IF NOT, PLAN FOR RESOLUTION:

_____
_____
_____
_____

KEY:
1. PATIENT
2. SYSTEM

PATIENT LEARNING CHECKLIST page 1 of 1

DIAGNOSIS PNEUMONIA

ADDRESSOGRAPH

INTERVENTION CODES
A. QUESTIONS ANSWERED.
B. INFORMATION PROVIDED. LIST WRITTEN MATERIALS.
C. TASK DEMONSTRATED.
D. MULTIDISCIPLINARY REFERRALS. SPECIFY.
E. REFER TO CLASS.

PATIENT/SIGNIFICANT OTHER CODES
A. NEEDS INSTRUCTION/REINFORCEMENT.
B. DEMONSTRATES VERBAL UNDERSTANDING.
C. RETURNS DEMONSTRATION.
D. SEE FLOW RECORD.

TEACH/DEMONSTRATE	CODE	DATE	TIME	INITIAL	CODE	DATE	TIME	INITIAL	COMMENTS
A. Signs and symptoms of respiratory infection or bronchospasm: 1. elevated temperature 2. changes in character of sputum 3. increased respiratory rate 4. shortness of breath 5. wheeze or stridor									
B. Dietary regimen: 1. Nutritional Services Consultation									
C. Activity progression regimen: 1. Pace activities during day to avoid fatigue. 2. Arrange activities after respiratory treatment.									
D. Do not smoke or allow smoking in the home: 1. Refer to Health Education Stop Smoking Program (372-3357).									
E. Breathing techniques: 1. Respiratory Care Services consult 2. pursed-lip breathing 3. minineb/MDI 4. Refer to Health Education (372-3314).									
F. Adult Immunizations 1. Discuss pamphlet 2. Refer to physician									
G. Establish your care with a personal physician.									

INITIAL	SIGNATURE	TITLE	INITIAL	SIGNATURE	TITLE

Used by permission of Kaiser Permanente Medical Center, Kaiser Foundation Hospital, Martinez, California.

ADULT PNEUMONIA CARE PATH*
PATIENT COPY

	ADMISSION		DISCHARGE
TESTS	• Receive diagnostic examinations as ordered by your physician.	• Measurement of the oxygen level in your blood stream if you are receiving oxygen. • Skin tests to rule out other causes of your illness if ordered by your physician.	
TREATMENT		• Discuss with your nurse the need to cough and deep breathe every 2 hours. • You will be instructed on the use of incentive spirometry.	
MEDICATIONS	• Intravenous fluids and antibiotics if ordered. • Oxygen if needed. • Respiratory Therapy will instruct you in the use of a Metered Dose Inhaler if indicated.	• Tylenol for fever if needed. • Discuss pain medication needs with your nurse. • Intravenous fluids will be discontinued if you are drinking adequate amounts of fluid. • IV entry port. • Discuss need for continued pain medication with your nurse. • Discontinue oxygen if indicated.	• Discontinue the IV entry port. • Intravenous antibiotics discontinued. • Discharge on oral antibiotics if ordered.
DIET	• Diet and fluids as tolerated.	• Regular diet. • Discuss with nurse the need to drink an adequate amount of fluids. • Regular diet. • Adequate fluid intake.	

Used by permission of Kaiser Permanente Medical Center, Kaiser Foundation Hospital, Martinez, California.

*Individual patient's course of therapy may vary from this guideline.

Continued.

COPD Clinical Pathway

Category/Day	Day 1/Unit	Day 2	Day 3	Day 4	Day 5
Diagnostic Testing	If test not done in ED, Test from ED/Day 1 as indicated	ABG or Pulse Ox ----------------------> or room air for Medicare	Theo level monitored for interacting medications (RN) --------> Antibiotics that interact with Theophylline: Erthromycin, Calrthromycin (Blaxin), Ciprofloxacin (Cipro), Ofloxacin (Floxin) CBC or <----------------------> CXR or <-----------> M7 (If on diuretics) Sputum results available on chart (lab)		
Patient Care and Treatments	RN/RT Assessment Safety Precautions (RN) Oxygen (RT) Vital Signs Q4 (RN) Admission weight (RN) Nebulizer (RT) Chest PT* Fan* I&O measured (RN) ---- Elimination evaluation maintained q shift (RN))	Vital Signs q_____ Daily Weight (RN) ---- ----------■ Measure output if needed (RN) -------- Bowel Assessment (RN) --	Vital Signs routine (RN) -----------------■ RN performs inhaler technique per protocol (see below) ----------------■ -----------------------■		 ■ -----------------■
Nutrition	Diet (type) Circle amount consumed: Breakfast: all 3/4 1/2 1/4 0 NPO Lunch: all 3/4 1/2 1/4 0 NPO Dinner: all 3/4 1/2 1/4 0 NPO Supplement (type) _____ frequency _____	Diet (type) Circle amount consumed (RN): Breakfast: all 3/4 1/2 1/4 0 NPO Lunch: all 3/4 1/2 1/4 0 NPO Dinner: all 3/4 1/2 1/4 0 NPO Supplement (type) _____ frequency _____	Diet (type) Circle amount consumed (RN): Breakfast: all 3/4 1/2 1/4 0 NPO Lunch: all 3/4 1/2 1/4 0 NPO Dinner: all 3/4 1/2 1/4 0 NPO Supplement (type) _____ frequency _____	Diet (type) Circle amount consumed (RN): Breakfast: all 3/4 1/2 1/4 0 NPO Lunch: all 3/4 1/2 1/4 0 NPO Dinner: all 3/4 1/2 1/4 0 NPO Supplement (type) _____ frequency _____	Diet (type) Circle amount consumed (RN): Breakfast: all 3/4 1/2 1/4 0 NPO Lunch: all 3/4 1/2 1/4 0 NPO Dinner: all 3/4 1/2 1/4 0 NPO Supplement (type) _____ frequency _____
Activity	BR with BRP with assistance	Plan ADL's around --------------------------------- patient's limitations Up to chair BID (RN)	Ambulate in room (RN)	Ambulate in hall (RN)	■ Discharge (MD)
Education	Orientation to hospital and unit (RN) Respiratory Therapy instructions as tolerated	Respiratory educational package for patient/ family to include (RT): – Smoking cessation – COPD video – Inhaler technique	Follow–up teaching (RT) -------■ Patient feedback (RT) ---------■ Consider diet instructions (RD) Reinforcement of MDI instruction technique (RN)		Discharge instruction information reviewed with patient/family (RN)
Consults	Pulmonologist* Discharge Planning Counseling: – Coping Mechanics – Pulmonary Rehab – Self–esteem	Initial Assessment completed & D/C options communicated (PFS) Dietitian Nutrition Screening/Needs Assessment Consider Calorie Count (RD) Pastoral Care* Counselor		Discharge Plan in place (PFS)	
Medications	Theophylline IV/PO ---- Steroids IV/PO -------- Anxiety meds Antibiotics IV/PO ----- Expectorants ---------- Cough Suppressant ---- Diuretics* IV/Med Lock ---------- Vitamin/Mineral Supplement*	-------------------------- -------------------------- -------------------------- -------------------------- -------------------------- -------------- Med Lock----■	Consider change to PO meds (MD)----------------------------------- Consider move to MDI's (MD)-----------------------	 ■ ■ ■	Relabel MDIs for home use (RP) RN insturcts patient that serevent inhaler is not used for acute bronchi spasm

NOTE: CLINICAL PATHWAYS ARE GUIDELINES FOR CONSIDERATION WHICH MAY BE MODIFIED ACCORDING TO INDIVIDUAL PATIENT NEEDS.

NOTE: * If patient condition indicates service is necessary

KEY TO DISCIPLINES PERFORMING SERVICES

RN – Registered Nurse	MD – Physician
RT – Respiratory Therapist	RP – Registered Pharmacist
RD – Registered Dietitian	Lab – Laboratory
PFS – Patient and Family Services	US – Unit Secretary
CM – Case Manager	PT – Physical Therapist

Protocol for MDI Administration "Without" Spacer
* Shake inhaler
* Hold inhaler in front of your mouth, do not close lips around mouthpiece
* Exhale completely
* Inhale slowly while you depress inhaler
* Hold your breath for 5 – 10 seconds
* Exhale normally
* If second dose is needed, wait 2 minutes between puffs

Protocol for MDI Administration "With" Spacer
* Remove cap from MDI and spacer
* Insert inhaler mouthpiece into opening at end of spacer
* Holding spacer with inhaler, shake 3 – 4 times
* Exhale normally, place mouthpiece of spacer in mouth and close lips
* Spray only one puff from inhaler into spacer and immediately begin to inhale slowly through your mouth until a full breath has been taken
* Hold breath for 5 – 10 seconds. Exhale
* If second dose is needed, wait 2 minutes between puffs

Form Date: June 14, 1995
Form Revision Date: August 16, 1995

COPD Clinical Pathway

PATIENT'S NAME:

OUTCOMES	Day 1/Unit	Day 2	Day 3	Day 4	Day 5
	Patient Age Appropriate Safety precautions taken		Patient lab values are returning to base line		
	Appropriate level of oxygen maintained		Patient exhibits no signs of Theophylline toxicity (1)		
			Patient is tolerating PO meds	Patient is independent on MDIs	Patient receives MDIs as relabeled for home use
		Patient activity level increased	Patient activity level increased	Patient activity level increased	Patient activity level increased
	Patient/Family aware of Clinical Path	Patient aware of educational material on disease manage-ment	Patient/Family education retained		Patient/Family aware of signs/symptoms that require patient to contact MD
	Patient/Family aware of activity expectations				
	Patient/Family aware Rex is smoke−free				Patient/Family under-stands instructions for medications
		Patient exhibits bowel function per patient's routine or Bowel Protocol initiated − − − − − − − −	− − − − − − − − − − − − − − − − − −	− − − − − − − − − − − − − − − − − −	− − − − − − − − ■
		Patient/Family under-stands anticipated LOS and D/C options			
	Patient/Family under-stands importance of patient consuming adequate nutrition				Patient nutritional consumption is adequate

Daily Variance Tracing

Variance Type/Date Occured	Initials	Reason/Comment	Initials	Action Taken/Date Resolved
1.				
2.				
3.				
4.				
5.				
6.				
7.				
8.				
9.				
10.				

NOTE: * If patient condition indicates service is necessary.

Form Date: June 14, 1995
Form Revision Date: August 16, 1995

(1) The following antiobiotics interact with Theophylline: Erythromycin, Clirthromycin (Biaxin), Ciprofloxacin (Clpro), Ofloxacin (Floxin), Norfloxacin (Noroxin)

NOTE: CLINICAL PATHWAYS ARE GUIDELINES FOR CONSIDERATION WHICH MAY BE MODIFIED ACCORDING TO INDIVIDUAL PATIENT NEEDS

Digestive System

Gastrointestinal Assessment

● Subjective Data

Mouth, gums, tongue, lips
  Painful
  Tender
  Sores, lesions
Teeth
  Dentures
  Loose teeth
Dysphagia
Eructation
Anorexia, weight loss/gain
Indigestion
Pyrosis (heartburn)
Fullness after eating
Pain, discomfort after eating certain foods
Nausea, vomiting; regurgitation without vomiting; hematemesis
Abdomen
  Painful
  Tender
  Cramping
Fatigue, malaise
Change in eating or bowel habits
Change in color, character, or frequency of stools or urine
Flatulence
Constipation
Diarrhea
Hemorrhoids, bleeding
Painful defecation
Use of laxatives or enemas
Change in skin color or texture; rash or itching
Edema of extremities

Discourage tobacco use *because it increases LES*

EXPECTED OUTCOMES

Patient's calorie and fluid intake is optimal
Electrolytes are within normal limits
Weight is maintained

● **NDX:** Risk for aspiration related to impaired swallowing

Assist and teach patient to cough and deep breathe q4h
Monitor breath sounds q4h
Elevate head of bed 30 to 45 degrees after meals and at bedtime *to prevent regurgitation*
Avoid supine position *to aid digestion*
Provide planned rest periods
Assist with feeding as needed
Administer oral hygiene qid

EXPECTED OUTCOMES

Patient demonstrates correct coughing and breathing techniques
Presents normal breath sounds

● **NDX:** Pain related to esophageal inflammation and/or heartburn

Provide calm, nonstressful environment
Reinforce physician's explanation of disease process
Administer and monitor antacids for effectiveness, side effects
Administer cholinergics and H_2 receptors *to reduce LES pressure*
Provide soothing back rubs *to promote comfort*
Change patient's position in small ways *to promote comfort*
Encourage activities and self-care *to decrease discomfort*

EXPECTED OUTCOMES

Patient reports a decrease in heartburn
Maintains activities at optimal level
Reports no pain or discomfort after eating

Patient/family teaching

Reinforce physician's explanation of disease and treatment goals
Discuss with patient and/or significant other(s) the importance of diet and diet restrictions
Explain need to avoid foods that cause dysphagia
Provide and review high-calorie, high-protein diet instruction sheet if applicable
Encourage increased fluid intake
Advise patient to avoid tobacco, aspirin, phenylbutazone, and excessive intake of high-fat foods

Advise elevating head while sleeping
Discuss methods of avoiding stress
Explain reasons why bending and stooping should be avoided
Discuss methods of avoiding constipation
Recommend high-fiber foods if tolerated
Encourage natural laxatives: bran, prunes, psyllium powder

Home care considerations

Discuss need to avoid weight gain, straining, and/or wearing tight clothing such as belts, girdles
Increase patient's activities to tolerance
Discuss medications: name, dosage, time of administration, purpose, and side effects
Explain importance of follow-up care with physician
Discuss symptoms of recurrence or progression of disease to report to physician (see Assessment p. 345)

● Bleeding Esophageal Varices

A condition usually associated with cirrhosis and portal hypertension in which the small esophageal veins become distended and rupture as a result of the increased pressure in the portal system; may be controlled medically, but surgery may be required

Assessment

Subjective data

Restlessness
Confusion
Anxiety

Objective data

Character, frequency, and amount of hematemesis
Respiratory distress
Altered vital signs
Aspiration of emesis
Disorientation
Dehydration
Electrolyte imbalance
Abdominal distention
Melena
Jaundice

Diagnostic tests

Esophagoscopy
Mesenteric angiography

Sclerotherapy
CBC, platelets, PT, arterial blood gases (ABGs), electrolytes
Blood alcohol
AST, ALT, LDH, alkaline phosphatase
Liver function tests
Guaiac stools for blood

Potential complications

Aspiration pneumonia
Hemorrhage
Shock
Hepatic coma
Death

Collaborative management

Therapeutic management

NPO
Esophagogastric tamponade with suction and pressures to be maintained
Gastric lavages
Parenteral fluids with electrolytes
Fresh whole blood
Indwelling urinary catheter with hourly measurements
Orotracheal suctioning
Oxygen therapy
Central venous pressure (CVP) line or Swan-Ganz catheter
Paracentesis
ABGs
Saline enemas
Vasopressin (Pitressin), neomucin, vitamin K, lactulose
Analgesics, usually phenobarbital
Histamine receptor antagonists (Tagamet, Zantac, Prilosec, Propulsid)
Esophageal sclerotherapy
Surgical intervention
Diet, activity

Nursing management

PATIENT PROBLEMS/NURSING DIAGNOSES

● **NDX:** Risk for aspiration related to esophagogastric tube, impaired swallowing

Maintain bed rest in quiet environment
  Position patient on side during vomiting episodes *to prevent aspiration*
  Elevate head of bed 30 degrees
Perform orotracheal suctioning prn

Auscultate chest for breath sounds q1h to 2h *to prevent respiratory compromise*
Administer oxygen therapy by mask or catheter
Assist and teach patient to turn and deep breathe qh; instruct patient not to cough *because it increases portal pressure*
Administer oral hygiene q1h to 2h; keep mouth and nares well lubricated with petroleum jelly *to promote comfort and skin integrity*

EXPECTED OUTCOMES
Patient presents normal breath sounds
Manages secretions adequately
Demonstrates turning and deep breathing exercises accurately

● **NDX:** Altered tissue perfusion, cardiopulmonary, cerebral, gastrointestinal, renal, peripheral related to hypovolemia

GI system
  Monitor bowel sounds; report changes to physician
  Monitor stools for melena
  Maintain esophagogastric tube
    Sengstaken-Blakemore tube (p. 352)
    Linton tube (p. 352)
    Monitor for signs of complications: aspiration, occlusion of airway, esophageal rupture
  Monitor character and amount of gastric drainage q1h to 2h
  Administer lavages via tube *to decrease bleeding*
  Maintain NPO
Cardiopulmonary system
  Assess for signs of hypovolemia: tachycardia; tachypnea; cold, clammy skin
  Replace blood as needed; monitor for reaction: rash, fever, tachypnea
  Monitor breath sounds
  Provide oxygen prn
  Maintain parenteral fluids with electrolytes, using large-bore catheter *to facilitate blood transfusion*
  Monitor hemoglobin (Hgb), hematocrit (Hct), serum electrolytes, and PT/INR
  Monitor CVP line or Swan-Ganz catheter
  Monitor ABGs
  Monitor BP, R, and apical P q15min to 30min
  Take rectal T q2h while esophagogastric tube is in place
Renal system
  Maintain urinary catheter to gravity drainage
  Measure intake and output qh; if urine output is <50 ml/hr, report to physician
  Monitor specific gravity of urine
  Monitor serum pH, BUN, and creatinine

Cerebral system

Assess level of consciousness (LOC) and mental acuity

Establish baseline neurologic assessment

Orient to time, date, and place as needed *to prevent confusion*

Ensure safety with siderails and restraints as needed

Encourage family to sit with patient *to provide support/protection*

Administer lactulose *to prevent encephalopathy*

Peripheral system

Monitor pedal pulses

Encourage active/passive range of motion (ROM) exercises *to promote circulation*

Maintain warmth of extremities

Apply antiembolic hose *to assist in venous flow*

Elevate legs *to increase venous flow*

Monitor medication administration; observe for effectiveness, side effects

Antibiotics

Vitamin K

Vasopressin

Antacids

EXPECTED OUTCOMES

Patient's gastric drainage is clear or clearing

Vital signs are normal

Electrolytes are within normal limits

Intake and output are balanced

Pedal pulses are palpable

Skin is warm and dry

Mental acuity is normal

● **NDX:** Pain related to invasive procedures and therapeutic treatments

Maintain position of comfort within limits of ongoing treatments

Administer skin care and back rubs q2h to 4h *to promote comfort*

Keep patient warm and dry

Perform passive ROM exercises q4h

Assess pain intensity level

Medicate according to pain scale

Provide diversional activities where possible

Provide alternate pain management techniques: imaging, deep breathing

Assess effectiveness of pain relief measures

Increase activity as tolerated

EXPECTED OUTCOMES

Patient reports reduction in pain/discomfort

Demonstrates relaxed affect

● **NDX:** Anxiety related to uncertainty and threat to bodily health

Remain with patient at onset of bleeding as much as possible

Use restraints if applicable

Keep siderails up

Monitor mental acuity and for signs of ensuing coma

Plan care to provide rest periods *to prevent fatigue*

Orient patient to place, date, and time frequently

Explain each procedure as much as time allows

Reinforce physician's explanation of disease process

Maintain nonstressful environment

Dim lights when possible

Discourage loud talking and noises

Encourage verbalization of fears and anxieties *to decrease stress*

Promote relaxation techniques: deep breathing, imaging, relaxation techniques

Discuss past successful coping behaviors to identify positive coping abilities

Involve in self-care as much as possible

Promote support by family/significant other(s)

EXPECTED OUTCOMES

Patient expresses understanding of cause of anxiety

Demonstrates ability to cope independently with stress

ADDITIONAL NURSING DIAGNOSES TO CONSIDER

Altered nutrition: less than body requirements related to anorexia, nausea, vomiting, diarrhea

Activity intolerance related to fatigue and anemia

Patient/family teaching and home care considerations

Explain diet restrictions of carbohydrates, fats, and proteins

Consult nutritionist/registered dietitian for low-roughage diet plan

Discuss importance of avoiding alcohol

Explain about available counseling

Alcoholics Anonymous

Al-Anon, Al-Ateen

Chemical dependency agencies

Instruct patient in a mild exercise-to-tolerance program with planned rest periods

Reinforce physician's explanation of effects of alcohol on disease process

Discuss medications: name, purpose, dosage, time of administration, and side effects; caution patient not to take over-the-counter medications (especially aspirin compounds) without checking with physician

Explain symptoms of recurrence or progression to report to physician

Discuss importance of follow-up care with physician

● Hiatal Hernia With Esophageal Reflux

A common condition in older adults, affecting females more than males; it is a protrusion of the stomach through the diaphragm at the normal esophageal hiatus; there are two types: in a sliding hernia the gastroesophageal junction and a portion of the stomach are above the diaphragm and in a periesophageal hernia the gastroesophageal junction is normal, but a portion of the stomach is above the diaphragm and lies adjacent to it. A hiatal hernia becomes more significant if it is accompanied by gastroesophageal reflux disease (GERD) in which the gastric juices reflux into the esophagus and in turn cause irritation, scar tissue, and possible stricture.

Assessment

Subjective data

Gradual onset of symptoms
Burning sensation in throat after eating; increases in supine position
Regurgitation without vomiting
Dull substernal, epigastric pain; may radiate to shoulder
Dysphagia except for water
Nausea
Belching
Borborygmus
Pyrosis (heartburn)
Fear and anxiety: symptoms similar to MI and peptic ulcer

Objective data

Abdominal distention
Tachypnea

Diagnostic tests

CBC, urinalysis, electrolytes
Motility studies
Electrocardiogram (ECG) to rule out heart disease
Esophageal manometry
Esophagraphy (barium swallow)
Chest radiologic study
Endoscopy with biopsy and cytology
Stool for occult blood

Potential complications

Esophageal stricture
Malnutrition
Electrolyte imbalance
Aspiration pneumonia
Hemorrhage

Collaborative management

Therapeutic management

Antacids
Histamine receptor antagonists: cimetidine (Tagamet), ranitidine (Zantac), Prilosec, Propulsid
GI stimulants: metoclopramide (Reglan)
Cholinergics: bethanechol chloride (Urecholine)
Stool softeners
Diet, bland
Activity
Surgical intervention (fundoplication)

Nursing management

PATIENT PROBLEMS/NURSING DIAGNOSES

● **NDX:** Altered nutrition: less than body requirements related to dysphagia and discomfort following meals

Maintain bed rest
  Place patient in sitting position *to facilitate swallowing*
  Avoid supine position *to prevent regurgitation*
Measure intake and output *to ensure balanced nutrition*
Administer GI stimulants *to increase gastroesophageal emptying* and cholinergics *to increase motility*
Assist with and teach patient to turn and deep breathe qid
Provide bland diet; small, frequent feedings *to prevent gastric distention*
Encourage water with meals *to cleanse esophagus and facilitate swallowing*
Maintain sitting position after meals for 1 to 2 hr *to aid digestion and prevent reflux*
Collaborate with nutritionist/registered dietitian for meal planning
Discourage smoking, alcohol, and spicy foods
Avoid constipation with stool softeners, natural laxatives *to prevent straining*
Encourage ambulation; caution against bending from waist
Discourage eating 1 to 2 hr before bedtime *to avoid heartburn/reflux*
Explain importance of weight loss if obese *to reduce pressure on gastroesophageal junction*

EXPECTED OUTCOMES

Patient's nutritional intake is adequate
Understanding of restrictions in diet and position are demonstrated

● **NDX:**   Pain related to reflux

Administer antacids after meals and hs *to decrease gastric acidity/discomfort*
Discuss importance of avoiding restrictive clothing: girdles, belts, longline bras
Provide diversional activities *to decrease attention on pain*
Explain association between food and discomfort
Provide list of foods that may cause pain

EXPECTED OUTCOMES

Patient expresses increasing comfort with diet and position restrictions
Understands purpose/side effects of antacids

Patient/family teaching and home care considerations

Instruct patient to elevate head of bed on 4-inch blocks and where to purchase needed supplies
Discuss and provide dietary plan and the need to avoid fats, spicy foods, alcohol, chocolate, peppermint, caffeine, tobacco
Encourage patient to eat slowly; chew foods well; take small bites; and have small, frequent meals
Stress importance of exercise and weight reduction if applicable; some modification of activities may be needed
Explain disease process and symptoms to report to physician
Discuss stool softeners and natural laxatives as alternatives to cathartics/laxatives
Outline medication management as to name, dosage, purpose, time of administration, and side effects
Discuss importance of avoiding certain medications: anticholinergics, diazepam, nitrates, calcium blockers, β-adrenergic antagonists
Stress importance of continuing follow-up care

● Esophageal Surgery

fundoplication for hiatal hernia: Fundus of the stomach is wrapped around the lower 3 to 4 cm of the esophagus to produce an area of higher pressure; a thoracic approach may be used
perforated esophagus repair: Perforation is closed and the bleeding controlled
esophageal diverticulum: Outpouchings are repaired and the lumen of the lower esophagus reduced to normal size

Assessment

Subjective data

Location and character of pain

Objective data

Decreased breath sounds
Splinting with respirations
Tachypnea
Bradypnea
Function of chest tubes (thoracic approach)
Character and amount of gastric drainage and urine output

Diagnostic tests

CBC and electrolytes
Chest radiologic study

Potential complications

Respiratory distress
Electrolyte imbalance
Gastroesophageal anastomosis leak
Hemorrhage
Shock
Tracheoesophageal fistula
Suture line infection
Pneumothorax (thoracic approach)
Pneumonia

Collaborative management

Therapeutic management

Analgesics
NPO
Parenteral fluids with electrolytes
Whole blood if required
Nasogastric tube and urinary catheter
Oxygen per mask or catheter as required
Incentive spirometer
Gastrostomy tube and type of feeding if appropriate
Diet, activity

Nursing management

PATIENT PROBLEMS/NURSING DIAGNOSES

● **NDX:**   Risk for aspiration related to anesthesia and nasogastric tube

Assess ability to swallow
Auscultate chest for breath sounds q2h to 4h

Elevate head of bed 35 to 45 degrees *to promote coughing and prevent aspiration*

Teach and assist patient to turn, cough, and deep breathe q2h to 4h; splint chest as needed

Maintain oxygen and/or use incentive spirometer qh *to aerate the lungs and prevent atelectasis*

EXPECTED OUTCOMES

Patient presents normal breath sounds

Performs turning, deep breathing adequately

● **NDX:** Fluid volume deficit related to abnormal fluid loss, NPO state, and nasogastric tube

Maintain NPO; assess for signs of dehydration: poor skin turgor, fever

Maintain parenteral fluids with electrolytes *to replace volume loss*

Monitor serum electrolytes

Measure intake and output

Monitor vital signs q4h

Maintain nasogastric tube or gastrostomy tube to intermittent suction or gravity drainage *to promote patency/correct functioning*

Monitor placement of nasogastric tube; tape in place; if tube is dysfunctional, notify physician; *do not reposition because it may disrupt suture line*

Monitor character and amount of gastric drainage q8h

Monitor wound for excessive drainage/bleeding prn; report excess to physician

Encourage movement of legs, feet *to promote venous return*

After nasogastric tube removal

Initiate oral fluids in small amounts *to assess tolerance and sphincter function*

Progress to soft, bland diet as tolerated

Report pain, retching, or vomiting to physician because it may indicate dysfunctioning gastroesophageal sphincter

For gastrostomy tube: administer tube feedings (p. 59)

EXPECTED OUTCOMES

Patient's intake and output are balanced

Electrolytes are within normal limits

Vital signs are normal

● **NDX:** Pain related to surgical intervention

Assess type, location, and intensity of pain; use pain rating scale

Administer analgesics to maintain comfort; assess effectiveness of pain relief measures

Collaborate with physician to initiate patient controlled analgesia (PCA)

Turn and change position q2h to 4h *to reduce fatigue, discomfort*

Provide back rubs and skin care *to promote comfort*

Maintain planned rest periods *to prevent fatigue*

Splint incision when coughing

Discuss alternate pain management techniques: deep breathing, imaging, relaxation techniques

Provide diversional activities *to decrease attention on pain*

EXPECTED OUTCOMES

Patient reports reduction in or absence of pain

Demonstrates more relaxed affect

● **NDX:** Anxiety related to surgical procedure and possible changes in lifestyle

Reinforce physician's explanation of surgical procedure and expected outcome

Encourage and allow time for verbalization of concerns; involve significant others

Discuss stress management techniques: breathing, relaxation, imagery

Provide quiet, nonstressful environment

Explain nursing care plan and all procedures *to alleviate apprehension and increase awareness*

Assess present coping patterns; assist patient with identifying alternate and positive ways of coping

Explain needed changes in lifestyle in nonthreatening and positive manner *to assist patient in problem-solving techniques*

EXPECTED OUTCOMES

Patient demonstrates progress in developing positive attitudes toward needed change in lifestyle

Uses family/significant other(s) for support group

Patient/family teaching

Provide and discuss diet and dietary restrictions

Eat small, frequent meals

Chew foods well and eat slowly

Drink water with meals

Elevate head of bed at night

Explain procedure for gastrostomy feedings (p. 59)

Discuss need to avoid smoking

Home care considerations

Explain importance of balancing activity and rest

Discuss need to avoid constipation with natural laxatives

Demonstrate wound and dressing change care
Explain signs of wound infection: pain, redness, fever, drainage
Provide information on needed supplies and where to purchase them
Reinforce stress management techniques
Discuss importance of follow-up care with physician

Endoscopy: Esophageal, Gastric, Duodenal

Insertion of a fiberoptic scope into the esophagus, stomach, or duodenum to determine pathological conditions and/or obtain tissue specimens for diagnostic studies; also used to remove foreign bodies (Figure 6-2)

Preendoscopy care

Encourage and allow time for verbalization of fears and concerns
Reinforce physician's explanation of procedure
Maintain NPO
Remove dentures and partial plates
Administer oral hygiene
Administer premedications

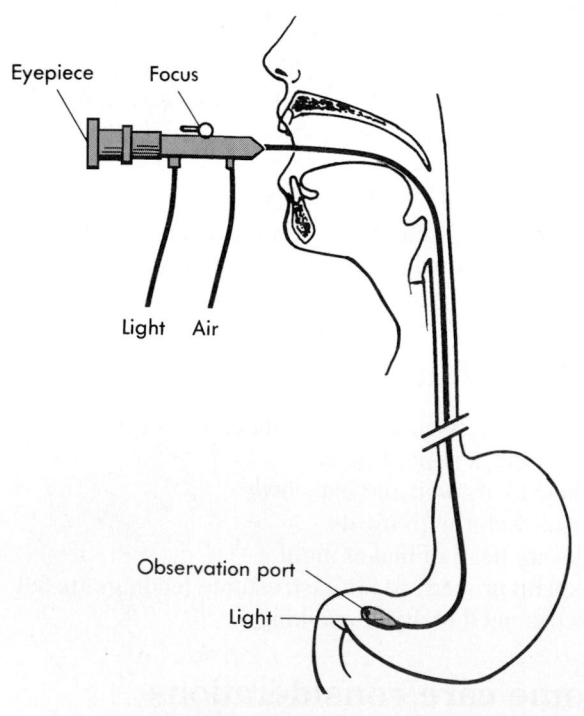

Figure 6-2 Stomach may be visualized by means of a fiberscope. (From Phipps WJ et al: *Medical-surgical nursing: concepts and clinical practice,* ed 5, St Louis, 1995, Mosby.)

Postendoscopy assessment

Subjective data

Sore throat

Objective data

Level of consciousness and vital signs
Swallow and gag reflexes present
Respiratory rate and depth
Hoarseness

Potential complications

Respiratory distress
Esophageal, gastric, or duodenal perforation
Dysphagia
  Subcutaneous crepitus in neck
  Extreme pain: increases with respirations or neck or shoulder movement
  Hematemesis

Interventions

Assist and teach patient to turn and deep breathe q2h *to maintain airway and aerate the lungs*
Administer warm saline gargles prn *to soothe sore throat*
Provide warm liquids until patient is able to swallow without discomfort, then increase diet as tolerated
Administer oral hygiene prn
Explain signs and symptoms to report to physician: increased pain, bleeding, difficulty breathing
Discuss deep-breathing exercises and oral hygiene
Encourage ongoing outpatient care

● Sengstaken-Blakemore Tube or Linton Tube

Sengstaken-Blakemore tube: Nasoesophagogastric tube with three lumens and two pressure balloons: two lumens are used to inflate the balloons, and the third is for gastric drainage; used to control esophageal hemorrhage (Figure 6-3, A)
Linton tube: Three-lumen nasogastric tube for control of gastric hemorrhage: two lumens suction esophageal and gastric contents, and the third lumen inflates the gastric balloon (Figure 6-3, B)

Preinsertion assessment and care

Assess patient's ability to swallow and mouth breathe; maintain patent airway

Explain purpose of tube and procedure

Observe amount and color of emesis after stomach contents have been aspirated

Check tube for patency of each lumen and strength of balloon(s)

Tube should not be more than 1 year old
  Use sphygmomanometer for balloon inflation of Sengstaken-Blakemore tube
  Use 50 ml syringe for balloon inflation of Linton tube
  Lubricate and chill tube according to manufacturer's instructions

Postinsertion care

SENGSTAKEN-BLAKEMORE TUBE

Tube is inserted through nose into stomach

Balloons are inflated to 20 to 40 mm Hg each or as ordered (Figure 6-3, *A*)

Lumens are securely clamped and labeled from each balloon

Gastric suction tube is labeled and attached to intermittent suction apparatus

Traction (¼ to 1 lb) is applied to gastric balloon as ordered

Tube is securely taped to nose or traction sponge

LINTON TUBE

Tube is inserted through nose into stomach

Gastric tube and esophageal tube are labeled and connected to separate intermittent suction apparatuses

Balloon is inflated with 100 to 200 ml of air or as ordered, and lumen is securely clamped and labeled (Figure 6-3, *B*)

Tube is taped to traction sponge and traction applied

Potential complications

Respiratory distress
Aspiration pneumonia
Chest pain
Abdominal distention

Interventions

Maintain prescribed balloon pressure

Release traction, deflate balloon(s) q8h to 12h *to prevent necrosis of tissues*

Irrigate only gastric lumen of tubes

Tape tube comfortably and securely to cheek *to prevent pressure on oral/nasal tissues*

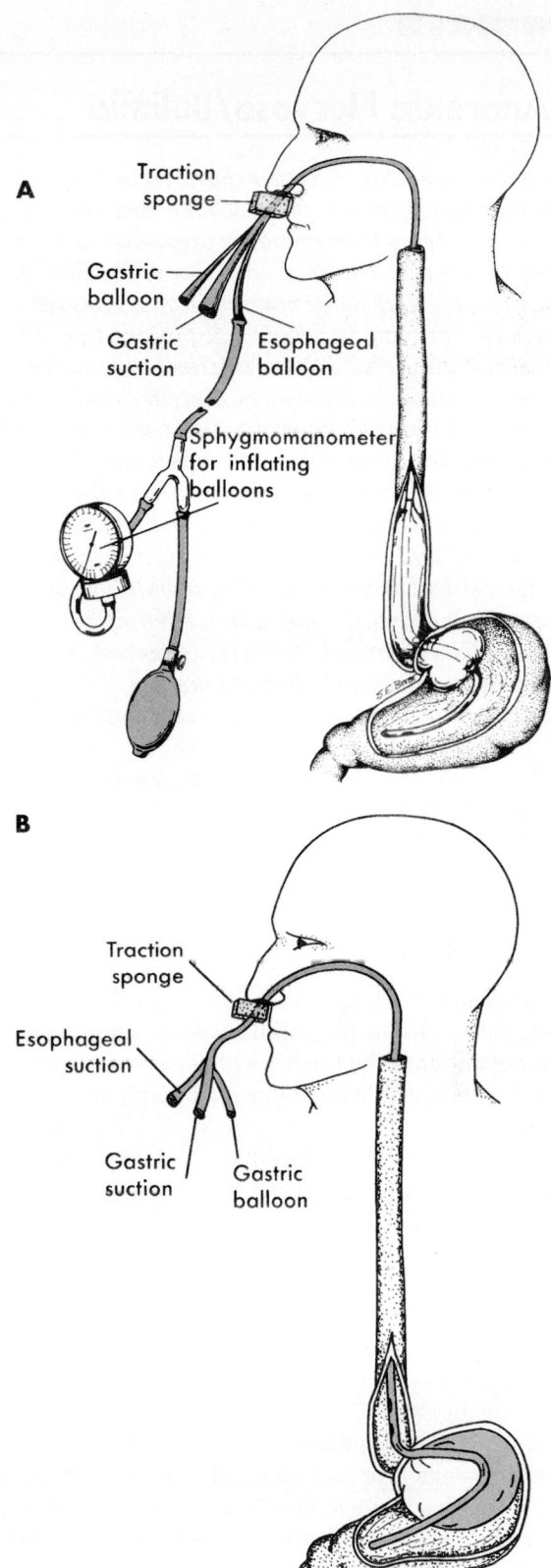

Figure 6-3   **A,** Sengstaken-Blakemore tube. **B,** Linton tube.

Stomach

● Anorexia Nervosa/Bulimia

anorexia nervosa: Disorder characterized by emaciation occurring as a result of self-inflicted starvation; etiology appears to be primarily psychological (severe body image disturbance/morbid fear of obesity), but it may include underlying organic factors; subtypes include restricting type and binge-purging type

bulimia: Eating disorder characterized by excessive overeating and use of laxatives, diuretics, and/ or self-induced vomiting to purge intestinal tract of food; subtypes include purging type and nonpurging type

Persons with either of these disorders believe strongly that they can attain control of self and others, autonomy, and competence by dieting and losing weight; severe disorders manifest a multitude of physiologic changes: bradycardia, electrolyte imbalances, neurologic problems (seizures), amenorrhea, decreased testosterone and musculoskeletal maturation, and hypotension

Usual age: adolescence; predominantly females
Peak ages: 12 to 13 years; 19 to 20 years and into young adulthood

Assessment

Middle- to upper-class socioeconomic level
Conservative philosophy, high personal standards
Often dependent relationship with a passive father
Often dependent relationship with a dominant mother
Family members closely fused
Personal boundaries not respected
Mind reading prevalent
Sense of independence sabotaged
Expressions of anger, anxiety, or aggressiveness blocked
Arguments not allowed
Togetherness prized
Loyalty exaggerated
Excellence as the standard
Anorectic seeks love and approval, becomes perfectionistic, cannot achieve it, develops physical symptoms
Family attention focuses on and reinforces weight loss and poor eating

PRODROMAL PERIOD

Increasing irritability
Eczema may develop
Abdominal discomfort

Headaches
Hyperactivity
Depression
Anxiety
Social withdrawal from friends
High level of investment in schoolwork and high-energy sports or high-stress employment

ORGANIC SYMPTOMS

Severe weight loss
Secondary amenorrhea
Bradycardia
Lowered body temperature
Decreased pH
Cold intolerance
Dry skin, poor turgor
Brittle nails
Lanugo hair
Decreased appetite
Feelings of satiety
Breasts atrophied
Axillary and pubic hair reduced
Sleep disturbances
Constipation
Increased susceptibility to infection

AFFECT/BEHAVIOR

Academically, professionally high achiever
Conforming behavior
Conscientious
Increased energy levels
Relentless pursuit of thinness and fear of fatness
Anorexia frequently precipitated by adolescent crisis
History of normal weight
Fear of developing feelings of sexuality
Disturbed body image of delusional proportions
  Defends emaciation as normal
  Feels rewarded by achieving and maintaining emaciated state
  Is fearful of weight gain
  Interprets others' concerns as attempts to make patient fat
  Admires emaciated self in mirror
Inaccurate and confused perception and interpretation of inner stimuli
  Does not recognize signs of nutritional need
  Is unable to assess amount of food taken
  Derives pleasure from refusal of food
  Hides food; may secretly flush it down toilet
  May induce vomiting after eating
  May use laxatives to speed passage of food
  Is preoccupied with food and related activities; may plan and prepare meals for others, collect recipes, count calories
  Increases activity to counteract weight gain

May conceal weights on body before being weighed
May hoard food, especially candy and nonnutritive
  foods
Paralyzing sense of ineffectiveness
  Behaves with defiance and rebellion but is over-
    whelmed by sense of ineffectiveness
  Feels he or she responds only to demands and wishes
    of others
  Doubts ability of or right to self-assertion

Diagnostic tests

CBC with differential: leukopenia, lymphocytosis,
  anemia
Blood serum studies
  Hypoglycemia, hypocholesteremia, hypoproteinemia,
    hypokalemia, hyponatremia
  Decreased estrogen levels, elevated BUN
  Fasting blood sugar; hypoglycemia
  Thyroid, pituitary studies
  ECG, T wave inversions
Urine studies: decreased urinary 17-ketosteroids, pres-
  ence of ketones

Potential complications

Cardiac dysrhythmias

Collaborative management

Therapeutic management

Determination of extent of nutritional deprivation
If severe, nasogastric feedings are ordered if food is re-
  fused by patient
Parenteral fluids with electrolytes/hyperalimentation
  for dehydration or life-threatening malnutrition
Medications: cypropheptadine (Periactin) to stimulate
  appetite, tricyclic antidepressants (Elavil), antianxiety
  agents: alprazolam (Xanax)
Daily weights when ordered
Referral to psychotherapist with family therapy approach to care, behavior modification therapy

Nursing management

PATIENT PROBLEMS/NURSING DIAGNOSES

● **NDX:** Altered nutrition: less than body requirements related to anorexia, self-induced vomiting, laxative abuse, and/or distorted perception of body

Encourage patient's own selection of foods *to increase
responsibility*

Limit mealtimes to 30 to 40 min *to prevent dawdling*
Six small meals may be required *to prevent gastric
  distention*
Diminish distractions during mealtimes
Encourage patient to eat slowly and relish the taste of
  food
Supervise patient following meals *to prevent vomiting*
Explain that food will not cause obesity at this time but
  will help patient maintain a normal weight
Avoid power struggles over food by minimizing attention paid to it
Be consistent in your own behavior *to increase patient
  confidence*
If tube feedings or TPN become necessary because
  oral intake is not adequate, explain the rationale in a
  calm, sensitive manner *to prevent patient from feeling
  a loss of control*
Monitor frequently to prevent patient from dislodging
  tube or needle
Involve nutritionist/registered dietitian in explaining
  meal planning, needed nutrients, and rationale for
  eating a variety of foods *to assist patient in feeling in
  control*
Monitor intake carefully *to ensure adequate nutrition*
Maintain strict calorie count after each meal
Provide at least 1200 to 1500 calories/day *to ensure balanced nutrition*
Obtain accurate weights to ensure slow, steady weight
  gain
  Encourage feeling of responsibility for weight gain
  Discourage patient from frequent self-weighing
Explain to patient that rehabilitation will be a long-term
  process

EXPECTED OUTCOMES
Patient expresses understanding of nutritional needs
Ingests caloric intake adequate to maintain a slow,
  constant weight gain
Resumes eating pattern consistent with desired weight
  gain

● **NDX:** Fluid volume deficit related to dieting/
  purging

Monitor intake and output and maintain accurate
  records
Include patient in scheduling fluid intake times *to encourage compliance*
Explain and discuss methods to avoid use of laxa-
  tives/diuretics *to maintain fluid balance*
Monitor parenteral fluids with electrolytes/TPN as
  needed; accompany patient to bathroom to prevent
  emptying of IV fluids
Monitor vital signs q4h *to evaluate adequate fluid volume*
Assess for hypotension, bradycardia

EXPECTED OUTCOMES

Patient's hydration is maintained adequately

Intake and output are balanced

Understanding of causative factors and behaviors is progressing

● **NDX:** Body image disturbance related to inaccurate perception of self as fat; poor self-esteem

Assess patient's feelings about self, body

Give positive support and praise for things well done *to increase feelings of self-worth*

Foster successful experiences

Begin with tasks easily accomplished *to increase compliance and confidence*

Focus on positive traits *to assist patient to view body accurately*

Encourage patient to verbalize thoughts about self and body *to increase confidence*

Have patient draw picture of self and discuss perception of self

Encourage wearing loose clothing to avoid focusing on body, weight, appearance

Encourage good hygiene and grooming for feeling of well-being

Respond factually and consistently to patient's questions concerning diet and nutrition

Encourage and reinforce constructive physical activity (bed making, helping other patients) *to assist patient in viewing self as worthwhile*

EXPECTED OUTCOMES

Patient begins to verbalize positive thoughts of self and self-worth

Begins to perceive self as thin and as an individual

Shows progress in accepting responsibility for actions

● **NDX:** Ineffective individual coping related to feelings of loss of control, fear of growing up, and/or personalized response to family dysfunction

Encourage ventilation of feelings; assist in identifying fears associated with bingeing, starving, and so on *to help patient deal with loss of control*

Observe and record responses to stress

Encourage speaking with staff when stressed *to promote patient's self-support*

Discourage (withdraw your attention from) rituals or emotional associations with meals, food, and so on

Support patient's attempts at self-determination, especially when with family, *to foster positive feelings about self and set realistic expectations*

Promote stress-reduction techniques: imaging, relaxation exercises, diversional activities

Encourage support by significant others

Discuss and teach problem-solving method *to promote positive communication skills*

EXPECTED OUTCOMES

Patient begins to exhibit positive coping skills

Maintains weight during stressful periods

Seeks appropriate support and resources

● **NDX:** Ineffective family coping related to inability to communicate and inability to meet the needs of all family members

Assess patient/family on knowledge of eating disorder and altered communication skills *to facilitate the needed changes*

Encourage patient and family to verbalize thoughts, perceptions, and feelings

Point out areas where patient and family members disagree *to foster positive behaviors*

Determine each family member's perception of what another has said *to reinforce listening skills*

Emphasize with patient and family members importance of using "I" statements and taking responsibility only for self

With family members present, be patient's advocate and support attempts at self-determination and control

Redirect control conflicts between patient and parents/significant other(s) away from food and onto issues related to curfews, school activities, job satisfaction, and so on

Refer family to community resources for psychologic counseling as needed

EXPECTED OUTCOMES

Patient begins to recognize needs of others

Identifies areas where needs and expectations are unmet

Responds positively to provided support

Seeks assistance as needed

ADDITIONAL NURSING DIAGNOSES TO CONSIDER

Constipation related to laxative misuse

Powerlessness related to a feeling of loss of control over life

Impaired skin integrity, related to malnutrition

Patient/family teaching

Reinforce nutritional guidelines and how to manage diet

Discuss with patient the need to reassess caloric requirements q2wk to 4wk

Reinforce use of stress-management techniques

Promote regular exercise program but discourage overexertion

Reinforce use of problem-solving and assertiveness skills to maintain sense of control over life

Discuss importance of socialization and other activities

Home care considerations

Encourage patient to seek assistance in sexuality problems as needed

Refer to home health social worker as needed

Encourage patient to keep physician, nutritionist/registered dietitian, and psychotherapist appointments

Refer to:

National Eating Disorders Organization
445 E. Granville Rd.
Worthington, OH 43085-3195
(614) 436-1112 FAX: (614) 785-7471

● Gastritis Attributed to *Helicobacter Pylori*

An infection of the mucosal lining of the stomach caused by the H. pylori *bacteria, formerly known as* Campylobacter pylori; *if diagnosed and treated early, the risk of progression to peptic ulcer disease is greatly reduced*

Assessment

Subjective data

Epigastric fullness, discomfort
Nausea
Abdominal tenderness
History of alcohol, aspirin ingestion
Anorexia, weight loss

Objective data

Vomiting, eructation
Hematemesis
Melena

Diagnostic tests

Serology assay/urease test
Breath tests to measure presence of bacteria
Biopsy

Collaborative management

Therapeutic management

Tetracycline (or Achromycin V) 500 mg qid for 14 days
Metronidazole (or Flagyl) 250 mg qid for 14 days
Pink bismuth tablets (bismuth subsalicylate, Pepto-Bismol) two tablets qid for 14 days
H_2-receptor antagonist (H2RA) (Tagamet, Zantac) if being taken previously for hyperacidity
Diet restrictions

Nursing management

Discuss importance of taking all medications as prescribed to ensure cure

Reassure patient that pink bismuth tablets may be taken with the tetracycline in this instance

Instruct patient to chew pink bismuth tablets thoroughly before swallowing

Stress importance of the following:
Take medications with a large glass of water
Do not take with milk
Take antacids and/or iron products, including vitamins with iron, 2 hr before or after the three prescribed medicines
Do not drink alcohol, beer, or wine or use tobacco products while taking the three medications
Avoid long periods in the sun or under sun lamp during the 2 wk period
Explain that symptoms may not improve immediately but will improve when treatment is finished
There may be some harmless side effects such as darkening of the tongue and/or urine/stool, or metallic taste in the mouth; these are temporary

Notify physician if any of the following symptoms are present and bothersome:
Diarrhea, nausea, abdominal pain
Vaginal discharge, itching
Skin rash

Encourage patient to keep follow-up appointments with physician for laboratory tests *to ensure cure*

● Peptic Ulcer Disease (Gastric and Duodenal)

Peptic ulcer disease includes both gastric and duodenal ulceration of the gastric mucosa caused by an imbalance of acid and pepsin; however, the incidence, physiology, and some etiology are different for each

gastric ulcer: Causative factors include medications (aspirin, antiinflammatories), chemicals (tobacco, alcohol); usually located in the distal portion of the stomach at the lesser curvature; the mucosa is normally protected by maintaining a neutral pH with release of mucus and bicarbonate; if this balance is altered, ulcer formation begins

duodenal ulcer: *Causative factors include hypersecretion of gastric acid (40%) and decreased pepsin in gastric juices (60%); usually located at the pylorus end of the stomach and in the duodenum; ulceration occurs when acid secretion exceeds the protective ability of the mucosa, or when the pH of the duodenal juices is reduced and the pepsin damages the mucosa; genetic factors, stress, and medications may also be contributing causes*

Assessment

Subjective data

GASTRIC ULCER

Left to midepigastric pain; may radiate to back
Pain may or may not be relieved by antacids, food

DUODENAL ULCER

Right epigastric pain; may radiate to back or thorax; pain usually relieved by antacids, food

COMMON DATA

Pyrosis (heartburn)
Fullness after eating
Eructation
Nausea
Bloating
Anorexia
Gnawing-type pain; not food related

Objective data

Abdominal distention
Vomiting

Diagnostic tests

Endoscopy with biopsy and cytology
Barium studies
Abdominal radiologic studies
Gastric analysis
Hgb, Hct, blood pepsinogen, gastrin levels
Stool for melena

Potential complications

Electrolyte imbalance
Gastric, duodenal hemorrhage
Perforation
Pyloric stenosis
Shock

Collaborative management

Therapeutic management

Analgesics
Aluminum-magnesium antacids: Delcid, Mylanta-II
Cimetidine (Tagamet)
Ranitidine (Zantac)
Sucralfate (Carafate)
Diet

Nursing management

PATIENT PROBLEMS/NURSING DIAGNOSES

● **NDX:** Altered nutrition: less than body requirements related to discomfort, anorexia

Assess patient's nutritional status: present diet, eating patterns, foods usually eaten, weight loss or gain
Assess patient's medication history: aspirin, steroids, vasopressors, antiinflammatories
Monitor vital signs q4h
Monitor intake and output q8h
Maintain nonstressful environment
Provide high-calorie, high-protein diet in small, frequent meals *to help neutralize the gastric acid*
Monitor effectiveness, side effects of antiemetics, antacids
Weigh as needed *to ensure maintenance of normal weight and assess loss or gain*

EXPECTED OUTCOMES

Patient tolerates diet without discomfort
Maintains balanced intake and output

● **NDX:** Pain related to irritation, disruption of gastric mucosa

Assess pain: location, type, frequency, and duration; sudden severe pain may indicate gastric, duodenal perforation
Monitor effectiveness, side effects of analgesics/antacids
Provide diversional activities *to reduce attention on pain*
Administer back rubs, changes in position *to promote comfort*
Discuss and teach relaxation techniques: deep breathing, imaging

EXPECTED OUTCOME

Patient reports reduction in or absence of pain

Patient/family teaching and home care considerations

Discuss relationship of causative agents to peptic ulcer disease

Provide and review written instructions concerning medications including name, purpose, dosage, time of administration, and side effects; instruct patient to take only antacids prescribed by physician and to avoid aspirin, steroids

Discuss dietary plan: importance of eating meals at regular times, necessity of not missing a meal, and benefits of small, frequent meals; avoid coffee, tobacco, and alcohol

Explain signs and symptoms of perforation: extreme epigastric pain and hematemesis

Describe importance of nonstressful environment, especially at mealtime

Discuss methods of stress management: relaxation, exercise, meditation

Encourage follow-up care with physician

● Gastric Hemorrhage

Condition in which ulceration of the mucosa has progressed to the vasculature of the stomach or duodenum; may be insidious or acute

Assessment

Subjective data

Nausea, vomiting
Abdominal tenderness, pain

Objective data

Decreased blood pressure
Elevated pulse
Abdominal distention
Hematemesis
Melena
Hyperperistalsis
Increased bowel sounds
Dehydration
Chills, fever
Anxiety/fear

Diagnostic tests

Endoscopy
GI series
Stools for occult blood
CBC, electrolytes, BUN

Potential complications

Electrolyte imbalance
Gastric perforation
Hemorrhage
Shock

Collaborative management

Therapeutic management

Analgesics
NPO
Nasogastric tube or Linton tube, depending on bleeding site
Parenteral fluids with electrolytes and vitamins
Whole blood or packed red blood cells (PBCs)
CVP line, Swan-Ganz catheter
Urethral catheter
Cimetidine intravenously
Antacids via nasogastric tube
Gastric lavage (norepinephrine bitartrate [Levophed] may be added to produce vasoconstriction)
Endoscopy: endoscope electrocoagulation
Vasopressin arterially
Surgical intervention: repair or resection
Diet: nutritionist/registered dietitian consultation
Exercise, rest

Nursing management

PATIENT PROBLEMS/NURSING DIAGNOSES

● **NDX:** Altered tissue perfusion: cardiopulmonary, GI, peripheral, and renal related to blood loss

Cardiopulmonary system
Auscultate chest for breath sounds q2h to 4h *to assess possible aspiration of emesis*
Maintain bed rest with head of bed elevated 30 degrees *to facilitate breathing*
Assess acuteness of bleeding and for signs of hypovolemia and shock: hypotension, tachycardia, tachypnea, decreased urine output
Monitor vital signs q15min to 30min until stable; take apical pulse
Maintain parenteral therapy: electrolytes, volume expanders, whole blood, packed cells *to prevent hypovolemia*
Monitor CVP line or Swan-Ganz catheter if appropriate
Balance treatments with rest periods *to prevent fatigue*
GI system
Auscultate abdomen for bowel sounds q4h
Monitor for abdominal distention
Monitor stools for melena
Maintain NPO

Monitor nasogastric tube and intermittent suction apparatus; measure gastric output q4h to 8h
Perform iced saline or water or tap water lavage with measured amounts of solution *to decrease bleeding*
Measure intake and output
Monitor electrolytes, Hgb, and Hct
Prepare for endoscopy; explain procedure *to reduce fear/anxiety*

Peripheral system
Monitor pedal pulses, capillary refill, and temperature of feet
Elevate legs *to increase venous flow*
Apply antiembolic stockings; remove daily
Maintain warmth of feet
Encourage active ROM of extremities *to promote circulation*

Renal system
Weigh patient daily: same time, clothing, and scale
Maintain indwelling urethral catheter; monitor hourly output; if output is <50 ml/hr notify physician
Monitor urine pH and specific gravity
Monitor serum BUN, creatinine

EXPECTED OUTCOMES

Patient's vital signs are normal
Intake and output are balanced
Gastric drainage is clear or clearing
Pedal pulses, capillary refill are normal

● **NDX:**   Altered nutrition: less than body requirements related to altered diet patterns, anorexia

When bleeding subsides and nasogastric tube is removed, initiate fluids in small amounts as tolerated
Progress to blended or soft foods in small, frequent meals
Collaborate with nutritionist/registered dietitian to provide high-calorie, high-protein diet; avoid increased calories if patient is overweight
Continue monitoring intake, output, and stools for melena
Monitor for complaints of fullness, nausea/vomiting *to avoid distention*
Administer saline enemas to clear bowel of old blood
Prevent constipation with natural laxatives: bran, prunes, psyllium powder
Assess effectiveness, side effects of antacids, vitamin K, cimetidine

EXPECTED OUTCOMES

Patient tolerates diet well, and weight is stable
Tolerates medications

● **NDX:**   Pain related to disruption of gastric mucosa

Administer analgesics (e.g., morphine); meperidine is usually avoided because it can cause nausea and vomiting

Assess effectiveness of pain relief measures
Assist and teach patient to turn and deep breathe q2h to 4h
Administer back care and oral hygiene *to promote comfort*
Discuss and teach alternate pain relief measures: imaging, relaxation techniques
Change patient's position frequently *to provide comfort*
Keep patient warm and dry
Provide planned rest periods
Ambulate patient with assistance when tolerated *to decrease discomfort*
Provide diversional activities *to decrease attention on discomfort*

EXPECTED OUTCOMES

Patient expresses reduction in or absence of pain
Appears relaxed and comfortable

● **NDX:**   Anxiety related to altered health status

Maintain quiet environment
Explain all procedures and treatments *to increase knowledge and reduce stress*
Encourage and allow time for verbalization of concerns
Assess level of anxiety/fear and current coping styles *to begin to help patient reduce anxiety* by using successful past coping behaviors
Discuss alternate coping behaviors and stress management techniques
Encourage communication with significant other(s) *to provide a support system*

EXPECTED OUTCOMES

Patient demonstrates positive coping behaviors
Expresses a reduction in anxiety
Uses stress management techniques appropriately

Patient/family teaching and home care considerations

Discuss nutritional plan, stressing importance of the following:
Small, frequent meals at regular intervals
Chewing food well and eating slowly
Avoiding caffeine, alcohol, tobacco, and aspirin
Reinforce physician's explanation of relationship of causative factors to disease process
Explain use of antiinflammatories and their relationship to ulcer formation
Always take with food
Take 1 hr after taking antacid *to avoid malabsorption of medication*

Reinforce stress management techniques

Provide medication instructions: name, dose, purpose, time of administration, and side effects; instruct patient to take only antacids prescribed by physician

Explain signs and symptoms of further bleeding: hematemesis, abdominal distention, tarry stools, fainting, dyspnea

Discuss importance of balancing exercise and rest periods

Encourage follow-up visits with physician

● Gastric Surgery

gastric resection: Removal of a gastric ulcer, leaving the stomach intact

subtotal gastrectomy: Removal of part of the stomach, usually the distal end, to prevent reformation of ulceration; the remaining part is anastomosed to the small bowel

Billroth I: Reshaping of the remaining stomach to reduce the curvature in order to merge it with the duodenum during the anastomosis

Billroth II: Following resection of part of the stomach and duodenum, the remaining stomach is anastomosed, side by side, to the remaining duodenum

total gastrectomy: Removal of the stomach, usually for cancer; the distal esophagus and proximal duodenum are also removed and an esophagojejunostomy is performed

vagotomy: Surgical interruption of the gastric vagal nerve to decrease gastric secretion and motility

pyloroplasty: Surgical procedure performed with a vagotomy to enlarge the gastric outlet and promote gastric emptying

Preoperative assessment and care

Assess respiratory status

Discuss and explain pain management

Reinforce physician's explanation of procedure

Teach patient to turn, deep breathe; methods of incisional splinting for coughing; use of incentive spirometer

Discuss placement of tubes, drains that may be present postoperatively

Insert nasogastric tube as ordered

Allow time for verbalization of concerns

Postoperative assessment

Subjective data

Location, character of pain

Nausea

Objective data

Splinting with respirations

Decreased breath sounds

Tachypnea

Bradypnea

Character and amount of gastric drainage

Vomiting

Urinary output

Abdominal distention

Diagnostic tests

Hgb, Hct, electrolytes

Potential complications

Dehydration, anemia

Electrolyte imbalance

Atelectasis

Anastomosis leak

Shock

Thrombophlebitis (p. 107)

Dumping syndrome (p. 363)

Paralytic ileus (p. 379)

Wound evisceration, infection

Postprandial hypoglycemia

Gastrojejunocolic fistula

Collaborative management

Therapeutic management

NPO until bowel sounds return

Parenteral fluids with electrolytes until diet is allowed

Nasogastric suction

Analgesics

Antiembolic stockings

Diet and activity

Nursing management

PATIENT PROBLEMS/NURSING DIAGNOSES

● **NDX:** Fluid volume deficit related to altered digestive process, absorption, and nasogastric tube drainage

Maintain NPO; assess hydration status

  Maintain nasogastric tube to intermittent suction apparatus

  Monitor color and amount of gastric output q4h and include in total output

  Do not reposition tube

  Maintain patency of tube by irrigation with measured amounts of saline *only* if ordered

Note that after gastrectomy, drainage will be minimal
Report excessive bleeding to physician
Administer frequent oral hygiene with petroleum jelly; keep nares well lubricated *to prevent dryness from mouth breathing and irritation from tube*
Monitor electrolytes, Hgb, and Hct
Maintain parenteral fluids with electrolytes *to ensure adequate hydration*
Measure intake and output q4h to 8h
Weigh q2 days: same time, clothing, scale

EXPECTED OUTCOMES
Patient's intake and output are balanced
Hydration is adequately maintained
Weight is maintained near normal

● **NDX:** Altered nutrition: less than body requirements related to altered gastric functioning/absorption

Auscultate bowel sounds and passage of flatus q8h
When bowel sounds return, administer small amounts of water via nasogastric tube as ordered
  Aspirate stomach 2 hr after last feeding of the day; contents should be <100 ml, and no pain, distention, or nausea should be present
  Report to physician if amount is >100 ml and/or the above symptoms occur
Initiate oral fluids when nasogastric tube is removed
  Offer 5 to 10 ml of warm water qh as ordered
  Increase amounts until 90 to 120 ml is tolerated qh
Progress to small, frequent meals of soft foods; avoid milk because it may cause dumping syndrome
Discontinue feedings if pain, nausea, distention, or vomiting occur and notify physician
Continue measuring intake

EXPECTED OUTCOMES
Patient tolerates increasing diet without discomfort
Ingests adequate calories to maintain normal weight

● **NDX:** Ineffective breathing pattern related to location of surgical incision

Assess respirations, observing for signs of distress
Maintain bed rest with head of bed elevated 30 degrees *to facilitate breathing*
Auscultate chest for breath sounds q4h
Assist and teach patient to turn, cough, and deep breathe q2h to 4h; provide support to incision *to reduce pain*
Administer incentive spirometer q4h *to aerate lungs adequately*
Provide pain medication before deep breathing exercises *to reduce discomfort*

EXPECTED OUTCOMES
Patient demonstrates breathing techniques accurately
Exhibits normal respirations

● **NDX:** Altered tissue perfusion: peripheral, cardiopulmonary, renal related to risk of hypovolemia

Peripheral system
  Check extremities for temperature, color, and sensation
  Monitor pedal pulses q4h
  Do not gatch knees *because it may interrupt venous flow*
  Apply antiembolic stockings and remove daily to inspect skin for redness, tenderness
  Encourage ROM leg exercises qh *to promote venous return*
Cardiopulmonary system
  Monitor vital signs q4h
  Auscultate chest for breath sounds q4h
  Monitor CVP/Swan-Ganz readings qh and prn
  Monitor ABGs *to assess adequate arterial flow*
Renal system
  Measure intake and output qh *to assess adequate kidney function;* if output is <30 ml/hr report to physician
  Monitor urine specific gravity and serum BUN, creatinine

EXPECTED OUTCOMES
Patient's vital signs are normal
Urine output is adequate and balances with intake
Laboratory values are within normal limits

● **NDX:** Risk for infection related to surgical incision, inadequate primary defenses

Monitor dressings and incision for drainage and bleeding q4h
Change dressings prn and observe healing process
Observe for signs of wound infection: redness, drainage, pain, odor; report these to physician

EXPECTED OUTCOMES
Patient's incision is clean, dry, and intact
Wound is healing adequately

● **NDX:** Pain related to surgical intervention

Assess location, type, and intensity of pain; use pain rating scale
Assess effectiveness of analgesics; collaborate with physician regarding patient-controlled analgesia PCA (p. 92)

Change position often and support with pillows *to decrease discomfort*

Administer skin care and back rubs q4h *to promote comfort*

Maintain quiet environment *to allow for adequate rest*

Schedule rest periods between treatments

Discuss alternate pain relief measures: imaging, relaxation techniques, deep breathing

Provide diversional activities *to decrease attention on pain*

EXPECTED OUTCOMES

Patient reports a tolerable level of pain/discomfort

Appears more relaxed

● **NDX:** Anxiety related to change in health status

Explain all procedures and treatments

Reinforce physician's explanation of surgical procedure and treatment

Encourage and allow time for verbalization of feelings

Assess present coping behaviors and support positive responses

Teach stress management techniques

Encourage communication with significant other(s) *to promote support*

EXPECTED OUTCOMES

Patient expresses and identifies anxieties

Uses stress management techniques appropriately

ADDITIONAL NURSING DIAGNOSIS TO CONSIDER

Diarrhea related to malabsorption

Patient/family teaching

Discuss and explain dietary plan and restrictions according to type of surgery performed

Eat small, frequent meals at regular intervals; avoid high-fiber foods, sugar, salt, caffeine, alcohol, milk, and tobacco

Take fluids between meals, not with meals

Eat slowly and chew foods well

Measure weight q2h to 4h

Provide instructions and demonstrate wound care; identify signs of wound infection

Reinforce importance of avoiding stressful situations, especially at mealtimes

Reinforce stress management techniques

Explain symptoms of dumping syndrome see following section: epigastric pain, weakness, nausea, vomiting after eating

Discuss medications: name, dosage, time of administration, purpose, and side effects; instruct patient to avoid over-the-counter medications, especially those containing aspirin

Discuss importance of adequate rest and exercise with planned rest periods

Explain use of natural laxatives to avoid constipation

Encourage follow-up care with physician

Home care considerations

Be certain that patient has names and phone numbers of home health care team

Discuss where and what to purchase for dressing changes

Provide information on community organizations for meal delivery, home health care aides as needed

● Dumping Syndrome

Postgastrectomy, gastroduodenostomy, gastrojejunostomy, or pyloroplasty syndrome caused by loss of the pyloric valve, allowing food and fluid to pass too rapidly into the small bowel; this causes blood sugar level to rise and increases insulin production, which in turn can cause hypoglycemia; appears 1 to 3 wk after surgery

Assessment

Subjective data

Time of onset of symptoms: usually after meals

Epigastric fullness

Nausea

Malaise

Palpitations

Vertigo

Urge to defecate

Objective data

Vomiting

Abdominal distention

Profuse diaphoresis

Tachypnea

Hypotension

Increased bowel sounds

Decreased blood sugar level (hypoglycemia)

Potential complications

Syndrome becomes chronic

ECG changes

Collaborative management

Therapeutic management

Diet: high-protein, high-fat, low-carbohydrate plan
Anticholinergics, pectin powder
Surgery to alter dumping rate

Nursing management

PATIENT PROBLEM/NURSING DIAGNOSIS

● **NDX:** Altered nutrition: less than body requirements related to inability to absorb nutrients

Collaborate with physician and nutritionist/registered dietitian about diet
  Provide six small meals a day
  Do not give liquids with meals
  Provide dry foods such as toast, crackers, and cereals
  Provide diet low in carbohydrates and salt, moderate in fat, and high in protein
  Avoid refined, concentrated carbohydrates *because they pass into intestines rapidly and cause increased insulin release*
  Include foods containing pectin: citrus fruits, yellow vegetables, bananas, apples, apricots, cherries, beans
  Avoid extreme temperatures in foods
Administer pectin powder; thoroughly mix with water: patient may experience a sense of oral dryness if mixture is not adequately liquefied
Provide liquids only between meals *to avoid increased dumping into intestine*
Administer anticholinergics 30 min before meals; assess for effectiveness
Monitor glucose levels *to assess for hypoglycemia*
Measure intake and output q8h
Position patient in recumbent position after meals *to allow foods to pass more slowly into intestine*

EXPECTED OUTCOMES

Patient tolerates diet without experiencing discomfort, distention, or nausea
Maintains weight and adequate nutritional status

Patient/family teaching

Discuss importance of dietary plan; stress small, frequent meals, foods to avoid, and foods to eat
Stress importance of eating slowly and chewing foods well

Explain that syndrome is usually only temporary, but its continuance after 2 to 3 wk needs to be reported to the physician
Instruct patient to lie down after meals and to avoid stressful situations, especially at mealtimes
Reinforce stress management techniques
Encourage follow-up visits with physician

Home care considerations

Provide dietary plan with foods high in protein and fat and low in carbohydrates
Stress importance of not drinking liquids with meals
Provide names and phone numbers of home health care team members
Refer to community agencies for assistance with meals as needed
Stress importance of maintaining normal weight

● Surgical Intervention for Obesity

Insertion of two rows of staples across upper one tenth of the stomach to reduce capacity and ensure early satiety; performed for patients highly motivated to lose weight and where medical management of obesity has been unsuccessful; two types of surgery are performed:
gastric bypass: *Anastomosis of jejunum to upper one tenth of the stomach, bypassing the remaining stomach (Figure 6-4, A)*
gastroplasty/vertical banding: *Small opening left in rows of staples, allowing small amounts of food to pass into stomach (Figure 6-4, B)*

Preoperative assessment

Observations/findings

Nutritional history
  Previous eating patterns and types of foods eaten
  Present weight >100 lb over ideal body weight
Medical history
  Absence of renal, cardiac, bowel, or liver disease
  No history of hypertension, diabetes, or arthritis
  No signs of upper respiratory infection or anemia
Psychologic adjustment to procedure
  Motivation to lose weight
  Weight loss minimal or absent after many attempts
  Presence of positive coping behaviors

Diagnostic tests

Renal and liver function studies
Abdominal and chest radiologic studies

Cholecystogram
Intravenous pyelogram
Barium enema
Pulmonary function test
Serum glucose, insulin, cholesterol, triglycerides, creatinine, protein, iron, CBC, urinalysis
Baseline ABGs

Collaborative management

Therapeutic management

Preoperative medication
Parenteral fluids with heparin
Nasogastric tube and indwelling urethral catheter

Nursing management

PATIENT PROBLEMS/NURSING DIAGNOSES

● **NDX:** Anxiety related to hospitalization, procedures, surgery, and altered health status

Attempt to maintain nonstressful environment
Discuss stress management techniques
Orient patient to surroundings and provide comfortable armless chair
Encourage and allow time for verbalization of concerns
Assess coping skills and promote positive, successful past behaviors

Reinforce physician's explanation of preoperative and postoperative care and surgical procedure
Perform activities in an unhurried manner, explaining each as it occurs
Encourage verbalization with significant other(s)

EXPECTED OUTCOMES
Patient expresses anxieties/concerns
Exhibits positive coping skills

● **NDX:** Knowledge deficit related to lack of information about preoperative and postoperative care

Discuss with patient and teach
  Use of trapeze bar and how to get in and out of bed
  Method for turning, coughing, and deep breathing with incisional support
  Use of incentive spirometer and diaphragmatic breathing procedure
  Procedure for sipping from a cup, 30 ml in 5 min
  Active ROM exercises, especially legs and feet
Explain that early ambulation (2 to 4 hr after surgery) will be required, and trapeze bars will be in place
Explain that preoperatively a nasogastric tube and indwelling urethral catheter will be inserted
Discuss postoperative dietary management: small sips of water increasing to 30 to 60 ml/hr as tolerated
Explain that IV line will be in place preoperatively, and an anticoagulant will be administered

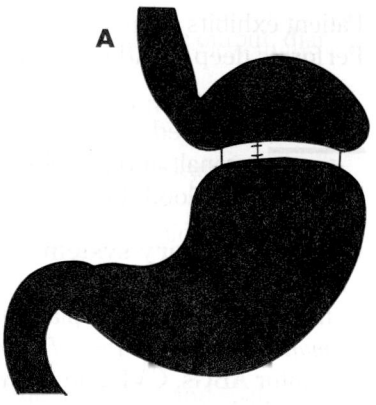

Gastric banding

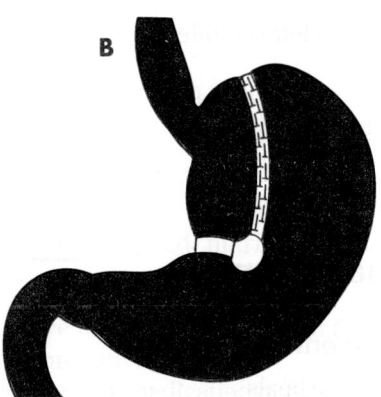

Vertical banded gastroplasty

Figure 6-4 Examples of gastric-restriction procedures. **A**, Gastric banding. **B**, Vertical banded gastroplasty. (From Beare PG, Myers JL: *Principles and practice of adult health nursing,* ed 2, St Louis, 1994, Mosby.)

Progress to clear liquids, using 1 oz cup, until soft, high-protein, low-fat diet is tolerated

Assess tolerance of foods and fluids as they are introduced: *nausea may occur if stomach becomes overextended*

Instruct patient to heed feeling of satiety to avoid nausea or vomiting

Administer vitamin supplements including vitamin B$_{12}$, folate, and calcium *to prevent anemia from reduced oral intake*

EXPECTED OUTCOMES

Patient tolerates frequent feedings adequately

Maintains desired weight loss

● **NDX:** Diarrhea related to induced malabsorption

Provide diet high in bulk with moderate fluid intake *because excess contributes to diarrhea*

Observe for signs of dumping syndrome (p. 363): nausea, distention, vertigo, palpitations

Provide perianal care after bowel movement; apply protective ointments as needed

Observe frequency, color, amount, and consistency of stools

Monitor electrolytes *because increased fluid loss may alter electrolyte balance*

Administer antidiarrheals

EXPECTED OUTCOMES

Patient expresses understanding of rationale for diet regimen

Verbalizes factors causing diarrhea

Has bowel elimination that is returning to normal

● **NDX:** Risk for impaired skin integrity related to obesity, fluid deficit

Monitor incision for healing, drainage

Administer frequent skin care, especially in folds or on pressure points

Provide special air or foam mattress as indicated

Promote frequent position changes *to increase comfort;* support incision

Place clear skin barrier on heels and elbows *to prevent shearing*

EXPECTED OUTCOMES

Patient's incision is healing and surrounding skin is clean, dry, and intact

Skin integrity is maintained without evidence of any stage of dermal ulcer

Patient/family teaching

Discuss importance of following eating regimen

Eat and drink slowly and chew foods well

  Always sit up while eating or drinking

  Do not overeat: stomach will expand and void surgical procedure

  Eat small amounts of all food and heed satiety feeling

  Avoid drinking 30 min before and after meals

  Eat with family, significant other(s)

  Use small plate and glass to make portions appear larger

  Do not snack between meals

  Avoid carbonated beverages

  Eat only two meals a day or as prescribed by physician

Explain importance of diet management

  Refer to nutritionist/registered dietitian as indicated; provide dietary list of foods to eat and avoid

  Have patient avoid high-calorie, high-carbohydrate foods and drinks, as well as gas-producing foods

  Maintain well-balanced, high-protein diet, 300 to 500 calories per day or as prescribed

  Discuss signs of hypokalemia: lower extremity muscle weakness, diarrhea, irregular pulse

Be accurate in measuring all food allowances

  Use 30 ml medication cup or 1½ tablespoon measuring scoop

  Maintain 1500 ml/day fluid intake or as prescribed

Add new foods to diet one at a time; intolerances can occur, especially with meat and poultry

  Discuss methods of processing foods with blender for gastroplasty patients

  Discuss availability of high-protein liquid supplements

Measure urine output daily

Keep accurate record of daily intake

Take chewable multivitamins daily

Weigh weekly because weight loss will be more noticeable

Instruct patient regarding rest and exercise

  Avoid heavy lifting and strenuous exercise

  Walk daily with goal of 1 to 2 miles per day within 4 wk

  Maintain planned rest periods

Demonstrate incisional and perianal care

Explain symptoms to report to physician

  Elevated temperature

  Wound drainage

  Persistent nausea and/or vomiting

  Hematemesis

  Abdominal tenderness and/or pain

  Abdominal distention

  Urine output of <750 ml/day for 3 consecutive days

  Constipation or continuing diarrhea

Reinforce stress management techniques
Explain importance of avoiding over-the-counter medications without first consulting physician
Encourage follow-up visits with physician, nutritionist/registered dietitian, including laboratory testing as ordered

Home care considerations

Provide information on what and where to purchase needed supplies: dressings, high-calorie supplements, blender
Explain signs of dumping syndrome: weakness, diaphoresis; may occur 2 to 3 wk following surgery
Refer to community support groups to augment coping with altered lifestyle
Discuss maintaining a positive self-image by wearing attractive, comfortable clothing, and to avoid purchasing smaller-sized clothing until ideal body weight is achieved
Encourage patient to dispose of "fat clothes" so they are not available to convey the message that the weight loss will not be permanent
Discourage patient from seeking liposuction until ideal body weight is attained

● Nasogastric Tubes

nasogastric tube: Tube used for gastric decompression, such as Levin or Salem sump (Figure 6-5), or for administration of food, fluid, or medication; a Levin tube must always be connected to intermittent suction; a Salem sump tube is usually connected to low continuous suction (because it is air vented) but may also be connected to intermittent suction

Preinsertion assessment and care

Assess patient's ability to swallow and mouth breathe
Assess nasal patency; observe for deviated septum, fracture
Check tube for patency
Lubricate and chill tube according to manufacturer's instructions
Explain purpose of tube and procedure

Postinsertion assessment

Character and consistency of gastric output
Patency of tube
Patency of sump if Salem tube is used

Placement for optimal drainage
Tube taped securely and comfortably to nose
Amount of pressure of suction apparatus
Nasal irritation

Potential complications

Dehydration
Electrolyte imbalance
Aspiration pneumonia

Interventions

Elevate head of bed 40 to 60 degrees *to reduce risk of aspiration or reflux*
Maintain NPO
Monitor character, amount, and consistency of gastric contents q4h; monitor gastric pH; if pH is <3.5, notify physician
Auscultate stomach for placement of tube prn by (1) inserting small amount of air in tube and listening for the air going into the stomach; use air vent on Salem tube and (2) aspirating tube and testing liquid for pH (gastric fluid has pH <3)
Connect tube to low, intermittent suction apparatus as ordered; irrigate with measured amounts of normal saline solution as ordered; *do not use tap water because it can alter electrolyte balance of stomach*
Salem sump tube
  Maintain patency of sump (air vent): keep opening higher than gastric tube and do not plug
  Sump tube may be irrigated, but instill 20 to 30 ml of air after irrigation to maintain patency
  If nausea occurs, tube is usually obstructed and relief is obtained with irrigation
  If vomiting occurs, turn patient on side to prevent aspiration; check for placement and obstruction
  Avoid dislodgment: tape securely to nose and allow enough tube for freedom of movement
  Apply lip balm or lubricant to nares and mouth prn
  Check tape holding tube prn; observe for reddened area

● Esophagostomy, Gastrostomy, Duodenostomy-Jejunostomy Management

esophagostomy: Surgically constructed stoma used to drain saliva and other secretions in patients with esophageal carcinoma, stricture, dysphagia, or atresia; may be used to administer tube feedings for these conditions; this procedure is similar to gastrostomy

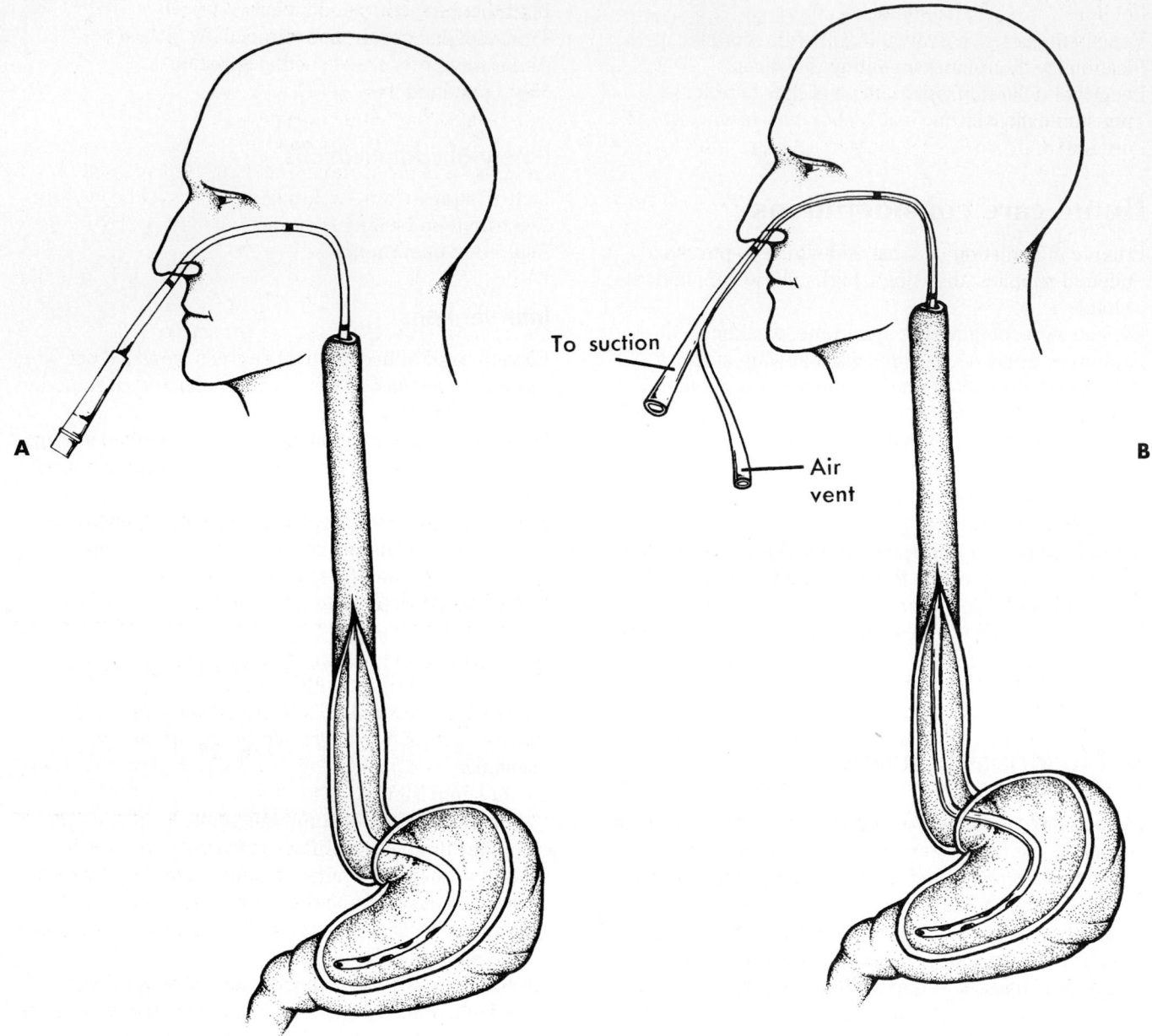

Figure 6-5 **A**, Levin tube. **B**, Salem sump tube. (From Given BA, Simmons SJ: *Gastroenterology in clinical nursing*, ed 4, St Louis, 1984, Mosby.)

except a longer catheter is used; the stoma may be permanent or temporary

gastrostomy: *Surgically constructed stoma or opening for a catheter in patients with esophageal carcinoma, stricture, trauma, atresia, and dysphagia; used for tube feedings or decompression and drainage; the ostomy is usually permanent, whereas the catheter is either temporary or permanent*

percutaneous endoscopic gastrostomy: *Feeding tube insertion using a gastroscope; the stomach is inflated with air and a cannula is inserted into*

the abdominal wall; a suture is threaded through and picked up by the scope and brought out through the mouth; the feeding tube is attached to the suture and drawn down into the stomach, out the abdominal wall, secured, and capped; this procedure is more cost effective and causes fewer complications

duodenostomy-jejunostomy: *Surgical incision for placement of a catheter for the feedings or decompression and drainage in patients when oral intake is prohibited or after gastrointestinal-esophageal surgery; may be permanent or temporary*

Assessment

Type and patency of stoma or catheter
Placement of dressing or stoma appliances
Length of catheter from incision to distal end
Taping of catheter
Pressure delivered by low, intermittent suction
   apparatus
Placement of closed gravity drainage system, clamp, or
   other collecting device
Character, color, and amount of drainage
Skin integrity around catheter or stoma
Condition of lips and mouth
Weight
Urinary output and specific gravity
Abdominal distention
Diminished bowel sounds
Character and color of stool

Potential complications

Dehydration
Nausea, vomiting
Electrolyte imbalance
Aspiration pneumonia
Wound infection
Hemorrhage/shock

Interventions

Measure intake and output q8h
For catheters
   Check color and consistency of drainage q4h; mea-
      sure amount q8h
   Maintain catheter to suction apparatus or gravity
      drainage
   Measure length of catheter q8h
   Tape securely to abdomen or neck; allow sufficient
      tubing for freedom of movement
For ostomy
   Monitor dressings and observe for drainage, color,
      and consistency
   Place stoma appliance over ostomy
When bowel sounds return or drainage is <300 to 500
ml/day
   Clamp catheter or cover ostomy
   Teach patient signs of retention and bowel obstruc-
      tion
      Nausea
      Abdominal distention
      Abdominal pain
   If these symptoms occur, notify physician immedi-
      ately, unclamp catheter, and connect to gravity
      drainage system

Initiate tube feedings as indicated (p. 59)
Provide skin care around surgical site q4h to 8h
   Wash area gently with soap and water
   Rinse and pat dry
   Apply skin barrier as needed
   Reapply dressings and appliance prn
Discuss with and demonstrate to patient and significant
   other(s) procedure of tube feeding and tube feeding
   preparation, as well as amount and times of feeding
   (p. 59)
Discuss and demonstrate ostomy care (p. 394) and skin
   care around the tube sites
Demonstrate dressing change procedure
Explain importance of weighing q2 days to 3 days
Provide information on symptoms of bowel obstruction
   and wound infection
Demonstrate medication preparation via tube feeding;
   discuss name, dose, purpose, time of administration,
   and side effects
Encourage follow-up appointments with physician

Intestine

● Inflammatory Bowel Disease: Regional Enteritis (Crohn's Disease, Ileocolitis) and Ulcerative Colitis

*regional enteritis: Chronic, recurrent nonspecific
   inflammation of unknown etiology affecting the entire
   intestine, usually the terminal ileum; it involves the
   mucosa and surrounding musculature and can lead to
   deep fissure formation*
*ulcerative colitis: Inflammatory intestinal disease of
   unknown cause, usually affecting the mucosal lining of
   the colon but may involve the entire large intestine;
   may be mild, chronic, or acute*

Assessment

Subjective data

Regional enteritis: cramplike abdominal pain; often in
   right lower quadrant with frequent diarrhea containing melena and/or steatorrhea
Ulcerative colitis: colicky abdominal cramps; pain is
   usually minimal; diarrheal stools are frequent and
   contain mucus, melena, and pus
Anorexia
Weight loss
Fever

Nausea
Generalized malaise

Objective data

Vomiting
Increased peristalsis
Anxiety, depression
Decreased muscle tone, skin turgor
Dry mucous membranes
Hypotension

Diagnostic tests

Barium studies of intestine
Sigmoidoscopy, colonoscopy
Biopsy, cytology
Radiologic study of abdomen
Serum iron, decreased
Serum electrolytes, decreased potassium
Albumin, decreased
Liver function tests
Hematologic studies: anemia, leukocytosis
Stools for melena, fat
ESR, elevated indicating inflammation

Potential complications

Electrolyte imbalance
Dehydration, malnutrition, anemia
Intestinal obstruction, perforation
Hemorrhage, shock
Fistula, peritonitis
Perianal abscess, fistula, fissure
Depression

Collaborative management

Therapeutic management

Anticholinergics: Donnatal, Probanthine
Immunosuppressants
Corticosteroids
Antibiotics
Antidiarrheals
Sedatives, analgesics
Parenteral fluids, elemental diet, TPN (depending on
  severity of disease)
Nasogastric suction; NPO
Sitz bath
Activity, rest, diet
Surgical interventions: ileostomy, colostomy,
  resection

Nursing management

PATIENT PROBLEMS/NURSING DIAGNOSES

● **NDX:**   Risk for fluid volume deficit related to abnormal fluid loss (diarrhea)

Maintain NPO; assess hydration status
Maintain parenteral fluids with electrolytes and vitamins
Monitor for signs of circulatory overload
Measure intake and output including emesis q8h
Monitor electrolytes *to determine replacement needs*
Weigh patient daily: same time, clothing, and scale
Monitor vital signs q4h; avoid taking temperature rectally
Administer antiemetics, antipyretics *to reduce fluid loss*

EXPECTED OUTCOMES

Patient's vital signs are stable
Hydration is adequate as evidenced by normal skin turgor and moist mucous membranes
Intake and output are balanced

● **NDX:**   Diarrhea related to inflammation of bowel

Maintain bed rest *to reduce intestinal motility and conserve energy*
Assess and monitor stools for amount, frequency, consistency, and color
Monitor stools for occult blood
Auscultate abdomen for bowel sounds q8h *to evaluate reduced peristalsis*
Monitor effectiveness and side effects of antidiarrheal, antibiotic, and steroid therapy
Balance rest with activity
Provide odor-free environment; keep covered bedpan within easy reach; empty, clean, and return promptly
Monitor for signs of bowel perforation: fever, tachycardia, lethargy, pain

EXPECTED OUTCOMES

Patient expresses reduction in frequency of stools
States stool returning to normal consistency

● **NDX:**   Altered nutrition: less than body requirements related to diarrhea and altered absorption

Assess nutritional status and assist patient with identifying irritating foods such as raw fruits and vegetables, whole grains, carbonated beverages, whole milk
Provide diet high in calories, protein, and minerals; low in residue, fat, and fiber

Prepared elemental diets are available
TPN as indicated *to allow intestinal tract to rest*
Six small meals are beneficial
Encourage patient to participate in meal planning *to provide sense of control and increase intake*
Maintain intake record and avoid foods that cause cramping, diarrhea
Administer anticholinergics *to reduce motility and increase absorption*
Administer vitamin B$_{12}$ *to correct malabsorption*
Encourage patient to eat slowly, chew well, and take small bites
Serve food attractively in a well-ventilated room
Monitor Hgb and Hct
Administer oral hygiene *to increase desire to eat and enhance taste of foods*

EXPECTED OUTCOMES

Patient maintains normal weight
Presents laboratory values that are within normal limits

● **NDX:** Risk for impaired skin integrity related to fluid/nutritional deficit and irritation from diarrhea

Assess perirectal area for inflammation, abscess, or fistula
Administer perirectal skin care after each bowel movement
  Wash gently with soap and water
  Pat dry and apply soothing protective ointments
Administer sitz baths *to reduce pain and irritated perianal tissue*
Provide skin care to bony prominences as needed *to reduce risk of skin breakdown*
Provide frequent position changes

EXPECTED OUTCOMES

Patient's perirectal tissue remains clean and intact
Skin turgor and color are normal

● **NDX:** Pain related to bowel inflammation and irritation

Assess character, intensity, and location of pain
Assess effectiveness, side effects of sedatives, analgesics, and rectal suppositories and ointments
Change patient's position frequently and administer back rubs *to relieve discomfort*
Provide diversional activities *to reduce attention on discomfort*
Ambulate patient with assistance as tolerated
Encourage and teach alternate pain management

methods: imaging, deep breathing, relaxation techniques
Balance rest and activity

EXPECTED OUTCOMES

Patient demonstrates a more relaxed affect
Verbalizes a tolerable level of pain

● **NDX:** Ineffective individual coping related to multiple stressors and needed lifestyle changes

Assess present and past coping patterns *to increase ability in managing present problems*
Provide time for and encourage communication with significant other(s) *to provide a support system*
Establish a supportive relationship with patient and/or significant other(s)
  Explain all procedures and treatments
  Involve patient and/or significant other(s) in plan of care and realistically reinforce physician's explanation of disease process
  Maintain quiet, nonjudgmental, and nonstressful environment
  Encourage use of stress management techniques
  Provide undisturbed rest periods
  Accept patient's dependency and encourage independent activities as strength returns
Provide information about support groups such as the following:
United Ostomy Association
36 Executive Park
Suite 120
Irvine, CA 92714
    1-800-826-0826
    (714) 660-8624
FAX: (714) 660-9262

Crohn's and Colitis Foundation of America, Inc.
386 Park Avenue South
New York, NY 10016-8804
    1-800-932-2423
    (212) 685-3440
FAX: (212) 779-4098

EXPECTED OUTCOMES

Patient expresses feelings/concerns more readily
Demonstrates understanding of needed lifestyle changes
Exhibits appropriate coping skills and behaviors

● **NDX:** Sexual dysfunction related to altered body function and lack of knowledge

Explore patient's knowledge of sexuality and current sexual practices and behaviors

Explain to patient and/or significant other that sexual activity needs to be curtailed only while perineal area is inflamed or fistulas or abscesses are present

Encourage patient and significant other to read about alternate sexual positions and techniques

Provide supportive and private environment

EXPECTED OUTCOMES

Patient expresses understanding of needed changes in sexual practices

Verbalizes feelings and concerns

Patient/family teaching

Assess understanding of disease process and the cause/effect relationships of precipitating factors

Provide instructions in diet management, stressing foods to avoid: raw fruits and vegetables, alcohol, chocolate, and gas-producing foods

Discuss importance of introducing new foods one at a time

Discuss importance of avoiding stress during meals, need to chew food well and eat slowly

Explain causal relationship of stress to disease process and symptoms of recurrence or progression of disease to report to physician

Provide information about medications including name, dosage, purpose, time of administration, side effects, and interactions; explain need to avoid over-the-counter medications unless first discussed with physician

Encourage follow-up appointments with physician

Home care considerations

Demonstrate procedure for perianal skin care

Stress importance of keeping area clean and dry

Discuss side effects of steroids: facial edema, ulcers, and reduced immune response to infection

Provide information about what and where to purchase needed supplies

Provide information on TPN if needed and discuss good aseptic technique

Discourage smoking

Provide names of community resources: VNA, nutritionist/registered dietitian, and social services

● Peritonitis (Secondary)

Inflammation of the peritoneal cavity caused by infiltration of intestinal contents from such conditions as a ruptured appendix, gastric or intestinal perforation or trauma, and anastomotic leaks

Primary peritonitis is a bacterial infection of the peritoneal cavity not associated with bowel conditions; seen mostly in children with renal disorders and in patients with ascites

Assessment

Subjective data

Abdominal pain and rigidity over area of inflammation
  Rebound tenderness
  May refer to shoulder
Anorexia
Nausea

Objective data

Vomiting
Abdominal distention
Decreased-to-absent bowel sounds
Failure to pass flatus or stool
Chills, fever
Tachycardia
Hypotension
Leukocytosis
Anxiety
Thoracic breathing: rapid, shallow
Fecal emesis

Diagnostic tests

CBC, electrolytes, WBC increased
Radiologic examination of abdomen
Peritoneal aspiration

Potential complications

Electrolyte imbalance
Dehydration
Metabolic acidosis
Respiratory alkalosis
Shock

Collaborative management

Therapeutic management

Parenteral fluids with electrolytes, antibiotics, and vitamins
Analgesics
Nasogastric suction, NPO
ABGs

CVP lines
Oxygen therapy, incentive spirometer
Peritoneal lavage with antibiotics
Surgical intervention

Nursing management

PATIENT PROBLEMS/NURSING DIAGNOSES

● **NDX:** Fluid volume deficit related to increased blood flow to peritoneum, vomiting, and/or gastrointestinal perforation

Assess hydration status
Maintain NPO *to decrease intestinal motility*
Monitor vital signs and CPV qh or prn; observe for signs of shock
Maintain parenteral fluids with electrolytes, antibiotics, and vitamins
Weigh patient daily: same time, clothing, and scale
Measure intake and output q1h to 2h; measure urine output hourly; if <50 ml/hr notify physician; *may indicate renal complications*
Assist with peritoneal aspiration/lavage, drainage
  Connect drain to gravity drainage as ordered
  Include drainage in output amount
  Send specimen for culture
Monitor electrolytes, blood gases, Hgb, and Hct
Perform passive or assist with and teach active ROM exercises q4h *to increase circulation*

EXPECTED OUTCOMES
Patient's hydration is adequate as evidenced by normal skin turgor and moist mucous membranes
Vital signs are stable
Intake and output are balanced

● **NDX:** Ineffective breathing pattern, secondary to abdominal pain and distention

Assess respiratory status; monitor for shallow, rapid respirations
Maintain bed rest in quiet environment with head of bed elevated 35 to 45 degrees *to increase lung expansion*
Monitor oxygen therapy or incentive spirometer
Assist and teach patient to turn and cough q4h and deep breathe q1h to 2h
Auscultate chest for breath sounds q4h

EXPECTED OUTCOMES
Patient exhibits normal respirations and breath sounds
Demonstrates ability to perform breathing exercises

● **NDX:** Altered nutrition: less th ments related to vomiting

Monitor nasogastric tube or naso-oral connect to low, intermittent suction
  Monitor character, amount, color, an drainage
Provide frequent oral and nasal hygiene
Monitor for passing of flatus
Auscultate abdomen for bowel sounds q8h
Monitor TPN as indicated (see p. 64)
When bowel sounds return and nasogastric-intestinal tube is removed, provide clear liquid diet as tolerated
If surgery is performed, see Intestinal surgery (p. 382)

EXPECTED OUTCOMES
Patient states absence of nausea/vomiting
Tolerates diet adequately

● **NDX:** Pain related to inflammation and distention

Assess type, location, and severity of pain
Administer analgesics only after diagnosis has been made, *because they mask signs and symptoms*
Assess effectiveness of pain relief measures
Maintain position of comfort *to minimize stress on abdomen*
Change positions in small ways *to reduce discomfort*
Provide planned rest periods
Discuss and teach alternate pain management techniques: visualizing, imaging, deep breathing
Provide diversional activities *to reduce attention on pain*

EXPECTED OUTCOMES
Patient verbalizes a tolerable level of pain
Exhibits improving ability to use alternate pain relief measures

● **NDX:** Anxiety related to situational crisis

Assess anxiety level (p. 35)
Assess present coping skills
Encourage and allow time for verbalization of feelings
Explain all treatments and procedures
Reinforce physician's explanation of illness and treatment
Assist with and teach relaxation techniques
Provide periods of undisturbed rest
Encourage support of family/significant other(s)

EXPECTED OUTCOMES
Patient expresses feelings and concerns and understands positive ways of coping
Appears more relaxed and comfortable

...ient/family teaching

Assess level of understanding of disease process
Discuss pain management and use of relaxation
techniques
Stress importance of signs and symptoms to report to
physician
Provide information about diet; increase to normal diet
as tolerated; avoid irritating foods and introduce new
foods one at a time
Discuss medications, side effects, and need to take all
medications as prescribed
Encourage follow-up appointments with
physician

Home care considerations

Demonstrate wound care and importance of sterile
technique
Provide information on what and where to purchase
needed supplies
Provide names of community resources to assist
with home care: visiting nurse, social services, home
health aides

● Short Bowel Syndrome

*Malabsorption following small bowel resection; severity
depends on the amount and portion of small bowel
removed; the loss of >3 meters of the small bowel
will affect the body's ability to absorb nutrients
and vitamins, especially if the ileocecal valve is
removed*

Assessment

Subjective data

Diarrhea
Weight loss
Fatigue
Weakness

Objective data

Frequent, watery diarrhea; may contain fat
Rapid dehydration resulting from malabsorption
Purpura, generalized bleeding
Anemia
Malabsorption of fat and fat-soluble vitamins
(A, D, E, K)

Diagnostic tests

Barium enema
Serum studies: reduced iron, vitamins B_{12} and A, cal-
cium, folate, magnesium, electrolytes, CBC, carotene,
cholesterol
PT/INR: increased
Stool for fat and culture
Lactose intolerance, elevated D-lactate level, decreased
xylose tolerance

Potential complications

Malnutrition
Electrolyte imbalance
Osteoporosis, osteomalacia
Night blindness
Tetany
Confusion, stupor

Collaborative management

Therapeutic management

Antidiarrheals
Anticholinergics
Antibiotics
Antacids
Vitamin B_{12}, folate, multivitamins
Histamine receptor antagonists (cimetidine)
TPN, parenteral fluids (p. 64)
Elemental diet progressing to low-lactose, high-calorie
diet

Nursing management

PATIENT PROBLEMS/NURSING DIAGNOSES

● **NDX:** Fluid volume deficit related to profuse diarrhea and fluid loss

Monitor parenteral fluids with electrolytes and
vitamins
Assess for signs of dehydration and shock; check LOC
q2h
Monitor vital signs q2h to 4h
Measure intake and output q8h
Weigh patient daily: same time, clothing, and scale
Monitor serum electrolytes, Hgb, and Hct

EXPECTED OUTCOMES
Patient's vital signs are normal
Intake and output are balanced
Skin turgor is adequate
Electrolytes are within normal limits

● **NDX:** Diarrhea related to decreased intestinal absorption

Assess effectiveness, side effects of antidiarrheals, antacids, histamine receptor antagonists
Monitor stools for color, consistency, amount, and frequency
Provide perineal care after each bowel movement; keep environment free of odor
Auscultate abdomen for bowel sounds q4h

EXPECTED OUTCOMES

Patient's stools are less frequent
Stool consistency is more normal

● **NDX:** Altered nutrition: less than body requirements related to loss of absorptive surface of intestine

Maintain TPN as indicated (see p. 64)
  Monitor urine for sugar and acetone qid
  Monitor blood glucose
  Observe central IV line for infection
  Institute elemental diet (Vivonex, Precision LR), usually when weight gain is apparent and diarrhea is less frequent
  Administer diet through nasogastric tube or orally, depending on patient's appetite: 300 to 350 ml q2h
  When given orally, provide a straw because the taste may be unpalatable to some patients
  Discuss with and assist patient and significant other(s) with accepting revised nutritional plan, which may be necessary for a long period
  Collaborate with nutritionist/registered dietitian on diet and nourishments
  Assess effectiveness and monitor side effects of antacids and anticholinergics
  Measure intake after each meal; maintain calorie count

EXPECTED OUTCOMES

Patient maintains weight at level normal for patient
Demonstrates understanding of changes needed in dietary regimen

Patient/family teaching

Discuss and provide written information about nutritional plan, usually low-lactose, high-calorie diet; introduce milk slowly and observe tolerance
Instruct patient and/or significant other(s) concerning signs and symptoms to report to physician: nausea, vomiting, diarrhea, or other intestinal problems

Discuss medication: name, dosage, purpose, time of administration, and side effects
Encourage follow-up visits with physician

Home care considerations

Discuss and provide information on TPN if it is to be given at home (p. 64)
Involve nutritionist/registered dietitian and provide referral to home health services
Stress importance of signs of dehydration: poor skin turgor, dry mucous membranes, weakness
Provide names, phone numbers of home health team members

● Intestinal Obstruction

Blockage of the intestinal tract, which inhibits the passage of fluids, flatus, and food; may be mechanical or functional

Causes

Mechanical

Adhesions
Strangulated hernia
Abscess
Carcinoma
Volvulus
Intussusception
Obstipation

Functional

Paralytic ileus
Spinal cord lesions
Regional enteritis
Electrolyte imbalance
Uremia

Assessment

Specific data

Small bowel
  Severe, cramplike abdominal pain, increasing with distention
  Mild distention
  Nausea
  Vomiting: early contains undigested food and chyme; later vomitus is watery and contains bile; finally, dark and fecal
  Rapid dehydration: acidosis

Large bowel
  Mild abdominal discomfort
  Severe distention
  Latent fecal vomiting
  Latent dehydration: rare acidosis

Common data

SUBJECTIVE DATA

Constipation
Nausea
Anxiety
Anorexia and malaise

OBJECTIVE DATA

Fever
Tachycardia
Diaphoresis
Pallor
Abdominal rigidity
Failure to pass stool or flatus rectally or per
  ostomy
Increased bowel sounds (early obstruction)
Decreased bowel sounds (later)
Urinary retention
Leukocytosis

Diagnostic tests

Serum electrolytes, CBC, amylase
Barium enema
Radiologic studies of abdomen

Potential complications

Dehydration
Electrolyte imbalance
Metabolic acidosis
Perforation
Shock

Collaborative management

Therapeutic management

NPO
Nasointestinal suction
Surgical intervention: see Intestinal surgery (p. 382)
Parenteral fluids with electrolytes, antibiotics, and
  vitamins
Analgesics
Oxygen therapy

Nursing management

PATIENT PROBLEMS/NURSING DIAGNOSES

● **NDX:** Fluid volume deficit secondary to nausea
  and vomiting, fever, and/or diaphoresis

Monitor vital signs and observe level of consciousness
  and for symptoms of hypovolemic shock
Maintain NPO; assess level of hydration
Monitor parenteral fluids with electrolytes, antibiotics,
  and vitamins
Insert and monitor nasointestinal tube and low, inter-
  mittent suction apparatus
  Measure drainage output q8h
  Observe contents for color, consistency
Position patient on right side, then left side to facilitate
  passage into intestine; do not tape nasointestinal tube
  to nose until tube is in correct position
Monitor tube for advancement qh
Indwelling urethral catheter may be inserted; report
  output of <50 ml/hr to physician
Monitor electrolytes, Hgb, and Hct
Prepare for surgery as indicated (p. 382)
If surgery is not performed, collaborate with physician
  and initiate oral fluids, either by clamping intestinal
  tube for 1 hr and giving measured amounts of water
  or tea or by giving these fluids after intestinal tube is
  removed
Open tube, if in place, at specified times as ordered to
  estimate amount of absorption
Observe abdomen for discomfort, distention, pain, or
  rigidity and report to physician
Auscultate bowel sounds tid, 1 hr after meals; report
  diminished/absent sounds to physician
Force fluids to 2500 ml/day unless contraindicated
Measure intake and output until adequate
Encourage ambulation *to stimulate peristalsis*
Observe initial stool for color, consistency, and amount;
  prevent constipation

EXPECTED OUTCOMES

Patient's vital signs are normal
Intake and output are balanced

● **NDX:** Pain related to distention, rigidity

Maintain bed rest in position of comfort; do not gatch
  knees
Assess location, severity, and type of pain; use pain rating scale
Assess effectiveness and monitor for side effects of
  analgesics; avoid morphine
Provide planned rest periods
Assist with and teach active or perform passive ROM
  exercises q4h *to prevent fatigue*

Change position frequently and administer back rubs and skin care *to promote comfort*

Auscultate bowel sounds; note increased rigidity or pain; give gentle enema if ordered

Provide and teach alternate pain relief measures

EXPECTED OUTCOMES

Patient verbalizes decreased discomfort; states pain is at tolerable level

Appears relaxed

● **NDX:** Ineffective breathing pattern related to abdominal distention and/or rigidity

Assess respiratory status; observe for shallow, rapid breathing

Elevate head of bed 40 to 60 degrees *to increase lung expansion*

Monitor oxygen or incentive spirometer therapy

Assist and teach patient to turn and cough q4h and deep breathe qh

Auscultate chest for breath sounds q4h

EXPECTED OUTCOMES

Patient demonstrates ability to perform breathing exercises

Exhibits respirations that are deep and slow

● **NDX:** Anxiety related to situational crisis and altered health status

Assess present coping behaviors and encourage use of past successful skills

Encourage and allow time for verbalization of anxieties and fears; provide quiet reassurance

Explain procedures and treatments and reinforce physician's explanation of illness, treatment, and prognosis

Maintain quiet, nonstressful environment; encourage support of family and significant other(s)

EXPECTED OUTCOMES

Patient expresses understanding of present illness

Demonstrates positive coping skills in dealing with anxiety

Patient/family teaching

Discuss dietary management, stressing importance of eating slowly, chewing food well, and eating at regular intervals

Explain need to prevent constipation
  Use natural laxatives or stool softeners
  Maintain fluid intake of 2500 ml/day
  Increase activity as tolerated

Provide instructions on symptoms to report to physician: abdominal pain, cramps, distention, and/or nausea and vomiting

Encourage follow-up care with physician

If surgery was performed, see Intestinal surgery (p. 382)

Home care considerations

Encourage patient to perform ROM exercises at home *to increase strength*

Promote increasing activity slowly but steadily *to increase bowel function*

Encourage short walks outdoors

Stress importance of adequate daily fluid intake

● Paralytic Ileus

Temporary decrease in or absence of intestinal motility after intestinal or abdominal surgery or in connection with any severe metabolic disease; cause may be neuromuscular, resulting from lack of potassium, or gastrointestinal, resulting from gastric inactivity and air swallowing

Assessment

Subjective data

Nausea

Feeling of fullness

Abdominal tenderness and distention

Objective data

Absent or diminished bowel sounds

Vomiting

Lack of flatus

Decreased urinary output

Fever

Diagnostic tests

Electrolytes (decreased potassium)

Abdominal radiography series

Potential complications

Dehydration

Electrolyte imbalance

Shock

Perforation of ileum
Peritonitis (p. 374)
Circulatory failure
Respiratory distress

Collaborative management

Therapeutic management

NPO
Parenteral fluids with electrolytes
Nasointestinal, nasogastric aspiration
Oxygen therapy
Medications to promote peristalsis: dexpanthenol
  (Ilopan), bethanechol (Urecholine), neostigmine
  (Prostigmin), metoclopramide (Reglan)
Activity, diet
Enema, rectal tube

Nursing management

PATIENT PROBLEMS/NURSING DIAGNOSES

● **NDX:** Ineffective breathing pattern related to abdominal distention and rigidity

Maintain bed rest in position to facilitate respirations;
  do not gatch knees
Assess respiratory status
Auscultate chest for breath sounds q4h
Monitor oxygen therapy
Assist and teach patient to turn and cough q4h and
  deep breathe qh
Balance activity and rest
Monitor vital signs q4h
Ambulate when tolerated *to increase peristalsis*

EXPECTED OUTCOMES

Patient demonstrates ability to perform breathing exercises
Exhibits normal respirations and breath sounds

● **NDX:** Fluid volume deficit related to vomiting and
  distention

Maintain NPO; assess level of hydration
Maintain parenteral fluids with electrolytes
Maintain nasointestinal tube to low, intermittent suction
  apparatus (p. 369)
  Do not tape tube to nose; position patient to facilitate
    passage of tube into intestine
  Monitor advancement qh
Monitor character, amount, and color of intestinal
  drainage q4h; report any change to physician
Nasogastric tube may be inserted in lieu of intestinal
  tube; connect to low, intermittent suction apparatus

Tape securely to nose
Irrigate with measured amounts of normal saline
Monitor color and amount of drainage
Measure intake and output; report urine output of <50
  ml/hr to physician
Monitor electrolytes
Collaborate with physician when intestinal or gastric
  output decreases and bowel sounds return to initiate
  feeding schedule
Clamp tube
Administer liquids (warm tea, carbonated beverages)
  in measured amounts
Monitor for pain, distention, nausea, and cramps; un-
  clamp tube if these signs occur
Remove tube and progress to previous diet
Continue measuring intake and output until adequate
  for patient

EXPECTED OUTCOMES

Patient's vital signs are normal
Hydration is normal as evidenced by skin turgor
Intake and output are balanced
Bowel sounds are normal
Electrolytes are within normal limits

● **NDX:** Constipation related to decreased intake

Assess effectiveness of and monitor for side effects of
  medication used to increase peristalsis
Auscultate abdomen for bowel sounds q4h; monitor for
  return of flatus and normal bowel elimination
Promote high-fiber diet and increased fluid intake as
  tolerated
Encourage ambulation

EXPECTED OUTCOMES

Patient understands causative factors of constipation
Defecates soft, formed stool

● **NDX:** Knowledge deficit related to lack of information about illness and its outcome

Reinforce physician's explanation of cause of paralytic
  ileus and that it is a temporary condition
Explain all procedures and treatments
Demonstrate technique for swallowing without ingesting air
Stress importance of increased fluid intake and activity
  to maintain peristaltic action

EXPECTED OUTCOMES

Patient verbalizes understanding of disease
  process
Participates in treatment regimen

● Diverticular Disease of Colon

Herniation (pocket formation) along the mucosa of the large intestine caused by low-fiber diets and weakened intestinal wall (diverticulosis); an inflammatory process may occur when a diverticulum ruptures or feces become impacted in the diverticulum (diverticulitis); the incidence increases with age (60% of people older than 60 years of age have the condition) and is most commonly found in the sigmoid colon

Acute diverticulitis

Subjective data

Cramplike pain and tenderness in left lower quadrant
Anorexia
Nausea

Objective data

Low-grade fever
Irregular bowel function
  Constipation
  Diarrhea
  Mucus, blood in stool
  Increased flatulence
  Abdominal distention
  Decreased bowel sounds

Diagnostic tests

Water-soluble contrast enema
Sigmoidoscopy, colonoscopy with biopsy
Ultrasonography
WBC, ESR: increased
Urinalysis, stool examination
Examination of surrounding organs (kidney, bladder)
  for possible involvement

Potential complications

Leukocytosis
Dehydration
Intestinal obstruction, perforation
Peritonitis
Fistula, abscess
Hemorrhage

Collaborative management

Therapeutic management

Bed rest
Parenteral fluids with electrolytes and antibiotics

Nasogastric aspiration (severe vomiting, distention)
Analgesics, anticholinergics
NPO increasing to high-fiber diet
Surgical intervention (resection, colostomy)
Diet, activity

Nursing management

PATIENT PROBLEMS/NURSING DIAGNOSES

● **NDX:**   Risk for fluid volume deficit related to nausea, diarrhea, anorexia, risk of hypovolemia

Maintain NPO; assess level of hydration
Maintain parenteral fluids with antibiotics and electrolytes
Monitor electrolytes
Collaborate with physician, nutritionist/registered dietitian; when pain and fever subside and/or nasogastric tube is removed, provide clear liquid diet and progress to soft diet until high-fiber diet can be tolerated
Force fluids to 2500 ml/day unless contraindicated
Assess and monitor amount of bleeding; check stools for occult or frank blood
Monitor vital signs q4h and Hgb, Hct as needed
Monitor blood transfusions or PBCs
Assist with exercises of legs and feet q4h *to increase venous return*
Measure intake and output; report output of <50 ml/hr to physician

EXPECTED OUTCOMES

Patient's hydration is adequate as evidenced by normal skin turgor
Intake and output are balanced
Vital signs are within normal limits

● **NDX:**   Constipation related to anorexia, low-fiber diet, and immobility

Monitor nasogastric tube and low, intermittent suction apparatus
  Maintain tube patency
  Irrigate with measured amounts of normal saline
  Measure gastric output q8h
Auscultate abdomen for bowel sounds q4h
Monitor stools for consistency, color, amount, and frequency; check for impaction
When nasogastric tube is removed, administer hydrophilic colloid laxative or psyllium (Metamucil) as tolerated *to promote defecation*
Ambulate as tolerated *to increase intestinal motility*

EXPECTED OUTCOMES

Patient tolerates increasingly high-fiber diet
Defecates soft, formed stool

● **NDX:** Pain related to inflammation, irritation of bowel

Maintain bed rest in position of comfort
Assess location, character, and severity of pain
Administer analgesics; avoid morphine; assess effectiveness of pain relief measures
Assist and teach patient to turn and deep breathe q2h; administer back rubs *to promote comfort*
Maintain planned rest periods
Change position frequently *to prevent pressure and fatigue*
Encourage and teach alternate pain management methods: relaxation techniques, imaging, deep breathing

EXPECTED OUTCOMES

Patient reports a tolerable level of pain
Appears relaxed

Patient/family teaching

Assess level of understanding of diverticular disease
Provide written dietary instructions and discuss relationship of diet to disease process
Include listing of high-fiber foods: bran, fruits, vegetables, nuts
Explain importance of regular meals, eating slowly, and chewing well
  Avoid large meals, extremely cold foods, and alcohol
  Increase fluid intake to eight glasses per day unless contraindicated
Discuss importance of elimination
  Establish regular bowel habits
  Avoid constipation, straining, enemas, and harsh laxatives
Use psyllium (Metamucil) or high-fiber wafers or powder
Encourage regular visits to physician

Home care considerations

Discuss bowel training and establishing regular elimination habits
  Set aside a daily time for bowel movement
  Avoid anxiety and interruption
  Drink plenty of fluids and exercise regularly
  Maintain a high-fiber diet
Explain signs and symptoms of recurrence of condition to report to physician

Pain, cramps in left lower quadrant
Diarrhea, constipation
Blood in stool

● Intestinal Surgery With or Without Fecal Diversion

Any surgery performed on the intestine from the jejunum to the colon for such conditions as carcinoma, obstruction, acute enteritis or colitis, benign tumors, trauma, appendicitis, incarcerated hernia, and diverticulitis; some of these conditions may require a fecal diversion, either an ileostomy or colostomy

Preoperative assessment and care

Assess respiratory status
Monitor potassium level
Prepare bowel
  Low-residue, clear liquid diet
  Magnesia preparations, oral antibiotics
  GoLytly bowel preparation
  Enemas until clear; avoid depleting debilitated or elderly patients with multiple enemas at one time
  Nasogastric/nasointestinal tube insertion
Provide patient with information regarding drains, tubes, and so on that may be present postoperatively (nasogastric tube, urinary catheter, or wound drains)
Teach patient to turn, cough, and deep breathe
Demonstrate methods for incisional support
Discuss importance of moving after surgery, especially feet and legs
Explain and discuss fecal diversion if appropriate including purpose and placement of stoma

Postoperative assessment

Subjective data

Location, type of pain
Nausea

Objective data

Character and amount of gastric or intestinal drainage
  Urinary output
  Ostomy drainage, if applicable
  Wound drainage
Vomiting
Abdominal distention
Placement of nasogastric tube

Decreased, shallow respirations
Decreased breath sounds

Diagnostic tests

Electrolytes, Hgb, Hct
BUN, creatinine
Stool for guaiac
Urine culture after indwelling catheter is removed
Wound culture; suspected infection

Potential complications

Dehydration
Electrolyte imbalance
Atelectasis
Hemorrhage
Shock
Peritonitis
Paralytic ileus
Pulmonary embolus
Thrombophlebitis
Wound evisceration
Wound infection

Collaborative management

Therapeutic management

Parenteral fluids with electrolytes
Nasogastric aspiration
Indwelling urethral catheter
NPO progressing to prescribed diet
Analgesics, antibiotics, vitamins
Histamine inhibitors (Cimetidine), antacids
Patient controlled analgesia (p. 92)
Oxygen therapy, incentive spirometer
Activity, antiembolic stockings

Nursing management

PATIENT PROBLEMS/NURSING DIAGNOSES

● **NDX:** Ineffective breathing pattern related to placement of incision and/or pain, anesthesia

Assess respiratory status: type, frequency, and character of respirations
Elevate head of bed 35 to 45 degrees *to promote lung expansion*
Auscultate lungs for breath sounds q2h
Assist and teach patient to turn and cough q2h and deep breathe qh; support incision
Provide incentive spirometer 10 times per hour
Administer pain medication before treatments as applicable *to reduce discomfort*

EXPECTED OUTCOMES

Patient exhibits normal respiratory rate and rhythm
Presents breath sounds that are clear

● **NDX:** Risk for fluid volume deficit related to gastric suction, diarrhea

Maintain NPO, assess hydration status: skin turgor, moist mucous membranes, capillary refill
Maintain parenteral fluids with electrolytes, vitamins, and antibiotics
Monitor vital signs q2h to 4h
Monitor dressings for excessive drainage, hemorrhage
Place temporary appliance on ostomy if applicable; measure drainage q8h
Monitor nasogastric/intestinal tube and low, intermittent suction
  Measure output q8h
  Test pH to evaluate acidity; <5 may indicate stress ulcer formation
  Check color and consistency of drainage
  Irrigate with measured amounts of normal saline
Measure intake and output q8h and monitor for fluid shift: edema, weight gain, rales
Monitor serum electrolytes and urine specific gravity
Encourage position changes *to stimulate circulation*
Monitor indwelling urethral catheter and closed gravity drainage system; measure output hourly; if <50 ml/hr, report to physician
Perform guaiac test on stool for signs of intestinal bleeding
Observe for abdominal distention and monitor bowel sounds for 2 to 3 days postoperatively
Monitor peripheral pulses, signs of edema, capillary refill
Apply antiembolic stockings and remove daily for skin care
Encourage movement of legs and feet *to promote venous circulation*

EXPECTED OUTCOMES

Patient's vital signs are normal
Intake and output are balanced
Hydration is adequate as evidenced by normal skin turgor and capillary refill
Peripheral pulses are palpable

● **NDX:**   Pain related to surgical intervention

Maintain bed rest in quiet environment
Monitor location, character, intensity of pain; use pain
   rating scale
Assess effectiveness of pain relief measures and ob-
   serve for side effects
Initiate patient controlled analgesia (p. 92) if pre-
   scribed
Encourage patient to take pain medication as pre-
   scribed for 48 hr
Encourage ambulation *to reduce discomfort from intesti-
   nal gas*
Coordinate care to allow for planned rest periods
Change position frequently; administer back rubs *to
   promote comfort and ease fatigue*
Discuss and teach alternate pain relief techniques as
   needed: guided imagery, deep breathing

   EXPECTED OUTCOMES
Patient reports a tolerable level of discomfort
Appears more relaxed, comfortable

● **NDX:**   Risk for impaired skin integrity related to increased wound drainage, altered circulation,
   nutrition

Administer nasal and oral hygiene frequently and keep
   nares and mouth moist
Change dressings as needed; use nonallergenic tape or
   Montgomery straps
   Assess healing process
   Monitor drainage for signs of infection; obtain culture
      prn
   Keep skin around incision clean and dry
Provide splinting of incision when coughing *to prevent
   dehiscence*
Maintain permanency of tubes and catheters by taping
   comfortably and securely
Initiate a wound pouching system if drainage is profuse
Assess color and condition of stoma and peristomal
   skin integrity if applicable (see Ostomy management
   p. 394)
Monitor perianal area if rectum was closed
   Keep skin clean and dry
   Change dressings as needed
   Observe for increase in drainage
Encourage ambulation *to promote circulation and healing*

   EXPECTED OUTCOMES
Patient's wound heals without incident
Surrounding tissue is clean, dry, and intact

● **NDX:**   Bowel incontinence related to surgical manipulation, immobility, altered nutritional intake

Administer antiemetics *to prevent vomiting* and antacids
   or histamine inhibitors *to neutralize acids*
Assess preoperative bowel habits and nutritional intake;
   explain cause of alteration
Observe for passage of flatus
Auscultate abdomen for return of bowel sounds q8h; *indicates normal bowel function or possible paralytic ileus
   if sounds do not return*
Observe first postoperative bowel movement: assess
   color, consistency, amount, and frequency
Administer vitamin K *because bowel preparation may inhibit absorption*
Administer stool softener *to promote peristaltic
   action*
Demonstrate and teach ostomy irrigation and appliance
   application if appropriate (p. 394)

   EXPECTED OUTCOMES
Patient understands causative factors of altered elimina-
   tion
Defecates soft, formed stool

● **NDX:**   Altered nutrition: less than body requirements related to NPO status, nasogastric
   suction

Collaborate with physician, nutritionist/registered di-
   etitian; after bowel sounds return and nasogastric/
   intestinal tube is removed or clamped, initiate clear
   liquids in measured amounts; observe for tolerance
   and discomfort or distention
Progress to soft or regular diet as tolerated
Assist patient in selection of high-protein, high–vitamin
   C foods *to promote healing*
Monitor for malabsorption syndrome after surgery of
   small intestine: steatorrhea, diarrhea, weight loss
Weigh patient daily: same time, clothing, and scale
Monitor intake and output until adequate for age and
   weight

   EXPECTED OUTCOMES
Patient maintains normal weight
Tolerates diet without discomfort

Patient/family teaching

Provide written dietary instructions and restrictions
Demonstrate dressing changes, wound care, aseptic
   technique
Discuss signs of wound infection: pain, redness,
   swelling, odor
Reinforce ostomy care if applicable (p. 394)
Explain importance of preventing constipation and us-
   ing natural laxatives or those prescribed

Discuss activities allowed and need for rest, mild exercise, and not lifting heavy objects (more than 5 to 10 lb) for 6 to 8 wk

Reinforce physician's explanation of surgical procedure and outcome expected

Discuss medications: name, dosage, purpose, time of administration, and side effects

Encourage follow-up visits with physician

Home care considerations

Discuss dietary plan to follow
  Foods high in protein and vitamin C
  Eat six small meals *to reduce feeling of fullness*
  Drink plenty of fluids *to promote healing*
  Eat slowly and chew foods well
Provide information on what type of and where to purchase needed dressings
Have patient return demonstrate sterile technique, handwashing procedure, and dressing change
Discuss signs and symptoms of problems to report to physician
  Tenderness, drainage, redness around incision
  Increased pain, eructation, or distention
  Bleeding from incision
  Nausea, vomiting
Refer to community resources for assistance with food preparation, personal care, transportation

● Continent Ileostomy (Kock's Pouch)

Surgical removal of the rectum and colon (proctocolectomy) with construction of an internal ileal reservoir, nipple valve, and stoma, allowing intermittent drainage of ileal contents; it is often performed in two stages, depending on age and physical condition of patient; performed for patients with ulcerative colitis, familial polyposis, or existing ileostomy diversion (Figure 6-6); obesity is considered a contraindication to this procedure

Preoperative care

Administer prescribed bowel preparation
  Oral antibiotics
  Mild laxatives
  Colonic irrigations
  Ileostomy irrigation
Bowel preparation will depend on the following:
  Age and nutritional status

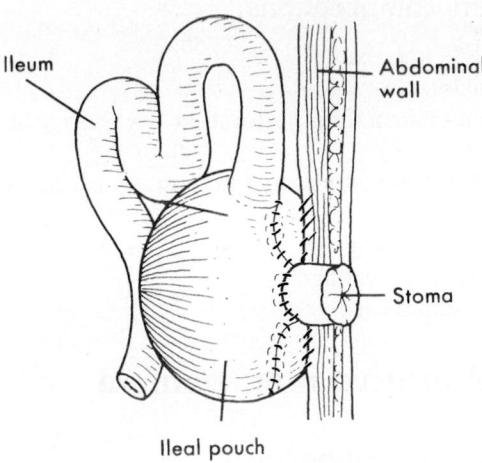

Figure 6-6   Continent ileostomy (Kock's pouch).

  Extent of disease process in colon
  Presence of existing ileostomy
  Stoma site selected
Insert nasogastric tube and indwelling urethral catheter as ordered
Involve enterostomal therapist in preoperative education; visit from a patient with a successful pouch is often beneficial
Reinforce physician's explanation of surgical procedure and postoperative care

Postoperative assessment

Subjective data

Location and character of pain
Nausea
Abdominal cramps

Objective data

Patency and placement of plastic ileal reservoir catheter
Patency of nasogastric tube
Placement of suture holding catheter in place
Color and amount of the following:
  Ileal reservoir drainage
  Gastric drainage
  Urine output
  Wound drainage
Color of stoma
Vomiting
Abdominal distention
Diminished breath sounds

Diagnostic tests

Electrolytes, Hgb, Hct

Potential complications

Electrolyte imbalance
Atelectasis
Intestinal obstruction, perforation
Peritonitis
Wound infection: stoma and rectum
"Pouchitis"
Bloody diarrhea, fever
Valve prolapse, leakage
Pouch perforation

Collaborative management

Therapeutic management

Parenteral fluids with electrolytes
Nasogastric/ileal reservoir aspiration
Irrigating solution
Indwelling urethral catheter
Sitz baths
Analgesics, antibiotics, vitamins
Diet management
Activity
Enterostomal therapy consultation

Nursing management

PATIENT PROBLEMS/NURSING DIAGNOSES

● **NDX:** Ineffective breathing pattern related to pain and risk of decreased lung expansion

Assess respiratory status and respiratory rate q2h to 4h
Assist and teach patient to turn and cough q2h to 4h and deep breathe qh; support incision
Auscultate chest for breath sounds q4h
Provide incentive spirometer q1h to 2h
Elevate head of bed 30 to 45 degrees *to increase lung expansion*

EXPECTED OUTCOMES

Patient exhibits normal respiratory rate and rhythm
Presents clear breath sounds

● **NDX:** Risk for fluid volume deficit related to increased ileal output

Assess for dehydration: decreased skin turgor, dry mucous membranes, slow capillary refill
Maintain NPO *to allow intestine to rest*
Maintain parenteral fluids with electrolytes
Measure intake and output q8h
Monitor vital signs q4h
Monitor nasogastric tube and low, intermittent suction

apparatus; irrigate gently with measured amounts of normal saline q2h to 4h
Monitor indwelling urethral catheter and closed gravity drainage system; report output of <50 ml/hr to physician; *may be indicative of hypovolemia*
Monitor serum electrolytes, Hgb, Hct, and urine specific gravity
Monitor for circulatory overload: tachycardia, neck vein distention, rales

EXPECTED OUTCOMES

Patient's vital signs are stable
Intake and output are balanced
Hydration is adequate as evidenced by normal skin turgor

● **NDX:** Risk for impaired skin integrity related to acidity of ileostomy drainage and surgical procedure

Monitor dressings q1h to 2h for 24 hr; then q4h for 48 hr
Change dressings as needed; include rectal dressing
Place dressing around reservoir catheter *to prevent tension and absorb drainage from stoma*
Report excessive bleeding to physician
Monitor color of stoma (pink-red is normal); report any change to physician
Administer wound and stomal care prn
  Wash around stomal catheter and wound with clear water, pat dry, and allow to air dry
  Apply skin sealant around stoma *to prevent irritation*
  Apply pouch if drainage is profuse or attach to bedside drainage bag
  Assess healing process
Administer sitz baths tid *to promote healing and comfort*

EXPECTED OUTCOMES

Patient's wounds are healing adequately
Surrounding skin is clean, dry, and intact

● **NDX:** Altered bowel elimination related to ileostomy and ileal pouch reservoir

Monitor ileal reservoir catheter and closed gravity drainage system
Avoid placing tension on suture and catheter
Irrigate gently with 20 to 30 ml of normal saline q3h and prn, as determined through collaboration with physician, *to slowly increase pouch capacity*
Observe return flow: should equal amount instilled plus ileal contents
  Measure return; if less than amount instilled, include in intake
  Monitor color and consistency of drainage
Auscultate abdomen for bowel sounds q4h

Observe and monitor for signs of reservoir catheter obstruction
  Feeling of fullness in lower abdomen or around catheter
  Nausea, vomiting
  Increased pain or cramps
If symptoms of reservoir catheter obstruction occur, perform the following procedure, if ordered, after discussion with physician
  Gently irrigate catheter with 20 to 30 ml of normal saline
  If there is no outflow, carefully remove skin suture
  Retain suture around catheter because it marks length of insertion
  Gently irrigate with 20 ml of normal saline and rotate catheter clockwise until outflow begins
  If no results occur, notify physician immediately
Ileal catheter should remain in place 14 to 21 days to allow reservoir healing
Continue irrigations q2h to 3h with 30 to 40 ml of normal saline; contents will thicken as diet increases
Increase fluid intake to 3000 ml/day unless contraindicated
Provide grape and prune juice to keep ileal content thin
If plugging occurs, gentle milking of catheter and rotation clockwise while irrigating may help; having patient cough and applying light pressure to lower abdomen may also help
Catheter may be removed, rinsed, and reinserted as ordered

EXPECTED OUTCOMES

Patient's understanding of ileal pouch's function is clear
Pouch remains patent, and output becomes more normal

● **NDX:** Altered nutrition: less than body requirements related to nasogastric aspiration and increased ileal output

Clamp or remove nasogastric tube as determined by physician when bowel sounds return or bubbles appear in ileal catheter
Provide water and clear liquids as tolerated; start with small sips and evaluate tolerance
Avoid carbonated beverages
Progress to soft, low-residue, low-fiber diet *to prevent catheter plugging*
Avoid gas-producing foods
Teach patient to chew foods well with mouth closed, eat slowly, and avoid talking while eating *to avoid swallowing air*
Have patient avoid drinking with straw *to prevent ingestion of air*
Consider patient's food preferences *to increase desire to maintain adequate diet*

EXPECTED OUTCOMES

Patient demonstrates understanding of diet regimen
Tolerates diet, and weight remains stable

● **NDX:** Pain related to surgical intervention

Maintain bed rest in quiet environment
Assess location, intensity, and character of pain; severe gas pains are usually present postoperatively
Administer analgesics and monitor effectiveness of pain relief measures; PCA may be beneficial for first 3 days
Assist with and teach active ROM exercises (especially for the feet and legs) q4h *to increase venous circulation*
Coordinate care to provide planned rest periods
Discuss and teach alternate pain relief measures
Change position frequently; administer back rubs *to promote comfort*
Provide diversional activities *to decrease attention on discomfort*
Ambulate with assistance *to increase peristaltic action and reduce gas discomfort*

EXPECTED OUTCOMES

Patient reports a reduction of pain
Presents a more relaxed affect

● **NDX:** Body image disturbance related to altered bowel function (ileostomy)

Encourage and allow time for verbalization of feelings and concerns; provide privacy
Encourage patient communication with significant other(s)
Assess present coping behaviors and strengths
Offer praise for accomplishments in discussing, viewing, or exploring stoma
Introduce to enterostomal therapist and/or support group
Encourage patient to view stoma and catheter and discuss their positive aspects
Reinforce physician's explanation of procedure and treatment; clarify misconceptions

EXPECTED OUTCOMES

Patient demonstrates understanding of fears/concerns
Begins to accept ileostomy as part of body
Uses positive coping skills to incorporate body changes into lifestyle

Patient/family teaching

Assist and teach patient to care for ileal reservoir catheter when patient is physically and psychologically able

Involve patient and significant other in plan of care

Set and explain daily goals, with ultimate goal being total patient management

Phase I

Familiarize patient with anatomy and physiology of ileal reservoir

Explain that drainage will depend on food ingested and emphasize importance of high-liquid intake

Teach patient to irrigate catheter: use 50 ml syringe, normal saline, and 500 ml graduate

Instill 30 to 50 ml of normal saline

Measure outflow

Make certain all irrigating fluid is returned

Reconnect catheter to closed gravity drainage system

Phase II

When ordered, clamp catheter for 1 hr, then release for 30 min and reclamp

Irrigate prn with normal saline if outflow is thick

Teach patient procedure in small segments until mastered

Explain that purpose of clamping procedure is to gradually increase reservoir capacity

Explain that clamping time will increase by 15 to 30 min daily until 3 to 4 hr is reached, usually in 5 to 6 days

Continue to connect catheter to closed gravity drainage system at night

See box above, right

Phase III

When ordered, remove catheter and teach patient reinsertion procedure using the following equipment and guidelines

Equipment

No. 28 plastic catheter with insertion tube

50 ml graduate

50 ml syringe

Normal saline

Water-soluble lubricant

Tissues

4 × 4 dressing

Nonallergenic tape

Guidelines

Have patient sit on side of bed

Remove dressings and catheter; disconnect catheter from drainage system

Rinse catheter with water and lubricate tip; place other end into graduate

Place graduate below stoma

Method for Increasing Ileal Reservoir Capacity

- Leave catheter in pouch with continuous drainage for first 3 wk
- Week 4
  Intubate and irrigate catheter every 3 hr during day
  Connect to gravity drainage at night
  Irrigate once at night
- Week 5
  Intubate every 3 hr and irrigate bid
  Connect to gravity drainage at night
  Irrigate once at night
- Week 6
  Intubate every 4 hr and irrigate bid
  Intubate at night only for discomfort or feeling of fullness
- Week 7 and thereafter
  Intubate pouch qid
  Irrigate once daily until return is clear

Modified from Thompson JM et al: *Mosby's clinical nursing,* ed 3, St Louis, 1993, Mosby.

Gently intubate stoma until resistance of nipple valve is felt (2 inches or 5 cm)

Slide catheter through valve with gentle pressure to insertion line

If catheter meets resistance, do not force

Have patient lie down, relax, and take deep breaths

Insert catheter through valve during exhalation

Drainage time is about 5 to 10 min unless fecal material is thick; irrigating with 30 ml of normal saline will thin material

Air bubbles in catheter are normal

When drainage is complete, remove catheter and wash with soap and water; rinse well and dry; store in plastic bag

Cleanse stoma and skin with warm water; pat dry and apply 4 × 4 dressing; secure with tape

Discuss importance of maintaining drainage schedule

Time between drainage periods will increase as reservoir capacity increases

Provide and discuss written schedule (see box above)

Explain importance of diet regimen

Eat well-balanced, low-residue diet

Avoid gas-producing foods: cabbage, cauliflower, carbonated beverages

Avoid foods that can clog catheter: corn, nuts, mushrooms, lettuce, fruit peels

Eat at regular times, chew food well, eat slowly, and avoid straws

Maintain fluid intake of 2500 ml/day; drink prune and grape juice to help liquefy drainage

Discuss signs and symptoms of "pouchitis" to report to physician

Inability to intubate stoma

Abdominal distention

Nausea, vomiting

Increased abdominal pain

Elevated temperature

Incontinence of stool and/or flatus (nipple valve dysfunction)

Explain need to wear nonirritating clothing until wound heals

Demonstrate care of surgical incisions

Encourage follow-up visits with physician

Home care considerations

Provide list of foods and fluids to eat and avoid

Observe and evaluate return demonstration of wound care, sterile technique

Stress importance of handwashing

Provide information on what and where to purchase needed supplies

Teach patient procedure for sitz bath, if applicable; be certain water is not too hot

Reinforce signs and symptoms of "pouchitis"

Refer to community resources (VNA) for assistance with ADLs, personal care as needed

● Ileoanal Reservoir

A surgical procedure anastomosing the ileum to an ileal reservoir constructed at the anus, allowing normal bowel elimination without an ileostomy (Figure 6-7); procedure may be performed in one, two, or three stages, depending on patient's age and physical condition

Stage I: colectomy, temporary ileostomy, and construction of ileal reservoir at anus

Preoperative assessment and care

Reinforce physician's explanation of surgical procedure and expected outcome; clarify misconceptions

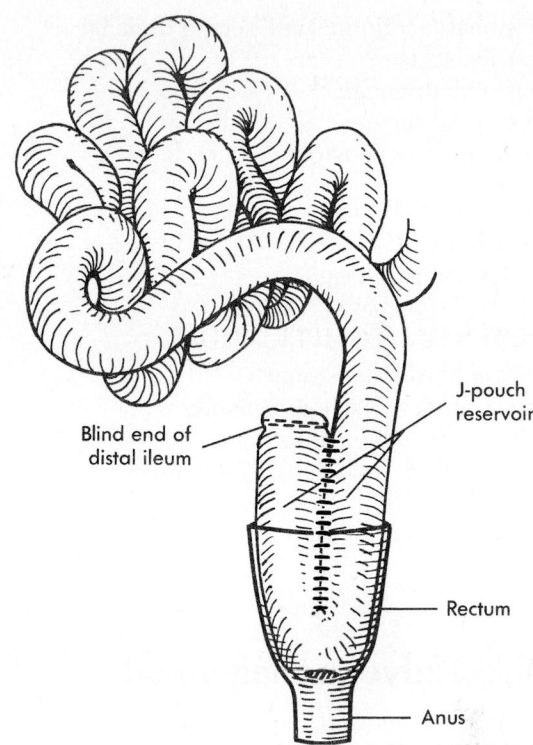

Figure 6-7 Ileoanal anastomosis with a valveless ileal reservoir. Side-to-side anastomosis of a J-loop of terminal ileum is incised at apex and anastomosed to anal sphincter; remaining rectal mucosa provides support. Defecation occurs through anus. (From Phipps WJ et al: *Medical-surgical nursing: concepts and clinical practice*, ed 5, St Louis, 1995, Mosby.)

Contact enterostomal therapist for preoperative assessment and teaching

Monitor baseline vital signs

Prepare bowel as ordered: tap water enemas, oral antibiotics

Encourage and allow time for expression of concerns and feelings; promote positive aspects of surgical procedure

Explain possibility of nasogastric tube, indwelling urethral catheter, and presacral drainage tube exiting from abdomen postoperatively

Postoperative assessment

SUBJECTIVE DATA

Location, intensity, character of pain

OBJECTIVE DATA

Presence of nasogastric tube, urethral catheter

Respiratory function

Location of ileostomy and presacral drain

Presence of nasogastric tube, urethral catheter

Color, character, and amount of drainage

Incisional (abdominal and rectal) drainage
Gastric drainage
Ileostomy drainage
Presacral drainage
Skin integrity of ileostomy and rectal area
Urine output

DIAGNOSTIC TESTS
Electrolytes, CBC, urinalysis

POTENTIAL COMPLICATIONS
Skin erosion from ileostomy
Reservoir abscess, ischemia, fistula
Intestinal obstruction, adhesions
Wound infection: "pouchitis" (inflammation of reservoir)
Cystitis, urinary retention
Phlebitis

Collaborative management

Therapeutic management

Antidiarrheals, bulk-forming agents
Analgesics, antibiotics, dermatologic creams
Parenteral fluids with electrolytes and vitamins
Nasogastric suction, NPO
Irrigation of reservoir
Presacral catheter drainage apparatus
Indwelling urethral catheter
Sitz baths
Diet, rest, ambulation, exercise
Enterostomal therapist

Nursing management

PATIENT PROBLEMS/NURSING DIAGNOSES

● **NDX:** Risk for fluid volume deficit related to risk of abnormal body fluid loss from ileostomy, gastric aspiration, and NPO status

Assess for signs of dehydration: poor skin turgor, dry mucous membranes, reduced capillary refill
Maintain NPO
Maintain parenteral fluids with electrolytes and vitamins
Monitor indwelling urethral catheter and closed drainage system; monitor hourly output for 12 hr; if <50 ml/hr, notify physician
Monitor nasogastric tube and low, intermittent suction apparatus; irrigate with measured amounts of normal saline to keep tube patent

Monitor ileostomy output; 800 to 1200 ml/day is not uncommon
Monitor presacral catheter, if applicable, and closed gravity drainage system; monitor output q2h for 12 hr, then q4h; include drainage in output
Calculate total intake and output q8h; assess for urinary retention
Monitor vital signs q2h until stable; then q4h
Weigh patient daily: same time, clothing, and scale
Monitor electrolytes, Hgb, and Hct
Collaborate with physician and, when nasogastric tube is removed, initiate liquids and progress to well-balanced ileostomy diet as tolerated; monitor for tolerance of new foods as they are introduced

EXPECTED OUTCOMES
Patient's vital signs are stable
Intake and output are balanced
Ileostomy output is within normal limits
Electrolytes are within normal limits

● **NDX:** Risk for impaired skin integrity related to ileostomy and rectal/anal drainage

Monitor perianal area for drainage and mucus; may be copious and odorous
Change dressings prn and clean area well; apply skin sealants and creams to promote healing, comfort, and skin integrity
Cleanse skin around presacral drain and change dressing as needed
Irrigate reservoir daily as ordered to remove mucus and other drainage and to prevent "pouchitis"
Provide absorbent pads to wear while ambulating or at night
Assist with and teach patient ileostomy and skin care (p. 394) as soon as tolerated physically and emotionally
Apply suitable appliance as soon as possible

EXPECTED OUTCOMES
Patient presents healing wounds, with surrounding skin clean, dry, and intact
Demonstrates increasing ability to manage ileostomy

Patient/family teaching

Reiterate ileostomy care and appliance change; observe return demonstration
Stress importance of and demonstrate skin care of perianal area and ileostomy site
Demonstrate prescribed daily reservoir irrigation

Discuss and teach patient Kegel exercises (squeezing and relaxing perineal muscles) to increase anal sphincter tone

Reinforce physician explanation of stage II procedure and clarify misconceptions

Explain that Gastrografin film of reservoir will be taken in about 6 to 12 wk to assess reservoir capacity and anatomic location

Explain that manometric studies of anal sphincter tone will also be performed

Stress importance of well-balanced diet, rest, and exercise

Instruct patient about signs and symptoms to report to physician: increasing diarrhea, drainage, abdominal distention, absence of feces, foul odor from anus

Encourage follow-up visits with physician

Stage II: ileostomy closure and anastomosis of ileum to anal reservoir

Preoperative assessment and care

See Stage I (p. 389)
Irrigation of reservoir is usually ordered

Postoperative assessment

SUBJECTIVE DATA
Location, intensity, and character of pain

OBJECTIVE DATA
Respiratory function
Color, character, and amount of drainage
  Incisional drainage (abdominal)
  Gastric drainage
  Rectal drainage
Urine output
Skin integrity (perianal area)

Diagnostic tests

Electrolytes, CBC, urinalysis

POTENTIAL COMPLICATIONS
Reservoir abscess, ischemia, fistula
Skin erosion (perianal area)
Intestinal obstruction
Wound or reservoir infection
Cystitis, urinary retention
Phlebitis

Collaborative management

Therapeutic management

Analgesics, antibiotics, antidiarrheals, dermatologic creams, ointments
Parenteral fluids with electrolytes and vitamins
Nasogastric suction, NPO
Ileal reservoir irrigation
Indwelling urethral catheter
Rest, ambulation, exercise
Sitz baths
Nutritionist/registered dietitian visits
Enterostomal therapist visits

Nursing management

PATIENT PROBLEMS/NURSING DIAGNOSES

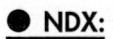 **NDX:** Risk for fluid volume deficit related to abnormal body fluid loss from NPO status, nasogastric suction, and ileoanal reservoir

Maintain NPO; assess for signs of dehydration: decreased skin turgor, urinary output

Maintain parenteral fluids with electrolytes and vitamins

Monitor nasogastric tube and low, intermittent suction apparatus; irrigate with measured amounts of normal saline to keep tube patent

Monitor indwelling urethral catheter and closed gravity drainage system; monitor hourly output; if <50 ml/hr notify physician

Measure intake and output q8h

Monitor vital signs q4h

Weigh patient daily: same time, clothing, and scale

Encourage patient to move feet and legs qh *to promote venous return*

Teach patient to turn, cough, and deep breathe qh *to increase cardiopulmonary function*

Monitor electrolytes, Hgb, Hct

Initiate voiding measures as needed after urethral catheter removal; observe for retention and signs of infection

EXPECTED OUTCOMES
Patient's vital signs are stable
Intake and output are balanced
Weight remains stable
Hydration is adequate as evidenced by normal skin turgor

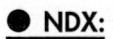 **NDX:** Risk for impaired skin integrity (perianal) related to diarrhea

Flush perianal area as needed with water or aluminum acetate (Domeboro solution) and dry thoroughly with soft cloth or cotton balls; avoid toilet tissue

Cover with skin barrier prn and use Tuck's pads *to reduce discomfort and pruritus*

Administer sitz baths

Irrigate ileal reservoir daily and monitor return solution for blood, foul odor

Involve enterostomal therapist

EXPECTED OUTCOMES
Patient's perianal wound is healing
Surrounding skin is clean, dry, and intact

● **<u>NDX</u>:** Bowel incontinence related to ileal output and lack of sphincter control

Monitor bowel movements for frequency and consistency; will be frequent initially (10 to 20 per day)

Collaborate with physician and provide well-balanced diet after nasogastric tube removal; introduce fresh fruits, spices, and dairy products one at a time to determine tolerance; refer to nutritionist/registered dietitian

Monitor for effectiveness, side effects of psyllium (Metamucil), diphenoxylate (Lomotil) to control diarrhea

Promote Kegel exercises qh *to increase sphincter tone*

EXPECTED OUTCOMES
Patient defecates fewer and more formed stools
Demonstrates ability to perform Kegel exercises

Patient/family teaching

Stress importance of protecting perineal area
  After urinating or defecating flush area with water and dry thoroughly, using hair dryer when possible; take sitz baths prn
  Apply skin sealants, lotions, and dermatologic creams prn
  Avoid harsh, perfumed soaps and nylon underwear
  Daily reservoir irrigation may be needed to prevent infection
Discuss bowel elimination; frequency will decrease (6 to 10 per day) and eventually drop to 3 to 4 per day
  Some incontinence may be noted at night; pads may be worn as protection
  Psyllium (Metamucil) and loperamide (Imodium) will help prevent diarrhea
    Use loperamide for only 48 hr; observe for abdominal distention
    Avoid laxative use
Provide information about diet and foods that cause diarrhea (spices, fresh fruit, and dairy products)

Instruct patient about signs and symptoms to report to physician: increasing diarrhea, drainage or foul odor from rectum, abdominal distention, absence of feces

Encourage follow-up visits with physician

Home care considerations

Continue with sphincter exercises
Reemphasize importance of keeping perianal area clean and protected with skin barriers, sealants
  Stress use of white, nonperfumed toilet paper and white cotton underwear
  Wear absorbent pads between buttocks to reduce moisture and prevent friction
Stress importance of taking only medications ordered by physician
  Avoid enteric-coated, large, and time-released medications because they may be incompletely digested
  Avoid crushing pills without permission from physician
Encourage medical alert identification

● Management of Naso-Oral Intestinal Tube (Cantor or Miller-Abbott Tube)

Cantor or Miller-Abbott tube: Intestinal tube, 6 to 10 ft (2 to 3.3 m) in length, that is passed through the nose or mouth into the stomach and intestine; a balloon for mercury is attached to the distal end; used for decompression and drainage in patients with bowel obstruction or paralytic ileus; tube is advanced manually, by peristaltic action, gravity, and weight of mercury (Figure 6-8)

Preinsertion assessment and care

Reinforce physician's explanation of procedure and its purpose

Assess patient's ability to swallow and willingness to cooperate

Assess abdomen for the following:
  Size, shape, softness
  Presence or absence of bowel sounds

Assess patient for presence of nausea, vomiting, and pain

Elevate head of bed 60 to 70 degrees; tilt head slightly forward to facilitate tube passage

Check tube for patency

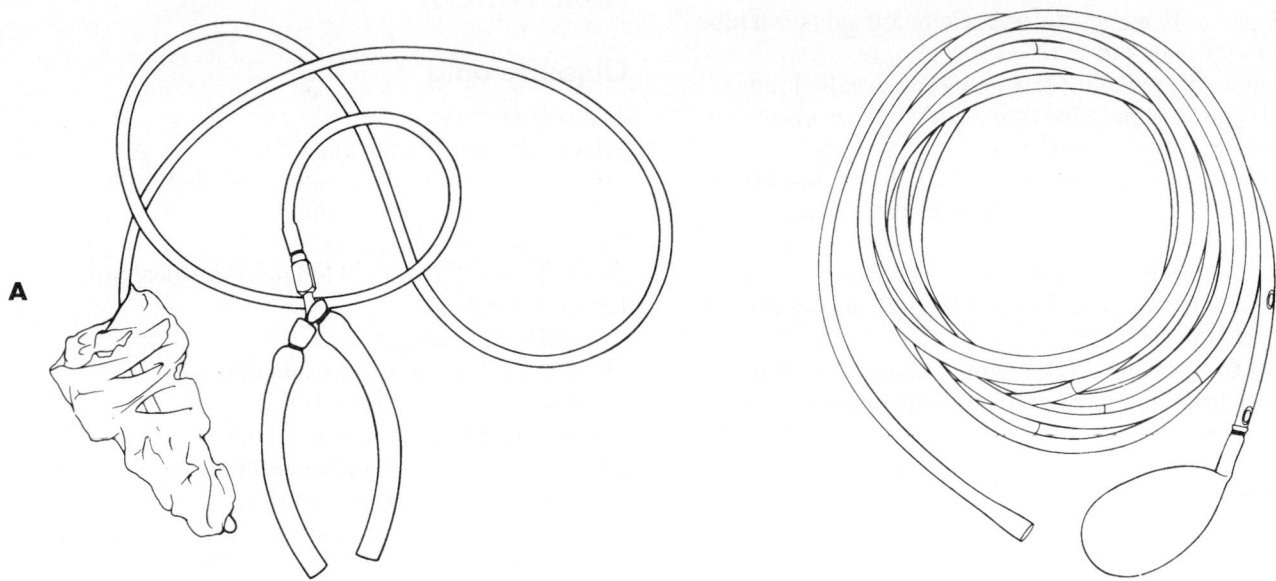

Figure 6-8 Intestinal tubes. **A**, Miller-Abbott tube. **B**, Cantor tube. (From Phipps WJ et al: *Medical-surgical nursing: concepts and clinical practice,* ed 5, St Louis, 1995, Mosby.)

Check that balloon is securely attached and test for leakage by inserting water into balloon via correct lumen with syringe

Prepare syringe with correct amount of mercury
   Cantor tube: mercury is injected into balloon via lumen before insertion
   Miller-Abbott tube: mercury is injected into balloon via lumen after insertion

Ice tube according to procedure and lubricate with water-soluble jelly before insertion

Insertion assessment

Heart rate and rhythm: *dysrhythmias may occur as a result of vagal stimulation*
Respiratory distress: *may occur if tube is inadvertently placed in trachea*
Vomiting

Postinsertion assessment

Subjective data

Nausea
Dysphagia
Sore throat

Objective data

Vomiting
Character and amount of drainage
Accurate placement of tube in stomach

Pressure delivered by intermittent suction apparatus
Patency of tube
Position of patient and tube to facilitate passage of tube
Abdominal distention, pain, or cramps
Increasing bowel sounds
Erosion of nares
Condition of mouth
Blockage of eustachian tube on insertion side

Potential complications

Dehydration
Electrolyte imbalance
Oliguria

Nursing management

Maintain NPO; assess for signs of dehydration
Insert prescribed amount of mercury into correct lumen of Miller-Abbott tube and label "mercury"
Connect nasointestinal tube to low, intermittent suction apparatus
Coil tube and pin to patient's gown; do not tape to nose; avoid placing tension on tube
Monitor color and consistency of intestinal drainage q4h
Irrigate tube gently with measured amounts of normal saline as ordered; if no return flow is obtained, include amount as intake
Auscultate abdomen for bowel sounds q4h; report increasing girth measurements

Turn patient to right side, to back, to left side until tube passes into intestine

Advance tube, usually 3 to 4 inches at specified times; lubricate intestinal tube thoroughly before advancing it

When bowel sounds return and/or flatus or stool is passed and after collaborating with physician

Clamp tube for 2 to 4 hr

Observe for signs of distention, cramps, or nausea

If these symptoms occur, unclamp tube and notify physician

If patient tolerates clamping procedure, administer small, frequent, measured amounts of water and observe tolerance

If patient tolerates fluids, tube is removed slowly, 2 to 3 inches at a time, or allowed to pass through rectum

Provide clear liquid diet and progress to regular diet as tolerated

Maintain bed rest in position of comfort: usually head of bed elevated 30 to 40 degrees

Administer oral hygiene q2h; provide lozenges or hard candy, if allowed, *to stimulate salivation*

Assess nares for irritation or dryness q2h; gently clean and apply lubricant as needed

Discuss advancement of tube and how to avoid dislodgment

Discuss signs and symptoms to report to physician

Ear pain or fullness on side of insertion

Nausea or vomiting

Increased abdominal pain or cramps

Feeling of abdominal fullness or pressure

● Ileostomy, Colostomy Management

ostomy: Surgical opening into the intestine to provide temporary or permanent passage of feces; necessitated by carcinoma, inflammation, trauma, or obstruction below the site of the ostomy; there are three types of colostomies:

end stoma: Bowel is cut and the distal end removed or sewn shut; the proximal end is pulled through the abdominal wall and a stoma made

double barrel: Bowel is cut and both ends pulled through the abdominal wall; proximal end will discharge effluent; distal end will drain mucous

loop: Bowel is not severed and a loop is pulled through the abdominal wall and supported with a rod until healing occurs; an opening is then made to discharge fecal material; this is usually temporary

Assessment

Objective data

Type of ostomy
 Ileostomy: usually permanent
 Colostomy: ascending, transverse, descending; may be temporary or permanent
Removal and closure of rectum
Level of patient's understanding of surgical procedure
Emotional status
 Acceptance of ostomy
 Understanding of ostomy function
 Ability to verbalize feelings
 Acceptance of body image change
Character, frequency, and amount of feces
Size, location, and color of stoma
Condition of skin around stoma
Appropriateness of appliance and size
Placement of stoma
Hydration

Diagnostic tests

Electrolytes, Hgb, Hct

Potential complications

Leakage under appliance
Signs of wound infection
Electrolyte imbalance
Dehydration
Intestinal obstruction
Hemorrhage
Stoma
 Prolapse
 Stricture
 Retraction
 Necrosis

Collaborative management

Therapeutic management

Diet management
Corticosteroid aerosol spray, nystatin powder
Odor-control preparation
Enterostomal therapy

Nursing management

 PATIENT PROBLEMS/NURSING DIAGNOSES

● **NDX:** Risk for impaired skin integrity (peristomal), secondary to ostomy drainage

Initiate peristomal care and apply ostomy appliance as soon as possible postoperatively

Measure stoma for correct appliance size at each appliance change; size should be ⅛ inch larger than stoma measurement

Change appliance prn and observe color, amount, and consistency of feces and color of stoma and surrounding skin

Maintain peristomal skin integrity

Wash with mild soap and water and rinse thoroughly with each appliance change; to avoid skin irritation, start with a drainable pouch

Pat skin dry with towel and apply effective skin barrier (Skin Prep, Stomahesive, Releaseal)

Instruct patient in caring for ostomy when physically and psychologically ready

Apply only clear appliance *to facilitate monitoring stoma*

Maintain a secure seal around stoma *to prevent leakage*

Involve enterostomal therapist if available

Control odor with deodorant drops or bismuth/chlorophyll preparations

EXPECTED OUTCOMES

Patient presents a healing wound, and surrounding skin is clean, dry, and intact

Expresses understanding of ostomy function

Demonstrates understanding of ostomy appliance system

● **NDX:** Body image disturbance related to presence of ileostomy, colostomy

Assist patient and significant other in accepting ostomy

Allow time for and encourage verbalization

Answer all questions and explain treatments and procedures

Provide care in a positive manner; avoid facial expressions connoting distaste

Observe for signs of inappropriate denial, grief, or anger

Provide privacy and a safe environment

Assess present coping patterns and explore strengths and resources

Encourage self-care and independence

Set goals with patient for the following:

Viewing stoma

Discussing self-care

Taking steps in performing self-care

Give positive reinforcement for each step taken

EXPECTED OUTCOMES

Patient expresses feelings and concerns

Demonstrates positive coping skills in dealing with presence of ostomy

Views stoma; discusses and performs some steps of care

● **NDX:** Sexual dysfunction related to ostomy and lack of knowledge

Assess stage of adaptation of patient to ostomy and explain its normalcy

Encourage communication with significant other and explain the need to share feelings

Explain that normal sexual activity can be resumed when allowed

Discuss methods of controlling odor, general hygiene

Provide information about alternate sexual techniques and positions

Encourage counseling if patient is unable to discuss sexuality

EXPECTED OUTCOMES

Patient verbalizes understanding of the information provided about sexual activity

Discusses feelings about sexuality with significant other

● **NDX:** Risk for fluid volume deficit related to increased fluid loss (ileostomy)

Assess for dehydration

Monitor intake and output and electrolytes q8h

Monitor stools for frequent, high-volume output, notifying physician if this occurs

Weigh patient daily: same time, clothing, and scale

Monitor vital signs q8h

EXPECTED OUTCOMES

Patient's vital signs are stable

Intake and output are balanced

Weight remains stable

Hydration is adequate as evidenced by normal skin turgor

● **NDX:** Constipation (colostomy) or high output (ileostomy) secondary to shortened bowel

Assess patient's previous bowel habits and lifestyle

Reinforce physician's explanation of surgical procedure and anatomy and physiology of ostomy

Colostomy feces will be more solid; ileostomy feces will be liquid to pasty

Colostomy may be irrigated to establish near-normal elimination; ileostomy should never be irrigated

Involve significant other when appropriate

Demonstrate irrigation procedure and have patient return demonstration until patient can perform it alone (see Colostomy Irrigation)

Provide information on where to purchase equipment and symptoms of intestinal obstruction or stomal prolapse to report to physician

Collaborate with physician and nutritionist/registered dietitian for diet instructions; each patient will differ in foods tolerated

Most ostomy patients are discharged on a general diet and given a list of foods that may cause gas or diarrhea

Follow these general rules

Ileostomates should have foods high in sodium and potassium: bananas, bouillon, citrus juices, tea, cola, rye flour, molasses

Ileostomates should avoid gas-producing, fried, rich, and highly seasoned foods, nuts, raisins, and all raw fruits except bananas

Colostomates should avoid gas-producing foods such as cabbage, beans, corn, broccoli, and cauliflower if gas is uncomfortable or embarrassing

Each patient will have to use a trial-and-error method to establish which foods can be tolerated

Introduce new foods one at a time

Stress adequate nutritional and fluid intake

Stress eating slowly, chewing food well, and eating regular meals

Advise avoiding carbonated beverages and extremes in temperature of foods

Involve patient and/or significant other(s) in meal planning

Auscultate abdomen for bowel sounds q8h; report absent sounds to physician

Discuss signs and symptoms of obstruction or stricture

Decreased drainage, constipation

Diarrhea

Cramps, abdominal distention

Nausea, vomiting

EXPECTED OUTCOMES

Patient expresses understanding of ostomy function

Begins to care for stoma and ostomy

Patient/family teaching

Explain and demonstrate stomal care step by step and have patient return demonstration

Discuss equipment used and where to purchase it; provide enough supplies to last a few days after discharge

Provide and explain written information on diet management

Provide information about outside support groups available and refer to home health care as needed

Discuss signs of wound infection, obstruction, prolapse to report to physician

Encourage follow-up visits with physician

Home care considerations

Discuss and provide written information about the following:

Normal stoma color is pink-red and any change must be reported to physician

Stoma will decrease in size and change shape during the first year

Measure size frequently to maintain good appliance fit

Many appliances are available, but it is best to use one that adheres to skin and only needs changing every 5 to 7 days

Change appliance when there is leakage or a burning sensation beneath or around appliance: *effluent can cause severe damage to skin*

Always use a skin barrier on the skin before applying pouch

Drink plenty of fluids to avoid dehydration because intake must compensate for output

Need to carry a medical alert card and names of medications patient should not take

Discuss changes in lifestyle that must be made: diet, some activities, but reassure patient that he or she is the same person he or she was before the ostomy

● Colostomy Irrigation

A procedure used by some colostomates to clear the bowel of fecal matter and to help establish an evacuation schedule; may not be applicable for all patients

Assessment

Objective data

Patient's emotional status

State of acceptance

Knowledge and understanding of procedure

Ability to comprehend

Tolerance of procedure

Size and color of stoma

Location of stoma(s)

Sigmoid colostomy

Descending colostomy

Hydration of patient

Temperature and amount of irrigating solution

Retention of irrigating solution; dehydrated patients may retain some fluid

Amount and character of return flow

Constipation

Diarrhea
Pain
Distention

Potential complications

Stomal bleeding
Perforation
Obstruction
Prolapse

Irrigating procedure

Usually irrigations are ordered whenever patient is
ready psychologically and physically
Explain procedure and equipment
May be done every day or every other day
Use equipment that will be used at home
Demonstrate procedure step by step
Assess patient's normal bowel habits
Involve patient in assisting with procedure as soon as
physically and emotionally able
Use commode as soon as possible for irrigations *to
provide a more normal environment*
Provide diversional activities after instillation of irri-
gating solution
During procedure observe these precautions
Have patient sit on commode when possible
Prepare 500 to 1000 ml warm tap water
Remove all air in tubing
Hold bag at shoulder level or 12 to 18 inches above
stoma
Apply irrigation sleeve over stoma; place end in com-
mode
Insert lubricated cone tip gently into stoma; avoid
using catheter, which may cause intestinal per-
foration
Allow solution to run into stoma slowly
Allow 45 min for return flow
Position change and/or abdominal massage will help
if return is slow
Irrigation sleeve may be folded and clipped and pa-
tient encouraged to ambulate
Stoma dilation may be ordered but is generally not
part of routine care
Using glove, lubricate finger closest to size of stoma
Insert finger gently into stoma, *never* force
Rotate finger gently for 1 min to dilate
Involve significant other when appropriate
Demonstrate procedure and have patient return
demonstration until he or she can perform it
unassisted
Provide information on where to purchase equipment
and symptoms of obstruction or prolapse to report
to physician

● Rectal Surgery

*Any surgery performed on the rectum necessitated by the
following:*
anorectal abscess: *Localized infection of area with
accumulation of pus in tissues of and around the
rectum*
anorectal fistula: *Abnormal opening between the
rectum and perineal area*
anal fissure: *A small tear in the lining of the anus*
hemorrhoids: *Collection of vascular tissue in the anus
(internal) or prolapsed (external)*

Assessment

Subjective data

Location, intensity, character of pain

Objective data

Character and amount of rectal drainage
Placement of drain
Urinary output

Diagnostic tests

Anoscopy
CBC, urinalysis
Digital rectal examination

Potential complications

Abdominal distention
Urinary retention
Hemorrhage
Infection

Collaborative management

Therapeutic management

Analgesic, topical anesthetic ointment
Ice packs, sitz baths, warm compresses
Stool softeners
Diet progression

Nursing management

PATIENT PROBLEMS/NURSING DIAGNOSES

● **NDX:** Pain related to surgical intervention

When on bed rest, turn patient side to side q2h
Administer analgesics as required; if ointments are

ordered, test first for allergic reaction; assess effectiveness of pain relief measures

Have patient avoid supine position if possible; place pillows between knees while on side

Monitor effectiveness of warm, wet compresses or ice bag

Ambulate with assistance; provide Gelfoam or flotation pads for sitting; avoid rubber rings, *which tend to spread buttocks and cause further discomfort*

Provide planned rest periods; have patient avoid sitting in chair for long periods

Administer analgesic before removing packing

Monitor sitz baths for effectiveness

EXPECTED OUTCOMES

Patient verbalizes increasing comfort level

Presents a more relaxed affect

● **NDX:** Constipation related to NPO status and painful defecation

Maintain NPO until nausea subsides

Provide low-residue, soft diet as tolerated

Increase fluids to 2000 to 2500 ml/day unless contraindicated

Monitor for bowel sounds q8h

Administer stool softeners; encourage defecation as soon as urge occurs; provide privacy

Monitor effectiveness of stool softeners

Encourage activity and ambulation as soon as possible

EXPECTED OUTCOMES

Patient's bowel sounds are normal

Bowel movements are soft and formed

● **NDX:** Altered urinary elimination, related to proximity of surgical procedure to bladder

Measure intake and output for 24 hr; observe for signs of urinary retention

Use voiding measures if necessary: run water nearby, pour warm water over lower abdomen, place hands in water

Assist patient with voiding: assist males to stand and void; for females, elevate head of bed or use commode

Promote and assist with ambulation *to increase urge to void*

EXPECTED OUTCOMES

Patient reports urine is clear and pale yellow and of adequate amount

Expresses ability to void without discomfort

● **NDX:** Risk for infection related to inadequate primary defenses

Monitor vital signs q4h

Observe dressings q2h to 4h: check for bleeding, drainage, odor, and packing

Change dressings prn; apply petroleum gauze

Cleanse perianal area after each bowel movement and keep area clean and dry

Assess for signs of healing

Shave area to prevent irritation, infection

Instruct patient in irrigating wound if applicable

EXPECTED OUTCOMES

Patient's wound is healing adequately

Surrounding tissue is clean, dry, and intact

Patient/family teaching

Discuss importance of diet management

  Maintain low-residue diet for 1 wk

  Increase roughage as tolerated

  Include fresh fruits

  Force fluids to 2500 ml/day unless contraindicated

Demonstrate care of incision and perirectal area

  Take sitz baths as ordered

  Use warm compresses

  Use petroleum gauze pads

  Cleanse perineal area well and dry thoroughly after each bowel movement

  Apply dressing

Discuss symptoms of wound infection and anal stricture to report to physician: redness, tenderness, swelling, drainage

Discuss maintaining soft bowel movements with use of stool softeners and natural laxatives

Explain importance of avoiding heavy lifting and straining

Encourage follow-up visits with physician

Home care considerations

Demonstrate wound irrigation if applicable; may use Water Pik, shower massager

Explain how to use a mirror to inspect area

Provide information of types of and where to purchase needed supplies

Inform patient that mesh panties are available to hold dressings, as well as sanitary belt and pads; men will find jockey shorts more effective

Gallbladder

● Biliary Obstruction (Stones, Infection)

Obstruction of the common and/or cystic bile ducts caused by stones, which inhibit the drainage of bile and cause an acute inflammatory process to occur

Assessment

Subjective data

Nausea
Weight loss
Anorexia

Objective data

Midepigastric colicky pain
Pain may radiate to shoulder
Vomiting
Chills
Fever
Dark, concentrated urine
Clay-colored feces
Tachycardia
Tachypnea
Abdominal distention

Diagnostic tests

WBC (elevated >12,000)
Serum bilirubin: elevated
Serum amylase: elevated
Ultrasound/radiologic abdominal series
Percutaneous transhepatic cholangiography
CT scan
Biliary scintigraphy
Cholecystogram (for chronic cholecystitis only)
Chest radiologic study (to rule out pneumonitis)
PT/INR: decreased

Potential complications

Jaundice
  Skin
  Sclera
Dehydration
Electrolyte imbalance
Bleeding tendencies (vitamin K deficiency)
Peritonitis if rupture occurs

Collaborative management

Therapeutic management

Analgesics, antibiotics, antiemetics, anticholinergics, vitamin K
NPO
Nasogastric suction
Parenteral fluids with electrolytes
Diet and activity
Surgical intervention: cholecystectomy with exploration of common bile duct or cholecystotomy (see p. 400)
Extracorporeal shock wave lithotripsy (ESWL) (see p. 402)

Nursing management

PATIENT PROBLEMS/NURSING DIAGNOSES

● **NDX:** Risk for fluid volume deficit related to abnormal loss of body fluids from NPO status, gastric suction, vomiting

Maintain NPO, assess for signs of dehydration: poor skin turgor, dry mucous membranes, reduced capillary refill
Monitor vital signs q4h or prn
Maintain parenteral fluids with electrolytes, vitamin K, antibiotics
Monitor nasogastric tube and low, intermittent suction apparatus; irrigate with measured amounts of normal saline prn
Auscultate abdomen for bowel sounds q8h
Administer oral hygiene prn *to reduce dryness of mucous membranes*
Assess for bleeding from gums, injection sites *(resulting from reduced PT)*, bile obstruction
Measure intake and output q8h; note color and consistency of urine, stools, and gastric contents
Monitor serum electrolytes to assess for depletion *caused by gastric suction, vomiting*
Observe for jaundice, pruritus, vitamin K deficiency and PT/INR results
Monitor stools for clay color or return of bile
Monitor skin turgor q8h
Administer antiemetics *to reduce nausea*

EXPECTED OUTCOMES

Patient's vital signs are stable
Intake and output are balanced
Electrolytes are within normal limits
Hydration is adequate as evidenced by normal skin turgor

● **NDX:** Pain related to disease process, presence of stones, infection

Assess character, location, and intensity of pain; use pain rating scale

Administer analgesics and anticholinergics; assess effectiveness of pain relief measures

Avoid morphine, *which may cause sphincter of Oddi spasms and increase discomfort*

Maintain bed rest in position of comfort: usually head of bed elevated 30 to 45 degrees *to increase respiratory function*

Teach alternate pain relief measures: imaging, deep breathing, relaxation techniques

Change position frequently in small ways *to promote comfort*

Provide diversional activities *to decrease attention on discomfort*

Administer skin care *to reduce itching and discomfort as needed*

EXPECTED OUTCOMES

Patient reports a reduction in pain intensity

Appears more relaxed

● **NDX:** Altered nutrition: less than body requirements related to vomiting and decreased nutritional intake

After removal of nasogastric tube, collaborate with physician to initiate clear liquid diet and progress to low-fat, soft diet *to reduce stimulation of the gallbladder and consequent pain and possible recurrence*

Perform a calorie count after each meal *to assess nutritional deficiencies*

Monitor bowel sounds; observe for abdominal distention

Monitor serum BUN, albumin

Encourage fluids to 2500 ml/day unless contraindicated

Monitor for food intolerances

Discuss food preferences

Provide quiet, nonstressful environment at mealtimes

Encourage activity and ambulation *to stimulate gastric, intestinal motility*

Weigh patient daily: same time, clothing, and scale

EXPECTED OUTCOMES

Patient maintains desired weight

Tolerates prescribed diet

Patient/family teaching

Review and discuss disease process as outlined by physician; allow time for questions

Review signs and symptoms to report to physician: fever, nausea/vomiting, pain, jaundice, itching, dark urine, bleeding from mucous membranes, blood in stools/urine, clay-colored stools

Provide and discuss written dietary instructions on low-fat diet: avoid ice cream, butter, whole milk, gravies, fried foods

Avoid gas-producing foods: cabbage, cauliflower, beans, carbonated beverages, brussel sprouts

Avoid spicy foods, caffeine, citrus fruits that irritate gastric mucosa

Advise patient and/or significant other(s) to increase fat in diet slowly

Discuss need for weight loss if appropriate

Discuss importance of rest, especially after eating

Stress importance of activity as tolerated

Encourage follow-up visits with physician

Home care considerations

Discuss importance of following dietary plan; involve nutritionist/registered dietitian to assist in explanation of reduced fat diet and weight loss program, if appropriate

Explain the need to rest in semi-Fowler's position following meals *because it increases bile flow*

Discuss importance of nonstressful environment at mealtimes

Encourage fluid intake of 2500 to 3000 ml/day unless contraindicated

Encourage walking and increasing level of exercise, *which stimulates digestion and improves gastric tone*

Refer to reputable weight loss clinic if needed

● Biliary Surgery

Surgery of the gallbladder
cholecystectomy: *Removal of gallbladder*
choledocholithotomy: *Removal of stones in common bile duct*
choledochojejunostomy: *Anastomosis of the common bile duct to the jejunum*

Assessment

Subjective data

Location, intensity, and character of pain

Objective data

Respiratory distress
Diminished breath sounds

Splinting with respirations
Tachypnea
Bradypnea
Character and amount
  Gastric drainage
  Bile drainage (T tube)
  Drainage from incision
  Urinary output

Diagnostic tests

Electrolytes, Hgb, Hct

Potential complications

Dehydration
Electrolyte imbalance
Hemorrhage
Shock
Peritonitis (p. 374)
Jaundice (3 to 4 days postoperatively)
Signs of wound infection
Thrombophlebitis (p. 107)
Atelectasis
Pulmonary embolus (p. 294)

Collaborative management

Therapeutic management

Analgesics, antibiotics, vitamin K
Nasogastric suction, NPO
Parenteral fluids with electrolytes
Oxygen therapy, incentive spirometer
Oral replacement of bile salts: florantyrone (Sancho),
  dehydrocholic acid (Decholin)
T tube drainage and clamping
Diet, activity, rest

Nursing management

PATIENT PROBLEMS/NURSING DIAGNOSES

● **NDX:** Ineffective breathing pattern related to decreased lung expansion and pain

Assess respiratory status; observe for splinting and
  shallow, rapid breathing *to prevent atelectasis*
Auscultate lungs for breath sounds q2h *to assess for congestion*
Administer incentive spirometer q2h to 4h
Administer pain medication to assist patient in moving
  and deep breathing
Assist and teach patient to turn and cough q2h and
  deep breathe qh; support incision *to reduce discomfort*

Elevate head of bed 20 to 30 degrees *to increase lung
  expansion*

EXPECTED OUTCOMES

Patient demonstrates ability to turn, cough, and deep
  breathe
Uses incentive spirometer correctly
Exhibits normal respirations and breath sounds

● **NDX:** Risk for fluid volume deficit related to NPO
  status and increased body fluid loss from nasogastric suction

Maintain NPO; assess for signs of dehydration: poor
  skin turgor, dry mucous membranes, decreased capillary refill
Maintain parenteral fluids with electrolytes and vitamin K
Monitor vital signs q4h
Monitor nasogastric tube and low, intermittent suction
  apparatus; irrigate prn with measured amounts of normal saline *to maintain patency*
Monitor intake and output q8h; observe for urinary retention
Monitor T tube and closed gravity drainage system if
  applicable; observe color and amount of drainage q8h;
  report drainage >500 ml/day to physician; *may indicate obstruction*
Replace bile salts *to aid in fat digestion*
Monitor serum electrolytes, Hct, and Hgb; PT/INR
Monitor stools for clay-colored feces and assess urine
  for presence of bile
Monitor for vitamin K deficiency: bleeding mucous
  membranes, injection sites
Weigh patient prn with same clothes and scale
Encourage movement of feet and legs *to increase venous return*

EXPECTED OUTCOMES

Patient's intake and output are balanced
Vital signs are stable
Hydration is adequate as evidenced by normal skin turgor

● **NDX:** Risk for impaired skin/tissue integrity related to tube drainage, altered nutritional
  state, and invasive procedure

Monitor incision q2h for 8 hr, then q4h for increased
  drainage, bleeding
Reinforce and change dressing prn
Report excess drainage or bleeding to physician
Cover "stab wound" drain with ostomy appliance or
  sterile dressing *to facilitate measuring of output;*
  change prn
Monitor vital signs q4h

Administer injections with small-gauge needle and apply more pressure longer *to prevent bleeding from injection site*

Provide swabs for oral hygiene if bleeding gums are noted

Assess patency of T tube q2h; observe for kinks in tubing

Anchor tubing to allow for freedom of movement

Assess skin around T tube q2h to 4h; clean prn with soap and water; rinse and pat dry

Apply petroleum jelly gauze or Skin Prep as needed *to prevent irritation*

Apply Montgomery straps as indicated *to prevent adhesive burns*

Observe skin and sclera for jaundice or pruritus, *which may indicate obstruction of bile flow*

Provide distracting activities and remind patient not to scratch skin if pruritus is present

Collaborate with physician and clamp T tube after meals; observe for distention, cramps, and pain; if symptoms occur, unclamp T tube and notify physician

Ambulate with assistance as tolerated *to increase circulation and healing process*

EXPECTED OUTCOMES

Patient's wound is healing well

Surrounding tissue is clean, dry, and intact

● **NDX:**   Pain related to surgical intervention

Assess location, type, and intensity of pain; use pain rating scale

Administer analgesics and assess effectiveness of pain relief measures

Collaborate with physician regarding patient controlled analgesia (see p. 92)

Maintain bed rest in quiet environment

Change position frequently; administer back rubs *to promote comfort*

Discuss alternate pain management techniques: imaging, deep breathing, relaxation

Provide diversional activities *to reduce attention on discomfort*

EXPECTED OUTCOMES

Patient reports a reduction of pain

Appears relaxed and comfortable

Patient/family teaching

Provide and review written diet instructions and restrictions; fats may be added as tolerated

Demonstrate care of incision and T tube (if applicable)

T tube requires draining of collection bag at prescribed times

Discuss medications: name, dose, administration time, and side effects

Explain that florantyrone (Sancho), dehydrocholic acid (Decholin) may be required to assist in fat absorption

Explain signs and symptoms to report to physician: increased epigastric pain, dark urine, clay-colored stools, jaundice

Discuss importance of increasing activity as tolerated and planned rest periods

Explain that bowel movements may be loose for a while because of increased bile

Encourage follow-up visits with physician

Home care considerations

Stress importance of aseptic technique for dressing changes, T tube management

Demonstrate handwashing technique and correct procedure for cleaning wound

Cleanse area with mild soap and water

Rinse well and pat dry

Apply Skin Prep around incision to protect skin

Maintain Montgomery straps as needed

Stress importance of draining T tube collection bag periodically *to reduce strain on tube*

Provide flow sheet for record keeping

Discuss importance of diet, eating slowly, and chewing foods well

Provide list of high-fat foods: whole milk, ice cream, butter, fried foods

Provide information on types of and where to purchase needed supplies

Refer to community resources for assistance with home care, ADLs as needed

● Biliary Lithotripsy

extracorporeal shock wave lithotripsy: Noninvasive procedure performed under analgesia, using high-energy shock waves to disintegrate gallstones, allowing them to pass through the common bile duct into the intestine

Assessment

Subjective data

Abdominal tenderness

Biliary colic; severe pain right upper quadrant (RUQ)

Location and character of pain

Nausea

Objective data

Condition of skin at treatment site: redness, bruising, hematoma
Hematuria
Vomiting

Diagnostic tests

Preprocedure: lipase, amylase, bilirubin, creatinine, PT/INR, APTT, Hgb, Hct, AST, ALT
Oral cholangiogram

Potential complications

Retained fragments causing common duct obstruction
Jaundice, severe abdominal pain
Fever, nausea, vomiting
Acute cholangitis

Collaborative management

Therapeutic management

Low-fat diet
Analgesics
Dicyclomine hydrochloride (Bentyl) for colic

Nursing management

PATIENT PROBLEMS/NURSING DIAGNOSES

● **NDX:** Ineffective breathing pattern related to decreased lung expansion

Assess respiratory status q4h to 8h
Monitor respirations for splinting and/or shallow, rapid breathing
Auscultate lungs for breath sounds q4h to 8h
Elevate head of bed 20 to 45 degrees *to increase lung expansion*
Assist and teach patient to deep breathe qh

EXPECTED OUTCOMES
Patient exhibits normal breath sounds
Demonstrates ability to perform breathing exercises correctly

● **NDX:** Risk for fluid volume deficit related to abnormal fluid loss from NPO status

Assess for signs of dehydration: poor skin turgor, dry mucous membranes, reduced capillary refill
Maintain parenteral fluids until fully reacted
Monitor vital signs q4h
Monitor intake and output q4h; observe for hematuria

Monitor for signs of jaundice
Encourage ambulation *to increase circulation*
Provide fluids to tolerance; 2500 to 3000 ml/day
Provide low-fat diet as tolerated

EXPECTED OUTCOMES
Patient's vital signs are stable
Intake and output are balanced
Tolerance for low-fat diet is without discomfort

● **NDX:** Pain related to corrective procedure and treatment

Assess location, intensity, and character of pain
Evaluate effectiveness of pain relief measures
Provide diversional activities *to decrease attention on discomfort*
Change patient position frequently *to promote comfort*
Discuss alternate pain relief measures: imaging, deep breathing, relaxation techniques
Notify physician if pain is severe and long lasting or does not respond to analgesics; *may indicate obstruction of bile*
Encourage ambulation *to increase circulation and healing*

EXPECTED OUTCOMES
Patient reports a decrease in pain or no pain
Presents a more relaxed affect

Patient/family teaching

Encourage returning to normal activities
Provide and review written dietary instructions
 Low-fat to regular diet depending on tolerance
 High-fat foods may cause discomfort; dicyclomine hydrochloride (Bentyl) usually relieves the pain
Discuss signs and symptoms to report to physician
 Severe nausea, vomiting
 Fever above 101°F (38°C)
 Severe abdominal pain, jaundice
Encourage follow-up visits with physician for ultrasonography and laboratory tests

● Laparoscopic, Endoscopic Laser Cholecystectomy

Removal of the gallbladder without a surgical incision; four small punctures are made in the abdominal wall, and, with the use of a laparoscopic laser, the gallbladder is removed; 4.5 L of CO_2 is instilled in the

abdominal cavity to allow freedom of movement (this is usually the main cause of postoperative pain and complications)

Postoperative assessment

Subjective data

Nausea
Type, location, intensity of pain

Objective data

Respiratory function
Location of puncture wounds
Amount of drainage, bleeding
Vomiting
Placement of nasogastric tube and attending suction apparatus
Placement of indwelling urethral catheter

Diagnostic tests

Electrolytes
Urinalysis

Potential complications

Hemorrhage
Bile leakage into abdominal cavity

Collaborative management

Therapeutic management

Amount of pressure on nasogastric tube suction apparatus; irrigating instructions
Analgesics
Diet
Activity and exercise

Nursing management

PATIENT PROBLEMS/NURSING DIAGNOSES

● **NDX:** Ineffective breathing pattern related to decreased lung expansion and CO_2 inflation of the abdomen

Maintain bed rest until fully reactive
Place patient in Sims position (left side with right knee and thigh flexed toward chest and right arm along thigh) *to facilitate absorption of CO_2*
Assess respiratory status including breath sounds q4h to 8h

Assist and teach patient to deep breathe qh
Ambulate with assistance within 3 to 4 hr postoperatively

EXPECTED OUTCOMES

Patient exhibits normal breath sounds
Performs deep breathing qh

● **NDX:** Risk for fluid volume deficit related to risk of abnormal fluid loss from NPO status, nausea, and vomiting

Monitor vital signs q4h
Assess for signs of dehydration: poor skin turgor, dry mucous membranes, reduced capillary refill
Remove nasogastric tube when nausea decreases
Provide clear liquids as tolerated, avoiding carbonated beverages *to prevent distention*
Progress to regular or preprocedure diet as tolerated
Encourage fluids to tolerance unless contraindicated
Calculate intake and output q8h
Remove indwelling catheter when intake and output are balanced

EXPECTED OUTCOMES

Patient's vital signs are stable
Intake and output are balanced
Skin turgor is normal
Tolerance of diet and fluids is adequate

● **NDX:** Pain related to corrective procedure

Assess location, intensity, and character of pain
Assess effectiveness of analgesics; avoid IM medications *because they can cause drowsiness and decreased mobility*
Notify physician if pain is unrelieved, severe, or long lasting; *may indicate bleeding, obstruction*

EXPECTED OUTCOMES

Patient reports decreasing or absent pain/discomfort
Presents a more relaxed affect

● **NDX:** Altered protection related to abnormal blood profile caused by hemorrhage

Monitor dressings for bleeding or bile drainage; change prn
Assess abdomen for distention or severe pain
Monitor vital signs q4h; *tachypnea, hypotension may indicate abnormal bleeding*

EXPECTED OUTCOMES

Patient's dressing remains dry without evidence of bleeding

Vital signs are stable
Abdomen remains soft and nondistended

Patient/family teaching

Discuss care of puncture sites and signs and symptoms
to report to physician
 Wound drainage, redness, edema
 Abdominal distention
 Nausea, vomiting
 Increased pain
Instruct regarding prescribed activities, usually not lim-
ited after 2 to 3 days (normally discharged in 24 to 48
hr)
Discuss importance of maintaining diet and fluid intake

Home care considerations

Advise patient to remain on liquid diet on day of discharge and increase to light meals for 3 to 4 days
Stress importance of low-fat diet, avoiding ice cream,
butter, whole milk, and fried foods
Explain that showering may begin on second day and
dressings are to be removed at that time
Stress importance of not lifting heavy objects (>10 lb)

● T Tube Management

*T tube: Tube placed in the common bile duct to carry off
excessive bile, decrease the amount of bile flowing into
the intestine, and prevent backflow of bile into the liver
when the common bile duct has been explored (Figure
6-9)*

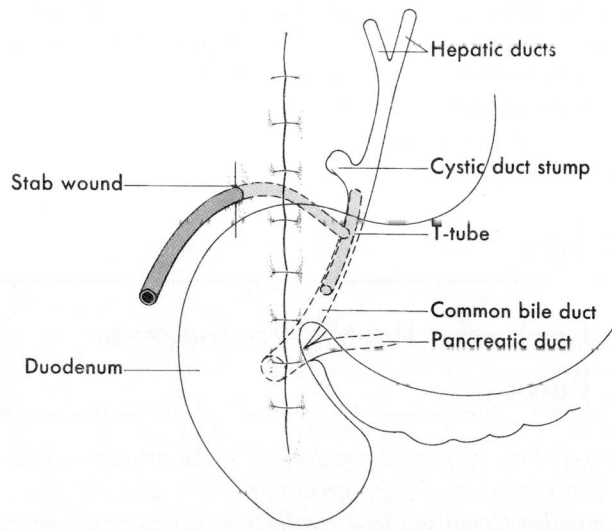

Figure 6-9 T tube. (From Beare PG and Myers JL: *Principles and
practice of adult health nursing,* ed 2, St Louis, 1994, Mosby.)

Assessment

Objective data

Character, color, and amount of bile drainage; <500
ml/day is within normal limits
Patency of tube
Leakage around tube
Tube taped securely to skin
Skin integrity around tube
Color, consistency, and frequency of stools

Potential complications

Jaundice: sclera, skin
Electrolyte imbalance
Abdominal distention
Fat-soluble vitamin (A, D, E, K) deficiency

Interventions

Connect T tube tubing to closed gravity drainage system placed well below incision
Secure connections with tape and allow enough tubing
to allow for freedom of movement
Place rolled 4 × 4 pads under T tube at exit site and
tape to skin to prevent tension
Monitor skin around T tube exit site; keep clean and
dry; use Stomahesive wafer or Skin Prep to prevent
irritation
Measure bile output q8h; report output >500 ml/day to
physician
Auscultate abdomen for bowel sounds q8h; report return to physician
Observe first stool for color, consistency, and amount;
should be dark (clay color may indicate bile duct
blockage)
Collaborate with physician to clamp tube and observe
for abdominal pain, distention, chills, fever, and nausea; if these occur, unclamp tube and notify physician
Increase time tube is clamped: usually before and after
meals to facilitate digestion

Patient/family teaching

Explain T tube cholangiogram (7 to 10 days postoperatively); T tube is removed after 24 hr if bile duct is
patent
Demonstrate care of skin, drainage system, and incision
Discuss measuring and clamping procedure of T tube
Discuss symptoms to report to physician: pain, increased drainage, distention, fever
Encourage follow-up visits with physician

● Transhepatic Biliary Decompression Catheter Management

A multivented catheter inserted through the abdominal wall, liver, and common bile duct and into the duodenum to allow bile to drain past the obstructed bile duct into the intestine; performed for hepatic dysfunction, biliary obstruction (jaundice), and inoperable malignancy of the biliary system

Assessment

Objective data

Location of catheter, type of drainage system
Character, color, and amount of drainage
Presence of stabilizing device or sutures
Decreasing jaundice and serum bilirubin
Color, frequency, and amount of stool and urine

Diagnostic tests

Catheter usually inserted in radiology department
Postinsertion x-ray examination, cholangiography
Serum bilirubin, electrolytes
Stool for occult blood
Urine for bilirubin

Potential complications

Biliary sepsis
Bleeding or increased retrograde flow of bile
Catheter obstruction
Hyponatremia, electrolyte imbalance

Interventions

Maintain catheter with closed gravity drainage system; place stopcock between catheter and tubing; keep stopcock open
Monitor and measure amount of drainage q2h for 8 hr, then q4h; observe for increased amount of drainage; if >1500 ml/day, notify physician immediately
Monitor catheter site for drainage, type of sutures, and dressing q2h to 4h; change dressing prn and apply antibacterial ointment *to prevent infection*
Collaborate with physician to irrigate catheter through external port of stopcock, closing off drainage bag
Aspirate a few ml to ascertain patency
Irrigate gently with prescribed amount of solution; this action may be painful for patient—explain before procedure

Do not force irrigation if resistance is met; notify physician because catheter may be obstructed
After instillation, open stopcock to allow irrigant to flow into drainage bag
Assess patient's tolerance and observe for increasing, continuous pain, cramping, or abdominal distention (peritonitis, catheter slippage)
Collaborate with physician to clamp catheter and observe patient for decreasing jaundice
Monitor stools, urine, skin, and sclera
Monitor serum bilirubin
Tape catheter comfortably to abdomen; cover with sterile dressing
Monitor electrolytes, especially for hyponatremia; observe for lethargy or altered mental status

Patient/family teaching

Demonstrate and observe return demonstration for catheter irrigation and care
Provide and review written instructions for irrigating procedure
Discuss signs and symptoms of malfunction to report to physician
Fever, chills, weakness
Bleeding, increased bile output
Increasing jaundice, abdominal pain, distention
Dislodgment of catheter
Food particles in catheter drainage
Explain need for prescribed visits to radiology department for evaluation of catheter position and function
Encourage follow-up visits with physician

Home care considerations

Provide written information on where and what equipment and supplies to purchase
Instruct patient and family or significant other(s) on aseptic technique and handwashing procedure
Evaluate care giver/patient ability to care for catheter
Provide names, phone numbers of home health care team members

Liver

● Cirrhosis: Portal, Postnecrotic, Biliary

Chronic liver disease characterized by the alteration and destruction of cells, progressive fibrosis, and eventual nodular formation that results from excessive alcohol intake (70% to 80% of patients), hepatitis, drug toxicity, biliary obstruction, metabolic disease, or CHF

Assessment

Subjective data

Right upper quadrant pain
Generalized malaise/weakness
Anorexia
Nausea
Weight loss or gain

Objective data

Vomiting
Abdominal distention
Irregular bowel function
  Clay-colored stools
  Flatulence
  Melena
Ascites
Elevated temperature
Pruritus
Decreased urinary output; dark urine
Foul breath
Spider angiomas
Jaundice: sclera, skin
Edema of extremities
Gynecomastia
Dysrhythmias, CHF, jugular venous distention
Clubbing of fingers
Dehydration
Altered mental status
History of substance abuse
History of hepatitis or biliary obstruction

Diagnostic tests

Electrolytes
Serum bilirubin (elevated, jaundice)
AST, ALT, LDH (elevated)
Serum albumin (decreased), ammonia (elevated)
CBC, PT/INR (prolonged), urinalysis
Endoscopic retrograde cholangiopancreatography
  (ERCP) (common bile duct obstruction)
Esophagoscopy (varices) with barium esophago-
  graphy
Liver biopsy, scans
Ultrasonography
Percutaneous transhepatic portography (visualizes por-
  tal venous system)
Paracentesis (ascites)

Potential complications

Electrolyte imbalance
Malnutrition
Pneumonia
Ascites
Oliguria
GI bleeding
Portal hypertension, esophageal varices, *caput medusae*
  (umbilical venous distention)
Hepatomegaly, splenomegaly
Coma

Collaborative management

Therapeutic management

Diuretics, analgesics, antibiotics, lactulose (ammonia
  detoxicant)
Digestants (Cotazym, Kanulase), vitamins K and C,
  iron, thiamin, folic acid, antifibrinolytics
Cholestyramine for pruritis
Stool softeners
Parenteral fluids with electrolytes
Fresh whole blood, fresh frozen plasma, or platelets
Nasogastric suction
Diet management according to disease process
Sodium and/or fluid restriction
Oxygen therapy, incentive spirometer

Nursing management

PATIENT PROBLEMS/NURSING DIAGNOSES

● **NDX:** Altered nutrition: less than body requirements related to inadequate diet, vomiting,
  and/or anorexia

Maintain NPO if indicated *to reduce stress on liver*
Administer TPN as indicated *to maintain caloric
  intake*
Maintain bed rest in quiet environment
Provide small, frequent feedings of prescribed diet;
  amount of fat, carbohydrate, and protein will depend
  on patient's ability to metabolize these nutrients; salt
  may be restricted
Maintain calorie count
Provide salt substitute; avoid those containing ammo-
  nium *to reduce risk of encephalopathy*
Assist and encourage patient to eat; consider prefer-
  ences in food choices
Provide oral hygiene prn, especially before meals
Weigh patient daily: same time, clothing, scale
Monitor for edema, ascites

EXPECTED OUTCOMES
Patient tolerates prescribed diet
Demonstrates understanding of needed diet
  changes
Gains optimum weight

● **NDX:** Risk for fluid volume excess related to compromised regulatory mechanism (malnutrition), excess fluid, sodium intake

Assess for hydration status: good skin turgor, moist mucous membranes
Monitor for jugular vein distention; *may indicate vascular congestion*
Assess for dependent edema
Maintain parenteral fluids with electrolytes and vitamins; restrict fluid intake as ordered
Measure intake, output; assess for output less than intake
Note consistency, color, and frequency of stools and urine
Monitor serum and urine electrolytes; observe for signs of sodium and/or potassium imbalance
Auscultate lungs for breath sounds q4h *for signs of pulmonary edema*
Administer salt-poor albumin/plasma *to increase circulating volume and decrease edema*
Monitor vital signs q4h; observe for elevated temperature, dysrhythmias, and signs of CHF
Weigh patient daily; same time, clothing, and scale
Assess for effectiveness/side effects of diuretics

EXPECTED OUTCOMES
Patient's vital signs are stable
Intake and output are balanced
Edema is decreasing; no jugular vein distention is present
Electrolytes are within normal limits

● **NDX:** Risk for impaired skin integrity related to edema, dehydration, and/or jaundice

Assess skin for breaks, reddened areas, pruritus, and jaundice
Provide sheepskin with alternating pressure mattress as indicated *to reduce tissue ischemia*
Administer skin care frequently; provide clean linen, use lotion, and clip nails as needed; administer cholestyramine for pruritus
Provide perineal care after urination and bowel movement; apply lotions *to prevent breakdown*
Turn patient q2h and administer back care; change position slightly prn *to promote comfort*
Perform passive or assist with active ROM exercises q4h *to increase circulation*

EXPECTED OUTCOMES
Patient demonstrates understanding of needed techniques to prevent skin impairment
Participates in these activities
Maintains adequate skin integrity

● **NDX:** Ineffective breathing pattern related to debilitated state and ascites

Elevate head of bed 45 to 60 degrees or as needed *to maintain ventilation*
Assist and teach patient to turn and cough q4h; deep breathe q½h
Auscultate lungs for breath sounds q4h
Assist and teach patient to use incentive spirometer q2h
Monitor blood gases, pulse oximetry for signs of atelectasis, pneumonia
Assess for signs of hypoxia (altered mentation)

EXPECTED OUTCOMES
Patient's blood gases are within normal limits
Respirations and mental acuity are normal
Breath sounds are clear

● **NDX:** Altered protection, hemorrhage related to risk of impaired blood coagulation or bleeding from portal hypertension

Monitor mucous membranes for signs of bleeding; avoid hard-bristled toothbrushes
Observe injection sites for prolonged bleeding; apply extra pressure and pressure bandage; use small-gauge needles
Monitor patient's use of razors and other sharp objects
Avoid straining during bowel movement and forceful nose blowing
Administer stool softeners
Monitor PT/INR and platelet count
Administer vitamin K and antifibrinolytic agents; assess for effectiveness/side effects
Observe for signs of bleeding: decreasing BP, increasing P, hematemesis, melena
Monitor vital signs, Hgb, Hct
Prepare for endoscopy if bleeding occurs
Monitor nasogastric tube and low, intermittent suction apparatus; measure gastric output qh and note color and consistency; irrigate, if ordered, with measured amounts of saline *to maintain patency*
Maintain parenteral fluids and/or transfusions
Administer vitamin K, vasopressin, and neomycin; avoid aspirin use

EXPECTED OUTCOMES
Patient demonstrates understanding and ability to perform needed changes in activities
Exhibits absent or controlled bleeding

● **NDX:** Altered thought processes related to increased serum ammonia and hepatic coma

Monitor frequently for changes in mental status, lethargy, drowsiness, and confusion
Monitor neurologic status for decreased motor ability
Avoid use of sedatives, tranquilizers, and narcotics
Provide safe environment: siderails up and bed in low position
Monitor serum ammonia levels
Monitor for possible violent behavior
Reduce environmental stimulus
Provide rest periods
Acknowledge feelings of anger or fear
Assist patient to redirect aggressive behavior to an adaptive activity
Orient patient to time and place as appropriate with each interaction
Teach and assist with stress-reduction measures: imaging, deep breathing, relaxation techniques
Help to focus on accomplishing self-care activities; assist with ADLs only as necessary
Provide high-calorie, low-protein diet if mental deterioration occurs *because protein metabolism produces ammonia*

EXPECTED OUTCOMES

Patient's mental acuity is improving or normal
Orientation to name, time, place is accurate
Ability to focus on and accomplish ADLs increases

Patient/family teaching

Provide and discuss written dietary instructions from nutritionist/registered dietitian, listing amount of protein, carbohydrate, fat, and salt allowed
Discuss and teach stress management techniques
Discuss with patient importance of avoiding stress during meals and need to eat small, frequent meals
Reinforce physician's explanation of relationship between alcohol and cirrhosis if applicable
Provide information about medications including name, purpose, dosage, time of administration, and side effects; caution against using any medicine not prescribed by physician
Explain importance of rest and exercise, avoiding exposure to infection
Discuss skin care if pruritus persists
Discuss signs of progression of disease to report to physician: hematuria, melena, abdominal distention, edema, fever, bleeding that does not subside, mental deterioration, personality changes
Encourage follow-up visits with physician
Ensure that significant other(s) know and understand symptoms of mental status change or behavior changes to report
Provide information about support groups in community

Home care considerations

Reinforce information on use of items that may deter mucous membrane bleeding; soft toothbrush or Water Pik, electric razors
Discuss methods of reducing itching from pruritus
  Keep nails short
  Apply lotions to keep skin moist
  Wear soft clothing, undergarments
  Try not to scratch
Encourage counseling, Alcoholics Anonymous, substance abuse programs
Provide information on where to purchase, rent alternating mattress, sheepskin
Stress importance of reducing salt/sodium intake, monitoring intake and output, and maintaining a balance

● Viral Hepatitis

virus A (HAV): Rapid onset of symptoms and destruction of liver cells caused by contaminated water or food; usually affects young adults (Table 6-1)
virus B (HBV): Slow onset of symptoms and destruction of liver cells caused by contaminated serum from needles and instruments; affects all age groups
virus C (HCV): Causes liver destruction following blood transfusion (formerly non–A, non–B)
virus D (HDV): Occurs in populations at risk for HBV infections
virus E (HEV): Occurs mostly in young adults in developing countries

Assessment

Subjective data

Nausea
Anorexia
Malaise
Headache
Tenderness and pain in right upper quadrant
Arthritic pain (HBV)

Objective data

Elevated temperature (HAV)
Jaundice
  Pruritus
  Urticaria
  Sclera
  Clay-colored stools
  Dark urine
Vomiting
Diarrhea

Table 6-1 Overview of Viral Hepatitis

	Hepatitis A	Hepatitis B	Hepatitis C	Hepatitis D	Hepatitis E
Occurrence	Worldwide; sporadic and epidemic, with a tendency toward cyclic recurrence; outbreaks in institutions	Worldwide; endemic; highest in young adults, homosexual men, heterosexuals with multiple sex partners, parenteral drug users, and health care and public safety workers	Worldwide; accounts for 90% of posttransfusion hepatitis in the United States	Worldwide; occurs epidemically and endemically in populations at risk for HBV infection	Epidemic and sporadic cases, particularily in developing countries; highest in young adults; rare in children or elderly
Etiologic agent	Hepatitis A virus (HAV)	Hepatitis B virus (HBV)	Hepatitis C virus (HCV)	A viruslike particle (HDV or the delta agent); coinfects with HBV	Viruslike particle (HEV)
Reservoir	Humans and captive primates	Humans and possibly captive primates	Humans, chimpanzees	Humans, chimpanzees	Humans, chimpanzees
Transmission	Person to person by fecal-oral route; contaminated food, water, shellfish	Direct and indirect contact with blood, saliva, and semen; sexual contact; perinatal	Percutaneous exposure to blood; person-to-person and sexual transmission have not been defined	Similar to HBV, including sexual contact	Contaminated water; person to person by fecal-oral route
Incubation period	15-50 days; average: 28-30 days	45-180 days; average: 60-90 days	2 wk to 6 mo; commonly 6-9 wk	2-10 wk	15-64 days; average: 26-42 days
Period of communicability	Latter half of incubation period to 1 wk after onset of jaundice	During incubation period and throughout clinical course of disease; carrier state may persist for years	From 1 or more wk before symptom onset, indefinitely during chronic and carrier states	Throughout acute and chronic disease	Not known; probably similar to HA
Susceptibility and resistance	Usually affects children and young adults; immunity after infection probably lasts for life; 45% of population has hepatitis A antibodies	All age groups; disease is mild in children; lifetime immunity follows infection if antibody to HBsAg develops and HBsAg is negative	All age groups; degree of immunity following infection is unknown	All persons susceptible to HB, HBV carriers; disease is severe in children	Unknown; no explanation for epidemics among young adults; pregnant women have highest fatality
Report to local health authority	Mandatory case report	Mandatory case report	Mandatory case report	Mandatory case report	Mandatory case report

From Thompson JM et al: *Mosby's clinical nursing,* ed 3, St Louis, 1993, Mosby.

History of blood transfusions, foreign travel (Asia, Africa)
History of recent anesthetic (Halothane)
History of IV drug use
History of accidental exposure to contaminated needles or instruments

Diagnostic tests

Serum AST, ALT, bilirubin: elevated
Alkaline phosphatase, lactic dehydrogenase: elevated
PT/INR (prolonged in severe hepatitis)
Stool and serology for HAV
Serum antigen/antibody tests for HBV
CBC, urinalysis, electrolytes, FBS
Liver biopsy
Liver function tests: abnormal
Serum albumin: decreased
HbsRg (positive type B)
anti–HAVlgM (positive type B)

Potential complications

Decreased urinary output
Dehydration and electrolyte imbalance
Altered mental status
Hyperglycemia or hypoglycemia
Hepatic coma

Collaborative management

Therapeutic management

Activity, rest
Sedatives, antiemetics, antacids, vitamin K
Antivirals, antibiotics
Diet according to tolerance of protein, carbohydrates, and fat
Parenteral therapy with electrolytes and vitamins for vomiting or GI bleeding
Antihistamines and cholestyramine for pruritus

Nursing management

PATIENT PROBLEMS/NURSING DIAGNOSES

● **NDX:** Activity intolerance related to weakness or fatigue secondary to infection

Maintain bed rest in quiet environment *to conserve energy;* assist patient in assuming position of comfort; bathroom privileges may be allowed
Assist and teach patient to turn q2h and deep breathe q½h *to prevent skin breakdown and increase lung expansion*

Change position frequently *to promote comfort*
Administer sedatives *to provide restful sleep and build energy level;* assess for effectiveness, side effects
Provide diversional activities
Assist with and teach active or perform passive ROM exercises q4h while patient is in bed *to maintain muscle tone*
Coordinate care to provide planned rest periods
Ambulate with assistance when tolerated
Assess response to increased activity
Reinforce progress toward independence

EXPECTED OUTCOMES
Patient expresses understanding of changes needed in activity levels
Increases activities as strength returns

● **NDX:** Altered nutrition: less than body requirements secondary to anorexia, vomiting, altered intestinal absorption

Collaborate with physician, nutritionist/registered dietitian and provide soft diet, monitoring intake of protein, fat, and carbohydrates
Offer small, frequent meals, attractively prepared
Encourage fluids to 2500 ml/day unless contraindicated; include fruit juices and carbonated beverages, which are easily digested
Assess for effectiveness, side effects of antacids and antiemetics; avoid Compazine and Thorazine
Weigh patient daily: same time, clothing, and scale
Provide oral hygiene as needed, especially before meals *to increase desire for food*
Monitor blood glucose: hypoglycemia or hyperglycemia may be present, requiring adjustment in dietary intake

EXPECTED OUTCOMES
Patient gains weight, progressing toward normal weight
Tolerates prescribed diet

● **NDX:** Risk for fluid volume deficit related to excessive loss of body fluids resulting from vomiting, fever, diarrhea

Maintain NPO if vomiting and/or anorexia are present
Maintain parenteral fluids with electrolytes and vitamin K
Assess for signs of dehydration: skin turgor, pedal pulses, dry mucous membranes

Measure intake and output q8h; include emesis/
diarrhea in output
Monitor stool and urine for color, consistency, and fre-
quency
Monitor for ascites, increasing jaundice, and mental de-
terioration
Monitor vital signs, electrolytes, Hgb, Hct
Monitor laboratory values for abnormal results

EXPECTED OUTCOMES

Patient's vital signs are stable
Intake and output are balanced
Skin turgor is normal

● **NDX:** Altered protection related to abnormal blood
profile/coagulation

Assess for signs of bleeding: mucous membranes, injec-
tion sites, emesis, stool
Monitor coagulation studies
Use small-gauge needles for injections and apply in-
creased pressure longer; rotate sites
Evaluate effectiveness of vitamin K administration

EXPECTED OUTCOME

Patient is free of bleeding as evidenced by clear skin,
absence of bleeding at gums and injection sites, no occult blood in urine and feces, normal coagulation studies

● **NDX:** Risk for impaired skin integrity related to
jaundice and ensuing pruritus

Administer frequent skin care; avoid soap or use superfatted soap
Provide shower or bath with baking soda or starch; apply lotions
Administer antihistamines *to control itching;* diphenhydramine (Benadryl)
Assess effectiveness of cholestyramine; *may cause nausea, constipation*
Offer frequent back rubs and changes in position *to
promote comfort*
Encourage short fingernails or use of gloves
Provide diversional activities *to decrease attention on
scratching*
Encourage patient not to scratch and to use knuckles if
the urge is persistent

EXPECTED OUTCOMES

Patient reports decreased pruritus/scratching
Participates in activities to maintain skin integrity

● **NDX:** Risk for infection related to inadequate secondary defenses and malnutrition

Maintain isolation techniques according to hospital
policy
Establish and explain blood and body fluid precautions
to prevent transmission to others
Ensure that all contacts are protected against hepatitis
Maintain stringent handwashing technique
Assess temperature and breath sounds q4h to 8h
Restrict visitors with infections, especially URIs
Provide nutritious diet with fluids to 2000 ml/day *to
promote cellular repair*
Administer antiviral medication: vidarabine (Vira-A),
acyclovir (Zovirax)

EXPECTED OUTCOMES

Patient demonstrates understanding of precautions by
following guidelines
Maintains normal temperature; respirations are clear;
no other evidence of infection

● **NDX:** Disturbance in self-concept related to disease process, hospitalization, and isolation

Encourage and allow time for communication of fears
and concerns *to promote a trusting relationship*
Reinforce physician's explanation of disease process
and treatment rationale
Explain purpose of isolation procedure to patient
and/or significant other(s)
Assess present coping patterns and be supportive and
understanding
Encourage communication with significant other(s)
Avoid making judgments about lifestyle *to promote self-
esteem*
Encourage bright colors (red, blue) in clothing *to offset
jaundice*

EXPECTED OUTCOMES

Patient uses adaptive coping measures as evidenced by
discussion of feelings
Uses diversional activities and maintains personal
grooming habits

Patient/family teaching

Discuss techniques to prevent transmission
  HAV: perineal care, handwashing after toileting, and
    disinfection of soiled articles of clothing
  HAV and HCV: caution not to share razors or tooth-
    brushes and to avoid serum or secretion contact
    with others
  Explain infectious nature of HAV, HBV, and HCV and
    the need to avoid infecting others (until laboratory
    values are normal); importance of not donating
    blood; need to avoid others with infections, espe-
    cially URIs

Provide information about drug rehabilitation program if appropriate

Stress importance of follow-up medical care for 1 year

   Regular laboratory tests as ordered

   Routine follow-up care with physician

Encourage family members and friends to seek injection of gamma globulin, ISG, HBIG, hepatitis B vaccine

Discuss symptoms of recurrence to report to physician

Provide instructions about medication including name, purpose, dosage, time of administration, and side effects; explain need to avoid medicines not prescribed by physician

Home care considerations

Reinforce physician's explanation of disease process so patient understands importance of the following:

   Diet instructions on amounts of protein, carbohydrate, and fat allowed

   No alcohol intake for at least 1 year

   Coordinating rest and exercise program to allow liver to regenerate

   Avoiding heavy lifting, contact sports

   Maintaining bowel function with adequate fluid intake, natural dietary bulk, stool softeners

Refer to community resources for assistance/counseling

Explain that it may require weeks to recuperate and to look for diversional activities to occupy the time

● Hepatic Surgery

Surgical removal or repair of portions of the liver resulting from trauma or carcinoma

Preoperative assessment and care

Assess cardiovascular, respiratory, cerebral, and renal status; obtain baseline vital signs; observe for jaundice

Prepare bowel as ordered: enemas, oral antibiotics, magnesium preparations; keep enemas to a minimum to prevent dehydration

Insert nasogastric tube and/or indwelling urethral catheter as ordered; monitor aspirate and/or urine for color and consistency

Administer vitamin K and/or blood transfusions

Reinforce physician's explanation of surgical procedure and postoperative care; explain that chest tubes may be present

Provide emotional support to patient and significant other(s)

Postoperative assessment

Subjective data

Nausea

Location, character, type of pain

Dyspnea

Objective data

Placement of chest tubes and drainage apparatus if applicable

Character and amount of the following:

   Chest drainage if applicable

   Gastric drainage

   Urinary output

   Wound drainage

Vomiting

Abdominal distention

Tachycardia

Tachypnea

Splinting of respirations

Decreased breath sounds

Elevated temperature

Diagnostic tests

Serum electrolytes, albumin, liver function studies

Electrolytes, CBC, glucose, PT/INR

Potential complications

Electrolyte imbalance

Decreased serum albumin levels

Hypoglycemia

Atelectasis (p. 305)

Pneumonia (p. 288)

Paralytic ileus (p. 379)

Hemorrhage

Shock

Subdiaphragmatic abscess

Jaundice

Ascites

Hepatic coma

Wound infection

Collaborative management

Therapeutic management

Analgesics

Nasogastric suction, NPO

Parenteral fluids with electrolytes and vitamin K
Antibiotics, albumin, transfusions
Connection of chest tubes to underwater seal
Oxygen therapy, incentive spirometer
Urethral catheter drainage

Nursing management

PATIENT PROBLEMS/NURSING DIAGNOSES

● **NDX:** Ineffective breathing pattern related to invasive procedure, chest tube placement, and/or pain

Elevate head of bed 30 to 45 degrees *to enhance lung expansion*
Assess placement of chest tubes and connect underwater seal to low, intermittent suction; monitor amount and color of aspirate q4h
Auscultate chest for breath sounds q2h; monitor respiratory rate and for signs of splinting
Assist and teach patient to turn and cough q2h and deep breathe q½h; support incision; medicate for pain before procedure when possible
Provide incentive spirometer q1h to 2h
Monitor pulse oximetry q8h, if applicable
Assist with ADLs *to conserve energy*

EXPECTED OUTCOMES
Patient exhibits normal respirations
Verbalizes understanding of need for breathing exercises
Uses incentive spirometer routinely

● **NDX:** Risk for fluid volume deficit related to increased body fluid loss resulting from NPO status and/or nasogastric suction

Maintain NPO; assess hydration status: good skin turgor, moist mucous membranes, normal capillary refill
Maintain parenteral fluids with electrolytes and/or antibiotics
Monitor nasogastric tube and low, intermittent suction apparatus; irrigate gently with measured amounts of normal saline to maintain patency
Monitor urethral catheter and closed gravity drainage system; monitor output qh; report output of <50 ml/hr to physician
Measure intake and output q8h
Monitor vital signs qh until stable, then q4h
Encourage lower extremity movement *to increase venous return*
Apply antiembolic stockings; remove daily to inspect skin for redness, breakdown
Monitor serum electrolytes, albumin, and glucose

Monitor Hct to assess hydration status; *may be elevated in dehydration*
Auscultate abdomen for bowel sounds q8h
Monitor for peripheral edema; assess pedal pulses q8h
Monitor for signs of hypoglycemia: nausea, shakiness, lethargy
Monitor mental acuity q4h

EXPECTED OUTCOMES
Patient's vital signs are stable
Intake and output are balanced
Electrolytes are within normal limits
Skin turgor is normal

● **NDX:** Altered protection related to abnormal blood profile, altered clotting factors resulting from hemorrhage

Monitor dressings and incision q2h for drainage or bleeding; reinforce and change dressings as needed
Monitor for signs of bleeding: tachycardia; hypotension; cold, clammy skin
Assess for bleeding tendencies resulting from reduced vitamin K: mucous membranes, injection sites
Use small-gauge needles; apply increased pressure longer to control bleeding
Monitor Hgb, Hct, and clotting times
Assess for effectiveness, side effects of vitamin K administration

EXPECTED OUTCOMES
Patient's blood profiles (Hgb, Hct, clotting time) are within normal limits
No evidence of bleeding at sites of injection or wound exists

● **NDX:** Pain related to surgical intervention

Maintain bed rest in quiet environment in position of comfort; usually with head of bed elevated 35 to 45 degrees
Assess type, intensity, and location of pain; use pain rating scale
Administer analgesics and assess effectiveness of pain relief measures; medicate as prescribed for first few postoperative days
Consider patient controlled analgesia (p. 92)
Change position frequently; administer back rubs *to ease muscle soreness and promote comfort*
Discuss alternate pain relief measures: deep breathing, imaging, relaxation techniques
Provide diversional activities *to decrease attention on discomfort*
Encourage balanced activity/rest pattern

EXPECTED OUTCOMES

Patient reports a decrease in pain
Appears relaxed and comfortable

● **NDX:**   Altered nutrition: less than body requirements related to NPO status, decreased energy

Collaborate with physician to remove or clamp nasogastric tube when bowel sounds return
  Provide small amounts of water or clear liquids and
monitor tolerance; *too much fluid may cause vomiting*
  Progress to soft diet as tolerated; amounts of fat, carbohydrate, and protein will depend on ability of liver
to metabolize these nutrients; involve nutritionist/
registered dietitian
  Measure intake and output *to assess for adequate
balance*
  Administer oral hygiene prn, especially before meals
  Encourage fluids to 2500 ml/day unless contraindicated
  Weigh patient daily: same time, clothing, and scale

EXPECTED OUTCOMES

Patient's weight is maintained or returning to normal
Prescribed diet is tolerated without discomfort

Patient/family teaching

Provide and review written diet instructions with
amounts of fat, carbohydrate, and protein allowed
Demonstrate care of incision and discuss signs of
wound infection to report: tenderness, redness,
drainage, fever
Provide information about signs and symptoms to re-
port to physician
  Decreased mental acuity, lethargy
  Abdominal distention, pain
  Jaundice, dyspnea, fever
Discuss medications: name, dosage, purpose, times of
administration, side effects, and importance of taking
only medicines prescribed by physician
Discuss need for balance between activity and rest
Encourage follow-up visits with physician

Home care considerations

Provide information on what types of and where to purchase needed supplies: dressings, tape, disposable
gloves
Review importance of handwashing technique
Explain necessity of taking all medications as
prescribed
Discuss importance of weighing once a week and reporting loss to physician

Provide information on community resources for
assistance at home with ADLs, meals, transportation

● Continuous Peritoneal-Vena Caval Shunt for Ascites

*A subcutaneous shunt to remove ascitic fluid from the
abdomen to the heart, and from there to reenter the
systemic circulation and be excreted by the kidneys;
there are two types used:*
*LaVeen shunt: Has a one-way, pressure-sensitive valve
that remains open as long as the thoracic pressure is
lower than the intraabdominal pressure*
*Denver shunt: Has either a single or double valve;
a fluid-filled pump is implanted close to the skin
and allows the patient to press and pump the device
to keep the fluid moving and maintain patency*

Preoperative care

Reinforce physician's explanation of surgical procedure
Monitor baseline vital signs
Monitor BUN, creatinine, Hgb, Hct readings
Administer antibiotics as prescribed
Prepare local anesthesia
Maintain IV line for IV analgesia

Postprocedure assessment

Increased or decreased abdominal distention
Dyspnea
Diminished breath sounds
Tachypnea
Tachycardia, hypertension
Right upper quadrant pain
Jugular vein distention
Ankle edema
Increased or decreased urinary output
Level of consciousness
Leakage of fluid from incision site
Electrolyte imbalance; hypokalemia
Increased clotting time
Elevated bilirubin
Decreased Hgb, Hct, BUN
Disseminated intravascular coagulation
Wound infection

Interventions

LaVeen shunt

  Maintain bed rest; elevate head of bed 60 to 90 degrees

Provide incentive spirometer *to increase intraabdominal pressure*

Apply abdominal binder *to increase pressure*

Denver shunt

Maintain bed rest; must remain flat 30 min out of each hr for first 24 hr *to encourage abdominal fluid to flow toward the heart*

Teach patient to apply pressure to chamber slowly *to maintain patency of catheter*

Pump chamber about 10 times per hr or as ordered

Common interventions

Check vital signs q4h until stable, then q8h

Check neurologic signs q2h to 4h and report changes to physician

Check incision for excess bleeding or drainage and neck for edema q2h for 24 hr; then q4h for 24 hr; report presence of these signs to physician

Measure intake and output; report decrease in output to physician

Maintain NPO as ordered

Administer parenteral fluids with electrolytes and vitamins as ordered

Monitor serum electrolytes and blood clotting time; report significant changes to physician

Weigh patient daily: same time, clothing, and scale; if weight increases, notify physician

Auscultate chest for breath sounds q4h; report diminished breath sounds to physician

Manage pain as indicated; assess effectiveness of pain relief measure(s)

Assist and teach active or perform passive ROM exercises q4h *to increase venous flow*

Assist and teach patient to turn, cough, and deep breathe q2h to 4h *to maintain lung expansion*

Administer skin care and oral hygiene q2h to 4h

Evaluate incisions and report signs of wound infection: redness, tenderness, discharge, fever

Patient/family teaching and home care considerations

Instruct patient on signs and symptoms of a clogged shunt: weight gain in excess of 2 lb, increased peripheral edema, and/or dyspnea

Stress importance of weekly weights

Provide rest and activity schedule *to maintain consistency and balance*

Encourage follow-up care with physician and laboratory tests

● Liver Biopsy

Introduction of a special needle into the liver to obtain a specimen for pathologic examination; other noninvasive diagnostic procedures have replaced the biopsy, but it is still used when other procedures fail

Prebiopsy care

Type and crossmatch for possible transfusion

Monitor baseline VS

Assess mental alertness and ability to cooperate

Explain procedure and follow-up care

Administer analgesics or sedatives as ordered

Monitor for allergy to local anesthetic

Teach patient how to inhale and hold breath during needle insertion

Monitor bleeding, clotting, and PT results; report abnormal results to physician

Place on NPO 4 to 8 hr before biopsy

Have patient void immediately preprocedure

Postbiopsy assessment

Intraperitoneal, intrahepatic hemorrhage

Pneumothorax

Interventions

Apply pressure to biopsy site for first 15 min after procedure *to prevent hemorrhage*

Maintain bed rest in supine position for 24 hr

Position patient on right side for first 6 hr *to keep pressure at site*

Monitor vital signs every 15 min ×4, then q30min ×4, then q4h or as ordered

Observe biopsy site q30min ×4 for bleeding, swelling, or increased pain

Monitor Hgb and Hct

Manage pain as indicated; epigastric pain or referred shoulder pain may occur

Report increased respiratory rate, severe shoulder pain, decreased breath sounds to physician; *indicators for pneumothorax*

Administer vitamin K as ordered

Assist patient with eating and other activities as needed for 24 hr

Pancreas

● Acute and Chronic Pancreatitis

acute pancreatitis: *Acute inflammatory disease in which autodigestion of the organ occurs as a result of* *obstruction of the pancreatic duct; exact cause is unknown, but various causative factors are thought to be stones, tumors, trauma, and excessive use of alcohol*

chronic pancreatitis: *Chronic, progressive disease that may or may not follow acute pancreatitis; causative factors include gallbladder disease, carcinoma, and excessive use of alcohol; pancreas becomes fibrotic and necrotic, and enzyme action is markedly decreased or nonexistent*

Assessment

Subjective data

Acute pancreatitis

Severe pain in upper left quadrant: dull, unrelenting, boring

Increases in supine position; may radiate to shoulder and thoracic vertebrae

Nausea

Chronic pancreatitis

Intermittent epigastric pain: steady, boring, dull, or sharp

Radiates to back

Relieved when leaning forward

Nausea, anorexia

Weight loss

Objective data

Acute pancreatitis

Fever, chills

Tachycardia, hypovolemia, hypotension

Respiratory impairment, tachypnea with or without dyspnea, splinting; adult respiratory distress syndrome (ARDS) may develop

Decreased urine output

Discoloration of abdomen and/or flanks

Mild abdominal distention

Vomiting, diarrhea

History of cholelithiasis, gastritis, gastric ulcers, trauma, Crohn's disease

History of excessive use of alcohol, steroids, some antihypertensives and antibiotics

Confusion, lethargy

Jaundice

Hyperglycemia

Chronic pancreatitis

Vomiting

Diarrhea, steatorrhea

Malnutrition

Minimal jaundice

Fat-soluble vitamin deficiencies

Symptoms of diabetes mellitus

Diagnostic tests

Acute pancreatitis

CBC, BUN, urinalysis, FBS

Arterial Po_2 <60 mm Hg

Serum calcium, albumin (decreased)

Serum LDH, AST, ALT (increased)

Amylase: serum, urine, lipase (elevated)

Electrolytes: potassium decreased

Chronic pancreatitis

CBC, urinalysis

Alkaline phosphatase: elevated

Serum amylase, lipase: normal

Acute and chronic pancreatitis

Endoscopy

Serum glucose: elevated

Radiologic abdominal films

Ultrasonography/CT scan

Upper GI series/cholangiography

Stool for fat

Potential complications

Electrolyte imbalance, hypocalcemia

Hyperglycemia

Respiratory, circulatory, renal failure

Paralytic ileus

Jaundice

Shock, hemorrhage

Collaborative management

Therapeutic management

Analgesics, antacids, cimetidine, antibiotics, anticholinergics

Hemodynamic monitoring

Parenteral fluids with electrolytes, vitamins, serum albumin, and/or dextran

Nasogastric suction, NPO

Diet, activity, TPN

Digestants (pancreatic enzymes) for chronic pancreatitis

Insulin for hyperglycemia

Paravertebral block for pain management

Nursing management

PATIENT PROBLEMS/NURSING DIAGNOSES

● **NDX:** Risk for fluid volume deficit related to abnormal body fluid loss resulting from vomiting, fever, and/or gastric aspiration

Maintain NPO, assess hydration status: skin turgor, moist mucous membranes, normal capillary refill

Maintain parenteral fluids with electrolytes, vitamins, albumin, and antibiotics or TPN if indicated

Monitor nasogastric tube and low, intermittent suction apparatus; irrigate with measured amounts of normal saline; measure gastric output q4h

Auscultate abdomen for bowel sounds q4h

Observe for distention, vomiting, and decreased sounds after nasogastric tube is removed

Weigh as indicated to assess for loss (hypovolemia) or gain (edema, ascites)

Monitor vital signs q2h to 4h; *hypotension may occur as a result of pancreatic ischemia;* check apical pulse

Monitor CVP or Swan-Ganz catheter; monitor ABGs and pulse oximetry

Monitor urine output qh; report output <50 ml/hr to physician; *may indicate renal compromise*

Calculate intake and output q8h; report deficits; include gastric aspirate/emesis in output

Monitor mental acuity for decreased sensorium as sign of hypovolemia, hypoxia

Monitor for calcium imbalance: tremors, twitching

Monitor electrolytes, glucose, liver function studies, PT, and calcium

Monitor for peripheral/dependent edema

Assess pedal P

Encourage patient to move feet and legs qh *to increase circulation*

EXPECTED OUTCOMES

Patient's vital signs are stable

Electrolytes are within normal limits

Skin turgor is adequate

Intake and output are balanced

● **NDX:** Risk for infection related to inadequate primary defenses, nutrition imbalance

Monitor respiratory status: breath sounds, cough, sputum, shallow breathing, fluid collection

Change dressings promptly using aseptic technique; assess wound for signs of infection: redness, tenderness, increased drainage; obtain culture if present

Maintain aseptic technique when handling IV lines, catheters, tubes, drains

Promote good handwashing technique

Assist and teach patient to turn and cough q2h and deep breathe q½h

Administer skin care and oral hygiene q2h to 4h; observe for reddened areas or breakdown

Observe for signs of jaundice: skin, sclera, urine

Monitor temperature for elevation; initiate cooling measures for temperature >101°F (38.2°C)

Monitor urine for infection

Administer antibiotics as indicated

Encourage small, frequent position changes *to enhance lung expansion*

EXPECTED OUTCOMES

Patient's condition is afebrile

Breath sounds are normal

Skin remains clean, dry, and intact

Urine is clear without signs of infection

● **NDX:** Pain related to obstruction of pancreatic, biliary ducts

Maintain bed rest in quiet environment in position of comfort

Assess type, intensity, and location of pain; use pain rating scale

Assess effectiveness of pain relief measures

   Avoid morphine; small, frequent doses of meperidine are beneficial

   Medicate before pain becomes severe

   Teach alternate pain management techniques: deep breathing, relaxation, imaging

Change position frequently; administer back rubs *to promote comfort*

Perform passive or assist with and teach active ROM exercises q4h *to promote circulation and healing*

Coordinate care to provide for rest periods

Ambulate with assistance when allowed

Promote diversional activities *to decrease attention on discomfort*

Administer antacids *to neutralize gastric acid and reduce pancreatic enzyme production*

Administer cimetidine (Tagamet) *to decrease HCl and pancrease stimulation/pain*

EXPECTED OUTCOMES

Patient verbalizes that pain is decreasing

Appears relaxed and comfortable

● **NDX:** Altered nutrition: less than body requirements related to anorexia, vomiting, and/or decreased digestive enzymes

Monitor for presence of bowel sounds *to determine return of peristaltic action*

Collaborate with physician, nutritionist/registered dietitian and provide liquid to soft diet when tolerated

Provide high-protein, high-carbohydrate, low-fat, or diabetic diet in small, frequent meals

Administer bile pancreatic replacement if ordered; avoid taking with hot food/fluid, *which may inactivate enzymes*

Avoid coffee, tea, stimulants, and gas-producing foods
Monitor for food tolerances
Provide frequent oral hygiene, especially before meals *to increase appetite*
Administer antacids, insulin, and anticholinergics; assess for effectiveness, side effects
Weigh patient daily: same time, clothing, and scale
Monitor stools for color, consistency, amount, frequency; test for presence of fat
Monitor urine for sugar/acetone *to assess for hyperglycemia/ketoacidosis*

EXPECTED OUTCOMES

Patient demonstrates progressive weight gain/loss towards target weight
Tolerates balanced diet
Presents normal urine/stool

Patient/family teaching

Provide and review written dietary instructions
Reinforce causal relationship of alcohol use to pancreatitis; promote outside counseling with rehabilitation centers
Explain and teach about diabetes, blood testing, insulin therapy, and symptoms to report to physician
Discuss medications: name, schedule, dosage, purpose, and side effects; explain importance of taking only medicines prescribed by physician; promote discriminate use of narcotics
Encourage follow-up visits with physician

Home care considerations

Discuss signs and symptoms to report to physician: fever, recurrence of pain, nausea/vomiting, abdominal distention
Explain importance of pancreatic enzyme replacement therapy, if applicable; do not take with hot liquids/food *because the heat destroys enzyme potency*
Reinforce signs of hyperglycemia: polyuria, polydipsia, weakness, weight loss

● Pancreatic Surgery

pancreatic duodenectomy (Whipple's procedure):
Radical procedure for cancer of the head of the pancreas; the proximal head of the pancreas, adjoining duodenum, distal part of the stomach, and distal portion of the common bile duct are resected and an anastomosis of the jejunum to the pancreatic duct, common bile duct, and stomach is performed (Figure 6-10)

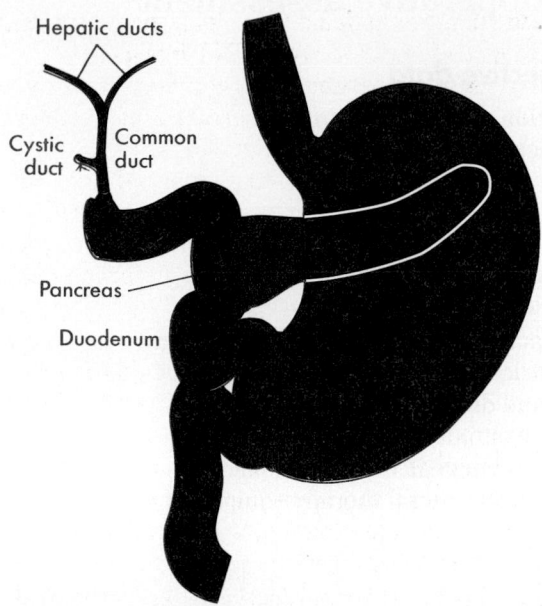

Figure 6-10 Whipple's procedure, or radical pancreas resection, entails resection of proximal pancreas, adjoining duodenum, distal portion of stomach, and distal segment of common bile duct. Anastomosis of pancreatic duct, common bile duct, and stomach to jejunum is done. (From Beare PG, Myers JL: *Principles and practice of adult health nursing,* ed 2, St Louis, 1994, Mosby.)

total pancreatectomy: Alternate procedure for cancer of the head of the pancreas; the pancreas and the spleen are removed, as well as the nearby lymph nodes; the jejunal stump is closed, and a proximal choledochojejunostomy and distal gastrojejunostomy or duodenojejunostomy is performed; pancreatic function is lost

Preoperative assessment and care

Assess respiratory, circulatory, and neurologic status; take baseline vital signs; observe for abdominal distention and peripheral edema
Assess nutritional status and history of substance abuse
Provide nourishing diet as tolerated
Administer parenteral fluids, TPN, and/or blood transfusions as ordered
Insert nasogastric tube and/or indwelling urethral catheter as ordered
Provide emotional support and reinforce physician's explanation of surgical procedure; clarify misconceptions
Administer vitamin K, salt-poor albumin, and antibiotics as ordered
Explain and teach about possibility of insulin and pancreatic enzyme therapy postoperatively

Postoperative assessment

Subjective data

Location and character of pain
Nausea

Objective data

Hypotension
Patency of nasogastric tube
Character and amount of the following:
  Gastric drainage
  Wound drainage
  Urine output
  Bile drainage if T tube is in place
Type of parenteral therapy equipment
  CVP line
  TPN line
Tachycardia
Splinting of respirations
Decreased breath sounds
Vomiting
Abdominal distention

Diagnostic tests

Electrolytes, PT/INR, FBS, Hgb, Hct
ABGs, pH, serum albumin
Serum and urine osmolalities

Potential complications

Oliguria
Dehydration
Electrolyte imbalance
Decreased serum albumin levels
Increased PT/INR
Hyperglycemia
Hypoglycemia
Atelectasis
Pneumonia
Elevated temperature
Jaundice
Subdiaphragmatic abscess, intraperitoneal infection
Paralytic ileus
Gastric/wound hemorrhage
Shock
Wound infection

Collaborative management

Therapeutic management

Analgesics, antibiotics, vasopressors, diuretics
Pancreatic enzyme therapy

Parenteral fluids with electrolytes, vitamins, and/or
  albumin
Blood transfusions
Nasogastric suction
Oxygen therapy, incentive spirometer
TPN
Stool softeners
Diet, activity

Nursing management

PATIENT PROBLEMS/NURSING DIAGNOSES

● **NDX:** Ineffective breathing pattern related to surgical incision, pain, and anesthesia

Elevate head of bed 30 to 45 degrees *to enhance lung expansion*
Monitor respiratory status q1h to 2h; observe for dyspnea and splinting
Auscultate chest for breath sounds q4h
Provide incentive spirometer qh
Monitor CVP or Swan-Ganz catheter and check ABGs and pH
Assist and teach patient to turn and cough q2h and deep breathe q½h; support incision and administer analgesics before procedure when possible *to reduce discomfort and increase lung expansion*

EXPECTED OUTCOMES

Patient exhibits normal respiratory rate
Performs deep breathing exercises correctly
Presents normal breath sounds

● **NDX:** Risk for fluid volume deficit related to abnormal body fluid loss resulting from nasogastric suction, NPO status, hypovolemia

Maintain NPO; assess hydration status: moist mucous membranes, good skin turgor, normal capillary refill
Maintain parenteral fluids with electrolytes, vitamins, and insulin
Monitor nasogastric tube and low, intermittent suction apparatus; irrigate with measured amounts of normal saline; measure output q4h
Monitor indwelling urethral catheter and/or T tube and closed gravity drainage system if applicable
Monitor urine output qh; report output of <50 ml/hr to physician *because urine volume decreases in hypovolemia*
Monitor urine for sugar and acetone q4h
Calculate intake and output q8h; report discrepancies and collaborate with physician to correct

Monitor vital signs qh until stable; report hypotension to physician

Encourage frequent movement of legs *to promote venous return*

Monitor electrolytes, glucose, and albumin levels

Monitor urine specific gravity; *>1.030 indicates hypovolemia*

Auscultate abdomen for bowel sounds q4h

Assess effectiveness, side effects of diuretics

EXPECTED OUTCOMES

Patient's vital signs are stable

Intake and output are balanced

Laboratory studies are within normal limits

Skin turgor is good

● **NDX:** Altered protection related to abnormal blood profile resulting from coagulation abnormalities and/or bleeding

Monitor incision and dressing q2h for bleeding or drainage; reinforce and change dressing as necessary

Monitor character and color of gastric aspirate and bile drainage for blood

Observe skin, sclera, and urine for jaundice

Provide measures to reduce itching and scratching if present

Monitor PT/INR and liver function levels

Monitor temperature for elevation q4h

Monitor Hgb and Hct

EXPECTED OUTCOMES

Patient presents laboratory values within normal limits

Shows no evidence of bleeding or jaundice

● **NDX:** Risk for infection, related to inadequate primary defenses

Maintain aseptic technique

Change dressings; observe for signs of infection (redness, swelling, tenderness) and healing process

Monitor temperature q4h

Administer and assess effectiveness of antibiotics and antipyretics

Collect urine specimen for culture/sensitivity when indwelling catheter is removed; initiate voiding measures when needed

Monitor breath sounds, signs of cough, sputum *to assess for pneumonia, atelectasis*

EXPECTED OUTCOMES

Patient's condition remains afebrile

Wound is healing adequately

Surrounding tissue is clear, dry, and intact

Lungs are clear

Urine shows no evidence of infection

● **NDX:** Pain related to surgical intervention

Assess type, intensity, and location of pain; use pain rating scale

Administer analgesics before pain becomes severe and before treatments

Collaborate with physician about PCA (p. 92)

Assess for effectiveness of pain relief measures

Change position frequently; administer back rubs *to promote comfort and relieve fatigue*

Discuss and teach alternate pain relief techniques: imaging, relaxation, deep breathing

Provide skin care and oral hygiene q4h *to relieve dryness and increase comfort*

Perform passive or assist with and teach active ROM exercises q4h

Ambulate with assistance when tolerated *to aid in decreasing gas discomfort*

Provide diversional activities *to reduce attention on pain*

EXPECTED OUTCOMES

Patient states that pain is decreasing

Appears relaxed

Demonstrates use of alternate pain relief measures

● **NDX:** Altered nutrition: less than body requirements related to malnutrition preoperatively, NPO status, and/or anorexia

Continue with TPN as indicated

Auscultate abdomen for return of bowel sounds

Collaborate with physician, nutritionist/registered dietitian and provide water and other clear liquids in small amounts after removal of nasogastric tube; monitor tolerance; progress to soft diet or diabetic diet as tolerated; provide small, frequent meals; measure intake

Administer and assess for effectiveness, side effects of insulin and pancreatic enzymes

Monitor serum glucose

Clamp T tube when ordered and observe for signs of pain, distention, and nausea (see p. 405)

Weigh patient daily: same time, clothing, scale

Monitor color, consistency, frequency of stools

Use stool softeners to prevent constipation; discourage straining

EXPECTED OUTCOMES

Patient tolerates prescribed diet/TPN

Demonstrates progressive weight gain

Presents serum glucose within normal limits

Patient/family teaching

Provide and review written dietary instructions for regular or diabetic diet as needed

Demonstrate insulin administration and blood testing procedures (p. 476)

Discuss signs of hypoglycemia and hyperglycemia (p. 482)

Demonstrate care of T tube if applicable (p. 401)

Discuss medications: name, schedule, dosage, purpose, and side effects; explain importance of taking only medicines prescribed by physician and need to use narcotics discriminately

Explain incisional care and signs of wound infection: pain, redness, swelling, discharge

Provide information about outside sources available for substance abuse rehabilitation

Demonstrate management of TPN if applicable (p. 64)

Discuss use of stool softeners, natural laxatives to prevent constipation

Discuss symptoms to report to physician
  Increased abdominal pain, distention
  Fever, jaundice
  Nausea, vomiting
  Gastric bleeding, tarry stools
  Mucosal bleeding
  Hypoglycemia/hyperglycemia

Encourage follow-up visits with physician

Home care considerations

Provide information on where and what supplies and equipment to purchase

Refer to social medicine for assistance with home care, meal planning, transportation

Demonstrate wound care and observe return demonstration for aseptic technique

Provide names, phone numbers of home health care team members

Evaluate home surroundings for comfort, safety requirements

Encourage patient to seek professional assistance with substance abuse if indicated

BIBLIOGRAPHY

Angelucci D, Todaro A: Reversing acute dehydration, *Nursing '93* 23(6):33, 1993.

Beachley M, Farrar J: Abdominal trauma: putting the pieces together, *Am J Nurs* 93(11):26, 1993.

Beare PG, Myers JL: *Principles and practice of adult health nursing,* ed 2, St Louis, 1994, Mosby.

Bockus S: When your patient needs tube feedings, *Nursing '93* 23(7):34, 1993.

Brentin L, Sieh A: Caring for the morbidly obese, *Am J Nurs* 91(8):41, 1991.

Bryant GA: When the bowel is blocked, *RN* (55)1:58, 1992.

Butler RW: Managing the complications of cirrhosis, *Am J Nurs* 94(3):46, 1994.

Chase SL: Antacids, *RN* 56(8):46, 1993.

Chase SL: GI remedies, *RN* 56(10):30, 1993.

Cheney AM, Maquindang ML: Patient teaching for x-ray and other diagnostics, *RN* 56(4):54, 1993.

Cole-Arvin C et al: Identifying and managing dysphagia, *Nursing '94* 24(1):48, 1994.

Doenges ME et al: *Nursing care plans: guidelines for planning and documenting patient care,* ed 3, Philadelphia, 1993, FA Davis.

Doherty MM, Carver DK: New relief for esophageal varices, *Am J Nurs* 93(4):58, 1993.

Doughty DB: What you need to know about inflammatory bowel disease, *Am J Nurs* 94(7):24, 1994.

Faller N, Lawrence KG: Comparing low-profile gastrostomy tubes, *Nursing '93* 23(12):46, 1993.

Fromm CG, Metzler DJ: Preparing your older patient for surgery, *RN* 56(1):38, 1993.

Gardner SS, Messner RL: Upper GI bleeds, *RN* 55(12):42, 1992.

Grau PA: Are you at risk for hepatitis B? *Nursing '91* 21(3):45, 1991.

Greenberg L: Fast action for splenic rupture, *Am J Nurs* 94(2):51, 1994.

Heeg JM, Coleman DA: Hepatitis kills, *RN* 55(4):60, 1992.

Holmgren C: Abdominal assessment, *RN* 55(3):28, 1992.

Jackson MM, Rymer TE: Viral hepatitis, anatomy of a diagnosis, *Am J Nurs* 94(1):43, 1994.

Jess LW: Acute abdominal pain, revealing the source, *Nursing '93* 23(9):34, 1993.

Johns JL: When the patient has an ulcer, *RN* 54(11):44, 1991.

Kim MJ et al: *Pocket guide to nursing diagnoses,* ed 6, St Louis, 1995, Mosby.

Krasner D: The 12 commandments of wound care, *Nursing '92* 22(12):34, 1992.

Krasner D: Six steps to successful stoma care, *RN* 56(7):32, 1993.

Lancaster S, Stockbridge J: PV shunts relieve ascites, *RN* 55(8):58, 1992.

Leckrone L: Preparing your patient for surgery, *Nursing '91* 21(7):47, 1991.

Lockhart JS, Hoelsken R: Abdominal hemorrhage, *Nursing '93* 23(3):33, 1993.

Long L: Ileostomy care, overcoming the obstacles, *Nursing '91* 21(10):73, 1991.

Madda MA: Helping ostomy patients manage medications, *Nursing '91* 21(3):47, 1991.

Marchiondo K: When the dx is diverticular disease, *RN* 57(2):42, 1994.

Martin FL: When the liver breaks down, *RN* 55(8):52, 1992.

Marx JF: Viral hepatitis, unscrambling the alphabet, *Nursing '93* 23(1):34, 1993.

McCance KL, Huether SE: *Pathophysiology, the biological basis for disease in adults and children,* ed 2, St Louis, 1994, Mosby.

McConnell EA: Loosening the grip of intestinal obstructions, *Nursing '94* 24(3):34, 1994.

McFarland GK, McFarlane EA: *Nursing diagnosis and intervention: planning for patient care,* ed 2, St Louis, 1993, Mosby.

McGinnis C, Matson SW: How to manage patients with a Roux-en-Y jejunostomy, *Am J Nurs* 94(2):43, 1994.

Meissner JE: Caring for patients with ulcerative colitis, *Nursing '94* 24(7):54, 1994.

Meissner JE: Caring for patients with cirrhosis, *Nursing '94* 24(9):44, 1994.

Metzler DJ, Fromm CG: Laying out a care plan for the elderly postoperative patient, *Nursing '93* 23(4):67, 1993.

Ondrusek RS: Cholecystectomy: an update, *RN* 56(1):28, 1993.

Pagan P: How to use a disposable end-tidal CO_2 detector, *Nursing '94* 24(1):50, 1994.

Paulford-Lecher N: Teaching your patient stoma care, *Nursing '93* 23(9):47, 1993.

Renkes J: GI endoscopy, *Nursing '93* 23(6):50, 1993.

Rich J: Penetrating chest injury, *Nursing '93* 23(9):33, 1993.

Roberts MK: Assessing and treating volvulus, *Nursing '92* 22(2):56, 1992.

Rogers-Seidle FF: *Geriatric nursing care plans,* St Louis, 1991, Mosby.

Ross Laboratories: Caring for a gastrostomy, *Nursing '94* 24(8):48, 1994.

Smith A: When the pancreas self-destructs, *Am J Nurs* 91(8):38, 1991.

Surratt S et al: Troubleshooting a sump tube, *Am J Nurs* 93(1):42, 1993.

Thompson C: Managing acute pancreatitis, *RN* 55(3):52, 1992.

Thompson JM et al: *Mosby's clinical nursing,* ed 3, St Louis, 1993, Mosby.

Van Niel J: What's wrong with this peristomal skin? *Am J Nurs* 91(12):44, 1991.

Wardell TL: Assessing and managing a gastric ulcer, *Nursing '91* 21(3):35, 1991.

DATE INITIATED _____ DRG ___196___

BY _____ ALOS _____

ALLERGIES: _____

USC UNIVERSITY HOSPITAL
1500 San Pablo
Los Angeles, Ca 90033

MULTIDISCIPLINARY PLAN

LAPAROSCOPIC CHOLECYSTECTOMY

ADMISSION DATE _____ TIME _____ DISCHARGE DATE _____ TIME _____

DISCHARGE OUTCOMES	
PHYSIOLOGICAL	Absence of infection. Pain controlled c̄ p.o. analgesics. Tolerating reg. diet.
COGNITIVE	Aware of signs and symptoms to report to M.D.
PSYCHOLOGICAL	Express fears/concerns R/T hospitalization.

PLAN OF CARE DISCUSSED WITH

_____ PATIENT

_____ SIGNIFICANT OTHER

DATE	INITIAL	DATE	INITIAL

DISCIPLINE	PRE–ADMIT	DOS DAY ___ DATE ___	PO #1 DAY ___ DATE ___ SURGICAL	DAY ___ DATE ___	DAY ___ DATE ___	DAY ___ DATE ___	DAY ___ DATE ___
LOCATION		OR/SURGICAL	SURGICAL				
LAB		CBC, Chem PT, PTT Liver panel serum amylase					
CARDIO–PULMONARY		ECG (over 40 or prev. history) Incentive Spirometer →					
IMAGING/ NUCLEAR MEDICINE		CXR (if over 40)					
SOCIAL SERVICES D/C PLAN		Initiate Discharge planning assessment	Patient will need someone at home for 48°. Someone must drive for MD appt. on 1st, 2nd, 3rd, 7th day				
REHAB. SERVICES							
PHARMACY		Preop. Ancef ↑ gm. Postop. Pain mgmt.	→ Δ to oral analgesic				

Used by permission of USC University Hospital, Los Angeles, California.

MULTIDISCIPLINARY PLAN

DISCIPLINE	PRE-ADMIT	DOS DAY ___ DATE ___	PO #1 DAY ___ DATE ___	DAY ___ DATE ___	DAY ___ DATE ___	DAY ___ DATE ___	DAY ___ DATE ___
NUTRITION		NPO Post-op: Liquics	Advance to full diet				
PATIENT ACTIVITY		Post-op Dangle ambulate c̄ assist.	Independent ambulation				
EDUCATION		Teach I.S. D.B. Benefits of early amb. Splinting Rationale for IV	Activity Restrictions Wound care s-sx to report to MD: (infection, bleeding, N/V, GI disturbance				
COLLABORATIVE PT. PROBLEMS							
1		Pain					
2		Potential for in-effective breathing pattern.					
3							
4		Potential for fluid volume deficit.					
5							
6							
OUTCOMES							
1		Verbalize hosp. routines	Verbalize concerns re: hospitalization				
2		Verbalize pain control					
3		Demonstrate DB, IS, splinting	Returns to ADL				
4		Verbalize importance of early ambulation	Nutrition is adequate: No N/V				
5			Skin integrity maintained				
6							

NME 413-170 (4-91)

	DOS DAY	PO #1 DAY	DAY	DAY	DAY	DAY	DAY
	DATE ___	DATE ___	DATE ___	DATE ___	DATE ___	DATE ___	DATE ___
SERVICE ___	INTERVENTIONS: Pre-op Teach	Monitor pain management					
CASE MGR ___	NPO, consent	Abdomen and lung assessment					
PT/OT ___	Notify MD of abnormal labs	Assess incision for signs of infection					
DIETICIAN ___	Betadine scrub night before & morning of procedure						
SOCIAL SERVICE ___	INTRA & POST-OP						
ECF ___	Thromboguards Post-op I/O						
OTHER ___	Pain management						

MULTIDISCIPLINARY PLAN UPDATE

DATE	SIGNATURES	DATE	SIGNATURES	DATE	SIGNATURES

USC UNIVERSITY HOSPITAL

1500 San Pablo
Los Angeles, CA 90033

MULTIDISCIPLINARY PLAN

| DIAGNOSIS Familial Polyposis/Ulcerative Colitis or Colon CA | NAME _____ |
| SURGERY Colon Resection, Ileal Pouch Anal Anastomosis/Segmental/Laparoscopic Colectomy | ALLERGIES _____ MR# _____ |

DISCHARGE OUTCOMES   DRG _____   ALOS _____   ADMIT DATE _____

PHYSIOLOGICAL Bowel function returns. Fluids & electrolytes within normal limits. Able to eat regular diet with adequate caloric intake. Pain controlled by po analgesics. Skin intact, no breakdown. Wound healing by first intention.

COGNITIVE Verbalizes medical follow-up plan & signs and symptoms to report. Demonstrates wound & ostomy care with minimal or no assistance.

PSYCHOLOGICAL Anxiety/fear controlled as evidenced by active participation in ADLs and decisions with medical care. Verbalizes positive feelings with personal adjustment achieved by D/C.

DISCIPLINE	PRE-OP/ PRE-ADMIT	PRO-OP DATE ___ DAY 1	D.O.S. DATE ___ DAY 2	P.O. #1 DATE ___ DAY 3	P.O. #2 DATE ___ DAY 4	P.O. #8 DATE ___ DAY 5	P.O. #4 DATE ___ DAY 6
LOCATION		Med/Surg	Med/Sur→OR→DOU	DOU	DOU →Med/Surg	Med/Surg	Med/Surg (home if Laparoscopic)
LABS		CBC with diff Chem 20 UA Type & Cross PRBC	K+ level at 5 a. m. CBC in p. m. If clinically indicated, CBC in PAR		CBC Chem 7		
CARDIO-PULMONARY		ECG I.S. initial teach	I.S. q 2° W/A	Evaluate for self I.S.			
IMAGING/ NUCLEAR MEDICINE		CXR					
SOCIAL SERVICES D/C PLAN REHAB. SERVICES		D/C planning Home health evaluation E.T. consult Mark stoma ASAP			Re-eval for home health needs E.T. to evaluate & teach ostomy care	Oncology consult prn	
PHARMACY		Bowel prep K+ supplement prn IV to begin at 2400 Sleeper If on steriods within last 6 months, the steriods on call to OR	Epidural of PCA Antibiotics x 3 doses IV fluids	Epidural of PCA IV fluids	Epidural or PCA IV fluids until adequate po intake For Laparoscopic Colectomy: Convert to po analgesia		Convert to po analgesics
DIETARY/ NUTRITION		Clear liquids NPO after MN	NPO	Advance diet as tolerated when bowel function returns—passing flatus		Nutritional guidelines	

Continued.

USC UNIVERSITY HOSPITAL

DIAGNOSIS Familial Polyposis/Ulcerative Colitis or Colon CA	1500 San Pablo Los Angeles, CA 90033	NAME _____ ALLERGIES _____
SURGERY Colon Resection, Ileal Pouch Anal Anastomosis/Segmental/Laparoscopic Colectomy	MULTIDISCIPLINARY PLAN	MR# _____

DISCHARGE OUTCOMES	DRG _____ ALOS _____ ADMIT DATE _____
PHYSIOLOGICAL	Bowel function returns. Fluids & electrolytes within normal limits. Able to eat regular diet with adequate caloric intake. Pain controlled by po analgesics. Skin intact, no breakdown. Wound healing by first intention.
COGNITIVE	Verbalizes medical follow-up plan & signs and symptoms to report. Demonstrates wound & ostomy care with minimal or no assistance.
PSYCHOLOGICAL	Anxiety/fear controlled as evidenced by active participation in ADLs and decisions with medical care. Verbalizes positive feelings with personal adjustment achieved by D/C.

DISCIPLINE	PRE-OP/ PRE-ADMIT	P.O.#5 ____ DAY 7 ____ DATE	P.O.#6 ____ DAY 8 ____ DATE	P.O.#7 ____ DAY 9 ____ DATE	P.O.#8 ____ DAY 10 ____ DATE	P.O.#9 ____ DAY 11 ____ DATE	P.O.#10 ____ DAY 12 ____ DATE
LOCATION		Med/Surg	Med/Surg	Med/Surg→Home			
LABS							
CARDIO-PULMONARY							
IMAGING/ NUCLEAR MEDICINE							
SOCIAL SERVICES D/C PLAN REHAB. SERVICES	Confirm all home health arrangements						
PHARMACY							
DIETARY/ NUTRITION	Regular diet						

PATIENT NAME: _____ MEDICAL RECORD # _____

MULTIDISCIPLINARY PLAN

DISCIPLINE	PRE-OP/ PRE-ADMIT	PRE-OP DATE ___ (DAY 1)	D.O.S. DATE ___ (DAY 2)	P.O.#1 DATE ___ (DAY 3)	P.O.#2 DATE ___ (DAY 4)	P.O.#3 DATE ___ (DAY 5)	P.O.#4 DATE ___ (DAY 6)
PATIENT ACTIVITY		Up ad lib	BR Daily wt at 6 a.m.	OOB with assistance Daily wt at 6 a.m.	Ambulance TID to QID Daily wt at 6 a.m.	Progressive ambulation Daily wt at 6 a.m.	Daily wt at 6 a.m.
EDUCATION		**Pre Op Teach** Aggressive TCDB Presence/Purpose of tubes/drains. Pain management Kegel exercises Early ambulation to promote return of bowel function	**Ileostomy Teaching** Give ostomy handout	Return of bowel function Quality/Quantity of stool will vary Quality - loose/watery may have leakage at night. (Not permanent)	Perianal skin care	Teach S/Sx of small bowel obstruction If ostomy: • Encourage to look at stoma • Peristoma skin assessment • Clamp application/removal	If Ostomy/passing flatus, teach: Appliance application Empty/wash bag Return demo-clamp Perianal skin care

KEY

1. To initiate a problem or intervention, document under corresponding date.
2. Document outcomes under appropriate date for achieving the goal.
3. To discontinue an intervention or resolve a patient problem highlight, date, and initial.

COLLABORATIVE PROBLEMS

DATE	COLLABORATIVE PROBLEMS	DC DATE INIT	DATE	COLLABORATIVE PROBLEMS	DC DATE INIT
	1. Knowledge deficit R/T hospitalization, surgery.			7. Impaired skin integrity, perianal, ostomy R/T bowel diversion.	
	2. Fear/anxiety R/T hospitalization, post-op course.			8. Altered bowel elimination R/T surgery.	
	3. Fluid/electrolyte imbalance, potential R/T bowel preps & diversion.			9. Altered nutritional intake (less than body requirements) R/T surgery.	
	4. Alteration in comfort, pain R/T surgery.			10. Body image, altered R/T ostomy.	
	5. Potential for infection R/T surgery.			11. Self-care deficit R/T ostomy.	
	6. Potential for injury complication R/T surgery.				

OUTCOMES

1. Able to verbalize medical plan/hospital routine.
2. Fears, anxiety controlled as evidenced by ability to participate in care/education.
3. Electrolytes/fluids within normal limits.
4. Verbalize pain controlled within 30 min of intervention.
   Laparoscopic Surgery: Pain controlled by po analgesic.
5. No infection throughout hospitalization.
6. No complication throughout hospitalization.
7. Skin remains intact. Wounds heal by first intention.
8. Bowel output returns.
9. **Laparoscopic Surgery:** Caloric intake supports maintenance of wt/wound healing.
9. Caloric intake supports maintenance of wt/wound healing.
10. Verbalizes feelings R/T body image changes.
11. Participation in education.
4. Pain controlled by po analgesics.

Continued.

PATIENT NAME: _____ MEDICAL RECORD # _____

MULTIDISCIPLINARY PLAN

DISCIPLINE	PRE-OP/ PRE-ADMIT	P.O.#5 DAY 7 DATE ___	P.O.#6 DAY 8 DATE ___	P.O.#7 DAY 9 DATE ___	P.O.#8 DAY 10 DATE ___	P.O.#9 DAY 11 DATE ___	P.O.#10 DAY 12 DATE ___
PATIENT ACTIVITY		Progressive ambulation	Independent ambulation				
		Weight at 6 am	Weight at 6 am				
EDUCATION		D/C Instructions **If Ostomy:** Assessment care of stoma Return demo—emptying, washing Application of water, odor control	Medications/Weight control **If Ostomy:** Colostomy Irrigation Return demo—changing bag, application of water				

COLLABORATIVE PROBLEMS

DATE		COLLABORATIVE PROBLEMS	DC DATE INIT	DATE		COLLABORATIVE PROBLEMS	DC DATE INIT
	4.	Alteration in comfort, pain R/T surgery.					
	5.	Potential for infection R/T surgery.					
	6.	Potential for complication R/T surgery.					
	9.	Impaired skin integrity (perianal, ostomy) R/T bowel diversion.					
	10.	Body image, altered R/T surgery.					
	11.	Self-care deficit R/T surgery.					

KEY

1. To initiate a problem or intervention, document under corresponding date.
2. Document outcomes under appropriate date for achieving the goal.
3. To discontinue an intervention or resolve a patient problem highlight, date, and initial.

OUTCOMES

4. Pain controlled within 30 min of intervention by po analgesics.	10. Verbalizes positive feelings with personal adjustment.	11. Independent in ostomy care.		
5. No infection throughout hospitalization.	11. Pt will be able to care for self. Support for home care prepared.			
6. No complications throughout hospitalization.	11. Verbalizes s/sx to report to medical team.			
9. Skin remains intact.				

PLAN OF CARE DISCUSSED WITH	PRE-OP DAY 1 DATE____	D.O.S. DAY 2 DATE____	P.O. #1 DAY 3 DATE____	P.O. #2 DAY 4 DATE____	P.O. #3 DAY 5 DATE____	P.O. #4 DAY 6 DATE____
DATE INIT SO/P			**INTERVENTIONS**			
	– Orient to hospital environment/routine. – Review medical plan.	– Weight at 6 am. – Report abnormal lab K⁺.	– Weight at 6 am. – Inspect wounds, skin & document Q.shift.	– Weight at 6 am. – Aggressive pain management. Offer pain meds at ordered intervals before ↑ activity.	– Weight at 6 am. Ileal Anal/Segmental/Colon Surgeries: – Teach • Monitor how foods affect consistency of stool.	– Weight at 6 am. – Continued abdominal/wound assessment/care. – Continued pain management.
	– Bowel prep as ordered. – Provide time for verbalization of feelings/questions.	– Post Op. – Epidural PCA management. Assess.	– Consult ET/skin nurse prn.			
	– Monitor labs & report abnormals. – Pre-Op Teach • Respiratory care:	– pain, aggravating, relieving factors. – Assess respiratory function, TCDB. – I.S. q 2° W/A – Encourage leg exercises, compression	– Use skin barriers as ordered (& for all ileal-anal anastomosis) to prevent skin breakdown. – Assess abdomen, bowel sounds, passing flatus, distention, nausea & vomiting q shift & prn.	– Continued bowel assessment. – Continued foley care. If Laparoscopic, DE foley	– Prevent constipation, fluid intake. • Prevent diarrhea – eat foods that thicken stool.	– Continued assessment for post-op complication. – Monitor caloric intake. – Daily perianal skin assessment.
CASE MANAGER:	– TCDB/I.S. q 2° W/A • Pain control	boots. – NG tube management.		– Assess/monitor nutritional intake when diet resumed.	• Foods that are incompletely digested should be avoided	Laparoscopic Colon Surgery: – Reinforce D/C teaching.
CONSULTING MD:	• Presence of tubes/drains: foley – May have NG, abdominal drains. – Presence/purpose of compression boots.	– Foley cath – I & O – Record q 4° × 24° – Call MD if urine output <30cc/hr × 2 hr	– Assess for dehydration. Replace fluids/electrolytes prn. – Monitor & document stool output. – Pain management.	– Instruct to eat foods slowly and chew well. – Increase foods gradually. Teach to eat at regular times.	– Continued J.P. management. (Expected output ≤100cc.) – Continued abdominal/wound assessment/care.	– Teach: Dr. Bearr available from 2000-2100 for questions/concerns.
SOCIAL SERVICE:	RN required to know daily wt. & I/O.	– Report N/V to surgery team – JP's to low intermittent suction or as ordered (Expected output ≤400cc)	– Continued assessment for S/Sx of infection. – Allow time for expression of feelings. – Provide support prn.	– Encourage adequate fluid intake. – Continue respiratory care. – Continue monitoring for s/sx of infection & post op complication.	Laparoscopic Colon Surgery: – Teach routine follow-up care. – Ambulate at regular intervals. – Rest frequently.	
ANOINTING OF THE SICK DATE:		– Zinc oxide at bedside. Apply to anus for skin protection. – Chart each shift condition of wound, dressing drainage.	– Refer to MSW prn. – Continue strict I & O. – Encourage OOB & early ambulation.	– Consult RN coordinator if coping difficulties. – Continued JP's to low intermittent suction. (Expected output ≤200cc.)	– Increase activities slowly. – Report S/Sx of redness, pain, drainage. – Report N & V, cramping, inability to evacuate bowel.	
		– Keep wound clean, dry. Change dressing, cleansing old drainage from wound.	– Assess/monitor perianal skin. – Remove dressings after 24°. – Continue JP's to low intermittent suction. (Expected output ≤300cc.)		– Avoid heavy lifting 6-8 weeks.	

DATE	SIGNATURES	DATE	SIGNATURES	DATE	SIGNATURES

PLAN OF CARE DISCUSSED WITH	P.O.#5 DAY 7	P.O.#6 DAY 8	P.O.#7 DAY 9	P.O.#8 DAY 10	P.O.#9 DAY 11	P.O.#10 DAY 12
INIT SO/P	DATE ____	DATE ____	DATE ____	DATE ____	DATE ____	DATE ____
DATE		INTERVENTIONS				

Interventions:

Teach routine follow-up care:
- Ambulate at regular intervals.
- Rest frequently.
- Increase activities slowly.
- Keep incisions dry.
- Report S/Sx of redness, pain, drainage.
- Avoid heavy lifting 6-8 weeks.
- Splint abdomen, chest coughing/sneezing.
- Driving – consult MD.
- Routine exercises (i.e., walking/swimming).
- Time release meds will only be partially absorbed – consult MD.
- Contact MD for diarrhea >24° or food blockage >4-6°.
- Normal ileostomy output 500-1000 cc/day.
- Stress doing Kegel exercises. Hold stool & increase capacity of pouch.

Review/Reinforce:
- Ostomy care.
- Follow-up medical plan.
- S/Sx to report to healthcare team.
- Report N & V, cramping, inability to evaluate bowel.

Teach Patient:
- Dr. Beart available from 2000–2100 for questions/concerns.

J-Pouch Ileal anal with ileostomy coloanal with colostomy:
- Pouch irrigation starting 2 wks post-op with increasing amounts of saline will increase pouch capacity.

CASE MANAGER: ____

CONSULTING MD: ____

SOCIAL SERVICE: ____

ANOINTING OF THE SICK DATE: ____

MULTIDISCIPLINARY PLAN UPDATE

DATE	SIGNATURES	DATE	SIGNATURES	DATE	SIGNATURES	DATE	SIGNATURES

BARNES

CARE PATH® 550 MAJOR SMALL & LARGE BOWEL PROCEDURE

1

SERVICE		PHYSICIAN		
PRIMARY NURSE		PRIMARY NURSE		
DC DATE	ADM DATE	DATE OF SURGERY		

A-8

Problem Number	PATIENT PROBLEMS/NURSING DIAGNOSES
#1	ALTERATION IN COMFORT RELATED TO ABDOMINAL SURGERY
#2	ALTERATION IN BOWEL ELIMINATION RELATED TO ABDOMINAL SURGERY
#3	ALTERATION IN SKIN INTEGRITY RELATED TO ABDOMINAL INCISION AND RECOVERY FROM SURGERY
#4	LACK OF KNOWLEDGE RELATED TO HOSPITALIZATION AND SURGICAL PROCEDURE
#5	ALTERATION IN BODY IMAGE RELATED TO ABDOMINAL SURGERY AND OSTOMY

* IF APPROPRIATE

#	1, 2, 3	3, 4, 5	4	4	1, 4
	ASSESSMENT / MONITORING	CONSULTS	PROCEDURES / TEST	TREATMENT	ACTIVITY
DAY 1 PRE OP	Assessment: Nursing Admission lab results Monitoring: VS routine O_2 saturation x1 I & O	Nurse specialist (if ostomy is a consideration).	CBC, 6, 12, PT, PTT T & C x2 units (admission labs) ECG ≥ 40 years old CXR ≥ 50 years old UA with micro *Mark ostomy site	Antithrombolytic stockings Mechanical bowel preparation	UAL
DAY 2 DOS	Assessment: Wound/dressing q 4 hrs. Bowel function q 4 hrs. Stoma appearance q 4 hrs. Pulmonary status q 2 hrs. Comfort level q 2 hrs. Braden score x1 Patency of tubes and characteristics of drainage q 8 hrs. IV patency & site appearance q 8 hrs. Fall risk factors Monitoring: VS q 1 hr. x 2 q 2 hrs. x 2 then q 4 hrs. I & O q 4 hrs. O_2 saturation x1 x 2	Respiratory Therapy for O_2		Antithrombolytic stockings O_2 to maintain O_2 saturation ≥ 92% Oral care q 4 hrs. Assist with Incentive Spirometer and TCDB q 2 hrs. Gastric decompression and tube irrigation	Bedrest
DAY 3 POD 1	Assessment: Wound/dressing q 4 hrs. Bowel function q 4 hrs. Stoma appearance q 4 hrs. Pulmonary status q 2 hrs. Comfort level q 2 hrs. Braden score x1 Patency of tubes and characteristics of drainage q 8 hrs. IV patency and site appearance q 8 hrs. Fall risk factors Lab results **O_2 saturation ≥ 92%** Monitoring: VS q 4 hrs. I & O q 8 hrs. Room air O_2 saturation x1 x2	Social Work Respiratory (if O_2 or tx needed) Nurse specialist (if ostomy placed).	CBC, 6	Antithrombolytic stockings Oral care q 4 hrs. Assist with Incentive Spirometer q 2 hrs. Gastric decompression and tube irrigation d/c foley d/c O_2	Up in chair with assist x1 x2 x3 Ambulate in room with assist x1 x2 Bed bath
DAY 4 POD 2	Assessment: Wound/dressing q 4 hrs. Bowel function q 4 hrs. Stoma appearance q 4 hrs. Pulmonary status q 2 hrs. Comfort level q 2 hrs. Braden score x1 Patency of tubes and characteristics of drainage q 8 hrs. IV patency and site appearance q 8 hrs. Fall risk factors Lab results **Voiding without difficulty (UO ≥ 240 cc q 8 hrs.)** Monitoring: VS q 4 hrs. I & O q 8 hrs.	Dietary screening		Antithrombolytic stockings Oral care q 4 hrs. Assist with Incentive Spirometer q 2 hrs. Gastric decompression and tube irrigation *Abdominal wound wet to dry dressing Change TID	Up in chair with assist x1 x2 x3 Ambulate in room with assist x1 x2 Bed bath

SIGNATURE	INIT.	SIGNATURE	INIT.	SIGNATURE	INIT.

550

3100-93 (New 8/93)

Copyright 1993, Barnes Hospital - All Rights Reserved

Continued.

BARNES

CARE PATH® 550
MAJOR SMALL & LARGE
BOWEL PROCEDURE

CNS	DIETARY	RT
HOME HEALTH	OT	OTHER
PT	SW	OTHER

A-8

Problem Number	PATIENT PROBLEMS/NURSING DIAGNOSES

1, 4	4	2, 3, 4	2, 3, 4	1, 4, 5	INITIALS (SEE KEY AT BOTTOM)		
MEDS / IVS	NUTRITION	PATIENT / FAMILY EDUCATION	DISCHARGE PLANNING	PSYCHOSOCIAL/ EMOTIONAL/ SPIRITUAL NEEDS			
IVF Laxative Oral antibiotic Bowel preparation Prn medication for sleep	Clear liquids NPO after MN	Nursing: Disease process Surgical procedure Primary nursing Plan of care Pre-op booklet (gastric drain, Incentive Spirometer, IV, Foley, TCDB, O_2, freq. VS, abdomen incision/wound Antithrombolytic device post-op analgesia). *Ostomy teaching process	Pt./family verbalizes understanding of care path. Plan of care has been mutually set with pt./family.	Provide emotional support for pt./family. Provide privacy.			
SQ Heparin IVF IV Antibiotics IV H_2 Antagonist Analgesic (PCA, Epidural, IM)	NPO	Reinforce post-op teaching **Demonstrates/verbalizes appropriate use of analgesic** **Verbalizes understanding of post-op teaching.**		Provide emotional support for pt./family. Provide privacy.			
SQ Heparin IVF IV H_2 Antagonist Analgesic (PCA, Epidural, IM)	NPO	Reinforce Incentive Spirometer *Initiate ostomy teaching record		Provide emotional support for pt./family. Provide privacy.			
SQ Heparin IVF IV H_2 Antagonist Analgesic (PCA, Epidural, IM)	NPO	Reinforce importance of post-op activity *Ostomy teaching record	Nursing: Assess Home Health needs *Caregiver available	Provide emotional support for pt./family. Provide privacy.			

SIGNATURE	INIT.	SIGNATURE	INIT.	SIGNATURE	INIT.

#	1, 2, 3	3, 4, 5	4	4	1, 4
	ASSESSMENT / MONITORING	**CONSULTS**	**PROCEDURES / TEST**	**TREATMENT**	**ACTIVITY**
DAY 5 POD 3	Assessment: Wound/dressing q 4 hrs. Bowel function q 8 hrs. **Bowel sounds present** Stoma appearance q 8 hrs. Pulmonary status q 8 hrs. Comfort level q 4 hrs. **Low risk Braden score** Patency of tubes and characteristics of drainage q 8 hrs. IV patency and site appearance q 8 hrs. Fall risk factors Lab results Hemodynamically stable Monitoring: VS q 8 hrs. I & O q 8 hrs.	Physical Therapy (if not ambulating in halls.)	CBC, 6	Antithrombolytic stockings Oral care q 4 hrs. Encourage Incentive Spirometer q 2 hrs. NG or gastric drain to gravity. *Abdominal wound wet to dry dressing Change TID	Up in chair with assist x1 x2 x3 x4 Ambulate in halls with assist x1 x2 x3 Bath with assist
DAY 6 POD 4	Assessment: Wound/dressing q 8 hrs. Bowel function q 8 hrs. Stoma appearance q 8 hrs. Pulmonary status q 8 hrs. Comfort level q 4 hrs. **Lungs clear** **No atelectasis** IV patency and site appearance q 8 hrs. Fall risk factors Monitoring: VS q 8 hrs. I & O q 8 hrs. Patency of tubes and characteristics of drainage q 8 hrs.	Home Health (if need identified).		Antithrombolytic stockings Uses Incentive Spirometer independently d/c NG or G-tube clamped per MD order *Abdominal wound wet to dry dressing Change TID	Up in chair with assist x1 x2 x3 x4 Ambulate in halls with assist x1 x2 x3 x4 Bath with assist
DAY 7 POD 5	Assessment: Wound/dressing q 8 hrs. Bowel function q 8 hrs. Stoma appearance q 8 hrs. Comfort level q 8 hrs. IV patency and site appearance q 8 hrs. Fall risk factors Monitoring: VS q 8 hrs. I & O q 8 hrs.			Antithrombolytic stockings **Uses Incentive Spirometer** **independently** G-tube clamped *Abdominal wound wet to dry dressing Change TID	UAL with minimal assist Bath with assist
DAY 8 POD 6	Assessment: Wound/dressing q 8 hrs. Bowel function q 8 hrs. Stoma appearance q 8 hrs. Comfort level q 8 hrs. IV site appearance q 8 hrs. Fall risk factors Monitoring: VS q 8 hrs. I & O q 8 hrs.	**Consults** **completed**		d/c antithrombolytic stockings d/c Incentive Spirometer use *G-tube clamped *Abdominal wound wet to dry dressing Change TID	UAL with minimal assist Bath with assist
DAY 9 POD 7	Assessment: Wound/dressing q 8 hrs. **Abdominal incision/wound** **without signs of infection.** Bowel function q 8 hrs. Stoma appearance q 8 hrs. Stoma visible **No phlebitis** **Fluid balance adequate** **(PO fluid intake ≥ 1000 cc/day** **and UO ≥ 720 cc/day)** Monitoring: VS q 8 hrs. d/c I & O			*G-tube clamped *Abdominal wound wet to dry dressing Change TID	UAL Independent with bath
DAY 10 DISCHARGE	Assessment: Wound incision x1 Bowel function x1 Stoma appearance x1 **Abdominal incision/wound** **without signs of infection.** **Bowel function normal** **Stoma viable** **Pain controlled with PO analgesics** **No skin breakdown** **No IV phlebitis** **Fluid balance adequate** **No fall** **Afebrile VSS**	**Consults** **completed**	**Hemodynamically stable**	G-tube d/c by MD prior to DC **No pulmonary or circulatory** **complications.** **DC home with dressing or** **wound closed** **No gastric tube.**	**Ambulating** **independently**

SIGNATURE	INIT.	SIGNATURE	INIT.	SIGNATURE	INIT.

Continued.

1, 4	4	2, 3, 4	2, 3, 4	1, 4, 5	INITALS (SEE KEY AT BOTTOM)		
MEDS / IVS	NUTRITION	PATIENT / FAMILY EDUCATION	DISCHARGE PLANNING	PSYCHOSOCIAL EMOTIONAL/ SPIRTUAL NEEDS			
SQ Heparin IVF IV H$_2$ Antagonist Analgesic (PCA, Epidural, IM)	NPO	Reinforce importance of post–op activity and NPO *Ostomy teaching record	Social Work (High risk screening)	Provide emotional support for pt./family Provide privacy.			
SQ Heparin IV fluids IV H$_2$ Antagonist Analgesic (PCA, Epidural, IM)	NPO	Pt. to verbalize importance of post–op activity. Instruct dietary advances. *Ostomy teaching record.	*Home Health plans initiated	Provide emotional support for pt./family Provide privacy.			
SQ Heparin IVF IV H$_2$ Antagonist Analgesic (PCA, Epidural, IM)	Diet as prescribed by MD	Pt./family observe abdominal wet-dry dressing change if wound open. Reinforce dietary specifics. *Ostomy teaching record.		Provide emotional support for pt./family Provide privacy.			
SQ Heparin IVF to hep lock d/c H$_2$ Antagonist d/c PCA, Epidural or IM Analgesia PO Analgesic Assess need to resume pre-op meds.	Diet as prescribed by MD	Instruct pt./family in: Wound care (and dressing change procedure if indicated) s&sx infection and problems with bowel function. *Ostomy teaching record.	**DC plans finalized** **Pt./family able to verbalize DC plans.**	Provide emotional support for pt./family Provide privacy.			
d/c SQ Heparin d/c hep lock PO Analgesics **Pain controlled with PO analgesics**	Diet as prescribed by MD	Pt./family to demonstrate wet to dry dressing change (if indicated) MD: Instuctions for activity and follow-up. ***Ostomy teaching record completed.**		Provide emotional support for pt./family Provide privacy.			
No adverse drug reactions.	**Tolerating diet** **Tolerating prescribed diet**	DC instructions per MD, nursing and consults. **Pt./family able to identify support systems and resources if needed.** **Pt. able to verbalize activity restrictions, s&sx of infection, appropiate bowel function and MD follow-up.**	**Pt. discharged** **Home with appropriate level of care**	Pt./family verbalizes feelings R/T surgery and diagnosis.			
SIGNATURE	INIT.	SIGNATURE	INIT.	SIGNATURE			INIT.

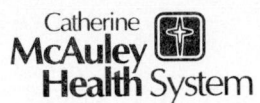

Catherine
McAuley
Health System

Nursing Service
5301 East Huron River Drive
P.O. Box 995
Ann Arbor, Michigan 48106

Nursing Care Plan Index

Diagnostic Conclusion Code:*
N - Nursing Diagnosis
C - Collaborative Problem

Primary Nurse _____   Associate Nurse _____

Primary Nurse _____   Associate Nurse _____

INDEX OF DIAGNOSTIC CONCLUSIONS

#	*DIAGNOSTIC CONCLUSION CODE	DATE IDENTIFIED	TITLE	SIGNATURE, TITLE	DATE RESOLVED
1	N		Knowledge Deficit R/T Preparation for Surgery and		
			Post-Op Recovery (N-K-077)		
			PER/OSTOMY		
2	N		Knowledge Deficit R/T Self Care Management of		
			New Ostomy (N-K-056)		
3	C		Post-Abdominal Surgical Procedure (C-A-091)		

SIGNIFICANT DATA	*(Safety level, cues needing followup, special considerations, patient assets/strengths, transfer dates)*	SIGNATURE, TITLE	DATE

PROJECTED DATE OF:

Transfer to _____ on _____

Discharge to _____ on _____

6102-001 N 2/93

REFERRALS MADE (Date, To Whom):

Dietary _____   Home Care _____   Other: _____

Social Service _____   Pharmacist _____   _____

Nursing _____   Pastoral Care _____   _____

Continued.

St. Joseph Mercy Hospital
Ann Arbor, Michigan 48106
**NURSING CRITICAL PATH
OSTOMY 148/149**

To be used with NMP:
- Knowledge deficit R/T Prep of pre-
  abdominal/ostomy surgery
- Post-abdominal surgery
- Knowledge deficit - Self Care of Ostomy

	PPT/Admission	OR	POD 1 Date_____	POD 2 Date_____	POD 3 Date_____	POD 4 Date_____
PHYSICAL ASSESSMENTS	Weight - on admit Lung sounds - on admit VS & Temp - BID I & O including ostomy Skin assessment	Implement Post abdom-inal Surg Procedure NMP Assess: Dressing q 4 hr GI Status q 8 hr Stomal Integrity q 8 hr Lung sounds q shift VS & temp q 4 hr I & O q shift	Dressings q 4 hr GI Status q 8 hr Stomal integrity q 8 hr Daily Wt. q shift q 4 hr q 8 hr Braden Scale	Dressings/Incisions q s⌐ GI Status q shift Assess stoma and peristomal skin ⌐ VS & temp q shift	── Continue ── BID/prn Lungs	── Continue
DIAGNOSTICS MD ORDERS	UA ECG LTES CEA TS CXR CHEM PROF		CBC,LYTES	LYTES	LYTES,CBC	
TREATMENTS	Bowel Prep Protocol IV Diet: Cl Liq Maintain comfort	ABX ⌐ IS, Cough, Deep Breathe IV Foley NG NPO Epidural/PCA ⌐	d.c ABX (if not ruptured) ── Continue ──	Soap and water wound care (ABX continue if ruptured) ── Continue──	──Continue── d/c Epidural	
ACTIVITY	ad lib	Turn q 2 hr, leg exercises, up in chair	Chair	Hall BID Chair	Hall TID	Hall TID
CONSULTS/ REFERRALS	Barb Boylan-Lewis, ET APS Cardiology prn					
DISCHARGE PLANNING	Assess home situation/ D/C Plan Identify primary caregiver		HHC prn Social Work/Consult prn: ECF Psychosocial needs			
PATIENT EDUCATION	Implement KD R/T Preparation for Surgery and Postoper-ative Recovery N-K-077 PER/Ostomy	Implement KD: Self Care Management of New Ostomy N-K-056 PER/New Ostomy		Bag change with pt-S/O Give clamp to practice Y N Open and close clamp Y N Visualize stoma Y N Special considerations: Verbalize and/or demonstrate 1. Colostomy Irrigation 2. Drainage per rectum expected 3. Mucous fistula care 4. Interest in ostomy association visitor 5. Special concerns, i.e., hygiene occupation	Teach soap and water wound care Y N Give closed wound care folder Y N Review Dietary Management - Flatus Blockage	Soap and water wound care per patient Y N Bag change - pt-S/O observed. pt-S/O prepare appliance Y N Teach emptying Y N Teach peristomal skin care T N
	RNSig_____	RNSig_____	RNSig_____	RNSig_____	RNSig_____	RNSig_____

St. Joseph Mercy Hospital
Ann Arbor, Michigan 48106
**NURSING CRITICAL PATH
OSTOMY 148/149**

To be used with NMP:
- Knowledge deficit R/T Prep of pre-abdominal/ostomy surgery
- Post-abdominal surgery
- Knowledge deficit - Self Care of Ostomy

POD 5 Date_____	POD 6 Date_____	POD 7 Date_____	POD 8 Date_____	POD 9 Date_____	POD 10 Date_____	Expected Outcomes
Incision q shift GI Status q 8 hr Stomal Assessment Peristomal skin Weight q day Lung Sounds prn VS & Temp q shift I & O q 8 hr	──Continue──	──Continue──	──Continue	BID VS		Passing stool flatus Y N Stoma intact Y N Peristomal skin intact Y N Lungs at baseline Y N VS - afebrile Y N Voiding Y N
		Braden				
		Check Pathology if indicated				
Soap and water wound care IV Foley DD IS & cough Diet NPO/liquids PCA/PO pain meds	d/c IV d/c foley - ISC q 6 hr if no void Liquids PO Pain Meds prn	(d/c ABX *if ruptured) General				Wound healing without symptoms of infection Y N Tolerating pre-op diet Y N Pain Mgmt with PO Meds Y N
Hall TID up ad lib						Achieves baseline activity Y N
Dietary Refer prn		Oncology if indicated by Pathology				**Pt-S/O states/demonstrates** Resources: HHC/ET Nurse Ostomy Assoc. Ostomy Folder Y N
Follow up HHC Begin after ABD surgery D/C sheet		Order D/C supplies Give a patient Rx for supplies		Review D/C sheet		Rx for ostomy supplies Y N supplier Y N supply list Y N
		Reinforce Dietary Management				Incision care: Symptoms to report to physician Y N Bag preparation Y N
	Bag change by pt-S/O with RN assist/observe Y N		Bag change by pt-S/O Y N			Bag change Y N Emptying and cleaning Y N
Review emptying Review skin care	Pt emptying own bag Y N Skin care by pt-S/O					Symptoms of skin problems/ treatment Y N Dietary Management Y N Thoughts R/T Ostomy: change in body image, incorporating ostomy into lifestyle Y N
RNSig_____	RNSig_____	RNSig_____	RNSig_____	RNSig_____	RNSig_____	RNSig_____

Continued.

St. Joseph Mercy Hospital
Ann Arbor, Michigan 48106

NURSING CRITICAL PATH OSTOMY 148/149

To be used with NMP:
- Knowledge deficit R/T Prep of pre-abdominal/ostomy surgery
- Post-abdominal surgery
- Knowledge deficit - Self Care of Ostomy

	POD 11 Date_____	POD 12 Date_____	POD 13 Date_____	POD 14 Date_____	POD 15 Date_____	Date_____	
PHYSICAL ASSESSMENTS Dressing GI Status Stomal Integrity Weight Lung Sounds Temp & Vital Signs I & O Skin Assessment							
DIAGNOSTICS MD ORDERS							
TREATMENTS							
ACTIVITY							
CONSULTS REFERRALS							
DISCHARGE PLANNING							
PATIENT EDUCATION							
RNSig_____	RNSig_____	RNSig_____	RNSig_____	RNSig_____	RNSig_____	RNSig_____	

Endocrine System

Endocrine Assessment

● Subjective Data

Change in stamina and ability to perform activities of daily living (ADLs)
Fatigue
Numbness
Tingling
Paresthesia
Bone pain
Change in mental status
Memory loss
Irritability
Anxiety
Nervousness
Depression
Headache
Syncope
Anorexia
Nausea
Abdominal pain
Change in body proportions
Palpitations
Shortness of breath (SOB)
Hoarseness
Anosmia
Decreased libido
Dysuria

● Objective Data

General appearance: body development, proportion (Figure 7-1, Table 7-1)
Vital signs (VS): blood pressure (BP), pulse (P), respiratory rate (R),
  temperature (T)

Skin
  Temperature
  Turgor
  Hydration
    Dry, scaly
    Excessive perspiration
    Excessive oiliness
  Texture
    Fine, smooth
    Coarse, leathery
  Color
    Increased pigmentation
      Gums
      Breasts
      Abdomen
      Scars/creases
    Yellow pigmentation
    Flushed
    Pale
    Cyanotic
    Purple striae over areas of fat
  Edema
    Face, eyelids
    Lower extremities
    Pitting/nonpitting
  Lipodystrophy
  Poor wound healing
Hair and nails
  Texture of nails
    Thick
    Brittle
    Thin
    Cracking
  Horizontal nail ridges
  Amount of hair
    Thin
    Increased
    Alopecia
  Distribution of hair
  Texture of hair
    Coarse, dry, brittle
    Fine, silky, soft
Musculoskeletal system
  Changes in height
  Changes in weight
  Fat distribution
    Central obesity
    Supraclavicular fat pads
    Dorsocervical fat pad (buffalo hump)
  Upper- to lower-body segment ratio
  Muscle mass and function
    Atrophy
    Development
    Dystonia
    Tremors
    Spasms

    Tetany
    Ataxia
    Weakness
    Paralysis
Central nervous system (CNS)
  Personality changes
    Complacent
    Dull
    Lethargic
    Confused
    Mood swings
    Depressed
    Labile
      Euphoric to depressed
      Manic behavior
      Frank psychosis
  Alterations in consciousness
    Drowsy
    Slowing of cognitive ability
    Memory loss
    Inappropriate response to questions
    Somnolence
    Stupor
    Confusion
    Coma
  Small, reactive pupils
  Position sense
  Response to touch, vibration, and pain
  Deafness
  Speech
    Monotonous
    Slowed
    Weak
    Hoarse
  Reflexes
    Hyperreflexia
    Hyporeflexia
    Trousseau's sign
    Chvostek's sign
  Seizures
Head and neck
  Mouth: brown pigmentation
  Tongue
    Color
    Size: enlarged
    Tremors
  Face
    Coarse
    Protruding
    Moon face
    Erythema
    Plethora
    Edema
      Wide, puffy eyes
      Wrinkled eyelids
  Broad, short, upturned nose

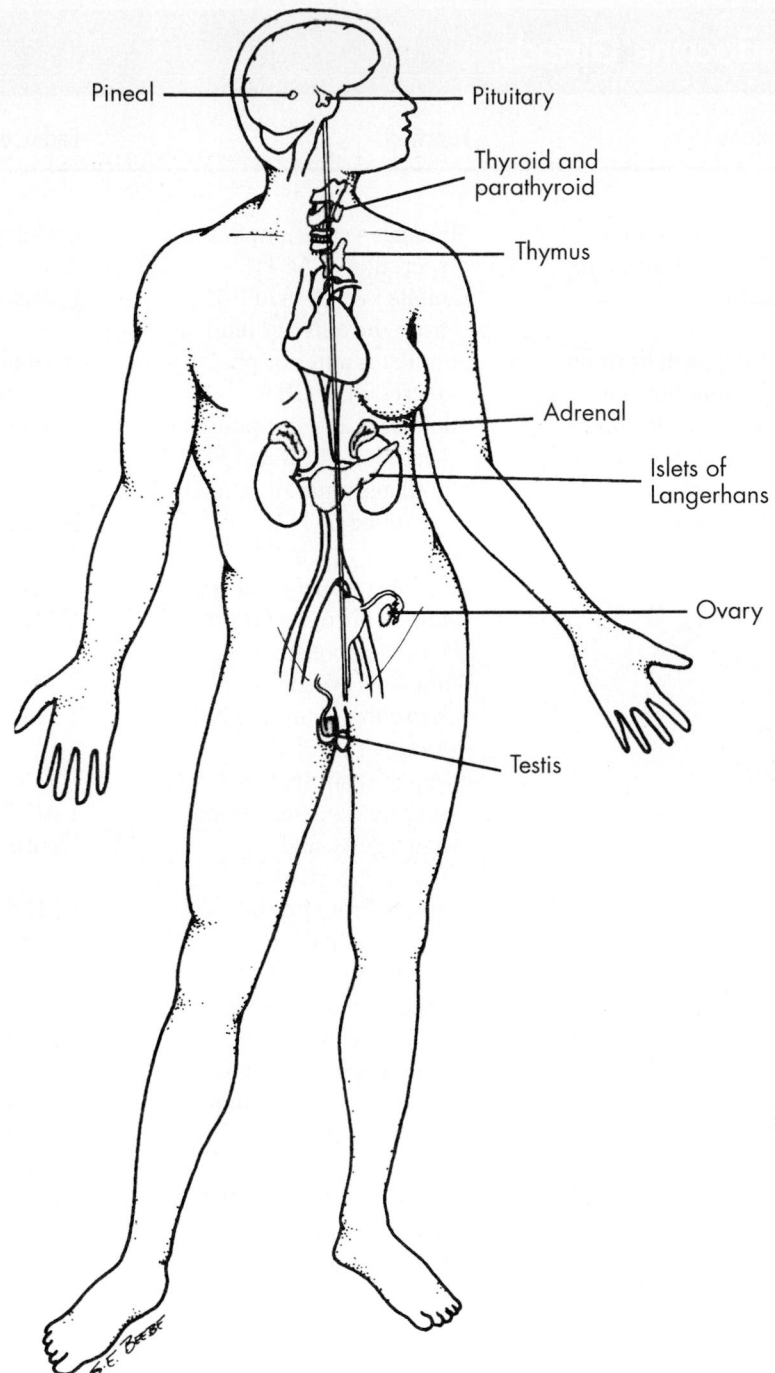

Figure 7-1 Endocrine system (male and female).

Enlarged lip
Enlarged nose
Anosmia
Eyes
   Visual acuity changes
   Visual field deficits
   Protruding eyeballs
   Drooping eyelids
   Cataracts

Periorbital edema
Ocular dysfunction
Microaneurysms
Hemorrhage
Exudates
Arteriolar narrowing
Thyroid
   Size
   Shape

Table 7-1 The Endocrine Glands

Endocrine Gland	Hormone	Function	Endocrine Disorders
Hypothalamus			
	CRH (Corticotropin releasing hormone)	Stimulates anterior pituitary secretion of ACTH	Cushing's syndrome Adrenal insufficiency
	Dopamine	Inhibits secretion of PRL from the anterior pituitary	Galactorrhea
	GRH (Growth hormone releasing hormone)	Stimulates anterior pituitary secretion of GH	Acromegaly Growth hormone deficiency
	GnRH (Gonadotropin releasing hormone)	Stimulates anterior pituitary secretion of LH and FSH	Hypogonadism
	TRH (Thyrotropin releasing hormone)	Stimulates anterior pituitary secretion of TSH	Thyrotoxicosis Hypothyroidism
Anterior Pituitary	GH	Promotes growth and retention of nitrogen for protein metabolism	↑ GH: Acromegaly, gigantism ↓ GH: Short stature
	TSH	Stimulates synthesis and secretion of thyroid hormones T_3 and T_4	↑ TSH: Graves' disease ↓ TSH: Secondary hypothyroidism
	ACTH	Stimulates adrenal cortex to secrete cortisol, adrenal androgens, and mineralocorticoids	↑ ACTH: Cushing's disease ↓ ACTH: Secondary adrenal insufficiency
	FSH	Women: Promotes follicular growth and development and secretion of estrogen	↑ LH, FSH: Precocious puberty
		Men: Stimulates Leydig cell of the testis to produce LH receptors; stimulates Sertoli cells to promote spermatogenesis	↓ LH, FSH: Delayed puberty, menstrual disorders, amenorrhea, infertility, impaired development of secondary sexual characteristics, Kallman's syndrome
	LH	Women: Promotes ovarian maturation and ovulation; regulates gonadal steroid production (estrogens and progesterone) by the ovary; maintains corpus luteum	
		Men: Regulates gonadal steroid production (testosterone) by the Leydig cell of the testis	
	PRL	Stimulates mammary glands of the breast to secrete milk	↑ PRL: Hyperprolactinemia galactorrhea, amenorrhea ↓ PRL: Failure to lactate

Key: ACTH (adrenocorticotropin hormone or corticotropin) FSH (follicle stimulating hormone)
CRH (corticotropin releasing hormone) LH (luteinizing hormone)
GnRH (gonadotropin releasing hormone) PRL (prolactin)
GRH (growth hormone releasing hormone) TRH (thyrotropin releasing hormone)
GH (growth hormone) TSH (thyroid stimulating hormone)

Table 7-1 The Endocrine Glands—cont'd

Endocrine Gland	Hormone	Function	Endocrine Disorders
Posterior Pituitary	ADH (Vasopressin)	Promotes reabsorption of water in the distal tubules of the kidney	↑ADH: Syndrome of inappropriate ADH (SIADH) ↓ADH: Diabetes insipidus
	Oxytocin	Stimulates uterine contractions at parturition, stimulates mammary contractions during suckling, promotes maternal behaviors	None known
Adrenal Cortex	Glucocorticoids (Cortisol)	Regulates metabolism of carbohydrates, fats, proteins; acts as antiinflammatory agent	↑Cortisol: Cushing's syndrome ↓Cortisol: Primary adrenal insufficiency
	Adrenal androgens (androstenedione, DHA, DHAS)	Masculinization of females	↑DHA: Hirsutism
	Mineralocorticoids (Aldosterone)	Balances sodium, water, and potassium concentration	↑Aldosterone: Primary aldosteronism Hypoaldosteronism
Medulla	Epinephrine Norepinephrine	Increases blood sugar; modulates vascular tone	↑Catecholamines: Pheochromocytoma
Pancreas Islets of Langerhans	Insulin (beta cells)	Promotes glucose entry into cells; initiates lipolysis	↑Insulin: Hypoglycemia, hyperinsulinism, insulin resistance ↓Insulin: Diabetes mellitus
	Glucagon (alpha cells)	Elevates blood glucose and stimulates lipolysis	
Thyroid	Thyroxine (T_4) Triiodothyronine (T_3)	Regulates metabolic rate	↑T_3, T_4: Hyperthyroidism, Graves' disease ↓T_3, T_4: Hypothyroidism
	Calcitonin	Decreases serum calcium levels, bone remodeling	Marker for medullary carcinoma of the thyroid
Parathyroid	Parathyroid hormone (PTH)	Regulates serum calcium concentration	↑PTH: Hyperparathyroidism, hypercalcemia, osteoporosis, renal calculi ↓PTH: Hypoparathyroidism, hypocalcemia, tetany
Gonads Ovaries	Estrogens	Induces secondary sex characteristics, sexual functioning	↓Estrogen (female): Delayed or failed puberty, osteoporosis ↑Estrogen (male): Feminization
	Progesterone	Prepares and maintains endometrium for implantation	Infertility, menstrual cycle disorders

Key: T_3 (triiodothyronine)
T_4 (thyroxine)

Continued.

Table 7-1 The Endocrine Glands—cont'd

Endocrine Gland	Hormone	Function	Endocrine Disorders
Testis	Testosterone	Induces secondary sex characteristics, sexual functioning	↓ Testosterone (male): Primary hypogonadism; feminization, infertility ↑ Testosterone (female): Hirsutism, virilization

Relationship Between Hypothalamic, Pituitary, and Target Gland Hormone Secretion

HYPOTHALAMUS	PITUITARY	TARGET	HORMONES
TRH	TSH	Thyroid	T_3, T_4
GRH	GH	IGF 1	
Dopamine	PRL	Breast	
CRH	ACTH	Adrenal	Cortisol
GnRH	LH	Ovary	E_2, progesterone
		Testis	Testosterone
	FSH	Ovary	E_2
		Testis	Inhibin, testosterone

The hypothalamus links the central nervous system with the endocrine system via the pituitary gland, which is stimulated to release hormones toward target cell membranes or organs. Hormones are released by some of the targets.

Key: ACTH (adrenocorticotropin hormone or corticotropin)
CRH (corticotropin releasing hormone)
GnRH (gonadotropin releasing hormone)
GRH (growth hormone releasing hormone)
GH (growth hormone)
FSH (follicle stimulating hormone)
IGF 1 (insulinlike growth factor)

LH (luteinizing hormone)
PRL (prolactin)
TRH (thyrotropin releasing hormone)
TSH (thyroid stimulating hormone)
T_3 (triiodothyronine)
T_4 (thyroxine)

Symmetry
Nodules
  Tenderness
  Systolic bruit
Gastrointestinal (GI) system
  Polyphagia
  Polydipsia
  Vomiting
  Diarrhea
  Steatorrhea
  Constipation
  Dehydration
  Weight change
  Increased abdominal girth
  Obesity
Cardiovascular system
  Easily bruised

Edema
Diaphoresis
Cold sweats
Tachycardia
Bradycardia
Hypotension: postural/orthostatic
Hypertension
Dysrhythmias
Cardiomegaly
Respiratory system
  Hoarseness
  Laryngeal stridor
  Tachypnea
  Kussmaul's respirations
  Acetone breath
  Stridorous respirations
  Supraclavicular retractions

Renal system
  Polyuria
  Oliguria
  Anuria
  Enuresis
  Dilute urine
  Colic
  Calculi
Reproductive system
  Upper- to lower-body segment ratio
  Menstrual cycle changes
    Amenorrhea
    Oligomenorrhea
  Galactorrhea
  Menorrhagia
  Impotence
  Female masculinization
  Changes in secondary sex characteristics
    Genital atrophy
    Breast atrophy

● Pertinent Background Information

Concurrent diseases or conditions

Cardiovascular disease
  Angina
  Hypertension
  Heart failure
  Pericardial effusion
  Myocardial infarction
Intestinal obstruction
Pulmonary edema
Psychological problems/stress
Pathologic fracture
Obesity

Previous surgery or illness

Cancer
Pancreatic disease
Burns
Renal disease
Cardiovascular disease
Transplant
Sarcoidosis
Trauma
Oophorectomy
Neck surgery
Adrenalectomy
Hypophysectomy
Gestational diabetes
Irradiation
Meningitis
Encephalitis

Family history

Diabetes mellitus
Thyroid disease
Hypertension
Pheochromocytoma
Rheumatoid arthritis
Short stature
Hirsutism
Bone disease
Infertility
Renal calculi

Social history

Physical environment
Psychological environment
Family structure/support
Occupation
  Exposure to hazards
  Shift work

Medication history

Corticosteroids
Diuretics
Medication for sleep, nerves, and/or anxiety
Alcohol

● Diagnostic Tests

Blood
  T_3 serum triiodothyronine
  T_3 resin uptake
  T_4 serum thyroxine
  Thyroid stimulating hormone (TSH)
  ^{123}I or ^{125}I (radioactive iodine uptake)
  Parathyroid hormone level (PTH)
  Adrenocorticotropic hormone (ACTH)
  Cortisol
  Ketones
  Testosterone or estrogen
  Cholesterol
  Triglyceride
  Creatinine phosphokinase (CPK)
  Catecholamine levels
  Potassium
  Sodium
  Calcium
  Phosphorus
  Phosphate reabsorption test
  pH
  CO_2
  Bicarbonate levels
  Blood urea nitrogen (BUN)

Fasting blood sugar (FBS)
Glucose tolerance test (GTT)
Thyroid stimulation test
Metyrapone test
Insulin assay
Urine
Calcium
Urinary-free cortisol
17-hydroxycorticosteroids
17-ketosteroids
Metanephrine
Specific gravity
Imaging studies
Bone x-rays
Thyroid scan/ultrasound
Computed tomography (CT) scans
  Thyroid
  Adrenal gland
  Parathyroid
Adrenal angiography
Adrenal venography
Inferior petrosal sinus sampling
Endocrine tests
Dexamethasone suppression test
ACTH stimulation test
Water deprivation test
Thyroid stimulation test
Thyroid suppression test

Poor appetite
Decreased libido
Paresthesia

Objective data

Neurologic system
  Lethargy
  Slow, monotonous, slurred speech
  Memory impairment
  Slow cognition
  Personality changes: complacent, dull, apathetic
  Nystagmus
  Night blindness
  Perceptive hearing loss
  Intention tremor
  Slowed deep tendon reflexes
  Ataxia
  Somnolence
  Syncope
Musculoskeletal system
  Muscle stiffness or aching
  Myalgia
  Arthralgia
  Fatigue
Cardiovascular system
  Intolerance to cold

Hypothyroidism: Myxedema

hypothyroidism: A condition characterized by decreased activity of the thyroid gland; caused by surgical removal of all or part of the gland, overdosage with antithyroid medication, decreased effect of thyroid releasing hormone secreted by the hypothalamus, decreased secretion of thyroid stimulating hormone by the pituitary gland, or atrophy of the thyroid gland itself
myxedema coma: A severe form of hypothyroidism; develops after a prolonged period of untreated or uncontrolled hypothyroidism

Assessment

Subjective data

Poor memory
Difficulty thinking clearly
Difficulty seeing at night
Sore muscles, aches, and pains
Feel cold
SOB

Gerontologic Considerations

● Diabetes mellitus is the most common endocrine disorder seen in older adults.
● Glucose tolerance decreases with aging, and blood glucose levels tend to increase.
● The classic signs and symptoms of diabetes may not be obvious in older adults.
● Dietary management may be complicated by a variety of social, economic, and financial factors.
● Hormone supplements must be administered with caution, because side effects are more likely to occur.
● Older adult diabetics are at increased risk for infection and should be counseled to receive proper immunizations and seek regular medical attention for even minor symptoms.

From Christensen BL, Kockrow EO: *Foundations of nursing,* ed 2, St Louis, 1995, Mosby.

Decreased sweating
Low BP, P, and T
Narrow pulse pressure
Diminished heart sounds
Precordial pain
Respiratory system
  Hoarseness
  SOB with mild exertion
GI/nutritional system
  Unexplained weight gain
  Anorexia
  Constipation
  Abdominal distention
  Ascites
Reproductive/sexual system
  Menorrhagia, metrorrhagia, amenorrhea
  Decreased libido
  Decreased fertility: spontaneous abortion
  Impotence
Integumentary system
  Skin: pale, cold, dry, coarse, scaling
  Nonpitting edema: hands, feet, periorbital area
  Upper eyelid droop
  Enlarged tongue and lips
  Coarse, thinning hair
  Nails: brittle, slow growing, thick

Diagnostic tests

Electrocardiogram (ECG): low-voltage, nonspecific ST segment changes, prolonged P-R interval, heart block, flat or inverted T wave
Blood
  Decreased serum T_4 and T_3
  Decreased serum sodium
  TSH levels: decreased if secondary hypothyroidism; elevated if primary hypothyroidism
  Increased serum: cholesterol, triglycerides, CPK, alkaline phosphatase
  Arterial blood gases (ABGs): hypoxia, elevated CO_2
  Normocytic, normochromic anemia
Cerebrospinal fluid: increased protein
Endocrine studies
  TSH test
  Radioiodide uptake test (suppressed response)

Potential complications

Angina, dysrhythmias
Heart failure
Myocardial infarction
Intestinal obstruction

Pleural/pericardial effusions
Stupor
Coma

Collaborative management

Therapeutic management

THR with synthetic L-thyroxine
Glucocorticoids if adrenal insufficiency diagnosis
IV fluids, albumin
High-protein, high-fiber, low-calorie, low-sodium diet
Restrict fluids
Diuretics
Stool softeners

Nursing management

PATIENT PROBLEMS/NURSING DIAGNOSES

● **NDX:** Fluid volume excess, extravascular, related to increased capillary permeability

Monitor intake and output q8h and prn
Monitor IV fluids, if administered, *to prevent overhydration*
Weigh patient daily and report significant gain to physician (significant gain is >0.5 kg daily)
Monitor for signs and symptoms *to identify excess extravascular volume*
  Periorbital edema
  Jugular vein distention
  Increasing abdominal girth
  Presence of abdominal fluid wave
  Dependent edema of extremities
  Pulmonary edema: dyspnea, orthopnea, and/or crackles in lungs; monitor chest x-ray results
Monitor serum albumin levels, electrolytes, creatinine
Maintain high-protein diet *to increase serum protein levels*
Restrict fluids as determined by collaboration with physician
Monitor VS q4h and observe for
  Increased pulse
  Labored respirations
  Development of S_3 gallop
Be cautious in administering sedatives, especially barbiturates, *because of increased sensitivity*
Notify physician of development or worsening of any of the previously mentioned signs or symptoms
Maintain patient on bed rest *to alleviate dyspnea and support edematous areas*

EXPECTED OUTCOMES

VS are stable; electrolytes are within normal range; weight is returning to normal range for patient; intake and output are balanced; edema is resolving

● **NDX:** Altered thought processes related to changed metabolic processes

Assess level of orientation q4h and reorient patient as necessary; explain procedures clearly and slowly; repeat as necessary; break down tasks into easy-to-accomplish segments

Help patient to focus on tasks and reach self-care goals

Provide a stable, calm, and nonstressful environment

Be consistent in timing and performance of activities and procedures

Restrict visitors as necessary

Avoid frequent changing of personnel

Prevent emotionally upsetting or confusing situations

Allow sufficient time for performance of procedures and activities

Plan care with patient *to engage patient as a partner in interventions designed to improve thought processes*

Allow sufficient time for patient to express needs and feelings

Assist patient to make choices and decisions

Provide diversional activities and materials

Assist significant other in acceptance of patient's slowness

EXPECTED OUTCOMES

Oriented to time, person, and place

Accomplishes planned self-care activities

Makes choices known to others

Discusses feelings and responses with significant other(s)

● **NDX:** Risk for trauma related to potential for changes in sensory perception and coordination

Assess for development or worsening of perception/coordination defects q8h

Assess muscle strength and mobility daily

Explain necessary safety precautions *to prevent accident/trauma*

Assist patient with ambulation as necessary; provide aids to ambulation (walker, cane) as needed

Monitor pulse rate, complaints of dyspnea or chest pain during activity

Balance periods of activity and rest

Place articles patient may wish to use frequently within easy reach

Arrange environment simply; avoid unnecessary clutter

Remove potentially hazardous objects from patient's environment

Place bed in low position

Face patient when speaking *to obtain patient's attention*

Speak slowly and clearly

Serve foods at tepid temperature *to prevent thermal injury*

Assist with bathing, shaving, and toileting as necessary

Use safety measures (e.g., jacket restraint; avoid wrist restraints) as necessary

Instruct patient to call for assistance when getting out of bed *to prevent a fall*

Keep call light within easy reach at all times

Provide nighttime lighting

Keep siderails up at all times

EXPECTED OUTCOME

Patient sustains no injuries

● **NDX:** Constipation related to decreased metabolic rate and/or decreased intestinal peristalsis and decreased dietary bulk and fluids

Maintain low-calorie diet that includes high-fiber foods

Administer fluids to tolerance; remind patient to drink fluids hourly if not restricted *to prevent constipation*

Monitor bowel pattern, consistency of color, odor of stool, and associated symptoms daily

Assess usual methods used *to prevent constipation*

Assess effectiveness of stool softener, laxatives administered

Provide privacy

Encourage exercise as tolerated

Teach patient to respond promptly to urge to defecate; avoid straining

Assist patient with recognizing activities that stimulate urge to defecate (drinking warm liquids)

Encourage patient to attempt defecation at same time each day *to establish a routine*

EXPECTED OUTCOME

Stool is normal in color, consistency, odor, and frequency

● **NDX:** Impaired skin integrity related to edema; dry, scaly skin; and immobility

Assess for redness or breakdown q24h; if patient is on bed rest, assess q8h

Administer skin care to pressure points four times daily and as necessary *to retain skin integrity*

Use superfatted soap for bathing; apply lotion after each bath or handwashing *to prevent dryness*

Use elbow and heel protectors *to prevent friction rub*

Place patient on decubitus-prevention mattress or bed

Elevate edematous extremities with pillows *to increase venous return*

Assist and encourage patient to make small position changes q½h to 1 h; turn q2h

Encourage ambulation when able; avoid sitting for long periods *to prevent venous stasis*

Encourage patient to avoid crossing legs *to prevent venous stasis*

Maintain optimal nutritional status

Conserve body temperature by use of blankets, warm clothing

EXPECTED OUTCOME

Skin turgor is good; skin is intact; patient uses preventive measures

Patient/family teaching

Explain basic concepts of the disease process and complications to report to physician

Explain reasons for physical and emotional changes

Teach name of medication, dosage, time and method of administration, purpose, side effects, and toxic effects

Emphasize that medication must not be discontinued without consulting physician

Emphasize importance of telling all health care personnel about disease and wearing medical alert band

Explain that condition is potentially reversible if treatment regimen is followed

Home care considerations

Explain need to avoid taking over-the-counter medications without consulting physician

Prepare for home by providing information about importance of
Ongoing outpatient follow-up
Understanding slowness and dullness
Increasing self-care
Avoiding very cold environments and stressful situations
Adequate periods of rest alternating with increasing activity/exercise
Maintaining balanced diet and adequate fluid intake
Preventing constipation

Discuss symptoms of infection to report to physician
Temperature above patient's normal
Cold or influenza symptoms
Redness or swelling around lesions
Frequency of or burning on urination

Hyperthyroidism: Thyroid Crisis (Storm, Thyrotoxic Crisis)

hyperthyroidism: Characterized by excessive action of thyroid hormone; causes may be classified as autoimmune (Graves' disease), viral, hyperplastic, genetic, or neoplastic (thyroid adenomas); or secondary to an acute systemic illness and factitious (excessive thyroid hormone treatment results in increased sympathetic tone, which is responsible for many of the assessment findings that follow)

Graves' disease: Most prevalent form of hyperthyroidism; most commonly seen in women during the third and fourth decades of life

thyroid crisis: A medical emergency caused by acute exacerbation of the symptoms of hyperthyroidism; usually precipitated by a stressful event such as surgery, infection, trauma, or acute cardiovascular disease

Assessment

Subjective data

Irritability/nervousness
Headache
Difficulty concentrating
Nausea
Abdominal pain
Increased thirst and/or appetite
SOB
Palpitations
Weakness

Objective data

Neurologic system
Hyperthyroidism
Tremors
Insomnia
Emotional lability
Diplopia
Brisk deep tendon reflexes
Muscle weakness or atrophy
Confusion
Memory loss
Easily distracted
Startled expression
Manic behavior
Thyroid crisis
Extreme restlessness
Confusion or disorientation

Psychosis
Apathy
Stupor or delirium
Coma
Eyes
  Conjunctival irritation
  Large, protruding eyes
  Lid retraction
  Periorbital edema
  Tremor of eyelids
  Weakness or paralysis of extraocular muscles
Cardiovascular system
  Hyperthyroidism
    Palpitations
    Rapid, bounding pulses
    Wide pulse pressure
    Irregular pulse/dysrhythmias
    Systolic cardiac murmur
    Edema
  Thyroid crisis
    Profuse diaphoresis
    Tachycardia disproportionate to change in BP
    Atrial fibrillation
    Weak pulses
    Hypotension
Respiratory system
  Hyperthyroidism
    Dyspnea
    Increased depth and rate of respiration
  Thyroid crisis: pulmonary edema
Musculoskeletal system
  Generalized muscle wasting
GI system
  Hyperthyroidism
    Weight loss
    Diarrhea
    Hyperactive bowel sounds
  Thyroid crisis
    Anorexia
    Protracted vomiting
    Severe abdominal pain
    Hepatomegaly
    Jaundice
Metabolic system
  Profuse sweating
  Sensitivity to heat
  Increased tolerance to cold
  Enlarged thyroid gland
  Bruit over neck
Integumentary system
  Skin: soft, warm, moist, shiny
  Reddened, hyperpigmented palms
  Hair: thinning, fine, straight (silky)
  Oily scalp
  Separation of nails from nail beds

Reproductive/sexual system
  Oligomenorrhea
  Amenorrhea
  Diminished libido
  Decreased fertility
  Gynecomastia in males

Diagnostic tests

Blood
  Elevated total and free T_3 and T_4
  Thyroid radioiodide uptake test (RAIU)
    Low uptake in thyroiditis or excess thyroid hormone medication (exogenous hyperthy-roidism)
    High uptake in Graves' disease
Serum
  TSH
    Increased with pituitary tumor
    Normal with thyroid hormone resistance
    Decreased with Graves' disease or factitious

Potential complications

Fever >106°F
Marked elevation in P and BP
Dangerous dysrhythmias
CHF
Pulmonary edema
Widespread tremors
Circulatory collapse
Shock
Death

Collaborative management

Therapeutic management

Medications
  Antithyroid medications
    Thioamides (PTU, ipodate agents, tapazole)
    β-adrenergic blockers (propanolol)
    Iodine (potassium or sodium iodide)
    Radioactive iodine
    Glucocorticoids
  Palliative medications
    Acetaminophen
    Eye lubricants
Dietary changes
  High calorie
  High protein
  High carbohydrate
  High vitamin B
  3 to 4 L fluid per day

Comfort measures: cooling (hypothermia blanket)
Surgical intervention: subtotal thyroidectomy
Thyroid crisis
  Glucocorticoids
  SSKI (saturated solution of potassium iodide)
  Thioureas (propylthiouracil)
  β-blockade
  Hyperthermia control (aspirin is contraindicated)
  Cooling measures
  Volume expanders and/or vasopressors for hypotension
  Total parenteral nutrition (TPN)
  Digoxin and/or diuretics for CHF

Nursing management

PATIENT PROBLEMS/NURSING DIAGNOSES

● **NDX:**   Altered thought processes related to increased stimulation of the sympathetic nervous system by high levels of thyroid hormone and sleep deprivation

Assess LOC, orientation, affect, and perception q4h to 8h; report negative changes
Discuss feelings and responses to situations and people; reinforce those that are appropriate
Provide a stable, calm, nonstressful, and nonstimulating environment *to minimize confusion*
  Control extraneous noise *to facilitate clarity of thought processes*
  Be consistent in timing and performing of activities and procedures *to minimize confusion related to activities*
  Restrict visitors as necessary *to minimize stress*
  Avoid frequent changing of personnel
  Prevent emotionally upsetting situations when possible
Plan care with patient; give clear, concise explanations *to facilitate concentration and understanding*
Anticipate needs to prevent hyperactive reactions
Inform patient that activities may be restricted *to minimize confusion*
Teach stress-reduction techniques and assess use by patient
Provide diversional activities and materials that decrease stimulation; avoid those requiring fine motor manipulation
Reorient patient to environment as needed and provide orienting cues: clock, calendar, familiar pictures
Monitor for adverse reactions to medications

EXPECTED OUTCOMES

Patient is oriented
Responds appropriately to situations and people

Uses stress-reduction techniques
Does not injure self, others, or property

● **NDX:**   Activity intolerance related to imbalance between oxygen supply and demand caused by increased resting metabolic rate and intolerance of heat

Assess baseline VS and prior activity level
Restrict activity to patient's level of tolerance by assessing physiologic response to activity (i.e., assess VS during activity and compare to baseline)
Allow patient to set priorities for care within limits
Space procedures *to allow adequate rest periods*
Provide needed equipment, supplies *to prevent expenditure of energy by patient before activity*
Discontinue activity at onset of signs of intolerance: dyspnea, tachycardia, fatigue
Assist patient with those activities patient is unable to perform because of weakness or tremors
Plan daily activity and rest pattern *to facilitate increasing tolerance for self-care*

EXPECTED OUTCOMES

Completes planned activities without evidence of intolerance
Asks for assistance only when needed

● **NDX:**   Sleep pattern disturbance related to an increased metabolic rate

Assess past and present sleep and activity patterns
Determine factors/techniques to induce sleep previously used by patient
Provide sleep aids requested by patient: warm drink, back rub, quiet music *to facilitate sleep and rest*
Discuss other sleep aids such as relaxation techniques
Discourage frequent daytime sleeping *to increase night sleeping;* provide nap times sufficient in length *to produce REM sleep*
Avoid intake of stimulants in diet *to avoid interference with sleep*
Assist patient with establishing a regular pattern of physical activity; reduce stimulating activities before sleep
Provide environment conducive to sleep: reduce lighting; close door to room; maintain quiet; maintain privacy
Avoid disturbing patient unnecessarily during the night for procedures *to allow uninterrupted periods of sleep and rest*
Schedule treatments and medications for daytime and evening hours when possible *to avoid interrupting sleep*
Assess effectiveness of sleep-promoting activities daily

EXPECTED OUTCOMES

Sleep pattern is normal for patient
Patient expresses feeling rested, alert, with energy to accomplish daily tasks

● **NDX:** Altered nutrition: less than body requirements related to diarrhea, nausea, abdominal pain, and/or hypermetabolic state

Provide high-calorie, high-protein, high-carbohydrate, high–vitamin B diet *to compensate for loss of calories, protein, glucose, and vitamins from bowel hypermotility and increased metabolism*
Offer frequent, small meals and between-meal supplements
Consult patient as to food preferences
Avoid stimulants: coffee, tea, colas, or other beverages with caffeine or theobromine *to prevent peristaltic stimulation and fullness from empty calories*
Avoid foods with large amounts of fiber or highly seasoned foods *to prevent stimulating bowel motility*
Encourage fluid intake to 2000 to 3000 ml/day; avoid juices that may cause diarrhea
Provide environment with congenial visitors if patient desires
Weigh patient daily; same time, scale, clothing *to evaluate effectiveness of diet and health care plan*
Monitor intake and output q8h
Assess effectiveness of medication for nausea and abdominal pain

EXPECTED OUTCOMES

Weight is increasing to that which is normal for patient
Takes prescribed diet without abdominal discomfort
Has no diarrhea
Intake and output are balanced

● **NDX:** Impaired tissue integrity (eyes) related to compromised protective mechanisms (inadequate tearing and lid closure)

Assess for eye changes: excessive tearing, feeling of foreign object, inability to close eyes, dryness, signs of infection, irritation, or abrasions q4h to 8h
Provide sunglasses during the day as necessary *to prevent injury from inadequate lid closure*
Administer artificial tears as ordered *to prevent injury to eyes from inadequate tearing*
Patch or tape eyes during sleep *to protect exposed cornea*
Prevent foreign bodies from contact with eyes (dirt, dust)
Assist and teach patient to perform eye motion exercises
Discuss feelings and techniques related to improving appearance

Ensure that patient understands that surgical intervention may be needed

EXPECTED OUTCOMES

Eyes remain moist without evidence of abrasions or infection
Patient uses methods to protect eyes and discusses feelings about appearance

● **NDX:** Hyperthermia related to hypermetabolic state

Maintain cool environment *to minimize discomfort related to hypersensitivity to heat*
Use light clothing and bed linens
Provide tepid sponge baths as necessary *to maintain normal body temperature*
Assess effectiveness of hypothermia blanket when in use; use measures to prevent skin breakdown
Administer acetaminophen as ordered (aspirin is contraindicated) *to control body temperature*
Increase fluid intake to 2500 ml/day *to cool body and prevent dehydration*
Monitor VS, LOC, urinary output q2h to 4h
Collaborate with physician in using additional cooling measures when condition indicates

EXPECTED OUTCOMES

Patient is alert and responsive
VS and urinary output are normal

● **NDX:** Risk for trauma related to potential for altered mental status

Remove potentially hazardous objects from patient's environment and arrange furniture *to prevent bumps or falls (e.g., bed in low position)*
Provide fluids for drinking and bathing that will not burn patient if spilled or used immediately
Assess muscle strength, mobility, and mental status q4h to 8h
Provide information about need to follow safety precautions *to decrease risk for trauma*
Assist patient with ambulating as needed
Instruct patient to call for assistance when getting out of bed; keep siderails up
Keep call light within easy reach of patient
Keep personal articles patient may wish to use frequently within easy reach
Encourage use of nonskid slippers
Provide night light

EXPECTED OUTCOMES

Patient is not physically injured
Understands safety precautions
Calls for assistance when needed

Patient/family teaching

Explain basic concepts of the disease process, signs and symptoms of recurrence, and complications to report to physician

Explain that symptoms of disease *may* be reversible if medical regimen is followed

Explain that nervous symptoms are part of the disease process and will decrease with treatment

Provide reasons for physical and emotional changes

Stress importance of discussing feelings about changes

Explain the need for a calm, stable environment

Explain to family members the importance of their role in minimizing patient's exposure to stress

Provide patient and family with information about eye protection

Teach name of medication, dosage, time and method of administration, purpose, side effects, and toxic effects

Home care considerations

Discuss with patient and family the need for the following:

A calm, stable environment to minimize patient's confusion

Family support to minimize the patient's potential for emotional upset

Planning daily activities and scheduling rest periods

Promoting an environment conducive to sleep

Diet to maintain weight and minimize bowel hypermotility

Eye protection and medical follow-up

Regulation of environmental temperature

Alterations in home environment and planning ADLs to minimize risk of injury to self, others, or property

Emphasize importance of planned rest periods of adequate duration

Emphasize importance of avoiding stressful situations and using stress-reducing techniques

Encourage high-calorie, high-protein, high-carbohydrate, and high–vitamin B diet with increased fluids until discontinued by physician

Discuss maintaining eye integrity: sunglasses, lubricants, protective coverings, and prescribed exercises

Explain need to avoid taking over-the-counter medications without physician approval

Emphasize importance of ongoing outpatient care

Instruct patient to inform health care givers (physician, dentist) of presence of disease and wear medical alert bracelet

Hypoparathyroidism

A rare condition characterized by a deficiency of parathyroid hormone (PTH); usually the result of damage to the parathyroid glands during thyroid or other neck surgery, radiation treatment, or parathyroidectomy; *the cause also may be idiopathic. The parathyroid glands fail to produce an adequate amount of PTH to maintain serum calcium levels. The reduced action of PTH on bone and kidney leads to hypocalcemia and hypophosphatemia. "Pseudohypoparathyroidism" refers to target organ resistance or unresponsiveness to PTH, not PTH deficiency.*

Assessment

Subjective data

Headache
Tingling
Irritability
Anxiety
Painful cramping
Stiffness
Fatigue
Palpitations
Abdominal pain
Depression

Objective data

Neurologic system
  Emotional lability
  Psychosis
  Paranoia
  Changes in LOC
  Papilledema
  Paresthesia: lips, tongue, fingers, feet
  Cataracts caused by calcification of lens
  Tremor
  Hyperreflexia
  Positive Chvostek's and/or Trousseau's signs
  Tetany
  Seizures
Musculoskeletal system
  Stiffness
  Twitching spasms
  Weakness
  Fatigue
  Dental abnormalities
Cardiovascular system
  Congestive heart failure caused by hypocalcemia
  Cyanosis
  Palpitations
  Cardiac dysrhythmias
  ECG changes: prolonged Q-T interval, peaked or inverted T waves, heart block
Respiratory system
  Hoarseness
  Laryngeal stridor
  Laryngeal edema

Gastrointestinal system
  Nausea, vomiting
  Diarrhea
Renal system: calculi formation
Integumentary system
  Dystrophic, dry, scaly skin and nails
  Cutaneous pigmentation
  Thinning hair
  Alopecia
  Horizontal ridges on nails
  Brittle nails

Diagnostic tests

Blood
  Serum calcium decreased
  Serum phosphorus increased
  Serum bicarbonate decreased
  Serum parathyroid hormone decreased or absent
Urine
  Hypocalciuria
  Hypophosphaturia

Potential complication

Renal calculi

Collaborative management

Therapeutic management

Calcium supplementation
Vitamin D supplementation
If acute tetany, IV calcium administration
Maintain serum calcium levels at 8 to 9 mg/dl to prevent hypercalciuria and nephrolithiasis
Respiratory therapy as indicated

Nursing management

PATIENT PROBLEMS/NURSING DIAGNOSES

● **NDX:** Risk for injury related to potential for seizures or tetany resulting from hypocalcemia

Monitor vital signs and reflexes
Monitor cardiac function if ECG abnormalities are present
Collaborate with physician *to manage early symptoms of tetany* by administering and monitoring effectiveness of parenteral fluids and calcium
Administer calcium cautiously *to prevent hypotensive thrombophlebitis*
Administer vitamin D and calcium supplements as ordered

Do not administer phosphate binders within 1 to 2 hr before or after calcium supplements or other medications
Monitor serum levels of calcium and phosphorus
When patient is on bed rest, pad rails and keep bed in low position *to prevent risk of injury if seizure occurs*
If seizure activity occurs when patient is out of bed
  Assist patient to floor
  Remove potentially harmful objects
Assess patient for injury after seizure
Inform patient of seizure and reorient if necessary

EXPECTED OUTCOMES
Patient has no injuries
Reflexes are normal
VS are stable
Takes diet and medications as prescribed

● **NDX:** Decreased cardiac output related to alterations in myocardial conduction

Assess vital signs
Monitor fluid balance, especially when nausea, vomiting, or diarrhea occurs
Monitor cardiac function: Q-T interval changes, abnormal T and P waves reflect hypocalcemic interference with conduction

EXPECTED OUTCOMES
Patient maintains adequate cardiac output
Vital signs remain stable

● **NDX:** Ineffective airway clearance related to laryngeal edema or seizure activity

Keep suction equipment and oral airway at bedside at all times
Have tracheostomy tray, oxygen, and manual resuscitation equipment readily available
Laryngeal edema
Assess respiratory efforts and voice quality
Auscultate for subtle laryngeal stridor
Report early symptoms to physician and collaborate *to maintain open airway*
Instruct patient to inform nurse or physician at first sign of tightness in throat or SOB
Position patient to optimize airway clearance: keep head in neutral position, midline
Seizure
If seizure occurs
  Maintain airway
  Clear immediate area *to avoid patient's self-injury during seizure*
  Monitor BP, P, R, and neurologic signs; check after seizure and prn

Note frequency, time, LOC, body parts involved, and length of seizure activity

Be prepared to collaborate with physician in treating status epilepticus: intubation, medications

Monitor patient during postictal period

Continue preseizure care as indicated

EXPECTED OUTCOMES

Respiratory rate, rhythm, and depth are normal for patient

Lungs are clear on auscultation

● **NDX:** Activity intolerance related to muscular weakness and/or fatigue

Assess past activity patterns

Assess for changes in musculoskeletal symptoms

Assess response to activity

Note changes in BP, P, R

Stop activity when changes occur

Increase participation in small increments as tolerance increases

Teach patient to monitor response to activity and alter, stop, or ask for assistance when changes occur

Plan care with patient *to determine activities patient desires to accomplish; schedule assistance from others*

Balance activity with rest *to prevent fatigue*

Keep articles and needed supplies within easy reach *to decrease energy expenditure*

EXPECTED OUTCOME

Activity level is increasing daily without dyspnea, tachycardia, or elevated BP; performs ADLs without effort

ADDITIONAL NURSING DIAGNOSES TO CONSIDER

Risk for fluid volume deficit related to diarrhea, nausea, or vomiting

Altered thought processes related to neurologic changes as evidenced by emotional lability, delirium, delusions

Risk for impaired skin integrity related to dry, scaly skin and immobility

Patient/family teaching

Explain basic concepts of the disease process

Discuss reasons for physical and emotional changes

Teach patient to check for and report early signs of tetany

Tingling sensations

Tremors

Positive Chvostek's and/or Trousseau's signs

Change in respiratory effort

Teach significant other(s) to recognize patient's seizure activity and determine course of action to take

Avoid restraining or interrupting behavior

Observe and record behaviors exhibited before and during seizure

Notify physician immediately

Remove hazardous objects; clear area around patient *to prevent injury*

Stress importance of daily activity and exercise to tolerance and reporting increasing muscle weakness or fatigue

Home care considerations

Discuss importance of maintaining safe home environment

Teach name of medication, dosage, time and method of administration, purpose, side effects, and toxic effects, and that medication needs to be taken for remainder of life

Explain need to avoid taking over-the-counter medications without consulting physician

Emphasize importance of ongoing follow-up care

Instruct patient to maintain high-calcium, high–vitamin D, low-phosphorus diet and increased fluid intake

The patient and significant other(s) should verbalize their understanding of disease process and principles of home and follow-up care and demonstrate method to check for Chvostek's and Trousseau's signs

Hyperparathyroidism

Hyperparathyroidism is the hypersecretion of parathyroid hormone (PTH) by one or more of the parathyroid glands, which leads to a state of hypercalcemia and hyperphosphatemia. Hyperparathyroidism may be due to primary or secondary causes; in primary hyperparathyroidism, hypertrophy of the gland is usually caused by a benign adenoma; secondary hyperparathyroidism is the result of excessive compensatory production of PTH that develops from conditions such as renal disease that cause a decrease in calcium levels.

Assessment

Subjective

Fatigue

Slow mentation

Mood changes

Memory loss

Depression

Easy fatigability
Painful joints
Difficulty urinating

Objective

Neurologic system
  Apathy
  Decreased cognitive function
  Drowsiness
  Hyperactive reflexes
Musculoskeletal system
  Muscular weakness (proximal)
  Bone pain with weight bearing
  Arthralgia
  Bone deformities, shortened stature
  Fractures
  Painful joints
  Hearing loss
Cardiovascular system
  Hypertension
  ECG changes: broad T wave, short or prolonged Q-T
    interval, bradycardia
GI/nutritional system
  Abdominal discomfort
  Polydipsia
  Anorexia
  Nausea and vomiting
  Weight loss
  Constipation
Renal system
  Polyuria
  Dysuria; difficulty urinating
  Dehydration
  Renal colic
  Uremia
  Calculi

Diagnostic tests

Blood
  Elevated PTH
  Elevated serum calcium
  Low serum phosphate
  Elevated serum chloride
  Low serum HCO_3
  Anemia
Urine
  Increased urine phosphate and urine calcium
  cAMP (cyclic adenosine monophosphatase) reflects
    concentration of biologically active PTH
Imaging
  CT scan: neck
  X-ray examination: subperiosteal bone resorption
  Ultrasound: enlarged parathyroid gland

Endocrine tests: elevated parathyroid hormone (PTH)
  radioimmunoassay

Potential complications

Renal failure
Pathologic bone fractures
Gastric ulcers
Pancreatitis
Stupor
Coma

Collaborative management

Therapeutic management

Fluid replacement: 2000 to 3000 ml/day
Parenteral hydration: usually with normal saline
Avoidance of thiazide diuretics
Medications
  Glucocorticoids
  Calcitonin
Treatment of choice: surgical removal of the gland(s)

Nursing management

  PATIENT PROBLEMS/NURSING DIAGNOSES

● **NDX:**   Risk for fluid volume deficit related to hyper-
         calcemia

Monitor IV and oral fluid intake *to promote adequate hydration*: 1000 ml/hr for short period may be given initially IV, then oral fluids to 3000 ml/day unless contraindicated
Monitor VS, central venous pressure (CVP), and
  breath sounds q4h as indicative of fluid volume imbalance
Monitor intake, output, and electrolyte values q4h *to
  assess hydration status*
Monitor cardiac rhythm for changes in T waves or Q-T
  intervals indicative of hypercalcemia
Assess muscle strength and mobility q4h *to evaluate
  effects of hypercalcemia*
Assess reflexes q4h *to evaluate for hyperreflexia*
Administer medications as ordered and observe for adverse reactions: hypotension with IV phosphates, extravasation with IV mithramycin
Weigh patient daily; same time, clothing, scale
Assess skin condition and turgor q8h *to evaluate hydra-
  tion status*
Maintain low-calcium, high-phosphorus diet
Collaborate with physician if any changes in physical
  condition are detected

EXPECTED OUTCOMES

VS are stable
Intake and output are balanced
Electrolytes are within normal range
Skin is warm and moist with good turgor

● **NDX:** Risk for trauma related to potential for pathologic fracture

Assess for pain; may be indicative of fracture
Maintain correct body alignment as indicated *to prevent fractures*
Assist patient with ambulation as needed *to prevent falls*
Provide aids to ambulation: walker, cane
Place articles that patient may require frequently within easy reach *to prevent injury*
Arrange environment simply; avoid unnecessary clutter
Provide night light *to facilitate mobility at night*
Place call bell within easy reach at all times
Instruct patient to call for assistance before getting out of bed
Keep bed in low position with siderails up *to prevent falls*
Assist with personal hygiene as needed
Use safety measures (e.g., jacket restraint) as necessary if patient is confused
Remove potentially hazardous objects from patient's environment

EXPECTED OUTCOMES

No physical injury occurs
Verbalizes no pain or increasing discomfort

● **NDX:** Altered thought processes related to slow mentation, depression, and/or drowsiness

Assess LOC and orientation q4h
Provide a stable, calm, and nonstressful environment *to prevent impaired cognitive operations*
  Be consistent in timing and performance of activities and procedures
  Restrict patient's visitors as necessary
  Avoid frequent changing of personnel
  Prevent emotionally upsetting or confusing situations if possible
Plan care with patient as appropriate *to promote cognitive mentation*
Anticipate patient's needs
Reorient patient to environment as necessary
Explain procedures slowly and clearly; repeat prn
Encourage patient to take active role in care
Avoid administration of narcotics or sedatives if possible

EXPECTED OUTCOME

Patient is alert, oriented, and accomplishes self-care as planned

Patient/family teaching

Instruct patient/family regarding low-calcium, high-phosphorus diet
Explain basic concepts of the disease
Discuss reasons for physical and emotional changes
Teach name of medication, dosage, time and method of administration, purpose, side effects, and toxic effects
Explain need to avoid taking over-the-counter medications without consulting physician
Instruct patient to maintain increased fluid intake
Emphasize importance of ongoing outpatient follow-up

Home care considerations

Discuss potential alterations to patient's home environment to facilitate ADLs and minimize potential for trauma
Discuss importance of avoiding risks
Stress importance of maintaining a safe environment to reduce risk of injury, need to report signs of fractures to physician

Adrenocortical Insufficiency

Hypofunction of the adrenal cortex; primary adrenocortical insufficiency, Addison's disease, results in a deficiency of mineralocorticoids and glucocorticoids; secondary insufficiency results in a deficiency of only glucocorticoids. Primary insufficiency (1 AI) is usually caused by idiopathic atrophy of the cortex, most likely autoimmune in nature. Secondary insufficiency (2 AI) is usually a result of suppression of pituitary function by exogenous glucocorticoid; pituitary tumor is a rare cause.

Assessment

Subjective data

Fatigue
Headache
Depression
Dizziness
Apathy
Nausea; loss of appetite
Decreased libido

Objective data

Musculoskeletal system
  Weakness
  Muscular atrophy
  Muscle and joint pain

Cardiovascular system
  Orthostatic hypotension
  Postural dizziness
  Decreased tolerance of cold or stress
  Hypovolemia
  Palpitations
  Diaphoresis
GI system
  Weight loss
  Anorexia
  Vomiting
  Abdominal pain
  Salt craving
  Diarrhea
Integumentary system
  Hyperpigmentation; bronze coloration
  Decreased body hair
  Vitiligo
Reproductive/sexual system
  Diminished secondary sex characteristics (especially females)
  Amenorrhea
  Premature menopause

Diagnostic tests

NOTE: (1 = primary AI); (2 = secondary AI)
Blood
  Decreased plasma cortisol
  Increased serum ACTH in primary; decreased in secondary
  Hyponatremia
  Hyperkalemia (1 AI)
  Normokalemia (2 AI)
  Metabolic acidosis
  Increased plasma renin levels (1 AI)
  Decreased plasma aldosterone (1 AI)
Urine: subnormal excretion of 17-hydroxycorticoids
Imaging: x-ray examination—small heart, adrenal calcification
Endocrine studies: ACTH stimulation test
  Cortisol response in 1 AI
  Normal/intermediate cortisol response in 2 AI

Potential complications

Adrenal (Addisonian) crisis: medical emergency involving intensification of symptoms of adrenal insufficiency; usually precipitated by infection, trauma, surgery, or excessive loss of body salts
Observations/findings in adrenal crisis include
  Profound weakness, fatigue
  Severe hypotension
  Nausea, vomiting
  Dehydration

Severe pain: back, abdomen, extremities
Severe headache
Fever
Shock
Cardiac arrest
Renal failure
Azotemia
Death

Collaborative management

Therapeutic management

IV fluid and sodium replacement
Glucocorticoids: corticosteroid replacement
Mineralocorticoids: fludrocortisone replacement
In crisis: vasopressors, plasma expanders, supportive therapy (e.g., oxygen)

Nursing management

PATIENT PROBLEMS/NURSING DIAGNOSES

● **NDX:** Risk for injury related to potential for adrenal crisis

Assess VS q4h and prn; report abnormal findings and severe hypotension to physician immediately *to prevent vascular collapse*
Monitor cardiac rhythm continuously if dysrhythmias occur *to recognize and treat hyperkalemia (initially), then hypokalemia*
Monitor intake and output q4h and prn; report output greater than intake; also watch for decreased urine output and water intoxication
Monitor neurologic status q4h; report increasing headache and confusion
Position patient *to promote cardiovascular and respiratory function*
Collaborate with physician if adrenal crisis develops to administer IV fluids, vasopressors, corticosteroids, and oxygen

EXPECTED OUTCOMES
VS are stable and within normal limits
Patient is alert, oriented
Intake and output are balanced

● **NDX:** Risk for injury related to potential for inability to tolerate environmental stresses

Select quiet, nonstimulating room with noninfectious roommate *to minimize stress and prevent infection caused by reduced inflammatory responsiveness*

Avoid exposure to cold: provide extra blankets; have patient wear bed socks and use warm robe when out of bed *to avoid stress from cold*

Administer steroid replacement therapy as ordered

Consult physician in situations in which increased doses of steroids may be indicated during periods of stress: surgery, infection, trauma

Always administer steroid therapy on time; do not discontinue or reduce dose abruptly

Medicate for pain or nausea as required

Encourage regular rest periods alternating with activity

Anticipate stressful situations and defuse if possible

Avoid discussing stress-producing topics; inform visitors

Monitor and restrict visitors if patient desires

Plan daily schedule with patient and avoid unexpected events *to prevent unnecessary stress*

EXPECTED OUTCOMES

Patient does not develop adrenal crisis

Begins to tolerate environmental stresses as evidenced by increased interest and participation in daily schedule and desire for visitors

Discusses disease process and asks questions

● **NDX:** Risk for infection related to inability of adrenal cortex to produce steroids in times of stress

Monitor for signs and symptoms of infection; report if detected (URI, UTI, wounds, IV, or infection sites) *to confirm and treat infection early*

Have patient turn, cough, and deep breathe q2h while on bed rest *to prevent respiratory infection from stasis*

Avoid unnecessary invasive procedures (urinary catheterization) *to prevent opportunity for infection*

Maintain sterile technique when caring for any skin lesions, tubes, drains, or IV lines *to prevent infection caused by contamination*

Culture suspicious wounds or secretions

Maintain optimal nutritional and fluid status

Avoid placing patient in room with other potentially infectious patients

Avoid having nursing personnel with infections care for patient

Screen visitors and restrict those with potential infections or instruct to wear mask and wash hands before visiting

EXPECTED OUTCOMES

Temperature is within normal range

No other signs of infection (respiratory, renal, or skin) present

● **NDX:** Activity intolerance related to fatigue and weakness

Assess present activity level

Allow patient to ambulate and increase strength at own pace; *muscle weakness will diminish as hormonal replacement is achieved*

Assist with ambulation as needed

Assist with active or perform passive ROM exercises while patient is on bed rest *to maintain muscle tone*

Provide patient with assistive devices: walker, cane, over-the-bed trapeze, siderails *to prevent injury caused by weakness and fatigue*

Anticipate need for help with ADLs: grooming, feeding, toileting

Restrict patient's activities to level of tolerance

Discontinue activity at first signs of intolerance: tachycardia, fatigue, dyspnea, cardiac dysrhythmias, drop in BP, complaints of vertigo

EXPECTED OUTCOMES

Performs ADLs without evidence of fatigue or weakness

Vital signs remain within normal limits during ROM exercises, ambulation, and ADLs

● **NDX:** Pain related to metabolic imbalance (headache, back, extremity, abdomen)

Provide hormonal replacement (hydrocortisone, fludrocortisone) as ordered

Identify with help of patient the location, severity of pain, and factors that increase or decrease pain

Assess need for and administer pain medication as ordered

Explore with patient available measures to reduce or relieve pain: positioning, use of pillows for support, warm or cold compresses, manipulation or massage of body part or area

Monitor effectiveness of interventions at routine intervals

Provide distraction (conversation, visitors, reading materials, quiet music) *to divert attention away from pain*

Assist patient with developing pain management techniques: progressive relaxation, guided imagery

EXPECTED OUTCOMES

Patient recognizes and reports onset of pain as a sign of adrenal crisis

Reports relief of pain

Exhibits relaxed body position and facial expression

Begins using relaxation techniques

● **NDX:** Fluid volume deficit related to inability of renal tubules to retain sodium and water

Monitor serum sodium levels q8h *to recognize and treat hyponatremia*

Measure intake and output q8h and prn; be aware of risk for decreased urine volume and renal shut-down

Weigh patient daily: same time, scale, and clothing; observe for weight loss

Recognize presyncopal signs of lightheadedness, postural dizziness, and visual changes

Encourage patient *to minimize postural dizziness* by changing positions gradually

Encourage fluid intake to 2500 ml/day or as ordered

Administer IV fluids and sodium replacement as ordered *to prevent dehydration*

Assess for signs and symptoms of hypovolemia or dehydration: poor skin turgor, weak pulses, tachycardia, thirst, low BP, cool skin, increased body temperature, dry mucous membranes, change in mental status

Report occurrence of any of these signs or symptoms to physician immediately

Administer antiemetics as ordered

Provide diet high in sodium *to compensate for sodium lost in renal tubules*

EXPECTED OUTCOMES

Intake and output are balanced

Skin is moist with good turgor

Mucous membranes and tongue are moist

Weight is stable within ideal range for body build and height

Patient/family teaching

Explain basic concepts of the disease process and symptoms of recurrence requiring medication dosage adjustment

Explain reasons for physical and emotional changes

Teach name of medication, dosage, time and method of administration, side effects, and toxic effects

Explain that hormone therapy must be continued throughout lifetime

Demonstrate to patient and significant other(s) method of administering IM injections

Teach patient to practice relaxation techniques daily

Explain need to avoid persons with infectious diseases (especially URIs)

Home care considerations

Provide patient with medical alert bracelet/identification and discuss its importance

Discuss plans to carry emergency medication

Discuss methods to incorporate diet, exercise, and rest periods into lifestyle

Remind patient of the need for lifelong hormonal replacement without interruption

Patient demonstrates ability to self-inject IM (hydrocortisone) before discharge

Discuss stressful situations that may require additional steroid replacement

Infection

Fever, persistent cough, influenza, or cold

Burning on urination

Wounds that are red and swollen

Injury (auto or other accident)

Surgery

Routine dental care

Profuse sweating in hot weather or during strenuous exercise

Emotionally charged situations

Positive or negative changes in lifestyle or relationships

Instruct patient to inform all health care providers of disease

Explain need for high-sodium, low-potassium diet with plenty of fluids

Instruct that emergency IM medication must be carried at all times for use in times of stress (trauma, illness)

Explain need to avoid taking over-the-counter medications without consulting physician

Emphasize importance of regular exercise alternating with rest periods and avoiding strenuous exercise

Cushing's Syndrome (Hypercortisolism)

Results from the overproduction of cortisol by the adrenal cortex; **Cushing's disease** *is caused by the overproduction of ACTH by a pituitary adenoma. There are two categories of hypercortisolism: ACTH dependent (involving hypersecretion of ACTH by the pituitary gland) and ACTH independent (involving hypersecretion of cortisol by the adrenal glands).*

ACTH-dependent *sources include Cushing's disease, ectopic ACTH (secretion of ACTH by nonpituitary tumor), ectopic CRH syndrome (secretion of CRH by nonhypothalamic tumor)*

ACTH-independent *sources include adrenal adenoma, adrenal carcinoma, micronodular adrenal hyperplasia, and exogenous steroid abuse*

Assessment

Subjective data

Anxiety

Paranoia

Irritability

Depression

Mood swings
Memory loss
Insomnia
Decreased energy
Decreased libido
Backache
Suicidal

Objective data

Neurologic system
  Impaired cognitive function
  Lability of moods
  Panic attacks
  Agitated depression
  Increased intraocular pressure
Musculoskeletal system
  Weight gain and distribution
    Central obesity (face, neck, trunk, abdomen)
    Supraclavicular fat pads
    Dorsocervical fat pad (buffalo hump)
    Facial rounding (moon face)
    Proximal muscle wasting (thin extremities)
  Weakness: unable to rise from squat or chair without
    assistance
  Activity intolerance
  Osteoporosis
  Fractures
  Vertebral compression
Cardiovascular system
  Hypertension
  Fluid retention with pitting edema
  Dependent edema
  Vascular fragility
    Increased bruisability
    Venipuncture difficulty
    Facial plethora
  CHF
Gastrointestinal system
  Polydipsia
  Polyphagia
  Glucose intolerance
Renal system
  Polyuria
  Hypercalciuria
  Calculi
Integumentary system
  Hyperpigmentation
  Impaired wound healing
  Abdominal striae
  Thin/coarse hair
  Thin, transparent, fragile skin
  Bruises (caused by loss of connective tissue)
  Cutaneous fungal infections (nails, chest, oral)
  Acne

Reproductive/sexual system
  (Findings resulting from androgen excess)
  Hirsutism (mostly facial)
  Oily facial skin, acne
  Thinning scalp hair/temporal baldness
  Oligomenorrhea
  Decreased libido
  Impotence

Diagnostic tests

Blood
  Cortisol increased; loss of diurnal variation
  ACTH increased or decreased
  Sodium increased
  Potassium decreased
  Glucose increased
  White blood cell count (WBC) increased
  Calcium and phosphorous normal
  Metabolic alkalosis
Urine
  24 hr urinary-free cortisol increased
  24 hr 17-hydroxycorticosteroids (17-OHCS) increased
  Calcium increased
Endocrine tests
  CRH test: administration of CRH to stimulate
    hypothalamic-pituitary-adrenal (HPA) axis
    Normal response: increased ACTH and cortisol
    Cushing's disease: highly increased ACTH and cor-
      tisol
  Dexamethasone suppression test: administration of
    dexamethasone to suppress HPA axis
    Normal response: decreased ACTH and cortisol
    Cushing's disease: no change in ACTH, cortisol
  Inferior petrosal sinus sampling (IPSS): to localize
    source of ACTH secretion by comparing *central*
    ACTH levels at the petrosal sinuses (pituitary gland)
    with *peripheral* levels of ACTH (arm); comparisons
    can be made before and after administration of CRH
Imaging
  CT scans
    Sella: pituitary macroadenoma or enlarged sella
      caused by adrenal hyperplasia
    Adrenal: enlargement or tumor
  X-rays
    Skull: sellar abnormalities
    Chest: cardiomegaly
  Bone densitometry: osteoporosis
  Inferior petrosal sinus sampling (IPSS)

Potential complications

Pathologic fractures
CHF
Peptic ulcers

UTI
Renal calculi
Steroid psychosis
Suicide

Collaborative management

Therapeutic management

Transsphenoid hypophysectomy (p. 492) of pituitary
adenoma
Medications
  Adrenocorticolytic agents (chemical adrenalectomy):
    mitotane (glucocorticoid replacement essential)
  Adrenal enzyme inhibitors
    Ketaconazole
    Trilostane
    Etomidate
  Metapyrone
Adrenalectomy (p. 490)

Nursing management

PATIENT PROBLEMS/NURSING DIAGNOSES

● **NDX:** Body image disturbance related to musculoskeletal, integumentary, and sexual/repro-
ductive changes

Encourage patient/family to provide old photographs *to
assist health care givers in assessment of physical
changes related to onset of disease*
Provide information about reversibility of symptoms
with treatment
Discuss feelings related to physical changes with patient
Assist patient with identifying and developing personal
strengths and coping mechanisms *for dealing with
physical changes*
Assist with grooming *to enhance appearance:* personal hygiene, hair removal measures, attractive
clothing
Respect patient's wishes for privacy
Be sensitive to needs
Set aside time each shift for active listening *to provide
emotional support*
Consult mental health nursing specialist

EXPECTED OUTCOMES

Discusses feelings about changes in appearance
Verbalizes knowledge that reversal of symptoms will
occur with treatment
Performs daily hygiene
Enhances appearance through judicious use of cosmet-
ics and clothing if appropriate

● **NDX:** Risk for infection related to impaired immune responses

Monitor T and for other signs or symptoms of infection
q4h *to enable early recognition and treatment of
infections*
Have patient turn, cough, and deep breathe q2h while
on bed rest *to prevent respiratory infection*
Avoid unnecessary invasive procedures (urinary
catheterization)
Use sterile technique when caring for any skin lesions,
tubes, drains, or IV sites *to prevent contamination and
subsequent infection*
Obtain culture for suspicious wound sites or secretions
Maintain optimal nutritional status
Avoid placing patient in room with other potentially infectious patient *to prevent contagious infection*
Avoid having personnel with URIs or other infections
care for patient; monitor visitors for signs of infection
and restrict as needed or explain importance of handwashing and wearing mask before visit *to prevent
transmission of infection*

EXPECTED OUTCOMES

Temperature within normal limits
No evidence of infection in integumentary, respiratory,
and renal systems

● **NDX:** Risk for impaired skin integrity related to
fragile capillaries and/or thinning of skin

Exercise caution with venipuncture; apply pressure to
venipuncture sites *to prevent hematoma formation*
Assess for redness or skin breakdown q8h; if patient is
on bed rest, assess q4h
Instruct patient regarding good skin hygiene routine
  Use oil or lotion in bathwater; rinse and dry well
  Avoid use of harsh soaps or rough towels
Use elbow and heel protectors and pull sheets
Place patient on decubitus-prevention mattress or bed
Assist and encourage patient to change positions fre-
quently; teach and assist with ROM exercises; ambu-
late as soon as possible; have patient avoid sitting po-
sition for longer than 1 hr
Instruct patient to exercise caution in ADLs *to avoid mi-
nor trauma*
Keep environment clear of obstructions *to minimize po-
tential for accidental trauma*
Instruct patient to wear protective clothing (socks and
shoes) *to prevent trauma*
Maintain optimal nutritional status

EXPECTED OUTCOMES

Interruptions in skin integrity are avoided
Skin is intact and without evidence of redness
Venipuncture does not produce hematoma

● **NDX:** Activity intolerance related to musculoskeletal weakness caused by increased protein catabolism

Allow patient to move at own pace; use siderails and overhead trapeze
Identify patient's priorities for energy expenditure
Alternate activity with rest periods *to aid in increasing tolerance*
Assist with and provide aids to ambulation (walker, cane, wheelchair) as necessary
Anticipate need for help with daily activities: grooming, toileting, feeding; provide needed supplies within reach *to reduce energy expenditure*
Restrict activities to patient's level of tolerance
Discontinue activity at first signs of intolerance: tachycardia, dyspnea, fatigue
Encourage patient to increase activity as tolerance increases but to seek assistance at appearance of symptoms of intolerance

EXPECTED OUTCOMES
Increases participation in self-care and activities daily
Reports decreased feelings of weakness and fatigue

● **NDX:** Altered thought processes related to impaired cognitive functioning and memory loss from hypercortisolism

Explain to patient and family the effects of hypercortisolism on cognitive function, mood, and memory and reversibility of symptoms with treatment
Evaluate past and present coping methods
Encourage discussion of feelings of loss of control
Discuss reactions that are out of proportion to event and methods for future coping
Explain that mood swings will abate with treatment
Teach and assist with relaxation techniques
Provide a stable, calm, and nonstressful environment *to avoid impaired cognitive operations*
  Be consistent in timing and performance of activities and procedures
  Restrict visitors as necessary
  Avoid frequent changing of personnel
  Prevent emotionally upsetting situations
Plan care with patient and anticipate needs *to promote cognitive functioning*
Provide diversional activities and materials of preference
Reorient patient to environment as needed
Explain procedures slowly and clearly; repeat prn
Assist with problem solving
Be aware of suicide potential

EXPECTED OUTCOMES
Patient is alert, oriented, and not confused about activities or health care procedures

Discusses feelings easily
Acknowledges inappropriate responses to situations and discusses plan for managing response
Practices relaxation techniques
Family recognizes effect of disease on patient's thought processes

● **NDX:** Fluid volume excess related to excessive secretion of cortisol causing sodium and water retention

Monitor electrolyte values and report abnormal findings to physician *to confirm and treat early signs of fluid overload*
Monitor intake and output q8h
Weigh patient daily: same time, scale, and clothing; report increasing weight
Avoid excessive fluid intake when patient is hypernatremic
Monitor ECG for abnormalities associated with electrolyte imbalances, usually hypernatremia and hypokalemia, *to allow early recognition and treatment of imbalances*
Monitor BP, P, and breath sounds q4h and report significant changes from patient's baseline
Assess dependent areas for edema: provide support and skin care for edematous areas, turn and reposition q2h
Maintain high-protein, high-potassium, low-sodium, decreased-calorie diet

EXPECTED OUTCOMES
VS and electrolytes are within normal range for patient;
Intake and output are balanced;
Weight is stabilized and within patient's normal limits;
No evidence of edema present

ADDITIONAL NURSING DIAGNOSES TO CONSIDER
Altered nutrition: less than body requirements related to charged CHO metabolism and hyperglycemia (see Diabetes mellitus, p. 472)
Risk for trauma related to potential for pathologic fractures
Risk for injury related to potential for hypertension
Risk for injury related to suicidal tendencies

Patient/family teaching

Explain the basic concepts of hypercortisolism and signs and symptoms with emphasis on emotional and cognitive impairments
Emphasize importance of family role in recognizing emotional and cognitive impairments, appropriate interventions in decision-making process, and provision of emotional support

Discuss reversibility of signs and symptoms with treatment of disease

Explain the need for dietary restrictions related to glucose intolerance, low fat due to lipolysis, and additional protein to promote catabolism

If indicated, provide information on adrenalectomy and prepare patient as needed

If indicated, provide information on pituitary radiation therapy

If indicated, provide information on transsphenoidal hypophysectomy

Home care considerations

Explain importance of maintaining a safe environment and balancing activity and rest

Teach name of medication, dosage, time and method of administration, purpose, side effects, and toxic effects

Explain that glucocorticoids must not be discontinued or reduced without consulting physician

If glucocorticoid replacement is indicated, discuss the importance of compliance and the potential need for doubling the dosage during times of stress; see Adrenal insufficiency (p. 459)

Patient should demonstrate ability to self-inject glucocorticoid IM

Avoid taking over-the-counter medications unless physician has been consulted

Emphasize importance of ongoing outpatient care

Explain importance of maintaining safe environment and balancing activity and rest during convalescence

Discuss the need for continued emotional support during convalescence and maintenance of reasonable expectations to avoid emotional crises

Discuss the potential for suicidal tendencies with depression

Primary Aldosteronism

Overproduction of mineralocorticoids (aldosterone) by the adrenal cortex caused by benign adenoma or, less commonly, carcinoma or hyperplasia of the adrenal cortex. Excess aldosterone leads to sodium reabsorption and hypovolemia causing hypertension; can be asymptomatic with spontaneous hypokalemia. Potassium depletion can lead to muscle weakness, fatigue, and alterations in cardiac conductivity resulting in metabolic alkalosis; most common cause is adrenal adenoma.

Assessment

Subjective data

Frontal headaches
Fatigue
Paresthesia
May be asymptomatic

Objective data

Neurologic system
  Muscle weakness
  Paralysis of arms and legs
  Autonomic dysfunction
Cardiovascular system
  Hypertension
  Postural hypotension without reflex tachycardia
  Increased pulse when squatting
  Cardiomegaly
Renal system
  Polyuria, especially nocturnal
  Polydipsia

Diagnostic tests

Blood
  Potassium, decreased
  Sodium, increased
  Aldosterone, increased
  Renin, decreased
Urine: potassium, increased
  Hypervolemia
  Metabolic alkalosis
Imaging/procedures
  ECG
    Depressed ST segments and T waves; appearance of U waves
    Premature ventricular contractions
  CT scan of adrenal glands to localize an adenoma to differentiate hyperplasia from adenoma
  Adrenal venous catheterization with measurement of plasma cortisol and aldosterone to distinguish between unilateral and bilateral source of hyperaldosteronism
Endocrine tests: failure to suppress aldosterone with usual maneuvers

Potential complications

Renal failure
Heart failure

Collaborative management

Therapeutic management

Unilateral adrenalectomy for adenoma
Spironolactone for hyperplasia
Low-sodium, high-potassium diet

Nursing management

PATIENT PROBLEMS/NURSING DIAGNOSES

● **NDX:** Fluid volume excess related to hypernatremia

Weigh patient daily: same time, scale, and clothing; re-
port to physician if gain >0.5 kg occurs
Measure intake and output q8h
Maintain low-sodium diet *to decrease fluid retention*
Monitor serum sodium levels q8h
Monitor for signs and symptoms of fluid overload: pul-
monary edema (dyspnea, orthopnea, crackles in lung
fields) *to allow early recognition and treatment of
overload*
Monitor chest x-ray examination results
Monitor VS q4h and prn; observe for increased
pulse, development of S_3 gallop, and labored
respirations
Notify physician of development or worsening of any of
the preceding signs or symptoms
Monitor pedal pulses q4h
Monitor effectiveness and side effects of diuretics

EXPECTED OUTCOMES

VS and breath sounds are within normal limits for
patient
Intake and output are balanced

● **NDX:** Altered tissue perfusion: cardiopulmonary,
related to dysrhythmias caused by hypokalemia

Maintain high-potassium diet: avocado, apricots, ba-
nanas, meat, poultry, potatoes, milk
Monitor serum potassium levels q8h and prn
Monitor for signs and symptoms of hypokalemia
ECG changes (ectopic beats, decreased T wave ampli-
tude, increased U wave amplitude)
Muscular weakness
Neurologic impairments
Administer potassium supplements as ordered *to cor-
rect electrolyte imbalance*
Collaborate with physician to alter development of any
of the preceding signs or symptoms
Anticipate need for assistance with ADLs *to prevent in-
jury and fatigue*

EXPECTED OUTCOMES

Plasma potassium levels are within normal range
ECG exhibits normal sinus rhythm
Exhibits no signs of muscle weakness or paresthesia

● **NDX:** Risk for injury related to potential for muscle
weakness, paresthesia, autonomic dysfunc-
tion, and/or tetany

Assess neuromuscular function q4h to 8h; report
changes indicative of potential tetany; increasing
weakness or paresthesia
Allow patient to move at own pace; encourage use of
siderails and trapeze for assistance
Assist with and encourage ambulation if patient is able;
instruct patient to call before getting out of bed *to prevent injury*
Keep call bell within reach at all times
Provide aids to ambulation such as a walker or cane
Encourage changing positions gradually
Anticipate postural hypotension when patient gets out
of bed or chair; if it occurs, have patient sit or lie down
with head lower than heart *to promote circulation to
head and prevent a fall caused by dizziness associated
with postural hypotension*
Keep bed in low position and siderails up
Use safety measures (padded siderails for tetany; oral
airway) as needed
Remove potentially hazardous materials and objects
from patient's environment

EXPECTED OUTCOME

Patient sustains no physical injury

Patient/family teaching

Explain basic concepts of the disease; signs and symptoms of hypokalemia, hypernatremia, and hypocalcemia to report to physician
Teach name of medication, dosage, time and method of
administration, purpose, side effects, and toxic effects;
if on spironolactone teach signs of hyperkalemia to
report
Discuss and prepare for adrenalectomy if planned
Emphasize importance of regular exercise alternating
with rest periods
Discuss and provide information about therapeutic low-
sodium, high-potassium diet

Home care considerations

Discuss importance of continuing medication until
physician indicates otherwise
Explain need to avoid taking over-the-counter medications without consulting physician

Emphasize importance of ongoing outpatient care
Emphasize importance of obtaining and wearing medical alert bracelet

Pheochromocytoma

A chromaffin cell tumor of the adrenal medulla that secretes an excess of the catecholamines: epinephrine and norepinephrine; the increased catecholamines cause severe hypertension, increased metabolism, and hyperglycemia

Assessment

Subjective data

Neurologic
  Anxiety/nervousness
  Feelings of impending doom
  Tremulousness
  Headache
  Nausea
  Sweating
  Palpitations
  Insomnia
  Paresthesia

Objective data

Episodes are intermittent and frequency can vary from every 2 months to 25 times per day
Cardiovascular system
  Persistent or paroxysmal hypertension
  Tachycardia
  Palpitations
  Flushing
  Excessive diaphoresis
Respiratory system: tachypnea
GI/nutritional system
  Hyperglycemia
  Vomiting
  Weight loss, occasionally gain
Renal system: decreased urine output
Integumentary system: sweating (excessive and inappropriate)
Precipitating risk factors
  Postural change
  Exercise
  Laughing
  Smoking
  Urination
  Change in body or environmental temperature
  Vasovagal stimulus
  Any event that increases pressure on tumor (pregnancy)

Diagnostic tests

Blood
  Serum catecholamines elevated
  Hyperglycemia
Urine: elevated urine metanephrines and/or normetanephrines
Imaging: abdominal CT scan or MRI showing tumor location
Endocrine tests: clonidine suppression test—failure of serum catecholamines to "suppress" after clonidine administration

Potential complications

Heart failure
Renal failure
Cerebrovascular accident (CVA)
Myocarditis
Dysrhythmias
Surgical morbidity or mortality

Collaborative management

Therapeutic management

Surgical removal of the tumor(s)
Medications
  α- and β-adrenergic blockers
  α-methylparatyrosine
  Catecholamine synthesis inhibitors

Nursing management

PATIENT PROBLEMS/NURSING DIAGNOSES

● **NDX:** Altered tissue perfusion: cardiopulmonary and renal related to hypertensive episodes caused by hypervolemia from excess catecholamines

Remain with patient during episodes of hypertension
  Monitor BP and pulse electronically q10min to 15min; use same arm consistently
  Be prepared to administer antihypertensive medications
  Position patient with head of bed elevated 30 degrees to minimize effects on ICP
  Perform neurologic checks; auscultate chest for heart sounds, rate, and rhythm
  Monitor breath sounds; observe for dyspnea
  Measure urinary output qh; report if <30 ml/hr
  Provide a calm, low-stimulus atmosphere
Monitor orthostatic VS; report if difference >10 mm Hg
Monitor intake and output q8h

Review events occurring before episode *to determine etiology;* discuss methods of avoiding precipitating events, if present, with patient

Keep bed dry and wrinkle-free if patient is diaphoretic

Provide quiet environment for adequate periods of rest

To minimize risk of hypertensive crisis:

  Do not palpate abdomen

  Avoid constrictive clothing

  Restrict activity

  Prohibit tobacco use

  Elevate head of bed

  Avoid Valsalva maneuver

  Identify and avoid factors that trigger hypertensive episodes

EXPECTED OUTCOMES

Orthostatic vital signs are within normal limits

Intake and output are balanced with output >30 ml/hr

Verbalizes no palpitation, nervousness, or headache

● **NDX:** Sleep pattern disturbance related to increased levels of circulating catecholamines

Assess usual sleep pattern and use of any aids

Provide sleep aids requested by patient: quiet music, warm drink

Discourage frequent daytime sleeping *to support regular sleep pattern at night*

Avoid intake of stimulants in diet

Assist patient with establishing a regular pattern of activity

Provide environment conducive to sleep: reduce lighting; close door to room; maintain quiet and privacy

Avoid disturbing patient at night for unnecessary procedures

Schedule treatments, procedures, and medications for daytime and evening hours when possible *to support regular sleep periods*

EXPECTED OUTCOMES

Reports feeling well rested after sleep

Maintains energy throughout day without need for naps

● **NDX:** Altered nutrition: less than body requirements related to increased metabolism and/or nausea

Assess nutritional status and food preferences

Assist patient to select daily menus and incorporate basic food groups *to promote appropriate dietary intake*

Provide several small meals if patient prefers

Ask patient's family to bring favorite foods from home, within limits of therapeutic diet

Assist patient with arranging meal tray and feeding if necessary

Provide dietary consultation *to reduce tyramine-containing foods in diet*

Monitor blood glucose; report if elevated

Monitor food intake daily

Weigh patient daily: same time, scale, and clothing

EXPECTED OUTCOME

Weight is increasing toward level required for body build and height

Patient/family teaching

Explain basic concepts of the disease process and potential risk factors

Discuss methods for avoiding hypertensive episodes

Provide written information about diet and reduction of tyramine-containing foods

Teach name of medication, dosage, time and method of administration, purpose, side effects, and toxic effects

Refer to Adrenalectomy (p. 490) for preoperative patient teaching if indicated

Home care considerations

Explain need to avoid taking over-the-counter medications without consulting physician

Emphasize importance of ongoing outpatient care

Provide information for obtaining medical alert bracelet and card

Hypopituitarism

Decreased or absent secretion of one or more of the anterior pituitary gland hormones; causes are varied and may include malignancies, other tumors, infection, vascular changes, or physical injury such as head trauma; hypopituitarism may be a disorder of the pituitary gland itself or may be caused by insufficient pituitary stimulation by the hypothalamus

Assessment*

Subjective data

Decreased libido

Weakness

Objective data

General

  Wrinkled, waxy skin

  Hypothermia

---

*Assessment depends on which hormonal deficiencies are present.

Low BP
Low serum glucose
Gonadotropin deficiency
  Incomplete secondary sex characteristics
  Impotence, infertility
  Loss of muscle tone
TSH deficiency: see Hypothyroidism (p. 448);
  symptoms will be less severe
ACTH deficiency
  See Adrenocortical insufficiency (p. 459)
  No hyperpigmentation
  No sodium depletion
Growth hormone deficiency
  Short stature
  Lack of development of secondary sex characteristics
  High-pitched voice
Prolactin deficiency: absence of lactation in postpartum
  women

Diagnostic tests

Deficiency of serum cortisol, thyroxine, testosterone,
  estrogen, and growth hormone
Lack of compensatory increased levels of serum
  ACTH, TSH, FSH, and LH
Endocrine studies: IGF-1, decreased
Imaging
  X-rays: Skull—sellar changes
  CT scan or MRI of head

Potential complications

Deficiencies are usually not severe (see specific disease entities)

Collaborative management

Therapeutic management

Hormone replacement
  Glucocorticoids
  Thyroxine
  Gonadal steroids
  Growth hormone in children
  Gonadotropin or GnRH therapy to restore fertility

Nursing management

PATIENT PROBLEMS/NURSING DIAGNOSES

● **NDX:** Body image disturbance related to changes
  in physical characteristics and capabilities

Encourage verbalization by patient of feelings related to
  physical changes

Assist patient with developing coping mechanisms *to
  deal with changes*
Reinforce patient's qualities that have positive effect on
  self-image
Answer questions and clarify misunderstandings regarding diagnosis and permanence or regression of
  changes
Assist patient with developing a plan *to incorporate any
  permanent changes into lifestyle*
Demonstrate acceptance of patient and encourage others to do the same
Reinforce behaviors that demonstrate acceptance of
  changes

EXPECTED OUTCOMES
Verbalizes feelings about physical changes to
  others
Discusses strengths and sets realistic goals

● **NDX:** Altered sexuality patterns related to hormonal deficiencies

Maintain privacy and confidentiality
Explore with patient and/or significant other usual patterns of sexuality and how current diagnosis may affect these patterns
Encourage patient and/or significant other to explore
  alternatives to usual patterns that consider limitations
  of the disease
Initiate referral to appropriate personnel if patient
  desires
Explore with patient and/or significant other alternatives to becoming parents if appropriate

EXPECTED OUTCOMES
Begins to discuss feelings about sexuality with partner
Verbalizes understanding of effect of diagnosis on sex-
  ual patterns
Accepts referral for counseling

Patient/family teaching

Provide and discuss information*
  Basic concepts of the disease process
  Name of medication, dosage, time and method of ad-
    ministration, purpose, side effects, and toxic effects

Home care considerations

Explain importance of the following:
  Regular outpatient follow-up
  Need to avoid taking over-the-counter medications
    without consulting physician

*For further interventions, refer to specific disease entity.

Importance of discussing feelings regarding body changes with significant other

Provide referral for sexual counseling when appropriate

Discuss alternatives to usual sexual patterns

Diabetes Insipidus

Disorder of hypothalamus or posterior pituitary that results in insufficient synthesis or secretion of vasopressin (antidiuretic hormone); consequently, the renal mechanism for concentration of urine is impaired and large amounts of dilute urine are excreted; causes may include head injury, neurosurgery, and hypothalamic tumors

Assessment

Subjective data

Unquenchable thirst
Preference for ice water

Objective data

Gastrointestinal system
  Polydipsia
  Weight loss
  Dehydration
  Constipation
Renal system
  Polyuria to 10 L daily
  Frequency
  Nocturia
Integumentary system
  Dry skin and mucous membranes
  Poor turgor

Diagnostic tests

Blood
  Serum osmolality >300 mmol/kg
  Increased sodium
Urine
  Specific gravity ≤1.005
  Osmolality ≤200 mmol/kg
Endocrine tests
  Dehydration test: water deprivation with close observation, paired measurements of serum and urine osmolality, and body weight measurements
  Normal response: urine becomes concentrated
  Central DI: urine remains dilute
  Nephrogenic DI: urine remains dilute

Psychogenic polydipsia: urine becomes concentrated (response may be slight if polydipsia is severe)
Dehydration followed by vasopressin administration:
  Normal response: slight increase in urine concentration
  Central DI: urine becomes concentrated
  Nephrogenic DI: no change
  Psychogenic polydipsia: urine becomes concentrated
Imaging/other tests
  CT scan of head: hypothalamic/pituitary lesions
  Visual field testing: defects related to hypothalamic/pituitary lesions

Potential complications

Severe dehydration
Hypotension
Shock

Collaborative management

Therapeutic management

Vasopressin: lysine vasopressin nasal spray
DDAVP (desmopressin acetate)

Nursing management

PATIENT PROBLEM/NURSING DIAGNOSIS

● **NDX:**   Fluid volume deficit related to inability of renal tubules to concentrate urine in absence of vasopressin

Provide sufficient fluid of patient's preference *to maintain equal intake and output for 24 hr*
Supplement oral intake with IV fluids as ordered
Monitor intake and output q2h; notify physician if output is >200 ml/hr and urine specific gravity is <1.005
Weigh patient daily *to assess fluid loss*
Check urine and plasma osmolality daily
Assess for signs and symptoms of dehydration: tachycardia, poor skin turgor, weak pulses, low BP, cool skin, increased body temperature, dry mucous membranes, changes in mental status, and weight loss
Report occurrence of any of preceding signs or symptoms to physician and initiate medical orders without delay
Administer vasopressin replacement therapy as ordered and monitor effectiveness
  Observe for side effects: hypertension, chest pain, uterine cramps, and increased peristalsis
  Monitor for overhydration: headache, changes in LOC, confusion
  Report abnormal findings

Monitor for hypoglycemia if taking chlorpropamide; give rapid-acting carbohydrates if symptoms present; report to physician

EXPECTED OUTCOMES

Intake and output are balanced
Intake is ≤2500 ml/day
Output is ≤100 ml/hr
Urine specific gravity is within normal limits
Skin is moist with good turgor
Weight is within patient's normal range
VS are within normal limits

Patient/family teaching

Explain basic concepts of disease process
Teach name of medication, purpose, time and method of administration, dosage, side effects, and toxic effects
  Demonstrate how to administer vasopressin; discuss special considerations related to intranasal administration
  Explain need to monitor for side effects and report if present
  Demonstrate how to monitor urine specific gravity and measure intake and output
  Discuss parameters for as-needed administration based on urine output
  Instruct to weigh daily; report loss or gain (symptoms of recurrence or fluid retention) indicating change needed in medication dosage
  Demonstrate injection method if medication is to be taken IM
Emphasize importance of maintaining fluid intake equal to output
Explain need to avoid liquids that may cause a diuretic effect: coffee, alcohol, tea
Provide information to obtain medical alert bracelet and card

Home care considerations

Emphasize importance of medical alert bracelet
Emphasize importance of monitoring output
Ensure understanding related to intranasal administration of DDAVP
Emphasize importance of regular outpatient follow-up
Explain need to avoid taking over-the-counter medications without consulting physician

Diabetes Mellitus

Diabetes mellitus is a disorder of hyperglycemia caused by inadequate insulin; cases of extreme insulin defi-ciency can lead to diabetic ketoacidosis; diabetes is characterized by polyuria, polyphagia, polydipsia, and weight loss accompanied by an elevation in plasma glucose

insulin-dependent diabetes mellitus (IDDM): *Deficiency of insulin production requiring exogenous administration of insulin to prevent acidosis (β-cell function is impaired)*

non–insulin-dependent diabetes mellitus (NIDDM): *Caused by a combination of insulin resistance and β-cell dysfunction*

Type I is used to describe diabetes resulting from autoimmune *destruction of beta cells; type II describes* nonautoimmune *forms of diabetes mellitus*

Assessment

Subjective data

Hunger
Thirst
Nausea
Headaches
Halos seen around lights

Objective data

GI system
  Polyphagia
  Polydipsia
  Weight loss
  Obesity
Renal system
  Polyuria
  Glycosuria
  Frequency
  Nocturia
Neurologic system
  Numbness and tingling of lower extremities
  Decreased sensations of pain and temperature in distal extremities
  Blurred vision
  Cataracts
Cardiovascular system
  Cold extremities
  Weak pedal pulse
Integumentary system
  Shiny skin and atrophic
  Hair loss on feet/toes
  Infections/ulcerations
  Dermopathy
Reproductive/sexual system
  Impotence
  Vaginal discharge
  Susceptibility to vaginal infections

Collaborative management

Therapeutic management
See Table 7-2
Nutritional therapy and education

Nursing management

PATIENT PROBLEMS/NURSING DIAGNOSES

● **NDX:** Fluid volume deficit related to absent or deficient insulin function

Assess VS q4h to 8h
Monitor intake and output q8h; check urine for ketones *as indicator of hyperglycemia*
Assess skin turgor, moisture and condition of mucous membranes q4h to 8h
Assess mental status
Monitor blood glucose before administration of insulin or oral hypoglycemics and meals, and/or according to a predetermined schedule, usually q4h initially
Begin teaching self-blood glucose monitoring (p. 478) *to promote self-care*
Monitor effectiveness of administration of insulin: usually rapid-acting ordered initially, then intermediate-acting in split doses with or without addition of rapid-acting (type 1); may need to use 70/30 insulin if patient has difficulty mixing the two different types of insulin
Monitor effectiveness of oral hypoglycemics if ordered for NIDDM
Assess for continuing signs of hyperglycemia (see Assessment, p. 472 and 474)
Assess for signs of hypoglycemia; blood glucose ≤60 mg/dl, dizziness, lightheadedness, tachycardia, sweating, shakiness, or altered LOC
Provide noncaloric fluids (as well as those allowed on ADA diet) to 2500 ml/day *to replace fluid loss from polyuria*
Monitor electrolyte and CO_2 laboratory values *for metabolic imbalance and acidosis*
Assess for disturbances in electrolyes and CO_2 (See Table 1-3, p. 68); be aware of potassium shift as fluid volume deficit improves
Assist with ADLs when patient is unable to complete because of weakness or malaise
Encourage self-care as condition improves

EXPECTED OUTCOMES

VS are stable and within normal limits for patient
Intake and output are balanced
Ketones are not present in urine; skin is moist with good turgor

Blood sugar, electrolytes, and CO_2 are within normal range
Patient completes ADLs without expression of fatigue or weakness

● **NDX:** Altered nutrition: less than body requirements related to diabetes mellitus, generally IDDM

Assess dietary intake pattern, preferences, and nutritional status
Provide dietary consultation *to instruct patient and family on ADA diet*
Assist patient to select daily menu based on ADA program prescribed; reinforce correct choices
Monitor daily food intake; assist at mealtimes when necessary because of fatigue; provide exchanges for foods not taken at mealtimes
Provide relaxing environment and allow ample time for meals; visiting by support person may be helpful
Stress importance of regular meal and snack times, eating all foods and snacks provided or exchanging; remind not to save exchanges for another meal
Collaborate with physician *to determine exercise program to meet patient's needs and lifestyle*
Begin first phase of program
Assist patient to check need for additional carbohydrates before exercise through use of self-blood glucose monitoring (Table 7-3)
Weigh patient daily: same time, scale, and clothing
Monitor blood glucose control
Monitor compliance with diabetes treatment regimen

EXPECTED OUTCOMES

Maintains stable weight or increases weight to that predetermined for body build
Selects menus based on ordered ADA diet and eats meals and snacks as scheduled
Monitors blood glucose
Determines type of snack and takes snack only if needed before exercise

● **NDX:** Altered nutrition: more than body requirements related to diabetes mellitus, usually NIDDM

Assess baseline nutritional status: height, weight, activity level, eating patterns and preferences, psychosocial concerns related to overeating
Teach relationship of obesity to diabetes
Provide dietary consultation for calculation of caloric requirements and instruction of ordered ADA diet
Assist to select daily menu based on low-calorie, low-fat, ADA diet; reinforce correct choices; encourage

Table 7-2 Two Major Classifications of Diabetes Mellitus

	Insulin-Dependent Diabetes Mellitus (IDDM)	Non–Insulin-Dependent Diabetes Mellitus (NIDDM)
DEFINITION		
Onset	<30 yr	>40 yr
Etiology	Postulated that beta cell destruction occurs resulting from infection (usually viral) and/or autoimmune response in genetically disposed persons	Interaction between heredity and environmental factors such as obesity, diet, and lifestyle is postulated
Insulin	Low	Normal or high
ASSESSMENT		
Observation/findings	Polyuria Polydipsia Polyphagia Weakness Fatigue Malaise Weight loss Irritability See Diabetic ketoacidosis (DKA) (p. 481)	Fatigue Polyuria Polydipsia Vision changes Tingling, numbness of extremities Slow healing of cuts Skin infections or pruritis Drowsiness See Hyperosmolar hyperglycemic nonketotic coma (HHNC) (p. 485)
DIAGNOSTIC TESTS		
Blood: fasting glucose	>140 mg/dl	>140 mg/dl
Oral glucose tolerance (first 2 hr)	>200 mg/dl	>200 mg/dl
Blood insulin level	Trace to absent	Normal to high
Serum osmolality	>300 mosm/kg	>300 mosm/kg
Plasma insulin	Absent	Low, normal, or high
Plasma pro-insulin	Not applicable absent to low	Low, normal, or high
Plasma C-peptide	Absent	Low, normal, or high
Urine: ketonuria	Usually present	Usually absent
COMPLICATIONS		
Acute	Diabetic ketoacidosis (DKA)	Hyperosmolar hyperglycemic nonketotic coma (HHNC)

Long term	Microangiopathies
	  Retinopathy
	  Nephropathy
	  Neuropathy
	Macroangiopathies
	  Cardiovascular
	  Cerebrovascular
	  Peripheral vascular
		Microangiopathies
		  Retinopathy
		  Nephropathy
		  Neuropathy
		Macroangiopathies
		  Cardiovascular
		  Cerebrovascular
		  Peripheral vascular

Table 7-2 Two Major Classifications of Diabetes Mellitus—cont'd

Insulin-Dependent Diabetes Mellitus (IDDM)	Non–Insulin-Dependent Diabetes Mellitus (NIDDM)
THERAPEUTIC MANAGEMENT	
Insulin preparations: rapid-acting, intermediate-acting, usually in split doses Diet, usually ADA exchange (usually three balanced meals and three snacks) Regular exercise program Self-blood glucose monitoring Treatment of existing complications	Diet, usually ADA exchange with decreased calories (usually three balanced meals and one high-protein snack) Oral hypoglycemic and/or insulin Regular exercise program Self-blood glucose monitoring Treatment of existing complications

patient to include foods high in complex carbohydrates (may assist in weight reduction)

Assess daily food intake; replace foods not eaten

Weigh patient daily: same time, scale, and clothing; give positive reinforcement for any weight reduction

Monitor blood glucose before meals and at bedtime or before bedtime snack

Collaborate with physician to determine exercise program to meet patient's needs and lifestyle; begin first phase of program

Discuss need to monitor dietary intake and exercise level using a diary *to increase accuracy*

Explore with patient ways to increase activity in daily routine and add exercise program

Refer to diabetic and/or weight reduction support group *to provide additional support and guidance*

EXPECTED OUTCOMES

Verbalizes understanding of relationship of obesity to diabetes

Selects meals and snacks based on ADA and/or decreased caloric guidelines

Takes all foods at mealtimes and snacks

Monitors blood glucose as scheduled

Keeps diary of dietary intake and exercise level

Identifies persons to use for support in making lifestyle changes

● **NDX:** Risk for impaired skin integrity related to reduced circulation and sensation in distal extremities

Instruct patient on risks of injury and potential for poor wound healing

Minimize environmental hazards

Keep skin clean and dry; encourage patient to inspect skin regularly

Observe for early signs and symptoms of infection

Emphasize importance of foot care

Encourage measures to increase circulation to extremities

EXPECTED OUTCOMES

Verbalizes understanding of risks and measures to avoid injury

Practices routine skin and foot care

Recognizes and reports early signs of skin lesions and infections

ADDITIONAL NURSING DIAGNOSES TO CONSIDER

Altered tissue perfusion: peripheral, cardiopulmonary, cerebral, or renal related to microangiopathy or macroangiopathy

Sensory/perceptual alterations: visual related to retinopathy

Sexual dysfunction related to neuropathy

Risk for infection related to hyperglycemia

Noncompliance with therapeutic plan related to difficulty of integration of therapy into lifestyle

Altered urinary elimination related to nephropathy

Patient/family teaching

Disease process

Explain diabetes mellitus specific to patient's type

Discuss control of disease through managing interrelationship among diet, maintenance of ideal weight, exercise program, medication if ordered, and blood sugar changes

Table 7-3 Before Exercise Snacks

Exercise	Blood Sugar Levels	Snack
SHORT WORKOUT		
Easy pace	less than 100	1 fruit or
Examples: 15 min		1 bread or
slow walk		4 oz milk
easy swim		
stretching	more than 100	no food needed
MODERATE WORKOUT		
Moderate pace	less than 100	1 meat, 1 bread,
Examples: 25-40 min		and 1 fruit
brisk walk		
stationary bike	100-160	1 milk, 1 fruit,
heavy housework		or 1 bread
aerobics class	161-300	no food needed
LONG WORKOUT		
Hard pace	less than 100	1 meat, 2 breads,
Examples: 1 hour		and 1 milk or
shoveling snow		1 fruit
skiing		
	100-160	1 meat, 1 bread,
		and 1 milk or
		1 fruit
	161-225	1 milk and 1 bread
	226-300	1 milk or 1 bread

More food may need to be added than is given here if patient works out 2 to 4 hr after taking short-acting insulin. In 2 to 4 hr this type of insulin peaks, and blood sugar can drop very quickly. Always carry carbohydrate snacks during exercise.

Prevention of complications

Acute
  Hypoglycemia (p. 486)
  Diabetic ketoacidosis (DKA) (p. 481)
Long term
  Microangiopathies, macroangiopathies
    Stress that maintaining control of blood glucose may decrease the risk of or minimize these complications
    Discuss need to do the following:
      Have regular medical follow-ups to check for early symptoms of complications: cardiovascular, peripheral, renal, neural, or visual
      Visit ophthalmologist, dentist, and podiatrist regularly
      Maintain control of BP and cholesterol
      Stop smoking and/or drinking alcoholic beverages
      Follow prescribed diet, exercise program; take medications; follow personal hygiene guidelines; and consult physician at first appearance of symptoms
    Teach symptoms of long-term complications to report to physician

Diet therapy

Reinforce explanation of prescribed ADA and/or calorie-reduction diet
Assist with setting realistic goals for weight reduction
Have patient and/or significant other calculate dietary needs and choose a sample diet, cutting down on foods with high cholesterol, saturated fats, salt, sugar, and alcohol
Discuss need to eat meals and snacks at regularly scheduled times every day
Stress need to determine additional food requirements before exercise by use of self-blood glucose monitoring; give samples to calculate snacks required
Stress that diet may be the only means of control for patients with NIDDM
Provide written material, names of personnel, and telephone numbers for questions and assistance with meal planning

Exercise

Discuss need for exercise program: positive effect on blood glucose control increases optimal functioning of body
Collaborate with physician and patient to plan program of progressive exercise based on patient's interest and physical condition
  Give details specifying exercise type, intensity, frequency, duration, warm-up and cool-down time
  Teach pulse-taking to monitor target HR during exercise
Explain need to exercise 1 to 2 hr after meal and how to adjust dietary intake as required
  Avoid exercise at peak insulin times
  Check blood glucose before and 30 min after exercise

Medications

  INSULIN
Provide information to patient and/or significant other about insulin
  Action of the type(s) of insulin to be used
  Time of day patient may expect to have reaction (peak action time; Table 7-4)
  Factors that precipitate hypoglycemia reaction

Table 7-4 Action of Insulin

Type	Company, Product	Species Source	Onset of Action (hours)	Peak of Action (hours)	Duration of Action (hours)
CONVENTIONAL INSULINS					
Regular	Lilly (Iletin I)	B-P*	½	2-4	6-8
	NovoNordisk	Pork	½	2½-5	6-8
Semilente	Lilly (Iletin I)	B-P	1-2	3-8	10-16
	NovoNordisk	Beef	½-1	5-10	12-16
NPH (Isophane)	Lilly (Iletin I)	B-P	1-2	6-12	18-26
	NovoNordisk	Beef	1-1½	4-12	24
Lente	Lilly (Iletin I)	B-P	1-3	6-12	18-26
	NovoNordisk	Beef	1-1½	7-15	24
Protamine zinc	Lilly (Iletin I)	B-P	4-6	12-24	26-36
	NovoNordisk	Beef	4-8	14-20	36
Ultralente	Lilly (Iletin I)	B-P	4-6	14-24	28-36
	NovoNordisk	Beef	4-8	10-30	36
PURIFIED INSULINS†					
Regular	Lilly (Iletin II)	Beef or pork	½	2-4	6-8
	NovoNordisk (Velosulin)	Pork	½	1-3	8
	NovoNordisk (Actrapid)	Pork	½	2½-5	8
Semilente	NovoNordisk (Semitard)	Pork	½-1	5-10	16
NPH (Isophane)	Lilly (Iletin II)	Beef or pork	1-2	6-12	18-26
			1-3	6-12	24-28
	NovoNordisk (Insulatard)	Pork	1½	4-12	24
	NovoNordisk (Protaphane)	Pork	1½	4-12	24
Lente	Lilly (Iletin II)	Beef or pork	1-3	6-12	18-26
	NovoNordisk (Monotard)	Pork	2½	7-15	22
	NovoNordisk (Lentard)	B-P	2½	7-15	24
Protamine zinc	Lilly (Iletin II)	Beef or pork	4-6	14-24	26-36
Ultralente	NovoNordisk (Ultratard)	Beef	4	10-30	36
Biphasic (30% regular, 70% NPH)	NovoNordisk (Mixtard)	Pork	½	4-8	24
HUMAN INSULINS					
Regular	Lilly (Humulin-R)	Bacteria	½	2-4	6-8
	NovoNordisk (Novolin-R)	Semisynthetic	½	2½-5	6-8
NPH (Isophane)	Lilly (Humulin-N)	Bacteria	1-2	6-12	18-24
	NovoNordisk (Novolin-N)	Semisynthetic	1½	4-12	24
Lente	Lilly (Humulin-L)				
	NovoNordisk (Novolin-L)	Semisynthetic	2½	7-15	24
Biphasic (30% regular, 70% NPH)	NovoNordisk 70/30	Semisynthetic	½	6-12	24

*B-P, mixed beef and pork insulin.
†The Food and Drug Administration recommends that purified insulins be used for all patients, and human insulins be considered for new patients.

Incorrect, increased dosage of insulin

Altered routine in mealtimes or exercise without planning

Stress

Other disease processes

Cold

Influenza

Nausea, vomiting

Infection

Dosage may be adjusted according to blood test results as ordered by physician

Provide information about care of insulin and equipment

Keep opened insulin vial currently in use at room temperature and away from sunlight; keep no longer than 2 months or expiration date

Have at least one unopened vial stored in refrigerator, not in freezer

Observe expiration dates

Be sure units marked on syringe are understood; ½ ml or ³⁄₁₀ ml syringes are in increments of 1 unit/line; 1 ml syringes are in increments of 2 units per line, 2 ml syringes in increments of 5 units/line

Handle syringe and needles carefully to avoid self-puncture

Maintain sterility of needle and syringe during procedure

Dispose of syringe and needle in safe container after use

Discuss use of special equipment for patients with vision problems or other handicaps

Provide instructions for preparing injection

Mix insulin by gently rolling bottle between hands; do not shake vigorously

Clean bottle top with alcohol

Read label and check expiration date

Insert air and withdraw exact dose

Withdraw rapid-acting insulin first if mixing two types of insulin (avoids contaminating rapid-acting with longer-acting insulin)

Read label again and check dosage

Discuss information about injection site with patient and significant other

Most rapid absorption occurs in abdomen, arms, and thighs

Importance of rotating site of injection with each dose of insulin to prevent atrophy, fibrosis, lipodystrophy, and decreased insulin absorption

Rotation within one body area (e.g., abdomen) may be recommended to ensure same length of absorption time

Need to avoid injection into extremities just before exercise

Need to use each site only once each month (Figure 7-2)

Need to record site used for each injection by location and number

Have patient and/or significant other demonstrate injection technique

Select site for injection

Clean skin with alcohol

Allow to air dry to prevent irritation

Hold syringe filled with correct insulin dosage as one would hold a pencil or a dart

Insert needle at 90-degree angle (45 degree if little subcutaneous tissue) and quickly push into tissue up to hub of needle

Withdraw plunger to check for entry into blood vessel; if blood returns, withdraw syringe and start procedure over

Inject medication

Withdraw needle and hold alcohol swab on area for a few seconds; do not rub

Record date and time given, type of insulin, dosage, and site of injection in diary

ORAL HYPOGLYCEMICS

Provide information about medications when ordered: action and dosage (Table 7-5)

Monitor blood glucose level at specific times; usually four times/day until effective dosage achieved; then two to three times/week with a complete profile one to two times/month (before and after meals, at bedtime, and once during night)

Take exact dosage before meal(s)

Observe for hypoglycemic reactions (p. 486); take 10 g carbohydrate (CHO) (p. 487) at first sign of reaction to raise blood glucose level in 10 to 15 min; then take longer-acting CHO to offset recurrence

Discuss other side or toxic effects to report to physician or nurse if they last longer than 24 to 48 hr

GI upset

Weakness

Paresthesia

Headache

Tinnitus

Skin rash

Jaundice

Photosensitivity

Intolerance to alcohol

Prolonged action of sedatives and hypnotics

Discuss planning for pregnancy with physician; notify immediately if pregnancy is suspected; oral hypoglycemic agents need to be stopped before pregnancy occurs and another regimen instituted in collaboration with physician

Self-blood glucose monitoring and urine testing

Give reasons for testing blood glucose

Maintain control of blood sugar

Reduce risk of complications

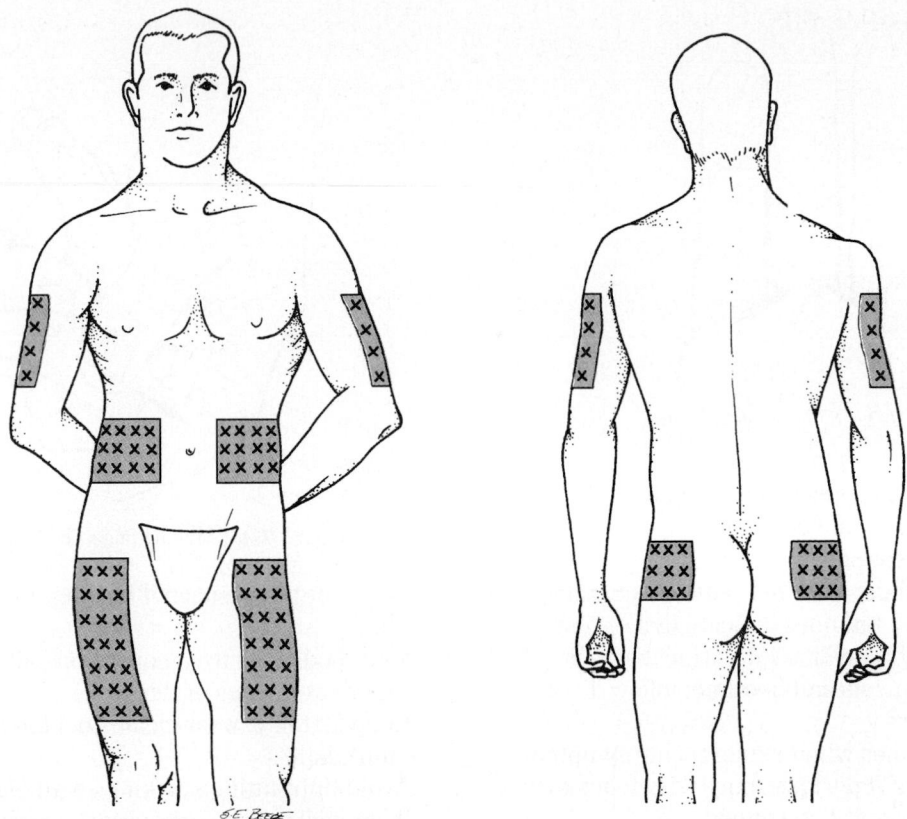

Figure 7-2   Rotation of insulin injection sites.

Table 7-5   Oral Hypoglycemics

Drug	Dosage Range (mg/day)	Onset (hr)	Duration (hr)	Serum Half-Life (hr)
Tolazamide	100-1000	4-6	10-18	7
Tolbutamide	250-3000	1	6-12	4-5
Acetohexamide	250-1500	1	8-24	6-8
Chlorpropamide	100-500	1	24-72	36
Glyburide	1.25-20	24	16-24	7-10
Glipizide	2.5-40	1-1.5	6-24	2-7

Instruct about blood glucose test
  Frequency of testing: usually before meals and exercise, 30 min after exercise, and to monitor any symptoms of hypoglycemia or hyperglycemia
  Need to rotate sites of finger punctures
    Use only sides of fingertips; produces less discomfort
    Use at least six sites on each finger (Figure 7-3)
    Advise that thumb and ring finger may have better blood flow
  Methods to increase blood flow

  Place hand in warm water for a few minutes
  Hold hand below heart level and "milk" finger (Figure 7-4)
Avoid using alcohol or povidone-iodine to clean finger because these products can interfere with test results
Need to wash, rinse, and dry hands well before beginning procedure
Procedure for using lancet and finger puncture device
Procedure to use and read reagent strips or use automated equipment

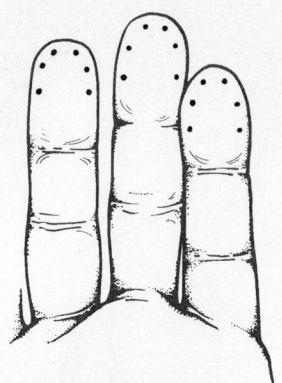

Figure 7-3 Finger puncture sites.

Care and storage of supplies and equipment
Disposal of lancets in safe container
Teach about urine testing
  Urine testing for sugar does not indicate amount of
    sugar in the blood but does indicate that excess
    sugar from blood is spilling into urine; ketones
  Test urine before meals and bedtime; follow direc-
    tions on container
  Test urine for ketones when experiencing symptoms
    of hyperglycemia; report presence of ketones to
    physician or follow predetermined plan
  Store urine testing supplies in dry, cool, dark area
    away from oral medications and children
  Record test results in diary; note any medications
    taken because some give false readings; e.g., sa-
    licylates or ascorbic acid give false-positive read-
    ings
Explain changes to make in diet, exercise, or medica-
  tion as a result of blood glucose or urine test as deter-
  mined through collaboration with physician
Discuss need to maintain diary to record
  Blood glucose/urine test
  Medication and dosage
  Exercise level
  Symptoms and interventions taken
  Missed meals or unusual situations

Personal care and hygiene

SKIN, FOOT, AND LEG CARE
Provide information about daily care
  Bathe daily using tepid water; check water tempera-
    ture with thermometer, especially when bathing feet
  Rinse and dry gently but thoroughly
  Apply lubricating lotion; do not leave skin wet
  Inspect body, especially feet, legs, and groin area
    daily; use mirror if unable to see any body part, e.g.,
    bottoms of feet
  Check for cuts, cracks, blisters, corns, boils, calluses,
    or ingrown toenails; if found, wash with mild soap
    and water, dry well, and cover with dry, sterile dress-

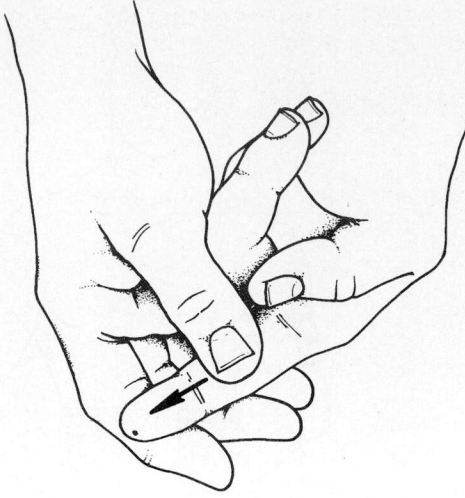

Figure 7-4 Milking finger to obtain blood sample.

ing; notify physician if healing does not begin in 24
  hr
Have podiatrist treat corns and calluses; do not use
  home remedies or devices
Keep feet dry; wear clean stockings (preferably cotton) daily
Avoid tight-fitting stockings with elastic
Wear well-fitting shoes; break in new shoes gradually;
  alternate two pairs of shoes; do not go barefoot
Exercise feet throughout the day; curl toes, rotate ankles, bend and stretch knees and hips; avoid one position for long periods; walk in place if standing,
  stand and walk if sitting
Do not use hot water bottles or heating pads on extremities
Wear protective clothing for warmth or sunshielding
Use sunscreen, at least SPF 15, daily
Use gloves when exposed to harsh soaps, gardening, using an oven, or handling heavy, rough
  objects
Be cautious when using machinery, tools, and equipment

CARE OF TEETH
Brush teeth or clean dentures after sleep and meals
  and before bedtime
Floss at least daily
Examine mouth for irritated gums, bleeding, or ulcers;
  report those that do not begin to heal in 24 hr
Schedule periodic dental examinations (usually every 6
  months)
Tell dentist about condition and check with primary
  physician before scheduling extensive dental care or
  surgery

CARE OF EYES
Explain that eye changes (vision) may be temporary if
  blood sugar is high

Schedule yearly examinations with an ophthalmologist; more often if vision changes are noted

URINARY AND GENITAL CARE

Drink six to eight glasses of water/day
Avoid urinary tract or vaginal infections
Avoid fluids with caffeine or alcohol
Urinate as soon as urge is felt
Wash and dry genital area daily
  Inspect for irritation and discharge
  Shower rather than take tub baths
    Wear underwear and/or pantyhose with cotton crotch
    Avoid douching except as ordered by physician
  Report to physician if following symptoms occur
    Urinary tract
      Difficulty in voiding
      Burning or pain on voiding
      Incontinence
    Vagina
      Heavy discharge
      Itching

Sick day rules

Explain that any illness, injury, or change in body functioning causes an increased need for glucose, which the body will automatically produce
Advise that a change in medication and food usually is required during these periods
Discuss signs and symptoms of illness, injury, or functional change that *may* require changes in medication or food
  Injuries
  Infections, including cold or influenza
  Nausea, vomiting
  Diarrhea
  Burns
  Dental care
  Surgery
  Pregnancy
  Emotional stress
  Unaccustomed physical activities: periodic jogging, swimming, tennis
Instruct to increase testing of blood glucose and urine ketones to every 4 hr or at least four times/day during this period
Explain importance of notifying physician when
  Blood glucose is 300 mg/dl or urine test results are 1% with or without ketones two successive times
  Experiencing an inability to take oral food/fluids
  Experiencing unusual thirst, increased urination, weakness, warm/flushed skin, blurred vision, or nausea and vomiting

Explain need to have blood or urine glucose and urine ketone record sheet nearby to report to physician when experiencing symptoms of high blood glucose
Instruct about action to take
  Drink a cup or more of broth, tea, nondietetic carbonated drinks, gelatin, or fluids with electrolytes
  Take insulin based on test results or discussion with physician

Travel tips

Discuss need to prepare for travel
  Inform physician
  Obtain immunizations well before trip when needed
  Have generic prescriptions in duplicate for
    Diabetic medications
    Syringes and needles
    Other medications needed
  Carry letter describing condition and treatment (in language of country visiting if possible)
  Buy and break in new shoes well in advance
  Obtain medical identification bracelet or necklace if patient normally carries a card
  Arrange for special meals while enroute
  Importance of carrying supply of insulin and syringes in hand luggage to prevent exposure to extreme temperature and prevent loss
  Need to take supply of emergency medication to prevent or treat possible travel complications
  Importance of carrying emergency carbohydrates and a meal
  Method to alter meal, medication, and activity needs when traveling to other time zones to maintain schedule
  Where to obtain emergency assistance and how to express needs in language of country visited*
  Importance of traveling with a companion when possible

Diabetic Ketoacidosis

Acute complication of diabetes mellitus, characterized by marked hyperglycemia, metabolic acidosis, increased plasma ketones, and severe dehydration

Assessment

See Table 7-6

*International Association for Medical Assistance to Travellers Directory of English Speaking Physicians Throughout the World, 417 Center St., Lewiston, NY 14092; (716) 754-4883.

Table 7-6 Comparison of Diabetic Ketoacidosis (DKA), Hyperosmolar Hyperglycemic Nonketotic Coma (HHNC), and Hypoglycemia

Assessment	Observations/Findings		
	DKA	**HHNC**	**Hypoglycemia**
Diabetes type	Usually IDDM	Usually NIDDM	IDDM, NIDDM, Dietary-related
Onset	Hours to days	Hours to days	Minutes to 1 hr
Renal	Polyuria; osmotic diuresis	Polyuria; osmotic diuresis	
	Dehydration	Dehydration	
Neurologic	Lethargy, drowsiness	Unconsciousness (50%)	Inability to concentrate
			Headache
	Paresthesia	Drowsiness	Lack of coordination
	Slowed reflexes	Confusion, disorientation	Numbness, tingling lips, tongue
	Confusion, disorientation	Seizures	Weakness; anxiety
		Hemiplegia (reversible)	Yawning, slurred speech
	Coma	Coma	Hyperreflexia, seizure activity
			Nighttime: nightmares, sleepwalking, restlessness
Respiratory	Tachypnea, Kussmaul's respiration	Tachypnea with shallow respiration	
	Sweet, fruity breath		
Cardiovascular	Hypotension	Orthostatic hypotension	Tachycardia
	Tachycardia	Tachycardia	Cool, clammy skin
	Weak pulses	Weak pulses	
	Warm to hot, dry, flushed skin	Warm to hot, dry, flushed skin	
	Decreased turgor	Decreased turgor	
		Hypothermia	
GI	Polydypsia	Polydypsia	Hunger
	Nausea, vomiting	Gastric distention	Nausea
	Abdominal pain	Hematemesis	
Risk factors	Undiagnosed IDDM	Undiagnosed NIDDM	Excessive insulin dosage, missed meal(s)
	Insufficient insulin dosage	Insufficient oral hypoglycemic agent	Unplanned increase in exercise program
	Stressors: surgery, injury, infection	Stressors: surgery, injury, infections	Vomiting
			Alcohol intake
	Sudden decrease in exercise program	Sudden decrease in exercise program	Drug interactions
	Pregnancy	High-protein, high-calorie enteral or parenteral feedings	Pregnancy
		Drug toxicities	
		Dialysis	
		Alcohol intake	
		Pregnancy	

Table 7-6 Comparison of Diabetic Ketoacidosis (DKA), Hyperosmolar Hyperglycemic Nonketotic Coma (HHNC), and Hypoglycemia—cont'd

	Observations/Findings		
Assessment	**DKA**	**HHNC**	**Hypoglycemia**
DIAGNOSTIC TESTS			
Blood:			
Serum glucose	200-800 mg/dl	800-2000 ml/dl	<60 mg/dl
Serum ketones	Elevated	Normal to slightly elevated	
Serum osmololity	300-350 mosm/L	>350 mosm/L	
pH	<7.38	7.30-7.42	
Sodium	<137	Elevated, normal, or low	
BUN	Elevated	Elevated	
Potassium	Normal or elevated then decreased	Normal or <3.5 mEq/L	
Urine:			
Urine acetone	Positive	Negative	Negative
POTENTIAL COMPLICATIONS			
	Shock	Thromboembolism	Seizure
	Renal failure	Shock	Shock
	Death occurs if untreated	Seizures	Delirium
		Coma	Coma
		Death occurs if untreated	Permanent brain damage
			Death occurs if untreated

Collaborative Management

Therapeutic management

Regular insulin IV bolus or continuous drip (5 to 10 units/hr)

Rapid IV hydration: 1 L/hr (approximately 6 L); normal saline initially, then as serum glucose decreases, glucose is added to infusion

IV potassium replacement as indicated

CVP

ABG

Monitor ECG

Insulin subcutaneously

Treatment of infection if underlying cause

Nursing management

PATIENT PROBLEMS/NURSING DIAGNOSES

● **NDX:** Fluid volume deficit related to osmotic diuresis

Monitor IV fluids; maintain large-bore IV *for rapid infusion*

Administer plasma expanders as ordered

Monitor BP, P, T, R q15min to 30min until stable for 1 hr then q½h until reactive and blood glucose controlled; then q4h to 8h

Assess for signs and symptoms of hypovolemic shock continuously, which include tachycardia; low BP; weak, thready pulses; cool skin; increased body temperature; change in LOC

Administer insulin; usually given IV initially

Rinse container and tubing with insulin per facility policy before adding prescribed dose *because insulin adheres to equipment and correct dosage may not be given*

Note that smaller doses are required for HHNC than for DKA

Assess effectiveness; report glucose level that continues to rise, falls too rapidly, or is 120 mg/dl or lower

Measure capillary blood glucose qh

Measure urine ketones qh in DKA

Monitor ECG for changes; report signs of hyperkalemia or hypokalemia

Monitor electrolyte and ABG levels; report changes and collaborate with physician *to adjust fluids, electrolytes, and HCO₃*

Monitor CVP if inserted

Insert nasogastric tube as indicated; monitor gastric drainage

Insert indwelling urinary catheter to straight drainage *for exact assessment of output*

    Monitor intake and output qh and report output <30 ml/hr

    Assess skin temperature, turgor, and capillary refill q2h

EXPECTED OUTCOMES

Patient's vital signs are stable

Intake and output are balanced

Skin turgor is good

Electrolytes are within normal range

Blood glucose is within patient's normal range

● **NDX:** Risk for injury related to confusion or seizures

Assess for presence of neurologic/sensory deficits and respiratory status q4h

Maintain oral airway at bedside

Keep bed in low position with padded siderails in up position when patient is on bed rest

Remove potentially hazardous materials from patient's immediate environment *to protect from injury*

Place articles frequently required within easy reach

Instruct patient to call for assistance before getting out of bed

Keep call light within patient's reach at all times

Be aware that patient's vision may be affected: assist with feeding, personal hygiene, and ambulation as needed

Maintain orientation to environment: assess LOC and orientation q4h and prn

Provide stimulation in the environment *that will assist in maintaining orientation:* pictures from home, calendar, clock, radio, television

Address patient by name; review day, date, time, and current events with patient as necessary

EXPECTED OUTCOMES

Patient sustains no physical injuries

Patient remains alert and oriented to time, place, and person

● **NDX:** Risk for infection related to increased susceptibility caused by hyperglycemia and protein depletion

Monitor for signs of infection q4h to 8h

    Sites of invasive lines

    Skin

    Respiratory and urinary systems

Maintain sterility of invasive sites (e.g., IV, catheters) *to avoid introducing infection;* provide meticulous, sterile daily care and rotate sites according to policy

Obtain culture for suspicious drainage *to identify source of infection and provide early treatment*

Teach and assist patient to turn, cough, and deep breathe q2h *to prevent respiratory infections*

Provide oral fluids to 2000 ml/day when allowed

Provide oral care q4h to 6h

Use aids *to promote circulation and prevent skin breakdown* when on bed rest

EXPECTED OUTCOMES

Temperature is within normal range

Cultures show no evidence of infection

Lungs and urine are clear

Skin is dry and clear with good turgor

● **NDX:** Altered nutrition: less than body requirements related to deficiency of effective insulin

Assess diet and fluid intake before DKA

Provide ADA diet and fluids as prescribed

Maintain food diary when necessary *to assist patient in determining intake*

Weigh patient daily: same time, scale, and clothing

Administer insulin; assess effectiveness by monitoring blood glucose; collaborate with physician to adjust medication dosage as necessary

Determine possible factors leading to DKA episode

    Not taking insulin

    Not observing diet

    Reduction in level of exercise

    Infection, stress, injury

EXPECTED OUTCOMES

Weight is stable or increasing toward predetermined level for patient's build

Blood glucose level is WNL

Patient/family teaching

Explain factors that predispose patient to ketoacidosis: increased food intake, omitted doses of insulin, failure to respond to increased need for insulin resulting from infectious process, decreased activity/exercise, stress, or pregnancy

Discuss early signs of DKA
Blood glucose 300 mg/dl or more
Ketones in urine
Unusual thirst
Increased urination
Hot, dry, flushed skin
Elevated temperature
Drowsiness
Nausea, vomiting, abdominal pain, diarrhea

Home care considerations

Teach action to take when early signs of DKA are noted
Continue diet and fluids; take broth or tea if unable to tolerate food
Have patient take insulin as scheduled or change dosage as indicated by tests, with physician approval, using algorithms
Test urine for presence of ketones
Notify physician if signs of DKA persist
Increase frequency of blood glucose testing when glucose >280 mg/dl
Assess knowledge of diabetes mellitus and management through patient's maintenance of ADA diet, exercise program, diabetic medication schedule, and blood glucose monitoring
See Diabetes mellitus (p. 472)

Hyperosmolar Hyperglycemic Nonketotic Coma

Metabolic disorder in which the blood sugar level is extremely elevated, increasing the serum osmolality and resulting in hypertonic dehydration; serum ketosis is usually not present

Assessment

See Table 7-6

Collaborative management

Therapeutic management

IV insulin administration
IV fluid administration, plasma expanders as needed
Electrolyte replacement as needed
Electrolyte, blood glucose, and bicarbonate levels
ABG
Monitor ECG

CVP
Insulin subcutaneously and/or oral hypoglycemics

Nursing management

See Diabetic ketoacidosis for the following diagnoses (p. 481):
Fluid volume deficit related to osmotic diuresis
Risk for injury related to confusion and/or seizures
Risk for infection related to increased susceptibility resulting from hyperglycemia and protein depletion
Altered nutrition: less than body requirements related to deficiency of effective insulin
See Diabetes mellitus for altered nutrition: more than body requirements related to diabetes mellitus usually NIDDM (p. 473)

PATIENT PROBLEM/NURSING DIAGNOSIS

● **NDX:** Altered tissue perfusion: peripheral, cerebral, cardiopulmonary related to risk of thromboembolism

Assess peripheral pulses q2h to 4h; report decreased amplitude or absence
Assess for thrombosis in extremities: vein—pain, swelling, tenderness, or Homan's sign; artery—mottling, cyanosis, coolness with delayed capillary refill
Teach active or assist with passive ROM exercises for extremities
Apply thromboembolic or pneumatic alternating-pressure stockings to lower extremities; remove daily, check condition of legs, then reapply
Assess VS, heart and breath sounds, and neurologic status q2h to 4h
Assist patient to assume position *to enhance cardiopulmonary effort*
Instruct patient to report sudden headache, chest pain, numbness in extremities

EXPECTED OUTCOMES

Vital signs are stable and within normal limits
Patient reports no headache, chest pain, numbness, or pain in extremities and is alert and oriented

Patient/family teaching

Explain factors that predispose to HHNC
Not taking oral hypoglycemic or insulin dosage
Sudden decrease in exercise program
Stressors: surgery, dental care, infections
Increase in food intake
Pregnancy
Review symptoms of HHNC; see Assessment, Table 7-6

Home care considerations

Assess knowledge of diabetes mellitus management including patient maintenance of ADA diet, adherence to exercise program, monitoring blood glucose, and taking of medications; see Diabetes mellitus (p. 472)

Teach action to take when signs of HHNC are noticed

Continue diet and fluids; take broth or tea if unable to tolerate food

Increase frequency of blood glucose monitoring

Take oral hypoglycemic as scheduled or change dosage as indicated by tests, with physician approval, using algorithm

Explain that insulin may be required during these situations

Notify physician if no improvement occurs

Hypoglycemia

An abnormally low serum glucose level, usually 60 mg/dl or less, caused by administration of too much insulin, excessive secretion of insulin by islet cells of pancreas, or dietary deficiency

Assessment

See Table 7-6

Collaborative management

Therapeutic management

10g fast-acting oral CHO
50% glucose IV bolus
IV fluids $D_{10}W$
Dietitian consultation

Nursing management

PATIENT PROBLEMS/NURSING DIAGNOSES

● **NDX:**   Risk for injury related to insufficient glucose to meet metabolic needs

Hypoglycemia *requires immediate intervention to prevent brain damage and death*

Obtain blood glucose stat and be prepared to administer 50% glucose IV if patient is a diabetic and is comatose; then initiate IV of $D_{10}W$ if prescribed *or*

Obtain capillary blood glucose and give 10 g of fast-acting CHO if patient is exhibiting early signs of hypoglycemia

Continue to monitor blood glucose q15min to 30min; slow-acting CHO may be needed *to prevent recurrence of symptoms*

Determine predisposing factor if possible
Decreased food intake
Increased exercise
Wrong medication, dosage
Consult physician, if no predisposing factor determined, for adjustment of insulin or oral hypoglycemic dosage
Monitor neurologic and cardiovascular status q30min until fully reactive

EXPECTED OUTCOMES

Blood glucose WNL after ingestion of CHO or IV glucose
VS are stable
Patient is alert and oriented

● **NDX:**   Risk for trauma related to rapid onset of altered LOC and seizure activity resulting from hypoglycemia

Keep oral airway and suction equipment at bedside
Pad siderails if patient is on bed rest *to prevent trauma* in the event of seizure activity
Assist to floor if patient is out of bed and remove hazardous objects *to reduce potential for trauma*
Note time, frequency, LOC, body parts involved, and length of seizure activity
Obtain stat blood glucose and administer IV glucose as ordered
Notify physician of seizure
Suction oropharynx as needed *to prevent aspiration*
Assess for injury
Check pulse and pupils
Reorient as necessary
Determine predisposing factor for hypoglycemia

EXPECTED OUTCOME

Patient is free of injury

Patient/family teaching

Involve significant other and/or peers from work setting in teaching because patient may not be able to intervene
Teach factors that may precipitate hypoglycemia: too much insulin or oral hypoglycemic medication, increased length of time between meals, omission of a meal or snack, unplanned exercise, extremely stressful situation

Home care considerations

Discuss symptoms of hypoglycemia
Mild: shaky, sweaty, cool feeling, irritable, weak, headache, nervous, drowsy, or personality changes

Moderate: nausea, faintness, disorientation, confusion
Severe: coma, seizure
Explain that hypoglycemic reactions may be different for each person; any unusual feeling or symptom must be considered; each patient must become familiar with initial reactions
Identify the time reactions will most likely occur; relate to type of insulin prescribed (see Table 7-4)
Teach action to take immediately: take 10 g of quick-acting carbohydrate
Avoid driving or any activities requiring clear thought processes and decision making
The following foods contain 10 g of quick-acting carbohydrate (CHO):

Orange juice	4 oz
Apple juice	4 oz
Grape juice	2 oz
Coca-Cola	3 oz
Ginger ale	4 oz
7-up	3 oz
Corn syrup	2 tsp
Honey	2 tsp
Granulated sugar	2½ tsp
Grape jam	2 tsp
Animal crackers	4
Space Food Stix	1
Gumdrops	10 small
Jelly beans	6
Hard candy such as Life Savers	5 or 6
Dextrose wafers or tablets as labeled	
Glucose paste, amount indicated on label	

Emphasize importance of always carrying fast-acting sugar in same pocket and keeping juice or other drink in same container in same place in refrigerator for easy, quick accessibility
Check blood glucose 15 min after taking quick-acting CHO; then take slowly digested carbohydrate such as milk, cottage cheese, bread, or peanut butter after response to fast-acting carbohydrate to offset a secondary reaction, if needed
Demonstrate method for glucagon administration to significant other; discuss action and dosage
Use if patient clamps mouth shut, is unable to swallow, or is unconscious; patient should respond in 5 to 15 min
Have patient eat slowly digested carbohydrate after responding
Follow physician's orders if no response
Telephone physician if further orders are not indicated
Give another injection of glucagon if ordered
Telephone for emergency help or take patient to emergency room of hospital
Demonstrate alternate method of glucagon therapy: oral glucose in tube; squeeze directly between cheek and gum area

Explain need to observe closely for further reaction for 1 to 1½ hr; avoid strenuous activity during this time
Determine predisposing factor after reaction is controlled
Emphasize importance of reporting frequent reactions to physician as directed
Give time of onset and duration until response to care
Discuss predisposing factor if known
Discuss prevention and early care
Always carry some form of quick-acting carbohydrate (see list); take when first symptoms appear
Eat correct diet regularly; remember between-meal nourishment when included in diet
Test blood regularly for glucose; anticipate probable reactions
Be aware of greater-than-normal activity or emotional stress; follow physician's directions to either notify physician, increase food intake, or decrease dosage of insulin
Discuss prevention of dosage errors
Check dosage of insulin or oral hypoglycemic with another person when possible
Record medication when it is taken to prevent duplication
Always wear medical alert band or chain and carry diabetic identification card
Determine ability to manage diabetes mellitus

Thyroidectomy

Surgical removal of part (subtotal thyroidectomy) or all of the thyroid gland to treat hyperthyroidism (Graves' disease, toxic adenoma, nodules, carcinoma); usually reserved for patient who does not respond to medical treatment with antithyroid drugs; treatment of choice to remove very large goiters or those compressing surrounding structures; may also be performed for men and women of child-bearing age for whom radiation exposure is unwanted, patients allergic to antithyroid medications, and pregnant women

Preoperative assessment

Assess baseline vital signs
Assess voice quality and ability to swallow

Postoperative assessment

Subjective data

Hypocalcemia
Numbness
Tingling

Incisional pain
  Intensity
  Location
Choking sensation
Dysphagia
Complaints of heaviness or fullness in throat
Complaints of tight dressing

Objective data

Increasing hoarseness
Change in tone or pitch of voice
Weak voice, inability to speak
Hypocalcemia
  Twitching
  Spasm, tetany
  Positive Chvostek's or Trousseau's sign
Incision site
  Color (redness)
  Pain: guarding of site
  Swelling
  Drainage, bleeding
Airway
  Stridorous respirations
  Retraction of neck muscles
  Cyanosis

Diagnostic tests

Blood
  Serum: total and free T_3 and T_4
  Calcium levels

Potential complications

Airway obstruction
Hemorrhage
Paralysis of recurrent laryngeal nerves
Hypothyroidism
Hypocalcemia; tetany

Collaborative management

Therapeutic management

IV fluids progressing to regular diet
Treatment of complications
Pain management including throat spray or lozenges
Incentive spirometer

Nursing management

PATIENT PROBLEMS/NURSING DIAGNOSES

● **NDX:**   Decreased cardiac output related to risk for hemorrhage

Monitor VS, LOC, orientation
Check dressing site every 10 for profuse bleeding (side of neck and back of head) *to identify signs of bleeding*
Keep dressing size minimized *to prevent impaired view of incision site*

EXPECTED OUTCOMES
Patient's vital signs are within normal limits
There is no evidence of hemorrhage

● **NDX:**   Ineffective airway clearance related to bleeding and/or laryngeal edema

Position patient on back with head of bed elevated 30 to 45 degrees *to promote ease in breathing*
Monitor for signs of respiratory distress or obstructed airway qh *to identify early signs of respiratory distress caused by tracheal edema:* stridor, wheezing, coarse airway crackles, dyspnea, cyanosis, labored respirations
Teach and assist patient to turn, cough, and deep breathe q2h and prn *to prevent pulmonary complications*
Keep suction equipment at bedside; gently suction oropharynx only when necessary
Have tracheostomy tray and oxygen immediately available *to use if patient experiences severe respiratory distress*
Notify physician if dressing requires reinforcement more than one time

EXPECTED OUTCOMES
Respirations and breath sounds are within patient's normal limits
No bleeding is present at surgical site

● **NDX:**   Risk for injury (tetany) related to hypocalcemia caused by parathyroid suppression or removal

Evaluate reflexes q4h to 8h; report neuromuscular irritability *to aid in early recognition and treatment of hypocalcemia*
Monitor calcium levels *to watch for hypocalcemia*
Maintain quiet environment with bed in low position and siderails padded *to prevent injury*
Collaborate with physician in treating symptoms of tetany: calcium and vitamin D supplementation

EXPECTED OUTCOME
Patient exhibits normal reflexes

● **NDX:**   Risk for infection related to invasive surgical procedure

Monitor VS and breath sounds q4h to 8h

Change dressing daily and prn when wet; observe for signs and symptoms of infection or impaired healing: redness, swelling, foul drainage, fever

Promote incision healing: prevent stress on suture line, cleanse site daily as ordered, and apply dry, sterile dressing

Use only necessary dressing and tape *to allow visibility of tissue around surgical sign* (edema, redness); remove tape toward incision *to prevent stress on suture line and possible interruption of wound healing*

EXPECTED OUTCOMES

Incision is dry and clean

VS are stable

Lungs are clear

● **NDX:** Impaired verbal communication related to damage and/or manipulation of laryngeal nerves

Monitor voice quality q2h *to evaluate damage to laryngeal nerves*

Monitor for edema at surgical incision and glottis

Discourage talking for first 48 hr *to prevent vocal cord edema*

Reassure patient that voice should return to normal after a few days

Provide alternate means of communication (e.g., pad and pencil or Magnadoodle)

Keep call bell within reach at all times

Report increasing hoarseness to physician

Anticipate patient's needs *to minimize patient's need to speak*

EXPECTED OUTCOMES

Uses alternate communication methods for 48 hr postoperatively

Communicates verbally without voice change

Has no edema at incision

● **NDX:** Pain related to surgical incision

Assess patient for verbal and nonverbal signs of pain

Have patient use pain rating scale *to indicate intensity of pain*

Discuss with patient factors that increase or relieve pain

Assist patient with finding physical position of comfort

Prevent tension on suture line; use pillows *to maintain head alignment;* use sandbags if pillows are insufficient

Prevent flexion or extension of head and neck *to prevent strain on sutures*

Teach patient to keep head in a neutral position

Instruct patient to use hands to support head during movement

Assist patient with using distraction *to control pain:* guided imagery, progressive relaxation, soft music, reading, visitors

Monitor effectiveness of pain medications

Administer analgesic throat spray or lozenges as ordered and as patient desires *to minimize pain*

EXPECTED OUTCOMES

Expresses feeling of well-being and comfort

Posture and face are relaxed

Patient/family teaching

Preoperative

Teach patient to support neck with towel to prevent strain on sutures and incision

Explain importance of not speaking postoperatively to prevent edema

Obtain pad and pencil for communicating postoperatively

Teach patient to turn and deep breathe; include use of incentive spirometer

Explain that hoarseness will subside after 4 to 5 days

Discuss pain management, use of pain rating scale

Reinforce physician's explanation of procedure; clarify any misconceptions; allow time for questions

Postoperative

Teach care of surgical incision

Emphasize importance of supporting incision until healed

Teach prescribed head and neck exercises: flexion, lateral movement, and hyperextension

Discuss symptoms of recurrent hyperthyroidism, hypothyroidism, or hypocalcemia to report to physician

Discuss symptoms of wound infection to report to physician

Emphasize importance of rest and relaxation

Home care considerations

Discuss with patient and family the importance of outpatient care and follow-up

Teach name of medication, purpose, time and method of administration, dosage, side effects, and toxic effects

Explain need to avoid taking over-the-counter medications without consulting physician

Manage stressful situations and emotional outbursts with stress management techniques

Discuss proper nutrition and fluid intake

Parathyroidectomy

Surgical removal of the parathyroid glands; if surgery is performed for adenoma, total removal of all involved glands is done; if the cause of hyperparathyroidism is hyperplasia, three total glands are removed and three

fourths of the fourth gland is removed, leaving sufficient gland to prevent hypocalcemia in most patients

Postoperative assessment

Subjective data

Pain: location, intensity
Choking sensation
Heavy/full feeling in throat
Tingling
Paresthesia (numbness)

Objective data

Signs and symptoms of hypocalcemia
  Stiffness
  Cramping
  Tremor
  Tetany
Respiratory system
  Hoarseness
  Laryngeal stridor
  Cyanosis
Incision site
  Redness
  Swelling
  Drainage
  Bleeding
  Dysphagia

Diagnostic tests

Blood
  Serum calcium
  Serum phosphorus
  Electrolytes

Potential complications

Hemorrhage
Hypocalcemia: seizures, tetany
Respiratory arrest

Collaborative management

Therapeutic management

IV fluids, progressing to diet as tolerated
Treatment of complications
Pain management

Nursing management

See Thyroidectomy (p. 487)

PATIENT PROBLEM/NURSING DIAGNOSIS

● **NDX:**   Altered nutrition: related to less than body requirements (hypocalcemia)

Assess Chvostek's and Trousseau's signs *to identify evidence of hypocalcemia*
Keep high-calcium snacks available to patient at all times *to treat symptoms of hypocalcemia*
Keep emergency calcium replacement available
Assess electrolytes *to monitor for fluctuations in calcium level*

  EXPECTED OUTCOME
Patient maintains adequate nutrition and appropriate calcium levels

Adrenalectomy

Surgical removal of the adrenal gland(s): unilateral removal is often indicated for treatment of benign adrenal adenomas or pheochromocytoma; bilateral adrenalectomy may be needed to treat ectopic ACTH-producing tumors or adrenal carcinoma.

Preoperative assessment and care

Assess baseline VS to determine control of predisposing disease factors (e.g., hypertension in pheochromocytoma or primary aldosteronism)
If scheduled for bilateral removal, explain that patient must take cortisone preparation throughout life; if unilateral, for only 6 months to 2 years
Monitor blood glucose for control of hyperglycemia
Teach patient to turn, cough, and deep breathe
Encourage questions and discussion of fears and anxiety
Administer preoperative steroid

Postoperative assessment

Subjective data

Pain
Restlessness

Objective data

Signs of adrenal crisis (p. 460)
  Falling BP
  Tachycardia; weak, thready pulses
  Elevated temperature
  Profound weakness
  Lethargy

Hypoglycemia
Electrolyte imbalance
Seizures
Dehydration
Flatulence
Site of incision
　Redness
　Swelling
　Drainage, bleeding
　Impaired healing
Respiratory distress
　Decreased breath sounds
　Tachypnea, bradypnea

Diagnostic tests

Decreased serum cortisol levels
Decreased serum aldosterone levels
Hyperglycemia
Hyperkalemia

Potential complications

Renal dysfunction
Atelectasis
Adrenal crisis
Coma
Cardiac arrest

Collaborative management

Therapeutic management

IV fluids progressing to regular diet when bowel
　sounds return
Incentive spirometer
Treatment of complications
Pain management

Nursing management

PATIENT PROBLEMS/NURSING DIAGNOSES

● **NDX:**　Risk for injury related to potential for adrenal
　　crisis

Administer IV fluids, vasopressors, and corticosteroids
　as ordered; assess effectiveness
Monitor cardiovascular, neurologic, respiratory, and re-
　nal function q4h
　Assess VS q4h and prn; report abnormal findings to
　　physician
　Monitor neurologic status q4h; report increasing
　　headache and confusion *to assess immediacy of risk
　　for injury*

Monitor cardiac rhythm continuously if dysrhythmias
　occur *because of electrolyte imbalances*
Monitor intake and output q4h and prn; report output
　that is greater than intake
Position patient to promote cardiovascular and respira-
　tory function

EXPECTED OUTCOMES
VS are stable and within patient's normal range
Intake and output are balanced
Patient is alert and oriented when reactive

● **NDX:**　Pain related to surgery (surgical incision)

Assess for verbal and nonverbal signs of pain; use pain
　rating scale
Administer pain medications and assess effectiveness
Discuss with patient factors that increase or decrease
　pain to identify those that can be used to reduce per-
　ception of pain
Assist patient with finding position of comfort
Assist patient with using distraction *to control pain:*
　guided imagery, progressive relaxation, soft music,
　visitors
Maintain support of surgical incision during movement
　or ambulation *to minimize tension at incisional site*
Increase ambulation as tolerated

EXPECTED OUTCOMES
Appears calm/relaxed
States pain is at tolerable level or absent
Uses learned pain control techniques

● **NDX:**　Risk for infection related to surgical incision
　　and abnormal cortisol levels

Change dressing daily and when wet; observe for signs
　of infection, impaired healing, dehiscence, redness,
　swelling, foul drainage, fever
Culture suspicious drainage *to identify any source of
　infection*
Promote incisional healing/avoid infection
　Prevent stress on suture line
　Remove sutures when ordered
　Use dry, sterile dressing when changing
　Use only necessary amount of tape and remove in di-
　　rection of incision
　Cleanse site daily
　Instruct patient to avoid touching incision site
Avoid unnecessary invasive procedures *to prevent po-
　tential for infection*
Assist patient to turn, cough, and deep breathe q2h
Monitor for signs of URI and UTI
Screen personnel and visitors for infections; restrict if
　present

EXPECTED OUTCOMES

Temperature is within normal range
Breath sounds are clear
Incision is healing
Urine is clear

● **NDX:**   Risk for fluid volume deficit related to unstable levels of circulating steroids

Maintain IV fluids to 2500 ml/day
Monitor serum electrolytes q8h and prn
Calculate intake and output q4h to 8h; report intake less than output
Weigh patient daily; observe for weight loss
Administer sodium replacement as ordered in diet or IV fluids if NPO *to maintain fluid volume*
Assess for signs and symptoms of fluid/electrolyte imbalance: poor skin turgor, weak pulses, tachycardia, thirst, low BP, cool skin, cardiac dysrhythmias, increased body temperature, change in mental status
Report any of the preceding signs or symptoms to physician without delay and carry out medical orders received
Check blood sugar via fingerstick q8h

EXPECTED OUTCOMES

Intake and output are balanced
Weight is stable
Skin is warm and moist with good turgor
VS are stable
Blood glucose is WNL

Patient/family teaching

Discuss symptoms of adrenal crisis to report
Emphasize importance of reporting risk factors to physician immediately for medication adjustment (increase steroids)
  Infection: fever, cold, influenza, persistent cough, burning on urination, wounds that do not heal
  Injury, surgery, dental care
  Profuse sweating
  Strenuous, unusual activity
  Emotionally charged events
  Infections, no matter how minor
Explain need to avoid persons with infections, especially URIs *to avoid contracting contagious diseases while immunosuppressed*
Teach name of medications, dosage, time and method of administration, side effects, and toxic effects
Demonstrate IM injection method to patient and significant other
Explain that if bilateral adrenalectomy was performed, steroid therapy will be needed for remainder of life

Teach care of incision and to report signs of infection
Emphasize importance of the following:
  Adequate rest
  Moderate exercise
  Good nutrition
Explain that if surgery was for Cushing's syndrome, symptoms of hypercortisolism will slowly recede

Home care considerations

Patient demonstrates ability to give IM self-injection
Emphasize importance of carrying injectable cortisol for administration in emergency
Patient and family understand situations that can require administration of additional steroids (see Adrenal insufficiency, p. 459)
Discuss importance of ongoing outpatient care and informing all physicians, dentists, other health care providers of surgery and prescribed medications
Emphasize importance of wearing medical alert band or chain and carrying identification card

Hypophysectomy

Surgical removal of pituitary gland to remove pituitary adenomas, craniopharyngiomas, and as palliative therapy in certain types of metastatic breast and prostate cancer; surgery is usually performed via transsphenoidal approach; often the treatment of choice for Cushing's disease

Preoperative assessment and teaching

Assess for upper airway infection (colds, sinus infection), report if present (surgery will be delayed)
Discuss and teach postoperative care and rationale
  Nasal packing
  Graft site, usually thigh
  Need for mouth breathing because of nasal packing
  No toothbrushing (oral hygiene by rinsing)
  Avoid coughing, sneezing, or noseblowing
  Decreased senses of smell and taste
Encourage questions
  Reinforce physician's explanation of procedure
  Allow time for discussion of fears and anxiety

Postoperative assessment

Subjective data

Pain
  Location
  Intensity

Objective data

Signs and symptoms of increased intracranial pressure
(ICP)
Increasing restlessness
Decreasing LOC
Unequal pupils
Visual changes
Widened pulse pressure
Bradycardia
Respiratory arrest
Gumline incision
Redness
Swelling
Edema
Drainage or bleeding
Nasal packing
Intact
CSF drainage (may be postnasal drip): frequent swallowing, coughing
Bleeding
Patent airway
Thigh, graft site
Redness
Swelling
Drainage

Diagnostic tests

Hormone levels
Electrolyte levels
Glucose levels

Potential complications

Cerebrospinal rhinorrhea
Diabetes insipidus (p. 471)
Meningitis
Hemorrhage
Adrenal crisis (p. 460)
Severe hypoglycemia (p. 486)
Decreased levels of pituitary hormones
(gonadotropins)

Collaborative management

Therapeutic management

Indwelling catheter
Incentive spirometer
Monitor intake and output
IV fluids progressing to oral diet
Treatment of complications
Pain management

Nursing management

PATIENT PROBLEMS/NURSING DIAGNOSES

● **NDX:** Risk for injury, related to potential for intracranial pressure

Assess for signs and symptoms of increased ICP qh for
first 24 hr, then q4h; check neurologic and vital signs
Notify physician at once if onset of restlessness or if
pupillary or VS change
Maintain head of bed elevated 30 degrees *to promote
circulation*
Avoid turning, extending, and flexing head for first 24 hr
Avoid having patient cough vigorously or use other Valsalva maneuvers for any reason *to prevent disruption
of graft;* use stool softeners if needed
Maintain calm, dimly lit environment *to prevent stimulation*
Pace care *to avoid excessive stimulation;* allow adequate
undisturbed rest periods

EXPECTED OUTCOMES
VS are WNL
Remains alert, oriented, with reactive pupils
Has no cough

● **NDX:** Ineffective airway clearance related to nasal
packing, postnasal drip, and/or dry oropharynx

Elevate head of bed 30 degrees *to avoid pressure at surgical site*
Assess for intactness of nasal packing q2h; determine
whether packing is slipping posteriorly
Patient must maintain mouth breathing; maintain oral
mucous membranes in moist condition
Provide oral care with saline solution or diluted mouthwash q2h and prn
Supply humidity to room or via face mask if necessary
Keep suction at bedside; gently suction oropharynx
only when absolutely necessary
Remind patient to deep breathe and turn q2h, *to avoid
forceful coughing*
Monitor for signs of respiratory distress: stridor,
wheezing, labored respirations, cyanosis
Check dressing and oropharynx for bleeding or CSF
leakage q2h to 4h prn

EXPECTED OUTCOMES
Breath sounds, respiratory rate and rhythm are within
normal limits
Nasal packing is intact without bleeding or postnasal
drip
Mucous membranes are moist
Color is good

● **NDX:** Risk for infection related to disruption in dura mater

Monitor incision *for signs and symptoms of infection* q4h
Evaluate drainage for CSF leakage (positive glucose reagent strip); report immediately
Assess for early signs of meningitis: chills, fever, malaise, headache, vomiting, nuchal rigidity; report immediately
Do not use toothbrush until incision is healed
Avoid foods that could irritate incision
Instruct patient not to touch dressing or packing; use sterile technique to change mustache pad each time it becomes damp

EXPECTED OUTCOMES
Temperature is within normal limits
Nasal packing negative for CSF
Incision is clean without signs of infection

● **NDX:** Risk for fluid volume deficit related to potential for surgically induced diabetes insipidus

Assess for signs of diabetes insipidus
    Monitor intake and output q2h during first 24 hr postoperatively
    Measure output qh; report if >200 ml/hr
    Report intake >3000 to 4000 ml per 24 hr
    Monitor urine specific gravity; report if <1.005
Collaborate with physician to correct condition if condition is present
Monitor VS, skin turgor, and mucous membranes q4h to 8h
Weigh patient daily: same time, clothing, and scale; monitor for weight loss *to identify/correct fluid volume loss*

EXPECTED OUTCOMES
Vital signs are stable
Intake is <2500 ml/day
Urine output is <100 ml/hr, and specific gravity is within normal range
Weight is stable
Skin turgor is good

● **NDX:** Pain at surgical site or headache

Assess patient for verbal and nonverbal signs of pain
Be aware that severe headache may be a sign of increased ICP
Discuss with patient factors that relieve pain; facilitate use of these measures if possible
Assist patient with finding position of comfort, maintaining neutral head position with head of bed elevated 30 degrees

Teach relaxation techniques *to reduce perception of pain*
Provide means of distraction from pain: guided imagery, soft music, visitors as tolerated
Administer pain medications as ordered; be aware that they may mask signs of increased ICP

EXPECTED OUTCOMES
Verbalizes increasing comfort and no headache
Face and body are relaxed
Uses relaxation techniques

Patient/family teaching

Explain that decrease in senses of taste and smell for several months is expected
Explain need to avoid persons with infections, especially URIs
Discuss symptoms of incisional or systemic infection to report to physician
Emphasize importance of avoiding vigorous coughing, straining, and noseblowing
Emphasize importance of ongoing patient care
Discuss signs and symptoms of hormonal imbalances to report to physician (see specific disease relating to hormone deficiency)
Teach name of medication(s), dosage, time and method of administration, side effects, and toxic effects

Home care considerations

Emphasize that hormone therapy may need to continue throughout lifetime
Explain need to notify care giver about unusual stress so medication dosages can be changed if needed
Provide information for obtaining medical alert bracelet and card

BIBLIOGRAPHY
American Diabetes Association. Position statement: insulin administration. *Diabetes care* 14(2):34-35, 1991.
Becker K: *Principles and practice in endocrinology and metabolism,* Philadelphia, 1990, Lippincott.
Kim MJ, et al: *Pocket guide to nursing diagnoses,* St Louis, ed 6, 1995, Mosby.
Kinney M, Packa D, Dunbar S: *AACN's clinical reference for critical care nursing,* ed 3, 1994, Bookmakers.
Kohler PO: *Clinical endocrinology,* New York, 1986, John Wiley & Sons.
Kreisberg R: Diabetic ketoacidosis. In Rifkin H and Porte D, editors: *Ellenberg and Rifkin's diabetes mellitus theory and practice,* ed 4, New York, 1990, Elsevier.
Loriaux, TC: Nursing care of clients with adrenal, pituitary and gonadal disorders. In Black JM and Matassarin-Jacobs E, editors: *Luckman and Sorenson's medical-surgical nursing: a psychophysiological approach,* ed 4, Philadelphia, 1993, WB Saunders.
Thompson JM et al: *Mosby's clinical nursing,* ed 3, St Louis, 1993, Mosby.
Wilson JD, Foster DW: *Williams textbook of endocrinology,* ed 8, Philadelphia, 1992, WB Saunders.
Wyngaarden JB, Smith LH: *Cecil textbook of medicine,* ed 18, Philadelphia, 1988, WB Saunders.

Musculoskeletal System

Musculoskeletal Assessment

● Subjective Data

Pain and/or edema in muscles, joints, or bones with or without movement
Weakness in extremities
Limited activity and movement
Sensory changes
Anorexia; weight loss
Insomnia
Tires easily, fatigue
Unsteady gait or stance
Frustration, anger at self

● Objective Data

General appearance
Age, (see Gerontologic considerations, p. 497)
Vital signs (VS): blood pressure (BP), temperature (T), pulse (P), and respiratory rate (R)
Weight
Joint(s) inflamed, edematous, and/or warm to touch
Impaired neurovascular status of each extremity
Deformities
Paralysis
Contractures
Posture
Abnormal body alignment
Limited ability or inability to move in bed

Abnormal gait; needs assistance
Decreased handgrip and range of motion
 (ROM)
Internal and external rotation of extremities
Ability to perform ROM exercises
Contusions, lacerations, scars
Wounds; amount and type of drainage
Facial and body gestures indicating pain
Loss of extremity
Pressure ulcers

Skin rashes
Allergies
Tenseness
Presence of casts, braces, prostheses, crutches, trac-
 tion, cane, or walker
Nutritional history
Ability to use trapeze in bed, sit up, and turn
Ability to perform activities of daily living (ADLs)
Constipation
Dependence, independence, and interdependence

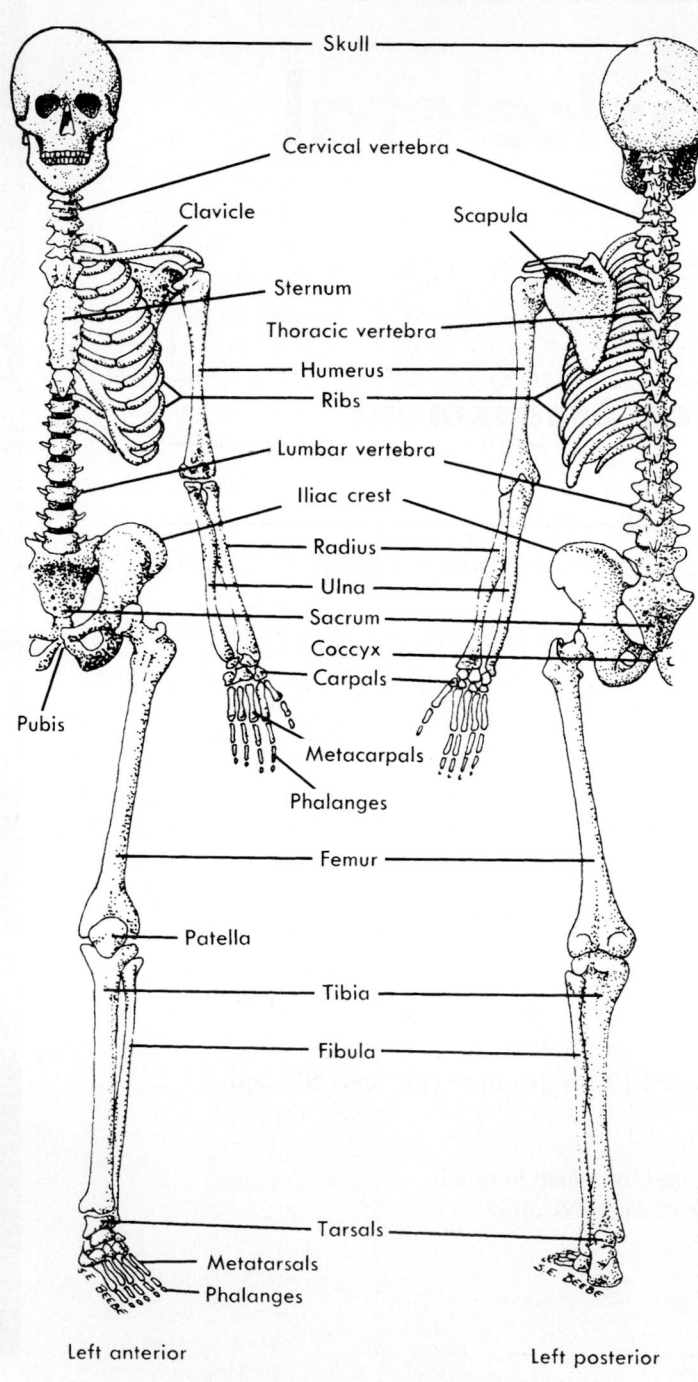

Figure 8-1   Musculoskeletal system.

● Pertinent Background Information

Concurrent diseases and/or conditions

Spinal cord injury, nerve impairment
Cerebrovascular accident (CVA)
Rheumatoid arthritis
Arthritis
Bursitis
Polyneuritis
Multiple sclerosis
Muscular dystrophy
Myasthenia gravis
Fracture
Ruptured disc
Ménière's disease

Labyrinthitis
Osteoporosis
Congenital conditions
Low back pain
Lupus erythematosus
Gout
Blood dyscrasias
Older adult (see Gerontologic Considerations box)

Previous surgery and/or illness

Orthopedic surgery
Spinal surgery
Poliomyelitis
Hemiplegia, paraplegia
Cerebral palsy
Parkinson's disease
Ataxia
Alcoholism
Syphilis
Impaired vision and/or hearing
CVA
Hyperparathyroidism
Osteoporosis
Rickets, osteomalacia
Tuberculosis

Family history

Carcinoma
Diabetes
Tuberculosis

Social history

Hazardous job or recreation (e.g., construction work or contact sports)
Safety measures used
Accident proneness
Alcohol, substance abuse, tobacco use

Medication history

Antiinflammatory agents: steroid and nonsteroid
Sedatives
Tranquilizers
Analgesics
Acetylsalicylic acid
Antimalarials
Antiemetics
Anticoagulants
Antidepressants
Insulin
Oral hypoglycemics
Psychotherapeutic agents

Gerontologic Considerations

- Physiologic changes of aging result in decreased joint flexibility and muscular strength.
- Changes in bone mass, particularly in older women, increase the risk of fractures. Hip fractures and compression fractures of the spine are most common.
- Degenerative joint disease related to "wear and tear" on joints is common. Joint replacement is increasingly common and has done much to improve mobility and the quality of life.
- Changes in the foot can occur from a lifetime of use, poorly fitted shoes, or heredity. Bunions and hammer toe are commonly seen in older adults. These may cause pain and lead to decreased mobility. Older adults should be encouraged to wear properly fitted shoes to reduce discomfort. If discomfort is severe, surgical correction may be necessary.
- The older adult's home should be checked for safety hazards such as rugs that could cause falls.
- Climbing unsteady or uneven surfaces should be avoided, because coordination and balance change with aging and falls may result.
- Older persons should be instructed in the correct use of assistive devices such as canes or walkers. They should be encouraged to use these measures regularly to prevent injury.

From Christensen BL, Kockrow EO: *Foundations of nursing*, ed 2, St Louis, 1995, Mosby.

Antibiotics
Antihypertensive agents

● Diagnostic tests

Serum
  Calcium
  Phosphorus
  Alkaline phosphatase
  Erythrocyte sedimentation rate (ESR)
  Creatinine clearance
  BUN
  Uric acid
  AST, ALT, creatinine phosphokinase (CPK)
  Coagulation studies
Urine
  Calcium
  Phosphorus
  Creatinine, uric acid

Procedures

X-ray examination of bones
Arthrogram
Arthroscopy
Myelogram
Fluoroscopy
Arteriogram
Venogram
Bone marrow aspiration
Bone, synovial fluid, or muscle biopsy
Incision and drainage of joint
Aspiration of joint
Electromyogram (EMG): muscle and nerve
  conduction studies
Bone scintigraphy (scan)
Computed tomography (CT) scan
Thermography
Magnetic resonance imaging (MRI)
Lumbar puncture
Discogram

Osteoporosis

Overall reduction in bone mass and density, as a result of bone formation being less than bone resorption, causing increased porosity and brittleness; suggested etiology-immobilization because of illness or aging process, decreased blood estrogen, increased ratio of blood estrogen, increased ratio of blood calcium to phosphorus, excessive steroid therapy, and people with red-blond hair and freckles; disease predisposes patients to fractures and/or deformities

Assessment

Subjective data

Backache, neck pain, decrease in height,
  kyphosis
History of steroid therapy or smoking

Objective data

Age and sex of patient (usually more than
  50 years of age and female)
History of inactivity or immobilization
Nutritional history
  Lack of vitamins C and D and calcium
  Diets high in acids, alcohol, and caffeine
History of endocrine disease
  Diabetes
  Hyperthyroidism
  Hyperparathyroidism
  Cushing's syndrome
  Acromegaly
  Hypogonadism
Anorexia nervosa
Hematologic malignancies
Alteration in self-concept
Decreased mobility

Diagnostic tests

Single-photon absorptiometry (SPA) (measures bone
  density)
Dual-photon absorptiometry (DPA)
Radiologic studies
Bone scan
Serum chemistries (low alkaline phosphatase)

Potential complications

Respiratory compromise
Fractures: lower radius, femoral neck,
  vertebrae
Increased immobility

Collaborative management

Therapeutic management

Diet
Calcium, vitamin D supplements, calcitonin
Estrogen therapy if postmenopausal or
  hysterectomy
Increased activity, exercise
Back corset, brace

Nursing management

PATIENT PROBLEMS/NURSING DIAGNOSES

● **NDX:** Impaired physical mobility related to disease process

Assess mobility, gait
Encourage ambulation with assistance; use walker or cane if indicated
Assist with and teach active ROM exercises q4h
Monitor and maintain body alignment; fractures can occur without patient's knowledge
Handle patient carefully and assist with and teach correct body mechanics *to prevent fractures*
Assist with and teach patient application of braces or corset as applicable
Administer calcitonin, estrogen, calcium, and vitamin D
Provide diet high in calcium and vitamins C and D
Monitor serum chemistries

EXPECTED OUTCOMES

Performs ROM exercises to tolerance
Uses walker, cane correctly
Demonstrates application of brace, corset correctly

● **NDX:** Body image disturbance related to lordosis and kyphosis

Encourage and allow time for verbalization of feelings; listen attentively
Clarify any misconceptions about disease process and treatment
Discuss ways of altering clothes to ensure a better fit and the use of scarves, color schemes *to enhance self-concept*
Assist patient in identifying strengths that were successful in the past
Identify present coping behaviors and praise for tasks accomplished
Encourage communication with significant other(s)

EXPECTED OUTCOMES

Appears more comfortable with self
Expresses desire to discuss clothing and ways to enhance self-image

ADDITIONAL NURSING DIAGNOSES TO CONSIDER

Impaired gas exchange related to kyphosis
Pain related to bone density loss in spine

Patient/family teaching

Stress importance of diet, activity, and rest; provide written aerobic exercise schedule; discourage jogging
Provide medication schedule including name, dosage, purpose, and side effects; discuss alendromate (Fosamax) therapy for bone replacement
Discuss importance of safe environment
　Use ambulatory devices as needed; avoid slippery areas
　Maintain awareness of possible falls or fractures; avoid small rugs; use hand rails
　Avoid activity after taking analgesics or muscle relaxants
　Avoid quick movements that may cause fractures
Encourage reduction of caffeine, alcohol intake, and smoking
Inform of risk of estrogen-related uterine cancer
Promote follow-up visits with physician for medication adjustments, serum calcium levels, Pap smears, and mammography

Orthopedic Sepsis: Acute Osteomyelitis

acute osteomyelitis: *Infection of the long bones and knee joint caused by acute local infection or bone trauma, usually caused by* Escherichia coli, Staphylococcus aureus, *or* Streptococcus pyogenes; *this condition may be asymptomatic for months, but once diagnosed, aggressive treatment is required with a long rehabilitation to prevent recurrence of the infection; surgical intervention may be required to drain infected areas*

Assessment

Subjective data

Pain, muscle spasms in affected joint
Headache
Weakness

Objective data

Redness and swelling in affected joint; increases with motion
Chills
Rapid elevation of temperature
Diaphoresis
Tachycardia
Restlessness
Irritability

Diagnostic tests

White blood cell count (WBC), blood cultures
Joint radiologic study
Culture of joint aspirate
Bone scan
MRI

Potential complications

Limited motion, contractures
Ankylosing of joint
Degenerative joint changes
Recurrence of infection
Chronic osteomyelitis

Collaborative management

Therapeutic management

Parenteral fluids with antibiotics
Antibiotics, analgesics
Irrigant solution
Immobilization of joint
Compresses: warm, moist, or alternate warm and cold
Diet, activity
Excision, aspiration, drainage, irrigation of joint
Physical medicine
  Physical therapy (PT)
  Occupational therapy (OT)

Nursing management

PATIENT PROBLEMS/NURSING DIAGNOSES

● **NDX:** Impaired physical mobility related to pain and swelling

Maintain bed rest; handle affected extremity gently
Immobilize joint/extremity with use of cast, splint, and/or pillows to maintain alignment; elevate *to reduce edema*
Assist with and teach active or perform passive ROM exercises to unaffected extremities q4h and deep breathe q½h
Involve in planning care and encourage self-care participation
Increase socialization; involve patient in unit activities and/or occupational therapy
Increase activity after fever and swelling subside or drainage decreases
Initiate ROM exercise of affected joint/extremity when tolerated
Monitor tolerance before increasing activity
Provide resistive exercises
Protect affected joint/extremity from trauma

Assist patient to chair; elevate affected extremity; limit to 30 min
Ambulate with crutches; advance to walker or cane as tolerated
Provide a safe environment
Instruct patient in weight bearing
Provide encouragement and support for each accomplishment

EXPECTED OUTCOMES

Mobility and joint use are improving with less discomfort
Participation in own care is increasing
Edema is diminishing

● **NDX:** Hyperthermia related to bacterial invasion and subsequent infection

Draw blood cultures immediately; monitor results
Maintain parenteral fluids with antibiotics
Administer antipyretics
Monitor for chills; check vital signs during and after chills
Monitor vital signs q4h; institute cooling measures as needed
Keep patient comfortable and dry following episodes of diaphoresis

EXPECTED OUTCOMES

Vital signs are stable
Temperature is approaching normal or is normal

● **NDX:** Pain related to inflammation and increased pressure at affected side

Assess location, intensity, and type of pain
Provide analgesics as indicated; assess effectiveness of pain relief measures
Assist patient with changing position frequently; support affected extremity; administer back rubs *to promote comfort*
Handle joint distal to site gently, because it may also be painful when extended
Provide diversional activities *to decrease attention on pain*
Discuss and promote alternate pain relief measures

EXPECTED OUTCOMES

Reports that level of pain is tolerable
Appears more relaxed, comfortable
Balances periods of activity with rest

● **NDX:** Impaired skin integrity related to infection, surgical intervention, drainage

Apply warm, moist compresses or alternate warm and cold compresses q2h to 3h
Collaborate with physician and prepare patient for excision and drainage if infected lesion present

Take cultures of aspirated fluid

Irrigate lesion if irrigating catheter is in place; continuous irrigation with antibiotics may be ordered

Monitor intake and output of irrigant

Do not allow irrigating bottle to run dry

Keep patient warm and dry

Observe for skin breakdown

Monitor incision for bleeding; change dressing as needed; maintain rigid aseptic technique

Provide high-calorie, high-protein diet as tolerated *to promote healing;* assist with meals as needed

Encourage fluids to upper limits for age and weight

Remove splints daily if ordered and monitor skin condition

Reposition patient q2h *to increase circulation to affected site*

EXPECTED OUTCOMES

Skin is clean, dry, and intact

Wound is closed with no signs of infection

WBC is within normal limits

ADDITIONAL NURSING DIAGNOSES TO CONSIDER

Altered tissue perfusion: peripheral related to site edema/infection

Body image disturbance related to extended treatment and rehabilitation

Patient/family teaching

Provide and discuss information on prescribed rehabilitation program: physical therapy and home instructions

Demonstrate incision care and stress importance of aseptic technique and a daily shower

Provide information about disease process and complications

Discuss signs and symptoms to report to physician

Tenderness, pain, discomfort

Fever, malaise

Drainage from incision

Provide medication schedule, including name, dosage, purpose, and side effects; instruct patient to take all prescribed medications

Stress importance of nourishing diet and increased fluid intake; avoid weight gain

Promote regular visits with physician

Home care considerations

Assess and continue with patient/family teaching and monitor the following:

Environmental/safety status

Care givers' ability to perform needed tasks

Accessible telephone and emergency numbers: physician, pharmacy, home health care team

Emergency call device to summon outside help

Absence of skatter rugs, unbacked carpets

Presence of stairs with hand rails

Grab bars at tub and toilet

Nonskid strips in tub

Adequate lighting for safe movement

Wide doorways to accommodate wheelchairs/walkers

Height of chair and bed for easy transfer on and off of each

Flashlights near bed and chair

Medications accessible and labeled

Availability of transportation to needed appointments

Needed supplies: what and where to purchase

Mobility status

Ability and desire to follow prescribed rehabilitation plan and exercises

Correct transfer techniques

Amount of weight bearing; reinforce wearing low-heeled, comfortable shoes

Correct use of walkers, canes, crutches

Ability to apply brace, corset, removable cast

Status of immobilizing device

Neurovascular status of each affected extremity

Condition of device: wet, loose, clean, soiled

Condition of skin under device: clear, red, tender

Nutritional status

Understanding of basic food groups and what to eat to provide optimal nutrition with no weight gain

Signs of weight loss, dehydration

Ability to prepare meals; refer to social agency to provide meals

Elimination status

Presence of elevated toilet seat

Use of stool softeners, natural laxatives, bulk in diet

Ability to be physically active

Amount of fluids taken per day: increase to upper limits for age and weight

Use of fracture pan/urinal/female urinal

Gouty Arthritis

Acute and/or chronic arthritis of the joints caused by either overproduction or insufficient production of uric acid, a byproduct of purine metabolism; it is thought to be hereditary; urate salts build up in body tissues because they are difficult to eliminate through the kidneys

Assessment

Subjective data

Joint pain, tenderness

Increased heat at site

Anorexia
Headache
Constipation

Objective data

Affected joint (usually metatarsophalangeal joint of
   great toe)
   Redness
   Swelling
   Shiny
   Vein distention
   Deformity
   Elevated temperature
   Chills
   Subcutaneous tophi: ears, joints, knuckles

Diagnostic tests

Serum and uric acid elevated, WBC, ESR
Microscopic examination of joint aspirate
X-ray examination of affected area

Potential complications

Decreased urine output
Hypertension
Renal calculi

Collaborative management

Therapeutic management

Antigout agents: colchicine (Colsalide), probenecid
   (Benemid)
Nonsteroid antiinflammatory agents: phenylbutazone
   (Butazolidin), indomethacin (Indocin), ibuprofen
   (Motrin), allopurinol (Zyloprim)
Analgesics, antipyretics
Cold packs
Dietary
   Low-calorie diet if overweight
   Low-purine diet

Nursing management

   PATIENT PROBLEMS/NURSING DIAGNOSES

● **NDX:**   Pain related to inflammation and edema

Assess intensity, location, and type of pain; use pain rating scale
Maintain patient in position of comfort with affected
   joint (initially foot) supported and in alignment; place
   cradle over foot; no weight bearing

Apply cold packs, ice bag to affected joint; avoid placing
   excess pressure on joint
Elevate affected area *to reduce edema and promote ve-
   nous return*
Administer analgesics and antigout and antiinflamma-
   tory agents; observe for side effects
   Colchicine: nausea, vomiting, bloody diarrhea, olig-
      uria, hematuria
   Phenylbutazone: nausea, vomiting, diarrhea, rash,
      edema, hypertension, leukopenia
Encourage fluids to 2500 ml/day *to increase elimination
   of urate salts*
Monitor serum uric acid levels

   EXPECTED OUTCOMES
Reports pain is at a tolerable level
Appears calm and relaxed
Exhibits lessening or absent edema

● **NDX:**   Impaired physical mobility related to joint
            pain and inflammation

Maintain bed rest with affected extremity elevated until
   edema and pain have lessened
Increase activity as pain and swelling subside
Ambulate with assistance; use walker or cane
Perform ROM exercise carefully to affected joint
Promote return to normal activities

   EXPECTED OUTCOMES
Performs ROM adequately in affected joint
Ambulates with walker or cane without discomfort

Patient/family teaching

Provide medication schedule including name, dosage,
   purpose, and side effects and explain necessity of taking colchicine hourly at onset of acute attacks
Report side effects of medications immediately; avoid
   salicylates if taking probenecid
Discuss importance of diet, exercise, and rest program
Provide list of high-purine foods (liver, kidneys, sar-
   dines, consomme, herring, anchovies, beer, alcohol);
   discuss foods to substitute (chicken, fish, vegetables,
   cheese, eggs, milk)
Emphasize importance of maintaining normal weight
Explain importance of high fluid intake (2500 ml/day),
   if not contraindicated
Encourage follow-up visits with physician

Fracture

*A break in bone continuity; types of fractures and their
causes are listed in Table 8-1*

Table 8-1 Types and Causes of Fractures

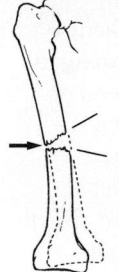

Angulated: Fracture with fragments at angles to each other   *Cause:* Direct or lateral force, causing break and loss of anatomic positions

Angulated

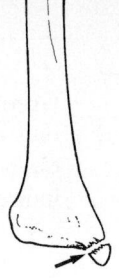

Avulsed: Fracture that pulls bone and other tissues from usual attachments   *Cause:* Direct energy or force, with resisted extension of bone and joint

Avulsed

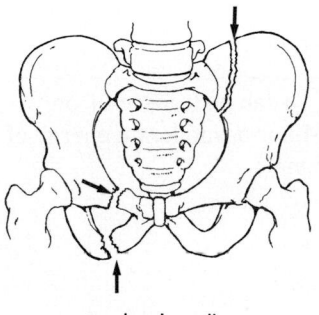

Bucket handle: Double vertical fractures of pelvis on same side, resulting in pelvic dislocation   *Cause:* Direct blow or anterior compression force, with or without sacral torsion

Bucket-handle

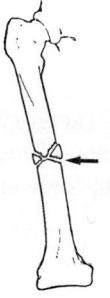

Butterfly: Butterfly-shaped piece of fractured bone, ususally accompanying comminuted fracture   *Cause:* Direct, indirect, or rotational force to bone.

Butterfly

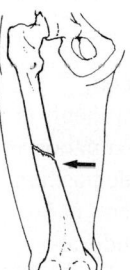

Closed: Skin intact over fracture *Cause:* Minor force or energy

Closed

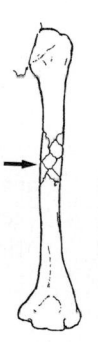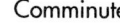

Comminuted: Fracture with more than two pieces; may have significant associated soft tissue trauma   *Cause:* Direct crushing injury or force to tissues and bone

Comminuted

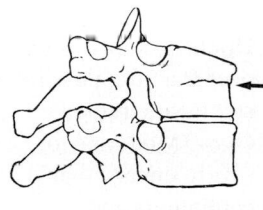

Compression: Fracture is squeezed or wedged together at one side   *Cause:* Compressive, axial energy or force applied directly from above fracture site

Compression

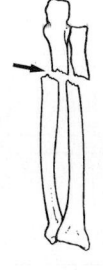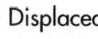

Displaced: Fracture with one, both, or all fragments out of normal alignment *Cause:* Direct energy or force to site

Displaced

From Mourad LA: *Mosby's clinical nursing series: orthopedic disorders,* St Louis, 1991, Mosby.

Continued.

Table 8-1   Types and Causes of Fractures—cont'd

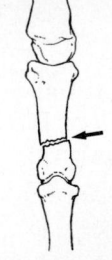

Extraarticular: Fracture near but outside a joint *Cause:* Direct energy above or below a joint

Extraarticular

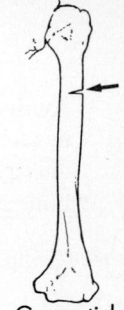

Greenstick: Break in only one cortex of bone *Cause:* Minor direct or indirect energy

Greenstick

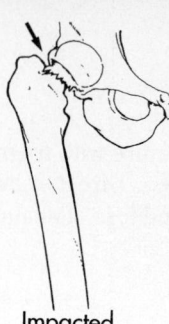

Impacted: Fracture with one end wedged into opposite end or inside fractured fragment *Cause:* Compressive axial energy or force directly to distal fragment

Impacted

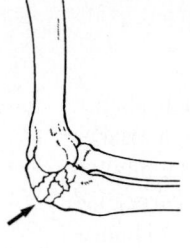

Intraarticular: Fracture involving bones inside a joint *Cause:* Direct or indirect energy or force to joint

Intraarticular

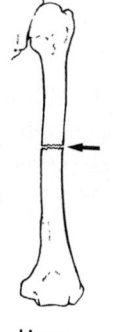

Linear: As a line, so can be transverse or oblique *Cause:* Minor or moderate energy of force directly to bone

Linear

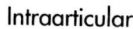

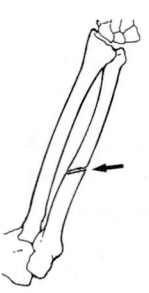

Nightstick: Fracture of ulna caused by blow to forearm elevated in defensive position *Cause:* Direct force or blow to forearm

Nightstick

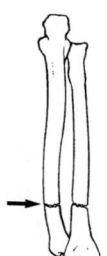

Nonangulated: Fracture with fragments in anatomic relationship to each other *Cause:* Minor force or energy

Nonangulated

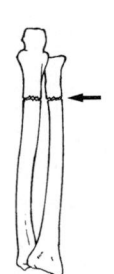

Nondisplaced: Fracture fragments in close approximation and anatomic position to each other *Cause:* Minor to moderate force or energy

Nondisplaced

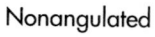

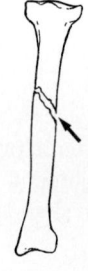

Oblique: Fracture at oblique angle across both cortices *Cause:* Direct or indirect energy, with angulation and some compression

Oblique

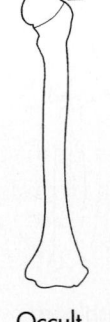

Occult: Fracture that is hidden or not readily discernible *Cause:* Minor force or energy

Occult

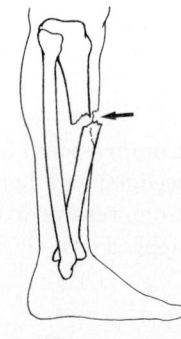

Open: Skin broken over fracture; possible soft tissue trauma *Cause:* Moderate to severe energy that is continuous and exceeds tissue tolerances

Open

Table 8-1   Types and Causes of Fractures—cont'd

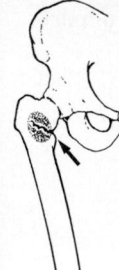

Pathologic: Transverse, oblique, or spiral fracture of bone weakened by tumor pressure or presence *Cause:* Minor energy or force, which may be direct or indirect

Pathologic

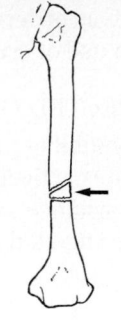

Segmented: Fracture with two or more pieces or segments *Cause:* Direct or indirect moderate to severe force

Segmented

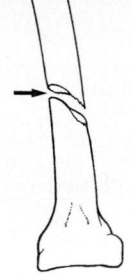

Spiral: Fracture that curves around cortices and may become displaced by twist *Cause:* Direct or indirect twisting energy or force with distal part held or unable to move

Spiral

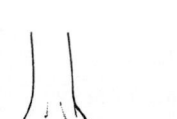

Stellate: Central fracture point from which fissures radiate *Cause:* Direct blow or force of moderate energy

Stellate

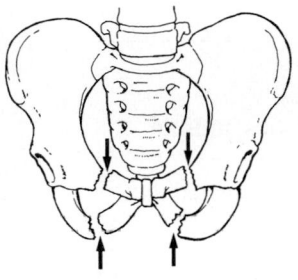

Straddle: Bilateral fractures of pelvic and pubic rami *Cause:* Fall that causes or results in straddling of hard object

Straddle

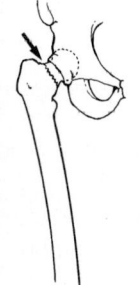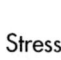

Stress: Crack in one cortex of bone *Cause:* Repetitive direct energy or force, as from jogging, running, or striking a lever, or from osteoporosis

Stress

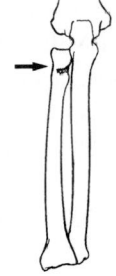

Torus: Fracture of one cortex of shafts of radius and ulna (one cortex of each bone), shown as wrinkle or buckle *Cause:* Direct blow to forearm or indirect compressive force, as from fall

Torus

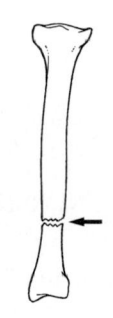

Transverse: Horizontal break through bone *Cause:* Direct or indirect energy toward bone

Transverse

Assessment

Subjective data

Fracture site
  Pain, tenderness
  Decreased sensation, numbness, tingling

Objective data

Fracture site
  Edema

Skin open or intact
Color and temperature of surrounding tissues
Presence/absence of pulse distal from break
Bleeding, hematoma
Restricted, limited mobility
Abnormal position of extremity
Signs of shock: hypotension, tachycardia
Signs of fat embolism: chest pain, dyspnea, changes in
  respiratory rate, decreased mental acuity

Diagnostic tests

Radiologic films of fracture
CBC, electrolytes

Potential complications

Malunion, delayed union, or nonunion of fracture
Thrombophlebitis
Fat embolism
Compartment syndrome (knee, elbow)
Infection
Nerve compression

Collaborative management

Therapeutic management

Open or closed reduction of fracture
Joint arthroplasty or total replacement
Analgesics, narcotics, sedatives, antibiotics, muscle
  relaxants
Application of cast, traction, splint, sling, external fixa-
  tion device
Ice application
Antiembolic stockings and/or antithrombic pump
Bed rest in specific position
Diet, activity, rest, mobility restrictions
Physical therapy
  Rehabilitation exercises
  Crutch walking

Nursing management

PATIENT PROBLEMS/NURSING DIAGNOSES

● **NDX:** Impaired physical mobility related to fracture and injury to surrounding tissues

Maintain bed rest in prescribed position *to facilitate
  healing*
Evaluate pressure points, change position q2h
Elevate affected extremity and apply ice bags as indicated *to reduce edema*
Support affected extremity above and below fracture
  when moving, turning, and lifting
Monitor cast, traction, and sling qh initially, then q4h;
  observe for cast integrity and position of traction
  weights and sling
Assist with and teach use of trapeze and other methods
  of moving and turning
Perform passive or assist with and teach active ROM
  exercises to unaffected joints *to maintain joint mobility*
Explain restrictions and limitations in activity

Encourage patient to perform ADLs within scope of
  limitations; provide supplies; assist as necessary
Assist with and teach patient use of urinal or bedpan for
  elimination; administer perineal care as needed
Ambulate as ordered; involve physical therapy department in use of crutches, walker, cane

EXPECTED OUTCOMES

Regains mobility to optimal level
Participates actively in treatment plan
Seeks assistance as needed
Verbalizes needed restrictions and understands ratio-
  nale

● **NDX:** Altered tissue perfusion: peripheral related
to location of fracture and risk of arteriovenous flow alteration

Monitor vital signs q2h to 4h
Monitor pulses distal from fracture q1h and observe for
  color, temperature, and sensation q2h
Assess capillary refill; report abnormal findings; com-
  pare with opposite extremity
Maintain body alignment and prescribed position *to en-
  sure adequate circulation*
Observe for signs of compartment syndrome (p. 535)
Apply antiembolic stockings: remove daily to inspect
  for pressure, pain, and redness
Encourage small movements of affected digits *to main-
  tain venous flow*

EXPECTED OUTCOMES

Pulses distal to fracture are present
Skin is warm
Capillary refill is normal (2 to 4 sec)

● **NDX:** Altered tissue perfusion: cerebral and/or
cardiopulmonary related to risk of fat embolus; *this dangerous complication requires immediate action; these emboli can occlude coronary arteries, pulmonary circulation, and
cerebral flow; death may ensue if not treated
promptly*

Assess cardiopulmonary status
  Monitor vital signs q2h to 4h; take apical pulse
  Monitor cardiac output, ABGs
  Observe for tachycardia, angina; instruct patient to re-
    port chest pain immediately
  Auscultate chest for breath sounds q4h; observe for
    diminished sounds
  Monitor respirations for tachypnea, dyspnea
  Assist with chest x-rays
  Assist and teach patient to turn and cough q2h and
    deep breathe qh
Assess cerebral status

Monitor level of consciousness (LOC), mental status orientation as to name, time, place q4h to 8h

Assess pupils for size, equality, and reaction to light

Instruct patient to report headache, dizziness, numbness/tingling of extremities immediately

EXPECTED OUTCOMES

Presents normal vital signs

Exhibits clear breath sounds

Presents laboratory values within normal limits

Remains alert, oriented

Reports no headache or chest pain

● **NDX:** Impaired tissue integrity related to surgical reduction, puncture wounds

Assess wound integrity and observe for signs of infection or drainage, especially at pin sites

Administer antibiotics and assess effectiveness, side effects

Monitor and change dressings prn using aseptic technique

Monitor temperature

Monitor traction/casts for pressure points

Provide frequent skin care to bony prominences and around cast/traction openings

Turn patient frequently; maintain body alignment

Maintain dry, wrinkle-free bed linen

Provide foam, air, or water mattress as needed; use bed cradle to prevent pressure

EXPECTED OUTCOMES

Tissue integrity is maintained

Temperature is normal

● **NDX:** Pain related to fracture and/or trauma

Assess location, intensity, and type of pain; use pain rating scale

Administer narcotics, analgesics, and muscle relaxants; avoid allowing pain to become severe; assess effectiveness of pain relief measures

Collaborate with physician regarding patient controlled analgesia (PCA)

Provide quiet environment initially and encourage diversional activities *to decrease awareness of discomfort*

Assist with and teach alternate pain management methods

Change position frequently and administer back rubs and massages *to promote comfort*

Encourage ambulation with assistance when tolerated

EXPECTED OUTCOMES

Reports a reduction in pain

Presents a relaxed manner

Participates in diversional activities

● **NDX:** Anxiety related to altered health/situational crisis

Monitor patient's level of anxiety (p. 35)

Reinforce physician's explanation of treatment and expected outcome; clarify misconceptions

Encourage and allow time for verbalization of feelings

Teach and assist with stress management techniques

Assess present coping behaviors and encourage use of behaviors that were successful in managing past experiences

Encourage interaction with significant other and friends, relatives

Explain all procedures and treatments; involve patient in plan of care; provide options; encourage safe decision making

EXPECTED OUTCOMES

Demonstrates relaxation techniques correctly

Verbalizes a feeling of less tension, apprehension

Appears calm and relaxed

Participates in activities appropriately

Patient/family teaching

Stress importance of prescribed rehabilitation plan of activity, rest, and exercise

Provide and review diet instructions regarding type and amount; need to avoid weight gain if applicable

Discuss medications: name, purpose, schedule, dosage, and side effects

Discuss signs and symptoms to report to physician: severe pain, changes in temperature, color, or sensation in extremity, foul odor or drainage from wound

Explain cast, splint, sling care as indicated (see Cast care p. 538)

Encourage follow-up visits with physician

Home care considerations

Assess and continue with patient/family teaching and monitor the following:

Environmental/safety status

Care givers' ability to perform needed tasks

Accessible telephone and emergency numbers: physician, pharmacy, home health care team

Emergency call device to summon outside help

Absence of scatter rugs, unbacked carpets

Presence of stairs with hand rails

Grab bars at tub and toilet

Nonskid strips in tub

Adequate lighting for safe movement

Wide doorways to accommodate wheelchairs/ walkers

Height of chair and bed for easy transfer on and off of each

Flashlights near bed and chair
Medications accessible and labeled
Availability of transportation to needed appointments
Needed supplies: what and where to purchase
Mobility status
  Ability and desire to follow prescribed rehabilitation
    plan and exercises
  Correct transfer techniques
  Amount of weight bearing; reinforce wearing low-
    heeled, comfortable shoes
  Correct use of walkers, canes, crutches
  Ability to apply brace, corset, removable cast
Status of immobilizing device
  Neurovascular status of each affected extremity
  Condition of device: wet, loose, clean, soiled
  Condition of skin under device: clear, red, tender
Status of wound
  Incision for healing, infection
  Signs of infection: redness, pain, swelling, fever,
    drainage
  Ability to care for wound; correct supplies and hand-
    washing technique
  Knowledge of where and what supplies to purchase
Nutritional status
  Understanding of basic food groups and what to eat
    to provide nutrition with no weight gain
  Signs of weight loss, dehydration
  Ability to prepare meals; refer to social agency to
    provide meals
Elimination status
  Presence of elevated toilet seat
  Use of stool softeners, natural laxatives, bulk in diet
  Ability to be active
  Amount of fluids taken per day; increase to upper
    limits for age and weight
  Use of fracture pan/urinal/female urinal

Maxillomandibular Fixation

Surgical procedure to reduce and repair jaw fractures or deformities, using wires and/or plate and additional fixation

Preoperative assessment and care

Assess respiratory status; observe for signs of upper
  respiratory infection
Explain purpose of wires after surgery and provide
  method of communication: pad and pencil, Magic
  Slate
Assist with and teach patient method for pushing secretions through clamped jaw (if possible) and demonstrate use of oral suction catheter

Discuss importance of oral hygiene and oral suctioning
  and teach procedure
Demonstrate feeding procedure using straw or syringe
Explain possibility of nasopharyngeal airway and/or
  nasogastric tube and aspiration postoperatively
Perform facial scrub and oral hygiene preoperatively
Administer prescribed antibiotics
Answer all questions and allow time for verbalization of
  fears and anxieties

Postoperative assessment

Subjective data

Location, character of pain
Nausea
Dyspnea
Apprehension

Objective data

Edema of the following:
  Face
  Base of tongue
  Front of neck
  Nose
Vomiting; aspiration of emesis
Elevated temperature
Drainage from mouth
Location of wire cutters or scissors

Diagnostic tests

CBC, electrolytes
Radiologic examinations for alignment of fracture

Potential complications

Respiratory distress
Aspiration pneumonia
Hemorrhage, shock

Collaborative management

Therapeutic management

Analgesics, sedatives, antibiotics, antiemetics
Parenteral fluids
Nasogastric aspiration or NPO if applicable
Oxygen therapy
Ice packs
Wire and band cutting procedure
Activity, rest
Dietary
  Diet (liquid) high in calories, protein, vitamins

Nutritious supplements: Ensure, milkshakes, Carnation instant breakfasts

Nursing management

PATIENT PROBLEMS/NURSING DIAGNOSES

● **NDX:**   Risk for aspiration related to wired jaws

Tape wire cutters or scissors to head of bed; if aspiration is imminent, cut wires as needed

Maintain bed rest with head elevated when reactive *to prevent aspiration*

Assess patient's ability to swallow *to prevent aspiration*

Perform oral suctioning prn; assist and teach patient to clear airway and perform suctioning

Provide and maintain suction apparatus at all times; observe for edema, drainage, and bleeding

Teach patient techniques to prevent vomiting: deep breathing, swallowing

Control with antiemetics prn

Monitor nasogastric tube and low, intermittent suction apparatus if applicable; maintain patency with normal saline irrigations prn

Apply ice bags *to reduce swelling*

Monitor vital signs, respiratory status q4h to 8h

Auscultate chest for breath sounds q4h to 8h *to monitor for possible aspiration*

Instruct patient to report immediately inability to manage self-suctioning or feeling of nausea

Maintain parenteral fluids and decrease amount as fluid intake increases

Provide clear liquid to full high-calorie liquid diet as tolerated after nasogastric tube has been removed

Assist and teach patient to use straw or feed with syringe; give small amount and wait for swallowing before continuing

Follow each feeding with water and mouth care

Provide small, frequent meals

Consult nutritionist/registered dietitian regarding alternatives in food selections (i.e., commercially prepared formulas)

Measure intake and output q8h

EXPECTED OUTCOMES

Performs self-suctioning to remove secretions

Ingests liquid diet without nausea

Presents clear breath sounds

Presents stable vital signs

● **NDX:**   Pain related to surgical procedure, edema

Assess type, intensity, and location of pain; administer prescribed analgesics; use pain rating scale; assess effectiveness of pain relief measures

Assist patient with changing position frequently while in bed *to promote comfort*

Maintain quiet environment *to provide adequate rest/sleep*

Administer back rubs *to promote comfort*

Offer diversional activities *to decrease attention on pain*

Administer frequent oral hygiene; use water jet, if available, or mouth swabs; keep lips well lubricated *to soothe irritated membranes*

Ambulate patient with assistance as needed *to change surroundings*

Assist with and teach alternate pain management techniques

Apply ice bags *to reduce edema/discomfort*

EXPECTED OUTCOMES

Reports a tolerable level of pain

Appears calm, relaxed

Adequately balances sleep with activities

● **NDX:**   Impaired verbal communication related to jaw wiring

Maintain call light within easy reach

Provide means of communication: pad and pencil, Magic Slate

Allow time for patient to write out thoughts and questions

Encourage patient to express fears and anxieties

Maintain equipment for communication and place within easy reach

EXPECTED OUTCOMES

Demonstrates ability to use alternate methods of communication

Appears comfortable with method selected

ADDITIONAL NURSING DIAGNOSES TO CONSIDER

Altered nutrition: less than body requirements related to anorexia

Impaired tissue integrity related to trauma from injury

Patient/family teaching

Provide and review diet instruction for full liquid diet and foods allowed: blended junior foods, eggnogs, and milkshakes; demonstrate use of straw or syringe; introduce spicy foods slowly

Discuss importance and purpose of small, frequent meals

Stress and teach oral hygiene and demonstrate use of Water Pic and dental wax *to keep lips moist*

Demonstrate method for cutting wires and under what circumstances to cut (wires will remain for 6 to 8 wk)

Discuss limiting strenuous activities/sports until wire removal
Explain signs and symptoms to report to physician: fever, increased pain, edema, foul odor from mouth
Discuss obtaining all medications in liquid form
Promote follow-up visits with physician

Home care considerations

Assess and continue with patient/family teaching and monitor the following:
Environmental/safety status
  Care givers' ability to perform needed tasks
  Accessible telephone and emergency numbers: physician, pharmacy, home health care team
  Medications accessible and labeled
Status of mouth/wires
  Correct oral hygiene procedures
  Wire-cutting procedure
  Condition of device: wet, loose, clean, soiled
  Condition of skin under device: clear, red, tender
Nutritional status
  Ability to prepare nourishing liquid diet
  Signs of weight loss or dehydration

Spinal Surgery

Surgery performed to relieve pressure on the spinal nerves and/or cord caused by a herniated disk, trauma, displaced fracture, incomplete vertebral dislocation from rheumatoid arthritis, osteoporosis; incision may be anterior or posterior in cervical, thoracic, or lumbar areas
laminectomy: *Removal of part of the disk lamina*
microdiscectomy: *Removal of part of the disk*
microsurgical dorsal root rhizotomy: *Severing of the sensory nerve root to the painful area; provides symptomatic relief and causes loss of sensation and possible motor damage; performed when other treatments have been unsuccessful*
facet joint rhizotomy: *Needle insertion into the facet joint with destruction of the nerve by microwave current; provides symptomatic relief*
laser therapy: *Percutaneous incision and insertion of laser to remove bulging disks; the laser destroys the disk*
chemonucleolysis: *Enzyme chymopapain is instilled into the disk to dissolve it; this procedure is not favored, because of anaphylactic reactions*

Preoperative assessment and teaching

Assess patient's neurovascular and respiratory status and location, intensity, and duration of pain

Discuss with and teach patient postoperative care and rationale
  Definition and importance of prescribed postoperative position and body alignment
  Methods for turning/log rolling, coughing, and deep breathing
  Use of trapeze and method for getting in and out of bed
  Necessary movement limitations and activities allowed
    ROM and isometric exercises
    Gluteal contractions, quadriceps setting
Explain that antiembolic stockings and sequential compression sleeves may be applied to lower extremities *to promote venous return*
Discuss and practice turning on side to eat and using a fracture bed pan
Discuss pain management and possible use of PCA; explain that discomfort may not be relieved at once following surgery because the nerves take time to heal
Encourage patient to ask questions; provide emotional support
  Reinforce physician's explanation of surgical procedure
  Allow time for and discuss patient's fears and anxieties

Postoperative assessment

Subjective data

Location and character of pain

Objective data

Neurovascular status of extremities
  Decreased sensation and motor activity
  Change in color, temperature, or pulse
Respiratory status (especially in cervical surgery)
  Difficulty in breathing
  Cyanosis
  Tachypnea
  Diminished cough
Body alignment: presence of immobilization devices
Character and amount of
  Wound drainage
  Urinary output

Diagnostic tests

CBC, electrolytes, clotting time
Spinal radiologic examinations
Urine for culture/sensitivity

Potential complications

Neurovascular damage, leaking spinal fluid
Hemorrhage

Shock
Urinary retention, infection
Abdominal distention
Paralytic ileus
Atelectasis, hypostatic pneumonia
Pulmonary embolus
Wound infection
Nonunion

Collaborative management

Therapeutic management

Analgesics, antibiotics, antiemetics, stool softeners
Parenteral fluids with electrolytes
Urinary drainage catheter
Oxygen therapy, incentive spirometer
Transcutaneous electrical nerve stimulation (TENS)
  unit (p. 94), patient controlled analgesia (p. 92)
Immobilization devices: brace, cast, corset
Diet, activity, rest
Antiembolic stockings
Physical therapy
  Rehabilitation evaluation and planning
  Ambulatory devices
  Strengthening exercises

Nursing management

PATIENT PROBLEMS/NURSING DIAGNOSES

● **NDX:** Ineffective breathing pattern related to anesthesia, surgical incision, and pain

Assess respiratory status q2h
Assist and teach patient to deep breathe qh
For cervical surgery
  Check respirations q½h for rate, rhythm, quality, and
    distress signs
  Maintain bed rest with head of bed elevated 30 to 45
    degrees
  Observe for diminished cough reflex
  Assess face and neck for edema qh
Maintain comfort with analgesics *to improve
  respiration*
Auscultate chest for breath sounds q2h
Monitor vital signs
Provide incentive spirometer qh to 2h
Encourage ambulation as soon as prescribed

EXPECTED OUTCOMES

Breath sounds are normal
Respiratory rate and rhythm are regular
Face and neck edema is absent

● **NDX:** Altered tissue perfusion: peripheral related
to surgical procedure and interruption of arterial flow

Monitor vital signs q2h to 4h
Assess neurovascular status of both legs; report
  changes in color, temperature, pulse, sensation, or
  motor activity to physician
  For cervical surgery: assess upper extremities for
    color, pulse, temperature, motor activity, and sensa-
    tion q2h; report changes to physician
Monitor for peripheral edema q4h
Apply antiembolic stockings *to increase venous return;*
  remove daily and inspect skin for pressure areas
Apply sequential compression sleeves as ordered
Monitor capillary refill on both feet q2h to 4h
Avoid heavy blankets over feet and extreme cold
  exposure
Encourage moving toes and feet *to promote venous
  flow*

EXPECTED OUTCOMES

Vital signs are stable
Capillary refill is within normal limits
Extremities are warm, of normal color, and pedal
  pulses are present
Motor activity and sensation are within normal limits

● **NDX:** Risk for infection related to invasive procedure and reduced primary defenses

Monitor temperature q4h; report elevation immediately
Monitor Hgb, Hct, WBC
Monitor dressing(s) for drainage q2h for 24 hr, then
  q4h; evaluate type of drainage; a clear or pink ring
  may indicate cerebrospinal fluid leakage; report to
  physician at once
Change dressings prn; physician may wish to do initial
  dressing; drainage is usually minimal
Report excess drainage, bleeding to physician
Obtain culture for suspicious drainage
Encourage adequate food and fluid intake *to promote
  wound healing*

EXPECTED OUTCOMES

Incision remains clean, dry, and intact
Temperature is normal
Laboratory values are within normal limits

● **NDX:** Altered urinary elimination related to anesthesia and/or bed rest

Measure intake and output q4h to 8h
If unable to urinate after 8 hr, catheterize per physician's order prn until voiding q.s

Encourage fluids to 2500 ml/day if not contraindicated *to promote elimination*
Assist with ambulation when allowed

EXPECTED OUTCOMES
Urinary output is normal for age and weight
Fluid intake is adequate

● **NDX:**   Impaired physical mobility related to musculoskeletal impairment and pain

Maintain bed rest, usually in supine or prone position with slight flexion of knees
Maintain immobilization of spine
Maintain body alignment throughout all procedures
  For cervical surgery, a soft cervical collar may be ordered if no immobilization device is present
  Do not flex head forward
  Elevate head of bed 40 to 60 degrees
Turn patient only as prescribed
  Administer pain medication 30 min before turning when possible
  Use log-rolling method
  Turn q2h from back to side to side
  While turning
    Support patient's legs with pillow between knees
    Support head with small pillow
    Roll in one continuous motion
    Support back with pillows
    Administer skin care with each turn; assess pressure points
Balance rest periods with activity
Increase activity as prescribed
  Initiate quadriceps setting and gluteal contractions
  Assist with and teach active or perform passive ROM exercises q4h as indicated according to surgical procedure
  Avoid sudden movements or twisting of extremities or neck
  Involve physical therapist if available
Ambulate with assistance when allowed
  Assist with and reinforce teaching of method for sitting up and getting out of bed
  Have patient wear supportive shoes
  Disconnect sequential compression device during ambulation
  Assist patient in walking
    Observe for vertigo, nausea, and hypotension
    Observe gait
    Avoid shuffling feet
  Place patient in straight-back chair with feet on floor
  Increase ambulation to tolerance; have patient avoid standing, sudden movements, and twisting
Encourage self-care as tolerated; assist with and teach modified ADLs as needed

EXPECTED OUTCOMES
Regains mobility to optimal level
Maintains proper body alignment
Participates in rehabilitation plan

● **NDX:**   Pain related to surgical intervention

Assess location, type, and intensity of pain; use pain rating scale and medicate as needed for continuous comfort
Administer analgesics; avoid morphine for cervical surgery patients; monitor for effectiveness, side effects
Assist patient with changing position frequently, maintaining correct body alignment *to promote comfort*
Provide and teach use of TENS unit if applicable
Discuss and teach alternate pain relief measures: back rubs, imaging
Instruct patient in use of PCA
Encourage diversional activities *to decrease attention on pain*

EXPECTED OUTCOMES
Reports that pain is at tolerable level
Appears relaxed and comfortable
Cooperates and attempts use of alternate pain management techniques

Patient/family teaching
Stress importance of prescribed activity, exercises, and restrictions
  Degree of activity and self-care allowed; ways to avoid overdependence
  Need to maintain good body alignment
  No heavy lifting, strenuous exercise, automobile driving or riding, stooping, or bending
  Methods of knee bending
  Need to avoid fatigue; exercise to tolerance with frequent rest periods
  ROM exercises as allowed
  Straight-backed chair for sitting; no knee crossing
  Convalescent period (may be an extended length of time: 2 to 9 months)
  Need to wear immobilization device as ordered: method of application, care, and removal of device; observance of device for areas that may cause skin irritation or breakdown
  Firm mattress with bedboard (essential)
Provide and review instructions on diet and fluid intake; explain ways to avoid weight gain and constipation
Discuss and demonstrate incisional care
  Signs and symptoms of wound infection
  Need to shower daily with mild soap and observe skin for signs of irritation; apply lotion as needed

Discuss signs and symptoms to report to physician
  Decreased motor activity and/or sensation in extremities
  Increased pain in surgical area
  Elevated temperature
Discuss medications: name, schedule, purpose, dosage, and side effects
Encourage follow-up visits with physician

Home care considerations

Assess and continue with patient/family teaching and monitor the following:
  Environmental/safety status
    Care givers' ability to perform needed tasks
    Accessible telephone and emergency numbers: physician, pharmacy, home health care team
    Emergency call device to summon outside help
    Absence of scatter rugs, unbacked carpets
    Presence of stairs with hand rails
    Grab bars at tub and toilet
    Nonskid strips in tub
    Adequate lighting for safe movement
    Wide doorways to accommodate wheelchairs/walkers
    Height of chair and bed for easy transfer on and off of each
    Flashlights near bed and chair
    Medications accessible and labeled
    Availability of transportation to needed appointments
    Needed supplies: what and where to purchase
  Mobility status
    Ability and desire to follow prescribed rehabilitation plan and exercises
    Correct transfer techniques
    Amount of weight bearing; reinforce wearing low-heeled, comfortable shoes
    Correct use of walkers, canes, crutches
    Ability to apply brace, corset, removable cast
  Status of immobilizing device
    Neurovascular status of each affected extremity
    Condition of device: wet, loose, clean, soiled
    Condition of skin under device: clear, red, tender
  Status of wound
    Incision for healing, infection
    Signs of infection: redness, pain, swelling, fever, drainage
    Ability to care for wound: correct supplies and hand-washing technique
    Knowledge of where and what supplies to purchase
  Nutritional status
    Understanding of basic food groups and what to eat to provide nutrition with no weight gain
    Signs of weight loss, dehydration
    Ability to prepare meals; refer to social agency to provide meals
  Elimination status
    Presence of elevated toilet seat
    Use of stool softeners, natural laxatives, bulk in diet
    Ability to be active
    Amount of fluids taken per day; increase to upper limits for age and weight
    Use of fracture pan/urinal/female urinal

Fracture or Dislocation of Cervical Spine

A condition of the cervical spine in which one or more vertebrae are fractured or dislocated; either condition may cause pressure on the spinal cord resulting in neurovascular dysfunction

Assessment

Subjective data

Neck pain, headache

Objective data

Signs of spinal cord compression
  Loss of mobility and sensation below compression
  Urinary retention
  Paroxysmal hypertension
  Bradycardia
  Dyspnea

Diagnostic tests

Radiologic examination of cervical spine
Baseline CBC, urinalysis, electrolytes

Potential complications

Respiratory distress
Abdominal distention, paralytic ileus
Decreased bowel and urine function
Complete paralysis of all extremities and trunk

Collaborative management

Therapeutic management

Immobilization devices: Halo traction, Crutchfield tongs, skeletal traction
Analgesics, muscle relaxants, stool softeners
Parenteral fluids with electrolytes

Diet, activity, rest
Physical therapy
    Rehabilitation planning
    Use of immobilizing devices and tilt table

Nursing management

PATIENT PROBLEMS/NURSING DIAGNOSES

● **NDX:** Impaired physical mobility related to musculoskeletal impairment and bed rest

Maintain bed rest in correct body alignment; have patient avoid lifting or twisting head; use sandbags until immobilization device is applied
Maintain and monitor immobilization device: Halo traction, cervical head halter, skeletal traction, Stryker frame, or Circolectric bed; maintain cervical spine in extension
Perform passive or assist with and teach active ROM exercises for all extremities q2h
Promote isometric exercises q2h to 4h
As fracture heals, traction is replaced with casts (Halo, Minerva) or neck brace; it is worn continuously; monitor for comfort and correct fit
Ambulate with assistance; monitor for vertigo and weakness; progress slowly

EXPECTED OUTCOMES

Participates in rehabilitation plan and activity schedule
Regains mobility to optimal level
Performs ROM exercises accurately

● **NDX:** Altered peripheral tissue perfusion related to injury, trauma

Monitor vital signs q2h to 4h
Assess neurovascular status q2h; monitor pulses, color, temperature, sensation, and mobility of all extremities
Apply antiembolic stockings; remove daily and monitor skin integrity
Encourage lower leg movement *to promote venous return*
Monitor extremities for edema and capillary refill

EXPECTED OUTCOMES

Vital signs are stable
Extremities are warm and of normal color
Capillary refill is normal
Motor activity and sensation are within normal limits

● **NDX:** Risk for impaired skin integrity related to pressure resulting from physical immobilization

Provide alternating pressure, gel, foam, air mattress *to maintain skin integrity*
Administer skin care q2h without turning if necessary
Change positions in small ways q1h to 2h *to decrease amount of pressure*
Apply lotions and provide massage and back rubs; *do not massage reddened areas*
Maintain wrinkle-free bottom sheets
Monitor bilateral skull dressings and tong placement of skeletal traction; observe amount of drainage and cleanse areas q4h with half-strength hydrogen peroxide or normal saline; allow to dry and redress
Monitor weights for correct amount and placement; *never release traction and keep weights off floor*

EXPECTED OUTCOMES

Maintains skin integrity around insertion sites
Moves about in bed frequently and maintains body alignment
Verbalizes understanding of needed immobilizing device

● **NDX:** Self-care deficit: feeding, bathing, toileting related to restricted positioning and trauma

Assess level of dependency
Plan care to meet needs as identified, e.g., provide total care only for those areas of self-care in which patient cannot participate
Feeding
    Maintain parenteral fluids with electrolytes until oral intake is adequate for patient
    Collaborate with physician and provide well-balanced diet when tolerated
    Initiate clear-to-full liquids and progress to soft or regular diet
        Provide foods easily chewed and swallowed
        Assist with feeding or feed prn
        Observe for signs of dysphagia
    Encourage patient to make own food selections *to promote independence*
    Serve food attractively arranged *to stimulate appetite*
    Provide oral hygiene before and after meals
Bathing
    Discuss and plan daily care and routines with patient
    Encourage self-care; instruct to avoid overexertion or fatigue
    Provide needed equipment for patient comfort and ADLs
    Assist as needed or perform total care if patient is dependent
    Promote increasing self-care as tolerated by patient
Toileting
    Measure intake and output; monitor for urine retention

Offer bedpan regularly or keep close at hand; fracture pan may be more comfortable

Encourage fluid intake of 2500 ml/day if not contraindicated

Provide privacy and perform perineal care as needed

Monitor bowel sounds: observe for decreased sounds, distention (paralytic ileus)

Prevent constipation with stool softeners, natural laxatives, high-fiber diet

EXPECTED OUTCOMES

Regains independence as activity and mobility increase

Participates in self-care to optimal level

Maintains weight normal for age, height

Experiences normal elimination patterns

● **NDX:** Pain related to fracture, trauma, edema

Assess location, type, and intensity of pain; use pain rating scale

Report any increase in pain to physician

Monitor devices for comfort

Administer analgesics and muscle relaxants; avoid morphine; assess effectiveness of pain relief measures

Collaborate with physician about PCA

Administer back rubs and massages *to promote comfort*

Encourage patient to change position slightly at frequent intervals *to promote comfort*

Reinforce correct body alignment

Provide diversional activities *to decrease attention on discomfort*

Discuss and teach alternate pain relief measures

EXPECTED OUTCOMES

Reports reduced level of discomfort

Seems relaxed; rest and sleep are adequate

Participates in diversional activities

ADDITIONAL NURSING DIAGNOSES TO CONSIDER

Ineffective breathing pattern related to location of fracture and frank spinal cord injury (see Spinal cord injury, p. 590)

Self-care deficit related to frank injury

Patient/family teaching

Stress importance of prescribed activity and immobilization device

Avoiding fatigue with planned rest periods

Signs and care of pressure points from device

Length of time device is to be worn

Demonstrate application and care of immobilization device

Discuss/explain the importance of good skin care around immobilization device

Explain importance of well-balanced diet; avoid weight gain

Avoid constipation with use of stool softeners; discuss importance of activity, exercise, and fluids

Discuss maintaining a safe environment *to prevent accidents and falls*

Provide information on resuming activities slowly and avoiding strenuous exercise

Encourage diversional activities

Provide phone numbers of home health care team

Encourage follow-up visits with physician

Home care considerations

Assess and continue with patient/family teaching and monitor the following:

Environmental/safety status

Care givers' ability to perform needed tasks

Accessible telephone and emergency numbers: physician, pharmacy, home health care team

Emergency call device to summon outside help

Absence of skatter rugs, unbacked carpets

Presence of stairs with hand rails

Grab bars at tub and toilet

Nonskid strips in tub

Adequate lighting for safe movement

Wide doorways to accommodate wheelchairs/ walkers

Height of chair and bed for easy transfer on and off of each

Flashlights near bed and chair

Medications accessible and labeled

Availability of transportation to needed appointments

Needed supplies: what and where to purchase

Mobility status

Ability and desire to follow prescribed rehabilitation plan and exercises

Correct transfer techniques

Correct use of walkers, canes, crutches

Ability to apply brace, corset, removable cast

Status of immobilizing device

Neurovascular status of each affected extremity

Condition of device: wet, loose, clean, soiled

Condition of skin under device: clear, red, tender

Status of wound

Incision for healing, infection

Signs of infection: redness, pain, swelling, fever, drainage

Ability to care for wound; correct supplies and handwashing technique

Knowledge of where and what supplies to purchase

Nutritional status

Understanding of basic food groups and what to eat
to provide optimal nutrition with no weight gain
Signs of weight loss, dehydration
Ability to prepare meals; refer to social agency to
provide meals
Elimination status
Presence of elevated toilet seat
Use of stool softeners, natural laxatives, bulk in diet
Ability to be physically active
Amount of fluids taken per day: increase to upper
limits for age and weight
Use of fracture pan/urinal/female urinal

Ankylosing Spondylitis

*A progressive inflammatory disease of the vertebral
column and surrounding tissues that begins in the
lower back and eventually causes ankylosing
(hardening or fusing) and deformity of the entire
spinal column; etiology is unknown but a heredity
factor (histocompatibility antigen HLA B27) is linked
to the disease*

Assessment

Subjective data

Vertebral pain and stiffness on arising; may radiate to
buttocks
Fatigue
Anorexia

Objective data

Limited mobility
Malaise, chest discomfort
Weight loss
Conjunctivitis, urethritis, polyarthritis
Kyphosis

Diagnostic tests

Radiologic examination of spine: indicates degeneration
and inflammation
Histocompatibility antigen HLA B27 (positive)
ESR: elevated

Potential complications

Neurologic damage
Respiratory dysfunction, depending on stage of progression
Thrombophlebitis
Fractured vertebrae
Polyarthritis

Collaborative management

Therapeutic management

Analgesics, antipyretics, nonsteroid antiinflammatory
agents, stool softeners
Bedboard, firm mattress, small pillow
Back brace, corset
Surgical intervention: cervical spinal fusion, osteotomy
Physical therapy
Exercise program
Occupational therapy
Social medicine: job change, assistance at home

Nursing management

PATIENT PROBLEMS/NURSING DIAGNOSES

● **NDX:** Impaired physical mobility related to musculoskeletal impairment and pain

Assess present mobility and observe for increased impairment
Assist with and reinforce prescribed exercise program
ROM exercises, ambulation, self-care, and ADLs as
tolerated
Discuss importance of making rest periods infrequent
because they are not beneficial
Provide diversional activities
Prepare bed with bedboard, firm mattress, and small
pillow; administer frequent back rubs and massages
Assess baseline vital signs
Assess neurovascular status: monitor peripheral pulses
and check extremities for color, warmth, sensation,
edema, and weakness q4h
Assist with and teach deep breathing exercises *to
promote respiratory and peripheral-vascular function*
Monitor skin and mucous membranes for irritation,
rashes, or breaks
Encourage Hubbard tank immersions *to relieve muscle
spasms and increase strength*
Administer antiinflammatory agents; observe for side
effects: gastric discomfort, diarrhea, constipation
Maintain elimination patterns *to promote normalcy*
Stool softeners
Adequate fluid intake
Promote ambulation; assist as needed

EXPECTED OUTCOMES

Participates in exercise program
Seeks assistance as needed
Maintains coordination and mobility at optimal level

● **NDX:** Pain related to inflammation/edema

Assess location, intensity, and type of pain; observe for
progression of pain to new areas

Administer analgesics; assess effectiveness of pain relief measures

Maintain back brace or corset in correct position

Encourage frequent, small position changes *to increase comfort*

Administer soothing backrubs

Promote diversional activities *to decrease attention on pain*

Teach and assist with alternate pain management techniques

EXPECTED OUTCOMES

Reports a reduction in discomfort

Presents a more relaxed behavior

Demonstrates learned pain-reducing skills with increasing success

● **NDX:** Body image disturbance related to altered body structure/function disturbance

Allow time for and encourage verbalization of feelings and concerns

Reinforce physician's explanation of disease process, treatment, and expected outcome; clarify misconceptions

Provide a supportive environment and assist patient with identifying positive coping styles

Provide realistic hope and set short-term goals to be attained; praise patient for each task accomplished or attempted

Encourage communication with significant other(s) and socialization with family and friends

Encourage self-care as tolerated *to promote independence*

Promote adherence to treatment plan *to postpone further development of deformities*

EXPECTED OUTCOMES

Verbalizes feelings/concerns and uses adaptive coping skills in dealing with altered image

Participates in treatment regimen and seeks assistance appropriately

Performs ADLs at optimal level

ADDITIONAL NURSING DIAGNOSIS TO CONSIDER

Self-care deficit related to increasing musculoskeletal impairment

Patient/family teaching

Stress importance and benefits of maintaining prescribed exercise program including swimming and other non–weight-bearing exercises as tolerated

Discuss medications: name, schedule, purpose, dosage, and side effects

Promote physical therapy activities: ROM, deep breathing; avoid excessive rest

Demonstrate application and care of brace or corset

Encourage nutritious diet and adequate fluid intake

Stress importance of safe environment *to prevent fractures*

Discuss signs and symptoms of disease progression: increased pain and immobility

Encourage follow-up visits with physician

Home care considerations

Assess and continue with patient/family teaching and monitor the following:

Environmental/safety status

  Care givers' ability to perform needed tasks

  Accessible telephone and emergency numbers: physician, pharmacy, home health care team

  Emergency call device to summon outside help

  Absence of scatter rugs, unbacked carpets

  Presence of stairs with hand rails

  Grab bars at tub and toilet

  Nonskid strips in tub

  Adequate lighting for safe movement

  Wide doorways to accommodate wheelchairs/walkers

  Height of chair and bed for easy transfer on and off of each

  Flashlights near bed and chair

  Medications accessible and labeled

  Availability of transportation to needed appointments

  Needed supplies: what and where to purchase

Mobility status

  Ability and desire to follow prescribed rehabilitation plan and exercises

  Correct transfer techniques

  Amount of weight bearing; reinforce wearing low-heeled, comfortable shoes

  Correct use of walkers, canes, crutches

  Ability to apply brace, corset, removable cast

Status of immobilizing device

  Neurovascular status of each affected extremity

  Condition of device: wet, loose, clean, soiled

  Condition of skin under device: clear, red, tender

Nutritional status

  Understanding of basic food groups and what to eat to provide nutrition with no weight gain

  Signs of weight loss, dehydration

  Ability to prepare meals; refer to social agency to provide meals

Elimination status

  Presence of elevated toilet seat

  Use of stool softeners, natural laxatives, bulk in diet

  Amount of fluids taken per day: increase to upper limits for age and weight

  Use of fracture pan/urinal/female urinal

Open Reduction with Internal Fixation

internal fixation: Surgical repair of bones and spine using such devices as a nail, pin, screw, wire, plate, rod, or a combination thereof. These surgeries include the following:

osteotomy: Alteration of bone structure to provide stability, straighten abnormal curvatures, or change weight-bearing surfaces

arthroplasty: Repair or remodeling of bones, cartilage, ligaments, or tendons to relieve pain, rectify traumatic injuries, or remove torn tissues

Harrington rod insertion: Procedure for correcting scoliosis

spinal fusion: Solidification of several vertebrae to strengthen, repair, or correct deformities

Preoperative assessment and care

Assess respiratory, neurovascular, nutritional, and integumentary status

Assess hearing, visual status and presence of other diseases

Monitor traction, braces if applicable

Discuss with and teach patient

  Method of coughing and deep breathing and use of incentive spirometer

  ROM exercises to unaffected extremities

  Postoperative position to be maintained

  Gluteal and abdominal contractions and quadriceps setting if applicable

  Dorsiflexion and plantar flexion of foot if applicable

  Monitor medications; especially be certain antiinflammatories and corticosteriods have been discontinued before admission if possible

  Method of log rolling

  Importance of leg abduction postoperatively; avoidance of adduction if applicable

  Use of trapeze, abduction brace, and pillow

  Method of bladder and bowel elimination

  Method of pain management

  Use of PCA (p. 92)

Discuss and assist patient in dealing with fears and anxieties

Reinforce physician's explanation of surgical procedure and follow-up care

Encourage communication with significant other(s)

Older adult patients may need instructions repeated with each task or procedure

Provide praise or encouragement for tasks attempted and completed

Postoperative assessment

Subjective data

Location and character of pain

Objective data

Correct placement of affected extremity, cast or brace
Neurovascular status of each affected extremity
Urinary output, vital signs
Color and amount of wound drainage
Mental alertness
Respiratory status

Diagnostic tests

CBC, electrolytes, blood gases
Radiologic examination of extremity/spine

Potential complications

Hemorrhage
Shock
Urinary retention, infection
Confusion if older adult
Decubitus ulcers
Atelectasis
Thrombophlebitis
Wound infection
Pin or prosthesis slippage
Extreme internal or external rotation
  Severe pain
  Localized edema of extremity
Malunion of fracture
  Severe pain
  Elevated temperature
  Severe muscle spasms
Fat embolus
  Difficulty in breathing
  Cough
  Chest petechiae
  Tachycardia
Compartment syndrome (p. 535)

Collaborative management

Therapeutic management

Position to be maintained
Immobilization devices
Analgesics, muscle relaxants, antibiotics
Parenteral therapy with electrolytes, urinary catheter
Oxygen therapy, incentive spirometer
Diet, activity, rest

Social medicine
  Postdischarge placement if indicated
  Home care assistance
Physical therapy
  Rehabilitation plan
  Exercises
Occupational therapy

Nursing management

PATIENT PROBLEMS/NURSING DIAGNOSES

● **NDX:** Impaired physical mobility related to surgical incision and temporary inability to bear weight

Maintain bed rest in prescribed position with firm mattress and trapeze
Assist and teach patient to cough and deep breathe qh
  Auscultate chest for breath sounds q8h
  Provide incentive spirometer
  Observe for dyspnea and chest pain
Turn patient on unaffected side q2h; maintain body alignment with pillow between knees and at back; turn on affected side if ordered
Ambulate with assistance; help patient with dangling legs at bedside, then with standing and pivoting on unaffected leg into chair (no weight bearing); involve physical therapy department if available
Maintain bed rest for 24 to 48 hr on spinal fusion patients; when allowed out of bed, must wear brace
Assist with and teach ROM exercises to unaffected extremities q4h, and with ROM exercises to knee, foot, and ankle of affected leg; passive continuous ROM machine may be ordered (p. 542)
Encourage and teach use of walker and increase ambulation and weight bearing as tolerated
Assist with ADLs as needed
Promote self-care as soon as patient is able
Balance rest periods with activity

EXPECTED OUTCOMES

Regains mobility and weight bearing to optimal level
Participates in rehabilitation plan
Progressively participates in own care

● **NDX:** Altered tissue perfusion: peripheral related to surgical procedure and interruption of A/V flow

Monitor vital signs q2h to 4h
Perform neurovascular checks on all extremities; monitor color, temperature, pulse, capillary refill, sensation, movement q2h to 4h
Monitor intake and output q4h

Administer parenteral fluids with electrolytes
Apply antiembolic stockings *to enhance venous return;* remove at least once daily to inspect skin
Encourage frequent movement of feet and legs *to promote venous return*
Administer anticoagulants as prescribed

EXPECTED OUTCOMES

Vital signs are stable
Neurovascular status and intake and output are within normal limits

● **NDX:** Risk for infection related to invasive procedure and lowered primary defenses

Assess incision for Hemovac placement; observe for increased drainage
Monitor incision for drainage q2h to 4h
Change dressings as needed; report bleeding, increased drainage to physician
Observe for signs of infection; obtain culture for suspicious drainage
Monitor temperature q4h
Provide well-balanced diet *to promote healing*
Monitor laboratory tests for increased WBC

EXPECTED OUTCOMES

Temperature is normal
Incision is healing
Surrounding tissue is clean, dry, and intact
Leukocyte count is within normal limits

● **NDX:** Pain related to surgical procedure and impaired mobility

Assess location, intensity, and character of pain using pain scale
Assess neurovascular status, especially for calf pain (thrombophlebitis)
Administer analgesics; assess effectiveness of pain relief measures
Reinforce instructions in use of PCA
Be alert for severe increase in pain caused by prosthetic slippage or malunion of fracture; report immediately
Provide frequent skin care and back rubs; change position slightly *to prevent skin breakdown and to provide comfort*
Monitor dosage of analgesics for the older adult patient because confusion and disorientation may result with normal dosage
Encourage and increase self-care activities as tolerated; medicate before activity
Provide diversional activities *to decrease attention on pain*
Teach and assist with alternate pain relief measures

EXPECTED OUTCOMES

Reports a reduction in pain level

Appears more relaxed and calm

Participates in self-care with less discomfort

ADDITIONAL NURSING DIAGNOSES
TO CONSIDER

Altered tissue perfusion: cardiopulmonary, cerebral related to fat embolus

Impaired skin integrity related to mechanical factors and/or physical immobilization

Patient/family teaching

Stress importance of following prescribed rehabilitation plan: amount of weight bearing, activities allowed, and correct body alignment; provide written material as a reference source

Discuss need for nutritious diet and fluids *to facilitate bone union and to maintain optimal circulation and elimination*

Prevent constipation with natural laxatives, stool softeners

If patient had arthroplasty surgery, discuss need to take antibiotics when having invasive procedures performed

Discuss signs and symptoms to report to physician: increased incision or leg pain, fever, decreased urinary output, signs of wound infection

Demonstrate incision care

Promote increasing self-care and ADLs as tolerated

Encourage follow-up visits with physician and physical therapist

Home care considerations

Assess and continue with patient/family teaching and monitor the following:

Environmental/safety status

Care givers' ability to perform needed tasks

Accessible telephone and emergency numbers: physician, pharmacy, home health care team

Emergency call device to summon outside help

Absence of skatter rugs, unbacked carpets

Presence of stairs with hand rails

Grab bars at tub and toilet

Nonskid strips in tub

Adequate lighting for safe movement

Wide doorways to accommodate wheelchairs/walkers

Height of chair and bed for easy transfer on and off of each

Flashlights near bed and chair

Medications accessible and labeled

Availability of transportation to needed appointments

Needed supplies: what and where to purchase

Mobility status

Ability and desire to follow prescribed rehabilitation plan and exercises

Correct transfer techniques

Amount of weight bearing; reinforce wearing low-heeled, comfortable shoes

Correct use of walkers, canes, crutches

Ability to apply brace, corset, removable cast

Status of immobilizing device

Neurovascular status of each affected extremity

Condition of device: wet, loose, clean, soiled

Condition of skin under device: clear, red, tender

Status of wound

Incision for healing, infection

Signs of infection: redness, pain, swelling, fever, drainage

Ability to care for wound: correct supplies and hand-washing technique

Knowledge of where and what supplies to purchase

Nutritional status

Understanding of basic food groups and what to eat to provide adequate nutrition with no weight gain

Signs of weight loss, dehydration

Ability to prepare meals; refer to social agency to provide meals

Elimination status

Presence of elevated toilet seat

Use of stool softeners, natural laxatives, bulk in diet

Ability to be active

Amount of fluids taken per day: increase to upper limits for age and weight

Use of fracture pan/urinal/female urinal

Total Joint Arthroplasty: Hip, Knee, Ankle, Shoulder, Elbow, Wrist, Finger

Replacement of a total joint with a prosthesis to provide stability and motion; performed on diseased or traumatized joints

Preoperative assessment and care

Assess medication history; be certain that antiinflammatories and corticosteroids were discontinued at least 10 days before admission, if possible

Assess respiratory, neurovascular, nutritional, and integumentary status

Assess hearing and visual status and presence of other diseases (diabetes, arthritis)

Discuss with and teach patient the following:
Method of coughing and deep breathing; use of incentive spirometer
ROM exercises to unaffected extremities
Postoperative restrictions or limitations; these may differ according to physician preference
Total hip arthroplasty (Figure 8-2)
Gluteal and abdominal contractions and quadriceps setting
Dorsiflexion and plantar flexion of foot
Hip hiking, isometric exercises
Use of trapeze and continuous passive motion device
Importance of leg abduction postoperatively
Total knee arthroplasty (Figure 8-3)
Quadriceps setting, gluteal contractions, and flexion-extension exercises
Straight leg lifts
Total shoulder arthroplasty
Presence of sling to support affected arm; no side elevation of arm
Prescribed exercises of fingers, wrist, and elbow
Total elbow arthroplasty
Presence of abduction humerus splint to prevent rotation
Elbow will be immobilized at 90 degrees of flexion

Prescribed wrist and finger exercises
Total wrist arthroplasty
Presence of volnar splint to prevent wrist flexion
Prescribed finger and arm exercises
Total thumb replacement
Presence of immobilizing splint or brace to provide wrist and thumb support but allowing for movement of fingers
Prescribed finger and arm exercises
Total finger arthroplasty
Presence of immobilizing splint or brace that provides involved finger support but allows movement of other fingers
Prescribed exercises for arm and unaffected fingers
Total ankle arthroplasty
Presence of posterior plaster cast and Hemovac suction apparatus
Method of crutch walking
Prescribed exercises for toes and knee
Involvement of physical therapy department in planning rehabilitation goals
Methods of bladder and bowel elimination
Methods of pain management: PCA (p. 92) or continuous epidural analgesia (CEA) (p. 92)
Administer antibiotics and anticoagulants
Measure for antiembolic stockings

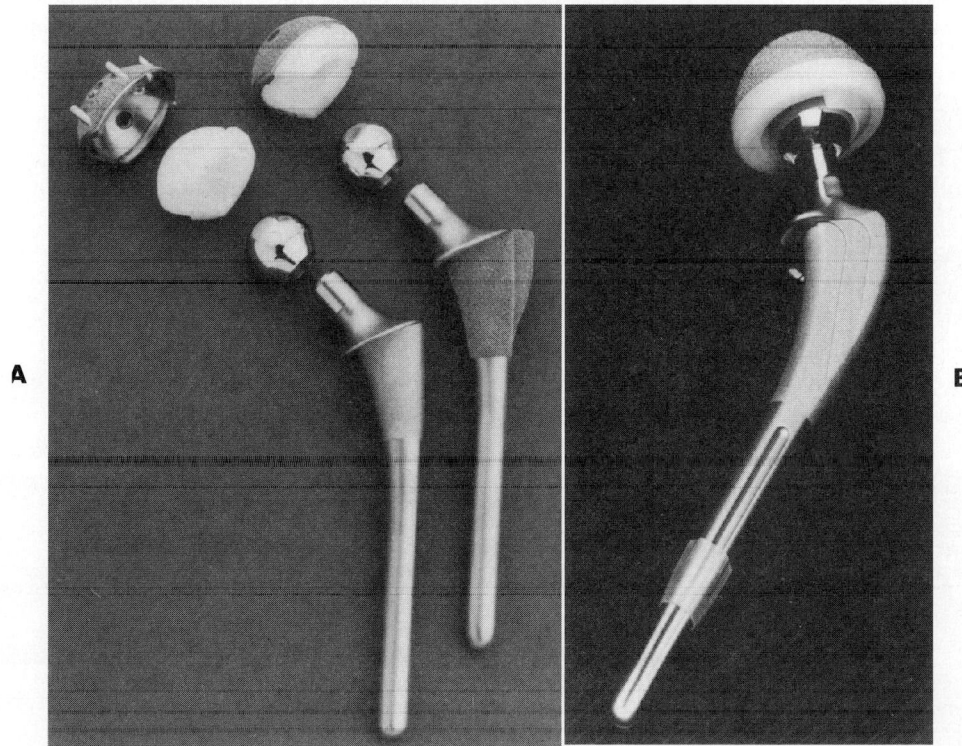

A

B

Figure 8-2 Several types of total hip replacement prostheses. (**A,** Courtesy Zimmer, Warsaw, IN. **B,** Courtesy Biomet, Warsaw, IN. From Mourad LA: *Mosby's clinical nursing series: orthopedic disorders,* St Louis, 1991, Mosby.)

Discuss sequential compression devices (athrombic pump)

Administer surgical scrub every q2days

Discuss and assist patient in dealing with fears and anxieties

Reinforce physician's explanation of surgical procedure and follow-up care

Encourage communication with significant other(s)

Repeat instructions as needed with each procedure or task for older adult patients

Provide praise and encouragement for tasks attempted or completed

Postoperative assessment

Subjective data

Location and character of pain

Objective data

Neurovascular status of involved extremity
  Peripheral pulse, pallor, cyanosis, edema
  Sensation, temperature, mobility
Site of incision; wound drains
  Hemovac
  Excessive bleeding or drainage
Respiratory status
Position of affected joint and extremity
Mental alertness

Diagnostic tests

Electrolytes, CBC, PT/INR
Joint radiologic study

Potential complications

Disorientation (older adult patient)
Tachycardia
Tachypnea
Chest pain
Atelectasis
Pneumonia
Thrombophlebitis
Pulmonary embolus
Hemorrhage
Shock
Fat embolus
Wound infection
Compartment syndrome (knee, elbow) (p. 535)

Collaborative management

Therapeutic management

Postoperative position of involved extremity
Parenteral fluids with electrolytes initially
Incision and draining apparatus care
Cast, splint, brace, sling: device depends on joint replaced
Analgesics, antibiotics, sedatives, antipyretics, anticoagulants, stool softeners, laxatives, antiinflammatory agents
PCA, TENS unit
Oxygen therapy, incentive spirometer
Antiembolic stockings, sequential compression device
Diet, rest, activity
Physical therapy
  Rehabilitation plan

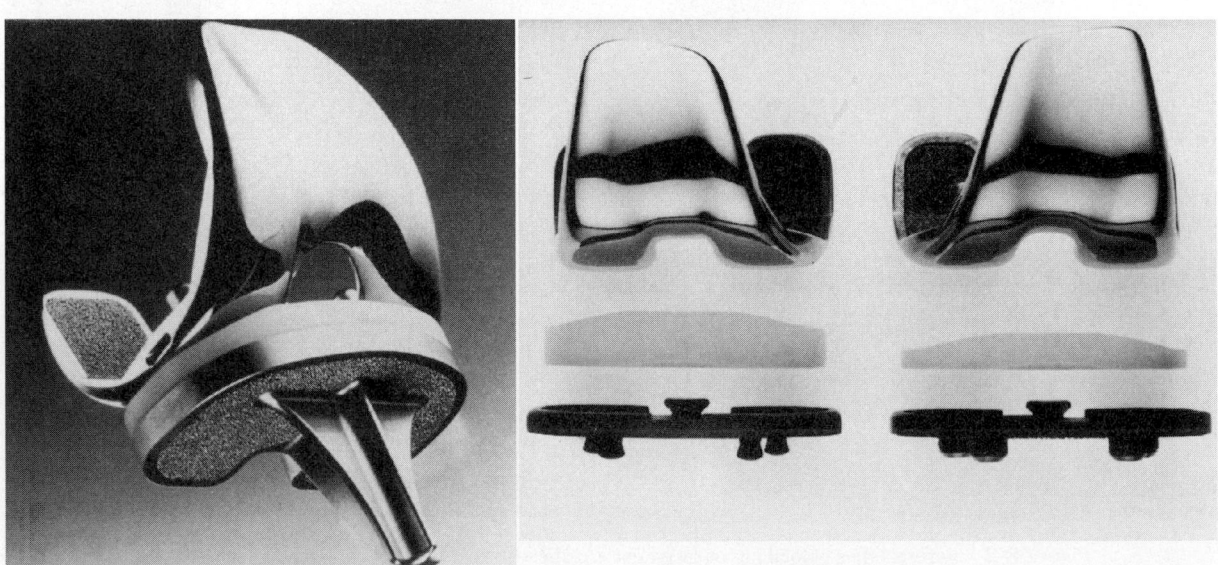

Figure 8-3   Several types of total knee replacement prostheses. (Courtesy Zimmer, Warsaw, IN. From Mourad LA: *Mosby's clinical nursing series: orthopedic disorders,* St Louis, 1991, Mosby.)

Occupational therapy
Crutch walking
Social medicine: follow-up placement, if needed

Nursing management

PATIENT PROBLEMS/NURSING DIAGNOSES

● **NDX:** Impaired physical mobility related to surgical procedure of joint involved and pain

Maintain bed rest with affected joint in prescribed position
Provide firm mattress, trapeze, and overhead frame
Maintain support of joint through use of splint, brace, sling, cast, or pillows
Perform passive or assist with and teach active ROM exercises to unaffected joints
Reinforce restrictions and limitations on affected joint *to prevent dislocation*
Assist with ADLs as needed
  Turn patient as ordered; support joint to maintain immobilization and body alignment
  Monitor skin for reddened areas; massage bony prominences prn
  Maintain wrinkle-free linens
Promote quadriceps, gluteal muscle sets and isometric exercises as indicated
Ambulate patient with assistance (duration of bed rest depends on joint replaced)
  Provide ambulatory aids as needed
  Observe weight-bearing restrictions
  Monitor for vertigo, weakness, and nausea
Continuous passive ROM machine may be ordered for affected extremity of hip and knee arthroplasty patients

EXPECTED OUTCOMES

Maintains proper body alignment in bed and while ambulating
Increases weight bearing as prescribed
Expresses understanding of and participates in rehabilitation regimen
Progresses toward self-care

● **NDX:** Altered tissue perfusion: peripheral related to reduced blood flow, tissue edema

Administer parenteral fluids with electrolytes *to increase tissue perfusion*
Monitor vital signs q2h to 4h and prn
Assess neurovascular status of affected extremity qh for 12 hr, then q4h; observe color, T, P, sensation, and mobility; observe for signs of venous thrombosis (p. 107) and compartment syndrome (p. 535)

Monitor antiembolic stocking or sequential compression device; remove stockings q2days to observe skin for redness, monitor pulses
Encourage foot flexion q2h to 4h *to promote venous return* if applicable
Apply ice bags to affected joint
Monitor CBC, electrolytes, and PT/INR
Maintain indwelling urethral catheter; monitor intake and output; observe for urinary retention; output may be less than intake for 24 to 48 hr
Administer anticoagulants *to prevent phlebitis;* assess effectiveness and for side effects

EXPECTED OUTCOMES

Vital signs are stable
Laboratory values are within normal limits
Extremities are warm and normal color, and pulse are palpable

● **NDX:** Risk for infection (wound, pneumonia) related to surgical intervention, immobility, and decreased primary defenses

Monitor incision and dressings for drainage and presence of drain or Hemovac *to keep surgical site clear of fluids*
  Monitor output for color and amount q4h; report excessive bleeding to physician
  Reinforce and change dressings prn; observe for signs of healing and wound infection
  Administer wound irrigation with antibiotics as indicated
  Obtain culture for any suspicious drainage
Assess respiratory status q4h; observe for pain, dyspnea, and tachypnea
Monitor T q4h; report any elevation to physician
Auscultate chest for breath sounds q4h; observe for diminished breath sounds
Initiate use of incentive spirometer q1h to 2h
Change position q2h while in bed *to prevent stasis of lung secretions*

EXPECTED OUTCOMES

Incision is clean, dry, intact
Temperature is normal
Respiratory rate and rhythm are regular
Breath sounds are normal

● **NDX:** Pain related to surgical intervention and impaired mobility

Assess location, intensity, and character of pain using pain rating scale
Administer analgesics, sedatives, and/or antiinflammatory agents; assess effectiveness of pain relief measures; monitor dosage for older adult patients *because prescribed dose may cause disorientation*

Monitor patient controlled analgesia or continuous epidural analgesia (CEA) as indicated

Change position frequently *to prevent fatigue and pressure on bony prominences;* administer back rubs as indicated

Provide diversional activities *to reduce attention on pain*

Discuss and teach alternate pain relief techniques

Promote self-care activities as tolerated

Monitor for severe chest or affected joint pain; may indicate emboli or displacement of joint

EXPECTED OUTCOMES

Displays more relaxed affect

States pain is at tolerable level

Participates in diversional activities

ADDITIONAL NURSING DIAGNOSIS TO CONSIDER

Risk for injury, related to dislocation of prosthesis

Patient/family teaching

Stress importance of and provide written instructions for prescribed rehabilitation program: daily exercises and/or ROM for affected joint, activity allowed, and position to be maintained; no adduction of extremity or >90 degree flexion

Discuss and demonstrate incision care

Provide medication schedule including name, purpose, dosage, and side effects; if patient is taking anticoagulants, explain need to have PT checked regularly, observe for bleeding, and avoid aspirin use

Explain need to use soft toothbrush, electric razor while on anticoagulant

Discuss need to take prophylactic antibiotics before invasive procedure including dental cleaning or procedure

Explain importance of high-protein, high-fiber diet and increased fluid intake *to facilitate healing and prevent constipation*

Discuss need for a safe environment

Discuss signs and symptoms of wound infection, dislodgment to report to physician: fever, inflammation, pain, immobility

Encourage follow-up visits with physician

Home care considerations

Assess and continue with patient/family teaching and monitor the following:

Environmental/safety status

Care givers' ability to perform needed tasks

Accessible telephone and emergency numbers: physician, pharmacy, home health care team

Emergency call device to summon outside help

Absence of skatter rugs, unbacked carpets

Presence of stairs with hand rails

Grab bars at tub and toilet

Nonskid strips in tub

Adequate lighting for safe movement

Wide doorways to accommodate wheelchairs/walkers

Height of chair and bed for easy transfer on and off of each

Flashlights near bed and chair

Medications accessible and labeled

Availability of transportation to needed appointments

Needed supplies: what and where to purchase

Mobility status

Ability and desire to follow prescribed rehabilitation plan and exercises

Correct transfer techniques

Ability to apply brace, corset, removable cast

Status of wound

Incision for healing, infection

Signs of infection: redness, pain, swelling, fever, drainage

Ability to care for wound: correct supplies and handwashing technique

Knowledge of where and what supplies to purchase

Nutritional status

Understanding of basic food groups and what to eat to provide nutrition with no weight gain

Signs of weight loss, dehydration

Ability to prepare meals; refer to social agency to provide meals

Elimination status

Presence of elevated toilet seat

Use of stool softeners, natural laxatives, bulk in diet

Ability to be active

Amount of fluids taken per day: increase to upper limits for age and weight

Use of fracture pan/urinal/female urinal

Amputation of Leg: Above or Below Knee

Surgical removal of part of the leg because of trauma, disease, tumors, or congenital anomalies; a skin flap is generally constructed to facilitate healing and use of prosthetic equipment

Preoperative assessment and care

Monitor neurovascular status, both extremities

Observe affected extremity for open, draining sites

Obtain baseline vital signs
Administer skin preparation as ordered
Encourage and allow time for verbalization of fears and anxieties
  Reinforce physician's explanation of operative procedure and phantom limb sensation
  Begin to deal with body image change, loss, and grief; listen carefully and support positive coping behaviors; assist patient with expressing feelings to significant other(s)
Explain process of and preparation for rehabilitation
  Strengthen muscles of upper extremities for crutch walking
    Push-ups from prone position
    Alteration of flexing and extending arms holding weights
    Sit-ups from seated position
  Practice crutch walking
  Practice quadriceps setting exercises, gluteal contraction exercises, and leg lift of affected extremity unless contraindicated
Practice use of overhead trapeze attached to frame
Explain types of prostheses available if appropriate
  Immediate postsurgical fitting (IPSF): for immediate or early ambulation and weight bearing; cast is applied to stump and prosthesis is attached to cast
  Delayed: dressing and elastic bandage are applied to stump; prosthesis is not made for 2 to 3 months

Postoperative assessment

Subjective data

Location, intensity, and type of pain

Objective data

Type of dressing or rigid plaster cast
Position of stump
Stump dressing, amount and color of drainage, presence of drains, Hemovac
Respiratory status, vital signs

Diagnostic tests

CBC, fasting blood sugar (for diabetics)

Potential complications

Hemorrhage, dehiscence
Wound infection
Phantom pain
Contractures
Abduction deformity

Collaborative management

Therapeutic management

Position of stump postoperatively
Type of dressing and/or postsurgical fitting applied
Analgesics, antibiotics, antipyretics, sedatives
Diet, activity, rest
Physical therapy
  Prescribed exercises and rehabilitation plan
  Occupational therapy for lifestyle changes
Orthotic technician: cast and prosthesis management
Social medicine: assist with home health care, placement as needed

Nursing management

PATIENT PROBLEMS/NURSING DIAGNOSES

● **NDX:**   Impaired physical mobility related to pain and musculoskeletal impairment

Maintain bed rest in prescribed position
Elevate stump *to prevent edema,* usually for 24 hr; avoid pillow unless it is removed for 30 min q2h to prevent contractures; avoid outward rotation; elevate head of bed no more than 30 degrees *to maintain alignment*
Turn from side to back to abdomen (after 24 hr) q2h *to prevent contractures*
Assist with and teach active or perform passive ROM exercises q4h to unaffected extremities *to maintain mobility*
Assist with and teach adduction and extension exercises to affected extremity q4h
Assist with ambulation
  Without prosthesis
    Avoid long periods of chair sitting *to prevent stasis of venous return*
    Provide ambulation devices: crutches, walker
    Encourage use of good walking shoes and maintain stump in normal position—relaxed and downward; involve physical therapy department
  With prosthesis
    Assist with measuring for prosthesis
    Provide ambulation device: crutches, walker
    Increase ambulation with prescribed amount of weight bearing; involve physical therapy department
Assist with and reiterate postoperative conditioning exercises: trunk flexion, sit-ups, hopping in place, hopping with walker *to maintain mobility*

EXPECTED OUTCOMES
Expresses understanding of treatment and exercise plan

Cooperates/participates in needed activities
Maintains correct body alignment
Exhibits no contractures

● **NDX:** Risk for fluid volume deficit related to increased drainage or bleeding at surgical site

Administer parenteral fluids and anticoagulants as indicated *to sustain hydration*
Monitor vital signs q2h to 4h
Measure intake and output q8h
Monitor dressings and incision for color and amount of drainage and for presence of drains or Hemovac; observe for bleeding; outline bleeding area on dressing with pen and write date and time
Apply pressure and elevate stump in case of hemorrhage; follow with use of tourniquet if hemorrhage not controlled
Monitor Hgb, Hct, PT/INR, and electrolytes
Monitor postsurgical cast for bleeding and mark area as discussed previously; observe for cast slippage and report to physician

EXPECTED OUTCOMES
Vital signs are within normal limits
Wound is healing
Skin is warm, dry

● **NDX:** Risk for infection related to surgical procedure and lowered primary defenses

Change stump dressing and elastic bandage *to produce shrinkage and prepare for prosthesis*
Wash and dry area; expose it to air before reapplying dressing
  Perform at least qod
  Observe for signs of infection and increasing edema
  Begin stump strengthening and conditioning; push against pillow and increase to firmer surface as tolerated
Change postsurgical cast dressing bid; wash and dry area; allow it to air dry
  Apply properly fitting stump sock prn, *to provide support*
  Observe incision and surrounding area for increasing edema and signs of wound infection
  Massage stump toward suture line as ordered: usually 1 wk postoperatively
  Reapply postsurgical cast
Maintain dry dressing; cover with plastic while using bed pan or if incontinent *to prevent soiling*
Begin teaching dressing change procedure
Monitor temperature q4h
Provide high-protein diet and encourage fluids to upper limits for age and weight *to promote healing*

Administer antibiotics and/or antipyretics: monitor for effectiveness, side effects

EXPECTED OUTCOMES
Participates in maintaining aseptic techniques
Remains afebrile with adequate wound healing

● **NDX:** Pain related to surgical intervention and immobility

Assess character, intensity, and location of pain; observe for compartment syndrome in below-the-knee amputation (p. 535)
Administer analgesics and sedative; assess effectiveness of pain relief measures
Assist patient with changing position slightly at frequent intervals *to reduce fatigue and pressure;* provide back rubs
Provide diversional activities *to reduce attention on pain*
Teach and assist with alternate pain relief measures
Monitor use of TENS unit (p. 94) or PCA (p. 92)
Discuss and explain phantom pain and that it is normal and usually temporary
Coordinate care to provide rest periods

EXPECTED OUTCOMES
States that pain is at a tolerable level
Appears calm, relaxed; is able to sleep and rest adequately
Understands phantom pain theory

● **NDX:** Body image disturbance related to loss of body part

Encourage and allow time for patient to express feelings of loss and grief
Assist in identifying positive coping behaviors and provide encouragement and praise for strengths observed
Provide praise for attempted and/or completed tasks
Encourage patient to discuss and view stump
Encourage patient to perform self-care activities and involve patient in stump care as soon as able; promote independence
Allow patient to wear own clothing *to increase self-esteem*
Promote communication with family and significant other(s)
Explain all procedures and treatments
Provide a supportive environment
Encourage socialization with another amputee

EXPECTED OUTCOMES
Begins using positive coping skills in dealing with loss of body part

Begins expressing feelings of acceptance of altered self
Participates in self-care activities, ADLs and stump care

ADDITIONAL NURSING DIAGNOSIS
TO CONSIDER

Risk for injury related to imbalance caused by loss of leg

Patient/family teaching

Stress importance of and review rehabilitation program; involve physical therapy department in daily exercises and stump strengthening and conditioning
Demonstrate dressing changes, incision care, skin care, and technique for massage of stump
Discuss and demonstrate care of IPSF as indicated; consult physical therapy department or provide referral for permanent prosthesis
Promote safe home environment; instruct patient to wear rubber-soled shoe as indicated
Discuss signs and symptoms to report to physician: fever, inflammation of incision, prolonged phantom pain, increasing edema of stump
Discuss importance of well-balanced diet, avoiding weight gain
Refer to support group
Encourage follow-up visits with physician/physical therapist

Home care considerations

Assess and continue with patient/family teaching and monitor the following:
  Environmental/safety status
    Care givers' ability to perform needed tasks
    Accessible telephone and emergency numbers: physician, pharmacy, home health care team
    Emergency call device to summon outside help
    Absence of skatter rugs, unbacked carpets
    Presence of stairs with hand rails
    Grab bars at tub and toilet
    Nonskid strips in tub
    Adequate lighting for safe movement
    Wide doorways to accommodate wheelchairs/ walkers
    Height of chair and bed for easy transfer on and off of each
    Flashlights near bed and chair
    Medications accessible and labeled
    Availability of transportation to needed appointments
    Needed supplies: what and where to purchase
  Mobility status
    Ability and desire to follow prescribed rehabilitation plan and exercises
    Correct transfer techniques

Reinforce wearing low-heeled, comfortable shoes
Correct use of walkers, canes, crutches
Status of wound
  Incision for healing, infection
  Signs of infection: redness, pain, swelling, fever, drainage
  Ability to care for wound: correct supplies, hand-washing technique, and application of bandage(s)
  Knowledge of where and what supplies to purchase

Arthroscopy

Management of various joint disorders using an arthroscope; a small surgical instrument is introduced via a trocar and scope into the joint, allowing visualization of the joint; this provides a means for diagnosing and performing needed surgery; most frequently scoped joints are the knee, elbow, and shoulder

Preoperative assessment and care

Determine presence of both pulses distal to the joint
Discuss with and teach patient
  ROM exercises to unaffected extremities
  Restrictions and limitations postoperatively
    These will vary with physicians and according to extent of surgery
    Usually patient is out of bed on evening of surgery but with no weight bearing if indicated
  Method of crutch walking if applicable
  Methods of pain management
  Purpose of NPO
Administer antiseptic scrub to affected joint
Reinforce physician's explanation of procedure

Postoperative assessment

Subjective data

Location and character of pain

Objective data

Position of joint and degree of elevation
Character and amount of drainage
Type of immobilization device (rarely used)
Neurovascular status of affected extremity: pulse, color, temperature, sensation, mobility

Potential complications

Edema
Hemorrhage

Thrombophlebitis (p. 107)
Infection
Postoperative arthrosis
Compartment syndrome (p. 535)

Collaborative management

Therapeutic management

Analgesics, antibiotics, sedatives
Position of joint postoperatively; exercises, ambulation
Ice bag to joint
Diet, activity, rest

Nursing management

PATIENT PROBLEMS/NURSING DIAGNOSES

● **NDX:** Altered tissue perfusion: peripheral related to arthroscopy and risk of altered arteriovenous flow

Elevate extremity *to promote venous return*
Monitor neurovascular status of affected extremity qh for 4 hr, then q4h; check pulse, color, temperature, sensation, and mobility
Monitor vital signs q4h
Apply ice pack to joint *to reduce swelling*
Monitor pressure dressing and observe for bleeding

EXPECTED OUTCOMES

Affected extremity is warm, dry, mobile
Vital signs are stable
Distal pulses are palpable

● **NDX:** Impaired physical mobility related to discomfort and prescribed immobilization

Maintain bed rest in position of comfort with involved joint elevated in slight flexion
Avoid excessive use of joint for 24 to 48 hr
Walking is permitted for knee arthroscopy
Encourage ROM exercises of unaffected extremities q2h
Ambulate with assistance, usually on evening of surgery
  Assist patient with getting out of bed, keeping affected extremity elevated until standing; no weight bearing until ordered
  Assist patient with use of crutches, walker as indicated
  Increase ambulation as tolerated
  Provide rest periods between ambulations
Initiate and assist with prescribed exercises; these de-

pend on physician's preference and extent of surgery
Involve physical therapy department if applicable
Teach dorsiflexion and plantar flexion of foot or wrist and increasing flexion of knee, elbow

EXPECTED OUTCOMES

Demonstrates increasing mobility
Participates in exercise program
Ambulates correctly with crutches

● **NDX:** Pain related to invasive procedure

Assess location, intensity, and type of pain; *severe unrelenting pain and edema may indicate compartment syndrome*
Administer analgesics and/or sedatives: assess effectiveness and for side effects
Provide diversional activities
Change position in small ways *to promote comfort*
Apply ice bag *to decrease edema/pain*

EXPECTED OUTCOMES

Reports a reduced level of discomfort
Exhibits relaxed facial expressions
Sleeps for longer periods at night

ADDITIONAL NURSING DIAGNOSIS TO CONSIDER

Risk for infection related to surgical procedure

Patient/family teaching and home care considerations

Stress importance and goals of prescribed rehabilitation program
  Knee
    Amount of weight bearing and knee flexion allowed
    Elevation of leg while sitting
    Avoiding twisting knee
    Dorsiflexion and plantar flexion exercises of feet
    Ambulation with crutches
    Swimming should be encouraged
  Elbow/shoulder
    Amount of flexion allowed
    Type of arm support needed (sling, cast) and care of device
    Activity permitted; avoid excessive use of joint
Discuss signs of wound infection to report to physician: fever, redness, pain, odor, edema at operative site
Importance of rest periods between exercises
Dates and times of physical therapy visits if applicable
Encourage follow-up care with physician

External Fixation for Complicated Fractures

A surgical procedure to immobilize and reduce complicated fractures; stabilizing pins or wires are inserted into and/or through the bone and attached to an external metal frame (Figure 8-4); may be applied to jaw, arm, leg, ribs, pelvis, fingers, or toes; one type of fixator is the Ilizarov external fixator (Figure 8-5; see box on p.530)

Preoperative assessment and teaching

Preoperative teaching may be limited depending on urgency of needed treatment

Assess neurovascular and respiratory status

Discuss with and teach patient the following:
  Methods of coughing and deep breathing and/or use of incentive spirometer
  Necessary ROM exercises, quadriceps setting, and gluteal contractions according to location of fracture
  Use of trapeze
  Necessary movement limitations and activities allowed
  Importance of external fixator
    Reinforce physician's explanation of procedure
    Fixator usually causes little pain or discomfort and allows for early ambulation
    Device is unsightly, but long-range results are the primary goal

Explain that extremity will be elevated postoperatively to reduce edema

Involve physical therapy department, if available, for crutch walking and exercises

Administer prescribed antibiotics and skin prep

Postoperative assessment

Subjective data

Location, intensity, and character of pain

Objective data

Elevation and position of extremity

Edema of extremity at operative site and below

Presence of supportive dressings

Character and amount of drainage from wound and pin sites

Neurovascular status of affected extremity: color, sensation, mobility, peripheral pulse, temperature

Diagnostic tests

CBC, PT/INR, chemistries

Radiologic examination of affected bone

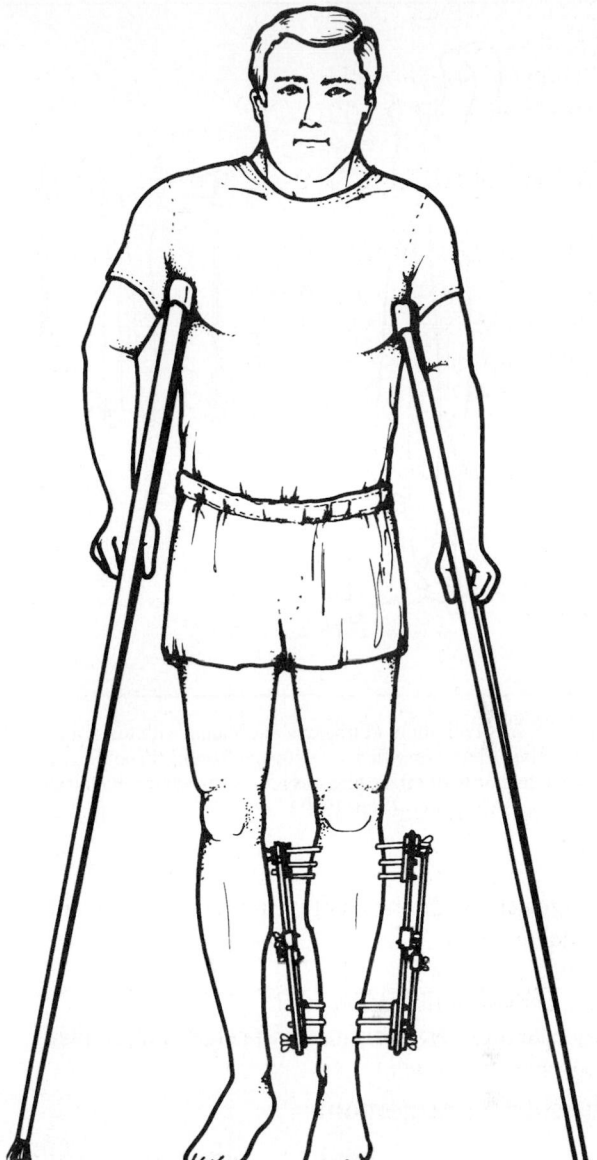

Figure 8-4   External fixation for complicated fractures.

Potential complications

Hemorrhage

Shock

Wound or pin site infection

Nonunion, malunion

Neuromuscular dysfunction

Compartment syndrome (p. 535)

Collaborative management

Therapeutic management

Position of affected extremity

Schedule for tightening nuts on fixator if applicable

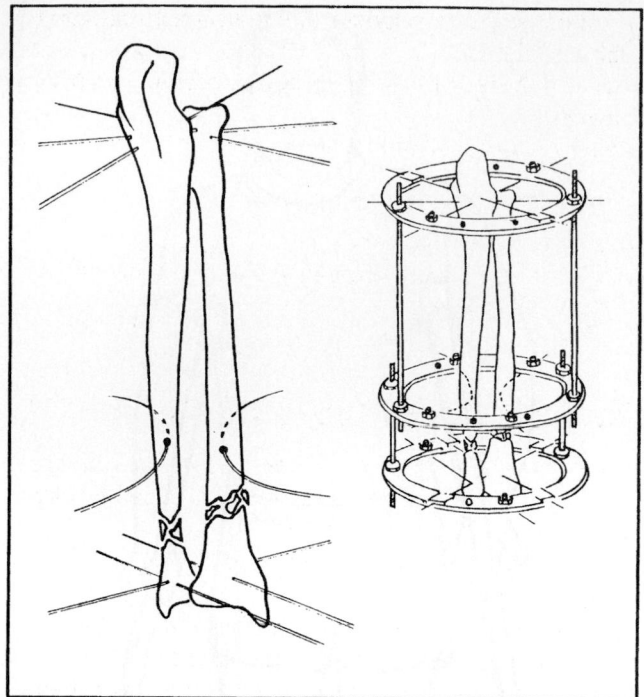

Figure 8-5 Treatment of fracture of the ulna with dislocation of the head of the radius using Ilizarov external fixator. (From Ilizarov external fixator general surgical technique brochure, Richards Medical Co, Memphis, Tenn, 1990.)

Ilizarov External Fixator

An external fixator, developed by Gauril Ilizarov, that allows control over a variety of bone disorders including rotation, angulation, translation, lengthening, and shortening. It preserves limb function and blood supply and promotes healing. Also known as a compression-distraction apparatus, it can be assembled in more than 600 different ways and, therefore, is very versatile (Figure 8-5).

Indications
  Open, closed fractures
  Nonunion, pseudoarthrosis of long bones
  Limb lengthening, shortening
  Correction of deformities, defects of bony or
    soft tissue
Postoperative care is essentially the same as for the external fixator on this page.

Analgesics, antibiotics, antipyretics, sedatives, antibacterial cream
Ice bag to area
Diet, activity, ambulation, rest
Physical therapy: exercises and rehabilitation plan

Nursing management

PATIENT PROBLEMS/NURSING DIAGNOSES

● **NDX:** Impaired physical mobility related to musculoskeletal impairment and pain

Maintain bed rest in position of comfort with extremity elevated
Assist with and teach active ROM exercises to unaffected extremities q2h to 4h; initiate quadriceps setting, gluteal contractions, or palmar or dorsal flexion as needed
Ambulate when edema of soft tissues has decreased
  Holding fixator with both hands, assist patient to sitting position on bed side; observe for vertigo and nausea
  Always support fixator, not extremity
  Assist patient to ambulate with crutches or sling as indicated
Do not change or adjust fixator bars (can cause misalignment)
No weight bearing until ordered

Physical therapy department should be involved where available
Elevate extremity while sitting up
Provide high-protein diet and fluids *to maintain muscle mass* for possible long rehabilitation

EXPECTED OUTCOMES

Demonstrates mobility returning to optimal level
Cooperates with and participates in exercise program
Uses supporting devices correctly

● **NDX:** Altered tissue perfusion: peripheral related to surgical procedure and interruption of arteriovenous flow

Monitor vital signs q2h for 8 hr; then q4h
Assess neurovascular status of affected extremity q2h; color, temperature, capillary refill, sensation, and mobility
Encourage moving joints below affected bone *to increase venous return*
Elevate extremity on pillow
Assist with coughing, deep breathing exercises *to increase oxygen intake;* provide incentive spirometer

EXPECTED OUTCOMES

Vital signs are within normal limits
Extremity is warm and normal color
Neurovascular checks are within normal limits

● **NDX:** Risk for infection related to pins and fixator insertion

Monitor pin sites, incision, and supportive dressing q1h to 2h for drainage and edema

Initiate pin site and incision care q2days

Assess for pain, tenderness, redness, and tension around each pin site

Obtain culture for drainage suggestive of infection

Cleanse around each pin site with hydrogen peroxide; rinse with normal saline

Apply antibacterial agent around each pin

Allow to air dry

Cover each pin head with cork or rubber tip *to prevent injury*

Cleanse fixator with sterile water

Assist with and teach patient wound, pin site, and fixator care as soon as patient is physically and emotionally able

Change incision dressings as necessary; observe for wound healing

Apply ice bags to areas *to reduce edema*

EXPECTED OUTCOMES

Tissue around pin sites remains clean and dry

Incision and surrounding area are healing

Demonstration of incision and pin care is adequate

T is normal

● **NDX:** Pain related to surgical intervention and immobility

Assess location, intensity, and character of pain; observe proximal joint for compartment syndrome signs: unrelenting pain, edema (p. 535)

Administer analgesics and sedatives: assess effectiveness of pain relief measures; encourage use of PCA (p. 92)

Assist patient with changing position frequently while in bed *to prevent fatigue and pressure*

Provide diversional activities *to decrease focus on discomfort*

Discuss and teach alternate pain management techniques

EXPECTED OUTCOMES

States pain is at a tolerable level

Appears more relaxed and calm

Reports ability to sleep and rest for increasing length of time

● **NDX:** Body image disturbance related to external fixator

Provide supportive environment *to allow for expression of feelings*

Promote and allow time for expression of feelings; encourage communication with significant other(s)

Assist in identifying positive coping patterns; acknowledge strengths *to provide encouragement*

Promote self-care activities and praise tasks attempted or completed

Stress that fixator is temporary and promote its positive aspects

Reinforce purpose of fixator

EXPECTED OUTCOMES

Attempts to express concerns/feelings

Begins to use positive coping skills in dealing with altered self-image

Seeks assistance appropriately

Patient/family teaching

Provide and review written goals, restrictions, and activities of rehabilitation program as outlined by physician and/or physical therapist

Demonstrate care of pins, fixator, and incision

Observe return demonstration

Stress importance of not tampering with fixator, which may alter alignment of fracture

Explain that showering is permitted but that patient needs to avoid swimming because chlorine and salt corrode metal

Stress importance of diet and elimination

Discuss signs and symptoms of wound infection to report to physician

Encourage follow-up visit with physician/physical therapy department

Home care considerations

Assess and continue with patient/family teaching and monitor the following:

Environmental/safety status

Care givers' ability to perform needed tasks

Accessible telephone and emergency numbers: physician, pharmacy, home health care team

Emergency call device to summon outside help

Absence of skatter rugs, unbacked carpets

Presence of stairs with hand rails

Grab bars at tub and toilet

Nonskid strips in tub

Adequate lighting for safe movement

Wide doorways to accommodate wheelchairs/walkers

Height of chair and bed for easy transfer on and off of each

Flashlights near bed and chair

Medications accessible and labeled

Availability of transportation to needed appointments

Needed supplies: what and where to purchase

Mobility status

Ability and desire to follow prescribed rehabilitation plan and exercises

Correct transfer techniques

Amount of weight bearing; reinforce wearing low-heeled, comfortable shoes

Correct use of walkers, canes, crutches

Status of wound

Incision for healing, infection

Signs of infection: redness, pain, swelling, fever, drainage

Ability to care for fixator: correct supplies and hand-washing technique

Knowledge of where and what supplies to purchase

Digital Replantation of Fingers, Thumb

Surgical reconnection of severed digit(s) after trauma by a sharp object, crushing blow, or avulsion; general criteria for replantation include thumb replacement, multiple digit replacement, or replacement if patient is a child or patient's occupation requires manual skills; surgery must be performed within 24 hr

Preoperative assessment and care

Preservation of digit(s)

Wrap digit(s) in gauze or dry cloth soaked with normal saline if available

Place in double plastic bags and seal

Place bags in ice

Never place digit directly on ice

Care of amputated stump: apply sterile pressure dressing and elevate hand as ordered

Administer parenteral fluids with antibiotics as ordered

Administer anticoagulant and tetanus toxoid as ordered

Assess respiratory, cardiovascular, and neurologic status

Determine presence or absence of further trauma or injury

Assess medication and medical history: diseases such as diabetes, chronic obstructive pulmonary disease (COPD), vascular disease, rheumatoid arthritis, osteoarthritis, and bleeding tendencies inhibit replantation success

Determine dominant hand

Assess emotional status where possible

Be alert for maladaptive behavior because functional return depends on patient's motivation, emotional acceptance, and willingness to adapt to alterations in body image and lifestyle

Reinforce physician's explanation of surgical procedure

Discuss and deal with fears and anxieties

Encourage communication with significant other(s)

Discuss with and assist patient to understand that nicotine and caffeine are potent vasoconstrictors and therefore are prohibited

Postoperative assessment

Subjective data

Location and character of pain

Objective data

Neurovascular status of digit

Sensation, color, temperature

Capillary refill, skin turgor

Edema

Anatomic position of digit, wrist, and elbow and elevation of each

Presence or absence of skin graft and graft site

Character and amount of drainage from incision

Diagnostic tests

CBC, PT/INR, chemistries

Radiologic examination of replantation

Potential complications

Hemorrhage

Shock

Vascular thrombosis or occlusion

Wound infection

Inappropriate or maladaptive behavior

Nonunion or malunion of digit(s)

Collaborative management

Therapeutic management

Position and immobilization of extremity and digits

Analgesic, antibiotics, anticoagulants

Leech therapy (see box on p. 533)

Fluorometry

Diet, activity, rest

Physical therapy: rehabilitation plan, exercises

Occupational therapy for change in lifestyle

Psychological social worker to evaluate and assist in acceptance of altered body image

Nursing management

PATIENT PROBLEMS/NURSING DIAGNOSES

● **NDX:**   Altered tissue perfusion: peripheral related to interruption of arteriovenous flow

Maintain bed rest in position of comfort within confines of prescribed position of affected arm

Maintain warm environment *to prevent vasoconstriction;* avoid topical pressure on affected limb

Apply heat *to promote vasodilation*

Elevate affected arm on pillow above heart level

Wrist and hand elevated 30 degrees

Forearm in prone position

Elbow flexion of no more than 10 to 15 degrees because further flexion may impair venous return

Maintain prescribed position of affected arm during repositioning

Assess neurovascular status of digit(s) qh

  Check sensation, temperature, color, pulse, skin turgor, and capillary refill qh

  Digit is pinker and capillary refill is faster immediately after surgery; accurate assessment and recording are imperative

  Report alterations in color to physician immediately

    Normal color to white or mottled: arterial occlusion

    Normal to dusky purple: venous congestion

    Leech therapy is used for venous congestion

    Initiate fluorometry readings as indicated

    Both nurses should assess status at change of shift

Monitor vital signs q4h for 24 hr, then qid; monitor BP on unaffected arm

Check dressing qh for drainage; report excess bleeding to physician; change dressing as indicated

Monitor Hgb, Hct, and PT/INR

Maintain parenteral fluids with antibiotics and anticoagulants: assess effectiveness and monitor for side effects of medications

Observe for occult bleeding: gums and injection sites if patient is on anticoagulants

Measure intake and output

EXPECTED OUTCOMES

Arteriovenous flow is maintained

Digit is warm and of normal color

Capillary refill, skin turgor, and sensation are within normal limits

Vital signs are normal

Laboratory values are within normal limits

● **NDX:** Risk for disuse syndrome related to surgical procedure with prescribed immobilization of hand

Teach active ROM exercises q4h to unaffected extremities while patient is in bed

Ambulate with assistance

  Maintain forearm and hand in sling

  Observe for vertigo and nausea

Leech Therapy

After microsurgery for digital replantation, a leech is introduced to the digit where venous congestion is present to drain the engorgement and restore normal venous circulation. The saliva of the leech contains an anticoagulant, a vasodilator, and an anesthetic to assist it in sucking out the blood. The procedure may be repeated every 4 hr until the digit returns to normal. A new leech is used for each treatment to prevent infection.

PRETHERAPY ASSESSMENT OF DIGIT

Venous congestion
  Skin color: pink, dusky purple
  Capillary refill: brisk
  Skin turgor: swollen, distended
  Temperature: cool

PRETHERAPY PREPARATION

Cleanse area with warm water

Explain procedure

Warn patient not to touch leech after it is applied

Place gauze or towels around site to prevent leech from escaping

Physician will apply leech to skin

INTRATHERAPY ASSESSMENT/CARE

After application of leech, monitor continually until leech is fully distended (10 to 15 min)

Leech will usually drop off once this occurs

If leech does not drop off, gently stroke it with an alcohol sponge

Never grasp leech with forceps because regurgitation might occur, resulting in a wound infection

POSTTHERAPY ASSESSMENT/CARE

Once the leech has dropped off the digit, gently pick it up and place it in alcohol-filled container and send it for disposal

Cleanse site and apply dressing because site will continue to drain and ooze for 24 to 48 hr

Assess digit for improved color, turgor, temperature

Involve patient and physical and occupational therapy departments in establishing rehabilitation goals according to physician's order

Individualize goals according to the following:

Healing process and progress

Patient's motivation to master manual skills

Patient's willingness to use replanted digit

Patient's acceptance of replanted digit into body image

Assist patient with and teach modified ADLs according to prescribed limitations dictated by surgery and if affected arm is dominant

Begin exercise program as planned

Encourage use of nondominant hand if appropriate

Allow time for completion of tasks

Encourage adequate fluid and food intake *to maintain normal elimination patterns*

Provide a supportive environment

Promote diversional activities *to increase focus on use of nondominant hand*

Encourage visitation *to promote feeling of well-being*

EXPECTED OUTCOMES

Undertakes using nondominant hand

Participates in activities, ADLs, rehabilitation program

Sets realistic goals for self and strives to complete tasks

● **NDX:**   Pain related to trauma and surgical procedure

Assess location, intensity, and character of pain; use pain rating scale

Administer analgesic; assess effectiveness of pain relief measures; encourage use of PCA

Assist patient with changing position frequently *to prevent pressure and fatigue;* maintain elbow flexion at prescribed amount

Discuss and teach alternate pain relief measures if applicable

Provide diversional activities *to reduce attention to pain*

EXPECTED OUTCOMES

Reports a tolerable level of pain

Presents a calm, relaxed facial affect

Sleeps/rests for longer periods

● **NDX:**   Body image disturbance related to replanted digit

Assess degree of acceptance of replanted finger

Provide time for and assist patient in expressing feelings, encourage communication with significant other(s)

Explain all procedures and treatments

Assess present and past coping behaviors and reinforce positive coping patterns that helped in the past

Stress positive aspects of replantation

Reinforce physician's explanation of expected outcome of surgical procedure; clarify misconceptions

Involve patient in self-care as soon as physically and emotionally able

Involve psychological social worker to evaluate needs and provide counseling

EXPECTED OUTCOMES

Begins to incorporate replanted digit into body image

Verbalizes concerns/feelings and begins to understand expected outcome

Participates appropriately in self-care

Patient/family teaching

Stress and review importance of prescribed rehabilitation program

Degree of movement of digit allowed and duration and times of exercise

Exercises for wrist, elbow, and arm

Position of arm, elbow, and hand during rest and ambulation

Stress that using and wanting to use the digit are the most important factors in function return

Paresthesia may last 4 to 6 months, whereas return of function may take a year

Replanted digit(s) may be shorter than opposing digits(s)

Demonstrate incision care and discuss signs of wound infection

Stress importance of well-balanced diet, fluid intake, rest, and daily exercise

Explain symptoms to report to physician

Changes in color and temperature of digit

Increased incision pain and/or edema

Wound infection

Discuss importance of physical therapy and follow-up visits with physician

Home care considerations

Assess and continue with patient/family teaching and monitor the following:

Rehabilitation/exercise plan

Correct positioning of hand

Willingness to perform exercises

Status of wound

Incision for healing, infection

Signs of infection: redness, pain, swelling, fever, drainage

Neurovascular status of replaced digit

Ability to care for wound: correct supplies and handwashing technique

Knowledge of where and what supplies to purchase

Compartment Syndrome

Increased arterial pressure in compartments of the forearm or lower leg after trauma; within compartments are muscles, blood vessels, and nerves, and any internal pressure (trauma, surgery, edema, bleeding) or external pressure (tight casts or dressings, IV infiltrations) can cause impaired circulation, nerve damage, and muscle weakness; if left unchecked, necrosis with loss of extremity and renal failure, acidosis, and shock (crush syndrome) can occur (Figure 8-6)

Assessment

Subjective data

Pain in compartment area: increasing, unrelenting, and unrelieved by narcotics
Pain with passive motion of fingers or toes
Paresthesia of hand or foot

Objective data

Swelling and localized redness
Absent P below compartment
Progressive loss of motor function

Diagnostic tests

Deep vein thrombosis (DVT) studies
Ankle or brachial index
Vascular occlusion studies
CBC, PT/INR

Potential complications

Neurovascular dysfunction of extremity
Muscle weakness
Necrosis, amputation
Renal failure, acidosis
Shock

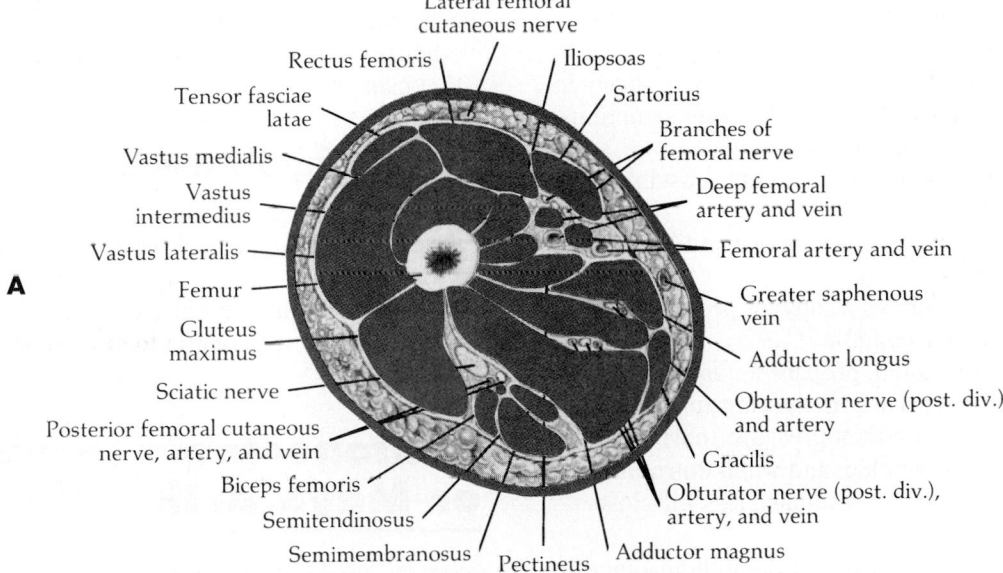

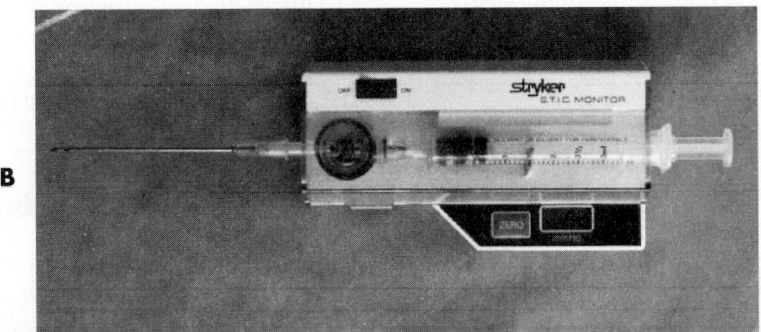

Figure 8-6 **A,** Compartments and cross section of the thigh. Each compartment contains muscle(s), nerve, artery, and vein. **B,** Equipment for measurement of interstitial venous pressure. (**A,** From Thompson JM et al: *Mosby's clinical nursing*, ed 3, St Louis, 1993, Mosby. **B,** Courtesy Stryker, Inc.)

Collaborative management

Therapeutic management

Analgesics, antibiotics
Dressing and cast removal; cast window made
Neurovascular check q½h
Tissue pressure monitoring, fasciotomy

Nursing management

PATIENT PROBLEMS/NURSING DIAGNOSES

● **NDX:** Altered tissue perfusion: peripheral related to interruption of arteriovenous flow, edema, trauma

Monitor and assess pain q½h if syndrome is suspected
Notify physician immediately if pain in extremity is any of the following:
  Increasing
  Unrelenting
  Unrelieved by narcotics
  Occurring during passive motion of fingers or toes
  NOTE: Be aware that this type of pain is the primary indicator of compartment syndrome; other symptoms may take longer to appear
Remove dressing or have windows cut in cast immediately as ordered
Assess neurovascular status of foot or hand bilaterally q15min to 30min
Measure forearm or calf bilaterally for presence of or increase in edema q1h to q2h
If no improvement is noted, prepare for and assist with interstitial venous pressure monitoring (p. 535), a means to measure interstitial pressure (normal pressure is about 0 to 30 mm Hg, and when this pressure nears 30 mm Hg, capillaries and arteries will close, causing occlusion)
Prepare for fasciotomy as ordered (longitudinal incision into fascia surrounding compartment to release pressure), if interstitial pressure is >30 mm Hg
Postoperatively, extremity will be immobilized in posterior cast or splint
Be aware that wound may be left open, with future grafting required; there may be more than one incision, depending on the number of affected areas in the compartment
Change dressings as needed; observe for altered alignment of extremity
Continue neurovascular monitoring qh; observe for return of color, T, and capillary refill
Assess pain and monitor effectiveness after analgesic administration

EXPECTED OUTCOMES
Compartment pressure is reduced as evidenced by palpable peripheral pulses, reduced muscle edema, minimal discomfort
Extremity is warm and dry, capillary refill is normal
Mobility is intact

● **NDX:** Anxiety/fear related to lack of knowledge of the syndrome and situational crisis

Reinforce physician's explanation of syndrome, procedure, outcome, and rehabilitation plan
Allow time for verbalization of fears and explain all treatments as much as possible
After procedure assist patient in identifying coping strengths and discuss ways of dealing with wound and possible skin grafting
Encourage communication with significant other(s)
Promote self-care activities
Provide diversional activities *to reduce anxiety/stress*

EXPECTED OUTCOMES
Begins to observe wound and discuss feelings about it
Participates in own care
Verbalizes understanding of treatment and rehabilitation plan

Patient/family teaching

Discuss and teach dressing change technique
Provide information on where to purchase needed supplies
Reinforce prescribed rehabilitation program
Promote return visits with physical therapist and physician

Bunionectomy (Keller or Mayo Arthroplasty)

Surgical correction of hereditary or acquired hallux valgus: acute angulation of the first metatarsophalangeal joint; a gap arthroplasty is performed, excising one of the bones and filling the space with a Silastic implant and also removing the bunion, the enlarged bursa, and knob of bone

Preoperative assessment/teaching

Observations/findings

Assess mobility and neurovascular status of toes
Discuss with and teach patient the following:
  Crutch walking
  Use of walker

Toe flexing
Quadriceps setting
ROM exercises

Postoperative assessment

Subjective data

Location and character of pain

Objective data

Neurovascular status of affected toes: color, temperature, sensation, edema
Site of incision for drainage and bleeding
Placement of plaster toe cap or splint

Potential complications

Fever
Wound infection
Recurrence of hallux valgus

Collaborative management

Therapeutic management

Analgesics, antipyretics
Type of immobilization device/positioning
Ambulation, weight bearing
Diet, activity, rest
Ice bags to affected site

Nursing management

PATIENT PROBLEMS/NURSING DIAGNOSES

● **NDX:** Impaired physical mobility related to musculoskeletal alteration

Maintain bed rest until fully reactive
Elevate foot of bed
  Place bed cradle over feet
  Monitor immobilization device for pressure areas and circulatory constriction
Ambulate with assistance, usually 24 to 48 hr postoperatively
Assist patient with performing ROM exercises q4h while in bed
Assist and teach patient to turn and deep breathe q2h to 3h while in bed; hold affected foot during turn and place on pillow after turn has been completed
Apply plaster walking boot if ordered
Initiate flexing exercises of toes five times qh when edema subsides and as ordered

EXPECTED OUTCOMES
Performs rehabilitation exercises correctly
Participates in self-care activities

● **NDX:** Altered tissue perfusion: peripheral related to surgical procedure and immobilizing device

Monitor vital signs q4h
Assess neurovascular status of toes q1h to 2h; check color, temperature, capillary refill, sensation, and mobility
Apply ice bags *to decrease edema*
Monitor toes for increasing edema
Encourage movement of legs *to increase venous return*
Elevate leg on pillow

EXPECTED OUTCOMES
Vital signs are normal
Extremity is warm and of normal color
Pulse, sensation, and mobility are normal

● **NDX:** Pain related to surgical intervention

Assess location, intensity, and character of pain; use pain rating scale
Administer analgesics; assess effectiveness of pain relief measures and monitor for side effects
Apply ice bag to area *to promote comfort*
Assist patient with changing position frequently while on bed rest *to relieve fatigue*
Provide diversional activities *to lessen concentration on discomfort*

EXPECTED OUTCOMES
States that pain is at tolerable level
Appears relaxed and calm
Sleeps for increasing number of hours

Patient/family teaching

Stress importance of and review foot and incision care and prescribed exercises
  Demonstrate dressing change
  Explain need for foot soaks in warm, soapy water after sutures are removed; need to dry feet well
  Discuss care of plaster boot if applicable
  Demonstrate toe and foot ROM exercises
  Explain importance of proper fitting footwear
Discuss activities allowed; encourage self-care and ADLs
Discuss signs of wound infection to report to physician: fever, pain, edema, redness
Encourage follow-up care with physician

Home care considerations

Assess and continue with patient/family teaching and monitor the following:

Environmental/safety status

Care givers' ability to perform needed tasks

Accessible telephone and emergency numbers: physician, pharmacy, home health care team

Emergency call device to summon outside help

Absence of skatter rugs, unbacked carpets

Presence of stairs with hand rails

Grab bars at tub and toilet

Nonskid strips in tub

Adequate lighting for safe movement

Wide doorways to accommodate wheelchairs/ walkers

Height of chair and bed for easy transfer on and off of each

Flashlights near bed and chair

Medications accessible and labeled

Availability of transportation to needed appointments

Needed supplies: what and where to purchase

Mobility status

Ability and desire to follow prescribed rehabilitation plan and exercises

Correct transfer techniques

Amount of weight bearing

Wearing proper fitting shoes

Correct use of walkers, canes, crutches

Ability to apply plaster boot if applicable

Status of immobilizing device

Neurovascular status of each affected extremity

Condition of boot if applicable: wet, loose, clean, soiled

Condition of skin under device: clear, red, tender

Status of wound

Incision for healing, infection

Signs of infection: redness, pain, swelling, fever, drainage

Ability to care for wound: correct supplies and hand-washing technique

Knowledge of where and what supplies to purchase

Traction Management

Method of providing a pulling effect to an extremity or body part while also maintaining a countertraction (pull in opposite direction) (see Table 8-2 for description and care and Figures 8-7 through 8-10)

Cast Management

Casts are applied to immobilize musculoskeletal tissues after trauma; they are made of plaster, fiberglass, plastic, or cast tape

Assessment

Subjective data

Location, intensity, and character of pain

Objective data

Type of cast applied, moistness

Neurovascular status of affected extremity

Integumentary status at edges and under cast

GI, renal, and/or respiratory dysfunction (body or cervical cast)

Potential complications

Neurovascular impairment

Skin impairment

Compartment syndrome (see p. 535)

Cast syndrome (reduced circulation through mesenteric artery caused by unnatural kinking from cast; may cause intestinal ileus)

Collaborative management

Therapeutic management

Type of cast applied

Positioning of cast

Ambulation

Ice bags to affected part

Diet, activity, rest

Analgesics, antibiotics

Physical therapy: rehabilitation plan if indicated

Occupational therapy if applicable

Nursing management

PATIENT PROBLEMS/NURSING DIAGNOSES

● **NDX:** Impaired physical mobility related to cast application

Maintain bed rest in position of comfort with extremity elevated

Assist with and teach ROM exercises to unaffected joints every 4 hours *to maintain strength*

Assist with and teach isometric exercises *to strengthen muscles above and below cast*

Begin ambulation as prescribed

Assist and teach crutch walking, use of cane, walker

Observe for vertigo or disequilibrium

Monitor use for correctness *to prevent further injury*

Involve patient in own physical care as tolerated *to promote independence*

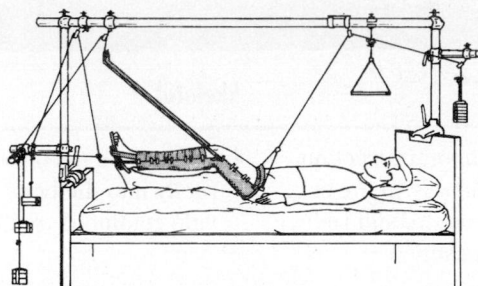

Figure 8-7   Balanced suspension with Thomas's splint and Pearson's attachment.

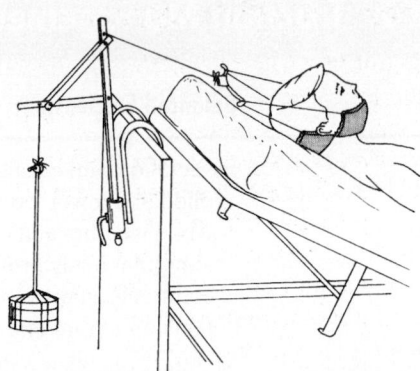

Figure 8-9   Cervical traction.

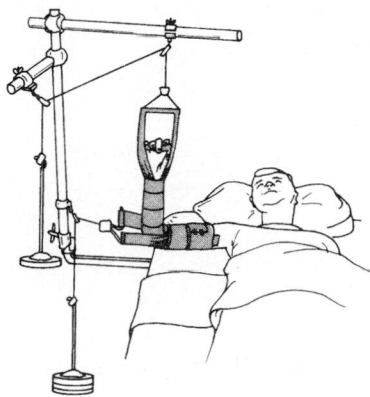

Figure 8-8   Traction of humerus.

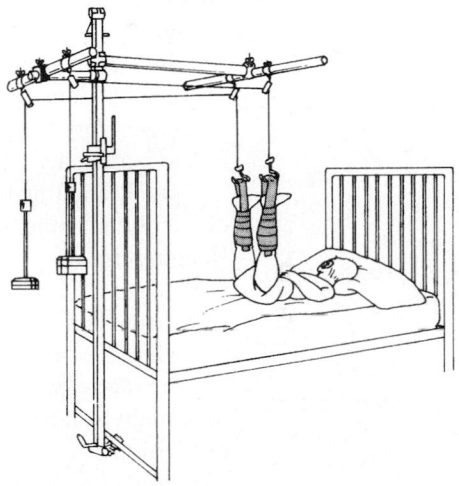

Figure 8-10   Bryant's traction.

EXPECTED OUTCOMES

Activity level is increasing
Performance of ROM exercises is adequate

● **NDX:**   Altered tissue perfusion: peripheral related to cast application and risk of interruption of arteriovenous flow

Monitor vital signs q2h to 4h until stable, then q8h
Monitor neurovascular status of affected extremity: assess color, temperature, pulse, capillary refill, sensation, and mobility
Elevate extremity on pillow, only to heart level, *to avoid delaying arterial flow*
Encourage movement of digits *to prevent venous stasis*
Assist with and teach deep breathing exercises *to increase oxygen level in the blood*

EXPECTED OUTCOMES

Vital signs are within normal limits
Neurovascular status is stable: color, temperature, capillary refill are normal and pulses are present; motion and sensation are adequate

● **NDX:**   Risk for impaired skin integrity related to cast application and/or trauma

Expose cast to air until dry; use only palms of hands when handling wet cast
Apply moleskin to edges of cast *to prevent irritation*
Massage under edges *to stimulate circulation and prevent skin breakdown*
Explain that skin under cast will feel warm until cast dries
Assist with and encourage small position changes *to relieve pressure*
Monitor cast for drainage: check stockinette, wadding beneath cast; call physician if drainage excessive

EXPECTED OUTCOMES

Skin under edges of cast is warm and dry
Cast is dry and intact

● **NDX:**   Pain related to cast application and/or trauma

Administer analgesics as prescribed
Monitor severity of pain to avoid complications, compartment syndrome (p. 535)
Provide analgesics often enough to ensure therapeutic blood levels, because pain may be severe; consider patient controlled analgesia

Table 8-2 Traction Management

Type	Balanced Suspension	Skin	Skeletal
Definition	Skeletal or skin traction applied to a lower extremity while weights and a splint simultaneously provide countertraction to and suspension of that extremity	Light or temporary traction applied directly to the skin to align fracture and reduce muscle spasm	Insertion of a pin or wire directly into the bone to provide continous traction

General interventions (same for all types of traction listed in this table)	Maintain constant pull in line with deformity
	Assess and maintain ropes and pulleys
	    Taut
	    Riding freely over pulleys
	    Free of bedding
	    Knots secure
	    Adequate space between pulley and traction
	Monitor and maintain weights
	    Hanging free
	    Off floor
	    Away from bed
	    NOTE: *Never remove weights; never lift weights*
	Monitor and maintain countertraction
	    Elevation of bed under part to which traction is applied
	    Pull exerted against fixed point
	    Pull exerted against traction in opposite direction		

Interventions for specific type of traction	Maintain anatomic position of extremity Maintain 20-degree angle between thigh and bed Have heel clear of sling under calf Maintain abduction of extremity Monitor femoral and popliteal pulses	Observe carefully for slippage and bunching up of bandage Replace bandage prn Observe for pressure areas at distal end of bandage (wrist or heel), especially if weight is > 7 lb Check neurovascular status q2h to 4h	Cover ends of pin with cord Observe site of insertion for redness, swelling, discharge, odor, bleeding Clean skin around puncture sites q8h with hydrogen peroxide soaked cotton swabs; allow to air dry; apply antibacterial ointment if ordered Monitor neurovascular status q2h to 4h

Pelvic	Side Arm	Cervical	Bryant's	Halo
Traction provided to lower back to reduce low back pain from fracture, herniated disks, muscle spasms	Skin or skeletal traction to the humerus to maintain alignment after open reduction procedure	Application of cervical halter with traction to relieve neck pain or when a cervical fracture is suspected	Treatment of fractures of femur shaft in young children	Metal brace inserted in the skull and iliac crest or femur with pins attached to four metal posts and a shoulder brace or body cast provides spinal support after spinal fusion or for preoperative treatment of scoliosis
Ensure that pelvic girdle is proper size for patient and that pelvic girdle fits snugly over iliac crests and pelvis Inspect skin areas over iliac crests for pressure points q4h Pelvic straps must be equal in length and unrestricted	Maintain position as directed by physician Check neurovascular status of affected arm q2h to 4h Notify physician immediately if any change is noted Apply chest restraint sheet for counter-traction prn	Position without pillows Monitor so weight and pulley are free of wall Observe for pressure areas Jaws, chin, and ears Side of head Back of head Pad as necessary for comfort	Raise buttocks slightly from mattress Observe bandages carefully for slippage and bunching over heel cords Observe for skin sloughing on both legs Check feet for color, P, T, and sensation q2h to 4h Use harness restraint to prevent turning over Avoid thick, wide diapers between legs	Cover ends of pins with cork to prevent injury Observe pin insertion sites for redness, swelling, drainage, odor, bleeding Clean skin around pin sites q8h with hydrogen peroxide soaked swabs; allow to air dry; apply antibacterial ointment if ordered Monitor straps for areas of constriction Pad pressure points as necessary for comfort Do not alter amount of traction applied Advise patient not to bend over, use reaching device

Encourage small movements and position changes *to promote comfort*

Administer back rubs *to increase circulation and promote comfort*

Discuss alternate pain management techniques

Apply ice packs over trauma site *to reduce swelling and pain*

EXPECTED OUTCOMES

Verbalizes a reduction in discomfort

Appears to rest and sleep adequately

Appears relaxed and talkative

ADDITIONAL NURSING DIAGNOSES TO CONSIDER

Altered elimination patterns related to cast and bed rest

Constipation related to inactivity

Patient/family teaching

Provide information on and stress importance of prescribed activities and rehabilitation exercises

Demonstrate turning procedure for patient in spica cast and reiterate crutch-walking procedure where appropriate

Discuss need to keep cast out of water; use plastic bag for showering

Notify physician immediately if cast becomes wet

Suggest clothing that can be put on easily

Discuss measures to ensure warmth of affected digits

Demonstrate neurovascular monitoring of each affected extremity as needed

Discuss signs and symptoms to report to physician
Fever; foul odor from cast
Increasing pain or decreased sensation

Demonstrate skin care around cast

Home care considerations

Assess and continue with patient/family teaching and monitor the following:

Environmental/safety status
Care givers' ability to perform needed tasks
Accessible telephone and emergency numbers: physician, pharmacy, home health care team
Emergency call device to summon outside help
Absence of skatter rugs, unbacked carpets
Presence of stairs with hand rails
Grab bars at tub and toilet
Nonskid strips in tub
Adequate lighting for safe movement
Wide doorways to accommodate wheelchairs/walkers
Height of chair and bed for easy transfer on and off of each

Flashlights near bed and chair
Medications accessible and labeled
Availability of transportation to needed appointments
Needed supplies: what and where to purchase

Mobility status
Ability and desire to follow prescribed rehabilitation plan and exercises
Correct transfer techniques
Amount of weight bearing
Correct use of walkers, canes, crutches

Status of cast
Neurovascular status of each affected extremity
Condition of cast: wet, loose, clean, soiled
Condition of skin under cast: clear, red, tender

Nutritional status
Understanding of basic food groups and what to eat to provide nutrition with no weight gain
Signs of weight loss, dehydration
Ability to prepare meals; refer to social agency to provide meals

Elimination status
Presence of elevated toilet seat
Use of stool softeners, natural laxatives, bulk in diet
Ability to be active
Amount of fluids taken per day: increase to upper limits for age and weight
Use of fracture pan/urinal/female urinal

Continuous Passive Motion Device

A patient-guided machine that provides passive exercise to the hip and knee after surgery or trauma; similar devices are available for ankle, shoulder, wrist, and fingers

Purpose

Facilitates early movement and increased flexion of joint

Prevents stiffness of joint and contractures of tissue

Enhances circulation and healing

Reduces pain of or psychological resistance to flexion and edema

Assessment/procedure

Physician's order to include the following:
Initial degree of flexion; number of degrees to increase flexion per hr and number of hr per day to use
Restrictions or special instructions for use

Assess patient's ability to operate and manage device

Explain purpose of machine and its advantages

Remove any splints before applying device as ordered

After machine is set up by physical therapist or cast or traction technician

Place extremity on device and check the following:

Lower buttock is against femur support

Knee is directly over center of frame

Foot is firmly against foot plate

Apply Velcro safety straps to extremity; check that they do not interfere with gear assembly

Set automatic flexion and/or extension motion as ordered by physician (usually at 10)

Increase flexion 1 to 5 degrees qh as ordered

Assess patient's tolerance before increasing flexion

Adjust speed as prescribed (maximum speed to flex joint from 0 to 110 degrees is about 1 min 40 sec; minimum speed is approximately 12 min; slow speeds are used initially and at night to facilitate sleep)

Set ROM limits as ordered by physician

Instruct patient in use of controls

Control has three settings: flexion, stop, and extension

Once device is operating, patient can control movement, stop, or reverse at any point within preset range limits

Each time machine is applied, reduce flexion 5 degrees for about 15 min and then increase to original setting

Encourage patient to use machine as much as possible and as tolerated

---

BIBLIOGRAPHY

Bailey MM, Michalski J: Close-up on clavicle fracture, *Nursing '92* 22(8):41, 1992.

Bailey MM, Michalski J: Close-up on scaphoid fracture, *Nursing '93* 23(3):49, 1993.

Bailey MM, Michalski J: Close-up on radial head fracture, *Nursing '93* 23(9):43, 1993.

Bailey MM, Michalski J: Close-up on posterior shoulder dislocation, *Nursing '93* 23(10):43, 1993.

Barkett PA: Obstructed airway with wire jaws, *Nursing '91* 21(12):33, 1991.

Botstein GR: Soft tissue rheumatism of the upper extremities: diagnosis and management, *Geriatrics* 45(11):30, 1990.

Bryant GA: When your patient needs back surgery, *RN* 55(7):46, 1992.

Doenges ME et al: *Nursing care plans: guidelines for planning and documenting patient care,* ed 3, Philadelphia, 1993, FA Davis.

Gluchacki BK: Recognizing compartment syndrome, *Nursing '91* 21(10):33, 1991.

Harris C: Osteoarthritis: how to diagnose and treat the painful joint, *Geriatrics* 48(8):39, 1993.

Jackson S: Assessing a femoral fracture, *Nursing '91* 21(11):57, 1991.

Kim MJ et al: *Pocket guide to nursing diagnoses,* ed 6, St Louis, 1995, Mosby.

Licata AA: Therapies for symptomatic primary osteoporosis, *Geriatrics* 46(11):62, 1991.

McCance KL, Huether SE: *Pathophysiology; the biological basis for disease in adults and children,* ed 2, St Louis, 1994, Mosby.

McFarland GK, McFarlane EA: *Nursing diagnosis and intervention: planning for patient care,* ed 2, St Louis, 1993, Mosby.

Monk HL: Fractures are never simple, *RN* 56(4):30, 1993.

Mourad LA: *Mosby's clinical nursing series: orthopedic disorders,* St Louis, 1991, Mosby.

Mulvey MA, Sharma PK: Traumatic amputation, *RN* 54(9):26, 1991.

North B et al: Living in a halo, *Am J Nurs* 92(4):55, 1992.

Nussman DS, Poole RC: Traumatic hip dislocation, *Am J Nurs* 91(11):34, 1991.

Peel K: Making sense of leeches, *Nursing Times* 89(27):34, 1993.

Pellino TA: How to manage hip fractures, *Am J Nurs* 94(4):46, 1994.

Present D, Shaffer B: Disease-associated fractures: detection and management in the elderly, *Geriatrics* 45(3):48, 1990.

Rogers-Seidle FF: *Geriatric nursing care plans,* St Louis, 1991, Mosby.

Strangio L: Leeches—when bleeding is exactly what you want, *RN* 54(9):31, 1991.

Thompson JM et al: *Mosby's clinical nursing,* ed 3, St Louis, 1993, Mosby.

Urrows ST et al: Profiles in osteoporosis, *Am J Nurs* 91(12):33, 1991.

Wainwright ST, Bacon ES: Traumatic amputation, *Nursing '93* 23(10):33, 1993.

USC UNIVERSITY HOSPITAL

1500 San Pablo
Los Angeles, CA 90033

MULTIDISCIPLINARY PLAN

DIAGNOSIS	NAME
SURGERY Total Hip Replacement (209)	ALLERGIES
Bilateral/Multiple Major Joint LE (471)	MR#

DISCHARGE OUTCOMES | DRG 209/471   ALOS 9.4/11.9 | ADMIT DATE:

PHYSIOLOGICAL Independent household ambulator. Absence of pain. Good/adequate circulation to affected extremity. Maintain total hip precautions.

COGNITIVE Demonstrates independence in home activity, hip precautions, and use of adaptive devices. Verbalizes follow-up medical plan.

PSYCHOLOGICAL Demonstrates realistic expectations of rehabilitation and adaptive coping patterns as evidenced by ability/willingness to participate in perioperative/recovery care activities.

DISCIPLINE	PRE-OP/ PRE-ADMIT	D.O.S. DATE ___ / DAY 1 / OR/Surgical	P.O.#1 DATE ___ / DAY 2 / Surgical	P.O.#2 DATE ___ / DAY 3 / Surgical	P.O.#3 DATE ___ / DAY 4 / Surgical	P.O.#4 DATE ___ / DAY 5 / Surgical	P.O.#5 DATE ___ / DAY 6 / Surgical
LOCATION		OR/Surgical	Surgical	Surgical	Surgical	Surgical	Surgical
LABS	CBC, PT, PTT U/A C+S Type & Cross √ on Autologous units	CBC in PAR	CBC Chem 7		CBC		
CARDIO-PULMONARY	ECG	I.S. Instruction & use q° WA	Continue I.S.	Evaluate for self I.S. use			
IMAGING/ NUCLEAR MEDICINE	CXR	AP and Lateral hip x-ray in PAR					
SOCIAL SERVICES D/C PLAN REHAB. SERVICES	P.T. eval Instruct hip precautions, equipment, crutch training. Initiate D/C planning.	Continue D/C planning. Assess home care needs. Initiate total hip precautions Consider Rehab eval P.T. hip protocol wt bearing/fixation Consult MSW prn	P.T. eval and exercise Confer with patient for activity instruction Assess home environment	Start progressive ambulation Wt bearing status per MD. O.T. eval & issue adaptive device. Demonstration of usage of adaptive equipment	Re-evaluate home care needs Consider Acute rehab transfer Arrange D.M.E. needs Include S/O in education to environment, i.e., stairs, rugs, pets, furniture, transfers P.T. training with lower extremity mgmt using equipment	Prepare for discharge Required minimal (25% or less) cues to maintain hip precautions Progress to crutches Demonstrates transfers Complying with lower extremity management	Reassess compliance with all activities Demonstrates energy conservation, work simplification Independent in activities, hip precautions, stairclimbing, car transfers Shower eval Discharge planning
PHARMACY		IV TKO when fully awake & when taking po fluids well. Epidural/PCA-pain mgmt Antibiotics x48° DO NOT DC until all drains/catheters DC'ed		Give one more dose of antibiotics after Foley is discontinued			
DIETARY/ NUTRITION	NPO after midnight	Post-op clear liquids Advance diet as tolerated					

USC UNIVERSITY HOSPITAL

1500 San Pablo
Los Angeles, CA 90033

MULTIDISCIPLINARY PLAN

NAME _____
ALLERGIES _____

MR# _____

DIAGNOSIS	
SURGERY Total Hip Replacement (209)	
Bilateral/Multiple Major Joint LE (471)	

DISCHARGE OUTCOMES	DRG 209/471	ALOS 9.4/11.9	ADMIT DATE: _____
PHYSIOLOGICAL			
COGNITIVE			
PSYCHOLOGICAL			

DISCIPLINE	PRE-OP/ PRE-ADMIT	P.O.#6 DATE	DAY 7	P.O.#7 DATE	DAY 8	P.O.#8 DATE	DAY 9	P.O.#9 DATE	DAY 10	P.O.#10 DATE	DAY 11	P.O.#11 DATE	DAY 12
LOCATION													
LABS													
CARDIO-PULMONARY													
IMAGING/ NUCLEAR MEDICINE													
SOCIAL SERVICES D/C PLAN REHAB. SERVICES													
PHARMACY													
DIETARY/ NUTRITION													

Continued.

MULTIDISCIPLINARY PLAN

DISCIPLINE	PRE-OP/ PRE-ADMIT	D.O.S. DAY 1 DATE	P.O.#1 DAY 2 DATE	P.O.#2 DAY 3 DATE	P.O.#3 DAY 4 DATE	P.O.#4 DAY 5 DATE	P.O.#5 DAY 6 DATE
PATIENT ACTIVITY	Betadine Shower TED hose apply to unoperative extremity.	HOB <45° Slings & Springs to operative leg. Avoid peroneal nerve pressure TED hose/sequentials encourage performance of isometric exercises, gluteal/ quad sets Ankle/toe pumps Encourage use of OHT	Activity to edge of bed, dangle & stand Any hip drainage-bedrest until clearance	Evaluate for ability to lift leg, get in and out of bed with minimal assist, stand to walk, and transfer to chair Encourage up in chair for meals	Ambulate or strengthening/ toilet transfer. If pt active, DC sequentials, and slings & springs BRP with assist	Ambulate/transfer maintaining hip precautions Shower	Stairs, climbing
EDUCATION	<u>Video</u> Pre-op clinic Pre-op teach D/C instructions. Begin Admission Assessment. Educational booklet provided to pt.	<u>Hip Precautions:</u> • Keep operative leg elevated • Do not cross legs • Do not use low chairs/toilets • No flexion >60° • No twisting • Instruct on use of OHT to turn		Explain stress/wt bearing restrictions Reinforce techniques on how to use ambulatory devices	D/C Training: • Hip precautions/activity restrictions • Sleep with pillow between legs. Sleep on back or on either side - teach why each side may be better for individual pt. • Sex education • Hygiene - use raised toilet seat. Lean toward operative side when performing toileting hygiene. BATHING - DO NOT sit in tub. • Signs & symptoms to report: wound infection, increase in pain, persistent swelling of leg (does not disappear after one hour of elevation), calf tenderness, sudden shortening of affected extremity.		

KEY
mgmt = management
OHT = overhead trapeze

	DATE	COLLABORATIVE PROBLEMS	DC DATE INIT	DATE	COLLABORATIVE PROBLEMS	DC DATE INIT
1. To initiate a problem or intervention, document under corresponding date.		1. Impaired physical mobility R/T disease/surgery.			7. Self care deficit R/T surgical procedure.	
2. Document outcomes under appropriate date for achieving the goal.		2. Alteration in comfort, pain R/T surgical procedure.				
3. To discontinue an intervention, or resolve a patient problem, highlight date and initial.		3. Potential for injury, i.e. displacement of prosthesis, infection, DVT R/T surgical procedure.				
		4. Tissue perfusion, alteration in R/T surgical procedure.				
		5. Fear/anxiety R/T hospitalization.				
		6. Knowledge deficit R/T activity/hip precautions.				

OUTCOMES

1. Demonstrates leg exercises as instructed by P.T.	1. Demonstrates wt bearing status and use of ambulatory devices.	1. Demonstrates ambulation & transfers with assistive device.
2. Verbalizes pain control within 30 min of intervention.	2. Pain controlled as evidenced by participation in activity.	1. Independent in activity, hip precautions, stairs, transfers, shower. Independent home exercise program initiated.
3. No injury/infection throughout hospitalization.	5. Apprehensions regarding hospitalization, continuum of health verbalized/controlled anxiety.	7. Minimal assistance required for self-care.
4. Tissue perfusion to affected extremity maintained throughout hospitalization.		7. Independent in self-care/or support system identified/able to provide for deficit.

PLAN OF CARE DISCUSSED WITH	D.O.S. DAY 1 DATE ___	P.O.#1 DAY 2 DATE ___	P.O.#2 DAY 3 DATE ___	P.O.#3 DAY 4 DATE ___	P.O.#4 DAY 5 DATE ___	P.O.#5 DAY 6 DATE ___
			INTERVENTIONS			
DATE INIT SO/P ___	Orient to room/environment. Explain purpose of equipment in use.	Transfuse 1 unit of autologous blood as ordered.	Monitor use of crutches/walker to determine proper use of aid/wt bearing activities.	Assess level of ability to participate in ADL.	Ensure home D.M.E. has been arranged prn.	Discharge Instructions: • Continue wearing TEDs for 1 month post surgery • Take ASA BID times 1 month • Continue exercise regimen • Reinforce hip precautions • Driving restrictions
	Assess location, type, severity of pain. Maintain Epidural/PCA.	Continued pain management.	Encourage isometrics & quad sets.	Assess level of support from family/friends.	Reinforce hip precautions.	
	Monitor respiratory status. Encourage use of I.S.	Reinforce hip precautions. Increase activity as ordered.	Nursing to assist pt in/out of bed maintaining hip precautions.	Ensure ADL equipment available.		
CASE MANAGER: ___	Monitor color, warmth, sensation, pulses of affected extremities.		Ensure po intake adequate to promote healing/maintain hydration.	BRP or BSC privileges by nursing maintaining hip precautions.		
CONSULTING MD. ___	Ice packs at surgical site to decrease edema daily after P.T.		Dietary consult as needed.	Discontinue sequential compression boots.		
SOCIAL SERVICE: ___	Observe hip wrap dressing every 2° for drainage. Reinforce prn.		Offer pain med 30 min prior to therapy. Encourage use as needed.	Discontinue springs & slings if pt able to SLR.		
ANOINTING OF THE SICK DATE: ___	Reinforce hip precautions. Record Hemovac output every 8°.		Discontinue foley 4 hrs after Epidural Catheter/PCA is removed.			
	Maintain foley.		May I&O catheterize every 8° if no void.			
	Apply TED hose. Remove BID x 30 min.					
	Sequentials.					
	Assess for signs & symptoms of DVT.					
	Assess bowel/bladder output. Consider laxative.					
	Encourage expressions of fears/anxiety.					
	Ensure initiation of P.T.					

MULTIDISCIPLINARY PLAN UPDATE

DATE	SIGNATURES	DATE	SIGNATURES	DATE	SIGNATURES

USC UNIVERSITY HOSPITAL
1500 San Pablo
Los Angeles, CA 90033 ©1991

SIDE 1   **MULTIDISCIPLINARY PLAN**

DIAGNOSIS _____   NAME _____
ALLERGIES _____

SURGERY   **Orthopedic Service-LAMINECTOMY / General Anesthesia**

DRG 215   ALOS 6.0   ADMIT DATE _____

DISCHARGE OUTCOMES

PHYSIOLOGICAL — Patient will have pain controlled at level < 3 on 1 - 10 scale c̄ p.o. meds, will ambulate c̄ steady gait independently, VS within normal limits & wound will be healing s̄ redness or edema.

COGNITIVE — Patient will verbalize spine precautions-no lifting, twisting, flexion, brace compliance & sitting only for meals & commode. Will verbalize s/sx of infection & when to call M.D.

PSYCHOLOGICAL — Patient will verbalize acceptance of lifestyle change to incorporate spine precautions into activities of daily living.

DISCIPLINE / LOCATION	PRE-OP/ PRE-ADMIT — OP CLINIC	DOS DAY 1 — SURGERY/PAR/DOU DATE	P.O.#1 DAY 2 — MED/SURG DATE	P.O.#2 DAY 3 — MED/SURG DATE	P.O.#3 DAY 4 — MED/SURG DATE	P.O.#4 DAY 5 — MED/SURG → HOME DATE	P.O.#5 DAY 6 DATE
LABS	CBC Chem 20 UA PT PTT	H & H					
CARDIO-PULMONARY	ECG May require PFT's ABG	I.S.					
IMAGING/ NUCLEAR MEDICINE	CXR						
SOCIAL SERVICES D/C PLAN REHAB. SERVICES	Psycho-social eval. P.T. eval & treat measure for brace	Initiate discharge planning Trapeze Rehab eval, if indicated	P.T. eval & teach bed mobility, logrolling, prone to stand transfer. Spine precautions	Home health eval if indicated Progressive ambulation	Identify D.M.E. requirements Instruct in stairs	Clearance by P.T. for discharge	
PHARMACY	General anesthesia	PCA in PAR - no pain management consult Ancef or Vanco IV TKO when taking po well. Decadron Zantac Vitamin C, Ferrous gluconate	D/C PCA D/C antibiotics when drains are out	Laxative or suppository prn			
DIETARY/ NUTRITION	NPO	Clear liquids Advance as tolerated					

MULTIDISCIPLINARY PLAN

PATIENT NAME: _____

DISCIPLINE	PRE-OP/ PRE-ADMIT	DOS DAY 1	P.O. #1 DAY 2	P.O. #2 DAY 3	P.O. #3 DAY 4	P.O. #4 DAY 5	P.O. #5 DAY 6
		DATE __	DATE __	DATE __	DATE __	DATE __	DATE __
PATIENT ACTIVITY		BR TED hose in PAR Bilateral leg squeezers in OR.	High rise toilet seat/BSC				
EDUCATION	Spine precautions Review pathway goals	Orient to room, unit & hospital routine. Teach &/or reinforce spine precautions	Reinforce lack of sitting (or as ordered by MD), except for meals & commode			Shower instructions: Water to flow on front of body only, no direct flow on back	

COLLABORATIVE PROBLEMS

DATE		DATE	
❶ Alteration in comfort, pain R/T surgery.		❼ Potential alteration in coping, anxiety R/T discharge planning.	
❷ Potential for infection R/T surgical procedure.		❽ Alteration in mobility R/T surgical procedure.	
❸ Potential alteration in elimination, bowel ileus R/T surgery.			
❹ Knowledge deficit R/T surgical procedure & spine precautions.			
❺ Potential for neurosensory impairment R/T surgery.			
❻ Potential alteration in coping, anxiety R/T hospitalization.			

OUTCOMES

❶ Pt. will have pain controlled at 4-5 on 1-10 scale by 4° post-op.	❶ Pt. will verbalize pain controlled at 3-4 on 1-10 scale.
❷ Pt. will remain free from s/sx of infection throughout stay.	❸ Pt. will resume bowel function.
❹ Pt. will verbalize spine precautions by 4° post-op.	❼ Pt. will verbalize feelings of assurance c̄ discharge plans within 8° of initiation.
❺ Pt. will remain free from neurosensory deficits during hospitalization.	❽ Ambulate to BR & hall c̄ assistance. Assisted self-care.
❻ Pt. will verbalize feelings of assurance c̄ hospital routine within 4° post-op.	

❹ Consistently demonstrates spine precautions.	❼ All DME equipment available.
❽ Supervised bed mobility, transfers. Independent self-care except shower.	❽ Independent ambulation all surfaces & stairs.
	❽ Independent shower.

Instructions

❶ To initiate a problem or intervention, document under corresponding date.

❷ Document outcomes under appropriate date for achieving the goal.

❸ To discontinue an intervention, or resolve a patient problem, highlight date and initial.

KEY

S/O	= Significant Other
Pt.	= Patient
A/E	= As evidenced by
I.S.	= Incentive spirometer
Δ	= Change
S/SX	= Signs & Symptoms
D.M.E.	= Durable medical equipment

Continued.

PLAN OF CARE DISCUSSED WITH

DATE	INITIAL	S.O.	Pt.

INTERVENTIONS

	DOS DAY 1	P.O. #1 DAY 2	P.O. #2 DAY 3	P.O. #3 DAY 4	P.O. #4 DAY 5	P.O. #5 DAY 6
DATE	___	___	___	___	___	___
	— Maintain patent IV c̄ PCA started in PAR. — Assess for edema & pain location, quality & duration.	— Encourage use of po pain meds at pain scale mid-point.	— Reinforce spine precautions.	— Assess bowel function & need for laxative or suppository.		
	— Notify M.D. if not controlled. — Orient to surroundings, unit & hospital routine.	— D/C foley. Assess bladder distension, urinary retention. I & O cath q̄4° PRN.	— Assess bowel function & need for laxative or suppository.	— Reinforce discharge plans. — Sitting per MD instructions.		
	— Assess for drainage, bleeding at surgical site. Notify M.D. if present & immediately if CSF noted. — Cold packs to surgical site x48°.	— Reinforce spine precautions: • sit only for meals/commode (or as MD orders) • avoid twisting, flexion or bending. • maintain back alignment when OOB.	— Introduce home health liaison for needs assessment.			
	— Assess bowel sounds, abdominal distension, flatus.	— Nursing to ambulate pt. c̄ back brace & continue p̄ cleared by P.T.				
	— Neuro ✓'s q1° x 12°, q4° x 12°. Notify M.D.'s if Δ occurs.	— Maintain sequential compression bilaterally while in bed.				
	— Log roll q2°. Keep spine in correct alignment c̄ pillow between legs.	— Maintain TED hose per policy.				
	— Notify M.D. if T > 101°.	— Assess orthostatic hypotension.				
	— Teach s/sx of infection, aseptic wound technique & good hand washing.					
	— Teach or reinforce spine precautions.					
	— Assess & record I & O until Regular diet tolerated along c̄ drains & foley out. — Check drains q̄4° & empty when 1/2 full.					

Case Manager: ___

Consulting MD: ___

Social Service: ___

Anointing of The Sick
Date: ___

MULTIDISCIPLINARY PLAN UPDATE

DATE	SIGNATURES	DATE	SIGNATURES	DATE	SIGNATURES

USC UNIVERSITY HOSPITAL
1500 San Pablo
Los Angeles, CA 90033 ©1991

DIAGNOSIS _____   NAME _____

SURGERY __**Orthopedic Service-LUMBAR FUSION WITH INSTRUMENTATION**__   ALLERGIES _____

SIDE 1   **MULTIDISCIPLINARY PLAN**   ADMIT DATE _____

DRG _214_ ALOS _10.1_

DISCHARGE OUTCOMES

PHYSIOLOGICAL
Patient will have pain controlled at level < 3 on 1 - 10 scale c̄ po meds, will ambulate c̄ steady gait independently, or c̄ D.M.E., VS within normal limits, improved neuro-sensory status & wound will be healing s̄ redness or edema.

COGNITIVE
Patient will verbalize spine precautions-no lifting, twisting, flexion & sitting as per M.D. instructions. Will verbalize s/sx of infection & when to call M.D.

PSYCHOLOGICAL
Patient will verbalize acceptance of lifestyle changes to incorporate spine precautions into activities of daily living.

DISCIPLINE	PRE-OP/ PRE-ADMIT	D.O.S. DAY 1	P.O. #1 DAY 2	P.O. #2 DAY 3	P.O. #3 DAY 4	P.O. #4 DAY 5	P.O. #5 DAY 6
		DATE	DATE	DATE	DATE	DATE	DATE
LOCATION	OP CLINIC	SURGERY/PAR/SICU	SICU → MED/SURG	MED/SURG	MED/SURG	MED/SURG	MED/SURG
LABS	CBC Chem 20 PT PTT UA		Hgb & Hct Lytes	Hgb & Hct			
CARDIO-PULMONARY	ECG	I.S.					
IMAGING/ NUCLEAR MEDICINE	CXR				AP & lat lumbar/sacral spine x-ray.		
SOCIAL SERVICES D/C PLAN REHAB. SERVICES	Psycho-social eval. R.T. eval, teach measure for brace	No Trapeze Orthomedics ☐ Lerman & Sons ☐	P.T. for all extremity ROM, passive assisted SLR Back brace fitting.	P.T. eval & teach bed mobility, logrolling, prone to stand transfer. OOB c̄ back brace If indicated, Home Health or D/C Planner for placement	Progressive ambulation c̄ assistive device prn	Continue ambulation Assess D.M.E. needs	
PHARMACY	MS PCA/ No pain management consult		Laxative or suppository prn		D/C Decadron, Zantac & PCA Begin po pain meds Ancef or Vanco D/C'd when drains are removed		
DIETARY/ NUTRITION		NPO until passing flatus	NPO until passing flatus	Clear liquids Advance diet as tolerated			

Used by permission of USC University Hospital, Los Angeles, California.

Continued.

MULTIDISCIPLINARY PLAN

PATIENT NAME: _____

DISCIPLINE	PRE-OP/ PRE-ADMIT	D.O.S. DAY 1	P.O. #1 DAY 2	P.O. #2 DAY 3	P.O. #3 DAY 4	P.O. #4 DAY 5	P.O. #5 DAY 6
		DATE ___	DATE ___	DATE ___	DATE ___	DATE ___	DATE ___
PATIENT ACTIVITY		BR Logroll q2° TED hose in PAR Bilateral leg squeezers begun in OR Gatch prn to any angle		OOB c̄ back brace High rise toilet seat			
EDUCATION	Spine precautions Review pathway goals	Spine precautions orient to room, unit & hospital routine	Instruct pt on rationale for I & O cath until complete return of bladder function	Reinforce sitting activity as per M.D. orders.			Shower instructions: Water to flow on front of body only, no direct flow on back

COLLABORATIVE PROBLEMS

DATE (D.O.S. DAY 1)	DATE (P.O. #3 DAY 4)
❶ Alteration in comfort, pain R/T surgery.	❼ Potential alteration in coping, anxiety R/T discharge planning.
❷ Potential for infection R/T surgical procedure.	❽ Altered mobility R/T surgical procedure.
❸ Potential alteration in elimination, bowel ileus R/T surgery.	
❹ Knowledge deficit R/T surgical procedure & spine precautions.	
❺ Potential for neuro-sensory impairment R/T surgery.	
❻ Potential alterations in coping, anxiety R/T hospitalization.	

OUTCOMES

D.O.S. DAY 1	P.O. #1 DAY 2	P.O. #2 DAY 3	P.O. #3 DAY 4	P.O. #4 DAY 5	P.O. #5 DAY 6
❶ Pt. will have pain controlled at 5-6 on 1-10 scale by 4° post-op.	❶ Pt. will verbalize pain controlled at 4-5 on 1-10 scale.	❶ Pt. will verbalize pain controlled at 3-4 on 1-10 scale.	❼ Pt. will verbalize feelings of assurance c̄ discharge plans within 8° of initiation.	❶ Pt. will verbalize pain controlled c̄ 3-4 on 1-10 scale c̄ po pain meds.	❽ Ambulates to BR & hall c̄ assistance. Assisted selfcare.
❷ Pt. will remain free from s/sx of infection throughout stay.	❸ Pt. will resume bowel function.				
❹ Pt. will verbalize spine precautions by 4° post-op.					
❺ Pt. will remain free from neuro-sensory impairment during hospitalization.					
❻ Pt. will verbalize feelings of assurance c̄ hospital routine within 4° post-op.					

Documentation instructions:

❶ To initiate a problem or intervention, document under corresponding date.

❷ Document outcomes under appropriate date for achieving the goal.

❸ To discontinue an intervention, or resolve a patient problem, highlight date and initial.

KEY

S/O	= Significant Other
Pt.	= Patient
A/E	= As evidenced by
△	= Change
S/SX	= Signs & Symptoms
D.M.E.	= Durable Medical Equipment
SLR	= Straight leg raises
I.S.	= Incentive spirometer

PLAN OF CARE DISCUSSED WITH | DATE | INITIAL | S.O. | Pt.

D.O.S. DAY 1	P.O.#1 DAY 2	P.O.#2 DAY 3	P.O.#3 DAY 4	P.O.#4 DAY 5	P.O.#5 DAY 6
DATE	DATE	DATE	DATE	DATE	DATE

INTERVENTIONS

D.O.S. DAY 1	P.O.#1 DAY 2	P.O.#2 DAY 3	P.O.#3 DAY 4	P.O.#4 DAY 5	P.O.#5 DAY 6
— Maintain patent IV c̄ PCA started in PAR.	— Assess bladder distension once Foley D/C'd. I & O cath q 4° prn.	— Reinforce spine precautions. — Teach back brace compliance when OOB.	— Introduce discharge planner, Home Health liaison for needs assessment.	— Encourage use of po pain meds at pain scale mid-point.	
— Orient to surroundings, unit & hospital routine.	— Reinforce spine precautions: • Sit only for meals & commode or as M.D. orders.	— Nursing to ambulate pt. c̄ back brace & continue p̄ cleared by P.T.		— Reinforce discharge plans.	
— Assess for edema & pain location, quality & duration. Notify M.D. if not controlled.	— Teach Pt. to avoid twisting, flexion or bending.	— Assess orthostatic hypotension.		— Reinforce mobility c̄ brace Reinforce Spine Precautions • No bending • No twisting	
— Assess for drainage, bleeding at surgical site. Notify M.D. if present & immediately if CSF noted.	• Maintain back brace compliance when OOB.	— Assess bowel function & need for laxative or suppository.		• No lifting • Keep spine in good alignment.	
— Cold packs to surgical site x 48°.	— Maintain leg squeezers bilaterally when in bed until discharge.			— D/C Foley I & O cath q̄ 4° PRN.	
— Assess bowel sounds, abdominal distension, flatus.	— Maintain TED hose per policy.				
— Neuro √'s q2° x 12°; q4° x 12°. Notify M.D. if Δ occurs.					
— Logroll q2°. Keep spine in correct alignment c̄ pillow between legs. — Notify M.D. if T > 101°.					
— Teach s/sx of infection, aseptic wound techinque & good hand washing.					
— Teach & reinforce spine precautions.					
— Assess & record I & O until Regular diet tolerated c̄ drains & foley out.					
— Cheek drains q4° & empty when 1/2 full.					

Case Manager: _____

Consulting MD: _____

Social Service: _____

Anointing of The Sick Date: _____

MULTIDISCIPLINARY PLAN UPDATE

DATE	SIGNATURES	DATE	SIGNATURES	DATE	SIGNATURES

Continued.

USC UNIVERSITY HOSPITAL
1500 San Pablo
Los Angeles, CA 90033 ©1991

SIDE 2   **MULTIDISCIPLINARY PLAN**

DIAGNOSIS _____   NAME _____
ALLERGIES _____

SURGERY **Orthopedic Service-LUMBAR FUSION WITH INSTRUMENTATION**   ADMIT DATE _____

DISCHARGE OUTCOMES DRG 214   ALOS 10.1

PHYSIOLOGICAL	Patient will have pain controlled at level < 3 on 1 - 10 scale c̄ p.o. meds, will ambulate c̄ steady gait independently or c̄ D.M.E., VS within normal limits, improved neuro-sensory status & wound will be healing s̄ redness or edema.
COGNITIVE	Patient will verbalize spine precautions-no lifting, twisting, flexion & sitting as per M.D. instructions. Will verbalize s/sx of infection & when to call M.D.
PSYCHOLOGICAL	Patient will verbalize acceptance of lifestyle change to incorporate spine precautions into activities of daily living.

DISCIPLINE	PRE-OP/ PRE-ADMIT	P.O.#6 DAY 7 DATE	P.O.#7 DAY 8 DATE	P.O.#8 DAY 9 DATE	P.O.#9 DAY 10 DATE	P.O.#10 DAY 11 DATE	P.O.#11 DAY 12 DATE
LOCATION		MED/SURG	MED/SURG → HOME				
LABS							
CARDIO-PULMONARY		I.S.					
IMAGING/ NUCLEAR MEDICINE							
SOCIAL SERVICES D/C PLAN REHAB. SERVICES		Clearance by P.T. for D/C.					
PHARMACY		PO pain medications					
DIETARY/ NUTRITION		Diet as tolerated					

MULTIDISCIPLINARY PLAN

PATIENT NAME: _____

DISCIPLINE	PRE-OP/ PRE-ADMIT	P.O. #6 DAY 7	P.O. #7 DAY 8	P.O. #8 DAY 9	P.O. #9 DAY 10	P.O. #10 DAY 11	P.O. #11 DAY 12
		DATE ___	DATE ___	DATE ___	DATE ___	DATE ___	DATE ___
PATIENT ACTIVITY		OOB c̄ back brace High rise toilet seat					
EDUCATION		Reinforce no direct spray from shower					

COLLABORATIVE PROBLEMS

DATE	DOC DATE / INIT			DOC DATE / INIT	DATE
❶ Alteration in comfort, pain R/T surgery.					
❷ Potential for infection R/T surgical procedure.					
❹ Knowledge deficit R/T surgical procedure & spine precautions.					
❼ Potential alteration in coping, anxiety R/T discharge planning.					
❽ Altered in mobility R/T surgical procedure.					

OUTCOMES

❷ Pt. will remain free from s/sx of infection throughout stay.

❹ Pt. will consistently verbalize/ demonstrate spine precautions.

❼ Pt. will verbalize/demonstrate feelings of assurance c̄ discharge plans.

❽ Supervised bed mobility, transfers. Independent self-care except shower.

❶ Pt. will verbalize pain controlled at <3 on 1-10 scale c̄ po pain meds.

❼ All D.M.E. available.

❽ Independent ambulation all surfaces & stairs. Independent shower.

---

❶ To initiate a problem or intervention, document under corresponding date.

❷ Document outcomes under appropriate date for achieving the goal.

❸ To discontinue an intervention, or resolve a patient problem, highlight, date, and initial.

KEY

S/O	=	Significant Other
Pt.	=	Patient
A/E	=	As evidenced by
Δ	=	Change
S/SX	=	Signs & Symptoms
D.M.E.	=	Durable Medical Equipment
SLR	=	Straight leg raises
I.S.	=	Incentive spirometer

Continued.

INTERVENTIONS

PLAN OF CARE DISCUSSED WITH				P.O.#6 DAY 7 DATE ___	P.O.#7 DAY 8 DATE ___	P.O.#8 DAY 9 DATE ___	P.O.#9 DAY 10 DATE ___	P.O.#10 DAY 11 DATE ___	P.O.#11 DAY 12 DATE ___
DATE	INITIAL	S.O.	Pt.						
				— Encourage use of po pain meds at <3 on 1-10 pain scale.					
				— Reinforce discharge plans.					
				— Reinforce proper body mechanics, no lifting.					
				— Reassess pt understanding of S/SX of infection & when to notify M.D.					
				— Limit sitting as per M.D. order.					

Case Manager: ___ ___

Consulting MD: ___ ___

Social Service: ___ ___

Anointing of
The Sick
Date: ___ ___

MULTIDISCIPLINARY PLAN UPDATE

DATE	SIGNATURES	DATE	SIGNATURES	DATE	SIGNATURES	DATE	SIGNATURES

Neurologic System

Neurologic Assessment
(Figures 9-1 and 9-2)

● Subjective Data

Dizziness
Vertigo
Weakness (bilateral or unilateral)
Paralysis
Headaches
Numbness
Bowel and/or bladder dysfunction
Pain
  Onset
  Duration and severity
  Location and radiation
  Character: throbbing, dull, prickling, tight
Memory loss, lapses
Tremors, tics
Nervousness
Syncope
Irritability
Drowsiness
Hallucination
Confusion
Disturbances in the following:
  Smell
  Taste
  Vision

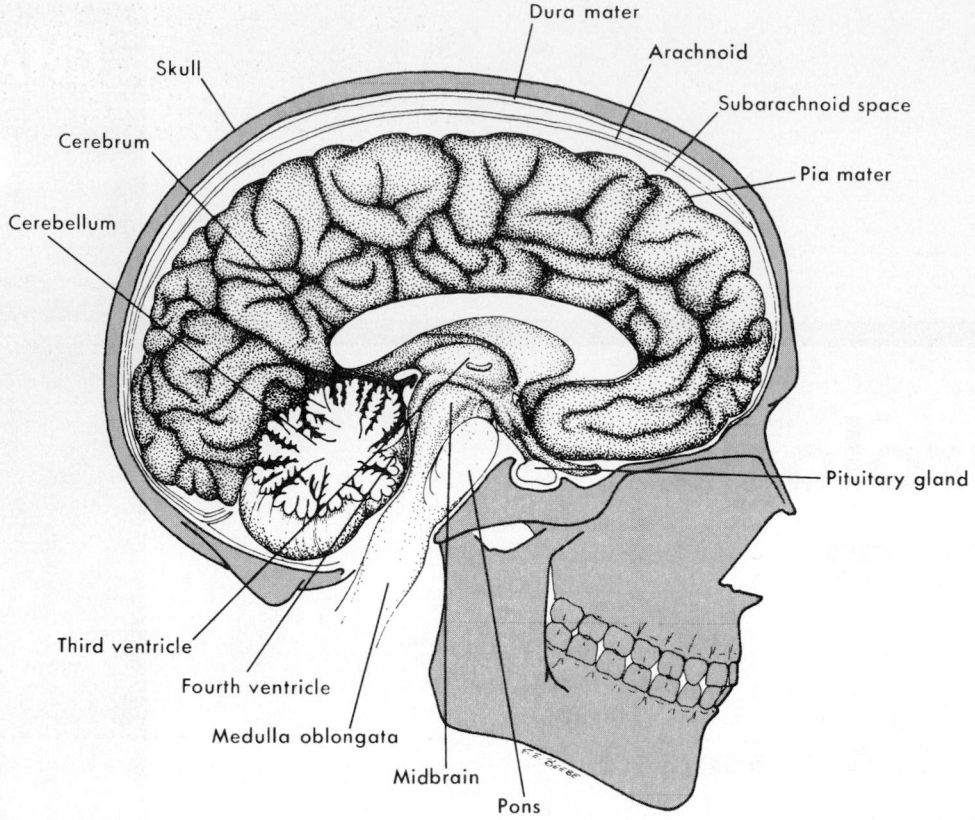

Dura mater
Arachnoid
Subarachnoid space
Pia mater
Skull
Cerebrum
Cerebellum
Pituitary gland
Third ventricle
Fourth ventricle
Medulla oblongata
Midbrain
Pons

Figure 9-1 Nervous system.

● Objective Data

Mental status
Level of consciousness (LOC) (Figure 9-3)
  See Glasgow Coma Scale (GSC) (Figure 9-4)
  Awake, alert, and oriented; able to maintain conversation
  Responds to verbal and/or painful stimuli
  Unexpected responses
  Drowsy, lethargic, sleeplike
  Able to follow commands
  Disoriented and stuporous
  Unable to respond to verbal or painful stimulus
  Comatose (Table 9-1)
Behavior
  General appearance
  Personal grooming
  Verbal expression
  Facial expression
  Ability to concentrate, express ideas
Intellectual or cognitive function
  Memory: immediate, recent, and past
  Abstract reasoning; insight
  Attention span

Emotional status
  Affect
  Mood and feelings
Level of dependence vs. independence in activities of
  daily living (ADLs)
Sensory dysfunctions
  Visual agnosia
  Tactile agnosia
Dysarthria
Language dysfunction
  Motor, expressive aphasia: Broca's aphasia
  Aphemia (pure word mutism)
  Sensory, receptive aphasia (Wernicke's aphasia)
  Auditory verbal agnosia (pure word deafness)
Apraxia
Meningeal signs
  Brudzinski's sign: to assess meningeal irritation—
    patient in supine position bends knees to avoid pain
    when neck is flexed
  Kernig's sign: to assess meningeal irritation—patient
    in supine position with hips flexed is unable to extend knees without pain
  Nuchal rigidity: stiff neck
Abnormal findings of particular gaits and postures
  (Figure 9-5; Table 9-2)

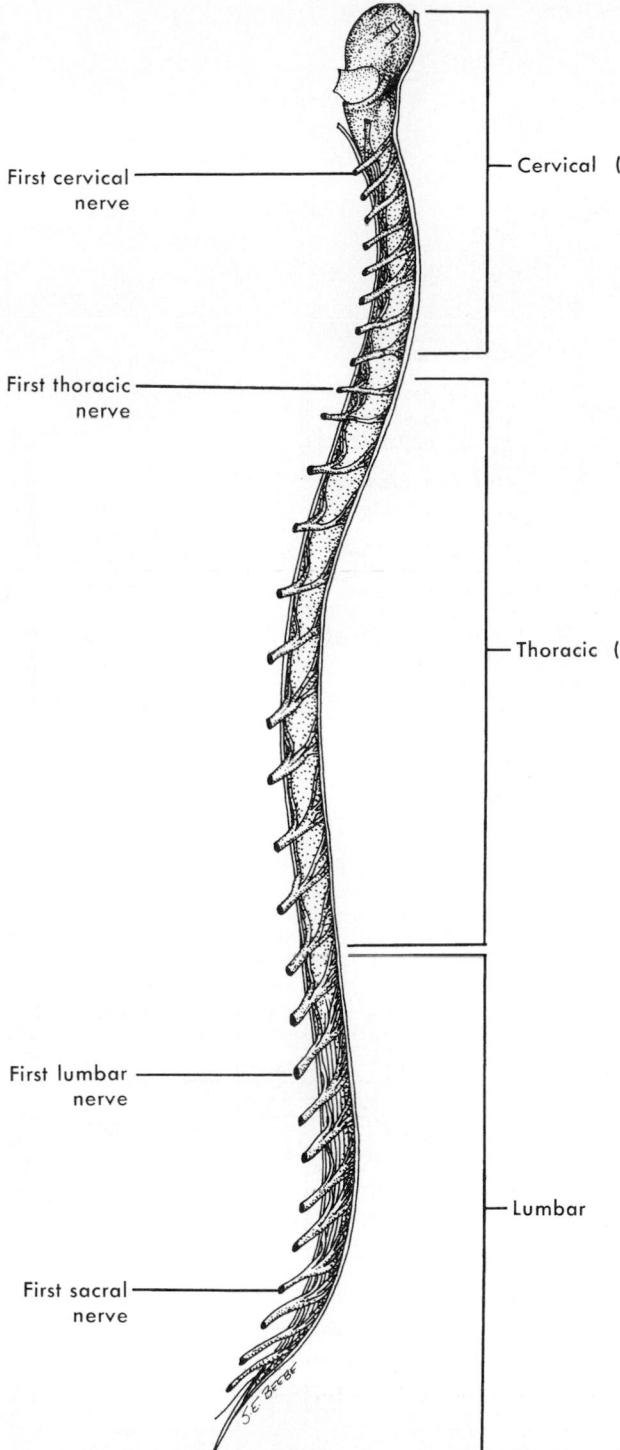

First cervical nerve

Cervical (8)

First thoracic nerve

Thoracic (12)

First lumbar nerve

Lumbar

First sacral nerve

Figure 9-2 Spinal column.

Table 9-1 Unexpected Levels of Consciousness

CONFUSION	Inappropriate response to question
	Decreased attention span and memory
LETHARGY	Drowsy, falls asleep quickly
	Once aroused, responds appropriately
DELIRIUM	Confusion with disordered perceptions and decreased attention span
	Marked anxiety with motor and sensory excitement
	Inappropriate reactions to stimuli
STUPOR	Arousable for short periods to visual, verbal, or painful stimuli
	Simple motor or moaning responses to stimuli
	Slow responses
COMA	Neither awake nor aware
	Decerebrate posturing to painful stimuli

From Seidel HM et al: *Mosby's guide to physical examination,* ed 3, St Louis, 1995, Mosby.

Angiomatous lesions
  Moles
Vital signs (VS)
  Blood pressure (BP)
    Both arms, standing, sitting
    Increased
    Decreased
    Widening pulse pressure
  Arterial pulses
  Respirations (Table 9-3)
    Rate
    Rhythm
    Quality
    Type of breathing pattern
    Chest movements
    Breath sounds
Eyes (Figure 9-6)
  Pupils
    Shape
    Equality
    Size
      Pinpoint
      Dilation
    Reaction to light, to accommodation
  Ptosis
  Nystagmus
  "Doll's eyes" (see Figure 9-7, p. 563)

General appearance
  Skin
    Temperature
    Color, discolored areas
    Turgor
    Rashes

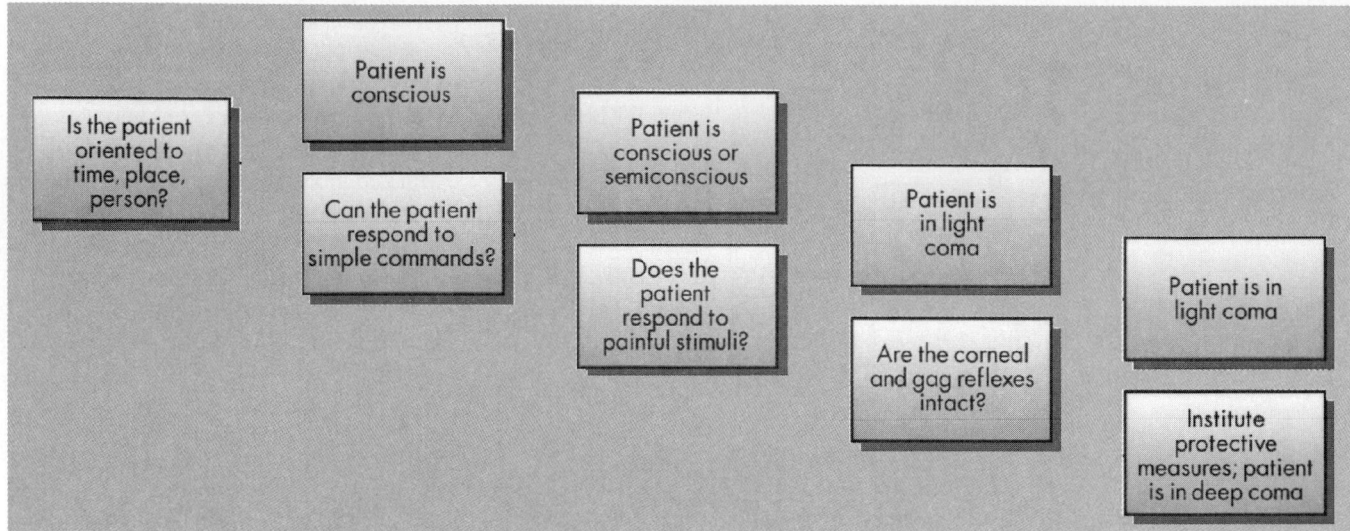

Figure 9-3   Procedure for assessing level of consciousness. (From Phipps WJ et al: *Medical-surgical nursing: concepts and clinical practice,* ed 5, St Louis, 1995, Mosby.)

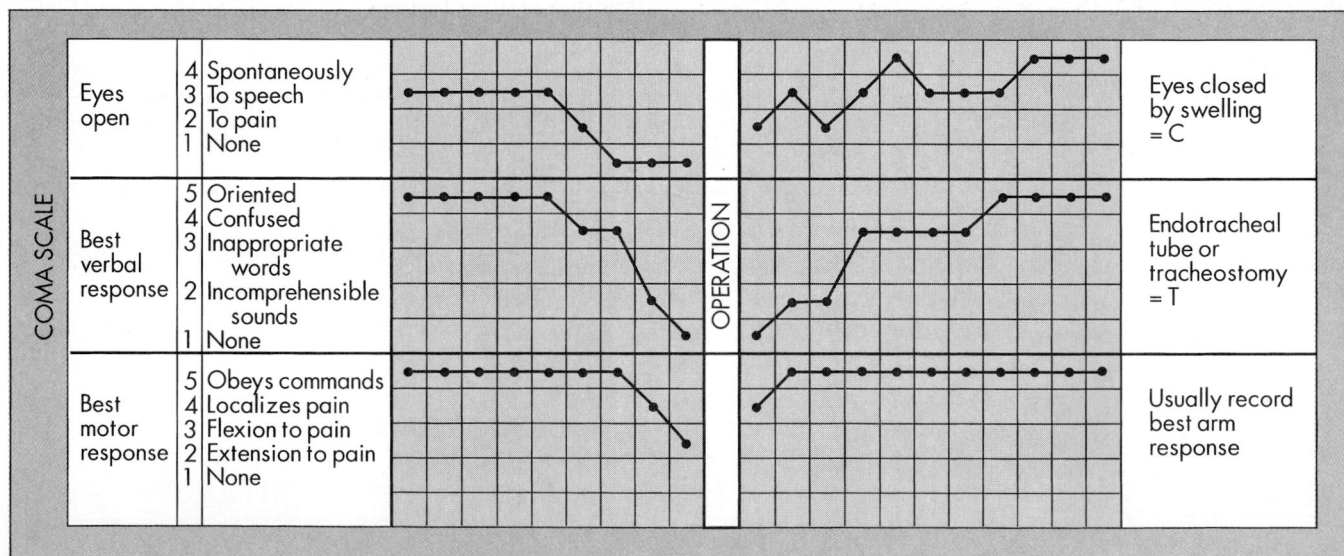

Figure 9-4   Glasgow Coma Scale, demonstrating measurement of level of consciousness. Notice change in patient's condition just before and after surgery. (From Phipps WJ et al: *Medical-surgical nursing: concepts and clinical practice,* ed 5, St Louis, 1995, Mosby.)

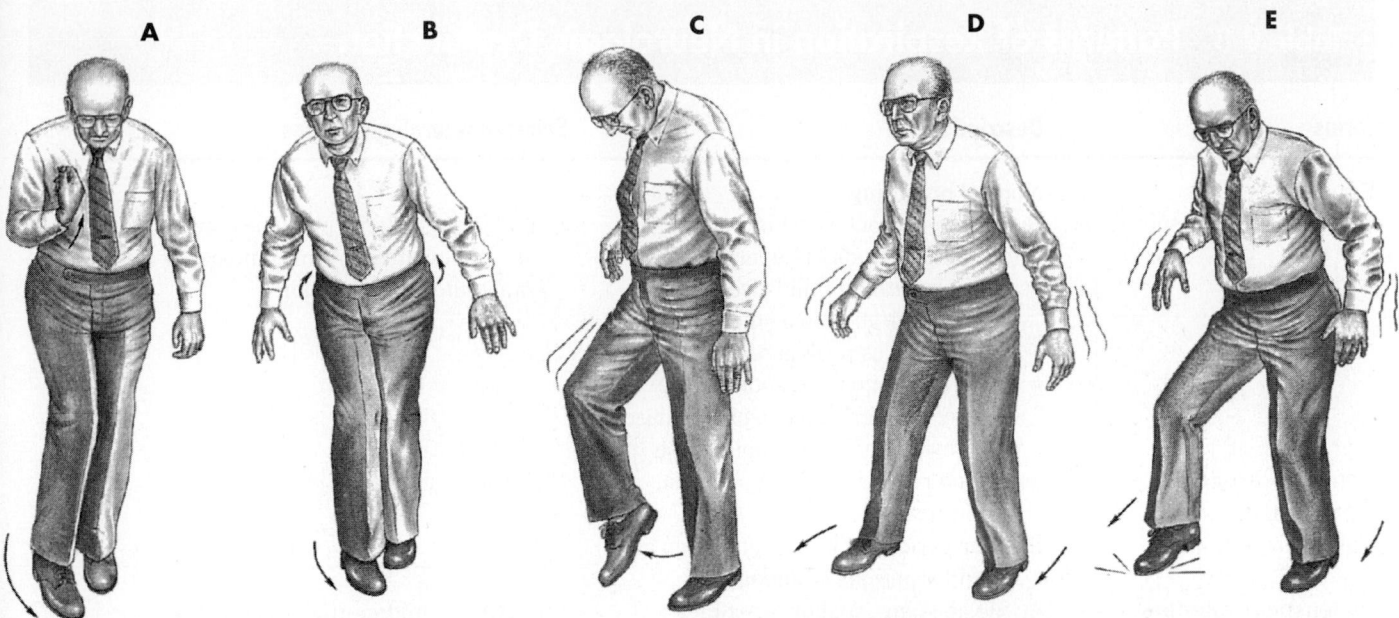

Figure 9-5 Unexpected gait patterns. **A,** Spastic hemiparesis. **B,** Spastic diplegia (scissoring). **C,** Steppage gait. **D,** Cerebellar ataxia. **E,** Sensory ataxia. (From Seidel HM et al: *Mosby's guide to physical examination,* ed 3, St Louis, 1995, Mosby.)

Table 9-2 Characteristics of Unexpected Gait Patterns

Gait Pattern	Characteristics
Spastic Hemiparesis	The affected leg is stiff and extended with plantar flexion of the foot. Movement of the foot results from pelvic tilting upward on the involved side. The foot is dragged, often scraping the toe, or it is circled stiffly outward and forward (circumduction). The affected arm remains flexed and adducted and does not swing (see Fig. 9-5, *A*).
Spastic Diplegia (scissoring)	The patient uses short steps, dragging the ball of the foot across the floor. The legs are extended, and the thighs tend to cross forward on each other at each step (see Fig. 9-5, *B*).
Steppage	The hip and knee are elevated excessively high to lift the plantar flexed foot off the ground. The foot is brought down to the floor with a slap. The patient is unable to walk on the heels (see Fig. 9-5, *C*).
Dystrophic	The legs are kept apart, and weight is shifted from side to side in a waddling motion. The abdomen often protrudes, and lordosis is common.
Tabetic	The legs are positioned far apart, lifted high and forcibly brought down with each step. The heel stamps on the ground.
Cerebellar Ataxia	The patient's feet are wide-based. Staggering and lurching from side to side are often accompanied by swaying of the trunk (see Fig. 9-5, *D*).
Sensory Ataxia	The patient's gait is wide-based. The feet are thrown forward and outward, bringing them down first on heels, then on toes. The patient watches the ground to guide his or her steps. A positive Romberg sign is present (see Fig. 9-5, *E*).
Dystonia	Jerky dancing movements appear nondirectional.
Ataxia	Uncontrolled falling occurs.

Modified from Burns, Johnson, 1980.
From Seidel HM et al: *Mosby's guide to physical examination,* ed 5, St Louis, 1995, Mosby.

Table 9-3 Patterns of Respiration in Neurologic Dysfunction

Terms	Description	Selected Neurologic Causes
Eupnea	Normal breathing	
Cheyne-Stokes respirations	Breathing characterized by regular, alternating periods of hyperpnea and apnea; breathing builds from respiration to respiration in a smooth crescendo and, as peak is reached, declines in an equally smooth decrescendo; ordinarily, hyperpneic phase endures longer than apneic phase	Deep bilateral diencephalic lesions, hypertensive encephalopathy, uremia, anoxia, or imminent transtentorial herniation
Central neurogenic hyperventilation	Sustained regular, rapid hypocapnic hyperpnea	Midbrain lesions
Biot's respirations	Regular periods of hyperventilation and irregular periods of apnea	
Apneustic respirations	Ataxic, gasping, shallow breathing	Infarction at midpontine or caudal pontine level, usually as a result of basilar artery occlusion
Posthyperventilation apnea	Respirations interrupted for up to 30 sec after five voluntary breaths in wakeful patients	Diffuse metabolic or structural forebrain disease
Cluster breathing	Breaths follow each other in disorderly sequence with irregular pauses between them	Low pons or high medulla lesion; may be result of expanding lesion in posterior fossa (cerebellar hemorrhage)
Ataxic breathing	Completely chaotic pattern with deep and shallow breaths occurring randomly; progressively leads to apnea	Dorsomedial medulla dysfunction; may appear in relation to meningitis or acute parainfectious demyelination

From Barber JM, Stokes LG, Billings DM: *Adult and child care: a client approach to nursing,* ed 2, St Louis, 1977, Mosby.

Ice water calorics (Figure 9-7)
Diplopia
Visual acuity
Visual fields
Ophthalmoscopic assessment
Motor function
  Balance
  Coordination of body movements
  Posture and gait
  Strength
    Hands, arms
    Lips, legs, ankles
  Muscle mass
    Size
    Tone
    Strength
Involuntary movement
  Tremors
  Tics
Seizure activity
Reflex responses (see box above, right; Table 9-4; Figure 9-8)
Autonomic functions

Reflex Responses

CLASSIFICATION		DESCRIPTION
0	(0)	Absent
1	(+)	Sluggish or diminished
2	(++)	Active or expected responses
3	(+++)	Slightly hyperactive or increased response
4	(++++)	Brisk with intermittent or transient clonus
5	(+++++)	Very brisk with sustained clonus

Bowel and/or bladder dysfunctions
Sexual dysfunction
Cranial nerve abnormalities (Table 9-5)
Nutritional assessment
  Weight, height
  Anthropometric measurements

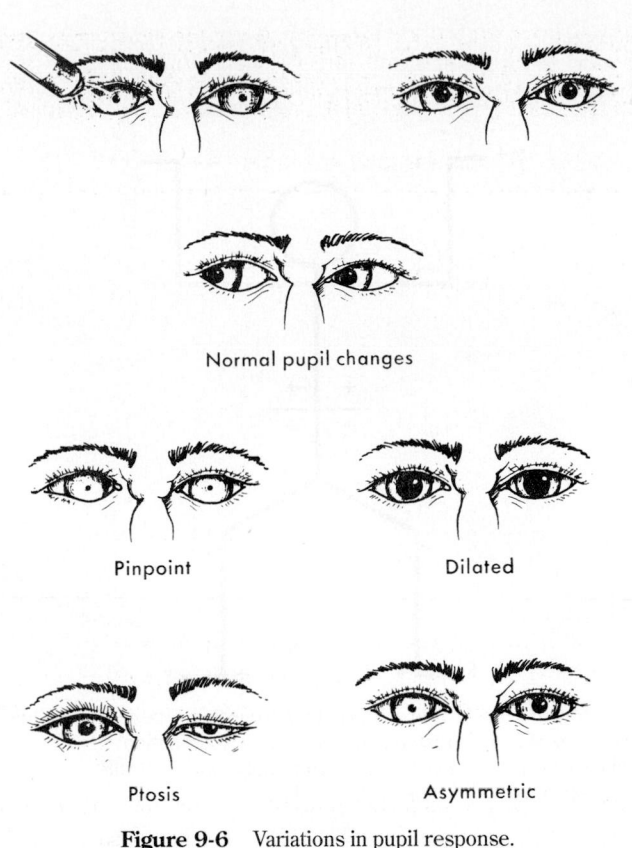

Normal pupil changes

Pinpoint   Dilated

Ptosis   Asymmetric

Figure 9-6   Variations in pupil response.

Triceps skinfold (TSF)
Arm muscle circumference (AMC)
Mid-upper arm circumference (MUAC)

● Pertinent Background Information

Description of past or concurrent neurological or muscular disorders
Recent operations or hospitalization
Epilepsy
Loss of consciousness
Headaches
Hypertension
Cancer
Coronary artery disease
Hyperlipidemia
Pernicious anemia
Diabetes
Coarctation of aorta
Allergies
Seizure disorders
Infections
Motor and/or sensory disturbances
Behavioral or emotional changes
Head trauma/spinal trauma
Drug abuse

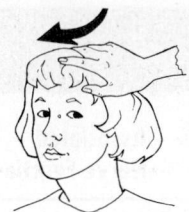
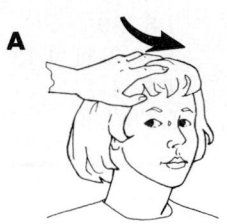
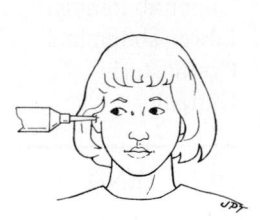

A

Doll's eyes   Ice water calorics
BRAINSTEM INTACT

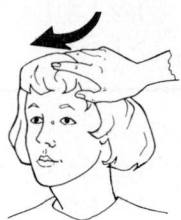
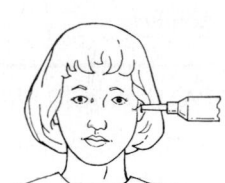

B

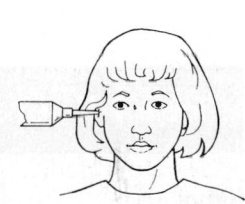

Doll's eyes   Ice water calorics
BRAINSTEM NOT INTACT

Figure 9-7   Ocular reflexes at different levels of consciousness. **A,** Response when brainstem is intact; eyes move in opposite direction of head movement. Nystagmus is present with ice water calorics. **B,** Response when brainstem is not intact; gaze remains fixed in direction of head movement. Nystagmus is not present with ice water calorics. (From Beare PG, Myers JL: *Principles and practice of adult health nursing,* ed 2, St Louis, 1994, Mosby.)

Dietary restrictions
Pregnancies

Family history

Hypertension
Seizure disorders
Neurologic disorders
Cancer
Strokes

Table 9-4　Reflexes

Reflexes	Associated Nerve Function
SUPERFICIAL	
Upper abdominal	T-8, T-9
Lower abdominal	T-10, T-11, T-12
Cremasteric	T-12, L-1
Gluteal	L-4 to S-3
DEEP TENDON	
Biceps	C-5, C-6
Triceps	C-6, C-7, C-8
Finger flexion	C-7 to T1
Brachioradialis	C-5, C-6
Patellar	L-2, L-3, L-4
Achilles	S-1, S-2
PATHOLOGIC FINDINGS	
Babinski sign (plantar)	L-4, L-5, S-1, S-2
Chaddock sign	L-4, L-5, S-1, S-2
Clonus	

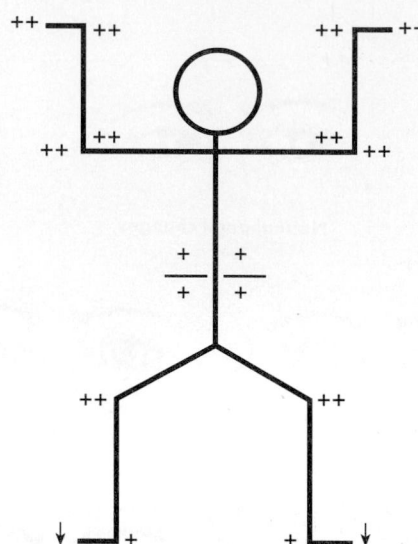

Figure 9-8　Stick figure drawing for recording reflexes. These are the reflexes usually tested in the screening examination; "+ +" values shown here are normal. (From Malasanos L: *Health assessment,* ed 4, St Louis, 1990, Mosby.)

Table 9-5　Cranial Nerve Function

Nerve	Findings
I. Olfactory	Smell
II. Optic	Visual acuity, visual fields; examination of fundi
III. Oculomotor	Pupillary reflex, external ocular muscles inducing upward, downward, and medial movements; involvement will cause ptosis, dilation of pupils
IV. Trochlear	Ocular movements; involvement will cause inability to look downward and laterally; nystagmus
V. Trigeminal	Sensory function: corneal reflex, skin of face and forehead, mucosa of nose and mouth; motor function: maxillary "jaw" reflex
VI. Abducens	Ocular movements; involvement will cause inability to look downward and laterally; nystagmus
VII. Facial	Motor function of upper and lower face; involvement will cause asymmetry of face and paresis; sensory function is tested by taste
VIII. Acoustic	Cochlear nerve test: hearing, lateralization, air and bone conduction; involvement will cause tinnitus, decreased hearing, or deafness
IX. Glossopharyngeal	Motor function: pharyngeal gag reflex, swallowing; vocal cord assessment: speak clearly without hoarseness
X. Vagus	
XI. Accessory	Strength of trapezius and sternocleidomastoid muscle; involvement will cause inability to elevate shoulder
XII. Hypoglossal	Motor function of tongue; involvement will cause lateral deviation, atrophy, tremor, inability to extend or move tongue from side to side

Mental retardation
Mental illness
Sudden, unexplained death

Social history

Sleep patterns
Exercise and activity level
Occupation: work patterns, exposure to toxic substances
Travel history, recent
Leisure activities
Dietary preferences
Smoking
Alcohol consumption
Psychosocial patterns
  Personality changes
  Relationships with family and friends
Social support system
School history; learning disorders

Medication history

Prescription medications
Over-the-counter medications
Use of controlled substances

Key aspects of neurologic examination*

Mental status
  LOC
    Glasgow Coma Scale
    Information obtained regarding mental status during history and physical examination
      Appearance
      Cognitive abilities
      Emotional stability
      Speech and language
Cranial nerves: II-XII commonly tested
Cerebellar function and proprioception
  Coordination and fine motor skills
  Balance
  Gait
Sensory function
  Perception of position sense
  Two-point discrimination
  Superficial touch and superficial pain
  Vibratory response to tuning fork
  Ability to identify familiar object by touch

Ability to identify number or letter drawn on body part
Superficial and deep tendon reflexes (DTR)
  Biceps
  Brachioradialis
  Triceps
  Patellar
  Achilles
  Abdominal reflexes
  Plantar reflex
  Ankle clonus
  Cremasteric reflex (in males)

● Diagnostic Tests

Cerebrospinal fluid (CSF) analysis
Complete blood cell count (CBC)
Erythrocyte sedimentation rate (ESR)
Gastric analysis with histamine
Blood chemistries
Arterial blood gases (ABGs) and pH
Blood glucose
Fluid and electrolyte levels
Enzyme studies
Skull films
Spinal films
Electroencephalogram (EEG)
Myelogram
Lumbar puncture
Cisternal puncture
Ventricular puncture
Electromyogram (EMG)
Tomogram
Echoencephalogram (EEG)
Pneumoencephalogram (PEG)
Evoked potentials (EP)
Ventriculography
Brain scan
Computed tomography (CT) scan
Positron emission tomography (PET) scan
Magnetic resonance imaging (MRI)
Digital subtraction angiography (DSA)
Cerebral angiography
Doppler scan: carotid and transcranial
Cerebral blood flow (CBF)
Biopsy
  Brain
  Nerve
  Muscle
Nerve conduction velocity determination
Caloric
Pulmonary function
  Vital capacity (VC)
  Minute ventilation
  Tidal volume (V_T)

---

*Modified from Seidel HM et al: *Mosby's guide to physical examination,* ed 3, St Louis, 1995, Mosby.

Surgical procedures

Craniotomy; burr holes
Cranioplasty
Craniectomy
Cordotomy
Sympathectomy
Laminectomy
Ventriculostomy
Ablative procedures
Vascular surgery

Diagnostic Procedures

Numerous procedures, both invasive and noninvasive, performed for neurologic diagnostics; general

Gerontologic Considerations

- As neurons are lost with aging, there is a deterioration in neurologic function, resulting in slowed reflex and reaction time.
- Tremors that increase with fatigue are commonly observed in adults.
- The sense of touch and the ability for fine motor coordination diminish with aging.
- Most older persons possess the ability to learn, but the speed of learning is slowed. Short-term memory is more affected by aging than long-term memory.
- The incidence of physiologic dementia or organic brain syndrome, including Alzheimer's disease, Pick's disease, and multiinfarct dementia, increases with aging.
- The incidence of cerebrovascular accident increases with age. The prognosis is affected by the location and extent of the cerebral damage. Rehabilitation potential after a stroke is often reduced by advanced age and coexisting medical problems.
- Nerve irritation resulting from arthritis, joint injuries, or spinal cord compression can cause chronic pain or weakness.
- Dementia is not a normal consequence of aging but may be a result of many reversible conditions including anemia, fluid and electrolyte imbalance, malnutrition, hypothyroidism, metabolic disturbances, drug toxicity, and hypotension.

From Christensen BL, Kockrow EO: *Foundations of nursing,* ed 2, St Louis, 1995, Mosby.

guidelines for preprocedure preparation and postprocedure observations/interventions are listed

Preprocedure preparation

For all tests or procedures patient and family or significant others should be fully informed of the nature of the procedure, its rationale, and risks involved
Reinforce physician's explanation
Explain procedure and any sensations or discomforts that will be experienced during and after procedure
Reinforce importance of cooperation and immobility of patient for appropriate procedures
Determine patient's allergies to iodine or procaine, or kidney function when indicated
Whenever possible, be present to provide physical and emotional support during procedure
Obtain signed informed consent as indicated

Postprocedure observations/interventions

Changes in LOC or orientation
Changes in any neurologic functions: speech, range of motion (ROM), visual acuity, sensory function
For vascular procedures: observe for hemorrhage, bleeding, and stability in vital signs
Maintain positioning postprocedurally as indicated
Restrict fluids and/or foods as ordered *to prevent aspiration*
Maintain bed rest as ordered
Measure intake and output *to monitor fluid status*
Control pain as indicated

Care of Patient with Altered Consciousness

altered consciousness (lowered): The state in which alteration in the interaction of the cerebral hemisphere and the reticular activating system (RAS) results in an inability of the individual to relate to self and environment

Assessment

Subjective data

Agitation, restlessness

Objective data

LOC: Glasgow Coma Scale (Figure 9-4)
Eye opening

Motor response
Verbal response
Eye movements (see Level of consciousness under
  Neurologic assessment, p. 557)
Motor function assessment
Motor function abnormalities
  Flaccidity
  Contractures
  Spasticity
  Abnormal posturing: decortication, decerebration
    (Figure 9-9)
Respiratory function
  Airway patency
  Secretions
  Respirations (Figure 9-10)
    Rate
    Patterns
      Cheyne-Stokes
      Apneustic
      Cluster
      Ataxic
  Breath sounds: equal or decreased
    Dullness
    Crackles
Cardiovascular function
  Heart rate, rhythm, quality
  Carotid, peripheral pulses: compare bilaterally
  BP
Temperature
  Hypothermia
  Hyperthermia
Skin
  Color
  Turgor

Nutritional assessment
  Dietary intake
  Weight loss, gain
  Decreases in anthropometric measurements

Diagnostic tests

Electrolytes, chemistry profile
  Fasting blood sugar (FBS)
  Sodium
  Chloride
  Potassium
  Calcium
  Phosphorus
  Magnesium
Serum ETOH (alcohol)
MRI
PET scan
CSF
ABG studies
Urine
  Toxicology screening
  Creatinine clearance
  Serum and urine osmolarity
Intracranial pressure (ICP) may be elevated
Skull x-ray examination; cervical and chest x-rays
CT scan
EEG

Potential complications

Respiratory system
  Aspiration, atelectasis
  Pneumonia

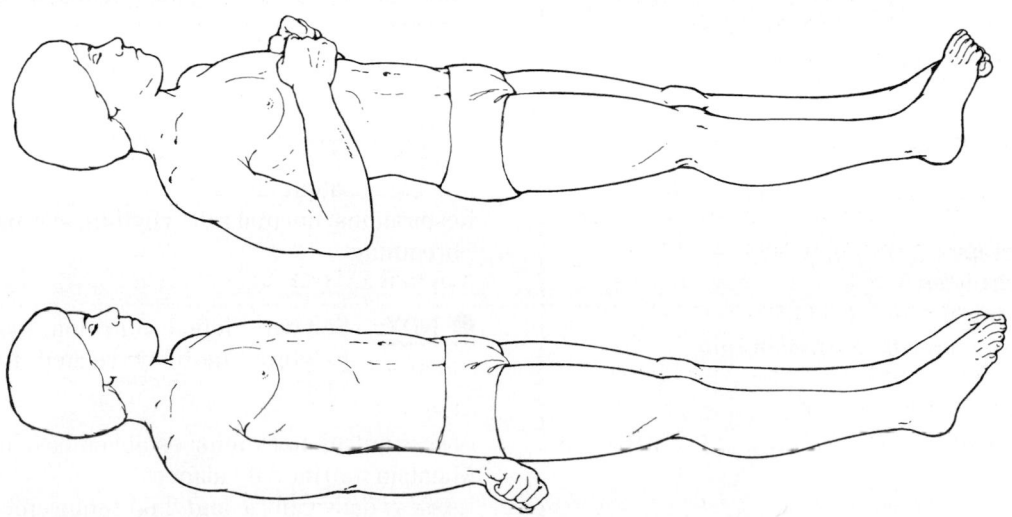

Figure 9-9   Decorticate and decerebrate posturing. (From Chipps E et al: *Mosby's clinical nursing series: neurologic disorders*, St Louis, 1992, Mosby.)

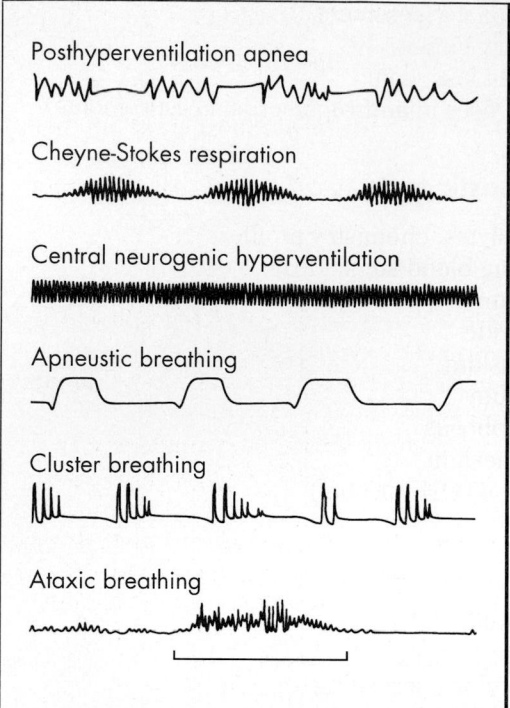

Posthyperventilation apnea

Cheyne-Stokes respiration

Central neurogenic hyperventilation

Apneustic breathing

Cluster breathing

Ataxic breathing

Figure 9-10 Breathing patterns at different levels of consciousness. (From Beare PG, Myers JL: *Principles and practice of adult health nursing,* ed 2, St Louis, 1994, Mosby.)

Neurogenic pulmonary edema
Adult respiratory distress syndrome (ARDS)
Increased ICP
Edema
Decubitus, constipation, contractures, malnutrition
Corneal ulceration
Dysrhythmias
Disseminated intravascular coagulation (DIC)
Urinary tract infection (UTI)

Collaborative management

Therapeutic management

Oxygen/ventilatory support (i.e., supplemental O_2; ABGs)
Respiratory therapy
Fluids and electrolytes
Temperature control
Cardiovascular/hemodynamic monitoring
Seizure control
ICP monitoring
Nutritional support
Medications
    ICP drugs
    Diuretics

Antidysrhythmics
Antihypertensives
Antibiotics
Anticonvulsants
Antacids
Stool softeners
Corticosteroids
Histamine antagonists
Artificial tears
Antipyretics

Nursing management

PATIENT PROBLEMS/NURSING DIAGNOSES

● **NDX:** Ineffective breathing pattern related to neurologic impairment

Assess and monitor respirations: rate, depth, and pattern; assess ventilation effort
Maintain patent airway, neck in midline position; avoid flexion of neck
Administer oxygen and humidification as indicated
Administer assisted ventilation
Assess for signs and symptoms of respiratory distress *to prevent hypoxia and decrease work of breathing*
Auscultate lung sounds q2h to 4h or as indicated
Insert oropharyngeal or nasopharyngeal airway to manage secretions
Monitor ABGs to manage respiratory status and acid-base balance
Monitor tidal volume
Elevate head of bed 30 degrees if possible *to maximize the following:*
    Breathing potential
    Cerebral venous drainage
Turn side to side and prone q2h *to optimize alveolar expansion*
Suction prn; hyperventilate 100% O_2 for 60 sec before and after suctioning

EXPECTED OUTCOMES

Maintains patent airway
Respirations: normal rate, rhythm, and pattern of breathing

● **NDX:** Self-care deficit: nutrition, hygiene/bathing, toileting, mobility related to alteration in LOC

Assess nutritional status; establish baseline weight
Maintain nutritional balance
    Assess daily caloric and fluid requirements
    Administer high-calorie, high-protein tube feedings

continuously or q2h as ordered; check tube place-
ment *to prevent aspiration;* check residual q8h
Initiate hyperalimentation or intralipid therapy as indi-
cated
Comb hair daily; shampoo every week as indicated
Keep nails clipped and clean *to prevent injury*
Administer oral hygiene q2h to 4h and prn *to prevent
drying of mucous membranes*
Remove dentures
Brush teeth tid
Clean mucous membranes with water and/or alka-
line mouthwash to prevent dryness and possible
ulceration
Keep lips moist with petroleum jelly or glycerin-type
lipsticks
Initiate oral lavages as indicated
Inspect tongue daily for cuts or crusting
Perform eye inspection and care q4h *to prevent cor-
neal ulcerations, keratitis, inflammation, or irrita-
tion*
Remove any formed crusts
Cleanse with eyedrops to provide lubrication
Close eyes and apply eye shield as necessary
Apply topical ointments as indicated
Avoid positioning patient on side with eyes open *to
prevent corneal ulceration*
Administer nose care q4h to 5h
Remove any formed crusts *to prevent obstruction*
Apply ointment to nares *to minimize drying*
Change nasal tube q72h as ordered; alternate nares *to
prevent breakdown of mucous membranes*
Inspect ears q4h to 6h for signs of dry or fresh drain-
age
Report any fresh drainage to physician
Remove crusts as ordered
Ensure elimination
Connect indwelling catheter to closed gravity
drainage as ordered *to monitor fluid status*
Monitor urinary output; assess for clarity, sedimen-
tation
Monitor fluid intake
Use external catheters as ordered
Care for catheter q8h and prn *to prevent urosepsis*
Monitor daily bowel movement; if none, check for im-
paction q2d to 3d
Initiate bowel program *to prevent constipation and possi-
ble impaction*
Give stool softeners daily
Give mild cathartics q2d to 3d
Give enemas as ordered

EXPECTED OUTCOME
Patient's needs for hygiene, nutrition, elimination, and
toileting are met

● **NDX:** Risk for impaired skin integrity

Assess and monitor skin integrity q4h to 8h *to prevent
breakdown*
Inspect ears, elbows, heels, and all pressure points
carefully
Administer skin care q2h to improve circulation
Use air mattress or egg crate mattress
Apply heel and elbow guards *to minimize irritation to
these pressure points*
Massage back and pressure points with lanolin-based
lotions *to increase circulation*
Apply cottonseed oil over feet and hands *to prevent
loss of cutaneous oil*
Keep bed linen taut, dry, and wrinkle free
Turn and reposition patient q2h *to minimize pressure
points on skin*
Remove and clean skin around any tubes (nasogastric
or endotracheal) daily *to minimize risk of breakdown caused by prolonged pressure at insertion
sites*

EXPECTED OUTCOME
Patient's skin integrity is maintained

● **NDX:** Impaired physical mobility related to neurologic impairment

Assess muscle mass and joint motion daily
Monitor for signs of joint contractures
Perform passive ROM exercise to all extremities q2h
to 4h and prn; involve large (arms, legs) and small
(fingers, toes) muscle groups *to prevent contractures*
Maintain body in proper alignment; reposition q2h; use
rolls, pillows as necessary
Apply splints as necessary *to prevent contractures and
maintain joint mobility*

EXPECTED OUTCOMES
Remains free of joint contractures; muscle is main-
tained
Demonstrates full ROM and joint mobility
Level of physical mobility is appropriate for physical
status

● **NDX:** Risk for injury related to neurologic impairment

Assess mental and physical status *to determine potential
for injury*
Initiate strategies *to prevent injury that are appropriate
for physiologic and psychological status*
If patient is unattended, maintain bed in low position
with siderails up *to prevent injury*

If patient is restless or agitated, pad siderails to prevent falls

To protect patient from self-injury, provide hand mittens as indicated; remove q8h for hand care

Provide soft restraints; contraindicated if seizures occur

Speak softly to patient, reassuring and explaining procedures and activities to promote understanding and facilitate reality orientation

EXPECTED OUTCOME
Patient is free of injury

● **NDX:**   Sensory/perceptual alterations related to neurologic disease or trauma

Assess LOC q4h to 8h; monitor and record level of mental awareness

Speak to patient; orient to person, day, hour, and location

Explain all activities and procedures *to facilitate understanding*

Encourage family, friends to talk to and touch patient

Assess environmental stimuli; eliminate as much as possible noises that are excessive or disturbing *to minimize anxiety and potential for restlessness or agitation*

Keep environment appropriate to time of day: open shades during day, turn out lights at night

Structure routine activities *to minimize anxiety*

Provide items around bed that will increase meaningful stimuli: clocks, calendars, personal favorite objects to facilitate reality orientation

Provide alternate methods of communication as indicated (e.g., picture boards, writing pads)

EXPECTED OUTCOME
Patient demonstrates stabilization of emotions and/or absence of signs of agitation/distress

● **NDX:**   Ineffective family coping related to situational crisis and/or prolonged disability that exhausts supportive capacity

Provide correct and updated information *to promote clarity and understanding*

Assist family to have a realistic perception of patient's condition and prognosis to promote understanding and acceptance

Assist family members to identify potential role changes necessary to maintain family integrity

Provide emotional support for family or significant other (e.g., allow to express feelings of loss, anger)

Encourage verbalization of feelings of death and loss *to minimize anxiety*

Permit and encourage participation in patient care as desired *to promote increased self-confidence*

Allow family to do small tasks for patient: combing hair, applying lotion, ROM exercises *to decrease feelings of helplessness*

Encourage use of resources to help in adjusting to situation (e.g., clergy, counseling) *to strengthen coping patterns*

EXPECTED OUTCOMES
Family (member) does the following:
Demonstrates ability to deal with situation
Verbalizes feelings
Seeks information to understand situation
Displays decreased anxiety regarding patient's presence

ADDITIONAL NURSING DIAGNOSES TO CONSIDER
Ineffective airway clearance
Impaired gas exchange
Risk for infection: urinary, respiratory

Patient/family teaching

Teach family how to assess the neurologic status of the patient and what findings require notification of the nurse, physician, or emergency room; notify nurse or physician of any seizure activity

Provide patient/family with discharge instructions, time and date of next outpatient appointment

Refer patient/family to local educational and support groups

If patient is taking multiple medications, suggest the purchase of a small, portable, multidose medication container; initiate and schedule teaching sessions for medication information

Stress importance of the patient wearing a medical alert tag at all times

Home care considerations

Altered LOC
Activity
Stress the importance and proper use of mobility devices: wheelchair, cane, walker to patient/family
Assist family to identify local community agencies that can help in providing such devices
Assist family to learn ways of adapting the home for accessibility
Stress the need for initial home health referral to do the following:
Teach family members proper body mechanics and how to protect their backs
Assist in learning safety measures to prevent falling

Teach the patient to change positions slowly to prevent untoward postural changes in blood pressure

Stress importance of implementing and maintaining daily exercise program with planned rest periods; active ROM exercises should be maintained

Diet

Stress the need to continue monitoring intake and output to prevent further cerebral edema and neurologic deficits; family may need to monitor urine osmolarity

Continue high-calorie, high-protein diet at home

Refer patient/family to community agencies that may provide home meals or nutritional counseling, if indicated

General instructions

Assist family members to recognize the signs and symptoms of seizure activity to report to nurse or physician

Ensure that family members are able to initiate seizure precautions as indicated

Encourage family to support independence but remember that patient may require assistance in maintaining medication regimen

Seizure Disorder (Convulsions, Epilepsy)

Paroxysmal episodes in sudden and violent involuntary motor movements of a group of skeletal muscles; generally are transitory and often involve disturbances in consciousness, behavior, sensation, motor-sensory, and/or autonomic functions (Table 9-6)

Assessment

Observations/findings

Assess patient for characteristics before, during, and after seizure activity

Document time, length, and body parts involved

Loss of or alteration in consciousness

Table 9-6 International Classification of Epileptic Seizures

Traditional Terminology	New Nomenclature

Focal motor; jacksonian seizures (occasionally become secondarily generalized)	I. Partial seizures (seizures beginning locally)
	  A. Simple (without impairment of consciousness)
	    1. With motor symptoms
	    2. With special sensory or somatosensory symptoms
	    3. With autonomic symptoms
	    4. With psychic symptoms

Temporal lobe or psychomotor seizures	B. Complex (with impairment of consciousness)
	    1. Simple partial onset followed by impaired consciousness—with or without automatisms
	    2. Impaired consciousness at onset—with or without automatisms
	  C. Secondarily generalized (partial onset evolving to generalized tonic-clonic seizures)
	II. Generalized seizures (bilaterally symmetric and without local onset)

Petit mal	A. Absences
Minor motor	B. Myoclonic seizure
Limited grand mal	C. Clonic seizure
	D. Tonic seizure
Grand mal	E. Tonic-clonic seizure
Drop attacks	F. Atonic seizure
	G. Infantile spasm III. Unclassified seizures (because of incomplete data) IV. Status epilepticus (prolonged partial or generalized recovery between attacks)

From McCance KL, Heuther SE: *Pathophysiology: the biological basis for disease in adults and children*, ed 2, St Louis, 1994, Mosby.

Motor activity
  Tonic, clonic
  Jerking, patting, rubbing movements
  Sudden, brief contractions of muscle groups
  Fluttering of eyelids
  Facial jerking
  Lip smacking
Movements may be confined to one area or may spread
  from one side to the other
Head and eyes deviate to the side
Respiratory function
  Tachypnea
  Apnea
  Difficulty in breathing
  Occluded airway

Diagnostic tests

Cerebral angiography
EEG
Echoencephalogram
CT scan
Magnetic resonance imaging (MRI)
Urine screening
Serum chemistries
  Hypoglycemia
  Increased BUN
Serum ETOH

Potential complications

Physical trauma, self-inflicted injury
Aspiration pneumonia
Respiratory impairment
Status epilepticus
Cerebral hypoxia
Death

Collaborative management

Therapeutic management

Airway management and ventilation
Medications (Table 9-7)
  Anticonvulsants
  Sedatives
  Barbiturates
Diet
  Regular
  Ketogenic
Surgery
  Resection of irritable (epileptogenic) focus
  Stereotactic lesions (corpus callostomy)

Nursing management

PATIENT PROBLEMS/NURSING DIAGNOSES

● **NDX:**   Risk for injury/trauma related to rapid onset
           of altered state of consciousness and seizure
           activity

Preconvulsive care (preictal stage)
  Pad siderails
  Maintain bed in low position
  When patient is on bed rest, raise padded siderails
  If patient is not on bed rest, maintain wheelchair in
    locked position at all times *to prevent injury and falls*
  Assist patient to identify auras
  Call light within reach at all times *to promote patient's
    feelings of security*
Convulsive care
  If out of bed during seizure activity, ease patient to
    floor and remove objects of potential harm; loosen
    constrictive clothing *to prevent injury to self*
  Turn head to side *to maintain patent airway*
  Note frequency, time, LOC, body parts involved, and
    length of seizure activity *to identify type of seizure ex-
    perienced*
  Provide privacy to maintain self-esteem
  Administer medications as ordered (see Table 9-7)
  Have suction equipment at bedside *to prevent airway
    obstruction*
  Administer supplemental O_2 as indicated *to prevent
    cerebral hypoxia*
Postconvulsive care (postictal stage)
  Assess and monitor patient carefully after seizure
  Maintain effective patent airway *to provide for ade-
    quate oxygenation and gas exchange*
  Assess patient for injury carefully, inspecting oral
    cavity
  Check BP, P, and R and do neurologic check immedi-
    ately after seizure and prn
  Assess for the following:
    Altered LOC
    Malaise
    Nausea, vomiting
    Muscular soreness, backache, or back weakness
    Aspiration
      Choking, difficulty in breathing, cyanosis
      Decreased or absent breath sounds
      Tachycardia
      Tachypnea
    Suction as indicated to prevent aspiration
Provide emotional support *to decrease anxiety and mini-
  mize feelings of shame or guilt*
Inform patient of seizure and reorient if necessary
Resume routine activity
Administer oral care as indicated

Table 9-7 Drugs Used in Seizure Disorders

Drug	Plasma Therapeutic Levels	Average Daily Dose	Side and Toxic Effects
Acetazolamide (Diamox)		1-3 g 750 mg	Drowsiness; aplastic anemia; headache; paresthesia
Carbamazepine (Tegretol)	4-10 μg/ml	450-700 mg (maximum dose 1200 mg); children: 20-30 mg/kg	Skin rash; blurred vision; ataxia; bone marrow depression
Clonazepam (Clonopin)	40-100 μg/ml	1.5-20 mg; children: 100-200 μg/kg/day	Drowsiness; ataxia; anorexia; behavior changes
Diazepam (Valium)		8-30 mg	Drowsiness; ataxia
Ethosuximide (Zarontin)	40-90 μg/ml	500-1500 mg; children: 20-40 mg/kg	Drowsiness; aplastic anemia; headache; lethargy
Mephenytoin (Mesantoin)		200-600 mg; children: 100-400 mg	Nystagmus; ataxia; skin rashes; serious toxicity common; pancytopenia
Methsuximide (Celontin)		300-600 mg	Drowsiness; ataxia; anorexia; aplastic anemia
Paramethadione (Paradione)		300-900 mg	Nephrotoxicity; neutropenia
Phenobarbital (Luminal)	20-40 μg/ml	80-120 mg; adults: 60-250 mg; children: 3-6 mg/kg	Drowsiness; ataxia; nystagmus
Phenytoin, sodium diphe-nylhydantoin (Dilantin)	10-20 μg/ml	300 mg or 4-7 mg/kg/day	Drowsiness; ataxia; nausea; rash; gingival hyperplasia; nystagmus; anemia
Primidone (Mysoline)	7-15 μg/ml	750-1500 mg; children: 10-25 mg/kg	Drowsiness; ataxia
Trimethadione (Tridione)		900-1200 mg/day; children: 900 mg/day	Bone marrow depression; dermatitis; photophobia; irritability
Valproic acid (Depakene)	50-100 μg/ml	1000-3000 mg; children: 15-60 mg/kg	Nausea; hepatotoxicity

Assist patient to a position of comfort and turn head to side to maintain patent airway

EXPECTED OUTCOME
Patient is free of injury

● **NDX:** Ineffective breathing pattern related to neurogenic impairment

Preconvulsive care
Keep oral airway at bedside
Have suction equipment readily available
Administer oxygen *to prevent cerebral hypoxia and decrease work of breathing*
Postconvulsive care
Maintain patent airway
Suction oropharynx as indicated to maintain patent airway

Administer oxygen as ordered *to minimize cerebral hypoxia*

EXPECTED OUTCOMES
Demonstrates patent airway
Lungs are clear
Respiration rate and depth are clear

● **NDX:** Social isolation related to lack of friends, groups because of stigmatization associated with seizure (epilepsy) disorders

Assess past experiences with social contacts, degree and amount of discrimination, ostracism of patient by family, friends, classmates, coworkers
Establish trust

Discuss feelings of loneliness; validate normality of feelings *to improve self-esteem and decrease sense of isolation*

Assist patient to identify barriers, actual or perceived, in establishing meaningful relationships

Offer support and encouragement to engage in social activities *to minimize feelings of isolation*

Assist in identifying diversional activities

Refer to and encourage participation in support groups

EXPECTED OUTCOMES

Verbalizes feelings of isolation

Identifies barriers to interaction with others

Seeks participation in social groups

Engages in conversation

ADDITIONAL NURSING DIAGNOSES TO CONSIDER

Ineffective airway clearance

Self-esteem disturbance related to repeated negative interpersonal experiences

Patient/family teaching

Assist patient and family to recognize auras, type of seizure activity involved, and course of action to take

Discuss importance of not restraining or interrupting behavior

Observe and record behaviors exhibited during pre-ictal and convulsive phases

Instruct patient and family about the nature of disorder and need to attempt to adopt positive attitude toward patient's life and treatment

Dispel and clarify common fears and myths about convulsive disorders

Epilepsy is not a form of insanity

Epilepsy does not get progressively worse

Emphasize importance of communication between patient and family regarding feelings of shame and humiliation associated with epilepsy

Explain importance of identifying aura and course of action to take

Explain need to identify and avoid stimuli that can stimulate onset of seizure activity

Flickering lights

Certain sounds

Certain types of food

Full bladder

Discuss medications: name, dosage, frequency of administration, purpose, side effects, and toxic effects

Stress importance of taking medication as ordered, not skipping dose

Explain need to avoid taking over-the-counter medications without physician approval

Explain importance of maintaining regular diet, exercise, and activity

Explain importance of well-balanced diet; avoid use of alcohol

Discuss importance of avoiding overexertion

Explain to family the following:

Need to encourage patient to continue with normal routines such as work, recreation, and other outside interests

Need to avoid being overprotective; assure patient and family that activity often inhibits seizure occurrence

Discuss need to avoid excessive physical and emotional excitement or stress; need to avoid stimulants

Instruct patient to wear or carry medical alert band or card

Discuss available agencies for use as references such as Epilepsy Foundation of America*

Educate patient regarding possible limitations or restrictions of driving privileges

Home care considerations

Activity

Seizure precautions are implemented as indicated

Assist patient to sit or lie down

Do not attempt to restrain patient or stop the seizure activity

Protect patient from physical injury

Provide privacy

Observe and record involved body parts, time and duration of the seizure activity

Report all seizure activity to the physician and home health nurse

Maintain regular exercise program

Maintain normal routine and avoid overprotection and social isolation

Diet

Avoid excessive use of stimulants

Avoid alcohol ingestion

Maintain a well-balanced diet; incorporate dietary restrictions as indicated

Maintain ketogenic diet if prescribed

General instructions

Stress the need for correct body mechanics when transferring patient or assisting during seizure activity

Assist family in making home environment as accessible and risk-free as possible

---

*Epilepsy Foundation of America, 4351 Garden City Dr., 5th Floor, Landover, MD 20785.

Cerebrovascular Disruptions

Alterations in cerebrovascular circulation; may be classified as ischemic or hemorrhagic

ischemic disruption: *Disruption of cerebral blood flow caused by thrombosis, embolus, or hemorrhage*

subarachnoid hemorrhage (SAH): *Bleeding into the subarachnoid space caused by ruptured cerebral aneurysm, hypertensive hemorrhage, ruptured arteriovenous malformation*

intracerebral hemorrhage: *Bleeding into cerebral tissue; caused by hypertensive rupture of cerebral vessel*

Assessment

Objective data

ISCHEMIC

Altered LOC
  Vertigo
  Drowsiness
  Stupor
  Mental confusion
  Disorientation
  Irritability
  Coma
Visual disturbances
  Diplopia
  Ptosis
  Monocular blindness
  Photophobia
Sensory disturbances
  Tingling
  Numbness
  Tinnitus
Motor disturbances
  Paresis
  Weakened reflexes
  Hemiplegia
Dysphasia
Aphasia
Nausea, vomiting
Elevated T and BP
Tachycardia
Tachypnea
Positive Kernig and Brudzinski signs (indicating meningeal irritation)

HEMORRHAGIC
Subarachnoid hemorrhage (SAH)
  Symptoms generally abrupt in onset

Increasing ICP
Altered LOC
  Headaches (may be severe)
  Vertigo
  Mental confusion
  Stupor
  Coma (common)
Ocular disturbances
Hemiparesis or hemiplegia
Seizures
Nausea, vomiting
Sweating and/or chills
Meningeal irritation
  Nuchal rigidity
  Positive Kernig or Brudzinski signs
  Photophobia
  Blurred vision
  Irritability, restlessness
  Elevated T
  Most commonly associated with head trauma
Intracerebral hemorrhage
  Altered LOC
    Mental confusion
    Stupor
    Coma (common)
  Severe hypertension
  Coagulopathy
  Respiratory distress
  Meningeal irritation
Arteriovenous malformation
  Headaches
  Seizure activity
  Motor/sensory deficits
  Aphasia
  Dizziness
  Fainting

Diagnostic tests

CT scan or MRI
Lumbar puncture and CSF evaluation (may not be performed because of elevated ICP)
  Elevated pressure
  Xanthochromic to grossly bloody
  Elevated protein (80 to 130 mg/100 ml)
  Elevated WBC
  Decreased glucose
Clotting studies
Cerebral angiography
Echoencephalography
Skull x-ray examinations
Brain scan
Regional cerebral blood flow studies (CBF)
Carotid Doppler flow studies (B-mode ultrasound)
Doppler ultrasonography

Potential complications

Cerebral vasospasm
  Focal neurologic deterioration
  Cerebral ischemia
  Cerebral infarction
Hydrocephalus
Rebleeding

Collaborative management

Therapeutic management

ISCHEMIC

Parenteral therapy
Medications
  Anticonvulsants
  Antiplatelet aggregation
  Antihypertensives
  Corticosteroids
  Diuretics
  Antihistamines
  Narcotic analgesic
Ventilatory support when indicated
ABGs (serial)
Cardiac monitoring
Seizure precautions
ICP monitoring
Nutritional support
Nasogastric tube
Foley or indwelling catheter

HEMORRHAGIC

Ventilator/oxygen support
ABGs (serial)
Complete activity restriction
Elevation of head of bed
ICP monitoring
Parenteral therapy
Medications
  Antihypertensives
  Corticosteroids (dexamethasone)
  Antifibrinolytics (aminocaproic acid)
  Stool softeners
  Antipyretics
  Analgesics (codeine)
Hyperventilation
Hypothermia as indicated
  Cardiac monitoring
  Seizure precautions
  Elastic stockings
  Foley or indwelling catheter
  Nasogastric tube

Surgery
  Aneurysm: clipping, ligation
  Arteriovenous malformation (AVM): embolization, surgical excision of AVM
Treatment of vasospasm
  Hypervolemic-hypertensive therapy: fluid and volume expanders
  Medications
    Serotonin antagonists (reserpine)
    Kanamycin sulfate
    Calcium-blocking agents (nifedipine, verapamil)
    Barbiturates
  Hemodynamic monitoring

Nursing management

PATIENT PROBLEMS/NURSING DIAGNOSES

● **NDX:** Altered tissue perfusion: cerebral related to vasospasm secondary to hemorrhagic injury

Assess neurologic status q15 min to 30 min or as indicated
Monitor for signs of increased ICP *to prevent changes in cerebral circulation*
Monitor for changes or signs of cerebral vasospasm
Maintain bed rest with head of bed elevated 15 to 40 degrees *to facilitate cerebral venous drainage*
Check BP, P, and R q15 min to 30 min
Report any sudden changes in BP, pupillary, or neurologic status immediately
Assess and monitor respirations and ventilation; provide oxygen as indicated *to decrease work of breathing*
Monitor ABGs as ordered to assess acid-base balance
Check rectal T q2h to 4h; hypothermia or cooling measures may be indicated
Initiate subarachnoid precautions (see box below)
Maintain strict intake and output

Subarachnoid Precautions

Provide private room with dim artificial lighting
Ensure complete bed rest
Maintain quiet environment
Reduce environmental stimuli
Limit visitors
Provide all nursing care
Administer stool softeners

Initiate treatment for vasospasm as ordered *to prevent further cerebral ischemia and injury*
Auscultate lung sounds q4h to 8h *to detect adventitious breath sounds*
Monitor PCWP, PAD, SVR, and BP to achieve and maintain within prescribed parameters

EXPECTED OUTCOMES
Patient demonstrates effective cerebral perfusion; is oriented to time, person, place
No alteration in consciousness
VS are WNL

● **NDX:** Altered tissue perfusion: cerebral related to increased ICP secondary to hemorrhagic injury

Assess neurologic status q15min to 30min or as indicated
Check BP, P, and R q15min to 30min
Monitor for signs and symptoms of increasing ICP (p. 624); report any changes in BP, P, or neurologic status immediately; maintain potency and sterility of ICP monitoring devices, if used
Elevate head of bed 30 to 40 degrees *to facilitate cerebral venous drainage*
Maintain head and neck in midline position
Monitor strict intake and output
Observe for signs of overhydration or dehydration
Report increase in systolic BP >20 mm Hg with widened pulse pressure
Initiate monitoring of ICP as ordered; report increase >15 mm Hg lasting 15 to 30 min
Administer medications as ordered
If steroids are administered: check stools, urine, and gastric contents for occult blood

EXPECTED OUTCOMES
Patient demonstrates effective cerebral perfusion; is oriented to time, person, place
No alteration in consciousness
ICP ≤15 mm Hg
No clinical signs of increased ICP

● **NDX:** Pain (headache, nuchal rigidity) related to irritation of meninges secondary to subarachnoid hemorrhage

Assess type, location, and severity of pain
Monitor for signs of increasing pain or discomfort; report any changes in character of pain

Administer medications as ordered: analgesics *to minimize discomfort*
Maintain quiet environment; remove or modify any stimuli that may heighten pain or discomfort; dim lights
Explain all procedures and treatments *to minimize anxiety and facilitate understanding*
Organize care *to maximize periods of quiet and rest to allow for sufficient REM sleep*
Move or reposition patient gently; avoid excessive movement
Implement relaxation techniques
Pace activities and plan ahead
Encourage open communication about feelings of discomfort

EXPECTED OUTCOMES
Reports pain relief
Achieves comfort level
Appears comfortable; sleeps and rests quietly

ADDITIONAL NURSING DIAGNOSES TO CONSIDER
Anxiety related to perceived and actual biologic threat
Ineffective breathing pattern related to neurologic impairment
Unilateral neglect secondary to cerebrovascular accident

Patient/family teaching

Provide explanation of primary clinical disorder, causes, and treatment as indicated
Encourage questions; correct any misconceptions
Discuss medications: name, dosage, frequency of administration, purpose, side effects, and toxic effects
Explain need to avoid taking over-the-counter medications without consulting physician
Explain need to increase activities as ordered; physical activity as tolerated
Explain need for planned rest periods
Discuss symptoms of progression of condition to report to physician
Explain importance of ongoing outpatient care
If patient is taking multiple medications, suggest the purchase of a small, portable, multidose medications container
Stress the importance of wearing a medical alert tag at all times
Alert the patient to change positions slowly to prevent postural changes in blood pressure
Provide patient/family with discharge instructions, time and date of next outpatient appointment
NOTE: Stroke victims, see p. 578.

Home care considerations

Activity
  Stress the importance and proper use of mobility devices (wheelchair, cane, walker) to patient/family
  Assist family to identify local community agencies that can help in providing such devices
  Assist family to learn ways of adapting the home for accessibility
  Stress the need for initial home health referral to do the following:
    Teach family members proper body mechanics and how to protect their backs
    Assist in learning safety measures to prevent falling
  Maintain regular exercise program including active and passive ROM exercises to all joints
  Continue planned rest periods to prevent fatigue and agitation
Diet
  Offer small portions frequently and supplemental feedings if indicated
  Avoid foods such as soft breads, mashed potatoes, semicooked vegetables, and large pieces of meat that may cause choking
General instructions
  Assist family, as indicated, to develop competency in
    Home ventilation
    Suctioning
    Tracheostomy care
    Parenteral or enteral home nutrition therapy
    Positioning techniques
  Assist family to recognize and report signs and symptoms of stroke including the following:
    Headaches
    Nausea and vomiting
    Restlessness and lethargy
    Changes in LOC
    Feelings of impending doom
    Pupillary changes
    Changes in VS
      Increased systolic BP
      Decreased pulse rate
  Implement speech exercises on a regular basis

Cerebrovascular Accident (Stroke)

Onset of neurologic deficits related to decreased cerebral blood flow caused by occlusion or stenosis of blood vessels from embolism, thrombosis, or hemorrhage, resulting in ischemia of the brain (NOTE: Symptoms depend on location and size of lesion)

Assessment

Subjective data

Generalized weakness
Visual deficits
  Blurred vision
  Partial loss of vision

Objective data

Symptoms may be rapid in onset or take several min or hr to complete
Altered LOC
Loss of sensation and reflexes
  Usually unilateral
  May be temporary or permanent
Flaccid or spastic muscle tone
Pupil inequality
Ptosis of eyelid
Drooping mouth
Elevated BP
Paralysis: may be unilateral or bilateral
Communication dysfunction
  Motor and sensory aphasia
  Apraxia
  Agnosia
Dysphagia
Bladder and bowel incontinence
Nausea and vomiting
Bruits: carotid, femoral, iliac arteries or abdominal aorta

Diagnostic tests

Lumbar puncture and CSF (performed with caution if increased ICP)
  Normal or elevated CSF
  Elevated protein level in CSF
CT scan
MRI
PET scan
Cerebral arteriography
EEG
Brain scan
B-mode ultrasound
Skull x-ray examination
Echoencephalography
Doppler ultrasonography
ECG

Potential complications

Increased ICP
Herniation of brain

Hypertension/hypotension
Aspiration, atelectasis
Respiratory failure
Seizure activity
Cardiac dysrhythmias
Malnutrition
Contractures, ankylosis
Deep vein thrombosis (DVT)
Pulmonary embolism
Subsequent CVAs
Bowel/bladder incontinence

Collaborative management

Therapeutic management

Airway patency support
  Oxygen-assisted ventilation
  Tracheostomy
Serial ABG analysis
Bed rest
Nutritional and fluid management
  Nasogastric tube
  Peripheral or central IV
Medications
  Antihypertensives
  Antifibrinolytics
  Antispasmodics
  Anticonvulsants
  Anticoagulants
  Antipyretics
  Corticosteroids
  Diuretics
  Antiulcer agents
  Vasodilators
  Stool softener
  Calcium channel blockers
ECG and cardiac monitoring
Hypothermia
ICP monitor
Indwelling urinary catheter
Neurologic rehabilitation

Nursing management

PATIENT PROBLEMS/NURSING DIAGNOSES

● **NDX:** Ineffective airway clearance related to impaired cough and inability to handle secretions

Assess and monitor respirations, cough reflex, and secretions

Position body and head *to prevent obstruction of airway and provide optimal secretion removal*
Suction secretions prn: hyperoxygenate in 100% O_2 for 60 sec before and after suctioning *to minimize hypoxemia;* limit suctioning to <15 sec at a time
Insert oropharyngeal or nasopharyngeal airway *to maintain airway patency*
Auscultate chest for breath sounds q2h to 4h *to detect adventitious breath sounds*
See Care of patient with altered consciousness (p. 567)
Administer oxygen/humidification as ordered *to decrease work of breathing and minimize potential for drying of mucous membranes*
Provide mechanical ventilation as ordered *to prevent/ minimize respiratory distress*
Monitor serial ABGs and hemoglobin (Hgb) as indicated *to assess oxygenation status*

    EXPECTED OUTCOMES
Demonstrates patent airway
Chest expansion is symmetrical
Breath sounds are clear to auscultation
ABGs and vital signs are within normal limits
No signs of respiratory distress

● **NDX:** Impaired physical mobility related to impaired neurophysiological function

Assess functional ability and extent of impairment; record and monitor changes and improvements
Maintain body alignment; use bedboard, air mattress, or footboard as indicated (Figure 9-11) *to lessen muscle fatigue*
Turn and reposition q2h *to facilitate comfort*
Elevate affected limbs on pillows *to prevent swelling*
Use pull sheet when indicated *to minimize tissue trauma*
When patient is on side, support with pillows; may use hand rolls and arm splints *to maintain patient in functional position* (see Figure 9-11)
Perform active and/or passive ROM exercise to all extremities q2h to 4h and prn (Figures 9-12 and 9-13) *to help relieve muscle soreness and weakness*
Assist and encourage patient to perform quadriceps setting and gluteal exercises q4h
Encourage hand, finger, and foot exercises
  Have patient squeeze rubber/sponge ball
  Perform flexion
  Perform extension of fingers, legs, and feet
Assist patient with using supportive devices as indicated: overhead trapeze, braces, wheelchair, canes, walker
Apply antiembolic stockings *to prevent venous stasis*

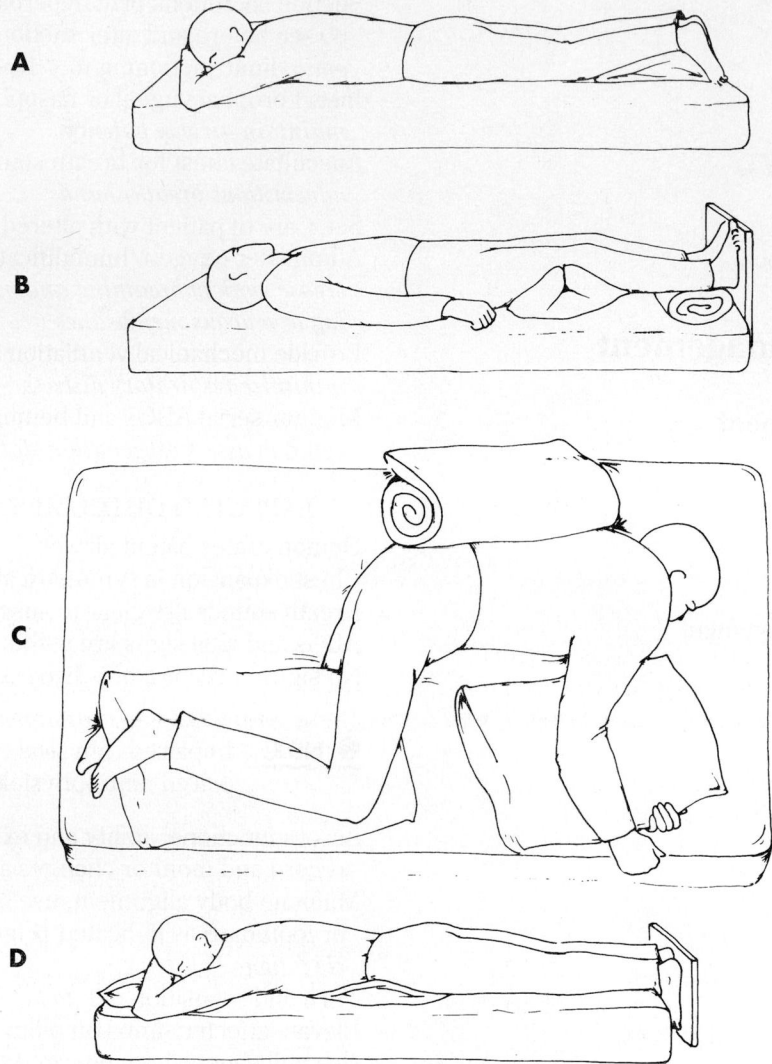

Figure 9-11 Various body positions to maintain correct alignment. **A,** Prone position. **B,** Supine position. **C,** Side-lying position. **D,** Prone position with support of feet.

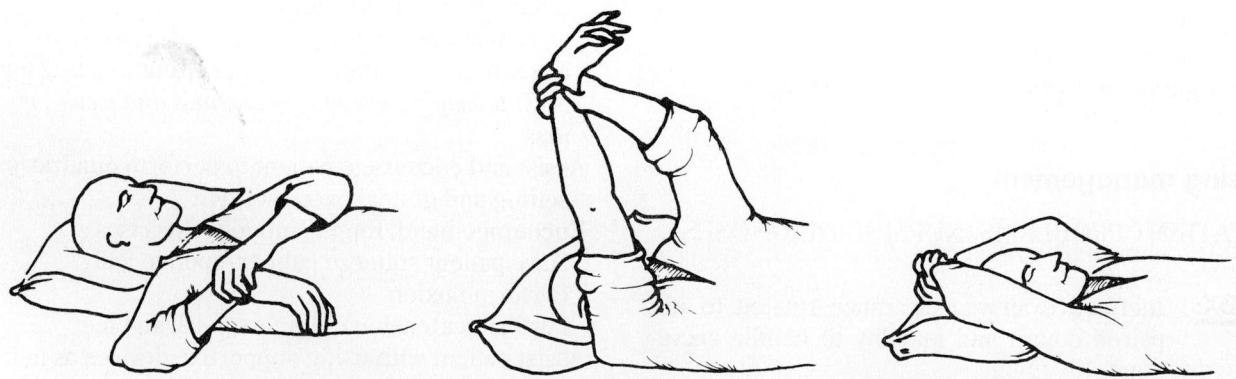

Figure 9-12 Range of motion of affected shoulder and elbow.

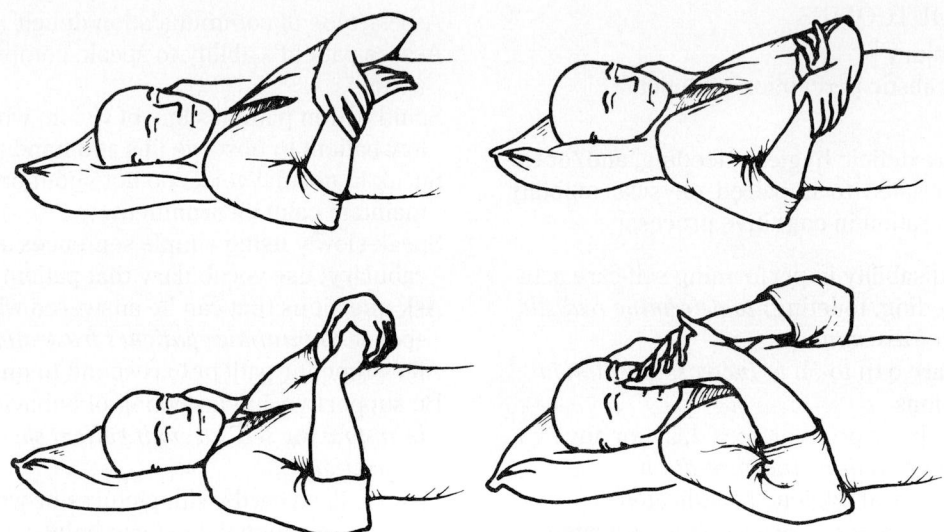

Figure 9-13 Range of motion of affected wrist and hand.

Encourage use of involved side when possible

Instruct patient to use healthy extremity to support weaker side (e.g., lift involved left leg with good right leg or lift involved left arm with good right arm) to increase mobility

Encourage patient to perform basic ADLs as soon as possible using unaffected side *to increase self-sufficiency*

Bathing

Brushing teeth

Combing hair

Eating

Begin progressive ambulation as ordered; assist to balanced sitting position; begin with transfer procedure from bed to chair to regain position sense

Consult with physical and occupational therapy departments regarding activity program to establish effective team approach

EXPECTED OUTCOMES

Demonstrates optimal physical mobility and function within physiologic limitations

Exhibits behaviors and skills necessary for resumption of activities

● **NDX:** Unilateral neglect related to right/left cerebral hemisphere lesions secondary to neurologic illness and trauma

Assess degree of neurologic deficit and patient's perception and awareness of deficit

Orient patient to environment on regular basis *to reestablish reality orientation*

Provide realistic feedback

Provide a safe environment *to minimize potential for injury*

Remove unnecessary furniture and equipment

Place call bell, bedside stand, and personal items on unaffected side within reach

Keep siderail up on affected side; lock rails up if patient is impulsive

Observe and anticipate needs

Structure environment to decrease environmental hazards

Approach and speak to patient from unaffected side

Assist patient to recognize and deal with perceptual deficit

Initially: arrange environment within perceptual field

After initial stress: promote increased attention to neglected side

Encourage patient to look at affected side *to assist in recovery*

Stay with patient, touching or stroking affected side; encourage patient to handle affected limbs

Instruct and remind patient to include affected limbs when performing simple tasks *to decrease weakness on affected side*

Use tactile stimulation to reintroduce patient to affected limbs; use scented lotions or differently textured materials *to stimulate different sensations*

Consult with rehabilitation team to design a rehabilitation program

Encourage patient to participate in ADLs; begin by teaching individual components of an activity; later, integrate components into total activity

Encourage activities that will force patient to look at or involve affected side (e.g., place food closer to affected limb)

EXPECTED OUTCOMES
Patient is free of injury
Demonstrates a realistic perception of deficit

● **NDX:** Self-care deficit: hygiene, feeding, and/or toileting related to impaired physical mobility and alteration in cognitive process

Assess degree of disability in performing self-care activities (bathing, feeding, toileting) *to determine realistic amount of required assistance*
Administer skin care q4h to 5h *to increase circulation*
  Use oil-based lotions
  Inspect area over bony prominences daily for any breakdown *to prevent decubitus formation*
Provide for total physical hygiene as indicated
  Comb hair daily; shampoo every week as indicated
  Keep nails clipped and clean to prevent self-injury
  Administer oral hygiene q4h to 8h; brush teeth; clean mucous membranes with water and/or alkaline mouthwash *to prevent drying of mucous membranes*
Assess and monitor nutritional status
Administer tube feedings as ordered; check tube placement to prevent aspiration
Initiate oral feedings as indicated to maintain caloric intake
  Begin with clear liquids *to prevent nausea*
  Assist with feedings as necessary
  Observe for difficulty in swallowing *to prevent aspiration*
  Position on side with head of bed elevated *to prevent aspiration* if feeding patient in bed
Encourage fluid intake to 2000 ml/day unless contraindicated to aid in elimination
Ensure regular elimination
  Connect indwelling catheter to closed gravity drainage system as ordered; provide catheter care q8h and prn *to prevent infection and possible urosepsis*
  Use external catheters as ordered
  Offer bedpan/urinal q2h to 4h if catheter is not used
  Monitor daily bowel movement; if none, check for impaction q2d to 3d
  Give stool softeners or enema as ordered *to prevent impaction*

EXPECTED OUTCOME
Patient's needs for hygiene, nutrition, elimination, and toileting are met

● **NDX:** Impaired verbal communication related to injury to cerebral speech center

Assess type of communication deficit (see box below)
Assess patient's ability to speak, comprehend, read, or write
Stand within patient's line of vision; when speaking, allow patient to observe lips and hands
Speak in normal voice; do not shout or speak loudly; maintain calm environment
Speak slowly using simple sentences and common vocabulary; use vocabulary that patient understands
Ask questions that can be answered with a *yes* or *no* response *to minimize patient's frustration level*
Allow time for patient to respond to questions
Be supportive and accepting of behavior *to assist in improving self-esteem if patient shows signs of frustration*
Provide flash cards with pictures or words of common objects to which patient can point
Consult with speech therapist to identify an appropriate means of communication

EXPECTED OUTCOME
Patient is able to communicate basic needs

ADDITIONAL NURSING DIAGNOSES
TO CONSIDER
Risk for impaired skin integrity
Self-esteem disturbance: body image
Powerlessness

Patient/family teaching

Assess understanding level of adjustment to disability
Explain to family the following:
  Need to encourage as many independent activities as possible; be alert to limitations
  Need to set realistic, achievable goals
  Need to avoid being overprotective
  Need to praise any tasks accomplished
  Importance of dealing with body image changes and behavioral changes

Communication Deficit

Expressive aphasia (Broca's aphasia): inability to express oneself verbally
Receptive aphasia (Wernicke's aphasia): inability to understand the spoken word
Global aphasia: combination of expressive and receptive aphasia

Need to allow patient to be expressive
Encourage diversional activities
  Reading to patient
  Watching television
  Listening to radio
Plan regular rest periods to prevent fatigue
Encourage verbalization and communication between patient and family to promote acceptance and understanding
Be sympathetic to emotional upsets but firm in following regimen
Reinforce physician's explanation of medical management
Stress importance of ongoing outpatient care and follow-up visits
Stress importance of continuation of rehabilitation program
Instruct patient and significant other in proper dietary and fluid needs
Stress importance of safety measures: siderails, ramps, low-heeled shoes, removal of scatter rugs to prevent injury

Home care considerations

Activity
  Stress the importance and proper use of mobility devices (wheelchair, cane, walker) to patient/family
    Assist family to identify local community agencies that can help in providing such devices
    Assist family to learn ways of adapting the home for accessibility
    Stress the need for initial home health referral to do the following:
      Teach family members proper body mechanics and how to protect their backs
      Assist in learning safety measures to prevent falling
  Maintain regular exercise program including active and passive ROM exercises to all joints
  Continue planned rest periods to prevent fatigue and agitation
Diet
  Offer small portions frequently and supplemental feedings if indicated
  Avoid foods such as soft breads, mashed potatoes, semicooked vegetables, and large pieces of meat that may cause choking
General instructions
  Assist family, as indicated, to develop competency in the following:
    Home ventilation
    Suctioning
    Tracheostomy care
    Parenteral or enteral home nutrition therapy
    Positioning techniques

Assist family to recognize and report signs and symptoms of stroke including the following:
  Headaches
  Nausea and vomiting
  Restlessness and lethargy
  Changes in LOC
  Feelings of impending doom
  Pupillary changes
  Changes in VS
    Increased systolic BP
    Decreased P
Implement speech exercises on a regular basis

Brain Tumors

Abnormal growths of primary, metastatic, or developmental origin occurring within the brain or supporting structures

Assessment

Subjective data

Headache: localized or general; may increase with activity (early and common symptom)
Dizziness occurring with position change; vertigo

Objective data

Altered LOC
Seizures
  Focal/simple
  Psychomotor/complex
  Generalized
Decreased response to verbal and painful stimuli
Inability to follow commands
Mental or personality changes
  Irritability
  Forgetfulness
  Loss of memory
  Impaired judgment
  Depression
Pupils: unequal response to light
Papilledema
Diplopia, loss of visual acuity
Ptosis
Tinnitus
Loss of hearing
Weakness or paralysis of face and/or extremities
Uncoordination of extremities
Paresthesia or anesthesia
Gait
  Staggering

Uncoordinated
 Wide-based walking
Difficulty in chewing with dysphagia
Vomiting with or without nausea
Aphasia
Agraphia (inability to express oneself in writing)
Obesity

According to location

FRONTAL LOBE

Inappropriate affective responses; forgetfulness
Lack of concern; loss of social graces
Facetiousness
Poor judgment
Impaired sphincter control
Focal motor seizures
Headaches

TEMPORAL LOBE

Recent memory loss
Visual phenomenon: "déjà vu"
Auditory disturbances: "auditory agnosia"
Psychomotor seizure
Olfactory or gustatory hallucinations
Sensory aphasia

OCCIPITAL LOBE

Visual disturbances
 Central blindness
 Cortical blindness and anosognosia
 Visual hallucinations

CEREBELLUM

Uncoordination: ataxia
Loss of equilibrium
Nausea, vomiting
Vertigo

PARIETAL LOBE

Sensory loss/agnosia
Apraxia
Body perceptional disorders

According to type

GLIOMAS (ASTROCYTOMAS)

Occurring in cerebral hemispheres
Headache
Vomiting
Personality changes; irritable, apathetic

ACOUSTIC NEUROMAS

Vertigo
Ataxia
Parasthesia and weakness of face (cranial nerves V, VII)
Loss of corneal reflex
Decreased sensitivity to touch or pain (cranial nerves V, XI)
Unilateral hearing loss

MENINGIOMAS

Seizures
Unilateral exophthalmos
Extraocular muscle palsy
Visual disturbances
Olfactory disturbances
Paresis

PITUITARY ADENOMAS

Acromegaly
Hypopituitarism: decreased thyroid, pancreatic, and gonadal function
Cushing's syndrome
Female: amenorrhea, sterilization
Male: loss of libido, impotence
Visual disturbances
Diabetes mellitus
Hypothyroidism
Hypoadrenalism
Diabetes insipidus
Inappropriate antidiuretic hormone (IADH)

Diagnostic tests

Physical and neurologic examination
Visual fields examination
MRI
Skull x-ray examination
Lumbar puncture; CSF: elevated protein
EEG
Echoencephalography
CT scan
PET scan
Cerebral angiography
Serum glucose, prolactin levels
Chest x-rays

Potential complications

Herniation
Elevated BP
Seizure activity
Neurologic deficit: mild to severe
Increased ICP

Cerebral edema
Alteration in respiratory function
Hydrocephalus
Alteration in consciousness
Personality change

Collaborative management

Therapeutic management

Surgical excision
  Microsurgery
  Laser surgery
Medications
  Corticosteroids
  Anticonvulsants
  Antacids
  Laxatives
Radiation therapy
Chemotherapy
Fluid/electrolyte therapy
Oxygenation/ventilatory support
ICP monitoring
Neurologic rehabilitation

Nursing management

PATIENT PROBLEMS/NURSING DIAGNOSES

● **NDX:** Altered tissue perfusion: cerebral related to increased ICP secondary to tumor

Obtain and record baseline history of signs and symptoms, monitor for signs of progression
Assess LOC q2h to 4h and prn
Use Glasgow Coma Scale for rapid assessment (p. 560)
Assess quality and strength of facial muscles and extremities q4h to 5h
Monitor BP, P, and R and do neurologic check q2h to 4h and prn
Monitor for and intervene at signs of increasing ICP (p. 624)
Maintain seizure precautions
Maintain safe environment
  Use siderails with padding
  Use soft restraints
Maintain quiet environment
Check rectal T q2h to 4h; hypothermia or cooling measures may be indicated
Administer medications as ordered
Monitor for signs of mental and personality changes

EXPECTED OUTCOMES
Patient is alert and oriented
Demonstrates improved or normal cerebral tissue perfusion
Neurologic signs are within acceptable limits
No signs of ICP

● **NDX:** Self-care deficit: hygiene, feeding, toileting, and/or mobility related to perceptual, cognitive, and/or neurologic impairment

Assess for degree of disability in performing ADLs: bathing, feeding, toileting, and mobility
Monitor for signs of progressive disability
Assist with daily physical hygiene care as indicated
  Administer oral hygiene prn *to prevent infection*
  Administer skin care *to minimize potential for decubitus ulcer formation*
Familiarize patient with surroundings *to decrease anxiety if eyesight and/or visual fields are impaired*
Ensure elimination
  Use external or indwelling catheter as indicated
  Initiate voiding measures prn
  Have patient avoid constipation and straining through use of stool softeners or mild laxatives
Maintain diet as ordered to maintain nutritional status
Feed and assist with nutritional intake as needed
Ambulate as tolerated; assist as necessary with wheelchair, walker, or cane
If patient is unable to ambulate, assist and teach patient to turn, cough, and deep breathe q2h and prn
Elevate head of bed 30 to 45 degrees
Perform active and passive ROM exercises to all extremities q4h to 5h *to prevent fixed joints*

EXPECTED OUTCOMES
Patients self care needs are met

● **NDX:** Anxiety related to actual or perceived biologic or psychologic threat

Assess for signs and symptoms of fear and anxiety, noting verbal and nonverbal expressions
Explore feelings, encouraging patient to discuss fears and concerns regarding diagnosis and prescribed therapies
Provide emotional support
Offer simple explanations to questions
Assist patient to deal with anxiety, providing alternate methods for dealing with stress: guided imagery, relaxation techniques

EXPECTED OUTCOMES

Anxiety level is reduced
Patient appears calm and is able to verbalize feelings
and concerns

ADDITIONAL NURSING DIAGNOSES
TO CONSIDER

Pain (headache)
Impaired verbal communication
Risk for injury secondary to seizure activity

Patient/family teaching

Assess level of understanding regarding disease
process and prescribed treatments
Reinforce physician's explanation of the disease and its
causes, symptoms, and treatment
Encourage questions; assess for any misconceptions
Discuss medications: name, dosage, frequency of ad-
ministration, purpose, side effects, and toxic effects
Explain need to avoid taking over-the-counter medica-
tions without consulting physician
Teach importance of well-balanced diet
Explain need for ongoing rehabilitation therapy as
ordered

Home care considerations

Activity
  Stress the importance and proper use of mobility devices (wheelchair, cane, walker) to patient/family
  Assist family to identify local community agencies
  that can help in providing such devices
  Assist family to learn ways of adapting the home for
  accessibility
  Stress the need for initial home health referral to do
  the following:
    Teach family members proper body mechanics and
    how to protect their backs
    Assist in learning safety measures to prevent falling
  Alert the patient to change positions slowly to prevent
  postural changes in BP
  Maintain a regular exercise program with planned
  rest periods
  Implement safety measures such as siderails and
  ramps as indicated
Diet
  Maintain well-balanced diet
    Offer small portions; instruct patient to chew slowly
    Offer supplemental feedings
  Monitor intake and output
General instructions
  Encourage independent activities to tolerance
  Encourage socialization with friends and family
  members

Develop competence of family members, as indicated,
in the following:
  Home ventilation
  Suctioning
  Tracheostomy care
  Chest physiotherapy
  Coughing and deep breathing exercises
  Home parenteral or enteral nutrition therapy
  Bowel/bladder management
Refer to home health agencies as indicated
Develop knowledge base regarding signs and symp-
toms of seizure activity
Implement seizure precautions as indicated
Report potential signs and symptoms of increasing
ICP including the following:
  Restlessness, lethargy
  Changes in level of consciousness
  Nausea and vomiting (may be projectile)
  Pupillary changes
  Changes in vital signs
  Seizures
  Changes in breathing patterns

Craniocerebral Trauma

*Any sudden impact or blow to the head with or without
loss of consciousness; the following are types of head
injuries*
linear fracture: *A break in the continuity of bone
without displacing bone tissue*
comminuted fracture: *Multiple breaks leading to
fragmentation of bone*
depressed fracture: *Bone fragments displaced below
the surface of the skull*
compound fracture: *A fracture complicated by
laceration of surrounding scalp or membranes*
concussion: *Shock to brain soft tissue without bruising
or lacerations; accompanied by temporary memory
loss and amnesia lasting approximately 48 hr*
contusion: *Shock to brain soft tissue with bruising and
laceration; accompanied by loss of consciousness and
amnesia; patient may exhibit varying degrees of
consciousness: stupor, agitation, disorientation, coma*
coup-contrecoup phenomenon: *Brain injury
resulting from acceleration type of injury causing
contusion and laceration in areas remote or opposite
from the site of impact (Figure 9-14)*
subdural hematoma: *An accumulation of blood
between the arachnoid and dura mater resulting from
contusion or laceration of subdural blood vessels;
symptoms (headaches, increasing drowsiness, seizures,
unilateral pupil dilation) may not occur for weeks or
months*

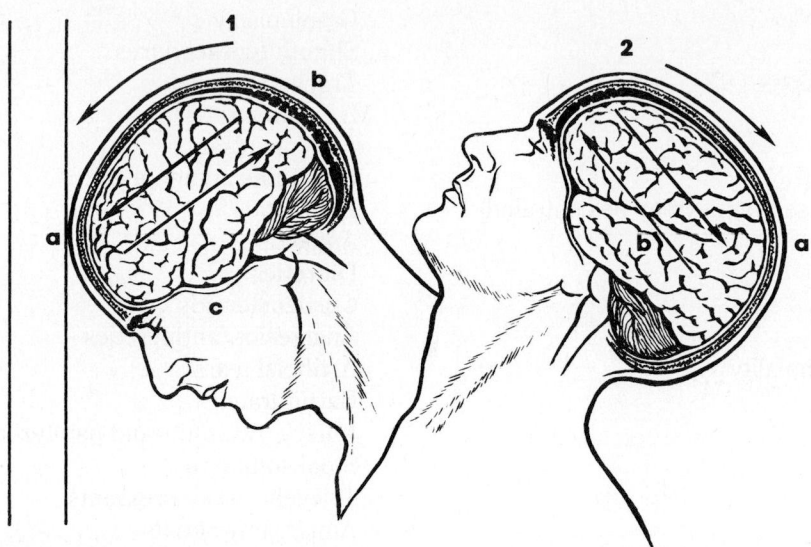

Figure 9-14 Coup and contrecoup head injury following blunt trauma. *1,* Coup injury: impact against object. *a,* Site of impact and direct trauma to brain. *b,* Shearing of subdural veins. *c,* Trauma to base of brain. *2,* Contrecoup injury: impact within skull. *a,* Site of impact from brain hitting opposite side of skull. *b,* Shearing forces through brain. These injuries occur in one continuous motion—the head strikes the wall (coup), then rebounds (contrecoup). (From Rudy EB: *Advanced neurological and neurosurgical nursing,* St Louis, 1984, Mosby.)

epidural hematoma: Bleeding in the epidural space between the skull and dura mater; usually involves a temporoparietal fracture, which results in a lacerated middle meningeal artery; transient loss of consciousness occurs and is followed by lucid periods; patient then lapses into unconsciousness again with signs of rapidly developing increased ICP; this is usually a surgical emergency

Assessment

Subjective data
Headache
Dizziness, vertigo

Objective data
Altered LOC; periods of consciousness followed by
  unconsciousness
Posturing
  Decorticate rigidity (see Figure 9-9)
  Decerebrate rigidity
  Motor and/or sensory movement of extremities: uni-
    lateral, bilateral
  Weakness, paresis, paralysis, stimulus, response
Mental changes
  Irritability

Restlessness
Confusion
Delirium
Stupor
Coma
Pupillary response
  Size, equality, response to light
  Corneal reflex
Brainstem integrity: EOM (extraocular movement),
  gag or swallow reflex
Airway patency
  Rate and rhythm of respirations
  Breathing pattern
  Secretion management
Unequal pupils and uncoordinated eye movement
Periocular edema, ecchymosis
Seizure activity
Hematemesis
Projectile vomiting
Lacerations and abrasions around head and face
Drainage from ears and nose
Elevated temperature
Elevated or decreased BP
Increased weakness
Facial asymmetry
Aphasia
Nuchal rigidity
Dehydration
Polyuria
Bruit over carotid artery

Diagnostic tests

Skull x-ray examinations
Cervical x-ray examinations
Chest x-rays
CT scan
MRI
Lumbar puncture; CSF sampling (may be contraindi-
  cated in ICP)
Pneumoencephalogram
Cisternogram
ABGs (serial)
Serum electrolytes, osmolality
CBC
EEG
Echoencephalogram
Urine osmolality

Potential complications

Increased ICP
Secondary head injury
Hemorrhage
Brain herniation
Aspiration
Respiratory failure: pneumonia
Neurologic deficit: mild to severe
  Paresis
  Paralysis
Extracranial dissection
Focal neurologic deficits
Neurogenic pulmonary edema
Cardiac dysrhythmias
Diabetes insipidus
Disseminated intravascular coagulopathy (DIC)
Syndrome of inappropriate secretion of antidiuretic hor-
  mone (SIADH)
Hydrocephalus
Hypertension/hypotension
Cerebral vasospasms
Hypopituitarism
Gastrointestinal (GI) hemorrhage
Contractures
Impaired nutritional status

Collaborative management

Therapeutic management

Respiratory management
Oxygenation/mechanical ventilation with volume venti-
  lation
Surgical repair
  Craniotomy
  Ventriculostomy

Cranioplasty
Shunting procedures
Tracheostomy
Medications
  Anticonvulsants
  Histamine antagonists
  Antibiotics
  Antacids
  Diuretics
  Corticosteroids
  Analgesics/antipyretics
  Artificial tears
  Barbiturates
  Muscle relaxants and paralyzers
  Stool softeners
  Tricyclic antidepressants
  Antianxiety agents
  Antihistamines
ICP monitoring
Cardiac monitoring/hemodynamic
Fluid and electrolyte management monitoring
Nutritional support
Physical therapy
Rehabilitation
Temperature control
Barbiturate coma therapy

Nursing management

PATIENT PROBLEMS/NURSING DIAGNOSES

● **NDX:** Altered tissue perfusion: cerebral related
to increased ICP secondary to acute head
injury

Assess neurologic status q15min to 30min as indicated;
  establish baseline parameters
Monitor and record signs of improvement or deteriora-
  tion: change in LOC; seizure activity
Assess for signs of increased ICP (p. 624)
Check BP, P, and R q15min to 30min, decreasing fre-
  quency as condition stabilizes
Initiate ICP monitoring as ordered; report increase of
  >15 mm Hg lasting 15 to 30 min
Elevate head of bed 30 degrees; maintain head in mid-
  line position *to promote venous drainage*
Maintain quiet environment
Avoid or minimize activities known to precipitate Val-
  salva maneuvers (e.g., prolonged suctioning)
Administer medications as ordered
Maintain normothermia
Monitor serial ABGs
Maintain strict intake and output *to monitor hydration*
  status; monitor specific gravity and color of urinary
  output

EXPECTED OUTCOMES

Patient is oriented to time, place, situation
Demonstrates no signs of increased ICP
No alteration in LOC
ICP of ≤15 mm Hg
No clinical signs of increased ICP

● **NDX:** Ineffective airway clearance related to impaired neurologic function

Avoid flexion of neck until cervical x-rays rule out neck injury
Assess and monitor respiratory function and secretions q30min to 60min
Maintain patent airway: endotracheal tube or tracheostomy as ordered; suction prn (hyperoxygenate with 100% O_2 for 60 sec before and after suctioning; suction <15 sec)
Monitor oxygen saturations *to ensure adequate oxygenation*
Position head *to prevent obstruction of airway and provide optimal secretion removal;* maintain neck in neutral position
Administer oxygen, humidification, or mechanical ventilation as ordered *to decrease work of breathing*
Auscultate lungs q2h to 4h *to detect adventitious breath sounds*
Obtain and monitor serial ABGs; maintain $PaCO_2$ as ordered *to prevent hypoxia and hypercapnia*
Assist in coughing and deep breathing when patient is conscious *to prevent atelectasis*
Maintain emergency needs at bedside
Elevate head of bed 30 degrees if patient is unconscious, unless contraindicated, *to maximize airway patency and control secretions*
Check BP, P, R, and Glasgow Coma Scale (p. 560) q15min to 30min; report any pupillary or mental changes immediately: changes may signal respiratory embarrassment
Maintain NPO status to prevent aspiration

EXPECTED OUTCOMES

Demonstrates effective breathing pattern
Clear breath sounds
ABGs and vital signs within normal limits
No sign of respiratory distress

● **NDX:** Sensory/perceptual alteration: cognitive, visual, auditory, kinesthetic related to neurologic trauma

Assess LOC, orientation, mood/affect, and thought process; monitor and record changes
Assess for any sensory deficits: responses to pain, touch; changes in vision including blurred vision, changes in visual field, depth and perception
Assess and monitor motor coordination, ability to locate body parts
Orient to reality: environment, situation, individuals interacting with patient *to decrease uncertainty*
Interpret sights, sounds, smells in environment *to prevent sensory overload*
Speak in calm voice with normal tone
Maintain eye contact
Provide meaningful stimuli: clocks, calendars
Place patient near window *to differentiate day and night*
Structure daily activities and routines
Place common and familiar object within field of vision *to assist in reality orientation*
Maintain safety precautions
  Bed in low position, siderail up *to prevent injury and falls*
  Assist with ambulation
  Remove potentially dangerous objects
Encourage decision making, exploration of environment to enhance competence and feelings of self-worth

EXPECTED OUTCOME

Patient demonstrates improved LOC, appropriate perceptual functioning

● **NDX:** Self-esteem/body image disturbance related to perceived changes in physical and personal self-image

Assess perception of body image and relate to degree of disability
Provide emotional support; allow patient to verbalize needs and participate in planning care
Encourage verbalization of feelings about body image and functional changes
Acknowledge and praise attempts to improve body image (e.g., wearing make-up, selecting clothing)
Assist patient to accept physical disability; assist patient to identify other physical characteristics that remain unchanged
Offer supportive counseling
Encourage participation in counseling and/or self-help group

EXPECTED OUTCOMES

Verbalizes positive expression of body image
Demonstrates signs of decreasing body image disturbance

ADDITIONAL NURSING DIAGNOSES
TO CONSIDER

Impaired physical mobility related to neurophysiologic function (see Cerebrovascular accident, p. 578)

Risk for unilateral neglect related to right cerebral hemisphere lesions secondary to neurologic trauma (see Cerebrovascular accident, p. 578)

Patient/family teaching

Discuss nature of disorder, treatment, and procedures; explain as they occur

Explain to family need to encourage verbalization about any body image change or limitations

Explain need to ambulate as tolerated

Teach about importance of planned rest periods

Discuss possible residual effects such as dizziness, headache, and memory loss, which may persist for 3 to 4 months after trauma

Discuss medications: name, dosage, frequency of administration, purpose, side effects, and toxic effects

Explain need to avoid taking over-the-counter medications without physician approval

Discuss symptoms of progression of condition to report to physician

Explain importance of ongoing outpatient care
Physician's visits
Physical therapy

Explain importance of diet as ordered; need to chew and swallow slowly

Discuss care of abrasions or lacerations as indicated

Home care considerations

Activity
Stress the importance and proper use of mobility devices (wheelchair, cane, walker) to patient/family
Assist family to identify local community agencies that can help in providing such devices
Assist family to learn ways of adapting the home for accessibility
Stress the need for initial home health referral to the following:
Teach family members proper body mechanics and how to protect their backs
Assist in learning safety measures to prevent falling
Alert the patient to change positions slowly to prevent postural changes in BP
Implement safety measures such as siderails and ramps as indicated
Maintain as much independence in ADLs as possible
Maintain a regular exercise program with planned rest periods
Refer to home physical therapy as indicated
Maintain socialization activities with friends and family
Diet
Maintain well-balanced diet

Maintain fluid intake of 2000 ml/day unless contraindicated
Maintain intake and output
Avoid use of alcohol
General instructions
Check stools for occult blood if patient takes corticosteroids
Report any seizure activity; maintain seizure precautions as appropriate
Report signs and symptoms of increasing ICP (see list in home care considerations for Intracranial tumors, p. 583)

Spinal Cord Injuries

cord injuries: Injuries in which the spinal cord is compressed by fractured or displaced vertebrae, bleeding, or edema
cervical cord injuries: Level of injury is located in the cervical spine C-2 to C-6
thoracic cord injuries: Level of injury is located in the thoracic spine T-1 to T-12
lumbar cord injuries: Level of injury is located in the lumbar spine L-1 to L-2
NOTE: Clinical descriptions of spinal cord injuries generally refer to deficits in terms of upper motor neuron (UMN) and lower motor neuron (LMN): UMN injuries involve the corticobulbar or corticospinal tract and result in muscle spasticity and increased tendon reflexes; LMN injuries involve anterior horn cells or nerve fibers after their exit from the spinal cord and result in muscle flaccidity, loss of reflexes, loss of tone, and muscle atrophy (Figures 9-15 and 9-16; Table 9-8)

Assessment

Observations/findings

CORD INJURIES

Loss of power, movement, and sensation of extremities below level of injury
Pain at level of injury
Urinary retention
Priapism
Absence of vasomotor tone and perspiration in cervical and upper thoracic cord injuries

CERVICAL CORD INJURIES

Paralysis of all extremities and trunk
Respiratory failure: hypoxemia
Bladder and bowel disturbances
Bladder retention, spasticity
Bowel incontinence

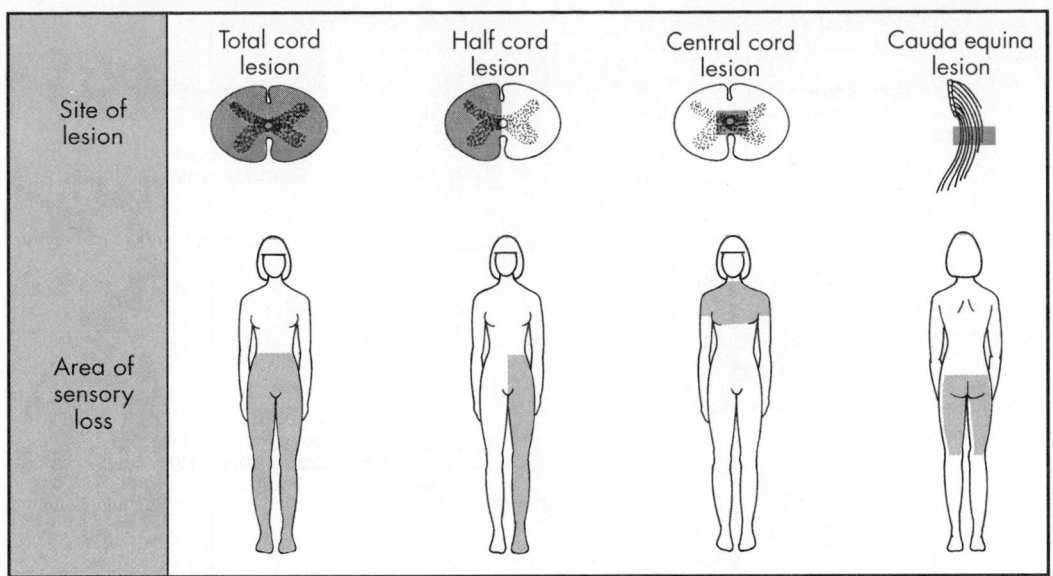

Figure 9-15 Common patterns of sensory abnormality. *Upper diagrams,* site of lesion; *lower diagrams,* distribution of corresponding sensory loss. (From Thelan LA et al: *Critical care nursing: diagnosis and management,* ed 2, St Louis, 1994, Mosby.)

Table 9-8 Clinical Manifestations of Upper and Lower Motor Neuron Lesions

Upper Motor Neuron	Lower Motor Neuron
Muscle spasticity, possible contractures	Muscle flaccidity
Little or no muscle atrophy	Muscle atrophy
Hyperreflexia	Loss of muscle tone
	Hyporeflexia or areflexia
	Fasciculations
Damage above level of brainstem will affect opposite side of the body	Muscle changes will be in muscles supplied by that nerve—usually muscle on same side as lesion

From Rudy EB: *Advanced neurological and neurosurgical nursing,* St Louis, 1984, Mosby.

Autonomic dysreflexia (Figure 9-16, B)
  Bradycardia
  Sweating above level of injury
  Elevated T
  Paroxysmal hypertension
  Headache
  Neurogenic shock

THORACIC CORD INJURIES

Paralysis of lower extremities; initially muscles are flaccid, later become spastic

Paralysis of bladder, bowel, and sphincters
Pain to chest or back
Abdominal distention
Loss of sexual function

LUMBAR CORD INJURIES

Paralysis of lower extremities, bladder, and rectum
  Flaccid muscles during spinal shock phase
  Spastic muscular activity
Loss of sexual function

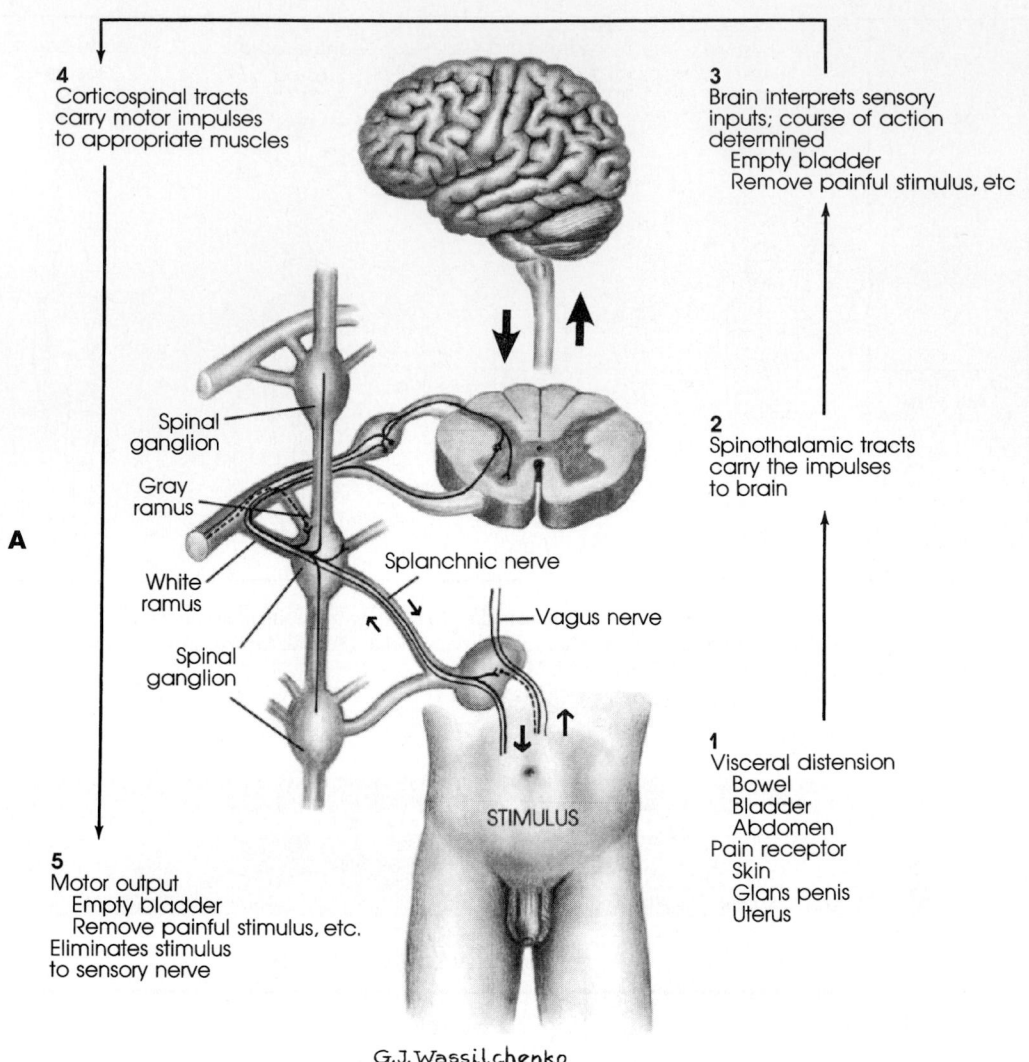

4
Corticospinal tracts
carry motor impulses
to appropriate muscles

3
Brain interprets sensory
inputs; course of action
determined
    Empty bladder
    Remove painful stimulus, etc

Spinal
ganglion

Gray
ramus

A

White
ramus

Spinal
ganglion

Splanchnic nerve

Vagus nerve

2
Spinothalamic tracts
carry the impulses
to brain

STIMULUS

1
Visceral distension
    Bowel
    Bladder
    Abdomen
Pain receptor
    Skin
    Glans penis
    Uterus

5
Motor output
    Empty bladder
    Remove painful stimulus, etc.
Eliminates stimulus
to sensory nerve

G.J.Wassilchenko

Figure 9-16 A, Normal response pathway.

Diagnostic tests

X-ray examination: vertebral fractures
CT scan
MRI
Serial ABGs
CBC with differential
Electrolytes
Myelography

Potential complications

Respiratory arrest: hypoxia
Pneumonia
Atelectasis
Spinal shock
  Complete transection

Flaccid paralysis below level of injury
Loss of reflexes below level of injury
Loss of proprioception, sensations of touch, T, and
    pressure below level of injury
  Orthostatic hypotension
Paralytic ileus
Loss of somatic and visceral sensations
Loss of ability to perspire below level of injury
Decreased BP
Urinary retention
Bowel dysfunction
Possible priapism
Bladder dysfunction
Fecal incontinence
Urinary tract infection
Autonomic dysreflexia
Sexual dysfunction

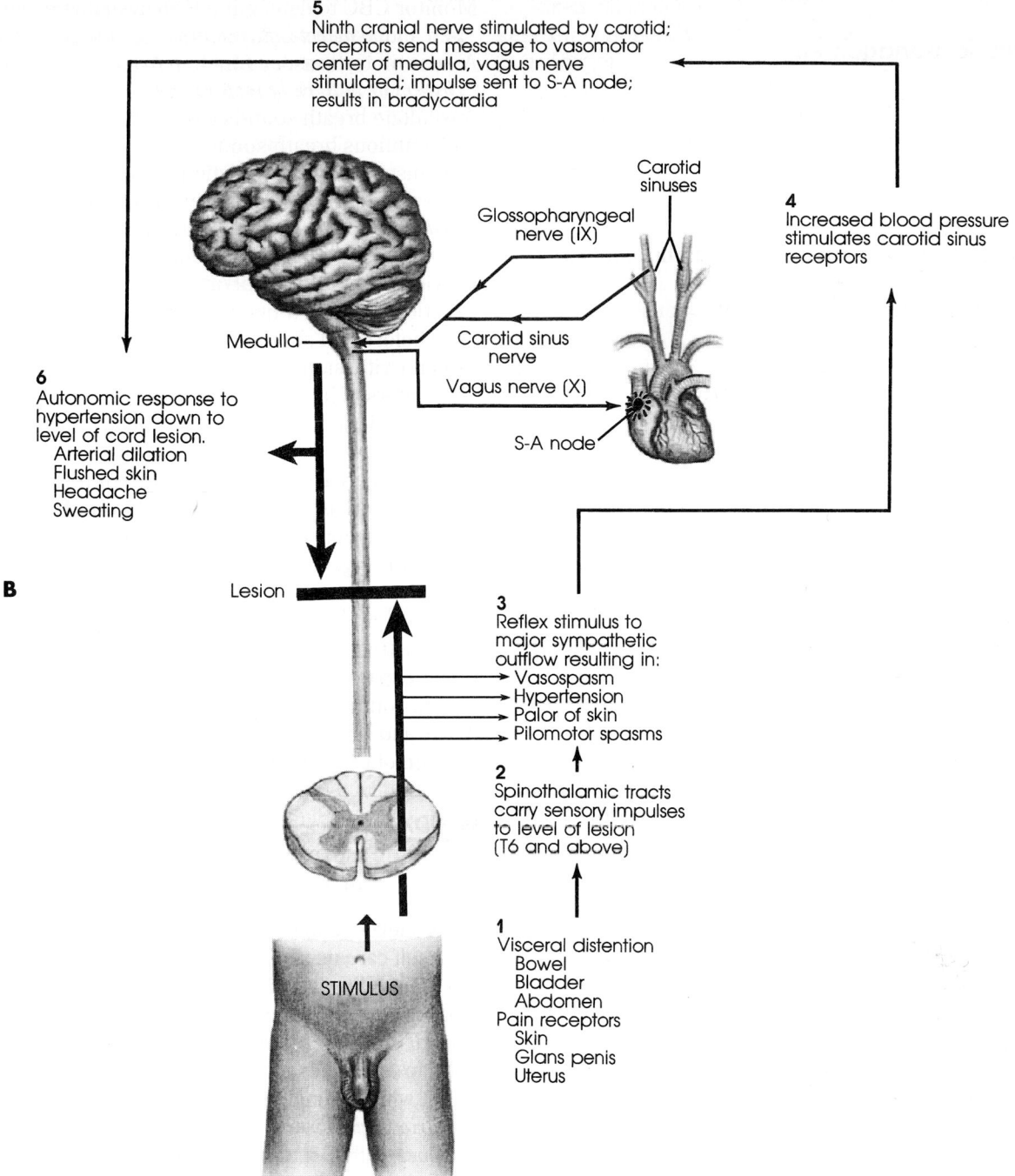

5
Ninth cranial nerve stimulated by carotid; receptors send message to vasomotor center of medulla, vagus nerve stimulated; impulse sent to S-A node; results in bradycardia

Carotid sinuses

Glossopharyngeal nerve (IX)

4
Increased blood pressure stimulates carotid sinus receptors

Medulla

Carotid sinus nerve

Vagus nerve (X)

6
Autonomic response to hypertension down to level of cord lesion.
　Arterial dilation
　Flushed skin
　Headache
　Sweating

S-A node

B

Lesion

3
Reflex stimulus to major sympathetic outflow resulting in:
→ Vasospasm
→ Hypertension
→ Palor of skin
→ Pilomotor spasms

2
Spinothalamic tracts carry sensory impulses to level of lesion (T6 and above)

1
Visceral distention
　Bowel
　Bladder
　Abdomen
Pain receptors
　Skin
　Glans penis
　Uterus

STIMULUS

Figure 9-16 cont'd.　B, Autonomic dysreflexia pathway. (From Rudy EB: *Advanced neurological and neurosurgical nursing,* St Louis, 1984, Mosby.)

Malnutrition: acute or chronic
Decubitus
Contractures, ankylosis
Spasms
Foot-drop, wrist-drop
Behavioral changes
　Anxiety

Grief reaction
　Acute depression
Heterotopic ossification
Severe bradyrhythmia
Deep vein thrombosis
Osteoporosis
Superior mesentoxic artery syndrome

Home care considerations

Activities
  Institute safety measures such as removing or nailing
    down area rugs to prevent falling
  Stress the importance and proper use of mobility
    devices (wheelchair, cane, walker) to patient/
    family
    Assist family to identify local community agencies
      that can help in providing such devices
    Assist family to learn ways of adapting the home for
      accessibility
    Stress the need for initial home health referral to do
      the following:
      Teach family members proper body mechanics and
        how to protect their backs
      Assist in learning safety measures to prevent falling
  Maintain quiet environment, reducing environmen-
    tal stimuli to minimum if patient is confused or agi-
    tated
  Assist with reality orientation as indicated
  Refer to home care services for potential in-home as-
    sistance
  Remove or disconnect door locks
  Avoid potentially dangerous tasks such as cooking or
    smoking
  Assist with daily hygiene as needed
  Maintain regular exercise program with planned rest
    periods
Diet
  Provide high-protein, low-calcium diet
  Encourage fluid intake to 2000 ml/day unless con-
    traindicated
  Assist in cutting food as needed
  Present one course of diet at a time (i.e., salad, then
    entrée)
  Establish routine voiding measures
  Establish regular bowel habits
  Avoid giving fluids before bedtime
  Monitor intake and output
General instructions
  Provide instructions on reporting any seizure activity
  Discuss need to maintain seizure precautions
  Provide skin care
  Encourage focus on remaining strengths and intact
    roles
  Encourage a sense of control
  Facilitate expression of emotions

Parkinson's Disease (Paralysis Agitans)

A progressive, degenerative disease of the brain's
  dopamine neuronal system, most commonly idiopathic
  in nature

Assessment

Objective data

Rigidity of limbs: arms lose natural swing and remain at
  side of body
Tremors
  Exaggerated by stress and anxiety
  Most severe when limb is resting; absent during sleep
  Fingers: pill-rolling movement
  Head: to-and-fro tremor
Movements
  Voluntary body movements become slower (brady-
    kinesia)
  Starting activities becomes difficult (akinesia)
Posture (Figure 9-17)
  Bent forward, head bowed
  Walking with slow, short, shuffling steps (festination)
  Breaking into run if pushed
  Propulsion
  Retropulsion
Uncoordinated and/or loss of muscular activity: im-
  paired writing (micrographia)
Blank facial expression (masked facies)
  Wide-eyed
  Infrequent blinking of eyes
Speech
  Slowed, soft, monotonous
  Dysarthric
  Slurred
Dysphagia
Excessive salivation and drooling
Emotional changes
  Generalized apathy
  Depression
  Nervousness
  Mood swings
  Social withdrawal
  Hallucinations
  Paranoia
  Dementia
Side effects of drugs
Autonomic manifestations
  Urinary incontinence
  Constipation
  Autostatic hypotension

Diagnostic tests

CSF
  Usually WNL
  May show slight increase in protein level
CT scan: normal results or may show cerebral atrophy
Mild microcytic anemia
GI studies
  Hypomotility
  Delayed emptying of stomach

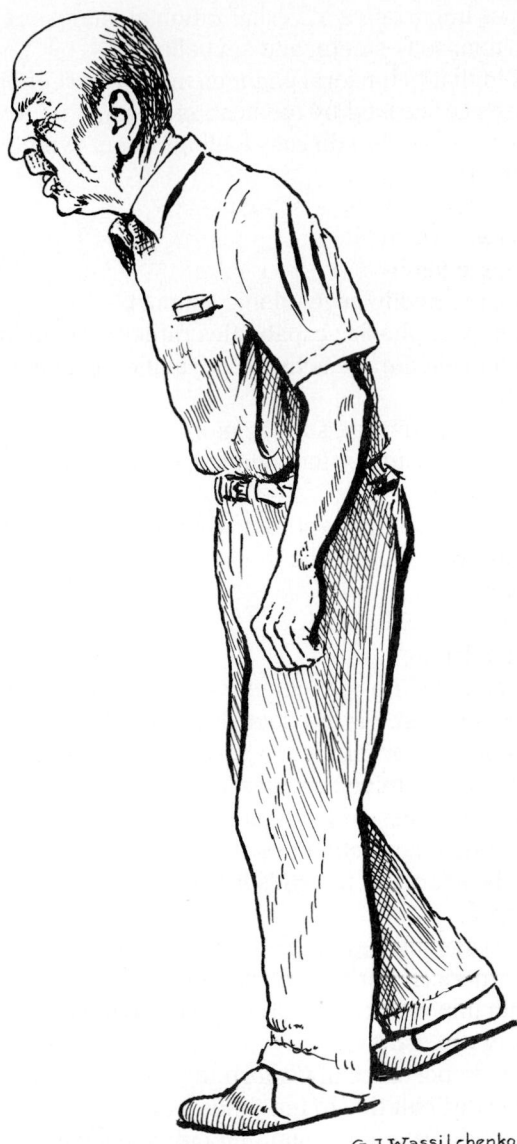

Figure 9-17 Posture and shuffling gait associated with Parkinson's disease. (From Rudy EB: *Advanced neurological and neurosurgical nursing,* St Louis, 1984, Mosby.)

Varying degrees of bowel distention
EEG
  Normal with minimal slowing
  Marked or moderate slowing and/or disorganization (with marked dementia or bradykinesia)
Skull x-rays
Cineradiographic study of swallowing

Collaborative management

Therapeutic management

Surgical stereotactic thalamotomy to relieve contra-lateral tremor and rigidity: neurotransplants

Medications
  Levodopa
  Carbidopa (Sinemet)
  Anticholinergics
    Benztropine mesylate (Cogentin)
    Trihexyphenidyl (Artane)
  Antiparkinsonian and antihistamine: orphenadrine hy-drochloride (Benadryl)
  Amantadine hydrochloride (Symmetrel)
  Ethopropazine hydrochloride (Parsidol)
  Nutritional therapy
  Physical therapy
  Occupational therapy
  Speech therapy

Nursing management

PATIENT PROBLEMS/NURSING DIAGNOSES

● **NDX:** Impaired physical mobility related to neuro-logic degenerative disorder

Assess level of disability
Encourage ambulation to tolerance *to improve mobility*
Assist to chair
Perform active or passive ROM exercises q4h to all ex-tremities *to increase muscle mass, tone, and strength*
  Neck
  Hands and fingers
  Wrists
  Elbows
  Knees
Evaluate effectiveness of drug therapy
Initiate gait-retraining program; consult with physical therapy department to increase ambulation
Provide physical therapy as ordered: massage and stretching exercises
Have patient practice lifting legs while walking rather than shuffling; try to maintain erect position
Maintain planned rest periods
Conduct occupational therapy as indicated by amount of tremors
Assist patient with turning q2h to 4h if unable to move self

EXPECTED OUTCOME

Patient demonstrates optimal level of mobility appropri-ate for physical disability

● **NDX:** Self-care deficit: feeding, hygiene

Assess functional disability related to self-care needs
Assess nutritional needs; consult with dietitian
Maintain well-balanced, soft diet
Avoid foods and medications that contain pyridoxine hydrochloride (vitamin B$_6$)

Maintain frequent, small feedings as indicated
Maintain fluid intake to 2000 ml/day unless contraindicated *to maintain adequate hydration*
Maintain supplemental high-calorie fluids such as eggnog, milk shakes, and malts
Use bibs and straws as indicated; place food and drinks within easy reach of patient
Initiate voiding measures as necessary
Institute bladder control program as indicated
Have patient avoid constipation through use of high-residue foods, stool softeners, and/or enemas
Provide or assist with general hygiene as indicated
Administer oral hygiene q4h to 6h and prn
Encourage self-care as tolerated: bathing, mouth care

EXPECTED OUTCOMES

Self-care needs are met
Demonstrates optimal nutritional intake
Demonstrates skin integrity

● **NDX:** Self-esteem disturbance related to actual or perceived changes in physical and personal self-image

Provide emotional support; allow patient to verbalize needs and participate in planning care *to foster feelings of self-worth*
Encourage verbalization of feelings about body image and functional changes
Acknowledge and support attempts to improve appearance
Permit expression of emotions
Encourage use of support groups

EXPECTED OUTCOMES

Experiences self-respect and self-confidence
Achieves goals that reflect awareness of abilities and limitations
Acknowledges and supports attempts to improve appearance
Permits expression of emotions
Uses support groups

ADDITIONAL NURSING DIAGNOSES TO CONSIDER

Impaired verbal communication
Risk for injury
Social isolation

Patient/family teaching

Assess level of understanding regarding disease and treatments prescribed
Reinforce physician's explanation of disease and its causes, symptoms, and treatment

Discuss importance of verbalization about loss of body function, self-esteem, and sexuality
Explain that behavioral changes may be part of disease process or caused by medications
Emphasize need to discuss feelings about symptoms
  Tremors
  Drooling
  Slurred speech
Explain to family
  Need to provide psychologic support
  Need to emphasize capabilities rather than limitations
  Need to encourage active participation in family activities
  Need to encourage socialization
  Need to encourage independence; avoid over-protection
  Need to permit patient to do things for self
    Self-care
    Feedings
    Dressing
    Ambulation
Explain that although patient may be physically disabled, he or she is intellectually normal
Discuss need for family to show security, love, need for patient, and patience with and understanding of patient's slowness and clumsiness
Explain that frustration over tremors and dependence may be source of patient's irritability and loss of self-interest
Discuss agencies available for use as resources such as the American Parkinson Disease Association*
Explain importance of daily exercise to delay progression of disease
Explain importance of performing any physical task that is difficult five to ten times a day
Explain importance of ongoing outpatient care
  Physician's visits
  Physical therapy
Discuss medications: name, dosage, frequency of administration, purpose, side effects, and toxic effects
Explain need to avoid taking over-the-counter medications without physician approval
Encourage patient to participate in activities to decrease attention on symptoms
  Reading
  Watching television
  Listening to radio
  Engaging in hobbies
  Painting
Prevent falls and injuries by clearing walkways of furniture and scatter rugs; build siderails on stairs and in tub or shower

---

*American Parkinson Disease Association, 116 John St., New York, NY 10038; National Parkinson's Foundation Hotline: 1-800-327-4545.

Provide supports as indicated when patient is ambulating with walker or cane

Provide speech therapy

Instruct patient to speak slowly and practice reading aloud slowly in an exaggerated manner

Provide electronic amplifiers as ordered for weak voice

Explain need for oral hygiene q2h to 4h and prn to control drooling

Have tissues easily accessible to patient (e.g., in pockets)

Have patient use bib while eating

Clean corners of mouth after eating and prn

Apply ointment if necessary

Explain importance of proper elimination

Conduct voiding measures as necessary

Conduct bladder control program as necessary

Provide raised toilet seat with siderails in home to facilitate sitting and standing

Home care considerations

Activity

Explain need for activity

Plan rest periods

Perform passive or active ROM exercises to all extremities

Encourage family or significant other(s) to participate in physical therapy exercise of stretching and massaging muscles

Give warm baths

Encourage daily ambulation outdoors except during extremely hot or cold weather

Encourage patient to practice lifting feet, using heel-toe gait, and swinging arms deliberately while walking

Place head of bed or back of chair on blocks to facilitate getting out of bed or chair; use pulleys such as sheets tied to end of bed

Have patient avoid sitting for long periods

Encourage patient to dress daily

Avoid clothing with buttons; use zippers instead

Avoid shoes with laces or small buckles

Provide diversional activities depending on extent of tumors or disability

Apply splints and braces as indicated

Diet

Explain need for well-balanced, soft diet; limit high-protein food, which may block effects of drugs

Cut foods for patient

Place all utensils within easy reach

Use blender for thick foods

Use braces for severe tremors occurring during meals

Maintain fluid intake to 2000 ml/day unless contraindicated

Serve frequent, small meals

Serve supplemental high-calorie fluids such as eggs and milk shakes

Use straws and bibs for excessive drooling

Avoid food high in vitamin B_6 (reverses effects of levodopa)

Instruct patient to swallow slowly and take small bites of food

Maintain intake and output

General instructions

Focus on strengths and intact roles

Reorient to time, person, and place as needed

Protect patient privacy

Monitor urinary and bowel habits

Multiple Sclerosis (Disseminated Sclerosis)

A chronic, progressive disease characterized by scattering of demyelinating lesions in the central nervous system (CNS), which affect the white matter of the brain and spinal cord

Assessment

Subjective data

Fatigue: may be increased by heat (e.g., hot bath or shower)

Sensory impairment

Numbness

Tingling

Loss of position sense: staggering gait

Weakness of extremities: facial palsy

Hyperactive reflexes

Decreased to absent superficial reflexes

Poor coordination

Ataxia

Spasticity of extremities

Tremors

Staggering gait

Dizziness, vertigo

Visual disturbances

Diplopia

Blurred vision

Dilation of affected pupil when light is shone into eye (Marcus Gunn phenomenon)

Nystagmus

Optic neuritis

Speech impairment: scanning speech
Muscular spasms
Positive Babinski sign
Weakness of throat muscles: difficulty in chewing and
  swallowing
Impotence
Fecal and/or urinary incontinence or retention
Mental changes
  Mood swings
  Depression
  Euphoria
  Irritability
  Apathy
  Inattention
  Lack of judgment
  Memory deficits

Diagnostic tests

CSF
  Usually normal
  Normal with low protein
  Increased white blood cell count (WBC)
  Increased gamma globulin level
MRI
Myelography
CT scan
PET scan
Evoked responses

Potential complications

Neurologic deficit: paralysis, quadriplegia
Visual disturbances; blindness
Sexual dysfunction
Spastic bladder, urinary retention
Bowel dysfunction
Respiratory failure; pneumonia
Infection
Decubitus ulcers
Thrombus formation
Speech deficits
Dementia

Collaborative management

Therapeutic management

Medications
  Antiinflammatory agents
  ACTH
  Corticosteroids
  Muscle relaxants
  Immunosuppressive agents
  Vitamin B

Antidepressants
  Antianxiety drugs/tranquilizers
  β-adrenergic blocking agents
Physical therapy
Occupational therapy
Rehabilitation
Psychotherapy/counseling
Nutritional therapy
Bowel and bladder management

Nursing management

PATIENT PROBLEMS/NURSING DIAGNOSES

● **NDX:** Impaired physical mobility related to neuro-
           muscular impairment

Assess and monitor degree of physical disability
NOTE: Limit activity level when patient is unduly tired,
  during periods of exacerbation
Maintain quiet, relaxing, and cool environment
Institute activity
  Massage and stretch muscles *to increase circulation
    and joint mobility*
  Perform resistive exercises to all extremities and
    joints
  Perform active or passive ROM exercises q4h to 5h
    and prn
  Instruct patient to avoid exercising when tired and on
    hot days
  Encourage ambulation to tolerance
  Encourage self-care activities *to promote perception of
    positive body image*
  Avoid use of heating pad; measure bathwater T (heat
    reduces muscle strength)
  Plan all activities to prevent fatigue
  Plan rest periods *to minimize fatigue*
  Encourage diversional activities during periods of ex-
    acerbation
    Reading
    Watching television
    Listening to radio and/or book recordings
If patient is confined to bed rest
  Position comfortably
  Turn q2h to 4h and prn *to prevent skin breakdown*
  Perform active or passive ROM exercises q2h to 4h *to
    promote circulation and joint mobility*
  Perform dorsiflexion of ankles and quadriceps q2h to
    4h
Help patient out of bed and into chair two or three
  times daily if allowed
  Observe for signs of thrombophlebitis
  Use antiembolic stockings
  Administer anticoagulation therapy as ordered *to min-
    imize thrombus formation*

Feed as necessary; hand braces may be indicated

Administer skeletal muscle relaxants to reduce spasticity (NOTE: Use with caution—may exacerbate general weakness and decrease mobility)

EXPECTED OUTCOMES

Demonstrates improved or minimal degree of physical immobility

Participates in activities that promote improved function

Verbalizes understanding of conditions that may exacerbate symptoms

● **NDX:** Altered elimination: bowel and bladder related to neuromuscular impairment

Assess degree of functional disability

Initiate bladder program as indicated

  Assess bladder function and voiding pattern (urgency, frequency, incontinence, nocturia)

  Teach perineal (Kegel) exercise to improve tone of urinary sphincter

  Measure intake and output

  Catheterize intermittently as indicated

  Teach self-catheterization whenever possible

  Plan bladder dysfunction program as appropriate for spasticity or flaccidity

Institute bowel control program

  Establish regular bowel routines

  Prevent constipation

Maintain high-fiber diet

Encourage fluids to 3000 ml/day, unless contraindicated, to promote adequate hydration

EXPECTED OUTCOMES

Maintains bladder and bowel elimination

Has stable intake and output

Evidences no bladder distention

Has regular bowel evacuation pattern

Does not experience fecal impaction

● **NDX:** Activity intolerance related to generalized weakness secondary to neuromuscular disease

Assess energy level and ability to carry out activities

Assess sleep and rest patterns; determine when patient feels strongest

Schedule nursing care, procedures, and tests *to permit maximal periods of rest*

Plan periods of uninterrupted rest to facilitate REM sleep

Assist patient to plan activities at level of ability

Instruct patient to avoid activities when tired or on days that are hot *to minimize fatigue*

EXPECTED OUTCOMES

Demonstrates improved activity tolerance

Verbalizes understanding of activity allowance and limitations

Verbalizes understanding of need to balance activities and periods of rest

● **NDX:** Self-esteem disturbance related to altered perception of self

Assess patient's perception of illness and physical disabilities

Encourage questions and verbalization of feelings *to promote understanding and acceptance*

Provide accurate explanation of disease process

Acknowledge and permit discussion related to actual and perceived changes to facilitate normal grieving process

Acknowledge concerns about body image *to enhance healthy adjustment to body changes*

Be supportive of patient's emotional changes and needs for improving image and self-esteem

Encourage expression of emotion *to facilitate normal grieving process*

EXPECTED OUTCOMES

Patient experiences self-confidence and demonstrates beginning of adaptation to physical changes

● **NDX:** Ineffective airway clearance related to motor weakness and/or immobility

Assess respiration: rate, depth, and pattern; assess degree of respiratory effort and cough reflex

Monitor serial ABGs to determine acid-base balance

Suction oropharynx as needed to maintain patent airway

Assist and teach patient to cough and deep breathe q2h to 4h and prn to minimize risk for atelectasis

Maintain patent airway and avoid flexion of patient's neck if immobile

Monitor oxygen saturation *to control peripheral oxygenation*

Auscultate breath sounds q2h to 4h and prn *to detect adventitious breath sounds*

Position patient for maximal respiratory expansion and control of respiratory secretions

Administer oxygen as indicated *to improve gas exchange and decrease work of breathing*

EXPECTED OUTCOMES

Demonstrates effective breathing pattern

Chest expansion is symmetrical

Breath sounds are clear to auscultation

ABGs and vital signs are within normal limits

No signs of respiratory distress

ADDITIONAL NURSING DIAGNOSES
TO CONSIDER

Sensory/perceptual alterations: visual
Altered role performance
Ineffective individual coping

Patient/family teaching

Assess level of understanding regarding disease
process

Explain nature of disease, emphasizing that it is not
hereditary

Explain that warm weather and hot baths may increase
weakness

Explain importance of avoiding fatigue and becoming
overworked or emotionally stressed, which may be
precipitating factors in exacerbation

Explain importance of exercising regularly, need to
maintain rest periods

Explain need to do muscle stretching exercises daily

Explain need for ROM exercises for patient with spasticity

Explain importance of daily routines for activities and
rest periods

Discuss need for patient support when ambulating with
walker, cane, or braces as indicated

Instruct patient to walk with a wide base, keeping feet
apart

Emphasize importance of speech therapy; instruct patient to speak slowly and practice reading aloud

Emphasize need for diversional activities
  Reading
  Watching television
  Listening to radio
  Knitting
  Playing quiet games

Explain importance of decubitus care if patient is confined to bed rest or wheelchair

Explain importance of regulating bathwater T; need to
avoid extremes of hot and cold because of loss of
temperature-change sense

Discuss symptoms of disease progression to report to
physician

Explain importance of avoiding persons with infections,
especially URIs

Discuss symptoms of cold or influenza to report to
physician
  Elevated temperature
  Chills
  Cough
  Extreme fatigue

Encourage activity as long as patient is able
  Recreational activities
  Work
  Household chores

Encourage verbalization

Allow time for patient to complete all activities and
deal with any body image changes and loss of self-
esteem

Encourage socialization with friends and family

Encourage independence and self-care to point of
tolerance

EXPECTED OUTCOME

Patient and/or significant other demonstrates knowledge necessary for home maintenance management

Home care considerations

Activities

  Institute safety measures such as removing or nailing
  down area rugs to prevent falling

  Stress the importance and proper use of mobility devices (wheelchair, cane, walker) to patient/family

  Assist family to identify local community agencies
  that can help in providing such devices

  Assist family to learn ways of adapting the home for
  accessibility

  Stress the need for initial home health referral to do
  the following:
    Teach family members proper body mechanics and
    how to protect their backs
    Assist in learning safety measures to prevent falling

  Alert the patient to change positions slowly to prevent
  postural changes in BP

  Encourage diversional activities such as the following:
    Reading or listening to recorded books
    Watching TV
    Listening to stereo or radio

  Maintain regular exercise program with planned rest
  periods

  Encourage daily ambulation outdoors except during
  particularly hot or cold weather

  Support patient during ambulation if needed

  Assist to walk with a wide base

  Encourage patient to dress daily
    Avoid clothing with buttons if possible
    Avoid shoes with laces or small buckles

  Assist with daily hygiene as indicated

  Administer skin care on regular basis to stimulate circulation and prevent skin breakdown

  Home speech therapy should continue as appropriate

  Apply splints or braces to minimize tremors

  Avoid individuals with respiratory infections

Diet

  Maintain well-balanced diet
    Offer small portions
    Offer supplemental feedings
  Monitor intake and output
  Weigh on a weekly basis

Administer oral hygiene before and after meals
Monitor and maintain routine elimination program:
  bowel and urinary output
Maintain regular bowel evacuations
Acidify urine with cranberry or orange juice

Myasthenia Gravis

A neuromuscular disorder characterized by muscular
weakness and fatigue resulting from a defect in
transmission of motor impulses at the neuromuscular
junction; probably a result of an autoimmune response

Assessment

Objective data

Fatigue
Expressionless facies/facial droop
Generalized weakness
  Increased with exercise
  May be confined to one area
  Weakness of face, jaw, neck, arms, hands, and/or
    legs
Difficulty in raising arms above head or extending fin-
  gers outward
Dysphagia/drooling
Choking; aspiration
Impaired swallowing
Difficulty in chewing
Weak, high-pitched, soft voice
Ptosis of one or both eyelids
Ocular palsy
Diplopia
Inability to walk on heels; may walk on toes
Strength decreases as day progresses
Stress incontinence
Anal sphincter weakness
Respirations
  Shallow
  Decreased vital capacity (VC)
  Use of accessory muscles
  Muffled cough
Brisk reflexes

Diagnostic tests

CT scan of chest or chest x-ray examination indicating
  thymoma
Tensilon test (edrophonium chloride)
Single-fiber electromyogram
Nerve conduction studies
Antiacetylcholine receptor (ACLR) antibody test (Cu-
  rare test)

Potential complications

Myasthenia crisis
Cholinergic crisis
Neuromuscular deficit: mild to severe
Pneumonia
Aspiration, atelectasis
Respiratory failure
Sepsis

Collaborative management

Therapeutic management

Surgery
Plasmapheresis
Thymectomy
  Suprasternal approach
  Transsternal approach
Tracheostomy
Mechanical ventilation/oxygen therapy
Bronchoscopy
Physical therapy
Occupational therapy
Medications
  Anticholinesterase
  Corticosteroids
  Pituitary hormones
Nutritional support

Nursing management

PATIENT PROBLEMS/NURSING DIAGNOSES

● **NDX:** Impaired verbal communication related to
  neuromuscular disease

Assess degree of speech impairment
Avoid rushing patient: provide sufficient time to re-
  spond to minimize patient anxiety and frustration
Provide for alternate communication methods if vocal-
  ization is impaired
  Magic Slate
  Pencil and pad
Provide handkerchief or tissues
Stand close to patient; listen carefully

EXPECTED OUTCOMES

Accepted method of communication is established
Verbalizes understanding of alternate methods of communicating needs

● **NDX:** Self-care deficit: feeding, hygiene related to
  decreased motor function

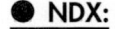

Assess severity of deficits

Initiate a self-care plan that permits patient maximal participation

Maintain regular diet as tolerated; with persistent dysphagia, tube feeding may be indicated; small, frequent feedings may be indicated

Administer oral hygiene q2h to 4h, after meals, and prn

Meet physical hygiene needs as indicated

Administer skin care q4h to 6h
  Turn patient q2h to 4h if patient is unable to ambulate
  Rub back

Administer eye care q4h to 5h
  Remove any formed crusts
  Place eye patch over affected eye *to prevent diplopia*
  Administer eyedrops as ordered

EXPECTED OUTCOME

Patient's self-care needs are met as evidenced by optimal nutritional status and skin integrity

● **NDX:** Impaired physical mobility related to neuromuscular weakness

Assess degree of physical limitations

Assess medications: check dosage, times taken

Work with patient to determine time of day patient is weakest

Increase activity to tolerance; plan treatments and major activities early in day or 30 min after medication is taken

Perform passive or active ROM exercises q4h to 5h and prn *to increase circulation and joint mobility*

Maintain planned rest periods *to minimize fatigue*

Administer medication as ordered
  Anticholinesterase: to be given 20 to 30 min before meals; note increase in muscular strength within 30 min of taking medication
  Medication should always be taken at scheduled time; never miss a dose (rationale: anticholinesterase maximizes physical mobility)

EXPECTED OUTCOME

Patient experiences optimal mobility

● **NDX:** Self-concept deficit: body image related to actual or perceived changes in physical and personal self-image

Assess patient's understanding and feelings about disease, and the effect it has had on physical appearance

Provide emotional support; allow patient to verbalize needs and participate in planning care

Encourage verbalization of feelings about body image and function changes

EXPECTED OUTCOME

Patient demonstrates positive strategies to deal with body image and functional changes

Patient/family teaching

Assess level of understanding regarding disease process

Explain to family the following:
  Need to encourage patient to deal with body image changes and fears of permanent disability, dying, or loss of body function
  Need to encourage verbalization
  Need to encourage independence and continued socialization

Discuss medications: name, dosage, time of administration, purpose, side effects, and toxic effects
  Anticholinesterase
    Importance of dosage
      Take at scheduled times
      Do not miss doses
      Take with milk, crackers, or bread
      Avoid taking with coffee, fruit or tomato juice
      Avoid taking with sedatives or tranquilizers
    Toxic side effects: muscular weakness, abdominal cramps, diarrhea

Discuss symptoms and first signs of drug toxicity to report to physician

Explain need to avoid taking over-the-counter medications without physician approval

Explain need to wear medical alert band

Discuss symptoms of recurrence or progression of disease or any complications, such as respiratory failure, to report to physician

Explain importance of avoiding persons with infections, especially URIs

Discuss symptoms of URI to report to physician
  Increased weakness
  Low-grade fever
  Chills
  Cough

Explain need to avoid use of tobacco and alcohol and prolonged exposure to hot or cold weather

Explain importance of ongoing outpatient care

Explain need to maintain regular diet according to patient's status
  Serve soft or solid food as tolerated
  Arrange foods and utensils so as to be easily managed by patient
  Instruct patient to chew small pieces of food well and eat slowly

Explain need for exercise to tolerance; to avoid strenuous activity
  Plan activities when maximal effect of medication is seen; patient will usually exhibit most strength in morning or after nap

Assist in planning ADLs in a manner in which patient will accomplish tasks without too many motions

Explain need for active or passive ROM exercises to all extremities

Explain need for planned rest periods and at least 8 hr of sleep at night

Emphasize need for diversional activities
  Reading
  Watching television
  Listening to radio
  Working puzzles

Emphasize importance of avoiding physical and emotional stress

Discuss need for speech therapy; instruct patient to speak slowly and practice reading aloud

Explain need to use eye patch over affected eye or frosted lens to increase clear vision if diplopia persists

Explain importance of avoiding constipation; may need to use stool softeners or mild laxatives

Explain need for adequate fluid intake: up to 2000 ml/day unless contraindicated

Discuss available agencies for use as references such as Myasthenia Gravis Foundation*

Refer patient and/or significant other to Visiting Nurses Association (VNA) or social service worker for obtaining any necessary equipment, such as suctioning equipment, for home use

Home care considerations

Activities
  Institute safety measures such as removing or nailing down area rugs to prevent falling
  Stress the importance and proper use of mobility devices (wheelchair, cane, walker) to patient/family
    Assist family to identify local community agencies that can help in providing such devices
    Assist family to learn ways of adapting the home for accessibility
    Stress the need for initial home health referral to do the following:
      Teach family members proper body mechanics and how to protect their backs
      Assist in learning safety measures to prevent falling
  Alert the patient to change positions slowly to prevent postural changes in BP
  Continue gait-training program and encourage patient to walk on heels
  Continue regular exercise program with planned rest periods
  Install safety devices such as siderails and ramps as indicated

---

*Myasthenia Gravis Foundation, 53 W. Jackson Blvd., Suite 1352, Chicago, IL 60604.

Encourage self-care activities to tolerance
Encourage patient to dress self daily
Diet
  Maintain well-balanced, regular diet as tolerated; administer tube feedings as ordered if dysphagia persists
  Offer small portions
  Offer supplemental feedings
  Provide oral hygiene before and after meals and as indicated
  Maintain bowel and bladder programs
General instructions
  Provide skin care q4h to 6h to prevent breakdown
  Administer eye care as indicated
    Remove formed crusts
    Place patch over affected eye
    Administer eyedrops as ordered
  Test stool for occult blood if corticosteroids are being administered
  Report any symptoms of cholinergic or myasthenia crisis; keep emergency equipment (airway, supplemental oxygen, atropine) readily available

Myasthenia Gravis Crisis, Cholinergic Crisis

myasthenia gravis crisis: Acute exacerbation of myasthenic process resulting in increased signs of weakness; usually a result of infection, surgery, or emotional upset

cholinergic crisis: Acute exacerbation of muscle paralysis resulting from an overdose of anticholinesterase

Assessment

Observations/findings

MYASTHENIA GRAVIS CRISIS

Respiratory distress progressing to periods of apnea and respiratory failure
Tachypnea
Extreme muscular weakness
Extreme fatigue
Restlessness
Anxiety
Irritability
Difficulty in handling secretions
Dysphagia
Inability to chew or move jaws
Facial weakness
Speech impairment
Elevated temperature
Ptosis of one or both eyelids

CHOLINERGIC CRISIS

Respiratory distress progressing to periods of apnea
  and respiratory failure
Dyspnea and wheezing
Vertigo
Blurred vision
Lacrimation
Salivation
Anorexia
Abdominal cramping
Nausea and vomiting
Dysarthria
Dysphagia
Muscular cramps and spasms (fasciculations)
Extreme weakness
Toxic effects of anticholinesterase
  Anorexia
  Abdominal cramps
  Nausea, vomiting
  Excessive salivation
  Sweating
  Diarrhea

Potential complications

Aspiration
Respiratory failure
Respiratory arrest

Collaborative management

Therapeutic management

Oxygen-assisted ventilation
Tracheostomy
Intake and output
Medication therapy: reduce or withdraw anticholinergic
  drugs
NPO as indicated

Nursing management

PATIENT PROBLEM/NURSING DIAGNOSIS

● **NDX:** Ineffective breathing pattern related to neuromuscular (respiratory) impairment

Assess respirations: rate, depth, pattern, and respira-
  tory effort
Maintain patent airway
Administer oxygen with assisted ventilation as ordered
Inspect and auscultate chest frequently *to monitor for
  adequate ventilation*
Monitor VC q2h to 4h as ordered
Assist and teach patient to turn, cough, and deep
  breathe q2h as possible

Suction q1h to 2h and prn with 100% O_2 before and af-
  ter suctioning; suction <15 sec
Monitor consciousness until breathing pattern is
  stabilized
Check rectal T q2h to 4h; cooling measures may be or-
  dered *to decrease work of breathing*
Maintain bed rest to maximize effective breathing
  Elevate head of bed 30 degrees as tolerated
  Maintain body alignment
Maintain neck in neutral position
Administer medication *to optimize ventilatory muscular
  activity*
  Reduce or withdraw anticholinergic drugs as ordered;
    may be given to differentiate type of crisis
    Myasthenia gravis crisis: patient worsens
    Cholinergic crisis: patient improves
  Keep atropine at bedside; *avoid use of morphine*
Maintain ventilatory support until crisis is resolved,
  then resume noncrisis management

EXPECTED OUTCOMES

Demonstrates effective breathing pattern without ventilatory support
Respiratory rate, rhythm, and pattern are WNL without
  mechanical support

ADDITIONAL NURSING DIAGNOSES
TO CONSIDER

Risk for injury related to neurologic deficit
Anxiety relate to fear of respiratory distress
Impaired swallowing related to dysphagia

Patient/family teaching and home care considerations

See Myasthenia Gravis (p. 607)

Amyotrophic Lateral Sclerosis

*A progressive lower motor neuron disorder of unknown
  etiology that results in muscular wasting and atrophy;
  commonly known as "Lou Gehrig's disease"*

Assessment

Observations/findings

Irregular muscular fasciculations
Uncoordination of movement of hands and fingers
Muscle wasting involving hands, arms, and
  shoulders
Spastic gait

Progressive weakness, flaccidity, and atrophy of legs
Dysarthria
Dysphagia
Excessive drooling
Loss of reflexes

Diagnostic tests

Elevated creatinine phosphokinase (CPK)
CSF: elevated protein
Myelography
CT scan: cerebral atrophy
Muscle biopsy
Electromyelogram
Nerve conduction studies

Potential complications

Neuromuscular deficit: mild to severe
Respiratory infection
Aspiration, atelectasis
Injury
Respiratory failure

Collaborative management

Therapeutic management

Cricopharyngeal myotomy to alleviate dysphagia
Cervical esophagostomy
Transtympanic neuroectomy
Medications
  Anticholinesterase
  Steroids
  Antibiotics
  Muscle relaxants
Oxygenation/ventilatory support
Cardiac monitoring
Parenteral fluids/nutritional support
Physical therapy
Occupational, speech therapy

Nursing management

PATIENT PROBLEMS/NURSING DIAGNOSES

● **NDX:** Ineffective airway clearance related to progressive neuromuscular impairment

Assess respiratory function and ability to handle secretions
Assess ability to swallow; maintain NPO if reflexes are weak
Maintain patent airway by the following:
  Proper body and head positioning
Suctioning q2h to 4h as indicated; hyperoxygenating with 100% O_2 before and after suctioning; suctioning <15 sec
Encouraging coughing and deep breathing as patient's condition permits
Observe for alterations in respiratory rate and pattern
Auscultate chest for breath sounds q2h to 4h
Administer oxygen, humidification, and ventilatory support as ordered *to promote oxygenation and decrease work of breathing*
Perform chest percussion and vibration *to loosen secretions*
Test muscular strength for respiratory effort by monitoring tidal volume and vital capacity

EXPECTED OUTCOMES
Demonstrates effective breathing pattern
Chest expansion is symmetrical
Breath sounds are clear to auscultation
ABGs and vital signs are within normal limits
No signs of respiratory distress

● **NDX:** Self-care deficit: feeding, bathing, and/or toileting related to progressive neuromuscular deterioration

Assess degree of self-care deficit
Encourage self-care as long as possible
  Bathing
  Feeding
Direct nursing care to promote self-care and prevention of complications according to severity of symptoms
Administer oral hygiene q4h to 5h
Provide physical hygiene as indicated
Check gag reflex
Modify eating patterns as gag reflex diminishes
Maintain high-calorie, high-protein, soft diet as tolerated
Initiate tube feedings as indicated
Administer skin care q4h and prn
  Use air mattress *to prevent breakdown at pressure points*
  Use footboard *to prevent foot-drop*
  Rub back *to stimulate circulation*
Anticipate and manage elimination needs
Help patient avoid constipation
  Encourage drinking fluids
  Use daily suppositories or stool softeners

EXPECTED OUTCOMES
Self-care needs are met
Fluid and nutritional needs are met
Elimination needs are met
Skin, oral, and eye hygiene needs are met

● **NDX:** Impaired physical mobility related to muscle weakness and wasting secondary to neuromuscular deterioration

Assess and document level of motor function
Consult with physiotherapist *to outline an appropriate exercise program*
Perform active or passive ROM exercises q4h to all extremities to maintain joint mobility
Apply necessary braces or splints *to support ankles and hands*
Turn q2h to 4h if patient is confined to bed *to prevent skin breakdown and mobilize respiratory secretions*
Encourage ambulation to tolerance
Avoid strenuous exercise to prevent fatigue
Administer or supervise physical therapy as ordered: massage and stretching exercises
Maintain planned rest periods
Test muscular strength of extremities q4h and prn

EXPECTED OUTCOMES
Maintains full ROM to affected limbs
Motor function is maintained
Demonstrates use of support devices

● **NDX:** Powerlessness related to perceived and/or actual lack of control over body function

Assess feelings and perceptions of physical deterioration
Assess expressions of dissatisfaction and frustration over inability to perform tasks
Provide emotional support; be aware that there is no cure
  Focus and support use of motor functions that still exist
  Encourage expression of feelings *to facilitate open communication*
Assist family and patient with accepting reality of progressive loss of bodily functions
Be supportive; encourage active listening and expression of feelings by patient and family members
Permit patient to participate in care as long as possible

EXPECTED OUTCOMES
Experiences an increased sense of control over life situation and prescribed activities
Verbalizes feelings of increased control
Participates in decisions regarding physical care and activities

ADDITIONAL NURSING DIAGNOSES TO CONSIDER
Ineffective breathing pattern related to neuromuscular degeneration
Impaired verbal communication
Risk for injury/trauma

Patient/family teaching

Assess level of understanding regarding disease
Reinforce physician's explanation of disease, symptoms, progression, and management
Emphasize that although activity is impaired, cognitive processes are not affected
Emphasize importance of verbalization of feelings about progressive muscular wasting and weakness
Emphasize need to discuss feelings about the following:
  Excessive salivation
  Weakening voice, hoarseness
  Dysphagia
Emphasize need for family to encourage active participation in family activities
Demonstrate use of electrolarynx to facilitate vocalization as tolerated
Discuss need to develop alternate methods of communication when voice becomes nonfunctional: use of eyes and eyelid blinking
Explain importance of ongoing outpatient care and physician's visits
Explain need for oral suctioning as disease progresses
Explain need for oral hygiene q2h to 4h and prn
  Have tissues easily accessible to patient
  Have patient use bib while eating
  Clean corners of mouth after eating and prn

Home care considerations

Activities
  Discuss use of braces, splints, and/or cervical collars as indicated for support of hands, ankles, and neck to increase self-care activities
  Maintain gait-retraining program
  Maintain regular exercise program to tolerance
  Maintain planned rest periods
  Maintain home physical therapy
  Encourage ambulation to tolerance
  Stress the importance and proper use of wheelchair, cane, or walker
  Assist family to learn ways of adapting the home for accessibility
  Explain need to avoid strenuous exercise/activity
  Explain need to perform ROM activities as tolerated
  Discuss agencies available for use as resources
  Explain importance of providing skin care frequently, turning patient q2h to 4h to alternate potential pressure areas
  Explain need to provide for and anticipate elimination needs
  Encourage regular coughing and deep breathing exercises
  Perform regular percussion and chest vibration *to mobilize secretions*

Diet
  Explain need for high-calorie, high-protein, soft diet as
    tolerated; assess swallowing reflex before feeding
  Assist patient in dealing with problems of swallowing
    Place puréed foods on posterior aspect of tongue
    Cut foods for patient
    Use wrist and hand braces
    May need to consider nasogastric or gastrostomy
      feedings
  Instruct patient to swallow slowly to prevent aspiration
  Administer oral hygiene before and after meals
  Administer tube feedings as ordered if patient is un-
    able to take oral nutrition
    Check tube feedings q4h or as ordered
    Elevate head of bed during tube feeding administration
Elimination
  Encourage fluid intake to 2000 ml/day unless con-
    traindicated
  Avoid constipation
    Encourage fluid intake
    Use stool softeners or suppositories as ordered
  Maintain urinary elimination program
    Perform intermittent catheterization
    Provide regular hygiene care for indwelling catheter
General instructions
  Encourage expression of emotions about changing
    body functions

Direct care to permit for maximal participation by the
  patient
Modify activities, diet, and care as symptoms increase
Maintain social interactions with family and friends

Guillain-Barré Syndrome (Acute Infectious Polyneuritis; Polyradiculitis)

A neurologic syndrome of acute ascending paralysis; etiology is unknown, but syndrome generally follows a recent infection; onset is rapid, and symptoms are generally reversible; characterized by widespread demyelination of ascending or descending nerves in the peripheral nervous system (Figure 9-18)

Assessment

Subjective data

Symmetrical muscular weakness of lower extremities,
  progressive to arms, trunk, head, and face

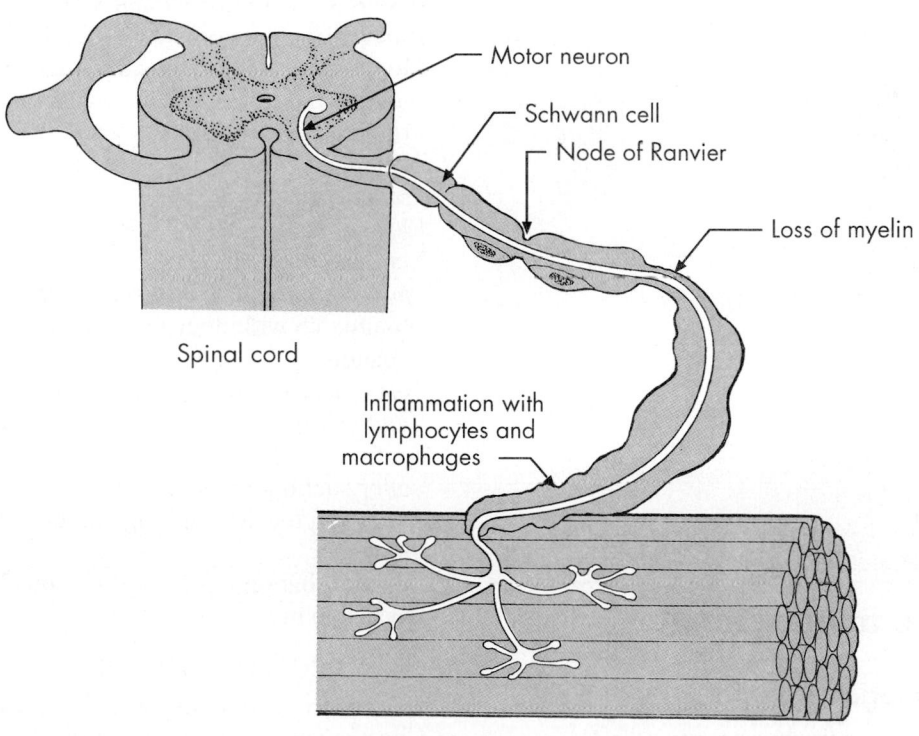

Figure 9-18   Demyelination of nerve segments in Guillain-Barré syndrome. (From Chipps E et al: *Mosby's clinical nursing series: neurologic disorders,* St Louis, 1992, Mosby.)

Dyspnea
Ascending paresthesia, pain, paralysis

Objective data

Paralysis of upper extremities may be partial, or complete quadriplegia may develop
Absent or diminished deep tendon reflexes
Unstable BP: hypertension (during acute phase), hypotension
Sinus tachycardia, bradycardia
Choking, tachypnea
Decreased or absent breath sounds
Dysphagia, difficulty in swallowing
Speech impairment
Low-grade fever
Urinary retention or infection

Diagnostic tests

Lumbar puncture: CSF
  Increased protein
  Normal WBC
Electromyography
Nerve conduction studies
Pulmonary function tests

Potential complications

Autonomic dysfunction
  Postural hypotension
  ECG changes: dysrhythmias
  Urinary, bowel incontinence
Aspiration, atelectasis
Respiratory failure
  Decreased VT
  Hypercapnia
Respiratory arrest
Neuromuscular deficit
  Atrophy
  Contractures
Infection: sepsis
Cardiac failure
Venous thrombosis
Pulmonary embolus
SIADH

Collaborative management

Therapeutic management

Endotracheal intubation; tracheostomy
Oxygen/mechanical ventilation
Serial ABGs
Chest physiotherapy

Physical and/or occupational therapy
Medications
  Antibiotics
  Immunosuppressive agents
  Propolactic antibiotics
  Analgesics (not opiates)
  Anticoagulant agents
  Pituitary hormones
Bed rest; monitoring of muscular strength
Parenteral therapy: enteral or oral nutrition with high-protein, high-calorie diet
Cardiac monitoring: hemodynamic monitoring
Plasmapheresis
Bowel and bladder management

Nursing management

PATIENT PROBLEMS/NURSING DIAGNOSES

● **NDX:** Ineffective breathing pattern related to neuromuscular impairment (ascending paralysis)

Assess respiratory function noting rate, depth, and pattern q1h to 2h and prn
Maintain patent airway, neck in neutral position
Administer oxygen, humidification, and assisted ventilation as ordered *to increase oxygenation and decrease work of breathing*
Assess and monitor VT and VC
Provide tracheostomy care if indicated (p. 319)
Monitor closely for signs of impending respiratory failure; do not leave patient unattended during periods of respiratory distress
Auscultate chest q2h to 4h *to detect adventitious breath sounds*
Elevate head of bed 30 degrees
Maintain body alignment and position *to increase comfort and maximize respiratory effort*
Monitor VS with neurologic signs q1h to 2h and prn for change
Test muscular strength q4h to 8h *to establish baseline and monitor for changes*
Suction prn: hyperoxygenate with 100% O_2 before and after suctioning; suction <15 sec
Assist and teach coughing and deep breathing as appropriate
Keep intubation equipment and mechanical ventilator available in acute phase

EXPECTED OUTCOMES

Demonstrates effective breathing pattern
Chest expansion is symmetrical
Breath sounds are clear to auscultation
ABGs and vital signs are within normal limits
No signs of respiratory distress

● **NDX:** Sensory/perceptual alterations related to neuromuscular paralysis: tactile, communication, visual

Assess and monitor signs of sensory alterations: inability to differentiate hot and cold, dull and sharp)
Record changes/improvement daily
Establish and maintain means of communication
 Call bell within reach *to increase patient's feelings of security*
 Magic Slate, pad and pencil, or word board at bedside
Administer eye care q2h to 4h; remove crusts, apply eye shields, and administer artificial tears *to prevent corneal ulceration*
Administer analgesics as indicated
Assist patient to differentiate tactile sensations: hot or cold
Protect patient from injury
 Test bath water and foods for appropriate temperature
 Keep all sharp objects out of reach
 Assist patient to turn q2h; observe for pressure points

EXPECTED OUTCOMES

Demonstrates increase in sensory stimulation
Sustains no injuries
Able to communicate needs

● **NDX:** Impaired physical mobility related to progressive weakness and paresthesia secondary to neuromuscular disease

Assess and document degree of functional ability
Maintain bed rest; place patient in position of comfort
Support extremities with pillows and footboards *to prevent edema and foot-drop*
Change position q2h to 4h; administer skin care q2h to 4h as indicated *to prevent skin breakdown*
Perform passive ROM exercises to all extremities
Increase frequency of nursing functions as patient's condition requires
Monitor for signs of thrombophlebitis
Encourage ambulation as tolerated
 Begin by having patient sit on bedside with support, progressing to chair bid to tid
 Later have patient walk in room or hall for 15 min qid
Administer analgesics as indicated
Administer anticoagulants as ordered
Consult with physical therapy department for structured exercise program
Maintain planned rest periods
Apply antiembolic stockings

EXPECTED OUTCOMES

Experiences optimal level of mobility
Performs passive and active ROM exercises

No complications related to immobility (e.g., contractures, decubiti)

● **NDX:** Altered nutrition: less than body requirements related to neuromuscular weakness

Assess and record ability to chew, swallow, and cough on daily basis *to prevent aspiration*
Monitor daily caloric intake
Consult with dietitian as indicated
Weigh daily *to establish baseline and detect any potential deleterious changes*
Administer diet as tolerated; progress from soft to solid foods
Supplement feedings with high-calorie, high-protein fluids such as eggnog and milk shakes
Administer enteral feedings as indicated
Encourage fluids to 2000 ml/day unless contraindicated
Maintain parenteral fluids as indicated and ordered *to maintain hydration status*

EXPECTED OUTCOMES

Nutritional and fluid needs are met
Weight is maintained or increased

● **NDX:** Powerlessness related to perceived/actual loss of body function imposed by progressive physical deterioration

Assess feelings of frustration, anxiety, and fear over loss of body function
Provide emotional support, thorough explanations, and reassurance
Be alert to emotional changes and mood swings
Encourage patient's participation and expression of needs and feelings
Encourage participation in self-care activities *to facilitate in increasing self-esteem*
Support and focus on existing body function (eating, dressing, shaving) as indicated
Consult and provide physical, occupational, and psychosocial support

EXPECTED OUTCOMES

Feels in control of or participates in as many routine activities as possible
Participates in decision making and activities related to care
Identifies need areas
Participates in self-care
Participates in diversional activities
Optimal communication is established

ADDITIONAL NURSING DIAGNOSES
TO CONSIDER

Functional incontinence
Altered urinary elimination
Risk for injury
Sensory/perceptual alterations

Patient/family teaching

Ensure that patient and/or significant other under-
stands that recovery may take up to 1 year or longer
Stress importance of dealing with body image changes
and fears of permanent disability, loss of function, and
dying
Explain to family the following:
 Need to encourage verbalization
 Need to encourage independence and socialization
 Need to encourage self-care as a strategy for health
 maintenance
 Importance of allowing patient to take meals with
 family
Discuss medications: name, dosage, frequency of ad-
ministration, purpose, and side effects
Explain need to avoid over-the-counter medications
without physician approval
Stress need to avoid individuals with infections, espe-
cially URIs
Encourage diversional activities: TV, reading, radio

Home care considerations

Activity
 Alert patient to change positions slowly to minimize
 orthostatic changes in BP
 Stress the importance and proper use of mobility de-
 vices (wheelchair, cane, walker) to patient/family
 Assist family to identify local community agencies
 that can help in providing such devices
 Assist family to learn ways of adapting the home for
 accessibility
 Stress the need for initial home health referral to do
 the following:
 Teach family members proper body mechanics and
 how to protect their backs
 Assist in learning safety measures to prevent falling
 Implement safety measures such as siderails and
 ramps
 Maintain regular exercise program with planned rest
 periods; perform regular passive ROM exercises to
 all extremities if patient is unable to exercise
 Encourage maximal participation in self-care activities
 Maintain home physical therapy program if indicated
 Provide regular skin care to promote circulation
 Use warm baths to alleviate/minimize stiffness and
 discomfort

Diet
 Maintain high-calorie, high-protein, regular or soft
 diet as tolerated
 Assess swallowing reflex before feeding/meals
 Modify diet if swallowing reflex diminishes
 Supplement diet with small, additional, high-calorie,
 high-protein snacks
 Encourage fluid intake to 2000 ml/day unless con-
 traindicated
 Monitor intake and output
 Weigh patient weekly
 Obtain home nutrition referral
 Maintain bowel and bladder programs
General information
 Encourage emotional expressions of anxiety, frustra-
 tions, and fears
 Maintain focus on remaining body functions

Neurologic Infections

*Those conditions in which a microorganism has gained
 entry into the body producing a reaction, brain
 abscess, or meningitis*
brain abscess: *Secondary to systemic infections or may
 be introduced through trauma; results in space-
 occupying lesions causing a potential for increased ICP*
meningitis: *Infection of the meninges, causing
 inflammatory reaction in the pia-arachnoid
 membrane; may be caused by bacteria or virus (acute
 aseptic meningitis)*
encephalitis: *Infection of the brain parenchyma*

Assessment

(NOTE: See box, p. 618, for specific findings)

Subjective data

Headache
Diplopia
Malaise
Anorexia

Objective data

History of recent URI, sinus or ear infection, penetrat-
ing trauma, or basal skull fracture
Elevated temperature
Meningeal irritation
 Nuchal rigidity
 Positive Kernig and Brudzinski signs
 Photophobia
Altered LOC: irritability, disorientation to coma

Cranial nerve dysfunction (III, IV, VI, VII, VIII)
  Ocular palsies
  Facial paresis
  Deafness
  Vertigo
Seizures: focal, generalized

Diagnostic tests

Lumbar puncture (contraindicated if increased ICP is
  suspected): CSF
  Protein level and pressure
  Glucose level
Serum blood cultures
CBC with differential
EEG
CT scan (serial)
X-ray examination
  Chest
  Skull
  Sinus

Potential complications

Increased ICP
Seizures
Neurologic deficit: paresis
Hydrocephalus
Herniation
Altered mentation
Pneumonia
Respiratory failure

Collaborative management

Therapeutic management

Institutional protocol for isolation or infection control as
  indicated by organism (identified)
Medications
  Antibiotic therapy
  Analgesics
  Glucocorticosteroids
  Anticonvulsants
  Antipyretics
Ventilatory/oxygenation support
Hypothermia
ICP monitoring
Fluid/electrolyte therapy
Serial CT scans
Temperature control
Bowel/bladder management
Nutritional support
Physical therapy

Nursing management

PATIENT PROBLEMS/NURSING DIAGNOSES

● **NDX:** Ineffective thermoregulation related to infectious process

Monitor T q2h to 4h or as indicated
Administer antipyretic medications as ordered
Maintain room temperature to 68°F or 20°C
Initiate cooling measures as indicated
  Give tepid sponge bath
  Remove excess bed linens
  Use hypothermia blanket
Encourage fluid intake
Monitor WBC as ordered

EXPECTED OUTCOME
Patient is normothermic; temperature is 98.6°F or 37°C

● **NDX:** Pain: headache related to cerebral tissue irritation

Maintain quiet environment; darken room if photophobia occurs
Maintain bed rest; assist patient in assuming position of comfort
Administer analgesics as ordered; monitor neurologic status
Administer comfort measures
  Elevate head of bed 30 degrees
  Put cool cloth over eyes
  Apply ice cap to head

EXPECTED OUTCOMES
Verbalizes absence of or improved headache
Appears to be resting quietly

● **NDX:** Ineffective breathing pattern related to increased ICP and depressed cerebral functioning

Assess and monitor respirations: rate, depth, and breathing pattern
Assess respiratory status q1h to 2h as indicated
Auscultate breath sounds
Monitor serial ABGs as ordered
Administer oxygen/ventilatory support as ordered
Position patient for optimal ventilation
Assist and instruct patient to turn and deep breathe q2h to 4h
Suction prn; hyperoxygenate with supplemental 100% O₂ before and after suctioning; suction <15 sec
Check BP, P, R, and LOC to indicate neurologic and respiratory stability

Specific Findings Associated with Bacterial Meningitis, Viral Encephalitis, Brain Abscess

BACTERIAL MENINGITIS

Elevated T (101°F to 103°F/38°C to 39.5°C)
Altered LOC
  Memory loss, disorientation to delirium to coma
Meningeal irritation
Oligenia
Muscle hepatoma, flaccid paralysis
Deafness
Petechial hemorrhage
Increased ICP

VIRAL ENCEPHALITIS

Altered LOC
Aphasia
Hemiparesis
Ataxia
Nystagmus
Ocular paralysis
Facial weakness

BRAIN ABSCESS

Acute
Chills and fever
Confusion
Drowsiness
Seizures: local or generalized
Motor or sensory deficits
Second Stage
Headache, recurrent and severe
Confusion to stupor
Increased ICP

DIAGNOSTIC TESTS

CSF
  Turbid
  Increased WBC
  Increased protein
  Decreased glucose
  Elevated CFS pressure (>180 mm H_2O)

CSF
  Increased WBC with mononuclear cells
  Increased (slightly) protein
  Normal glucose

CSF
  Increased WBC (lymphocytes)
  Increased (high) protein
  Normal glucose
  Elevated CSF pressure (200-300 mm H_2O)

EXPECTED OUTCOMES

Demonstrates effective breathing pattern
Chest expansion is symmetrical
Breath sounds are clear to auscultation
ABGs and vital signs are within normal limits
No signs of respiratory distress

Patient/family teaching

Discuss medications: name, dosage, frequency of administration, purpose, side effects, and toxic effects
Explain need to avoid taking over-the-counter medications without consulting physician
Explain to family need to encourage verbalization; help patient understand nature of disorder
Discuss symptoms of progression of condition to report to physician
Explain importance of ongoing outpatient care

Home care considerations

Activity
  Encourage self-care to tolerance
  Maintain regular exercise program with planned rest periods
  Report and record any seizure activity
  Maintain seizure precautions
  Assist patient to cough and deep breathe regularly
  Encourage ambulation to tolerance
  Maintain home physical therapy program if indicated
Diet
  Encourage fluid intake to 2000 ml/day unless contraindicated
  Monitor intake and output
  Weigh weekly
  Maintain well-balanced diet
General instructions
  Report any temperature elevations
  Administer antipyretics as ordered
  Administer antibiotics until all medication has been taken

Monitor stools for occult blood if glucocorticosteroid therapy is continued at home

Report any new or increased neurologic deficits

Substance Abuse (Drug Abuse and Intoxication)

NOTE: Care of the intoxicated patient will depend on the amount and type of drug ingested (see box p. 620); for severe drug overdose or intoxication refer to Care of patient with altered consciousness, shock syndrome, respiratory failure, and seizures

● Alcohol Intoxication

Assessment

Observations/findings

Acute intoxication
  Confusion
  Slurred speech
  Ataxia
  Depressed deep tendon reflexes
  Nystagmus
  Anxiety, restlessness
  Dilated pupils
  Stupor
  Coma
  Gastric irritation: vomiting
Withdrawal
  Anxiety
  Tremors
  Diaphoresis
  Nausea, vomiting
  Anorexia
  Confusion
  Moroseness
  Confabulation
  Delirium tremens
  Seizure activity
  Uncontrolled rage
  Hallucination
  Toxic psychosis
Chronic intoxication
  Mental confusion
  Cerebellar degeneration
    Ataxic gait
    Nystagmus
    Dysarthric speech
  Nutritional deficiencies
  Myopathy
  Hepatic coma

Seizure disorders
Marchiafava-Bignami syndrome (progressive organic dementia)
Wernicke syndrome
  Ophthalmoplegia
  Apathy, apprehension
  Confusion
  Coma
Korsakoff syndrome
  Disorientation to time and place
  Peripheral neuropathy
  Confabulation

Diagnostic tests

Serum ETOH (see Table 9-9)
Serum chemistries

Potential complications

Aspiration
Hypertension
Severe stages
  Hypoventilation
  Hypotension
  Hypothermia
  GI hemorrhage
  Myocardial infarction (MI)

Collaborative management

Therapeutic management

Acute
  Ventilatory support and management: oxygenation/ventilatory
  Fluid/electrolyte therapy

Table 9-9 Serum Alcohol Levels

Serum Alcohol Levels	Effects
Mild: 0.5 to 1.5 mg/ml	Muscular uncoordination, personality changes: talkative, morose, noisy
Moderate: 1.5 to 3 mg/ml	Marked ataxia, mental impairment, uncoordination, prolonged reaction time, nausea, vomiting, diplopia
Severe: 3 to 5 mg/ml	Dysarthria, amnesia, hypothermia, hypoventilation, coma

Drugs Commonly Abused

NARCOTICS

Opium
Heroin (horse, smack)
Oxycodone
Codeine
Methadone
Hydromorphone (Dilaudid)
Meperidine (Demerol)

HALLUCINOGENS

LSD (acid)
Mescaline
DMT
Scopolamine
Atropine
Phencyclidine: PCP (angel dust, crystal, dust
    mist, peace pill, superweed)
Psilocybin

ORGANIC SOLVENTS

Glue
Cleaning fluid

DEPRESSANTS

Alcohol
Barbiturates
Meprobamate
Chloral hydrate
Glutethimide (Doriden)

STIMULANTS

Cocaine (coke, rock, crack)
Amphetamines
Methylphenidate (Ritalin)

CANNABIS

Marijuana (grass, weed, joints)
Hashish (weed oil, hash)

Medications during withdrawal
    Phenothiazines
    Tranquilizers
    Barbiturates
    Anticonvulsants
    Thiamine
Respiratory therapy
Social services

Nursing management

PATIENT PROBLEMS/NURSING DIAGNOSES

● **NDX:** Ineffective breathing pattern (potential) related to CNS depression

Maintain patent airway; assisted ventilation as indicated
See Care of patient with altered consciousness (p. 560)
    and Respiratory failure (p. 309)
Position to optimize respiratory excursion, airway patency, and secretion removal
Monitor BP, P, and R q2h to 4h and prn
Provide oropharyngeal or nasopharyngeal tube as indicated to maintain patent airway
Suction prn: hyperoxygenate with 100% O_2 before and after suctioning; suction <15 sec
Auscultate breath sounds prn to detect adventitious breath sounds
Provide oxygenation/respiratory therapy
Monitor serial ABGs as indicated
Avoid use of sedatives, which may potentiate effects of alcohol
Provide soft restraints as indicated to protect patient from self-injury
    Keep restraints loose
    Position patient on side or stomach to prevent aspiration

EXPECTED OUTCOMES

Demonstrates effective breathing pattern
Chest expansion is symmetrical
Breath sounds are clear to auscultation
ABGs and vital signs are within normal limits
No signs of respiratory distress

● **NDX:** Ineffective individual coping related to inadequate coping methods

Maintain quiet, supportive environment; avoid punitive approach
Maintain safety precautions for anxious and restless patients
Provide supportive counseling services to patient when receptive
Ensure that patient and/or significant other is knowledgeable about effects of alcohol abuse

EXPECTED OUTCOMES
Demonstrates effective coping strategies
Discusses effects of alcohol abuse
Attends counseling/educational support groups

● Chemical Substance Abuse

*Intermittent or chronic use of stimulants or depressants
resulting in alterations in mental and physiologic
function*

Assessment

Observations/findings

DEPRESSANTS: NARCOTICS, OPIATES*
LOC
  Apathy
  Withdrawal
  Euphoria
  Coma
Airway obstruction
Stridor
Decreased BP
Tachycardia or bradycardia
Pupillary changes
  Pinpoint (opiates)
  Dilated (barbiturates)
Depressed gag and swallow reflexes
Respiratory distress, respiratory rate <8/min or
  >30/min
Seizure activity
Hypothermia
Method of administration
  Oral
  Subcutaneous: "skin popping"
  Nasal insufflation: "snorting"
  Intravenous
  Signs of withdrawal
    Abdominal and muscular pain
    Severe cramping

HALLUCINOGENS, STIMULANTS
General
  Anxiety progressing to pain
  Paranoid reaction
  Combativeness progressing to violence
  Insomnia
  Hallucinations
    Auditory
    Visual

---

*Refers to all drugs that possess some morphinelike activity.

Confusion
Ataxia
Depression: mild to severe
Suicidal tendencies
Anorexia
Nausea
Headache
Elevated BP
Elevated T
Tachycardia palpitations
Hypertension progressing to crisis
Pupillary changes: dilated
Photophobia
Diplopia
Horizontal and vertical nystagmus
Hot flashes
ECG changes
  Dysrhythmias
  ST-T wave changes
Decreased urine output
LSD, Mescaline
  Hyperactivity
  Pupil dilation
  Increased VS
  Low doses: euphoria
  High doses: hallucinatory psychosis
PCP: "Angel Dust"
  Low-to-moderate doses: effect begins within 5 min
    and peaks within 30 to 60 min
    Elevated systolic and diastolic pressures
    Tachycardia
    Increased deep tendon reflexes
    Small pupils
    Nystagmus: horizontal and vertical (persists for 4
      days)
    Tremors, clonus
    Euphoria
    Amnesia
    Agitation
    Image distortion
    Increased urine output
  High doses
    Slurred speech
    Drowsiness
    Depressed deep tendon reflexes
    Seizures
    Opisthotonos
    Bradypnea
    Decreased BP
    Disordered thought processes, hallucinations

Diagnostic tests

Serum chemical screening
Urinalysis

ABGs
ECG
Chest roentgenogram

Collaborative management

Therapeutic management

Depressants
  Respiratory support with oxygenation or ventilation
  Fluid/electrolyte therapy
  Emetics
  Gastric lavage
  Activated charcoal for ingested opiates
  Naloxone for opioid overdose
  Peritoneal dialysis
  Vitamins
Stimulants
  Decreased external stimuli
  Medications
    General
      Barbiturates, phenothiazines
      Sedatives, anticonvulsants
      Vitamins
    For LSD, mescaline
      Diazepam (oral)
      Avoid phenothiazine, which may potentiate psychotic action
    For PCP
      Haloperidol
      Diazepam
      Activated charcoal (high doses)
      Parenteral fluids
      Gastric suction for PCP
Psychiatric liaison
Social services

Nursing management

If patient arrives in coma refer to p. 560. If patient arrives in respiratory failure, refer to p. 309
Assess respirations q2h to 4h, noting rate, quality, and depth *to detect adventitious breath sounds*
Assess LOC and monitor q2h to 4h
Report any changes in consciousness or VS to physician to prevent further decline in neurologic status
Administer parenteral fluids as ordered *to maintain adequate hydration*
Understand that peritoneal dialysis may be indicated for long-acting barbiturates
Obtain accurate and detailed history regarding drug ingested: type, amount, time of ingestion, method of administration
Administer emetics as ordered; contraindicated in presence of depressed gag reflex, seizures, or coma

Administer gastric lavage as ordered (within 2 hr of ingestion); endotracheal tube is usually inserted before lavage in comatose patient
Keep patient physically active and stimulated
Provide patient with positive reassurance about condition; avoid punitive approach
Be firm, patient, and understanding
Administer medication as ordered: naloxone (Narcan) for opiate overdose; effects can be noted within 1 to 2 min if given intravenously
Give activated charcoal orally for ingested opiates
Check BP and P on admission and q4h as indicated by condition
Monitor cardiac status *for dysrhythmias*
Meet self-care needs as indicated

EXPECTED OUTCOMES

Demonstrates effective breathing pattern
Chest expansion is symmetrical
Breath sounds are clear to auscultation
ABGs and vital signs are within normal limits

● **NDX:**   Risk for violence self-directed or directed at others related to drug toxicity

Admit to private room when possible
Decrease external stimuli
  Use low lighting
  Avoid loud voices and rapid movements *to minimize further agitation*
NOTE: Administration of the following care may heighten patient's paranoid state and cause increased agitation; approach patient quietly, using friend to assist if required
Allow friend or family member to remain in room during all procedures to assist in "talking down"
Provide patient with support, reassurance, and reality-defining information
Instruct patient to avoid trying to differentiate between real perceptions and effects of drug; remind patient that effects of drug will end
Avoid mechanical restraints if possible
Approach cautiously; avoid whispering to others
Explain all procedures; allow same person to care for patient at all times
Administer medications as ordered
Avoid phenothiazine (may potentiate effect or produce anticholinergic crisis)
Administer parenteral fluids as ordered
Monitor BP, P, and R q2h to 4h or as indicated by level of consciousness

EXPECTED OUTCOME

Patient demonstrates calm and nondestructive behavior

ADDITIONAL NURSING DIAGNOSES
TO CONSIDER

Withdrawal related to decreased intake of drug/alcohol after long-term use

Ineffective individual coping related to chemical substance abuse

Altered nutrition: less than body requirements related to chronically poor dietary intake

Self-care deficit related to depressed mood or altered reality orientation

Altered family processes related to dysfunctional family relationships

Patient/family teaching

Explore patient's willingness to participate in self-help and support group experiences

Provide supportive, nonjudgmental approach to patient

Provide opportunity for participation in counseling and group support

Lumbar Puncture (Spinal Tap)

Puncture usually made at the junction of the third and fourth lumbar vertebrae to obtain CSF for purposes of measuring CSF pressure and laboratory examination

Preprocedure preparation

Explain procedure

Have patient empty bowel and bladder

Position patient on side with spine close to edge of bed; support soft mattress with bedboards

Maintain aseptic technique throughout procedure
　Handle specimen with care
　Verify specimen delivery to laboratory within 30 min to ensure diagnostic accuracy

Explain to patient that procedure may be uncomfortable

Explain importance of immobilization during procedure

Instruct patient to breathe normally; not to hold breath

Provide patient with physical and emotional support during procedure

Postprocedure assessment

Observations/findings

Altered LOC
Headache: mild to severe
Nuchal rigidity
Hypotension
Tachycardia
Tachypnea
Bleeding from site of puncture
Elevated temperature

Diagnostic tests

Normal adult CSF
　Pressure: 70 to 200 mm of water
　Color: colorless, clear
　Glucose level: 45 to 75 mg/100 ml
　Protein level (total): 20 to 45 mg/100 ml
　Red blood cells: none
　White blood cells: 0 to 5 cells/mm^3
　Microorganisms: none

Potential complications

Transient back pain
Paresthesia in legs
Headache
Infection
Elevated ICP
Coagulation abnormalities

Immediate postprocedure care

Maintain bed rest; place patient in supine position, keeping head of bed flat for 4 to 8 hr as ordered; if headache occurs, elevate feet 10 to 15 degrees above bed

Assist and teach patient to turn and deep breathe q2h to 4h

Check BP, P, and R q15min for four times, then qh for four times, then as ordered

Control pain as ordered

Observe site of puncture for redness, swelling, or drainage and report any symptoms to physician

Maintain diet as ordered

Force fluids unless contraindicated

Explain importance of keeping head and body position flat in bed

Ongoing care

Resume activities as ordered
Ambulate to tolerance

Hypothermia: Care of Patient

Controlled reduction and maintenance of body temperature to decrease the metabolic rate

Assessment

Observations/findings

PATIENT

Shivering
Decreased BP
Bradycardia
Bradypnea
Altered LOC
Medication reactions
Pupil inequality

EQUIPMENT

Cooling solution; amount in unit
Patency of connections
Pads

Potential complications

Dysrhythmias
Increased ICP
Respiratory failure
Decreased urinary output
Intestinal ileus
Frostbite and burns

Immediate care

Take and record T before starting treatment and q5min
  until desired T is reached, then q15min
Check BP, P, and R and do neurologic check q5min to
  10min while T is stabilizing
Observe for any change in skin color or presence of
  edema and induration; report any changes to physician immediately *to prevent peripheral ischemia*
Assist and teach patient to turn, cough, and deep
  breathe q1h to 2h *to facilitate*
Measure intake and output; measure output qh; report
  output <30 ml/hr to physician; specific gravity test
  may be ordered
Connect indwelling catheter to closed gravity drainage
  as ordered
Auscultate chest for breath sounds q1h to 2h
Administer medication for shivering as ordered
Test gag reflex before administering any oral fluids or
  food to patients with temperatures <90°F (32.2°C)
Perform naso-oral suction as indicated *to maintain
  patent airway*
Administer skin care q1h to 2h *to promote circulation*
  Lubricate skin before and during procedure with oil
    or lotion *to prevent dryness*
  Place bath blankets over thermal blankets
Maintain good body alignment
Perform passive or active ROM exercises q4h *to main-
  tain joint mobility*

Administer oral hygiene q1h to 2h; keep lips well lubri-
  cated *to prevent dryness*
Administer nose care q1h to 2h
Provide emotional support
  Remain with patient when anxious
  Anticipate needs

Ongoing care

Patient

Check BP, T, P, and R and do neurologic check q30min
  for four times, then q4h for 24 hr, then as ordered
Check any dressing and all skin surfaces q1h to 2h
  until patient's T is stable
Measure intake and output
Assist and teach patient to turn, cough, and deep
  breathe q2h
Resume care of disease as ordered

Equipment

Check for leaks or punctures in pads before applying to
  patient

Increased Intracranial Pressure

*Slow or sudden elevation in CSF pressure caused by
  edema, hemorrhage, or trauma; caused by increase in
  CSF or obstruction to outflow*

Assessment

Observations/findings

Deterioration in LOC
  Restlessness
  Instability
  Anxiety
  Confusion
  Lethargy
Headache: location, duration, severity
Visual disturbances
  Diplopia
  Blurring
  Decreased acuity
Motor weakness
Paresis
Progressive weakness or paralysis of extremities
Pupil dysfunction (ipsilateral to edema or lesion)
Papilledema
Vomiting (projectile), nausea

Changes in respiratory rate; Biot's or Cheyne-Stokes respirations
Elevated BP (systolic); widened pulse pressure
Pulse rate decreased to 50 beats/min or below
Elevated T
Seizure activity
After cranial surgery
  Swelling around surgical site
  Elevation of bone flap

Diagnostic tests

Lumbar puncture
Continuous ICP monitoring
Cerebral perfusion pressure
Serial ABGs
Serum studies
  Electrolytes
  Coagulation studies
  Anticonvulsant levels

Potential complications

Deterioration of neurologic function
Infection; sepsis
Respiratory failure
Cerebral hemorrhage
Herniation

Collaborative management

Therapeutic management

Management of ventilatory status
  Oxygenation
  Ventilatory support
  Hyperventilation
Medications
  Diuretics
  Osmotic diuretics
  Muscle relaxants
  Fluid restriction
  Steroids
  H_2 histamine blocker
  Anticonvulsants
  Barbiturate coma
  Antiinfectives
  Stool softeners, laxatives
  Antacids
Fluid restriction
Cardiac monitoring; hemodynamic monitoring
Surgical intervention
Ventricular drainage

Nursing management

PATIENT PROBLEM/NURSING DIAGNOSIS

● **NDX:** Altered tissue perfusion: cerebral related to sustained elevations in ICP

Assess and monitor LOC, reporting any changes immediately
Maintain patent airway *to facilitate oxygenation*
Elevate head of bed 30 degrees
Maintain bed rest *to minimize energy expenditures*
  Avoid semiprone or prone position
  Avoid flexion of neck
  Avoid compression of neck veins
  Avoid extreme hip flexion
Monitor BP, P, and R q30min; if possible take BP on same arm each time
Perform neurologic check q30min using Glasgow Coma Scale (p. 560); report scores of 8 or less or any significant changes
Check rectal T q2h to 4h and prn; perform cooling measures as indicated
Monitor ABGs q2h to 4h as indicated
Maintain parenteral fluids as ordered; hypertonic solutions may be ordered
Measure intake and output *to monitor hydration status*
Initiate specific medical management as indicated
Avoid Valsalva maneuvers: vomiting, retching, straining; initiate measures to avoid constipation as indicated
Avoid isometric muscular contractions; instruct patient to avoid pushing feet against bedboard
Perform passive ROM activities as ordered *to maintain joint mobility and promote circulation*
Avoid stress-producing procedures during rapid eye movement (REM) stages of sleep
Explain and prepare for diagnostic tests and/or return to surgery as ordered
See standard of care for primary condition

EXPECTED OUTCOMES
Patient remains free of injury
Demonstrates appropriate orientation and LOC
Demonstrates vital signs within normal limits
Demonstrates an effective breathing pattern
Demonstrates normal ICP
Demonstrates normal ROM

Intracranial Pressure Monitoring (Table 9-10)

Insertion of a catheter for purposes of monitoring ICP and/or removing CSF

Table 9-10 Comparison of ICP Monitoring Systems

System	Advantages	Disadvantages
Ventricular catheter	Reliable measurement within CSF Access for CSF drainage and sampling Access for determination of volume-pressure curve	Difficulty locating lateral ventricle Risk of intracerebral bleeding or edema at cannula track Risk of infection Need for transducer repositioning with head movement
Subarachnoid bolt/screw	Useful if ventricles are small No penetration of brain Decreased risk of infection	Unable to drain CSF Unreliable pressure when high ICP herniates brain into bolt Requires intact skull Need for transducer repositioning with head movement
Epidural sensor	Ease of insertion No dural penetration Lower risk of infection No adjustment of transducer needed with head movement	Unable to drain CSF Unable to recalibrate or rezero after placement Separate, large monitoring system required Questionable accuracy of sensing ICP through dura
Fiberoptic transducer-tipped catheter	Versatile system that can be placed in ventricle, subarachnoid space, or brain tissue Able to monitor intraparenchymal pressure Access for CSF drainage with ventricular system No adjustment of transducer needed with head movement	Catheter relatively fragile Unable to recalibrate or rezero after placement Separate monitoring system required

From Thelan LA et al: *Critical care nursing: diagnosis and management,* ed 2, St Louis, 1994, Mosby.

intraventricular (ventriculostomy): Placement of catheter into lateral ventricle; CSF may be removed for control of ICP or diagnostic evaluation

subarachnoid method: Screw or commercial bolt with stopcock that can be rapidly passed into subarachnoid space

epidural method: Placement of sensor through a burr hole between the skull and dura

fiberoptic method: System can be placed in three different areas—intraventricular, intraparenchymal (in subarachnoid space), and subdural space—to monitor intraparenchymal pressure; provides access for CSF drainage (with ventricular system); no adjustment of transducer is needed for head movement

Assessment

Observations/findings

PATIENT

Normal levels: 1 to 15 mm Hg
Moderate elevation: 15 to 40 mm Hg

High levels: >40 mm Hg
Cerebral perfusion pressure (CPP): 50 to 85 mm Hg
  Calculation of formula:

  CPP = MABP (mean arterial blood pressure) − ICP
  CPP <50 mm Hg: ischemia
  CPP <20 to 30 mm Hg: irreversible ischemia

Wave forms (Figure 9-19)
  A waves: large plateau formations characterized by varying increases and decreases of ICP ranging from 50 to 90 mm Hg and lasting 5 to 20 min; related to cerebral dysfunction
  B waves: occur more regularly—1½ to 1/min, ranging from 10 to 50 mm Hg
  C waves: rapid rhythmic oscillations at amplitudes to 20 mm Hg
Hemodynamic measurements
  Intraarterial pressure
  Pulmonary capillary wedge pressure (PCWP)
  Pulmonary artery diastolic pressure
  Cardiac output (CO)
Level of consciousness

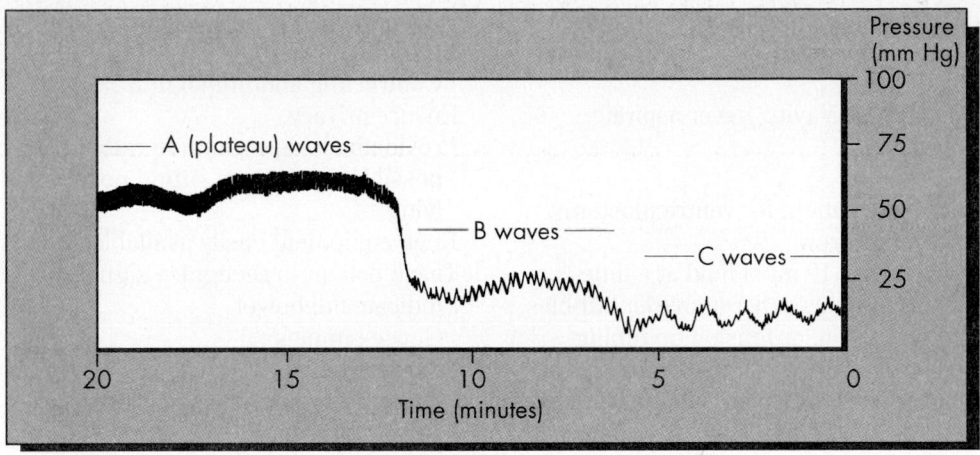

Figure 9-19   Intracranial pressure waves. Composite drawing of A (plateau) waves, B waves, and C waves. (From Chipps E et al: *Mosby's clinical nursing series: neurologic disorders,* St Louis, 1992, Mosby.)

Decreased blood pressure
Increased ICP: changes determined by baseline
  pressure
CSF
  Clear
  Cloudy
  Blood tinged
  Xanthochromic
Elevated temperature

EQUIPMENT

Flush solution (for *initial* tubing flush only)
  Ringer's lactated injection
  Normal saline solution
Pressure line tubing
Transducer
Pressure monitor

Potential complications

Meningitis
Hemorrhage: catheter insertion site
Infection
  Swelling
  Inflammation
  Redness
  Leaking of CSF

Preparation

PATIENT

Reinforce physician's explanation of procedure, duration, and equipment that will be used
Record baseline observations of patient and ICP at
  time of insertion

EQUIPMENT

Calibrate all equipment before insertion
  Transducer
  Recording display unit
Position transducer to eye of patient for ventriculostomy or at level of both for subarachnoid screw
Be aware that insertion must be done under sterile conditions

Ongoing care

PATIENT

Maintain head of bed elevated at 30 degrees with patient in supine position; avoid neck flexion, prone position, or extreme hip flexion
Assess pressures qh, prn, and after changes in body position or condition
Notify physician if plateau wave forms begin to increase steadily
Calculate CPP qh
Assess and report any changes in LOC or pressures to physician
Check BP, P, and R and do neurologic check q1h to 2h
Check rectal temperature q2h to 4h
Check dressing q1h to 2h
Change dressing qd
Never flush or irrigate ventricular cannula
Administer stool softeners as ordered; have patient avoid straining
See Increased intracranial pressure (ICP) (p. 624)
NOTE: The following items may change pressure readings
  Obstructed airway
  Suctioning
  Body position
  Valsalva maneuver

Report any changes in patient's condition to physician
Observe monitor during removal of CSF for precipitous
  drop in pressure
Remove CSF slowly and by gravity; never aspirate

  EQUIPMENT
Level transducer to eye of patient for ventriculostomy;
  to bolt for subarachnoid screw
Flush pressure tubings with 10 ml of fluid at a time
Check patency of pressure lines q4h; remove air bubbles
Prevent kinking, compression, or tension on tubing
Calibrate transducer q4h to 6h or as indicated by manu-
  facturer; never apply direct pressure to diaphragm of
  transducer
Change pressure tubing q24h

Bowel Training

Method of bowel evacuation by reflex conditioning

Assessment

Observations/findings

Impaction
Diarrhea
Bowel incontinence
Dehydration
Autonomic hyperreflexia (dysreflexia)
  Restlessness
  Chills
  Hypertension
  Diaphoresis
  Headache
  Elevated temperature
  Bradycardia
  Flushing

Patient/family teaching

Explain purpose and necessity of developing bowel reg-
  ulation
Encourage patient's participation in developing a program
Assess previous bowel habits
Establish regular bowel habits
  Time of day that will be convenient for patient once
    discharged: after breakfast
  Development of program to have bowel evacuation at
    same time each day or q3d
Administer medications as indicated
  Stool softeners
  Mild laxatives
Teach exercises that will help develop abdominal mus-
  cles and tone

  Pushing up
  Bearing down
  Contracting abdominal muscles
Ensure privacy
Provide bedside commode rather than bedpan when
  possible; encourage sitting position rather than
  lying
Keep equipment easily available at bedside
Teach patient to recognize signals or "cues" that may
  indicate full bowel
  Goose pimples
  Perspiration
  Raising of hair on arms or legs
  Sense of fullness
Instruct patient to eat diet high in fiber

Skull Tongs and Halo Traction

Methods of immobilizing the neck and stabilizing the spine

Assessment

Observations/findings

Site of insertion of tongs
  Redness
  Swelling
  Drainage
Skin condition: decubiti of scapula, coccyx, and heels
Alignment of head, pulleys, and weights: do not allow
  patient's head to touch head of bed
Weights
  Pounds ordered
  Off floor, hanging freely
Position of bed

Ongoing care

Inspect and clean site of insertion q1h to 2h; remove
  any formed crusts with hydrogen peroxide q6h to 8h
  and prn
Administer skin and scalp care q2h to 4h
  Use air mattress
  Give back rubs
  Keep bed linen dry and free of wrinkles
  Avoid powders
Perform passive ROM exercises to all extremities q4h
Apply antiembolic stocking
Check alignment of pulleys and weights q4h to 6h; sand-
  bags may be indicated for restlessness as ordered
Turn patient q2h as ordered
Maintain safety precautions
Assist and teach patient to deep breathe q2h

Establish means of communication and keep within easy reach of patient: call bell
Provide diversional activities
Assist with ambulation as indicated for patient with halo traction

Patient/family teaching

Explain purpose of tongs
Explain methods of turning when possible
Explain importance of keeping head straight

Stryker Frame

Metal frame bed used to facilitate administration of nursing care to patient with spinal cord injuries

Assessment

Observations/findings

PATIENT

Body position: straight body alignment
Place in center of frame
Body parts not resting on metal frame
Skin
  Temperature
  Color
Pressure areas
Pulse
Respirations
Lightheadedness
Numbness

EQUIPMENT

Canvas supports
Arm and foot supports
Locks
Frame
  Anterior
  Posterior

Preparation of unit

Check unit for security of bolts, locks, and frame before placing patient on Stryker frame
Prepare bed with linens, foam mattress, arm rests, and footboards before receiving patient

Ongoing care

Turn patient q2h during day
Turn patient q4h during night

Check P and R before and after turning
Free all excess tubing before turning
Secure all bolts tightly before turning
Reassure patient when turning
Administer skin care q2h to 4h and prn
Inspect pressure points q2h to 4h

General Rehabilitative Care of Neurologic Patient

May involve minimal to long-term chronic rehabilitative care; specialized settings have programs designed to meet special need areas; the following discussion describes general guidelines for observation and intervention in the care of the neurologically impaired patient

Conditions requiring rehabilitative approach

Cognitive impairment
  Alteration in memory
  Alteration in speech, auditory, or visual function
Sensory-perceptual impairment
Impaired physical mobility
Paralysis
Behavioral changes
Spinal cord injuries
Alteration in elimination function
Self-care deficit
Ineffective individual coping
Chronic pain

Rehabilitative approach

Reinforce physician's explanation of disorder and its limitations and allowances
Deal with behavioral response
  Allow patient to go through stages of grief over loss of body function
  Be supportive but firm in dealing with patient
Encourage verbalization of feelings and fears
Use positive and reassuring approach to patient
Encourage independence when possible; be alert to limitations
Involve family or significant other in care and instructions
Establish program for ADLs
Encourage patient's participation in developing a program
Establish daily routines of activity and rest periods

Sample

7:00 to 7:30	Morning care
7:30 to 8:30	Breakfast
9:00 to 9:30	Commode (bowel training)
9:30 to 10:30	Bath
10:30 to 11:00	Chair, stretcher
11:00 to 12:00	Bed rest; turn and position
12:00 to 12:30	Lunch
12:30 to 2:30	Bed rest; turn and position
2:30 to 3:00	Exercises
3:00 to 5:00	Bed rest
5:00 to 6:00	Chair, stretcher, dinner
6:00 to 9:00	Bed rest
9:00 to 9:30	Exercises
9:30 to 10:00	Evening care
10:00 PM to 7:00 A.M.	Bed rest

Turn and reposition to the following:
Right side
Left side
Prone position
Supine position
Attempt to avoid sensory deprivation by providing the
following:
Calendars
Clocks
Pictures
Include schedule for favorite television or radio pro-
grams, hobbies, and visiting hours
Explain all treatments and procedures as they occur
Alert staff to patient's emotional changes and mood
swings
Allow patient time to express needs
Refer to social service, VNA, and/or local rehabilitation
centers as ordered
Report symptoms of urinary tract infection to physician
Foul odor of urine
Sedimentation, pus, or blood in urine
Decreased output
Low-grade fever
Chills
Encourage participation in bowel and bladder training
Avoid constipation
Cleanse perineal region; wipe from front to back after
urination
Cleanse perineal region with soap and water after each
bowel movement
Give high-calorie, high-protein diet as ordered; avoid
high-calcium foods

Activities

Explain importance of exercise programs
Exercise to tolerance; avoid fatigue
Assist and instruct patient to use assistive devices as
ordered

Plan rest periods
Encourage patient to participate in self-care as indicated

Nutrition

Assess daily caloric needs
Maintain high-calorie, high-protein, low-residue diet as
ordered
Limit high-calcium and gas-producing foods

Elimination

Encourage fluids to 3000 ml/day unless contraindi-
cated
Have patient avoid constipation through use of stool soft-
eners, mild cathartics, suppositories, and/or enemas
Check for bowel movement q3d
Institute bowel and bladder programs
Avoid overdistention of bladder and bowel
Initiate intermittent catheterization as indicated

Patient/family teaching

Ensure that patient and significant other(s) know and
understand the following:
Importance of exercise programs
Need to exercise to tolerance; avoid fatigue
Importance of fluid intake; measure intake and output
Importance of turning q2h to 4h while in bed
Need to inspect skin and bony prominences for detec-
tion of skin breakdown
Importance of skin care q2h to 4h while in bed
Need to avoid constrictive clothing below level of le-
sion (e.g., garters, belts)
Need to avoid UTIs
Need to avoid overdistention of bladder; empty on
regular basis
Need for fluid to 3000 ml/day
Need to ensure daily bowel evacuation to avoid fecal
impaction; encourage participation in bowel training
Need for ongoing support and counseling services
Sexual counseling: patients can engage in some form
of satisfying sexual activity; limitations depend on
site of injury; incomplete injuries and high cord in-
juries allow for varying amounts of sensation and
sexual function—even if spinal reflexes are absent,
sensation of genital organs may endure
Female reproductive system usually remains intact;
patient can bear children—refer for family planning
counseling
Refer to appropriate support services
Vocational rehabilitation
Recreational rehabilitation
Home care

Paraplegia

Paralysis of the lower extremities resulting from injury to the spinal cord

Assessment

Observations/findings

Atrophy of nonfunctioning body parts
See Musculoskeletal assessment (p. 495)
Bladder distention
Dysuria
Bowel incontinence, impaction

Rehabilitation

Give praise for tasks completed
Avoid tasks that patient cannot complete
Provide diversional activities as indicated
  Reading
  Watching television
  Listening to radio
  Working puzzles
  Listening to tape cassettes
Establish means of communication
  Call bell within reach
  Calling out to nurse

Bed activities

Perform weight-bearing exercises
  Begin elevating head of bed, progressing to high-
    Fowler's position as tolerated when condition
    stabilizes
  Use tilt bed as ordered
    Begin elevating patient's head at 10 degrees for 10 to
      15 minutes tid, progressing to 15 degrees for 1 hr
      bid or tid
    Keep legs wrapped with elastic stockings as ordered
    Take BP before tilting patient and every 5 min at 10
      degrees; in absence of hypotension or dizziness,
      progress to 15 degrees as tolerated
    Gradually progress to 90-degree elevation as tolerated
Change position qh: maintain body alignment
  Prone position
  Supine position
  Rolling to side
  Sitting up
  Moving forward and backward
Check placement of lower extremities with each
  movement
Administer skin care q2h to 4h *to promote circulation*
  Use air mattresses
  Give back rubs with lanolin-based lotions

Put foam rubber pads on chairs
Keep bed linen dry and free of wrinkles
Place rubber sheet under bath blanket
Use body corset as ordered
Perform muscle-building exercises
  Active ROM exercise to support extremities
  Dumbbells: extending and flexing of arms
  Overhead trapezes
  Push-ups
  Sit-ups
  Hand-finger exercises
    Rubber sponge balls
    Extension and flexion
Teach method of turning self and pulling up in bed

Wheelchair activities

Get patient out of bed bid or tid
Demonstrate method of transferring from bed to wheelchair and from wheelchair to toilet or shower
Demonstrate management of wheelchair: moving forward, backward, turning, stopping, and locking

Self-care activities

Encourage self-care as tolerated
  Bathing
  Dressing
  Combing hair
  Shaving
  Oral hygiene
Encourage patient to wear own clothing: pajamas, slip-
  pers, or shoes

Motion activities

Use long leg braces as ordered
Perform physical therapy as ordered
  Weight-bearing exercises
  Parallel bar exercises
  Balancing exercises
  Crutch-walking exercises
To relieve spasticity
  Perform active or passive ROM exercises
  Wear long leg braces
  Give medications as ordered

Elimination

Perform urinalysis weekly as indicated
Check urine output for sedimentation or presence of re-
  nal calculi
Perform intermittent catheterization as ordered
Initiate bowel and bladder programs
Teach self-catheterization when appropriate

Quadriplegia

Paralysis of the upper and lower extremities resulting from injury to the spinal cord (thoracic and cervical regions)

Assessment

Observations/findings

Loss of sweating reflex
Bladder distention and incontinence
Mass reflex of bladder
  Muscular spasms
  Diaphoresis
  Elevated BP
  Headache

Rehabilitation

Encourage staff to allow time for patient care; do not rush patient
Provide diversional activities as indicated
  Reading
  Socializing with nursing staff
Provide means of communication
  Calling out to nurse
  Whistling

Bed activities

Maintain good body alignment to promote comfort
Turn and position patient q1h to 2h *to stimulate circulation and improve muscle mass, tone, and strength*
  Use supports: sandbags and pillows
  Avoid external rotation of lower extremities
  Position patient: supine, prone, and on side
Cough and deep breathe q1h to 2h *to prevent atelectasis*
Administer skin care q1h to 2h *to promote circulation and prevent skin breakdown*
  Use air mattress
  Use footboard
  Keep bed linen dry and wrinkle free
  Rub back and heels with lanolin-based lotions *to promote circulation*
  Change bed clothing prn
  Place rubber sheet under bath blanket to be used as draw sheet
  Assist with or provide perineal care after each voiding or bowel movement
  Begin elevating head of bed as condition stabilizes, progressing to high-Fowler's position as tolerated
Tilt table as ordered; begin raising head to 10 degrees for 10 to 15 min tid, progressing to 20 degrees for 1 hr bid to tid, on to 90 degrees for 1 hr bid to tid, on to 90 degrees as tolerated
Take BP before tilting patient and at 5 to 10 min intervals as head is being raised; in absence of hypotension or dizziness progress to 90 degrees
Apply elastic bandages or stockings as ordered

Wheelchair activities

Use three or four persons to transfer patient to stretcher chair or stretcher for 15 to 30 min bid to tid as ordered
Encourage wheelchair activity as ordered as condition stabilizes
Provide braces, splints, and other supports as ordered
Take safety measures
  Soft jacket restraints
  Soft abdominal binders
  Siderails when indicated

Self-care activities

Encourage patient to wear clothing from home and make selections

Motion activities

To relieve spasticity
  Perform gentle, passive ROM exercises
  Have patient wear braces
  Give medications as ordered
  Prepare for rhizotomy or chordotomy as ordered

Nutrition

Give tube feedings as indicated
Position patient with head of bed at 30 to 45 degrees
Feed patient
  Allow 30 to 45 min for feeding time
  Give small bites of food
Perform oral hygiene q4h and after meals
  Clean with hydrogen peroxide and water
  Gargle and mouthwash
  Brush teeth

Elimination

Provide indwelling or external catheter to closed gravity drainage as ordered
Instruct patient to develop exercise or signals that may help to stimulate urge to defecate
  Smoking
  Pressure on inner thigh
  Stroking anus
  Digital rectal stimulation

Drinking coffee

Massaging abdomen downward or right to left

Instruct patient to respond to "cues" promptly

Discuss importance of established, well-balanced diet that includes bulk and roughage

Discuss foods to avoid

Bananas

Beans

Cabbage

Foods that previously have been constipating

Encourage fluids to 3000 ml/day unless contraindicated

Include prune and orange juice and coffee in daily diet as preferred

Discuss possible programs to develop

Instruct patient to take 8 to 10 oz of prune juice 12 hr before time set for defecating; insert glycerin suppository high in rectum 15 to 20 min before set time, then place patient on bedpan, toilet, or commode

Insert lubricated glycerin suppository 2 hr before set time and position patient in sitting position or transfer to bedpan or commode

Instruct patient to drink 4 to 8 oz of prune juice each night

Instruct patient to drink a warm drink 30 min before set time

Water

Coffee

Milk

Insert laxative suppository for 2 to 4 days, then glycerin suppository for 2 to 4 days; note length of time between insertion and defecation; place patient on bedside commode at appropriate time; if no bowel movement, give small tap water enema

Instruct patient to recognize signs of impaction

No formed stool for 3 days

Semiliquid stools

Restlessness and increased feeling of discomfort

Discuss treatment for impaction

Laxative suppository

Tap water or oil-retention enemas

Manual clearing of bowel followed by enema

Beare PG, Myers SL: *Principles and practice of adult health nursing,* ed 2, St Louis, 1994, Mosby.

Bronstein KS et al: *Promoting stroke recovery: a research based approach in nursing,* St Louis, 1991, Mosby.

Campbell VG: Neurological system. In Thompson JM et al, editors: *Mosby's clinical nursing,* ed 3, St Louis, 1993, Mosby.

Chipps E: Myasthenia gravis: the patient in crisis, *Crit Care Nurs* 11:7, 1991.

Chipps E, et al: *Mosby's clinical nursing series: neurologic disorders,* St Louis, 1992, Mosby.

Conway BL: *Carini and Owens' neurological and neurosurgical nursing,* ed 8, St Louis, 1982, Mosby.

Davis J, Niason C: *Neurologic critical care,* New York, 1979, Van Nostrand Reinhold.

Glanze WD et al, editors: *Mosby's medical, nursing, and allied health dictionary,* ed 4, St Louis, 1994, Mosby.

Goodman G: *The pharmacological basis of therapeutics,* ed 7, New York, 1985, Macmillan Publishing.

Hickey F: *The clinical practice of neurological and neurosurgical nursing,* ed 2, Philadelphia, 1986, JB Lippincott.

Hodges K: Meningioma, ashocytoma and germinoma case presentation of 3 intracranial tumors, *J Neurosc Nurs* 21:2, 1989.

Johanson BC et al: *Standards for critical care,* ed 3, St Louis, 1988, Mosby.

Kim MJ et al: *Pocket guide to nursing diagnoses,* ed 6, St Louis, 1995, Mosby.

Krenzel JR, Rohrer LM: *Handbook of care of paraplegic and quadriplegic individuals,* Chicago, 1972, National Association of Paraplegia and Quadriplegia.

McCance KL, Heuther SE: *Pathophysiology: the biological basis for disease in adults and children,* ed 2, St Louis, 1994, Mosby.

Pagana K, Pagana T: *Mosby's diagnostic and laboratory test reference,* ed 2, St Louis, 1995, Mosby.

Phisler S, Bullas J: Acute Guillain-Barré syndrome, *Crit Care Nurs* 10:10, 1990.

Phipps WJ, et al: *Medical-surgical nursing: concepts and clinical practice,* ed 5, St Louis, 1995, Mosby.

Richmond TS, ed: Neurotrauma, *Nurs Clin North Am* 21(4):549, 1986.

Rudy E: *Advanced neurological and neurosurgical nursing,* St Louis, 1984, Mosby.

Seidel HM et al: *Mosby's guide to physical examination,* ed 3, St Louis, 1995, Mosby.

Snyder M: *A guide to neurological and neurosurgical nursing,* New York, 1983, John Wiley & Sons.

Taylor J, Ballenger S: *Neurological dysfunction and nursing intervention,* New York, 1980, McGraw-Hill.

Thelan LA, et al: *Critical care nursing: diagnosis and management,* ed 2, St Louis, 1994, Mosby.

Vogt G, et al: *Mosby's manual of neurological care,* St Louis, 1985, Mosby.

BIBLIOGRAPHY

Barker E: *Neuroscience nursing,* St Louis, 1994, Mosby.

Barry K, Texerian S: The role of the nurse in the diagnostic classification and management of epileptic seizures, *J Neurosurg Nurs* 15(4):243, 1983.

USC UNIVERSITY HOSPITAL
1500 San Pablo
Los Angeles, CA 90033 ©1991

NAME _____ SIDE 1 ALLERGIES _____

MULTIDISCIPLINARY PLAN

ADMIT DATE _____

DIAGNOSIS ____ Acoustic Neuroma ____

SURGERY ____ CRANIOTOMY ____   DRG __001__ ALOS __12.4__

DISCHARGE OUTCOMES

PHYSIOLOGICAL: Patient will have ADL needs met by self or c̄ assistance of other(s). Will be able to explain surgical site care, verbalize precautions to take for medication use. Complications/injury will be prevented or minimized, discomfort relieved/controlled & infectious process(es) resolving/absent.

COGNITIVE: Patient will be able to verbalize disease process/prognosis & therapeutic regimen & state the s/sx to report to health care team.

PSYCHOLOGICAL: Patient will verbalize acceptance of potential lifestyle changes & incorporate into ADLs. Able to verbalize fears/anxieties & demonstrate effective coping mechanisms A/E ability to participate in self-care decisions.

DISCIPLINE	PRE-OP/ PRE-ADMIT	DOS DAY 1	POD#1 DAY 2	POD#2 DAY 3	POD#3 DAY 4	POD#4 DAY 5	POD#5 DAY 6
LOCATION DATE		SURGERY/PAR/NSICU	NSICU	NSICU→DOU	DOU	DOU → MED/SURG	MED/SURG
LABS	CBC Chem 20 UA PT PTT T & C 2u PRBCs	Chem 7 ⟩ on arrival Hct ⟩ to unit	CBC Chem 7	CBC Chem 7	CBC Chem 7	CBC Chem 7	
CARDIO-PULMONARY	ECG R/O Arrhythmias	I.S. Pulse oximetry O$_2$ 40% face mask A-Line	DC A-Line	DC face mask & pulse oximetry			
IMAGING/ NUCLEAR MEDICINE	CXR 2 Views						
SOCIAL SERVICES D/C PLAN REHAB. SERVICES			Assess need for speech/swallowing consult Consider need for OT evaluation—self-care	Assess need for PT consult. Consider need for social worker services	Asses need for home health evaluation if indicated. Support adaptive group OT	Assess need for Rehab consult	
PHARMACY	IV of LR	IV fluids Corticosteroid Ocular lubricants Analgesics H$_2$ antagonist Antibiotic Vestibular Sedative	Stool softener Antiemetic	Convert IV to SL DC antibiotics			
DIETARY/ NUTRITION	NPO	NPO until awake, then ice chips	Advance to diet as tolerated if no swallowing difficulty, otherwise refer to speech/swallow consult recommendations				

Used by permission of USC University Hospital, Los Angeles, California.

PATIENT NAME: _____

MULTIDISCIPLINARY PLAN

DISCIPLINE	PRE-OP/ PRE-ADMIT	DOS / DAY 1 DATE ___	POD#1 / DAY 2 DOS DATE ___	POD#2 / DAY 3 POD #1 DATE ___	POD#3 / DAY 4 POD #2 DATE ___	POD#4 / DAY 5 POD #3 DATE ___	POD#5 / DAY 6 POD #4 DATE ___
PATIENT ACTIVITY		BR HOB ↑ 30 – 45° Leg squeezers begun in OR	OOB TO chair c̄ assistance only BID	Ambulate c̄ assist TID			DC leg squeezers
EDUCATION Baseline vestibular testing/pt education done re: dizziness Basic audiogram, c̄ air, bone, speech, middle ear testing	I.S. instruct C & DB. Teach reason for surgery, post-op restrictions & expected LOS	Orient to room, unit & hospital routine Pro-optic moisture eye chamber to affected eye Monitoring of dressing for drainage Discuss need for Foley	DC Foley I & O cath q 6° prn Review s/sx of CSF leak Discuss c̄ pt/family need for safety precautions due to pt's balance disturbances (up c̄ assist only). Move slowly when getting up & keep eyes open. May experience difficulty c̄ reading (nystagmus)	Review disease process, prognosis & understanding of therapeutic regimen during hospitalization. Teach self-application & care of eye moisture chamber	Review all previous teaching. Consult for placement of spring or gold weight by ophthalmology may be indicated.	Balance visit	Shower instructions: • Staples may become wet • Towel dry throughly p̄ showering • Avoid hot curls until hair has regrown Postop audiogram, balance lab visit, vestibular rehab will begin q d

COLLABORATIVE PROBLEMS

DATE		DATE	
❶ Potential for altered level of consciousness R/T postop cerebral edema &/or bleeding.		❼ Knowledge deficit R/T lack of exposure to hospitalization, misinterpretation of information received or limitation of cognitive ability; discharge planning.	
❷ Potential for infection R/T suppressed inflammatory response secondary to steroids or exposure to pathogens.		❽ Potential for inadequate corneal lubrication R/T facial nerve involvement.	
❸ Potential for injury R/T possible postop weakness, paresthesia, ataxia or vertigo.		❾ Impaired hearing R/T manipulation of cranial nerve VIII.	
❹ Alteration of comfort; pain R/T surgical procedure.			
❺ Potential for impairment physical mobility R/T ↓ strength, perceptual/cognitive impairment, pain or restriction in activity.			
❻ Potential anxiety/fear R/T situational crisis of hospitalization or change in health status & separation from support system.			

OUTCOMES

❶ Pt. will maintain usual or improved LOC & motor-sensory function.	❺ Pt. will regain &/ or maintain optimal physical mobility.	❽ Pt. will be able to apply care for & remove eye moisture chamber independently or c̄ S/O assistance.	❼ Pt. will be able to correctly perform procedures & explain reasons for actions.
❷ Pt. will demonstrate timely healing free from infectious spread.	❼ Pt. will verbalize understanding of condition/disease process.		❹ Pt. will verbalize pain controlled c̄ po pain medications.
❸ Pt. will remain free from injury during hospitalization.	❾ Pt. will verbalize understanding of hearing loss & will take measures to optimize present hearing.		❾ Pt. will verbalize under-standing of discharge plans.
❹ Pt. will verbalize pain controlled c̄ ordered medications. Displays relaxed posture & able to sleep &/or rest.			
❻ Pt. will acknowledge & discuss fears. Will appear relaxed & reports anxiety reduction to a manageable level.			

KEY

❶ Document outcomes under appropriate date for achieving the goal.

❷ To discontinue an intervention, or resolve a patient problem, highlight date and initial.

Continued.

PLAN OF CARE

PLAN OF CARE DISCUSSED WITH: S.O. ___ Pt. ___ DATE ___ INITIAL ___

INTERVENTIONS

DOS DAY 1	POD#1 DAY 2	POD#2 DAY 3	POD#3 DAY 4	POD#4 DAY 5	POD#5 DAY 6
DATE ___	DATE ___	DATE ___	DATE ___	DATE ___	DATE ___
– Assess neuro status per MD order, report △s to MD – Strict I & O – Monitor temp per unit routine – Assess respiratory status q 1° x 24° – Reposition frequently & encourage use of I.S. – Evaluate for s/sx of ↑ICP: • decreased response to stimuli • △s in VS • restlessness • weakness/paralysis of extremities • changes in vision or pupillary △s • worsening of headache – Monitor urine characteristics - color, odor, clarity – Assess for clinical signs of infection & report to MD if present – Note c/o pain location, intensity & duration – Medicate for pain as ordered & assess pain relief – If pt has headache, reduce bright lights & room noise if possible – Provide eye patch as ordered to ↓ eye strain – Assess pt &/or S/O level of anxiety – Answer questions & explain all procedures prior to initiation – Clarify misunderstandings of info & involve pt & S/O in decision making, care planning & evaluations – Assess ability to close eyelid. Notify MD if unable to do so – Avoid nose blowing or sneezing if preventable	– Assess for factors that impair physical mobility: • pain &/or nausea • fear of falling • vertigo • dislodging tubes • compromising surgical wound – Treat those items present above &/or educate pt as needed – Assure pt that activity ordered will enhance rather than compromise healing process – Provide praise & encouragement for all efforts to ↑ mobility – Reinforce need for assistance when getting OOB – Provide pt c̄ safe environment (seizure precautions may also be indicated) – Provide info to pt & S/O in short segments – Discuss expected length of recovery – Assess pt ability to swallow prior to advancing diet – If pt has hearing loss, speak distinctly. Note side of hearing loss & speak to unaffected ear – Discuss c pt the need to verbalize lack of hearing – Discuss need for eye moisture chamber, apply as ordered – Assess respiratory status q 2°	– Increase activity & participation in ADLs – Encourage S/O to assist c̄ ↑ activity – Assess for need of stool softener – Assess pt & S/O understanding of disease process, prognosis & understanding of therapeutic regimen – Discuss application, care for & removal of eye moisture chamber – Assess affected eye for irritation & drainage – Apply cool compresses to affected eye if ordered – Change VS c̄ neuro V/s to q 4° p̄ transfer – Continue strict I & O – Assess resp status q 4° – Continue use of I.S. – Assess for s/sx of CSF leak: • Worsening headache upon standing • Ask if pt experiencing frequent swallowing or feels fluid in the back of the throat • Have pt bend over & note drainage presence • If drainage noted, place a sterile pad under nose & observe for halo of blood surrounding clear or yellow colored ring of spinal fluid • If above present, notify MD immediately • Temp elevation may indicate meningitis • Reassess frequently	– Reassess pt &/or S/O level of anxiety – Support planning for realistic lifestyle p̄ hospitalization within limitations but fully using capabilities – Explore sources of support: • S/O • Clergy • Social Worker – Encourage use of po pain meds – Assess need for home health evaluation & outpatient therapies – Coutinue to monitor for CSF leakage	– DC leg squeezers once pt fully ambulatory – Reassess pt need for stool softner – Encourage increased activity – Continue to monitor for CSF leakage	– Instruct in showering technique

Case Manager: _____

Consulting MD: _____

Social Service: _____

Anointing of The Sick Date: _____

MULTIDISCIPLINARY PLAN UPDATE

DATE	SIGNATURES	DATE	SIGNATURES	DATE	SIGNATURES

USC UNIVERSITY HOSPITAL

1500 San Pablo
Los Angeles, CA 90033

©1991

SIDE 2

MULTIDISCIPLINARY PLAN

DIAGNOSIS — Acoustic Neuroma

SURGERY — CRANIOTOMY

NAME —

ALLERGIES —

ADMIT DATE —

DISCHARGE OUTCOMES	DRG 001 ALOS 12.4
PHYSIOLOGICAL	Patient will have ADL needs met by self or c̄ assistance of other(s). Will be able to explain surgical site care, verbalize precautions to take for medication use. Complications/injury will be prevented or minimized, discomfort relieved/controlled & infectious process(es) resolving/absent.
COGNITIVE	Patient will be able to verbalize disease process/prognosis & therapeutic regimen & state the s/sx to health care team.
PSYCHOLOGICAL	Patient will verbalize acceptance of potential lifestyle changes & incorporate into ADLs. Able to verbalize fears/anxieties & demonstrate effective coping mechanisms A/E ability to participate in self-care decisions.

DISCIPLINE	PRE-OP/ PRE-ADMIT	POD #6 DAY 7 DATE	POD #7 DAY 8 DATE	POD #8 DAY 9 DATE	POD #9 DAY 10 DATE	POD #10 DAY 11 DATE	POD #11 DAY 12 DATE
LOCATION		MED SURG	MED SURG → HOME				
LABS							
CARDIO-PULMONARY							
IMAGING/ NUCLEAR MEDICINE							
SOCIAL SERVICES D/C PLAN REHAB. SERVICES	Ordered therapies to assess pt discharge needs						
PHARMACY	DC S.L.		To be discharged c̄ po pain medications				
DIETARY/ NUTRITION	Regular diet						

Continued.

PATIENT NAME: _____

MULTIDISCIPLINARY PLAN

DISCIPLINE	PRE-OP/ PRE-ADMIT	POD #6 DAY 7	POD #7 DAY 8	POD #8 DAY 9	POD #9 DAY 10	POD #10 DAY 11	POD #11 DAY 12
		DATE ___	DATE ___	DATE ___	DATE ___	DATE ___	DATE ___
PATIENT ACTIVITY		Ambulate as much as tolerated					
EDUCATION		Teach s/sx to report to health care team. Instruct pt in care of surgical site. Discuss discharge medications. Reinforce safety precautions at home.	Staples to be removed 7-10 days postop. Discuss follow-up care regimen.				

COLLABORATIVE PROBLEMS

DATE	COLLABORATIVE PROBLEMS	DATE INIT	DATE	COLLABORATIVE PROBLEMS	DATE INIT
	❶ Potential for altered cerebral tissue perfusion R/T cerebral edema altering or interrupting cerebral blood flow.	⟋		❾ Impaired hearing R/T position of tumor.	⟋
	❷ Potential for infection R/T suppressed inflammatory response (medication induced) or exposure to pathogens.	⟋			⟋
	❸ Potential for injury R/T seizure activity, weakness, paralysis, paresthesia, ataxia or vertigo.				⟋
	❹ Alteration in comfort, pain R/T headache &/or surgical procedure.				⟋
	❼ Knowledge deficit R/T lack of exposure to hospitalization, misinterpretation of information received or limitation in cognitive ability; discharge planning.				⟋
	❽ Potential impaired corneal tissue integrity R/T inadequate lubrication.	⟋			⟋

OUTCOMES

KEY

❶ Document outcomes under appropriate date for achieving the goal.

❷ To discontinue an intervention, or resolve a patient problem, highlight date and initial.

❶ Pt will maintain usual or improved LOC & motor-sensory function.	❼ Pt & S/O will describe follow-up care regimen.	
❷ Pt will continue to demonstrate healing free from infectious spread.		
❸ Pt will demonstrate absence of seizure or injury.		
❹ Pt will verbalize pain controlled c̄ po pain medications.		
❽ Pt will be able to apply, care for & remove eye moisture chamber independently or c̄ S/O assistance.		
❾ Pt will verbalize if unable to hear any conversation involved in.		

	POD #6 DAY 7	POD #7 DAY 8	POD #8 DAY 9	POD #9 DAY 10	POD #10 DAY 11	POD #11 DAY 12
PLAN OF CARE DISCUSSED WITH	DATE ____	DATE ____	DATE ____	DATE ____	DATE ____	DATE ____
DATE INITIAL S.O. Pt.			INTERVENTIONS			

DAY 7 (POD #6):

– Teach s/sx that need to be reported to the health care team:
  • rhinorrhea
  • changes in vision
  • elevated temp
  • intense headache
  • drainage from surgical site
  • balance Δs
– Teach pt how to care for surgical site:
  • Avoid scrubbing
  • Dab very dry
  • Keep hair off wound × 72°
  • Avoid sun exposure
  • OK to shampoo p̄ staples out × 24°
– Instruct pt & S/O regarding discharge meds. Include name & purpose, route, dosage, frequency, time of administration & side effects.
– Explain safety precautions to maintain at home:
  • Assistance when ambulating in the dark
  • Assistance in performing ADLs as needed
– Continue to monitor for CSF leakage

DAY 8 (POD #7):

– Reinforce those s/sx that need to be reported to the health care team
– Encourage tips to recovery:
  • Return to normal social & physical activity
– Verbalization of concerns c̄ health care team
– Emphasize the importance of ongoing outpatient care & follow-up visits
– Review those medications pt will take home

Case Manager: _____

Consulting MD: _____

Social Service: _____

Anointing of The Sick
Date: _____

MULTIDISCIPLINARY PLAN UPDATE

DATE	SIGNATURES	DATE	SIGNATURES	DATE	SIGNATURES

Genitourinary/ Renal System

Genitourinary/Renal Assessment

● Subjective Data

Reported changes in voiding pattern
  Anuria
  Diurnal frequency
  Dysuria
  Hesitancy
  Force of urinary stream
  Frequency of urination
  Nocturia
  Oliguria
  Polyuria
  Urgency
  Incontinence (type/containment devices used)
Bladder spasm
Pain
  Back
  Flank
  Groin
  Colicky
  Lumbar
  Urethral
  Genital
  Perineal
  Abdominal
Sexual history
  Decreased libido
  Dyspareunia
  Impotence

Gastrointestinal (GI) status
  Anorexia
  Nausea/vomiting
  Constipation/diarrhea
  Thirst
  Hiccoughs
  Metallic taste in mouth
  Fatigue/malaise/weakness
  Restlessness
  Headache
  Inability to concentrate
  Pruritis
  Muscle cramps
  Paresthesias of lower extremities
  Visual disturbances/changes
  Lost sense of smell

● Objective Data

See Figure 10-1
Physical examination
  Kidney (abdominal mass, flank mass, costovertebral
    angle tenderness) (Figure 10-2)
  Bladder (presence of distention, pain)
  External genitalia (redness, sores, ulcers/lesions,
    rash, inflammation, pain) (Figures 10-3, 10-4, and
    10-5)
  Urethra (drainage, pain, inflammation)
  Vagina (drainage, discharge, redness, inflamma-
    tion)
  Testes/scrotum (enlargement, mass, tenderness)
    (Figure 10-6)
  Prostate via rectum (size, consistency, induration)

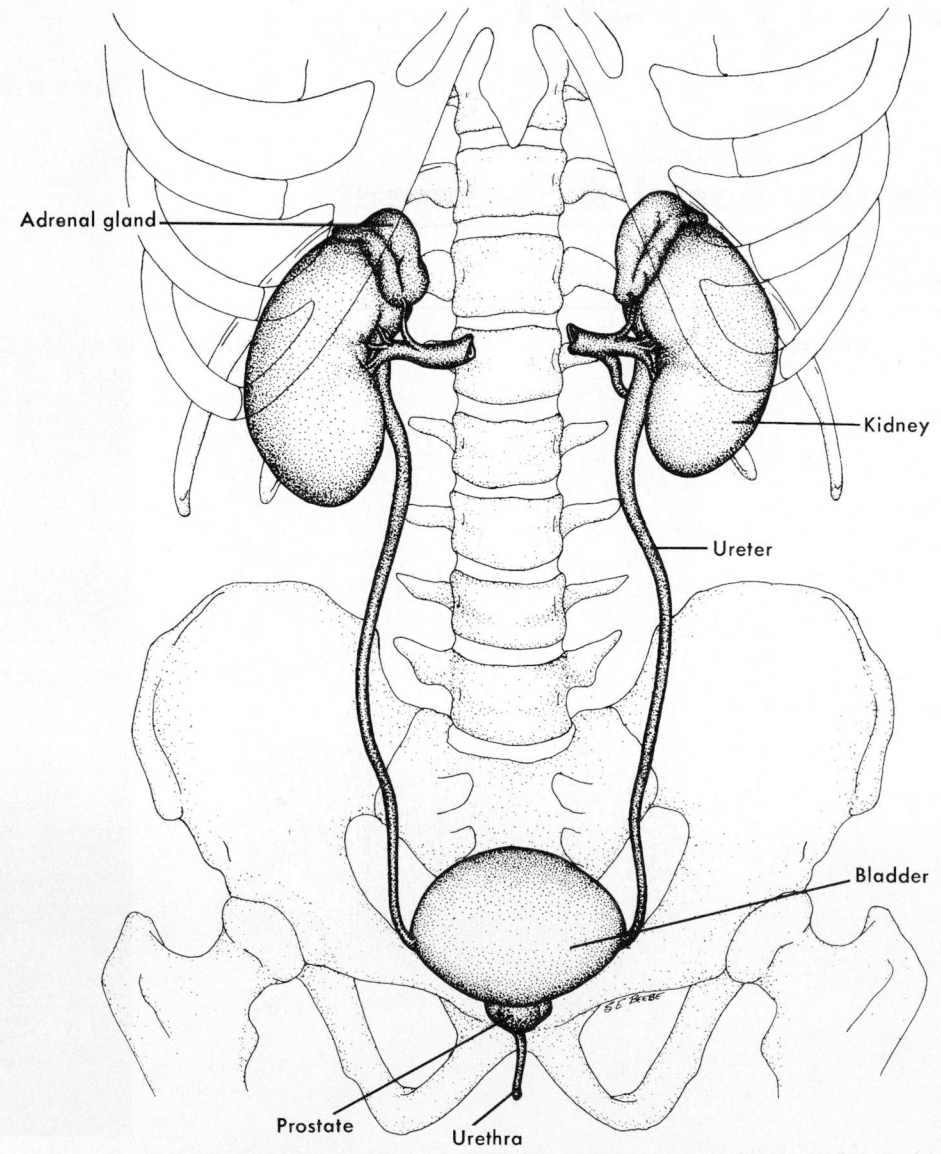

Figure 10-1   Genitourinary system.

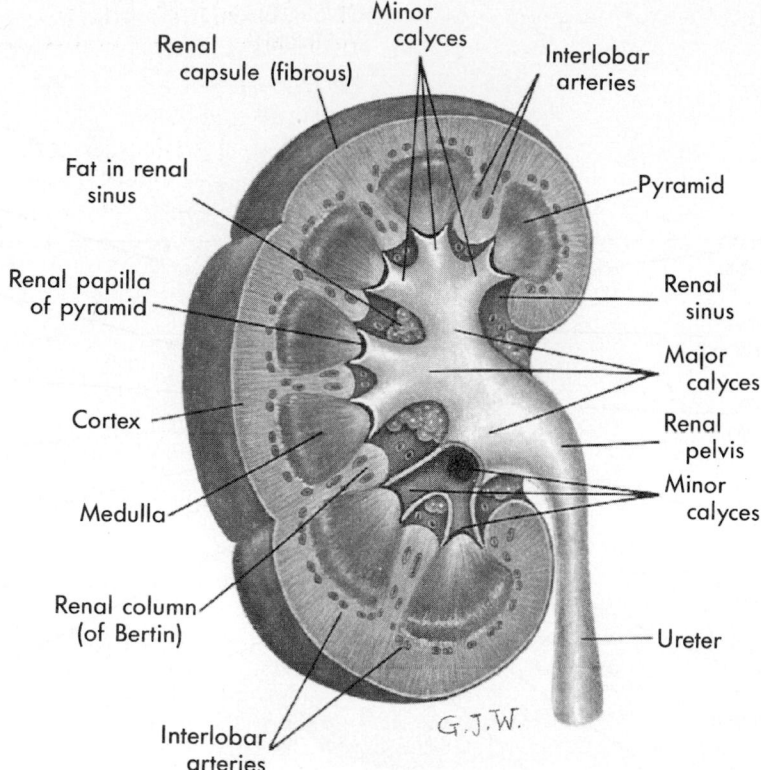

Figure 10-2 Cross-section of the kidney showing basic structures. (From Brundage DJ: *Mosby's clinical nursing series: renal disorders,* St Louis, 1992, Mosby.)

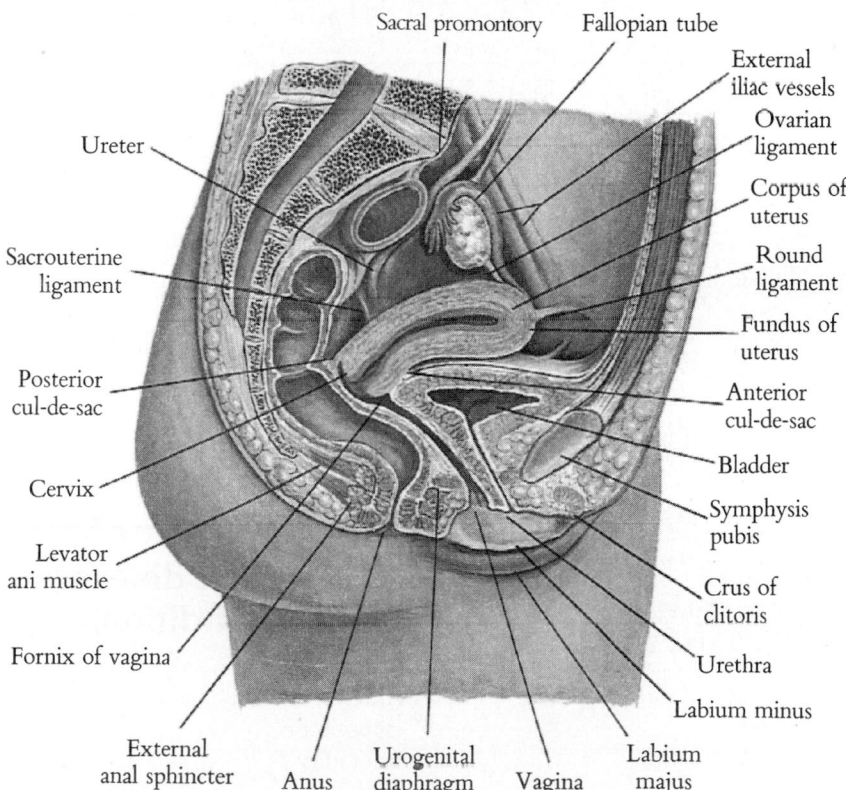

Figure 10-3 Midsagittal view of the female pelvic organs. (From Seidel HM et al: *Mosby's guide to physical examination,* ed 3, St Louis, 1995, Mosby.)

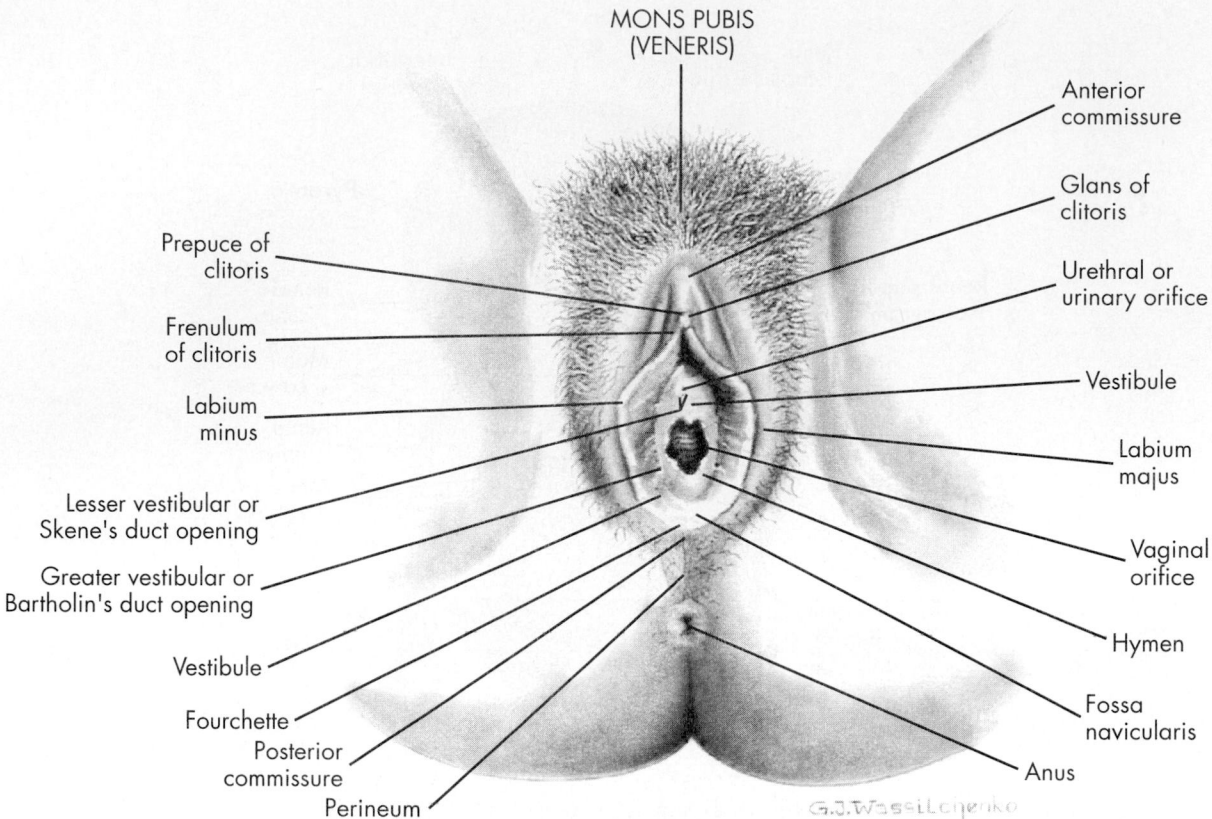

Figure 10-4 External female genitalia. (From Bobak IM: *Maternity and gynecologic care: the nurse and the family,* ed 5, St Louis, 1993, Mosby.)

Character of urine
  Color (clear, yellow, red, pink, rusty brown, tea, cola)
  Odor
  Amount
  Specific gravity
Indwelling catheter (type/date of insertion)
Vital signs
  Fever
  Tachycardia/bradycardia
  Hypotension/hypertension
Respiratory status
  Decreased breath sounds
  Crackles
  Rales
Mental status/behavior
  Disorientation/confusion
  Agitation
GI status
  Absent/decreased bowel sounds
  Abdominal distention/rigidity
  Weight (recent loss or gain >10 lb)
  Melena
  Hematemesis
  Urinelike odor to breath

Edema
  Generalized
  Positional
  Pitting
  Nocturnal
Mucous membranes
Jugular venous distention/flat neck veins
Skin turgor
Skin (dry, scaly, pale, black, yellow-tan)
Brittle nails

● Pertinent Background Information

Concurrent diseases and/or conditions

Anemia
Amenorrhea
Impotence
Infertility
Diabetes
Tuberculosis
Hormonal/endocrine imbalance

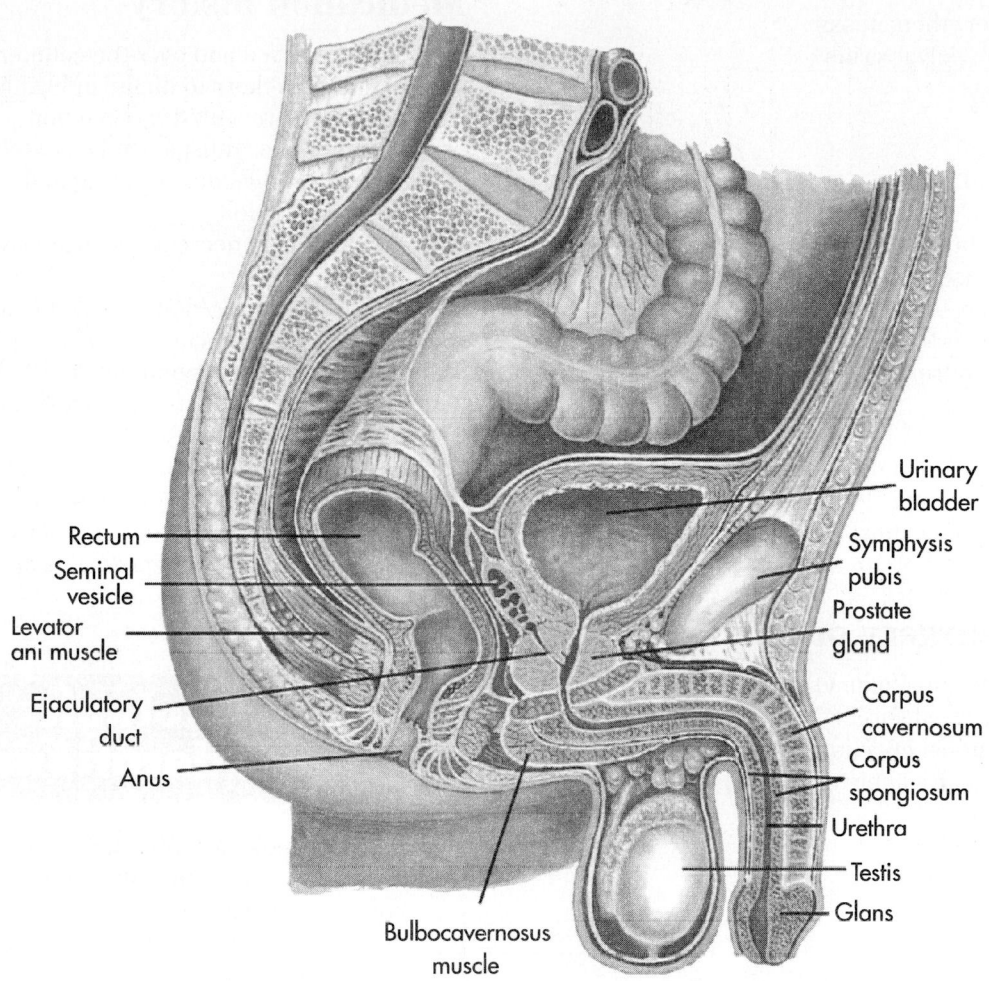

Urinary
bladder

Symphysis
pubis

Prostate
gland

Corpus
cavernosum

Corpus
spongiosum

Urethra

Testis

Glans

Rectum

Seminal
vesicle

Levator
ani muscle

Ejaculatory
duct

Anus

Bulbocavernosus
muscle

Figure 10-5 Male pelvic organs. (From Seidel HM et al: *Mosby's guide to physical examination,* ed 3, St Louis, 1995, Mosby.)

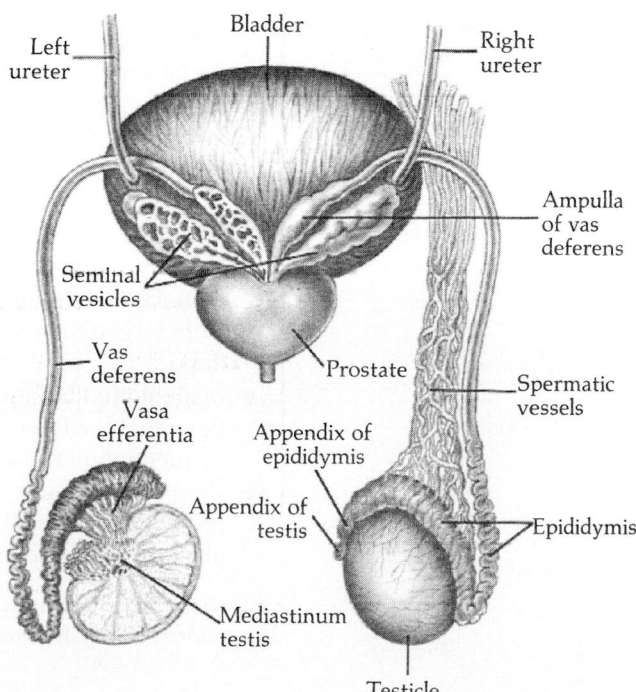

Bladder

Left
ureter

Right
ureter

Ampulla
of vas
deferens

Seminal
vesicles

Vas
deferens

Prostate

Spermatic
vessels

Vasa
efferentia

Appendix of
epididymis

Appendix of
testis

Epididymis

Mediastinum
testis

Testicle

Figure 10-6 Testes. (From Thompson JM et al: *Mosby's clinical nursing,* ed 3, St Louis, 1993, Mosby.)

Systemic lupus erythematosus
Vascular disease; polyarteritis
Sickle cell disease
Amyloidosis
Gout
Hyperparathyroidism
Cerebrovascular Accident (CVA)
Traumatic brain injury
Alzheimer's disease
Spinal cord injury
Transverse myelitis
Guillain-Barré syndrome
Hepatitis
AIDS
Cancer/leukemia (chemotherapy/radiation)
Dialysis (CAPD/hemodialysis)
Allergies (food, medication, environmental)

Previous surgery or illness

Genitourinary (trauma/injury)
Urologic and/or renal surgery
Urinary tract/vaginal infections
Gynecologic/obstetrical history (LMP, gravida para,
   forceps delivery)
Hepatitis
Tuberculosis
Neurologic disorders
Spinal cord disorders
Peripheral nervous system disorders

Family history

Renal and other types of cancer
Congenital anomalies/urologic disorders
Diabetes mellitus
Hypertension
Renal disease
Polycystic kidney disease
Lupus erythematosis

Social history

Marital status
Family structure
Employment status
Occupation
Exposure to chemicals
Sexual history (exposure to STDs)
Products used or hygiene (e.g., feminine sprays/soaps)
Use of caffeine
Use of illegal drugs
Smoking history

Medication history

Current prescribed and over-the-counter medications
   Adrenergic blockers to diminish bladder resistance
   Antibiotics to prevent/treat infection
   Anticholinergics/antispasmodics to relax smooth
      muscle in the bladder resulting in decreased invol-
      untary contraction
   Anticoagulants to decrease consistency of or thin
      blood
   Analgesics (narcotic/nonnarcotic to control pain)
   Alpha-adrenergic blockers to decrease bladder outlet
      resistance, manage symptoms of BPH
   Adrenergic agents to manage stress incontinence,
      enuresis, retrograde ejaculation
   Antidysrhythmics to regulate heart rate
   Antidepressants to manage depression associated
      with acute or chronic genitourinary conditions/
      diseases; tricyclic antidepressants also used to man-
      age incontinence

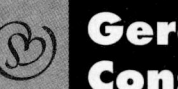

Gerontologic Considerations

- Urinary frequency, urgency, nocturia, and incontinence are common with aging. These occur because of weakened musculature in the bladder and urethra, diminished neurologic sensation combined with decreased bladder capacity, and the effects of medications such as diuretics.
- Urinary incontinence is a leading reason for institutional placement of older adults.
- Urinary incontinence can lead to a loss of self-esteem and result in decreased participation in social activities.
- Older women are particularly at risk for stress incontinence because of hormonal changes and weakened pelvic musculature.
- Older men are particularly at risk for urinary retention because of prostatic hypertrophy.
- Urinary tract infections in older adults are often associated with invasive procedures such as catheterization, diabetes, and neurologic disorders.
- Inadequate fluid intake, immobility, and conditions that lead to urinary stasis increase the risk of infection in the older adult.
- Frequent toileting and meticulous skin care can reduce the risk of skin impairment secondary to urinary incontinence.

From Christensen BL, Kockrow EO: *Foundations of nursing,* ed 2, St Louis, 1995, Mosby.

Antihypertensives to manage blood pressure (BP)

Chemotherapeutic agents to treat various types of cancer

Cholinergic agents to stimulate bladder contraction

Diuretics to increase renal excretion of water and solutes

Decongestants to decrease urinary output, manage incontinence

Erythrocyte-stimulating hormone to treat anemia resulting from chronic renal failure

Hormones to increase/decrease existing levels of hormones such as estrogens/androgens)

Immunosuppressive agents to reduce graft rejection after renal transplantation

Muscle relaxants to promote regular bladder emptying

Papaverine hydrochloride to manage erectile dysfunction

Stool softeners to decrease straining with bowel movements and therefore reduce pressure on genitourinary organs

Vasodilators to diagnose/treat impotence

Vitamins to replace/augment existing levels of vitamins/iron

Intravenous fluid/TPN therapy to replace/maintain necessary fluid volume, electrolyte levels

Blood transfusions to replace/maintain appropriate circulating blood volume

● Diagnostic Tests

Urinalysis
Color
Clarity
Odor
pH
Specific gravity
Osmolality
Sediment
Red blood cells (RBCs)
Pus
Bacteria
White blood cells (WBCs)
Casts
Crystals/calculi
Blood
Protein
Glucose
Creatinine
Urea
Uric acid
Electrolytes
  Sodium
  Potassium

  Chloride
  Calcium
  Phosphorus
  Magnesium
Urine culture and sensitivity
Urine collection (24 hr)
  Aldosterone
  17-hydroxycorticosteroids
  17-ketosteroids
  Catecholamines
    Norepinephrine
    Epinephrine
    Dopamine
  Stone analysis
    Oxylate
    Crystine
  VMA
  Calcium
  Phosphorus
  Uric acid
Urine clearance tests
  Inulin
  Creatinine
  Phenolsulfonphthalein (PSP)
Voiding diary
Blood analysis
  Osmolality
  Electrolytes
    Sodium
    Potassium
    Chloride
    Calcium
    Magnesium
    Phosphorus
    Alkaline phosphatase
  Blood urea nitrogen (BUN)
  Creatinine
  Uric acid
  Total protein
  Albumin
  Glucose
  Complete blood cell count (CBC)
  Coagulation factors
    Prothrombin time/INR (PT/INR)
    Activated partial thromboplastin time (APTT)
  Blood type and antibody screen
  Tissue compatibility testing
  Serum complement
  Antistreptolysin O-titer
  Hepatitis B and C antigens
  HIV antigen
  Tumor markers
    Prostatic specific antigen
    Alpha-fetoprotein (AFP)
    Human chorionic gonadotropin (HCG)

Wound/throat cultures
Radiographic studies
 Flat plate of abdomen
 Kidney, ureters, bladder (KUB)
 Excretory urogram
 Nephrotomogram
 Antegrade pyelogram
 Retrograde pyelogram
 Retrograde cystogram, voiding
  cystourethrogram
 Retrograde urethrogram
 Renal angiogram (renogram)
  Renal arteriogram
  Renal venogram
 Renal computed tomography (CT) scan
 Renal and prostate ultrasonography
Other tests
 Whitaker test
 Penile temescence tests
 Radionuclide imaging
 Endoscopic studies
  Cystoscopy
  Cystourethroscopy
  Ureteroscopy
  Percutaneous renal endoscopy (nephroscopy)
 Renal biopsy
 Urodynamic studies
  Cystometrogram
  Uroflowmetry
  Pressure flow study
  Urethral pressure profile
  Electromyography and electromyogram
  Dynamic infusion cavernosometry and
   cavernosography (DICC)
  Magnetic resonance imaging (MRI)
 Chest x-ray
 ECG
 Pulmonary function tests

Urinary Tract Infection

Infection, with or without symptoms, which occurs in the lower or upper urinary tract (Table 10-1); most urinary tract infections (UTIs) (80%) are caused by Escherichia coli; asymptomatic UTI is most common for persons over the age of 65; the percentage is increased for those in long-term care facilities or hospitals; risk and severity may be enhanced with conditions such as vesicoureteral reflux, urinary tract obstruction, urinary stasis, recent urethral instrumentation, septicemia, pregnancy, diabetes, and spinal cord injury

Assessment

See Table 10-1

Diagnostic tests

Urinalysis
 Cloudy
 Bacteria
 Pyuria
 WBCs
 RBCs may be present
Positive urine culture and sensitivity
Radiography
 KUB
 Excretory urography
 Cystoscopy
CBC: elevated WBC; often left shift

Potential complications

Dehydration
Bacteremia
Parenchymal scarring
Renal involvement
Urinary calculi
Abscess formation

Table 10-1	Symptoms of Urinary Tract Infection	
	Subjective	**Objective**
Lower UTI (cystitis, urethritis, prostatitis)	Suprapubic discomfort	Hematuria
	Lower back pain	Pyuria
	Bladder spasm	Malodorous urine
	Dysuria	Fever
	Urinary urgency	
	Urinary frequency	
	Nocturia	
Upper UTI* (pyelonephritis)	Flank pain	Enlarged kidney
	Malaise	Costovertebral tenderness
	Anorexia	Abdominal rigidity
	Nausea	Chill
		Vomiting
		Decreased urinary output

*Findings are in addition to those for lower UTI.

Collaborative management

Therapeutic management

Medications
  Antibiotics
  Antispasmodics
  Analgesics/antipyretics
Bed rest with gradual return to activities as tolerated
Oral or IV fluids
Cystoscopy/IVP
Urology consult
Infectious disease consult
Surgical intervention for obstruction
Follow-up cultures may be ordered
  Weeks one and four
  Every 3 to 4 months for 1 year for chronic UTI

Nursing management

PATIENT PROBLEMS/NURSING DIAGNOSES

● **NDX:** Infection related to presence of bacteria in the urinary tract

Assess temperature (T) q4h and report if >101°F (38.5°C), *which may indicate progressing infection*
Monitor character of urine and report if cloudy and malodorous, *which may indicate that present medication therapy is ineffective*
Collect repeat midstream urine for culture and sensitivity when no evidence of improvement is noted
Encourage high oral fluid intake *to promote systemic flushing of some bacteria* (unless fluid restriction is ordered/appropriate)
Offer cranberry juice *to prevent bacteria from sticking to bladder wall*
Instruct patient to void as soon as urge is felt and completely empty bladder; *these prevent overdistention of and decreased blood supply to the bladder and decrease chance for bacteria to colonize*
Encourage patient to shower rather than bathe; this promotes good hygiene without allowing bacteria to enter the urethra
Encourage good perineal hygiene by keeping perineal area clean and dry, *which discourages growth of bacteria*
Teach female patient to wipe perianal area from front to back *to decrease ability of bacteria to enter urinary tract*

EXPECTED OUTCOME

Exhibits no signs or symptoms of UTI (see Table 10-1)
Urine culture and sensitivity negative for bacteria

● **NDX:** Altered urinary elimination related to UTI

Monitor urinary output and report if <30 ml/hr, *which may indicate inadequate fluid volume*
Provide opportunities for patient to void q2h and prn (assist to bathroom and/or with urinal/bedpan)
Promote ability of patient on bed rest *to completely empty bladder* by assisting to upright position before patient voids
Advise patient to avoid drinking fluid for 2 to 3 hr before bedtime *to decrease nocturia*
Advise patient to avoid caffeine and alcohol, *which exacerbate irritative symptoms*

EXPECTED OUTCOMES

Maintains balanced fluid intake and output
Usual voiding pattern is resumed by patient
Reports absence of dysuria, urinary frequency and urgency, nocturia

● **NDX:** Pain related to UTI

Assess nature, intensity, location, duration, and precipitating and alleviating factors of pain *to establish baseline condition*
Provide bed rest *to promote healing and comfort;* increase activities as ordered/tolerated
Institute comfort measures (sitz baths, warm perineal soaks, relaxation techniques/guided imagery, diversional activities)
Encourage high oral fluid intake *to dilute urine and decrease dysuria*
Monitor and document response to efforts aimed at decreasing discomfort
Notify physician of unrelieved or increasing pain *to collaborate on alternate approaches*

EXPECTED OUTCOMES

Takes analgesics as needed
Verbal and nonverbal evidence of decrease in pain

ADDITIONAL NURSING DIAGNOSES TO CONSIDER

Self-esteem disturbance related to UTI
Altered sexuality patterns related to UTI
Impaired skin integrity related to bed rest/UTI

Patient/family teaching

Teach methods of preventing recurrence of UTI
  Force fluids to 2000 to 2500 ml/day unless restricted
  Avoid fluids that aggravate urinary tract (caffeinated beverages) and drink fluids that promote systemic flushing (e.g., water and cranberry juice)
  Empty bladder every q2h to 3h
  Shower rather than bathe and use antibacterial soap

Avoid using perfumed products in perineal area and
colored toilet tissue

Discourage douching unless ordered by physician

Keep perineal area clean and dry

Wipe from front to back when cleansing perineal
area

Void before and after sexual intercourse

Wear cotton underpants; avoid nylon underpants

Wear loose, nonrestrictive clothing

Teach about ordered medications: names, dosages,
schedules, purposes, and side effects; remind patient
taking Pyridium that urine may be orange in color

Home care considerations

Emphasize importance of ongoing outpatient care because of high incidence of recurrent infection

Teach symptoms of recurring UTI (e.g., dysuria, urgency, and frequency) and importance of reporting to
physician

Reinforce importance of completing prescribed medication therapy (patient with chronic infections may be
prescribed prophylactic medication after completion
of present antibiotic therapy)

Teach method and importance of obtaining midstream
specimen for culture and sensitivity after completion
of antibiotic therapy

Teach method of self-monitoring urine test for bacteria
(Microstix) (patient with chronic infections may be
asked to test frequently)

Advise patient to avoid taking over-the-counter medications without physician approval

Advise patient to take rest periods as needed during the
day

Urinary Calculi (Urolithiasis)

*Formation of stones in the kidney (pelvis or calyx) and
their passage in the path of urine flow; renal calculi
are classified according to their composition (usually
calcium, uric acid, cystine, phosphate, oxalate, or
struvite); urinary calculi may vary from a few
millimeters up to a size that occupies the entire renal
pelvis (Figure 10-7)*

Assessment

Subjective data

Pain (back, flank, abdominal, groin, colicky)
Nausea/vomiting
Chills
Dysuria
Frequency/urgency of urination

Objective data

Anxiety/distress
Hematuria (microscopic or gross)
Oliguria
Fever

Diagnostic tests

Serum BUN, creatinine, calcium, phosphorus, uric
acid: elevated results

Urinalysis: WBC, hematuria, abnormal color, bacteria,
crystals

Urine culture and sensitivity

Urine collection (24 hr): abnormal creatine
clearance/abnormal excretion of calcium, phosphorus, magnesium, uric acid, cystine,and oxalate

KUB: radiopaque stone

Renal ultrasound: stones identified

Renal CT scan: abnormalities of kidneys

Intravenous (IV) urogram: filling defects; ureteral dilation; hydronephrosis

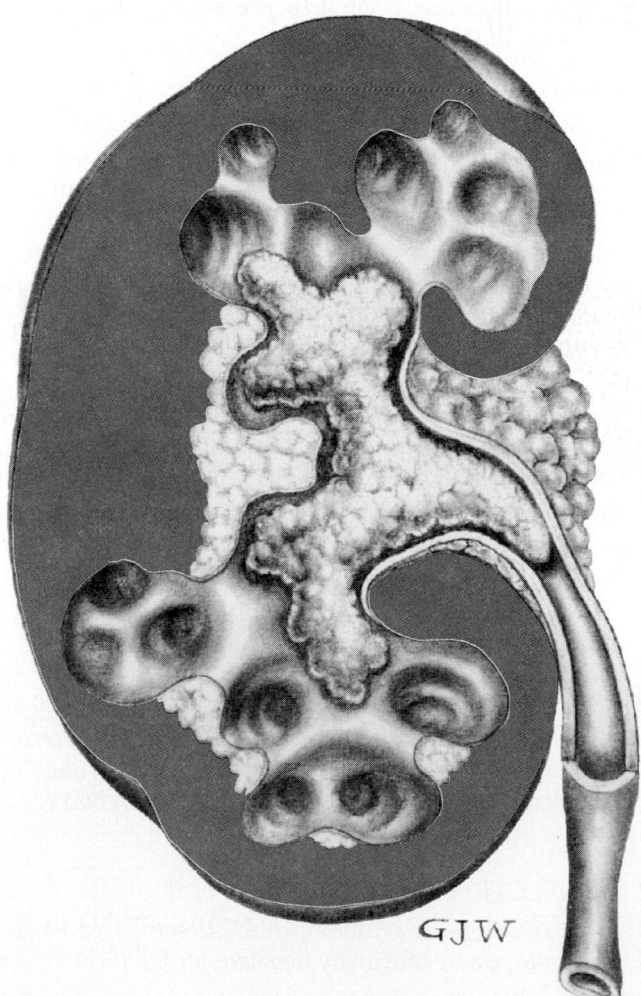

Figure 10-7 Staghorn calculus. (From Brundage DJ: *Mosby's
clinical nursing series: renal disorders,* St Louis, 1992, Mosby.)

Analysis of stones: constituents such as cystine, calcium, oxalate, uric acid

Potential Complications

Infection
Obstruction
Sepsis
Hydronephrosis
Renal failure
Kidney loss

Collaborative management

Therapeutic management

See Table 10-2 for treatment plan based on type of stone
Medications
  Analgesics
  Antispasmodics
  IV or oral fluids
Catheterization
Straining of all urine for stones and analysis
Urology consult
Endocrinology consult (to assess parathyroid function)
Dietary consult
Surgical interventions (Table 10-3)

Table 10-2 Therapeutic Management for Renal Calculi

TYPE OF STONE	TREATMENT PLAN
Calcium	Nonthiazide diuretics
	Low-calcium diet
	Oral phosphates
Uric acid	Allopurinol
	Sodium bicarbonate
	Sodium citrate
	Potassium phosphate
	Low-purine diet
Cystine	D-penicillamine
	Sodium bicarbonate
	Low-animal protein diet
Struvite	Penicillin
	Drugs to acidify urine

Table 10-3 Interventions for Urinary Calculi

STONE DISINTEGRATION

Extracorporeal shock wave lithotripsy (ESWL)
Carefully directed shock waves enter the body via a liquid medium, which surrounds the body and disintegrates the calculus

Laser lithotripsy
Endoscopy tube is threaded up the ureter to the stone, and laser energy is passed via a fine wire into the stone, breaking it into fine pieces

Percutaneous stone dissolution
Chemical agents are injected into the nephrostomy tube to dissolve the stone

Percutaneous ultrasonic lithotripsy (PUL)
Ultrasonic probe is inserted into renal pelvis, and pulses of ultrasound are administered to disintegrate the stone

STONE EXTRACTION

Endoscopic removal of stone
After tube is inserted via flank incision through the parenchyma into renal calyx, an endoscope is passed and the stone is extracted

Ureteroscopy and stone basket extraction
A flexible ureteroscope is passed transurethrally into ureter; a special collapsible wire basket instrument is inserted to snare the stone, which is then pulled out with the instrument

Pyelolithotomy
Removal of stone through an incision into the renal pelvis

Nephrolithotomy
Removal of stone through a longitudinal incision across the middle two thirds of the kidney

Ureterolithotomy
Removal of stone by incision into the ureter

Cystolithotomy
Removal of stone by incision into the bladder

Nephrectomy/partial nephrectomy
Removal of a kidney when extensive renal damage occurs

Nursing management

PATIENT PROBLEMS/NURSING DIAGNOSES

● **NDX:** Pain related to passage of renal stone(s) and/or surgical incision

Assess type, intensity, location, and duration of pain; document *so changes may be noted*

Identify verbal and nonverbal responses to pain

Monitor for syncopal episodes associated with renal colic

Offer analgesics, document effectiveness and tolerance *so treatment plan can be altered as needed*

Institute nonpharmacologic comfort measures
  Optimal positioning
  Restful environment
  Relaxation techniques/guided imagery
  Diversional activities

EXPECTED OUTCOMES

Patient is relaxed with no other evidence of pain

Reports increase in comfort level

● **NDX:** Altered urinary elimination, related to stone in path of urinary flow

Assess patient's usual voiding pattern and begin voiding diary *so changes can be noted*

Monitor for signs and symptoms of UTI (dysuria, frequency, urgency) and report to physician *for evaluation and treatment*

Maintain patency of catheters to *promote optimal flow of urine*
  Tubing below level of bladder *to allow for gravity flow*
  Assess for clamping/kinks in tubing
  Secure catheters while still allowing for patient movement
  Irrigate as ordered

Label each tube clearly and record drainage from each tube separately *to allow for accurate assessment of output from each system*

If nephrostomy tube in place
  Tape to flank
  Do not clamp
  Irrigate only with physician's order (may be continuous or intermittent)
  Have extra tube available at bedside
  Notify physician immediately if nephrostomy tube becomes dislodged

If double-J ureteral stent in place, check that suture from urinary meatus to stent is present (suture will be used to remove stent)

After urinary catheter is removed, institute measures *to facilitate voiding*
  Privacy

Comfortable positioning
  Running tap water
  Placing patient's hand in warm water
  Pouring warm water over perineum
  Relaxation techniques
  Applying oil of peppermint (a few drops in bedpan/ urinal or on cotton ball in front of urinary meatus)
  Stroking inner aspect of thigh gently with ice
  Offering analgesic
  Voiding 1 to 2 hr after fluid intake
  Double voiding (to empty bladder more completely)

Strain all urine for stones and send for analysis if found

Report, describe, and document passage of all stones

Encourage patient to drink at least 2500 ml/day (unless contraindicated) *to flush stones from system*

Monitor and report signs and symptoms of urinary retention (e.g., bladder distention) and report to physician

Monitor intake and output frequently *to identify imbalance requiring treatment*

EXPECTED OUTCOMES

Intake and output are balanced

All stones are passed

Regular voiding pattern is resumed

● **NDX:** Altered nutrition: less than body requirements related to nausea and vomiting

Identify factors contributing to nausea and vomiting; relieve as possible

Remove noxious sights/smells from room if possible

Monitor and document effectiveness/tolerance of ordered antiemetics

Instruct patient to change position slowly *to decrease GI upset*

Provide frequent oral hygiene *to decrease acidic taste in mouth, throat*

Encourage small, frequent meals *to prevent overdistention of the stomach*

Encourage patient to eat easily digestible foods (e.g., toast, crackers)

Encourage patient to eat slowly *for optimal digestion*

If emesis occurs, assess and document character and amount for physician evaluation

Request dietitian as needed

EXPECTED OUTCOME

Patient exhibits no nausea/vomiting

● **NDX:** Risk for impaired skin integrity related to wound drainage

Assess incisional site for signs and symptoms of infection (erythema, edema, pain, drainage) and report to physician

Change surgical dressings using sterile technique as
ordered

Inspect skin surrounding catheters and tubes and report redness, breakdown

Apply ostomy pouch and skin barrier around wounds
exposed to prolonged or copious urinary drainage *to
prevent excoriation*

EXPECTED OUTCOME

Skin is intact

Patient/family teaching

Explain purpose/procedure of ordered diagnostic
tests

Teach patient/family to care for incision and perform
ordered dressing changes; refer to home health
agency if needed

To help prevent UTI

Empty bladder every q2h to 3h

Drink 2000 to 3000 ml/day unless contraindicated;
(e.g., water, cranberry juice)

Avoid fluids that aggravate urinary tract (caffeinated
beverages)

Shower rather than bathe and use antibacterial soap

Keep perineal area clean and dry

Wipe from front to back when cleansing perianal area

Teach about ordered medications: names, dosages,
schedules, purposes, and side effects

Home care considerations

Emphasize importance of ongoing outpatient care

Teach patient and those in contact to use good handwashing techniques

Advise patient to take frequent rest periods during the
day and sleep 6 to 8 hr per night; increase activity as
ordered and tolerated

Encourage patient to avoid contact with persons who
have infections (e.g., colds, flu)

Encourage patient to report signs and symptoms of incisional infection (redness, swelling, pain, drainage)
to physician

Teach symptoms of UTI (dysuria, urgency, frequency,
foul-smelling urine, fever >101°F [38.5°C]) and encourage patient to report these findings to physician

Instruct patient to maintain ordered diet at home

Teach patient how to measure/strain urine; advise patient to save any passed stones or gravel and notify
physician when stones are passed

Advise patient to report abnormalities of urine to physician (e.g., frank hematuria)

Instruct patient how to collect 24 hr urine at home

Advise patient to avoid taking over-the-counter medications without physician approval

Acute Urinary Retention

*A condition in which the bladder becomes distended with
urine and the patient is unable to empty the bladder;
potential causes of acute urinary retention are
medications, constipation/fecal impaction, anxiety,
immobility from acute illness, obstruction, trauma,
postoperative complications, and muscle tension*

Assessment

Subjective data

Cessation of urination
Dribbling
Urinary frequency
Inability to start stream
Decrease in force of stream
Interruption of flow
Dysuria
Nocturia
Bladder/suprapubic tenderness
Restlessness
Anxiety

Objective data

Postvoid residual >100 ml
Output less than intake
Bladder distention
Diaphoresis

Diagnostic tests

Urinalysis: white/red blood cells, bacteria
Urine culture and sensitivity: bacteria
Serum electrolytes, BUN, creatinine: abnormal/
elevated results
KUB: abnormalities with kidneys, ureters, or bladder
Urodynamic studies: evidence of obstruction
Cystogram: obstruction/deficient contractility
IVP: obstructive uropathy

Potential complications

Urinary tract infection
Vesicoureteral reflex
Compromised/insufficient renal function

Collaborative management

Therapeutic management

Catheterization
Voiding schedule/program

Urology consult
Medications
  Antibiotics (if infection present)
  Cholinergics to stimulate bladder contraction
  Adrenergic blocking drug to diminish bladder
    resistance
  Analgesics
  IV fluids (for postobstructive diuresis syndrome)
Pharmacology consult
Surgical resection or laser ablation of obstructive lesion
Dilation of stricture or surgical repair of pelvic descent

Nursing management

PATIENT PROBLEMS/NURSING DIAGNOSES

● **NDX:** Urinary retention related to obstruction or neuromuscular dysfunction

Assess bladder frequently for distention/tenderness
  and document changes *so collaborative treatments can
  be instituted*
Monitor intake and output *to determine imbalances re-
  quiring interventions*
Institute measures that facilitate bladder emptying
  Privacy
  Comfortable positioning
  Running tap water
  Placing patient's hand in warm water
  Applying heat to suprapubic area (if ordered)
  Pouring warm water over perineum
  Relaxation techniques
  Applying oil of peppermint (a few drops in bedpan/
    urinal or on cotton ball in front of urinary meatus)
  Stroking inner aspect of thigh gently with ice
  Offering analgesic
  Voiding 1 to 2 hr after fluid intake
  Double voiding (to empty bladder more completely)
Monitor and document effectiveness/tolerance of med-
  ications *so changes can be made when required*
Apply ice to perineum *to decrease swelling when ordered*
Check postvoid residual *to determine whether bladder is
  emptying effectively;* report if >100 ml
Catheterize patient as ordered using sterile technique
  to minimize risk of infection
If unable to pass catheter (sign of obstruction) remove
  and report to physician
If bright red urine occurs after decompression (sign of
  tissue damage, irritation, or inflammation), notify
  physician
Monitor for and report postobstructive diuresis; urine
  output >200 ml/hr
Vital signs (VS), intake and output, and serum and
  urine electrolytes must be assessed frequently *for evidence of abnormalities*

EXPECTED OUTCOMES
Intake and output are in balance
Regular voiding pattern is established

● **NDX:** Pain related to bladder fullness and inability to void

Assess and document type, intensity, location, and dura-
  tion of pain
Identify factors that precipitate and alleviate pain
Offer analgesics, documenting effectiveness and
  tolerance *to determine need for treatment plan change*
Institute nonpharmacologic comfort measures
  Optimal positioning
  Sitz baths/warm perineal soaks
  Relaxation techniques/guided imagery
  Diversional activities

EXPECTED OUTCOME
Patient is relaxed, without other evidence of pain, and
  reports increased comfort

ADDITIONAL NURSING DIAGNOSES
TO CONSIDER
Risk for infection related to frequent home catheteriza-
  tion
Self-esteem disturbance related to need for home self-
  catheterization

Patient/family teaching

To help prevent UTI
  Empty bladder q2h to 3h
  Encourage patient to take fluids to 2000 to 3000
    ml/day (unless contraindicated) to flush bacteria
    from system
  Avoid fluids that aggravate urinary tract (e.g., caf-
    feinated beverages) and drink fluids that promote
    systemic flushing (e.g., water and cranberry juice)
  Shower rather than bathe and use antibacterial soap
  Keep perineal area clean and dry
  Wipe from front to back when cleansing perianal area
Teach about ordered medications: names, dosages,
  schedules, purposes, and side effects

Home care considerations

Teach/reinforce method of self-catheterization
  (Table 10-4)
Teach care of foley catheter and drainage units
Emphasize importance of ongoing outpatient care
Teach symptoms of UTI (dysuria, urgency, frequency,
  foul-smelling urine, fever >101°F [38.5°C]) and
  encourage patient to report these findings to physi-
  cian

Table 10-4 Instructions for Self-Catheterization

EQUIPMENT

Catheter
Soap/water
Water-soluble lubricant
Washcloth
Mirror
Pan/toilet
Measuring container
Storage container

PREPARATION

Try to urinate (measure output)
Wash hands thoroughly with soap and water
Assume appropriate/comfortable position
Position mirror if needed

PROCEDURE

Men
Wash and rinse end of penis with soap and water
  (pull back foreskin if not circumcised)
Lubricate first 2 inches of catheter
Hold penis in nondominant hand and extend out
  from body
Slowly insert catheter into urethra (7 to 10 inches)
  until urine begins flowing
Allow all urine to drain into measuring container
Slowly remove catheter; if urine begins to flow again,
  stop until drainage ends, then continue to
  remove catheter
Replace foreskin to normal position
Measure/record amount

Women
Separate vaginal folds with fingers of nondominant hand and
  cleanse perineal area with soap
Lubricate tip of catheter
Hold catheter in dominant hand
Using nondominant hand to keep vaginal folds open, insert
  catheter into urethra (about 3 inches) until urine begins
  flowing
Press down with abdominal muscles to help empty bladder
  into measuring container
Allow all urine to drain
Remove catheter when urine flow stops
Measure/record amount

AFTER PROCEDURE

Wash penis/perineal area to remove lubricant
Wash catheter in soap and water, rinse well
Dry catheter and wrap in clean towel
Place in clean container for storage in clean area
Wash hands

Instruct patient to measure urine after voiding and note
  character of urine, time, amount, and force of stream
  (use voiding diary if appropriate)
Advise patient to avoid taking over-the-counter medications without physician approval

Indwelling Urethral Catheter Management

*A catheter inserted through the urethra into the bladder
  to drain urine (Figure 10-8)*

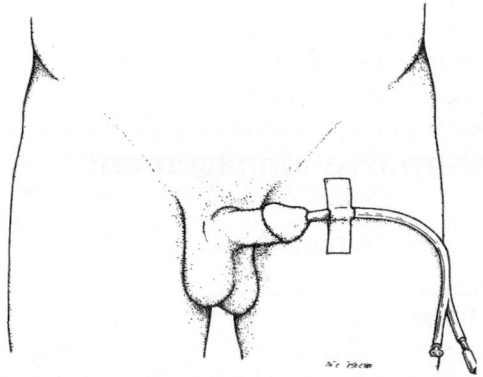

Figure 10-8 Indwelling urethral catheter.

Assessment

Subjective data

While catheter is in place
  Bladder spasms
  Sensation of needing to void
  Discomfort/pulling at catheter insertion site
After catheter removal
  Inability to urinate
  Difficulty initiating urine stream
  Small urinary stream
  Dysuria
  Frequency/urgency with urination

Objective data

While catheter is in place
  Distended bladder
  Fever
  Chills
  Pyuria
  Hematuria
  Edema of urethral meatus
After catheter removal
  Urinary retention with overflow
  Hematuria
  Dribbling
  Incontinence

Diagnostic tests

Urinalysis: cloudy, malodorous, WBC, RBC, bacteria
Urine culture and sensitivity: bacteria

Potential complications

Recurrent and/or progressive UTI
Septicema
Urinary tract calculi
Strictures
Urethral erosion
Epididymitis
Difficulty in voiding after removal

Collaborative management

Therapeutic management

Medications
  Antibiotics
  Local anesthetic agents
  Stool softeners
Periodic catheter change

Nursing management

PATIENT PROBLEM/NURSING DIAGNOSIS

● **NDX:**   Altered urinary elimination related to presence of indwelling urethral catheter

Monitor intake and output frequently *to determine imbalances that require treatment*
Palpate bladder *to determine whether distention is present*
Maintain patency of catheter *to promote optimal drainage*
  Avoid clamping or occluding catheter
  Irrigate catheter as ordered
  Keep catheter drainage unit and tubing below level of bladder
Maintain integrity of closed gravity drainage system at all times *to decrease risk of infection;* change system per policy (usually q4days)
Maintain tension-free catheter
  Tape drainage tubing to inner aspect of lateral thigh or use catheter strap (female)
  Tape catheter to abdomen or upper thigh or use catheter strap (male)
Cleanse periurethral area bid to promote hygiene and comfort
Apply anesthetic ointment to urethral meatus if ordered
Collect urine specimens only by aspirating urine through catheter collection port with sterile 10 ml syringe and 25-gauge needle
After urinary catheter is removed, institute measures to facilitate voiding
  Privacy
  Comfortable positioning
  Running tap water
  Placing patient's hand in warm water
  Applying heat to suprapubic area (if ordered)
  Pouring warm water over perineum
  Relaxation techniques
  Applying oil of peppermint (a few drops in bedpan/urinal or on cotton ball in front of urinary meatus)
  Stroking inner aspect of thigh gently with ice
  Offering analgesic
  Voiding every q1h to 2h after fluid intake
  Double voiding (to empty bladder more completely)
Report abnormalities in urine, residual volume >100 ml and/or retention of urine with overflow to physician

EXPECTED OUTCOMES
Patient experiences no symptoms of infection while catheter is in place or after removal

Voids without evidence of complications after removal of catheter

ADDITIONAL NURSING DIAGNOSES
TO CONSIDER

Body image disturbance related to presence of indwelling urethral catheter at discharge

Anxiety related to ability to care for indwelling urethral catheter

Patient/family teaching

Explain to patient that presence of catheter may cause urge to urinate

To help prevent UTI

Encourage patient to maintain fluid intake of 2000 to 3000 ml/day (unless contraindicated) to flush bacteria from system

Avoid fluids that aggravate urinary tract (caffeinated beverages) and drink fluids that promote systemic flushing (e.g., water and cranberry juice)

Teach about ordered medications: names, dosages, schedules, purposes, and side effects

Home care considerations

Teach/reinforce method of caring for indwelling urinary catheter (Table 10-5)

Emphasize importance of ongoing outpatient care

Teach patient how to cleanse periurethral area

Advise patient to report absence of urine, persistent leaking around catheter, accidental removal of catheter, and back pain to home health nurse or physician

Teach signs and symptoms of UTI (dysuria, urinary urgency and frequency, foul-smelling urine, fever >101°F [38.5°C]) and encourage patient to report these findings to physician

Advise patient to avoid taking over-the-counter medications without physician approval

Urinary Incontinence

Urinary incontinence is the involuntary loss of urine; incontinence affects more than 12 million people in this country: at some time, 26% of women between ages 30 and 59 are incontinent, 15% to 30% of the noninstitutionalized population 60 and older are incontinent; risk and severity of incontinence may be related to existing medical conditions and diseases, urinary or vaginal infections, surgical history, childbearing history, hormonal changes, sexual history, age, obesity, physical condition, and certain

medications; a variety of mechanisms may be involved, and incontinence may be classified into five types: functional, stress, reflex, urge, and total

functional incontinence: *The involuntary loss of urine that is unpredictable and occurs when continent people are unable or unwilling to get to the bathroom on time; there is no impairment of the urinary system*

stress incontinence: *The involuntary loss of 50 ml or less of urine occurring with increased intraabdominal pressure; this type of incontinence is associated with decreased tone of the pelvic floor muscles, damage to the internal sphincter bladder neck caused by surgery, trauma, or radiation, decreased estrogen levels, or UTI*

reflex incontinence: *The involuntary loss of urine at fairly predictable intervals; the detrusor contraction is stimulated by a full bladder; the bladder empties, but a large residual usually remains; this type of incontinence is associated with spinal cord lesions above S-2 to S-4, traumatic injuries, tumors, multiple sclerosis, other demyelinating diseases, and some cerebral lesions*

Table 10-5 Instructions for Care of Indwelling Urethral Catheter

PROCEDURE

Wash hands with soap and water before and after handling catheter or drainage unit

Care of collecting bags, leg bags, and tubing

Wash with soap and water

Soak for 15 min in a mild vinegar *or* bleach solution

Rinse with lukewarm water

Protect end of catheter with clean gauze square when disconnecting and before reconnecting catheter to clean drainage system

REMINDERS

Empty drainage bag once q8h or as soon as it fills

Avoid clamping or kinking tubing

Empty the bag by loosening the clamp on the end of the leg or bedside bag

Always keep the drainage bag lower than the bladder

Catheter should be changed when it becomes obstructed, falls out, or drainage tubing is coated with grit and sediment (some policies indicate q4wk)

urge incontinence: The involuntary loss of urine occurring after a strong urge is felt, but the patient is unable to hold the urine long enough to reach the bathroom or receptacle; this type of incontinence is associated with detrusor instability caused by disorders of the central nervous system such as CVA, Parkinson's disease, Alzheimer's disease, or brain tumors or trauma; bladder irritation caused by infection or ingestion of irritating fluids or overdistention of the bladder related to increased fluid intake or decreased intervals between voiding may also result in urge incontinence

total incontinence: The involuntary, unpredictable, or continuous loss of urine; this type of incontinence is associated with neurologic diseases or conditions, anatomic deficits such as fistulae or damage from surgery, trauma, or radiation

Assessment (all types)

Urinary incontinence is considered a symptom of an underlying problem or condition rather than a disease process in itself; Table 10-6 compares the five types of urinary incontinence

Diagnostic tests

Voiding diary
Nocturia
Urinary frequency (more often than q2h)
Urinary urgency
Leakage of urine after coughing, lifting, or exercising
Postvoid residual: urine remaining in the bladder (>50 ml) immediately after voiding
Urodynamic testing: reduced bladder and urethral sphincter function
Voiding cystourethrogram: bladder distends below inferior margin of symphysis pubis when patient is upright
IVP: normal unless complicated by UTI or other condition such as ectopic ureter
Cystoscopy: abnormalities in bladder and lower urinary tract
Urinalysis culture and sensitivity: infection, hematuria
Bladder biopsy: abnormal bladder cells

Collaborative management

Therapeutic management

See Table 10-6 for a comparison of the five types of urinary incontinence
Urology consult
Pharmacology consult/evaluation
Occupational therapy consult
Physical therapy consult: general and pelvic exercise programs

Dietary consult: weight reduction if necessary
Psychological consult/support

Nursing management

INCONTINENCE, ALL TYPES

PATIENT PROBLEMS/NURSING DIAGNOSES

● **NDX:** Impaired skin integrity related to urinary incontinence

Assess perineal area for redness, irritation, swelling, or breakdown and document initial findings *so subsequent changes may be identified and treated*
Cleanse skin with mild soap and water or nonrinse cleaners and dry well after each incontinent episode *to prevent irritation of skin surfaces*
Apply skin barrier, protective spray, or sealant q8h to 12h and after each episode of incontinence *to prevent breaks in integrity*
Keep bed linen dry and wrinkle free *to decrease shearing effect on skin surfaces*
Use absorbent products, briefs, shields, or underpants if incontinent episodes are frequent *to provide optimal protection from urine on skin surfaces*
Be certain plastic does not touch skin and *cause maceration from increased perspiration*
Apply external collection device to further protect skin if incontinence continues and skin shows signs of breakdown
  Males
    Condom catheter with drainage bag
      Check penis regularly *for excoriation or constriction* and condom *for twisting and pooling of urine*
    Retracted penis pouch with drainage bag
      Clip pubic hair and apply skin protective barrier film before applying
      Check regularly for excoriation and adherence
  Females
    Prepare skin and apply external device
    Check regularly for excoriation
    Connect external devices to collection system
    Coil tubing *to prevent dependent loops and urine stasis*
    Keep drainage bag below bladder at all times *to promote gravity drainage*

EXPECTED OUTCOME
Skin remains intact

● **NDX:** Body image disturbance related to urinary incontinence

Provide an accepting and supportive atmosphere *to maintain patient's self-esteem and promote verbalization of feelings, fears, concerns, and questions*

Table 10-6 Incontinence Assessment and Therapeutic Management

Factors	Functional Incontinence	Stress Incontinence	Reflex Incontinence	Urge Incontinence	Total Incontinence
SPECIFIC ASSESSMENT					
Character of voiding urge	Usually strong	Sudden, associated with increased abdominal pressure	None	Very strong with inability to delay voiding	None
Amount voided	Moderate to large	Small, usually <50 ml	Moderate	Small to large	Constant leakage
Nocturia (more than two times)	May be present	Not usual	Always	Common	Always
Frequency of urination (more than q2h)	Variable	Increased	Regular intervals related to volume	Increased	Constant, unpredictable
Awareness of incontinence	Aware	Aware	Unaware; however, sympathetic response may be present: diaphoresis, flushing of skin, "gooseflesh," nausea	Aware	Unaware
Precipitating factors	Inability to reach receptacle Environmental problems, e.g., lack of privacy, siderails up on bed Physical, mental disabilities	Increased intra-abdominal pressure Obesity Laughing Coughing Sneezing Lifting Exercise	Full bladder Bladder contraction or spasm	Sensation of full bladder and inability to reach receptacle on time Catheter use Increased fluids Increased urine concentration Alcohol, caffeine use	Unpredictable
THERAPEUTIC MANAGEMENT					
	Evaluate medication regimen and change as necessary and possible Behavioral therapy Evaluate and change environmental factors	Surgery Vesicourethral suspension Artificial urinary sphincter Periurethral injection Alpha-adrenergics Estrogen therapy Anticholinergics Skin care management	Intermittent catheterization External catheter drainage Surgery; continent diversion Indwelling catheter (last resort) Skin care management	Medications Anticholinergics Antispasmodics Treatment of infections Evaluate diuretic therapy and change when possible; e.g., schedule Reduced-calorie diet if obese Skin care management	Surgery Repair fistulas Correct congenital defect Artificial sphincter Urinary diversion External collecting devices Skin care management

Modified from McFarland GK, McFarlane EA: *Nursing diagnosis and intervention: planning for patient care*, ed 2, St Louis, 1993, Mosby.

Determine how incontinence has affected patient's daily activities and sexual activity in order *to provide emotional support* and suggest methods of problem management

Identify positive features of patient's life *to promote feelings of self-worth*

Offer assistance from other professionals (psychologist, sexual counselor) *to assist with the management of emotional changes*

Encourage communication with significant other(s) and/or members of support group *to decrease feelings of isolation*

EXPECTED OUTCOMES

Participates in ADLs at optimal level

Comfortably discusses feelings, fears, concerns, and questions

Identifies approaches for making positive changes in daily activities

Accepts assistance from professionals and support group

FUNCTIONAL INCONTINENCE

● **NDX:** Functional incontinence related to sensory, cognitive, or motor deficits or altered environment

In collaboration with physician and pharmacist, assess effect of medications and determine whether changes may decrease risk of incontinence

Monitor intake and output *to determine whether appropriate fluid balance is maintained*

Adjust fluid intake so that largest amounts are taken at time of day when patient feels attempts at continence will be successful

Advise patient to maintain fluid intake of at least 2000 ml/day (unless contraindicated) *to ensure adequate fluid intake and output*

Cognitive deficit

Assess and document cognitive deficit *so that individualized and appropriate voiding program may be established*

Plan a fixed voiding schedule (q2h) *to eliminate incontinence and assist patient with voiding as needed*

Document times of voiding *so that accurate records may be referred to as needed to update plan of care*

Positively reinforce successes in maintaining continence *to promote self-esteem and motivation*

Motor/sensory deficits

Identify and document sensory or motor deficits that may inhibit patient from reaching bathroom or receptacle in time to void *so that necessary assistance may be provided*

Provide equipment to enable patient to eliminate alone: bedpan or urinal within reach, trapeze or walkers for easy movement, bedside commode, elevated toilet seats, bar in bathrooms

Determine optimal interval between voiding to prevent incontinence *to establish individualized and appropriate voiding program*

Slowly increase intervals between voidings; optimal time to reach is q3h to 4h

Assess pain and comfort level so that analgesics or nonpharmacologic methods of pain control may be employed before established voiding times

Altered environment

Assess environment *to determine obstacles that may inhibit patient's ability to reach toileting facilities in adequate time*

Institute safety measures

Orient to location of bathroom and/or placement of toileting equipment

Remove obstacles (e.g., furniture, belongings) from path to bathroom

Keep bed in low position

Use night light or keep bathroom door ajar with light on

Maintain privacy so patient will be comfortable voiding

Place call light within reach and answer promptly *to promote success with voiding program*

Suggest bed clothes that permit easy removal before voiding

EXPECTED OUTCOMES

Exhibits no sign of injury

Fluid intake is at least 2000 ml/day (unless contraindicated)

Intake and output are balanced

Establishes and maintains voiding program

Remains continent

STRESS INCONTINENCE

● **NDX:** Stress incontinence related to weak pelvis and structure supports, overdistention between voidings, or high intraabdominal pressure

Observe urinary meatus to check for leakage when patient has a full bladder and document/report findings to determine effectiveness of treatment plan

Instruct patient to cough while in lithotomy position; if no leakage, repeat with patient at 45-degree angle; continue with patient standing if no previous leakage

Weak pelvic and structural supports

Instruct in techniques aimed at strengthening pelvic muscles (pubococcygeus)

Kegel exercises

Identify pelvic muscles by doing the following:

Tightening muscles around anus while sitting or standing

Starting and stopping urine flow while voiding
Keeping buttocks, thigh, and abdominal muscles relaxed
Perform quick Kegel exercises: tighten and relax pelvic muscles as rapidly as possible
Perform slow Kegel exercises: tighten muscle group and hold for count of 10, then relax
Pull in—push out exercises
Use pelvic and abdominal muscles to pull up pelvic floor as though trying to suck water
Push out or bear down to push imaginary water out
Daily schedule
Week 1: do 10 of each exercise (quick and slow Kegel exercises and pull in—push out exercises) qid
Each succeeding week increase exercises by five, completing four sets a day
Results should be seen in about 3 months
Teach method for using weighted cones *to increase muscle tone*
Insert weighted cone vaginally
Contract pelvic muscles to retain cone for 15 min
Perform bid
Increase weight of cone as ordered
Instruct patient to tighten pelvic muscles before coughing, laughing, or any activity that increases abdominal pressure to prevent leakage
Overdistention
Assess factors leading to overdistention: increased fluid intake, use of diuretics, or decreased frequency of urination resulting from immobility, unwillingness to ask for assistance
Assess abdomen for bladder distention immediately after an episode of incontinence *to determine whether urine is being retained*
Discuss reasons for voiding frequently (preventing bladder irritation, decreasing potential for UTI)
Plan a fixed voiding schedule
Set interval shorter than that in which incontinence occurs, such as q2h, to ensure sufficient time in which to prepare for voiding; assist with voiding as needed
Teach to double or triple void
Identify factors that may interfere with patient's attempts to maintain continence to amend plan of care as needed
Provide positive reinforcement for continent behavior
High intraabdominal pressure
Discuss with patient that weight reduction may decrease incidence of incontinence by reducing pressure on the bladder
Dietitian to counsel patient
Institute nutritionally sound weight-loss program
Patient to make daily menu selections within restrictions

Physical therapist to coordinate appropriate exercise regimen
Weigh weekly to determine effectiveness of reduction plan
Promote motivation and compliance by praising efforts to comply with treatment plan

EXPECTED OUTCOMES
Performs pelvic muscle exercises daily and experiences fewer episodes of incontinence
Voids on a regular schedule without bladder distention
Complies with diet/exercise program

REFLEX INCONTINENCE

● **NDX:** Reflex incontinence related to neurologic impairment

Assess for signs and symptoms patient may experience before incontinence (e.g., diaphoresis, flushing, pilomotor response, or nausea)
In collaboration with physician, identify acceptable residual urine volume
Perform catheterization with sterile technique *to decrease occurrence of UTI and bladder changes*
Report residual volume more than that determined acceptable and amend plan of care as needed (e.g., intermittent catheterization)
Before expected voiding, place patient in optimal voiding position
Assess for autonomic dysreflexia (hyperreflexia): pounding headache, blurred vision, hypertension, profuse diaphoresis above level of spinal injury, severe pilomotor response and pale skin appearing below injury level, nausea, restlessness, and nasal congestion; *if these findings exist,* elevate head of bed, empty bladder (to alleviate symptoms), and immediately notify physician
Help patient to identify activities that may stimulate voiding so that these may be avoided or used to initiate voiding when needed (e.g., stroking inner thigh, anal stimulation, stroking vulva or glans penis)
Encourage patient to initiate voiding or perform self-catheterization before social activities, trips
Advise patient to carry self-catheterization equipment for use when unplanned delays occur

EXPECTED OUTCOMES
Intake and output are balanced
Uses triggering mechanism to initiate voiding; residual volume is within prescribed limits *or*
Empties bladder via self-catheterization with a volume not >300 ml

URGE INCONTINENCE

● **NDX:** Urge incontinence related to decreased bladder capacity, bladder irritability, overdistention of the bladder, or neurologic deficits

In collaboration with physician and pharmacist, assess effect of medications and determine whether changes may decrease risk of incontinence
Motor/sensory deficits (see Functional incontinence p. 660)
Overdistention (see Stress incontinence p. 661)
Irritable bladder
  Assess for symptoms of UTI (e.g., dysuria, cloudy urine); obtain culture and report to physician
  Discuss need to avoid irritating fluids such as drinks with caffeine or alcohol

EXPECTED OUTCOMES
Remains continent and is able to increase interval between voidings without episodes of incontinence

TOTAL INCONTINENCE

● **NDX:** Total incontinence related to neurologic dysfunction; independent contraction of detrusor reflex caused by surgery, trauma, or radiation; or anatomical problems such a fistulae

Assess type of incontinence in collaboration with physician using voiding diary and checking for residual
Provide absorbent briefs, undergarments, and underpads; plan schedule for routine changes q1h to 2h during period when most fluids are being taken, q2h to 3h during sleep periods
Encourage patient to increase level of self-care when able

EXPECTED OUTCOMES
Wet garments are changed on a regular basis
Assumes increased responsibility for self-care

ADDITIONAL NURSING DIAGNOSES TO CONSIDER (FOR ALL TYPES OF INCONTINENCE)
Altered role performance related to inability to engage in usual ADLs
Isolation related to inability to communicate feelings and relate to others

Patient/family teaching

Assist patient in identifying urinary elimination pattern by explaining how to organize voiding diary and evaluate findings

Help patient identify how voiding schedule will be incorporated into daily activities
Discuss methods for preventing and managing unexpected incontinence
  Void before social activities, trips
  Carry a change of clothing for use when unexpected episodes of incontinence occur
  Plan sexual activity for times when bladder is empty *to decrease chances of incontinence during this time*
  Discuss availability of undergarments or shields with absorbent materials
Teach about ordered medications: names, dosages, schedules, purposes, and side effects

Home care considerations

Encourage patient to maintain voiding diary and schedule at home
Discuss need to perform ADLs and resume self-care within capabilities
Teach symptoms of UTI and encourage patient to report these to physician
Teach signs of skin impairment, early action to take, and when to report to physician
Encourage patient with weakened pelvic muscles to perform appropriate exercises (e.g., Kegel exercises) daily
Review techniques to control odor of urine
Discuss importance of maintaining fluid intake at 2000 to 2500 ml/day (unless contraindicated); explain that decreased fluid intake does not reduce episodes of incontinence
Reinforce need to evaluate episodes of incontinence for precipitating factors and to make changes as necessary; report continued incontinence
Encourage patient to continue communicating with others who are supportive: significant other(s) or support group
Emphasize need to keep regular laboratory and follow-up appointments
Reinforce need to continue weight reduction (if needed) and exercise program
Discuss care and storage of equipment: catheters, external collection devices
Help patient evaluate home environment for necessary modifications
Provide information about available resources for individuals with incontinence (see box on p. 663)

Surgery for Female Urinary Incontinence

Marshall-Marchetti-Krantz operation: A surgical procedure for correcting stress incontinence; the urethra and vesical neck of the bladder are suspended

Incontinence Information and Support

Alliance for Aging Research (bladder training)
2021 K Street, N.W.
Suite 305
Washington, DC 20006

Continence Restored, Inc.
785 Park Avenue
New York, NY 10021

Help for Incontinent People
P.O. Box 544
Union, SC 29379

SIMON Foundation for Continence
P.O. Box 835
Wilmette, IL 60091

to restore the normal vesicourethral angle by suturing the paraurethral anterior vaginal wall to the periosteum of the symphysis pubis and the lower rectal fascia via suprapubic incision
Pareya procedure: *A surgical procedure performed vaginally to restore the normal vesicourethral angle, thus decreasing stress incontinence; the urethra and vesical neck are suspended by suturing the anterior vaginal wall to the rectal fascia*
Other procedures include Pereya-Raz, Stame, and Buret

Assessment

Subjective data (postoperative)

After urinary catheter removal
  Dysuria
  Urinary frequency/urgency
  Inability to start urine stream
  Incisional pain

Objective data (postoperative)

Decreased urinary output
Unbalanced fluid intake and output
Cloudy, foul-smelling urine
Incisional erythema or edema

Diagnostic tests (preoperative)

Urinalysis: white/red blood cells, bacteria
Urine culture and sensitivity
Cystoscopy: abnormalities with bladder/urethra
Urodynamic testing: reduced bladder and urethral sphincter function
Urine flow rate measurement: abnormal urinary flow patterns
Urethral pressure profile: abnormal urethral pressure during bladder filling/micturation
Whitaker test: abnormal pressure between renal pelvis and ureterovesical junction

Potential complications

UTI and postoperative complications
  Atelectasis
  Thrombophlebitis
  Pulmonary embolism
  Paralytic ileas
  Wound infection

Collaborative management

Therapeutic management

Medications
  Antibiotics
  Analgesics
  Stool softeners
  IV fluids
NPO until bowel sounds present
Indwelling urethral catheter and/or suprapubic catheter
Voiding schedule/program (after catheter removed)
Intermittent self-catheterization

Nursing management

PATIENT PROBLEMS/NURSING DIAGNOSES

● **NDX:** Pain related to surgical incision and manipulation of organs

Assess and document type, intensity, location, and duration of pain *so changes can be noted and interventions implemented*
Identify verbal and nonverbal responses to pain
Ensure that urethral catheter and/or suprapubic tube are patent *to promote optimal drainage and prevent pressure from urinary backflow*
Tape catheters securely *to prevent pulling sensation and irritation*
Apply anesthetic ointment to swollen urethral meatus if ordered

Offer analgesics, document effectiveness and tolerance *so that pharmacologic changes may be made as needed*
Institute nonpharmacologic comfort measures
  Optimal positioning
  Relaxation techniques/guided imagery
  Restful environment
  Diversional activity
  Splint incision when turning, coughing, and deep breathing

EXPECTED OUTCOME

Patient is relaxed and verbalizes increased comfort

● **NDX:** Altered urinary elimination related to presence of urethral catheter and/or suprapubic catheter

Maintain patency of catheter *to promote optimal flow of urine*
  Tubing below level of bladder *to allow for gravity flow*
  Assess for clamping/kinks in tubing *to prevent urine stasis*
  Secure catheters *to prevent dislodging*
  Irrigate catheters as ordered
Monitor intake and output frequently *so that abnormal balance will be identified and treated*
Assess for bladder distention and report to physician
Cleanse periurethral area bid and prn *to prevent infection and promote patient comfort*
Document tolerance of clamping routine if ordered for residual checks and amend treatment plan as needed
After urinary catheter is removed, institute measures to facilitate voiding
  Privacy
  Comfortable positioning
  Running tap water
  Placing patient's hand in warm water
  Applying heat to suprapubic area (if ordered)
  Pouring warm water over perineum
  Relaxation techniques
  Applying oil of peppermint (a few drops in bedpan/urinal or on cotton ball in front of urinary meatus)
  Stroking inner aspect of thigh gently with ice
  Offering analgesic
  Voiding 1 to 2 hr after fluid intake
  Double voiding (to empty bladder more completely)
Report to physician abnormalities in urine; residual volume >100 ml; and/or retention of urine with overflow *so that collaborative changes can be instituted*

EXPECTED OUTCOMES

Intake and output are in balance
Urethral catheter and suprapubic catheter are patent
Able to void after catheter removal without evidence of urinary retention

● **NDX:** Risk for infection related to potential for UTI resulting from presence of indwelling urethral catheter and/or suprapubic catheter

Report temperature >101°F (38.5°C) to physician
Maintain sterile technique during catheterizations *to decrease risk of bacteria entering urethra*
Order urine culture and notify physician if cloudy and/or malodorous urine is noted; monitor results

EXPECTED OUTCOME

Temperature is within normal limits for patient

● **NDX:** Impaired skin integrity related to surgical incision

Assess incision q4h for presence of erythema, edema, tenderness, and drainage; document findings *so that changes can be identified and treated*
Report signs and symptoms of infection (fever/chills) to physician
Obtain wound culture as ordered to identify presence of bacteria *so that presence of bacteria may be identified*
Monitor for elevation of WBC, *which indicates presence of infection*
Administer and monitor tolerance of ordered antibiotics

EXPECTED OUTCOME

Incision is clean and dry

ADDITIONAL NURSING DIAGNOSES TO CONSIDER

Altered tissue perfusion: peripheral, cardiopulmonary, or gastrointestinal related to risk of stasis of blood as evidenced by thrombophlebitis (p. 107) pulmonary embolism (p. 294), or parlytic ileus (p. 379)
Body image disturbance related to need for continued urethral catheter and/or suprapubic catheter at discharge or dissatisfaction with surgical outcome

Patient/family teaching

Explain postoperative procedures/routines to patient; encourage questions
Develop plan with patient to increase participation in ADLs
Teach/demonstrate proper body mechanics (e.g., bend knees to pick up items from the floor)
Explain to patient that an urge to urinate may be felt when catheter is in place and not to be concerned about sensation
Reinforce importance of keeping hands clean and not touching incision *to prevent infection*

To prevent UTI

Empty bladder q2h to 3h

Encourage patient to maintain fluid intake of 2000 to 3000 ml/day (unless contraindicated) to flush bacteria from system

Avoid fluids that aggravate urinary tract (caffeinated beverages) and drink fluids that promote systemic flushing (water and cranberry juice)

Shower rather than bathe and use antibacterial soap

Keep perineal area clean and dry

Wipe from front to back when cleansing perianal area

Teach about ordered medications: names, dosages, schedules, purposes, and side effects

Home care considerations

Emphasize importance of ongoing outpatient care

Advise patient to avoid interacting with persons who have infections (e.g., colds, influenza) during recuperation period

Reinforce need to rest and increase activity as tolerated; avoid sitting or standing for long periods

Instruct patient to avoid heavy lifting (>5 lb) and heavy housework as indicated by physician

Encourage patient to ask physician when sexual activity may be resumed

Teach patient to perform wound care and dressing change as ordered

Teach symptoms of wound infection (fever, chills, redness, swelling, tenderness, and purulent and/or malodorous drainage from incision) to report to home health nurse or physician

Teach/reinforce method of self-catheterization as needed (see Table 10-4)

Teach symptoms of UTI (dysuria, urgency, frequency, foul-smelling urine, fever >101°F [38.5°C]) and encourage patient to report to physician

Advise patient to avoid taking over-the-counter medications without physician approval

Advise patient to avoid straining during bowel movements; ask physician to prescribe stool softeners/laxatives as needed

Urinary Diversion

A method of diverting urine away from the bladder so that it leaves the body through another route; urinary diversion may be used to manage bladder tumors, strictures/ trauma of ureters and urethra, pelvic malignancy, neurogenic bladder, chronic infection, and advanced cases of cystitis (Table 10-7)

Urinary diversion may either be ureteroenterocutaneous

Table 10-7	Common Urinary Diversion Procedures

URETEROENTEROCUTANEOUS DIVERSION

Conventional conduit

Ureters are transplanted to an isolated section of the terminal ileum (ileal conduit) and brought to one end of the abdominal wall (see Figure 10-9)

Continent ileal urinary reservoir (see Figure 10-10)

Ureters are anastomosed into a prepared segment of the ileum, forming a pouch that contains two nipple valves

Ureterosigmoidostomy

Ureters are introduced into the sigmoid colon

CUTANEOUS URINARY DIVERSION

Cutaneous ureterostomy (see Figure 10-11)

One or both ureters are implanted into an opening in the abdominal wall

Vesicostomy

Bladder is sutured to the abdominal wall, and a stoma is created through the abdominal and bladder walls

Nephrostomy

Catheter is inserted into the renal pelvis

(a portion of the intestine is used to create a urinary reservoir) or cutaneous (urine drains through an opening created in the abdominal wall and skin) (Figures 10-9, 10-10, and 10-11)

Assessment

Subjective data

Pain

Anxiety

Objective data

Decreased urinary output

Unbalanced fluid intake and output

Cloudy, foul-smelling urine

Skin excoriation surrounding stoma

Incisional erythema, edema

Diagnostic tests

Urinalysis: white/red blood cells, bacteria

Urine culture and sensitivity

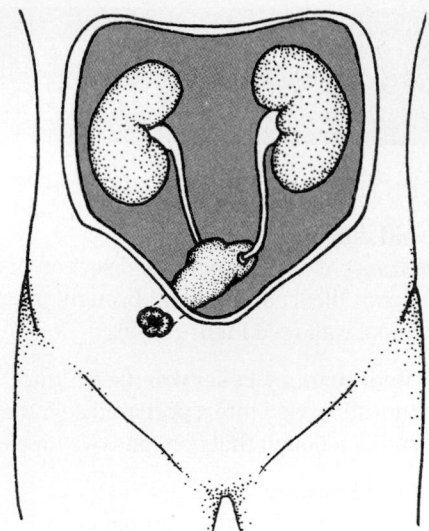

Figure 10-9 Ileal conduit.

Serum electrolytes, BUN, creatinine: abnormal/
  elevated results

Potential complications

Hemorrhage
Shock
Atelectasis
Thrombophlebitis
Pulmonary embolism
Electrolyte imbalance
Paralytic ileus
Peritonitus
UTI
Hydronephrosis
Renal failure

Collaborative management

Therapeutic management

Preoperative bowel preparation (enemas, laxatives, re-
  stricted diet)
Medications
  Antibiotics
  Analgesics
  Antipyretics
  Antiemetics
  Local antiinfective ointment/cream
  Stool softeners
  IV fluids
NPO until bowel sounds present
Enterostomal therapist
Dietitian

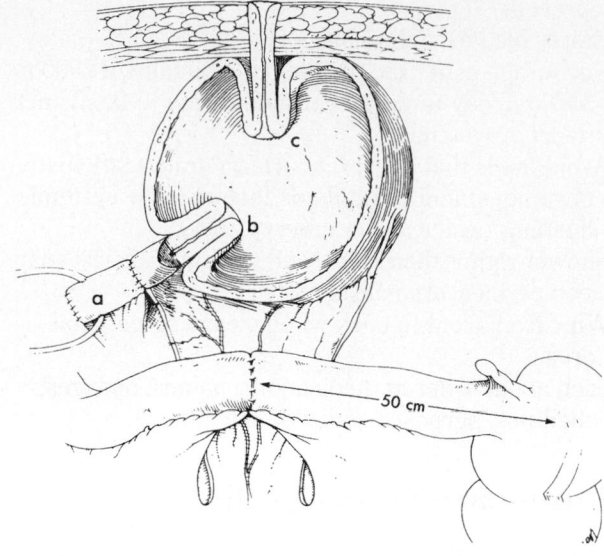

Figure 10-10 Kock continent ileal reservoir. *a,* Original ileal
conduit with implanted ureters; *b,* reflux-preventing nipple valve; *c,*
continence-maintaining nipple valve. (From Gerber A: *J Enterostom
Ther* 12:15, 1985.)

Psychological consult
Pharmacology consult
Sex therapist

Nursing management

PATIENT PROBLEMS/NURSING DIAGNOSES

● **NDX:** Pain related to surgical incision and/or urinary obstruction

Assess type, intensity, location, and duration of pain and
  document changes *so that changes can be notified and
  treatment initiated*
Identify verbal and nonverbal responses to pain
Ensure catheters/drains are patent and not causing dis-
  comfort related to obstruction of flow
Offer analgesics, documenting effectiveness and toler-
  ance *so that needed pharmacologic changes can be made*
Institute nonpharmacologic comfort measures
  Optimal positioning
  Relaxation techniques/guided imagery
  Restful environment
  Diversional activity
  Splint incision when turning, coughing, and deep
    breathing

  EXPECTED OUTCOME
Patient is relaxed and reports increased comfort

● **NDX:** Altered urinary elimination related to urinary diversion

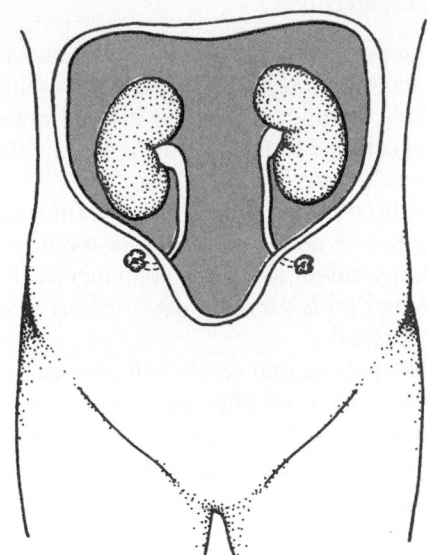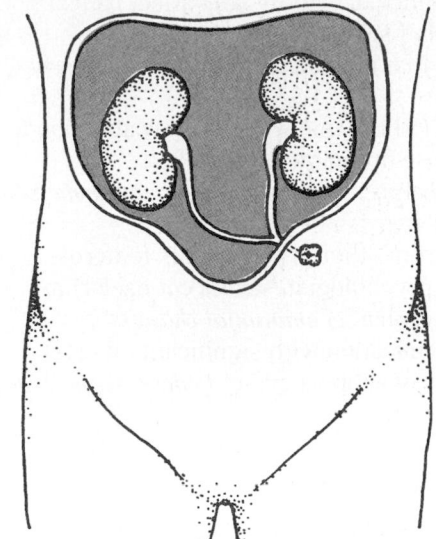

Figure 10-11 Cutaneous ureterostomies.

Monitor urine from all sources (ureteral stents, conduit catheters, reservoir catheters) and record color, clarity, and volume

Label each collecting container/catheter/stent (type, left or right) *to avoid errors when recording output*

Report urinary output of <30 ml/hr, *which may indicate altered fluid balance*

Pink-colored urine and mucus from conduit and continent diversions is expected for the first 24 hr postoperatively; report frank bleeding

Maintain patency of catheters/stents *to prevent backflow*
   Avoid kinking drainage tubing
   Keep drainage bag below level of patient's kidneys
   Position so that flow of urine is not impeded
   Tape ureteral stents securely

Assess size, shape, color, type, and placement of stoma/ureteral buds and record *so that changes can be reported promptly*

   EXPECTED OUTCOMES

Urinary output is >30 ml/hr; intake and output are balanced; urine is clear

● **NDX:** Impaired skin integrity related to incision/ostomy

Keep skin surfaces clean and dry

Change position *to prevent breakdown of skin surfaces*

Change dressings as ordered using sterile technique *to prevent infection*

Change dressings when wet *to decrease risk of excoriation;* use skin barrier around stoma; apply antiinfective ointments as ordered

Inspect skin around stoma and report signs of erythema, breakdown, and/or excoriation *so that any change can be evaluated and treated promptly*

Check color of stoma; report if other than pink

Check for leakage around appliance and, if noted, confer with enterostomal therapist to institute methods *to prevent urine contact with skin surfaces*

Change temporary appliance as needed in accordance with institutional policy and advice from enterostomal therapist; reapply/remeasure as needed

Monitor for signs and symptoms of incisional infection (fever, erythema, edema, malodorous drainage, pain) and report to physician for treatment; order culture of suspicious drainage and check results

   EXPECTED OUTCOMES

Skin surfaces are dry and intact

Stoma buds are pink and swelling is decreasing

● **NDX:** Body image disturbance related to loss of normal body function and presence of urinary stoma/bud on abdomen

Provide an accepting and supportive atmosphere *to maintain patient's self-esteem and promote verbalization of feelings, fears, concerns, and questions*

Assist patient in identifying coping measures used effectively in the past *so that these behaviors may be used to help patient to adapt to ostomy*

Offer opportunities to look at and touch ostomy; encourage participation in care

Explore how presence of ostomy may affect patient's normal activity and sexual functioning

Discuss activities that may be prohibited (e.g., heavy contact sports)

Identify types of clothing that will not draw attention to ostomy (e.g., loose-fitting garments)

Identify positive features of patient's life *to promote feelings of self-worth*

Offer assistance from other professionals (enterostomal therapist, psychologist, sexual counselor) *to assist with management of emotional changes*

Encourage communication with significant other(s) and/or members of support group *to decrease feelings of isolation*

EXPECTED OUTCOMES

Participates in ADLs and care of ostomy at optimal level

Comfortably discusses feelings, fears, concerns, and questions and identifies approaches for making positive changes in daily activities

Requests assistance from professionals and support group appropriately

ADDITIONAL NURSING DIAGNOSES TO CONSIDER

Ineffective breathing pattern related to pain or fatigue

Altered tissue perfusion: GI related to peritonitis

Altered urinary elimination related to UTI

Risk for fluid volume deficit related to potential for excessive losses and electrolyte imbalances

Ineffective individual coping related to fear of diagnosis, prognosis

Sexual dysfunction related to postoperative condition and self-consciousness about stoma

Patient/family teaching

Preoperative

Encourage verbalization of fears, concerns, and questions related to upcoming surgery

Provide information about equipment, tubes, and drains to expect postoperatively (depending on type of diversion)

Discuss purpose and type of bowel preparation

Determine whether significant other(s) will be involved in care postoperatively

Request enterostomal therapist consult (determines location of stoma in collaboration with patient and physician)

Offer visit from Ostomy Visitation Program (through American Cancer Society)

Postoperative

Encourage verbalization of fears, concerns, and questions related to ability to care for appliance

Include significant other(s) in teaching sessions

Enterostomal therapist meets with patient *to address special needs*

Explain/reinforce importance of thorough handwashing before and after caring for ostomy

Include patient in care of appliance early in postoperative period *to promote optimal level of self-care and independence*

Advise patient that stoma will decrease in size approximately 3 to 6 wk after surgery

Instruct patient about purpose of prescribed diet; dietary consult for special needs

Identify liquids that have diuretic effect (e.g., alcoholic beverages, tea, and coffee)

Encourage patient to maintain fluid intake of 2000 to 3000 ml/day (unless contraindicated) *to maintain adequate level of hydration*

Teach about ordered medications: names, dosages, schedules, purposes, and side effects

Home care considerations

Teach/reinforce method of changing/managing appliance

Emphasize importance of ongoing outpatient care

Reinforce need for rest and increased activity as tolerated

Provide patient with a list of instructions that includes places to purchase supplies and type/size of appliance needed

Instruct patient to shower daily *to promote hygiene;* avoid bathing *to prevent loosening of bag*

Instruct patient to empty appliance q2h to 3h or when >100 ml of urine accumulates to prevent bag from leaking or separating

Explain to ureterostomy patients importance of not irrigating ureteral buds

Instruct patient to attach appliance to bedside closed gravity system at night, keeping drainage apparatus lower than ostomy

Schedule follow-up care for patient with continent diversion who performs self-catheterization of reservoir

Offer to refer patient to sexual counselor as needed

Instruct patient to report the following symptoms to home health nurse and/or physician

Absence of urine

Hematuria; cloudy, foul-smelling urine

Pain in back or abdomen

Fever >101°F (38.5°C)

Incisional redness, pain, swelling, or drainage

Severe skin excoriation

Retraction of stoma
Malaise
Nausea/vomiting
Abdominal distention/pain
Encourage patient to avoid straining during bowel
movements, call physician to order stool softeners
and/or laxatives
Advise patient to avoid taking over-the-counter medications without physician approval

Artificial Urinary Sphincter (AUS)

A urological prosthetic device used to manage stress incontinence caused by sphincter incompetence; it consists of three major components: an abdominal reservoir, a periurethra cuff, and a pump mechanism (Figure 10-12)
The movement of fluid through a tubing network from the cuff to the abdominal reservoir operates the device; fluid normally remains in the cuff, promoting continence, until pumped into the reservoir; this action deflates the cuff and allows urine to pass through the urethra; the cuff automatically refills with fluid through hydraulic action. In females, the cuff is located near the bladder neck; in males, near the bladder neck or bulbous urethra.

Assessment

Subjective data (postoperative)

Bladder spasm
Pain

Objective data (postoperative)

Incontinence
Leakage of urine
Scrotal swelling
Labial swelling

Diagnostic tests

Urinalysis: cloudy, malodorous, WBC, RBC,
bacteria
Urine culture and sensitivity
See Urinary incontinence, p. 657

Potential complications

Patient's inability to operate AUS
UTI
Infection
Compromised bladder wall compliance
Progressive renal deterioration

Collaborative management

Therapeutic management

Urology consult
Medications
Antibiotics
Analgesics
Stool softeners
IV fluids
NPO until bowel sounds present
Psychological consult/support

Nursing management

PATIENT PROBLEMS/NURSING DIAGNOSES

● **NDX:** Pain related to low, transverse, deep surgical incision and bladder spasm

Assess type, intensity, location, and duration of pain and document *so that changes are noted and treatment plan altered*
Identify verbal and nonverbal responses to pain
Notify physician if scrotum/labia are swollen *so that care can be collaboratively initiated* (e.g., Trendelenburg position, ice)
Offer analgesics, document effectiveness and tolerance *so needed changes can be implemented*
Institute nonpharmacologic comfort measures
Optimal positioning
Relaxation techniques/guided imagery
Restful environment
Diversional activity

EXPECTED OUTCOME
Patient is relaxed and expresses increased comfort

● **NDX:** Altered urinary elimination related to presence of artificial urinary sphincter and bladder spasms

Locate pump qh and document findings; notify physician *immediately* if unable to palpate pump, *which may indicate its movement into inguinal canal*
Activate pump when ordered
Provide privacy while palapating or activating pump
Pump bulb q2h during the day and once midway through the night or as scheduled by physician
Deflate device when patient is asleep when ordered and connect to an external urine collecting device; may use pads for female, changing as necessary to maintain dryness
Report any leakage of urine to physician *so that source of leakage may be identified and treated*

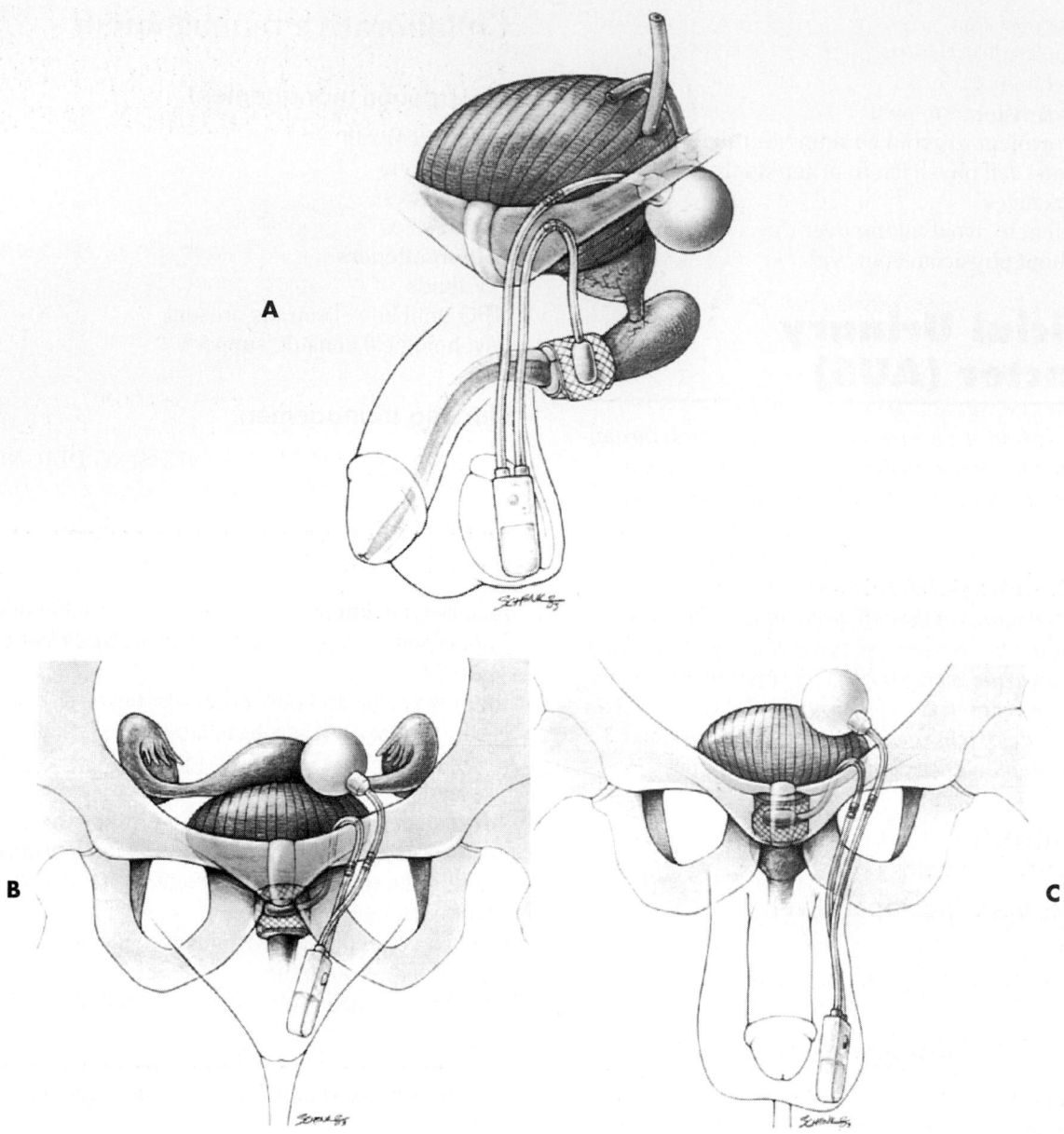

Figure 10-12 **A,** Placement of AUS cuff around bulbous urethra in male. **B,** Placement of AUS in female. Cuff is placed around bladder neck, balloon is placed in prevesical space, and pump is placed in labia. **C,** Placement of AUS in male. Cuff is placed around bladder neck, balloon is placed in prevesical space, and pump is placed in scrotum. (Courtesy American Medical Systems, Inc., Minnetonka, Minn. From Doughty D: *Urinary and fecal incontinence: nursing management,* St Louis, 1991, Mosby.)

Monitor intake and output frequently *to identify and treat imbalances*

  EXPECTED OUTCOMES
AUS operates successfully without leakage
Intake and output are in balance

● **NDX:**   Risk for infection (urinary and/or wound), and rejection of artificial sphincter related to implantation of foreign body surrounding urinary tract

Report signs and symptoms of infection to physician for treatment
Fever >101°F (38.5°C)
Erythema/edema/pain of wound or surrounding area
Purulent/malodorous drainage from wound
Obtain urine culture and notify physician if cloudy and/or malodorous urine is noted; monitor results
Report signs and symptoms of AUS rejection to physician for treatment
Erosion

Increasing pain
Abdominal tenderness
Swelling
Urinary retention
Monitor tolerance and effectiveness of antibiotics and
document *so that pharmacologic changes are made
when needed*

EXPECTED OUTCOME

Patient does not exhibit signs and symptoms of infec-
tion/rejection

ADDITIONAL NURSING DIAGNOSES
TO CONSIDER

Body image disturbance related to presence of AUS
Anxiety related to concern about care of AUS

Patient/family teaching

Explain surgical procedure; encourage questions and
verbalization of concerns and feelings
Explain that urethral catheter will be removed as ordered by physician
Teach about ordered medications: names, dosages,
schedules, purposes, and side effects

Home care considerations

Teach and reinforce method of caring for AUS
(Table 10-8)
Emphasize importance of ongoing outpatient care
To prevent UTI
Encourage patient to maintain fluid intake of 2000 to
3000 ml/day (unless contraindicated) to flush bacteria from system
Avoid fluids that aggravate urinary tract (e.g., caffeinated beverages) and drink fluids that promote
systemic flushing (e.g., water and cranberry juice)
Teach signs and symptoms of UTI (dysuria, urgency,
frequency, foul-smelling urine, fever >101°F
[38.5°C]) and encourage patient to report to
physician
Teach signs and symptoms of wound infection
(fever, chills, redness, swelling, tenderness, and
purulent and/or malodorous drainage from incision) and encourage patient to report to physician
Teach symptoms of AUS rejection (erosion, increasing
pain, abdominal tenderness, swelling, urinary retention)
Instruct patient to wear a medical alert tag at all times
*so that if patient is ever unconscious, the pump may be
activated and urine eliminated*

Table 10-8 Instructions for Care of AUS

PROCEDURE

Palpate pump and activate AUS
Locate AUS in labia or scrotum with thumb and
forefinger of dominant hand
Locate and gently support tubing above pump with
nondominant hand to prevent pump from slipping
away
Using thumb and forefinger of dominant hand, squeeze
pump until it reaches decompressed state, which
allows urine to flow
Within 1 to 3 min cuff will refill and compress urethra

TROUBLE SHOOTING

If urine does not flow
Move from supine to sitting or standing position
Cough
NOTE: Pump may need to be deflated twice to fully
empty bladder

REMINDERS

Follow prescribed pumping schedule
Do not leave AUS completely inflated while asleep unless
ordered
Report leakage of fluid to physician
Report if AUS goes flat
Some incontinence may occur with certain physical
activities

Benign Prostatic Hypertrophy/Hyperplasia

*The enlargement of the prostate gland, associated with
endocrine changes of aging, which may prevent the
bladder from emptying appropriately*

Assessment

Subjective data

Hesitancy in starting flow of urine
Diminished force/amount of urine stream
End-stream dribbling
Urinary frequency/urgency
Dysuria

Sense of not emptying bladder
Nocturia
Incontinence
Fatigue
Nausea/vomiting
Weight loss

Objective data

Enlarged prostate gland
Hematuria

Diagnostic tests

Urinalysis: WBC, RBC, sediment, bacteria
Urine culture and sensitivity
Serum BUN/creatinine: elevated
Serum WBC: elevated
Voiding diary: frequency, urgency, nocturia, incontinence
IVP/IVU: dilation of ureters with hydronephrosis; delayed excretion contrast medium; parenchymal thinning
Urinary flow study: poor flow pattern; prolonged voiding time; large postvoid residual
Prostatic ultrasound: bilateral enlargement of gland with no hypoechoic areas suspicious of malignant tumor

Potential complications

Acute urinary retention
UTI
Pyelonephritis
Hydronephrosis
Compromised renal function
Detrusor decompensation

Collaborative management

Therapeutic management

Medications
  Analgesics
  Antibiotics
  Antispasmodics
  A-adrenergic blocking drugs (antagonists)
  Endocrine therapy
  Estrogens, androgen antagonists, luteinizing hormone
  Stool softeners/laxatives
Catheterization: intermittent or long term
Surgeries
  Transurethral resection of prostate (TURP)

Open prostatectomy for very large gland
Balloon dilation of prostate
Laser ablation of prostate
Transurethral microwave therapy
Implantation of intraurethral prostatic stent

Nursing management

PATIENT PROBLEMS/NURSING DIAGNOSES

● **NDX:**   Altered urinary elimination related to BPH

Monitor intake and output frequently *so that imbalances can be reported and treated*
Implement voiding diary *to identify abnormal elimination requiring specific interventions*
Monitor serum BUN/creatinine levels for evidence of increase
After urinary catheter is removed (if used), institute measures to facilitate voiding
  Privacy
  Comfortable positioning
  Running tap water
  Placing patient's hand in warm water
  Applying heat to suprapubic area (if ordered)
  Pouring warm water over perineum
  Relaxation techniques
  Applying oil of peppermint (a few drops in bedpan/urinal or on cotton ball in front of urinary meatus)
  Stroking inner aspect of thigh gently with ice
  Offering analgesic
  Voiding 1 to 2 hr after fluid intake
  Double voiding (to empty bladder more completely)
If postvoid residual ordered, record/report findings

EXPECTED OUTCOMES
Intake and output are in balance
Voiding pattern is established

● **NDX:**   Pain related to hypertrophy of prostate

Assess type, intensity, location, and duration of pain and document *so changes can be made in plan of care*
Identify verbal and nonverbal responses to pain
Ensure that catheter is patent *to promote optimal drainage, prevent pressure from backflow*
Secure catheter *to prevent pulling sensation*
Offer analgesics, documenting effectiveness and tolerance *so changes in pharmacologic plan can be made*
Institute nonpharmacologic comfort measures
  Optimal positioning
  Relaxation techniques/guided imagery
  Restful environment
  Diversional activity

EXPECTED OUTCOME

Patient is relaxed; verbalizes increased comfort

● **NDX:** Risk for infection (UTI) related to BPH

See UTI, p. 648

ADDITIONAL NURSING DIAGNOSES
TO CONSIDER

Body image disturbance related to BPH

Sexual dysfunction related to BPH

Anxiety related to fear of cancer, embarrassment about symptoms, and concerns about effect on ADLs

Patient/family teaching

Explain method and reasons for voiding diary

Explain reasons for checking postvoid residual

Teach about ordered medications: names, dosages, schedules, and side effects

Home care considerations

Emphasize importance of ongoing outpatient care

Teach/reinforce method of self-catheterization (see Table 10-4)

Instruct patient to measure urine after each void and note character of urine, time, amount, and force of stream (use voiding diary if appropriate)

Reinforce methods of preventing UTI (see UTI, p. 648)

Teach symptoms of UTI (dysuria, foul-smelling urine, fever >101°F [38.5°C]) and encourage patient to report to physician

Provide accurate information concerning sexual function to dispel myths

Advise patient to avoid taking over-the-counter medications without physician approval

Advise patient to avoid straining during bowel movements and ask physician for stool softeners/laxatives as needed

Penile Implant

Surgical implantation of a prosthesis in the penis to restore erectile function; the two common types are semirigid (which maintains a continuous state of erection) and inflatable (which allows a flacid or erect penis) (Figures 10-13, 10-14, 10-15, and 10-16)

Assessment

Subjective data (postoperative)

Pain

Spasm

Anxiety

Objective data (postoperative)

Scrotal edema/discoloration

Incision: redness, swelling, drainage

Function of prosthesis

Change in character of urine (e.g., hematuria)

Fever

Diagnostic tests (preoperative for erectile dysfunction)

Medical, sexual history

Nocturnal penile temescence tests

Snap gauge device: evaluates rigidity of a single tumescent episode

NPT monitor: continuous monitoring of tumescence

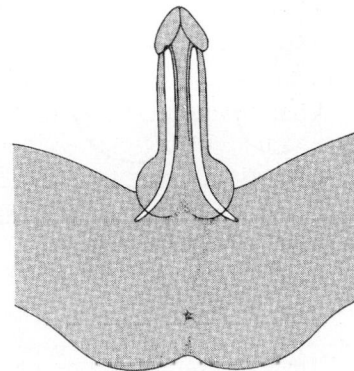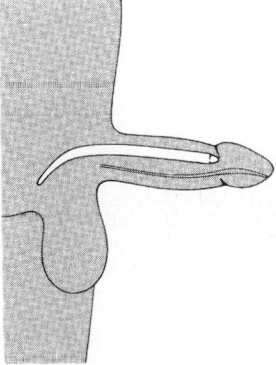

Figure 10-13   Semirigid intrapenile prosthesis. (From Beare PG, Myers JL: *Principles and practice of adult health nursing,* ed 2, St Louis, 1994, Mosby.)

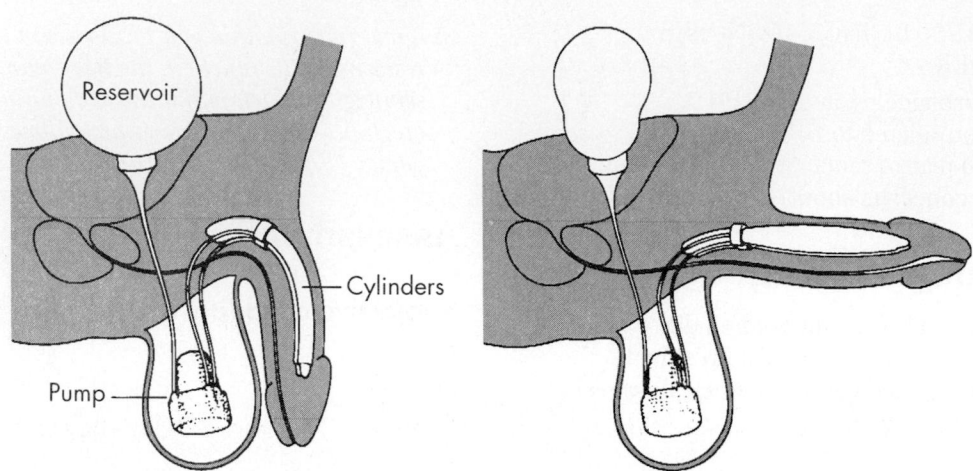

Figure 10-14 Scott inflatable penile prosthesis. (From Beare PG, Myers JL: *Principles and practice of adult health nursing,* ed 2, St Louis, 1994, Mosby.)

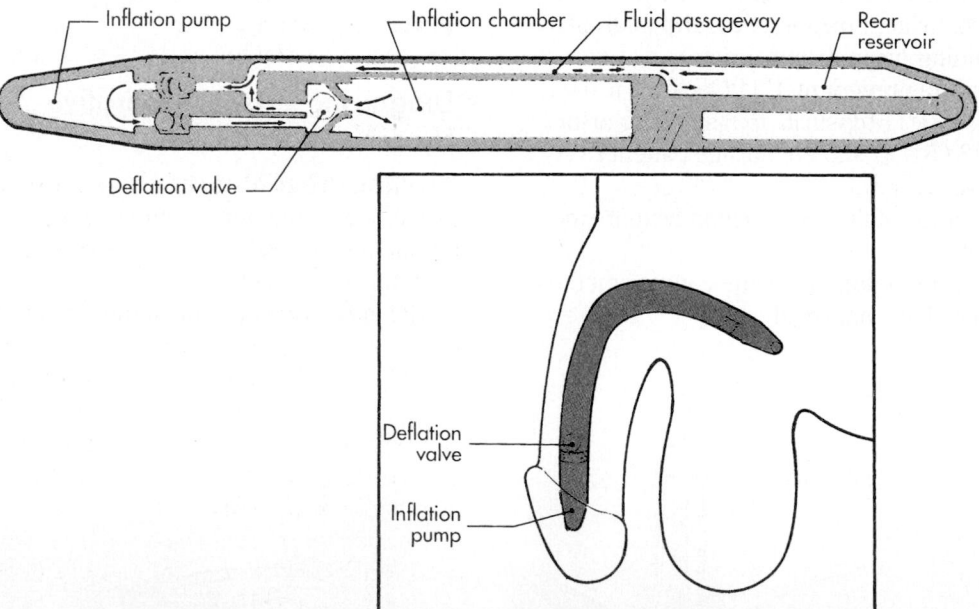

Figure 10-15 One-piece inflatable penile prosthesis. (From Gray M: *Mosby's clinical nursing series: genitourinary disorders,* St Louis, 1992, Mosby.)

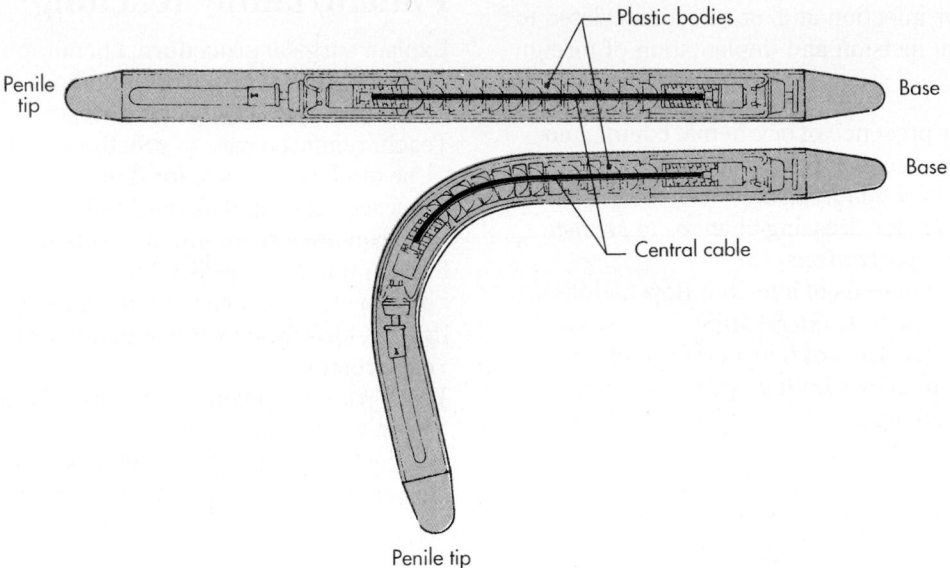

Figure 10-16   One-piece prosthesis with central cable that shortens plastic bodies to produce erection. (From Gray M: *Mosby's clinical nursing series: genitourinary disorders,* St Louis, 1992, Mosby.)

Rigiscan monitor: computer-based tumescence monitor that records penile tumescence and provides information on rigidity of tumescent episodes

Doppler studies for penile blood flow

Dynamic infusion cavernosometry/cavernosography (DICC): erectile dysfunction

Penile arteriogram: insufficient blood flow

Urinalysis: hematuria, WBC, RBC, sediment, bacteria

Urine culture and sensitivity

Glucose

Testosterone

Prolactin

Potential complications

Rejection

Mechanical failure

Extravasation of fluid from prosthesis reservoir into surrounding tissue

Urethral or glans erosion

Infection

Collaborative management

Therapeutic management

Medications
  Analgesics
  Antispasmodics
  Antianxiety agents
  Antibiotics

Hormonal therapy
Stool softeners/laxatives
IV fluids
Ice to scrotal area
Psychological consult
Sexual counseling

Nursing management

PATIENT PROBLEMS/NURSING DIAGNOSES

● **NDX:**   Pain related to surgical incision

Assess type, intensity, location, and duration of pain and document *so changes are noted and treated*

Identify verbal and nonverbal responses to pain

Offer analgesics, documenting effectiveness and tolerance *so pharmacologic interventions are updated*

Institute nonpharmacologic comfort measures
  Optimal positioning
  Restful environment
  Relaxation techniques/guided imagery
  Diversional activities

Elevate scrotum as ordered *to decrease discomfort from edema*

Apply ice to scrotal area as ordered *to decrease edema*

Use bed cradle *to decrease pressure from bed linen on surgical area*

EXPECTED OUTCOME

Patient is relaxed; verbalizes increased comfort

● **NDX:** Risk for infection and/or rejection related to surgical incision and implantation of foreign object

Assess incision for presence of erythema, edema, tenderness, and drainage; document findings *so that changes are identified and treated*

Use sterile technique for dressing changes *to prevent introduction of microorganisms*

Report signs and symptoms of infection (fever, chills) to physician *for immediate intervention*

Report signs and symptoms of rejection (stretched skin, appearance of device outline, pain over implant site, urinary retention) to physician **for immediate intervention**

Obtain wound culture as ordered *to identify bacteria*

Monitor for elevation of WBC, *which indicates presence of infection*

Administer and monitor tolerance of ordered antibiotics

   EXPECTED OUTCOMES
Temperature is within normal range for patient; incision is dry and without evidence of redness or swelling; outline of implant is not visible on penis

● **NDX:** Altered sexuality patterns related to penile implant

Provide an accepting and supportive atmosphere *to maintain patient's self-esteem and promote verbalization of feelings, fears, concerns, and questions*

Explore how penile implant may affect patient's sexuality

Encourage patient to look at and participate in care of dressings, location of pump

Offer assistance from other professionals (sexual counselor, clergy) *to assist patient to manage emotional changes*

Encourage communication with significant other(s) and/or persons with implants *to decrease feelings of isolation*

   EXPECTED OUTCOMES
Verbalizes fears, feelings, and concerns related to sexuality
Participates in care and activation of penile implant

   ADDITIONAL NURSING DIAGNOSES
   TO CONSIDER
Body image disturbance related to presence of penile prosthesis
Depression related to unrealistic expectations after penile implant

Patient/family teaching

Explain surgical procedure; encourage questions and verbalization of concerns, feelings
Teach name and type of prosthesis
Teach/reinforce care of prosthesis
   Use model or picture for demonstration
   Practice inflating/deflating pump as ordered by physician
   Explain prescribed inflation schedule
Explain that prosthesis restores erectile capability but has no effect on ejaculation, fertility, or orgasm
Provide for privacy when inflating or teaching patient to use prosthesis
Teach patient appropriate method for perineal care after bowel movement
Teach about ordered medications: names, dosages, schedules, purposes, and side effects

Home care considerations

Emphasize importance of ongoing outpatient care
Reinforce importance of good handwashing technique for patient and others in contact with patient
Reinforce need for rest, sleep
Advise patient to discuss with physician when sexual intercourse may be resumed
Explain that wearing loose clothing will disguise appearance of semirigid implants
Reassure patient that mechanical failure of pump usually can be corrected under local anesthetic
Advise patient to avoid strenuous activity, heavy lifting, jogging, or sports until approved by physician
Encourage patient to report the following findings to physician
   Incisional redness, pain, swelling, drainage
   Elevated temperature
   Inability to urinate
   Penile pain
Advise patient to carry medical identification in case of emergency
Advise patient to avoid taking over-the-counter medications without physician approval
Instruct patient to avoid straining during bowel movements and ask physician for stool softeners/laxatives as needed

Prostatectomy

Removal of part or all of the prostate gland. Indications for prostatectomy include cancer, obstructive uropathy, acute urinary retention, bladder complications, or urinary infections related to BPH (Figure 10-17); surgery is usually done transurethrally, but the prostate gland may also be removed via open procedure (Table 10-9)

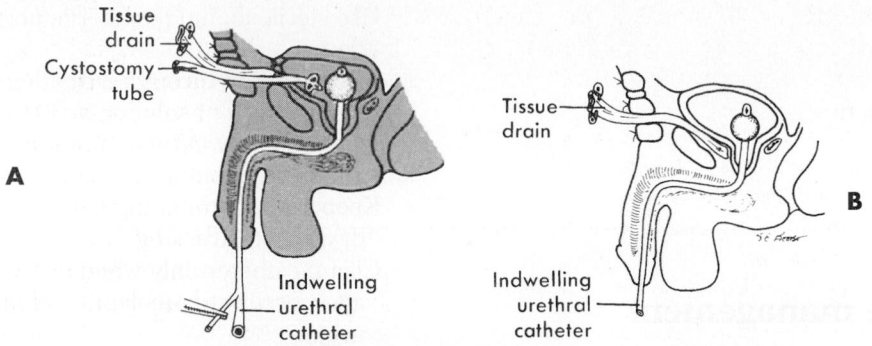

Figure 10-17 **A,** Suprapubic prostatectomy. **B,** Retropubic prostatectomy.

Table 10-9 Types of Prostate Surgery

Name	Description
Transurethral resection of prostate (TURP)	Removal of part or most of the prostate gland via resectoscope inserted through the urethra
Suprapubic prostatectomy (see Figure 10-17A)	Removal of the prostate gland through an incision made into the bladder
Retropubic prostatectomy (see Figure 10-17B)	Removal of the prostate gland via an incision in the lower abdomen through the anterior prostatic fossa without entering the bladder
Perineal prostatectomy	Radical removal of prostate gland through an incision between the scrotum and rectum
Radical retropubic prostatectomy	Removal of the prostate gland including the capsule, seminal vesicles, and adjacent tissue through an incision in the lower abdomen; the urethra is anastomosed to the bladder neck for prostatic cancer

Assessment

Subjective data

Pain
Bladder spasms

Objective data

Change in character and volume of urine (hematuria)
Distended bladder
Incision if present
  Redness
  Swelling
  Drainage
Removal of catheter
  Incontinence
  Frequent urination
Small urinary stream
Retention with overflow
Inability to urinate

Diagnostic tests

Urinalysis: hematuria, WBC, RBC, sediment, bacteria
Urine culture and sensitivity
Serum BUN/creatinine: elevated
Serum electrolytes: abnormal
CBC: decreased Hct/Hgb, elevated WBC
Cystoscopy: obstruction
IVP: obstructive uropathy

Potential complications

Hemorrhage
Acute urinary rentention

Stress incontinence
Erectile dysfunction
Fistula
Bladder neck contracture
Epididymitis
Infection
Paralytic ileus
Pelvic abscess

Collaborative management

Therapeutic management

Medications
  Analgesics
  Antispasmodics
  Antibiotics
  Stool softeners
  IV fluids
Blood transfusion
Psychologic consult
Sexual counseling

Nursing management

PATIENT PROBLEMS/NURSING DIAGNOSES

● **NDX:** Altered urinary elimination related to prostatectomy and bladder irrigation

Monitor intake and output frequently *so that imbalances
are noted for early treatment*
Monitor for signs and symptoms of dilutional hyponatremia (change in behavior/mental status, muscles
twitching, nausea/vomiting, SOB, elevated BP, decreased serum sodium) and report these findings to
physician for evaluation
Stop irrigation *if fluid excess is suspected* and notify
physician
Maintain patency of catheters *to promote optimal flow of
urine*
  Tubing below level of bladder to allow for gravity
  flow
  Assess for clamping/kinks in tubing
  Secure catheters while still allowing for patient movement
  Irrigate tubes as ordered
Avoid Fowler's position for long periods *to prevent vascular stasis in lower extremities*
Label each tube clearly and record drainage from tube
separately *to allow for accurate assessment of output
from each system*
Record amount of irrigant and urine output; subtract ir-
rigant from output and record
Maintain continuous bladder irrigation (CBI) if ordered

Use sterile technique/sterile normal saline for irriga-
tion
Instill irrigant through irrigating port of catheter
Regulate flow of solution at 40 to 60 drops/min or
enough *to establish and maintain clear urinary flow*
Maintain suprapubic catheter
  Keep area surrounding insertion site covered with
  dry, sterile dressing
  Clamp catheter only when ordered so patient can
  attempt to void; unclamp and measure residual
  urine
  Monitor tolerance and document
After urinary catheter is removed, institute measures to
facilitate voiding
  Privacy
  Comfortable positioning
  Running tap water
  Placing patient's hand in warm water
  Pouring warm water over perineum
  Relaxation techniques
  Applying oil of peppermint (a few drops in
  bedpan/urinal or on cotton ball in front of urinary
  meatus)
  Stroking inner aspect of thigh gently with ice
  Offering analgesic
  Voiding 1 to 2 hr after fluid intake
  Double voiding (to empty bladder more completely)
Monitor and report signs and symptoms of urinary reten-
tion (e.g., bladder distention) and report to physician
Assure patient that irritative voiding symptoms will di-
minish
Encourage fluid intake of 2000 to 2500 ml/day unless
contraindicated

EXPECTED OUTCOMES

Intake and output are balanced
Catheters remain patent while in place
Patient establishes regular voiding pattern after
catheter is removed (usually within 6 wk)

● **NDX:** Risk for fluid volume deficit related to hemorrhage

Monitor for signs and symptoms of hemorrhage (hypotension; tachycardia; dyspnea; cool, clammy skin;
syncope; hematuria) and report to physician for evaluation
Monitor abdominal/suprapubic dressing q2h *to assess
whether bleeding has occurred or increased*
Monitor urethral and suprapubic catheter drainage *to
assess whether color indicates bleeding* (i.e., change
from pink to red)
Maintain traction on catheter as ordered *to decrease risk
of hemorrhage;* release intermittently as ordered to decrease risk of bladder neck damage

Avoid manipulating rectum (e.g., taking rectal T), *which may place increased pressure on surgical area*
Monitor Hct/Hgb for evidence of decrease
Monitor blood transfusions according to institutional policy

EXPECTED OUTCOMES
Vital signs are stable and within patient's normal range
Incision is clean and dry when present
Catheter drainage remains pink-tinged changing to clear yellow

● **NDX:** Risk for infection (UTI/incisional) related to prostatectomy

Monitor for signs and symptoms of UTI (e.g., dysuria, frequency, urgency) and report to physician for evaluation and treatment
Obtain urine culture if urine is cloudy or malodorous *to identify bacteria*
Assess incision for presence of erythema, edema, tenderness, and drainage; document *findings so changes may be identified and treated*
Use sterile technique when changing dressing *to decrease risk of infection*
Report signs and symptoms of infection (fever, chills) to physician
Obtain wound culture as ordered *to identify bacteria*
Monitor for elevation of WBC, *which indicates presence of infection*
Administer and monitor tolerance of ordered antibiotics

EXPECTED OUTCOMES
Temperature is within normal limits for patient
Incision is dry and clean
Voids clear yellow urine without difficulty

● **NDX:** Pain related to prostatectomy

Assess type, intensity, location, and duration of pain and document changes
Identify verbal and nonverbal responses to pain
Ensure that catheters are patent; irrigate as ordered until urine is free of clots
Offer analgesics, documenting effectiveness and tolerance
Institute nonpharmacologic comfort measures
Optimal positioning
Restful environment
Relaxation techniques/guided imagery
Diversional activities

EXPECTED OUTCOME
Patient is relaxed and verbalizes increased comfort

● **NDX:** Altered sexuality patterns related to prostatectomy

Provide an accepting and supportive atmosphere *to maintain patient's self-esteem and promote verbalization of feelings, fears, concerns, and questions about incontinence, sexuality, and cancer*
Explore how having a prostatectomy has affected patient's sexuality
Offer assistance from other professionals (sexual counselor, clergy) *to assist in management of emotional changes*
Provide opportunities for communication with significant other concerning sexuality *to decrease feelings of isolation*

EXPECTED OUTCOMES
Patient seeks psychosocial support when needed
Patient verbalizes fears, feelings, and concerns related to sexuality

ADDITIONAL NURSING DIAGNOSES TO CONSIDER
Ineffective breathing pattern related to anesthesia
Altered tissue perfusion: renal, peripheral related to prostatectomy
Body image disturbance related to prostatectomy

Patient/family teaching

Explain surgical procedure; encourage questions and verbalization of concerns, feelings
Provide information about expectations of return of sexual functioning
Explain reason for urethral/suprapubic catheters
Explain reason for checking postvoid residual
Explain reason for ordered blood transfusion(s)
Explain importance of turning, coughing, and deep breathing q2h; instruct in use of incentive spirometer and splinting
Explain importance of early ambulation and activity
Demonstrate appropriate technique for handwashing
Teach exercises that strengthen pelvic floor muscles *to decrease/eliminate incontinence and enhance sexual function*
Teach about ordered medications: names, dosages, schedules, purposes, and side effects

Home care considerations

Emphasize importance of ongoing outpatient care
Reinforce importance of good handwashing technique for patient and others in contact with patient

Teach care of catheter and drainage units if present

Advise patient to avoid interacting with persons who have infections (e.g., colds/influenza)

Reinforce importance of adhering to dietary/fluid restrictions

Reinforce need for rest, sleep

Encourage gradual progression of activity and participation in ADLs as tolerated; restrict lifting and driving as advised by physician

Provide information about expectation of return of sexual functioning in collaboration with physician

Erection and orgasm usually the same as preoperatively unless nerves are damaged

Impotence from radical procedures

Retrograde ejaculation

Reinforce restrictions on sexual intercourse as ordered

Explain that urinary control will return, in phases, as surgical site heals

Teach signs and symptoms of UTI (dysuria, foul-smelling urine, fever >101°F [38.5°C]) and encourage patient to report to physician

Advise patient to report the following signs and symptoms to physician

Heavy urinary bleeding

Difficulty voiding

Incisional redness, swelling, pain, drainage

Elevated temperature

Pain when walking

Advise patient to avoid taking over-the-counter medications without physician approval

Advise patient to avoid straining during bowel movements and ask physician for stool softeners/laxatives as needed

Glomerulonephritis

A group of diseases that result in an inflammatory reaction and/or necrotizing lesion within the glomeruli; usually caused by an immunologic response (Figure 10-18)

Glomerulonephtritis (GN) may be a primary disease of the kidneys or develop secondary to a systemic disease such as systemic lupus erythematosus

Assessment

Subjective data

Headache
Malaise
Dyspnea
Low-grade fever
Low back, flank pain
Anorexia

Nausea/vomiting
Chills
Frequent infections
Visual disturbances

Objective data

Decreased urinary output
Dark brown or rust-colored urine
Fever
Hypertension
Edema (facial, sacral, ankle)
Weight gain
Jugular venous distention
Azotemia

Diagnostic tests

Urinalysis: hematuria, proteinuria, RBC, WBC, granular casts

Urine protein excretion (24 hr): elevated protein excretion

Serum complement: decreased

Antistreptolysin O-titer: increased

Hepatitis B antigen: present

Pulmonary function tests: abnormalities in respiratory function/capacity

ECG: abnormalities in cardiac function/capacity

Blood chemistries: decreased serum albumin, elevated BUN/creatinine, abnormal levels of electrolytes

Culture of throat/skin lesion: streptococcal organism

KUB: normal size kidneys, slight bilateral enlargement

Renal biopsy: diffuse endocapillary proliferation

Potential complications

Infection
Renal failure
Anemia
Hypertension
Encephalopathy
Cardiac failure
CHF

Collaborative management

Therapeutic management

Medications
Antibiotics (if infection present)
Corticosteroids/cytotoxic agent *to decrease immune system response and antibody formation*
Antihypertensives *to control BP*
Diuretics *to remove excess fluid*
Antacids

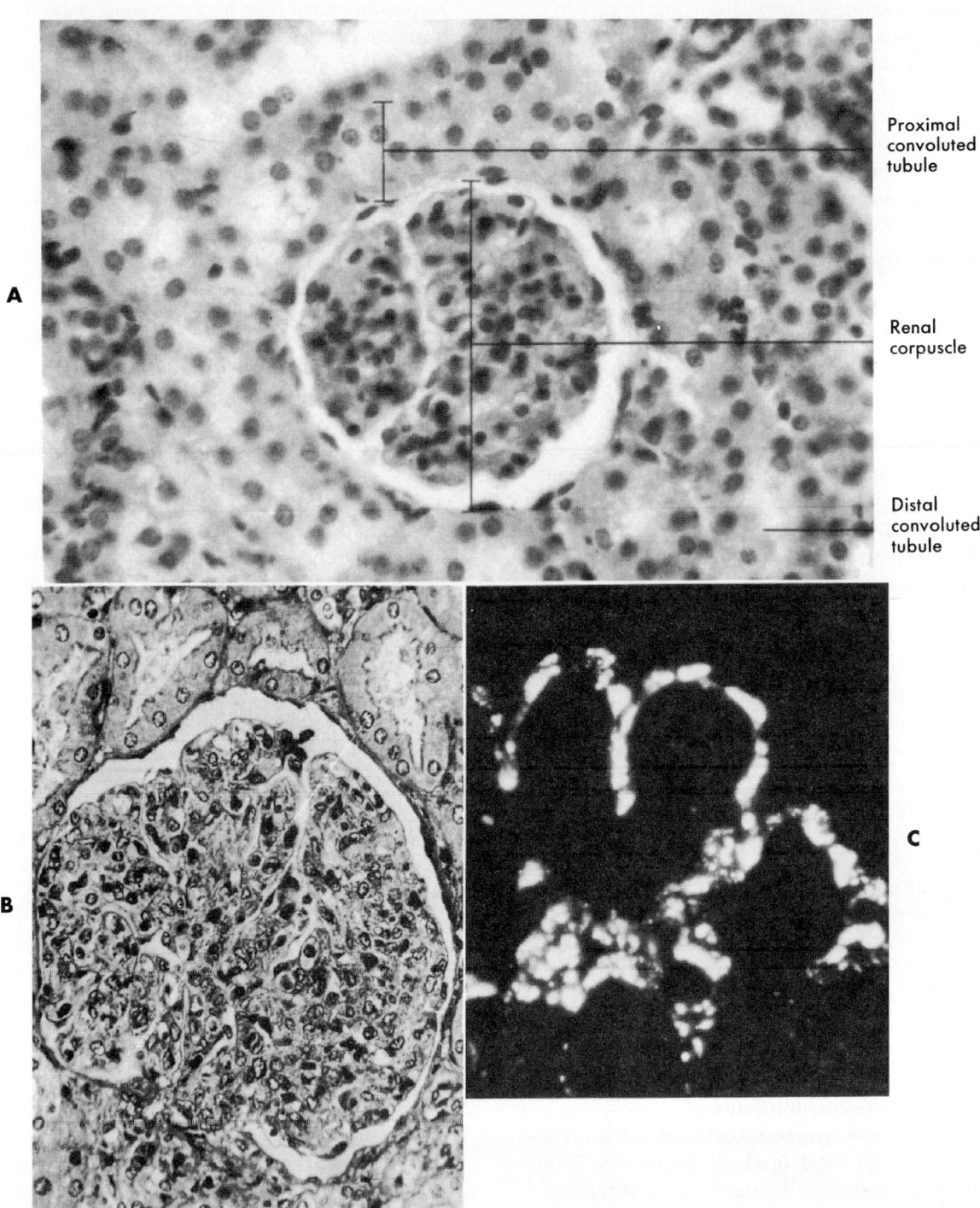

Proximal
convoluted
tubule

Renal
corpuscle

Distal
convoluted
tubule

Figure 10-18 **A,** Photomicrograph of kidney showing normal glomerulus surrounded by profiles of sectioned renal tubules (× 140). **B,** Acute poststreptococcal glomerulonephritis. Swollen, hypercellular glomerular lobules with few open capillaries (× 250). **C,** Acute poststreptococcal glomerulonephritis. "Humps" of immune complex stained with fluorescent antihuman complement (C) (× 1000). (Courtesy Dr. Claude Cornwall, Syracuse, NY.) (**A** from Thibodeau; **B** and **C** from Kissane. All from Brundage DJ: *Mosby's clinical nursing series: renal disorders,* St Louis, 1992, Mosby.)

H_2 blockers
Plasmapheresis to remove antibodies
Hemodialysis/peritoneal dialysis (chronic or rapidly
  progressive disease)
Fluid/sodium/potassium/protein restriction
Increased calories
Fluid replacement according to fluid loss
Bed rest
Dietitian recommended as necessary
Psychological consult

Nursing management

PATIENT PROBLEMS/NURSING DIAGNOSES

● **NDX:** Activity intolerance related to protein depletion and/or renal dysfunction

Explain reasons for ordered bed rest
Provide exercise within prescribed activity restriction
  (e.g., ROM exercises) *to decrease risk of muscle atrophy*
Plan rest periods between activities *to conserve energy*
Monitor blood chemistries for evidence of body deple-
  tion of protein (e.g., proteinuria)

EXPECTED OUTCOMES

Patient adheres to and tolerates prescribed activity plan
BP remains within patient's normal limits without excessive protein excretion as activity increases

● **NDX:** Altered tissue perfusion: renal related to immunologic injury to kidney

Monitor intake and output to determine whether fluid
  balance is appropriate, report urinary output of <30
  ml/hr to physician
Replace fluids as ordered according to fluid loss
Offer ice chips, if ordered, to control thirst; include in
  intake measurement
Monitor for signs and symptoms of fluid excess (CHF,
  hypertension, weight gain, edema, decreased urine
  output, S_3 and S_4 heart sounds, distended neck veins)
  and report to physician for treatment
Monitor for signs and symptoms of hypertensive crisis
  (elevated BP, tachycardia, bradycardia, confusion, decreased LOC, headache, tinnitus, nausea, vomiting,
  seizures) and report to physician for evaluation and
  treatment
Monitor BP and note response to and tolerance of antihypertensive medications
Monitor electrolytes and report abnormal laboratory
  values and signs and symptoms of electrolyte imbalance
  Hypokalemia: abdominal cramps, lethargy, dysryth-
    mias

Hyperkalemia: muscle cramps and weakness
Hypocalcemia: neuromuscular irritability
Hyperphosphatemia: hyperreflexia, paresthesias,
  muscle cramps, itching, seizures
Elevated BUN and creatinine: uremia (confusion,
  lethargy, restlessness)
Assess effectiveness of electrolytes administered par-
  enterally and orally *to detect and treat changes in
  condition*
See nursing diagnosis of Fluid volume excess under
  Renal failure (p. 685)

EXPECTED OUTCOMES

Intake and output are in balance
BP, P, and weight within normal range for patient
Patient is alert and oriented

● **NDX:** Risk for infection related to depressed immune system

Assess effectiveness, tolerance of immunosuppressive
  medications and cytotoxic agents
Monitor serum WBC, antibodies, and T cell values; report abnormal laboratory results to physician
Monitor for signs and symptoms of systemic infection
  (fever >101°F [38.5°C]), chills, flushed skin, sore
  throat, productive cough) and report to physician for
  evaluation and treatment
Monitor for signs and symptoms of UTI (see UTI, p.
  648) and report to physician for evaluation and treatment
Avoid instrumentation and/or catheterization of urinary tract if possible; maintain closed gravity drainage
  system if urethral catheter present *to decrease risk of
  introducing organisms*

EXPECTED OUTCOME

Temperature and laboratory studies are within normal
range for patient

● **NDX:** Altered nutrition less or more than body
requirements

Weigh patient daily: same time, clothing, and scale
Refer to dietitian *to plan appropriate diet for patient*
  Protein of 0.8 to 1.0 g/kg/day adjusted based on blood
    level *to decrease excretory load on the kidneys and
    possible accumulation of potassium and hydrogen ions*
  Reduced sodium/fluid intake *to decrease fluid reten-
    tion/edema*
  High-calorie, high-carbohydrate diet

EXPECTED OUTCOME

Dietary intake meets identified nutritional needs as evidenced by stable weight and laboratory studies

Patient/family teaching

Encourage coughing and deep breathing at least q2h *to prevent respiratory tract infections*

Encourage turning, changing position, and ambulating at least q2h *to prevent respiratory tract infections and promote optimal skin integrity*

Reinforce dietary and fluid restrictions (e.g., high-carbohydrate, low-protein, low-sodium diet)

To prevent UTI

Empty bladder every q2h to 3h

Shower rather than bathe and use antibacterial soap

Keep perineal area clean and dry

Wipe from front to back when cleansing perineal area

Teach about ordered medications: names, dosages, schedules, purposes, and side effects

Home care considerations

Emphasize importance of ongoing outpatient care

Reinforce importance of good handwashing technique for patient and others in contact with patient

Advise patient to avoid interacting with persons who have infections (e.g., colds/flu)

Reinforce need for adequate rest, sleep

Encourage patient to report to physician the following signs and symptoms of recurrence and progression of disease

Edema, puffy eyes, swollen extremities

Lethargy

Decreased urinary output

Instruct patient to weigh self daily: same time, clothing, and scale; report weight gain to home health nurse and/or physician

Encourage patient and/or significant other to monitor BP daily and report elevation to physician

Encourage patient to report symptoms of infection to physician (e.g., fever, sore throat, flu, cough)

Encourage patient to observe character of urine after each void and report abnormalities (e.g., hematuria) to physician

Teach symptoms of UTI (dysuria, foul-smelling urine, fever >101°F [38.5°C]) and encourage patient to report to physician

Advise patient to avoid taking over-the-counter medications without physician approval

Advise patient to avoid straining during bowel movements and ask physician for stool softeners/laxatives as needed

Polycystic Kidney Disease (PKD)

A genetically transmitted disorder in which normal kidney tissue is replaced with grapelike clusters of cysts (Figure 10-19); surrounding cells are destroyed over time because of compression

Assessment

Subjective data

Family history of polycystic kidney disease (PKD)

Abdominal fullness

Flank, abdominal, or lumbar pain

Frequent infections, UTI

Psychological problems (e.g., hopelessness, depression)

Objective data

Palpable abdominal mass

Hypertension

Variable urine output

Hematuria

Diagnostic tests

CBC: elevated WBC, anemia

Urinalysis: white/red blood cells, proteinuria, pyuria, bacteria

Urine culture and sensitivity

Serum electrolytes, BUN, creatinine: abnormal/elevated levels

Urine electrolytes: abnormal levels

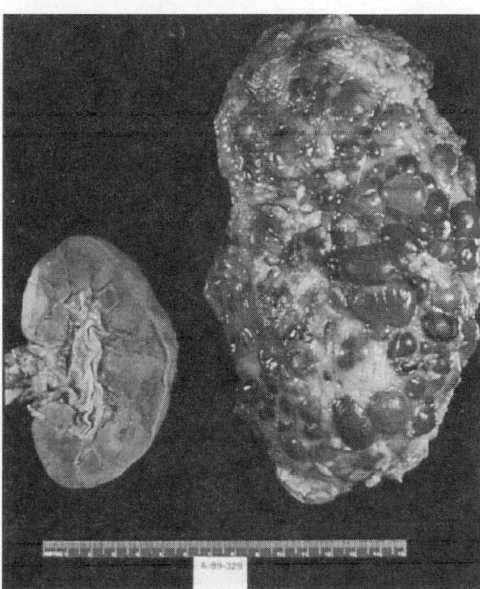

Figure 10-19 Polycystic kidney. **Left,** cross-section. **Right,** whole kidney showing cysts. (From Brundage DJ: *Mosby's clinical nursing series: renal disorders,* St Louis, 1992, Mosby.)

Urine creatinine clearance: decreased kidney function
KUB/renal ultrasonography: enlarged kidneys
Renal biopsy: abnormal kidney cells, tissue
Renal ultrasound: abnormalities of kidney(s)
Intravenous urogram: irregular outline and distortion of calyceal pattern; presence of cysts, nephrocalcinosis, or obstruction of the collecting system

Potential complications

Ruptured cysts
Infection
Calculi
Liver cysts
Renal bleeding
Obstruction
Malignancy
Salt-wasting defect
End-stage renal disease

Collaborative management

Therapeutic management

Medications
    Antihypertensives
    Diuretics
    Antibiotics
    Analgesics
Fluid restriction, parenteral IV fluids
Dietary restriction of protein and sodium
Dialysis and renal transplant when renal failure occurs (see Renal failure, p. 685)
Genetic counseling
Dietitian as recommended
Psychologic consult

Nursing management

PATIENT PROBLEMS/NURSING DIAGNOSES

● **NDX:** Pain related to renal cysts

Assess type, intensity, location, and duration of pain and document *so that changes can be noted and interventions started*
Identify verbal and nonverbal responses to pain
Offer analgesics, documenting effectiveness and tolerance *so that pharmacologic changes can be made as needed*
Institute nonpharmacologic comfort measures
    Optimal positioning
    Relaxation techniques/guided imagery
    Restful environment
    Diversional activity

EXPECTED OUTCOME
Patient is relaxed and expresses increased comfort

● **NDX:** Altered tissue perfusion: renal related to replacement of normal renal tissue with cysts or incompetence of kidney

Monitor intake and output *to determine whether fluid balance is appropriate*
Monitor for signs and symptoms of fluid deficit (e.g., hypotension, poor skin turgor, decreased urinary output, thirst, dry mucous membranes, weight loss) and report to physician for treatment
Monitor for signs and symptoms of fluid excess (e.g., CHF, hypertension, weight gain, edema, decreased urine output, S_3 and S_4 heart sounds, distended neck veins) and report to physician for treatment
Weigh patient daily: same time, clothing, and scale
Monitor BP and note response to and tolerance of antihypertensive medications
Monitor for signs and symptoms of hypertensive crisis (e.g., elevated BP, tachycardia, bradycardia, confusion, decreased LOC, headache, tinnitus, nausea, vomiting, seizures, dysrhythmia) and report to physician for treatment
Monitor blood test results *to identify decrease in renal function*

EXPECTED OUTCOMES
Intake and output are in balance
Weight is stable and within normal range for patient
Vital signs are within normal range for patient

● **NDX:** Risk for infection (UTI, local, systemic) related to disease process, depressed immune system, and/or presence and rupture of fluid-filled cysts

Monitor for signs and symptoms of systemic infection (e.g., fever >101°F [38.5°C], chills, flushed skin, sore throat, productive cough) and report to physician for evaluation, treatment
Monitor for signs and symptoms of UTI (see UTI, p. 648) and report to physician for evaluation and treatment
Avoid instrumentation and/or catheterization of urinary tract if possible; maintain closed gravity drainage system if urethral catheter is present

EXPECTED OUTCOMES
Temperature is within normal range for patient
Urine is clear yellow to amber in color
Breath sounds are clear

● **NDX:** Dysfunctional grieving related to loss of kidney function, changes in lifestyle, decision of having no children, and life-threatening prognosis

Provide an accepting and supportive atmosphere *to maintain patient's self-esteem and promote verbalization of feelings, fears, concerns, and questions*
Explore how having PKD has affected patient's daily activities/lifestyle *to provide support and suggest methods of problem management*
Observe for behavioral and emotional signs of grieving (e.g., denial, anger, crying, withdrawal, noncompliance, dependency) and help patient explore these feelings
Assist patient in identifying coping measures used effectively in the past *so that these may be used to adapt to PKD*
Identify positive features of patient's life *to promote feelings of self-worth*
Reinforce adaptive behaviors and set limits on maladaptive coping mechanisms that interfere with well-being
Provide answers to questions about treatment for PKD
Offer assistance from other professionals (psychologist, sexual counselor, geneticist, clergy) *to help manage emotional changes and decisions concerning pregnancy*
Encourage communication with significant other(s) and/or members of support group *to decrease feelings of isolation*

EXPECTED OUTCOMES
Participates in ADLs at optimal level
Comfortably discusses feelings, fears, concerns, and questions
Identifies approaches for making positive changes in ADLs, lifestyle
Requests assistance from professionals and support group when needed

ADDITIONAL NURSING DIAGNOSIS TO CONSIDER
Altered family processes related to genetically transmitted disease

Patient/family teaching

Encourage coughing and deep breathing using schedule *to prevent respiratory tract infections*
Encourage turning, changing position, and ambulating using a schedule *to prevent respiratory tract infections and promote optimal skin integrity*
Reinforce dietary and fluid restrictions
To help prevent UTI
Empty bladder q2h to 3h (if able to void)

Shower rather than bathe and use antibacterial soap
Keep perineal area clean and dry
Wipe from front to back when cleansing perianal area
Teach about ordered medications: names, dosages, schedules, purposes, and side effects

Home care considerations

Emphasize importance of ongoing outpatient care
Reinforce importance of good handwashing technique for patient and others in contact
Advise patient to avoid interacting with persons who have infections (e.g., colds/influenza)
Reinforce need for rest, sleep
Advise patient and/or significant other to monitor BP and report elevation to physician; teach BP procedure
Encourage patient to observe character of urine after voiding and report abnormalities (e.g., hematuria) to physician
Teach symptoms of UTI (dysuria, foul-smelling urine, fever >101°F [38.5°C]) and encourage patient to report to physician
Advise patient to avoid taking over-the-counter medications without physician approval

Acute Renal Failure

A sudden and severe impairment of renal function resulting in an acute uremic episode; primary causes of acute renal failure (ARF) are impeded blood flow to the kidney, damage to renal tissue, and disrupted urinary flow

Assessment

Subjective data

Change in voiding pattern
Headache
Inability to concentrate
Weakness
Thirst
Metallic taste in mouth
Nausea
Pruritis

Objective data

Anuria
Oliguria
Bladder distension (in obstruction only)
Anemia
Fever
Hypotension

Hypertension
Dry mucous membranes
Decreased venous filling and skin turgor
Kussmaul respirations
Mental status changes
Edema (eyes, legs, hands)
Jugular venous distention
Bruising
Pallor
Weight loss or gain
Vomiting

Diagnostic tests

Urine studies: decreased pH, abnormal findings with
  osmolality, specific gravity, sodium, creatinine, and
  urine sediment
CBC: increased WBC, decreased Hgb, Hct, increased
  BUN/creatinine, phosphate, magnesium, calcium,
  potassium, sodium
KUB: normal or enlarged kidney
Renal ultrasound: obstruction, abnormally sized or
  shaped kidney
Retrograde pyelography: obstruction
Intravenous urogram: obstruction, strictures, or
  masses
Renal scan: cysts, tumors, or impaired perfusion
Renal biopsy: abnormal cells, tissue
ECG: dysrhythmias

Potential complications

Hypervolemia
Acidosis
Hyperkalemia
Hyperphosphatemia
Hypertension
Anemia
Infection
Cardiovascular/respiratory failure

Collaborative management

Therapeutic management

Medications
  Alkalinizing agents
  Potassium-lowering agents
  Antihypertensives
  Diuretics
  Antiinfective agents
  Phosphate-binding agents
  H_2 blockers
  Multivitamins
  Ferrous sulfate

Sodium bicarbonate
Antiemetics
IV fluids
Bed rest
Restraints (only when all other measures fail)
Daily weights
Blood transfusions
Total parenteral nutrition (TPN)
Dialysis
Transplantation
Dietary consult

Nursing management

PATIENT PROBLEMS/NURSING DIAGNOSES

● **NDX:** Fluid volume excess related to inability of
  kidney to adequately process water and
  sodium

Monitor intake and output frequently *so that abnormal
  fluid balance is identified and treated*
Monitor for signs and symptoms of fluid excess
  Hypertension
  Weight gain
  Edema
  Jugular venous distention
Monitor serum electrolyte levels *for abnormalities asso-
  ciated with fluid volume excess* (hyperkalemia, hyper-
  phosphatemia, hypermagnesemia, hypocalcemia)
Monitor effectiveness and tolerance of medications or-
  dered to decrease fluid volume (e.g., diuretics)
Monitor ECG for dysrhythmias, *which may be associ-
  ated with increased/decreased levels of serum potassium*

EXPECTED OUTCOMES
Intake and output are in balance
Weight is stable and within patient's normal range
Heart and breath sounds and electrolytes are within
  normal limits for patient

● **NDX:** Altered nutrition: less than body requirements related to GI disturbances and/or
  restricted dietary intake

Dietitian to assist with developing appropriate meal plan;
  include patient in planning *to increase compliance*
Encourage small, frequent meals *to promote digestion of
  foods*
Weigh patient daily: same time, clothing, and scale
Monitor for conditions that increase loss of needed nu-
  trients (e.g., nausea, vomiting, anorexia)
Monitor effectiveness and tolerance of antiemetics *so
  pharmacologic changes can be made as needed*
Monitor laboratory studies *that may indicate whether*

protein intake is adequate (e.g., serum protein, lipids, potassium, calcium)

Offer oral hygiene regularly *to improve taste in mouth*

EXPECTED OUTCOMES

Patient's dietary intake meets identified nutritional needs as evidenced by stable weight and laboratory studies

Patient participates in developing and complies with nutritional plan

● **NDX:** Fluid volume deficit related to diuretic phase of disease process and/or hemorrhage

Monitor intake and output frequently

Monitor for signs and symptoms of inadequate fluid volume

  Hypotension

  Tachycardia

  Weight loss

  Decreased venous filling and skin turgor

  Dry mucous membranes

  Hemoconcentration; note electrolyte levels (e.g., sodium)

Monitor effectiveness and tolerance of medications ordered *to enhance renal blood flow and systemic circulating volume* (e.g., vasoconstrictors/electrolyte replacements)

Institute measures to decrease hemorrhage

  Use smallest gauge needle possible for venipuncture, injections

  Apply pressure to all injection sites until bleeding stops

  Advise patient to move slowly and carefully to decrease likelihood of bruising, trauma

Monitor for signs and symptoms of hemorrhage

  Hypotension

  Petechiae

  Prolonged bleeding with venipuncture

  Bleeding gums

  Increased abdominal girth

EXPECTED OUTCOMES

Patient's intake balances output

Skin turgor is good

Evidence of bleeding is absent

● **NDX:** Risk for injury related to mental status changes from chemical abnormalities

Assess mental status at admission and document changes

Orient to time, place, and person as needed

Instruct patient to call for assistance when getting out of bed

Observe for changes in behavior *that may indicate alterations in brain function*

Institute seizure precautions

  Airway/suction readily available in room

  Pad siderails

  Restrain only when other measures fail *to protect patient*

EXPECTED OUTCOME

Patient sustains no injuries

ADDITIONAL NURSING DIAGNOSES TO CONSIDER

Risk for infection related to compromised immune system

Risk for impaired skin integrity related to decreased activity, uremia, and edema

Self-care deficit related to fatigue/mental status changes

Altered family processes related to health crisis

Patient/family teaching

Explain cause of the ARF episode when known

Encourage turning, changing position, and ambulating at least q2h *to prevent respiratory tract infections and promote optimal skin integrity*

Explain reasons for dietary and fluid restrictions

Teach about ordered medications: names, dosages, schedules, purposes, and side effects

Teach about BP procedure

Home care considerations

Emphasize importance of ongoing outpatient care

Reinforce importance of good handwashing technique for patient and others in contact with patient

Advise patient to avoid interacting with persons who have infections (e.g., colds/influenza)

Reinforce need for rest, sleep

Advise patient to weigh self daily: same time, clothing, and scale and report changes in weight of 2 lb or more to home health nurse and/or physician

Advise patient to measure urine with each void and report to physician decrease in urine and/or inability to urinate

Instruct patient to check BP at same time each day and report changes to physician; teach procedure for taking BP

Encourage patient to report signs and symptoms of infection to physician (e.g., fever, sore throat, influenza, cough)

Advise patient to avoid taking over-the-counter medications without physician approval

Advise patient to avoid straining during bowel movements and ask physician for stool softeners/laxatives as needed

Chronic Renal Failure

An irreversible, slowly developing condition of impaired renal function; potential causes of chronic renal failure (CRF) are polycystic kidney disease, chronic glomerulonephritis, chronic pyelonephritis, chronic urinary obstruction, hypertensive nephropathy, diabetic nephropathy, and gouty nephropathy

Assessment

Subjective data

Headache
Pruritus
Metallic taste in mouth
Loss of sense of smell
Nocturnal leg cramping
Paresthesia of lower extremities
Blurred vision
Anorexia
Nausea/vomiting
Hiccoughs
Diarrhea
Constipation
Thirst
Fatigue
Bone pain
Insomnia
Amenorrhea
Decreased libido

Objective data

Anuria
Oliguria
Anemia
Hypertension
Dysrhythmia
Kussmaul respirations
Urinelike odor to breath (ammonia)
Mental status changes (drowsiness, confusion, stupor, coma)
Edema
Jugular venous distention
Bruising
Pallor
Dry skin
Brittle nails
Uremic frost
Hematemesis
Melena
Weight gain/loss

Diagnostic tests

Urinalysis: acidic pH, WBCs, RBCs
Urine (24 hr): normal volume (early), no or low volume, proteinuria, decreased creatinine clearance
CBC: decreased Hct/Hgb/platelets
Blood chemistry: abnormal levels of BUN, creatinine, potassium, calcium, phosphorus
KUB
  Small/contracted kidneys
  Very large with polycystic disease
Renal ultrasound: small/contracted kidneys

Potential complications

Anemia
Hypertension
Hyperkalemia
Congestive heart failure
Pulmonary edema
Pericarditis
Accelerated atherosclerosis
Peptic ulcer disease
Osteodystrophy
Metabolic encephalopathy
Peripheral
Neuropathy

Collaborative management

Therapeutic management

Medications
  Alkalinizing agents
  Anticonvulsants
  Antihypertensives
  Diuretics
  Antiinfective agents
  Phosphate-binding agents
  H_2-receptor agents
  Anabolic agents
  Antianemics
  Antiemetics
  Antipruritics
  Laxatives/stool softeners
  Electrolytes/minerals
  Vitamins
Bed rest
Dietary consult
Daily weight
Dialysis
Renal transplantation

Nursing management

PATIENT PROBLEMS/NURSING DIAGNOSES

● **NDX:** Fluid volume excess related to inability of kidney to adequately process water and sodium

Monitor intake and output frequently *so that abnormal fluid balance will be identified and treated*
Monitor for signs and symptoms of fluid excess
  Hypertension
  Weight gain
  Edema
  Jugular venous distention
Monitor serum electrolyte levels for abnormalities, *which may be associated with fluid volume excess (hyperkalemia, hyperphosphatemia, hypermagnesemia, hypocalcemia)*
Monitor effectiveness and tolerance of medications ordered to decrease fluid volume (e.g., diuretics if some kidney function is present)
Monitor ECG for dysrhythmias, *which may be associated with increased/decreased levels of serum potassium*

EXPECTED OUTCOMES

Weight is stable
Breath and heart sounds are normal
Electrolytes are within normal range for patient

● **NDX:** Altered nutrition: less than body requirements related to GI disturbances and/or restricted dietary intake

Dietitian to assist with developing appropriate meal plan; include patient in planning *to increase compliance*
Encourage small, frequent meals *to promote digestion of foods*
Weigh patient daily: same time, clothing, and scale *to ensure accurate and reliable data*
Monitor for conditions that increase loss of needed nutrients (e.g., nausea, vomiting, anorexia) *so that a plan may be implemented to resolve these problems*
Monitor laboratory studies that *may indicate whether protein intake is adequate (e.g., serum protein, lipids, potassium, calcium)*
Offer to provide oral hygiene regularly *to improve taste in mouth*

EXPECTED OUTCOMES

Patient's dietary intake meets identified nutritional needs as evidenced by stable weight, serum albumin, total protein, iron, Hgb and Hct

Patient collaborates in developing and complies with nutritional plan

● **NDX:** Risk for injury related to mental status changes from chemical abnormalities

Assess mental status at admission and document *so that changes will be noted*
Orient to time, place, and person as needed
Explain procedures, treatments, use of equipment; clarify as needed
Observe for changes in behavior, *which may indicate alterations in brain function*
Provide clutter-free environment
Observe frequently if patient is unable to call for assistance
Institute seizure precautions
  Airway, suction readily available in room
  Pad siderails
Restrain only if other measures fail *to protect patient*

EXPECTED OUTCOME

Patient is free of injury

ADDITIONAL NURSING DIAGNOSES TO CONSIDER

Risk for infection related to compromised immune system
Risk for impaired skin integrity related to decreased activity, uremia, and edema
Self-care deficit related to fatigue/mental status changes
Altered family processes related to chronic disease process
Sexual dysfunction related to effects of uremia
Body image disturbance related to altered renal function
Ineffective individual coping related to chronic disease process

Patient/family teaching

Explain details of CRF to patient/family
Discuss treatments aimed at combating the effects of CRF (e.g., renal dialysis/transplantation)
Encourage turning, changing position, and ambulating at least q2h *to prevent respiratory tract infections and promote optimal skin integrity*
Explain reasons for dietary and fluid restrictions
Teach about ordered medications: names, dosages, schedules, purposes, and side effects

Home care considerations

Emphasize importance of ongoing outpatient care
Reinforce importance of good handwashing technique for patient and others in contact

Advise patient to avoid interacting with persons who have infections (e.g., colds/influenza)

Reinforce need for rest, sleep

Advise patient to weigh self daily: same time, clothing, and scale; report changes in weight of 2 lb or more to home health nurse and/or physician

Advise patient to measure urine with each void and report decrease in urine and/or inability to urinate to physician

Instruct patient to check BP at same time each day and report changes to physician

Encourage patient to report signs and symptoms of infection (e.g., fever, sore throat, influenza, cough) to physician

Advise patient to avoid taking over-the-counter medications without physician approval

Advise patient to avoid straining during bowel movements and ask physician for stool softeners/laxatives as needed

Care of Patient After Hemodialysis

Hemodialysis is one form of treatment for acute or chronic renal failure; an external dialyzing system is used to *remove toxic wastes and excess water/fluid and correct electrolyte imbalances; types of access for hemodialysis include external (temporary) arteriovenous cannula (shunt) (Figure 10-20), internal (permanent) arteriovenous fistula, and internal (permanent) arteriovenous graft (Figure 10-21)*

Assessment

Subjective data

Muscle cramps
Pruritis
Headache
Nausea/vomiting

Objective data

Anuria
Vascular access problems (bleeding/clotting/infection)
Hypervolemia
  Hypertension
  Tachycardia
  Jugular venous distention
  Postural edema
  Weight gain

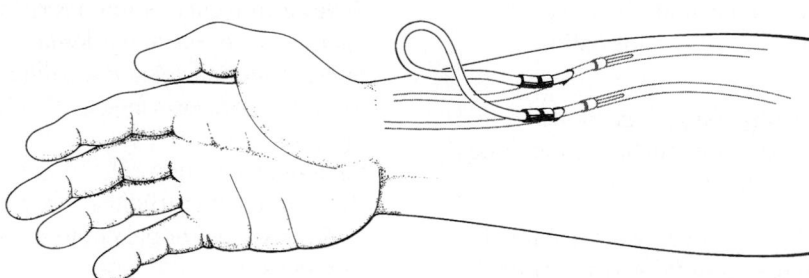

Figure 10-20   External arteriovenous shunt. (From Beare PG, Myers JL: *Principles and practice of adult health nursing,* ed 2, St Louis, 1994, Mosby.)

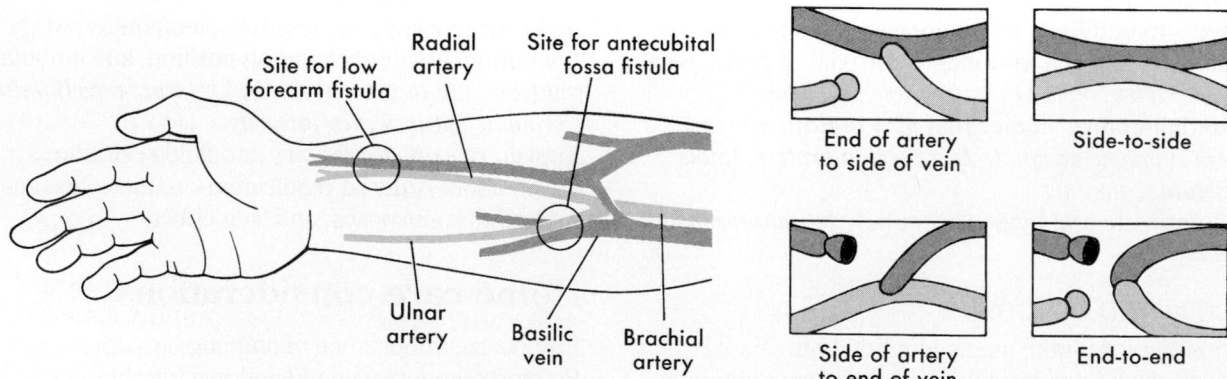

Figure 10-21   Internal arteriovenous fistula. Types of fistula construction. (From Beare PG, Myers JL: *Principles and practice of adult health nursing,* ed 2, St Louis, 1994, Mosby.)

Hypovolemia
  Hypotension
  Bradycardia
  Flat neck veins
  Weight loss
  Dry mucous membranes
Confusion
Seizures
Agitation

Diagnostic tests

Serum electrolytes: abnormal levels
Serum BUN/creatinine: elevated levels expected
Coagulation studies: abnormal PT, PTT, platelet count
Hct/Hgb: decreased levels expected
See Chronic renal failure (p. 688)

Potential complications

Hemorrhage
Air embolism
Severe hypotension
Hepatitis
Septicemia
Hemodynamic problems
Infection
Metabolic problems
Mechanical problems

Collaborative management

Therapeutic management

Medications
  Analgesics
  Antacids
  Antibiotics
  Anticoagulants
  Antidysrhythmics
  Antiemetics
  Antihypertensives
  Antiinflammatories
  Antimicrobials
  Sedatives
  Vitamins
  Ferrous sulfate
  Diuretics
  Calcium
  Sodium bicarbonate
Fluid restriction
Daily weight
Dietary restrictions (dietitian recommendations)
TPN
Guaiac GI tract fluids

Blood transfusions
Psychologic consult

Nursing management

PATIENT PROBLEMS/NURSING DIAGNOSES

● **NDX:** Altered tissue perfusion: peripheral related to risk of vascular access clotting/disconnection

Monitor and document patency of access device frequently *so that changes will be identified* (see Figures 10-20 and 10-21)
  Auscultate for bruits (use doppler as needed)
  Palpate for thrills
  Evaluate patency of exposed area of device (shunt should be wrapped securely with gauze, exposing only a portion of loop)
  Observe color of blood and condition of surrounding skin
  Observe for leakage
  Inspect fistula needle puncture sites after dialysis (if bleeding noted, apply pressure until bleeding subsides)
Report signs and symptoms of clotting of access device to physician
  Dark or separated blood within shunt
  Site cool to touch
  Absence of bruits and/or thrills
Monitor and report signs and symptoms of inadequate peripheral perfusion
  Sudden, unrelieved pain
  Numbness
  Tingling
  Decreased capillary refill time
  Cool skin temperature of extremity distal to access site
Avoid taking BP and performing venipuncture in arm with fistula or cannula *to decrease risk of infection/clotting*
Do not wear jewelry or identification band on extremity with access site
Avoid cutting off dressings at access site *so that puncturing of access will not occur*
Institute measures to manage potentially emergent situations with shunt, subclavian or femoral line
  Keep smooth, rubber-tipped clamps and tourniquet at bedside in case of line disconnection
  If disconnection occurs, clamp tubing and notify physician immediately
  If tubing is pulled out, apply pressure to site and place tourniquet above site; notify physician immediately

EXPECTED OUTCOMES

Access devices are intact as evidenced by presence of bruits, thrills, and blood circulation

Site of access and distal extremity are warm with capillary refill time of 1 to 2 sec

● **NDX:**   Fluid volume excess related to fluid accumulation/inadequate dialysis

Monitor intake and output frequently *so that abnormalities with fluid balance will be identified and treated*
Restrict fluid as ordered
Monitor for signs and symptoms of fluid accumulation (caused by inadequate dialysis)
  Weight gain (check daily same time, using same scale and clothing)
  Elevated BP
  Dyspnea
  Distended neck veins
Monitor blood work *for abnormalities associated with fluid volume excess*
  Elevated BUN/creatinine (nitrogenous waste build-up)
  Elevated sodium/potassium/pH (electrolyte accumulation)
  Anemia (continuing problem with chronic renal failure and blood loss)

   EXPECTED OUTCOME

Patient does not have symptoms of excess fluid after treatment

● **NDX:**   Fluid volume deficit related to rapid removal of body fluid during treatment

Monitor intake and output frequently *so that abnormalities with fluid balance will be identified and treated*
Replace fluid as ordered
Monitor for signs and symptoms of fluid deficit
  Weight loss (check daily at same time, using same scale and clothing)
  Lowered BP
  Nausea
  Muscle cramps

   EXPECTED OUTCOME

Patient has decreased weight after treatment

● **NDX:**   Risk for infection related to presence of access site and invasive procedure

Institute measures to decrease risk of infection
  Use sterile technique when caring for access site(s)
  Cleanse access area gently with hydrogen peroxide or alcohol wipes; cover with dry, sterile dressing
Report signs and symptoms of infection to physician for evaluation: temperature elevation above patient's normal, erythema, edema, drainage at access site
Monitor WBCs for elevation (may indicate infection)

   EXPECTED OUTCOMES

Temperature remains within patient's normal range
No signs or symptoms of infection are noted at access site

● **NDX:**   Body image disturbance related to presence of access device for hemodialysis

Provide an accepting and supportive atmosphere *to maintain patient's self-esteem and promote the verbalization of feelings, fears, concerns, and questions*
Explore how having hemodialysis, access catheter has affected daily life and activities *to provide emotional support and suggest methods of problem management*
Identify positive features of patient's life *to promote feelings of self-worth*
Offer assistance from other professionals (psychologist, sexual counselor) *to assist in management of emotional changes*
Encourage communication with significant other(s) and/or members of support group *to decrease feelings of isolation*

   EXPECTED OUTCOMES

Patient uses psychosocial support systems
Feels comfortable verbalizing fears, feelings, and concerns
Complies with treatment plan

   ADDITIONAL NURSING DIAGNOSES
   TO CONSIDER

Pain/discomfort related to dialysis process
Altered thought processes related to dialysis disequilibrium syndrome or dialysis dementia
Ineffective individual/family coping related to diagnosis of chronic illness
Noncompliance to prescribed treatment regimen (e.g., dietary restrictions)

Patient/family teaching

Explain procedure for surgery to place access device for hemodialysis and hemodialysis procedure; encourage questions, verbalization of concerns and feelings
Explain purpose of prescribed medical regimen
Explain reasons for dietary/fluid restrictions
Teach about ordered medications: names, dosages, schedules, purposes, and side effects

Home care considerations

Emphasize importance of ongoing outpatient care
Reinforce importance of good handwashing technique for patient and others with whom patient comes in contact; maintain aseptic technique when cleansing access site(s)

Advise patient to avoid interacting with persons who have infections (e.g., colds/flu)

Provide written medication schedule for patient; review which medications should be held until after dialysis treatment (to promote optimal absorption)

Reinforce care of access device

Palpate for thrill qd; report absence of thrill to physician

Report presence of dark, separated blood to physician

Report pain, numbness, tingling, change in color of affected extremity to physician

Avoid having blood pressure and/or blood taken from affected extremity

Always carry clamps to stop bleeding in case shunt separates

Advise patient to institute measures that decrease risk of trauma to or bleeding of access device

Keep sterile dressing on site

Wear loose sleeves

No lifting of heavy objects or carrying heavy purse on arm with access

Wear plastic covering on affected extremity if exposed to water

Encourage patient to report redness, pain, swelling, or drainage from access site(s) to physician

Reinforce importance of adhering to dietary/fluid restrictions; record daily intake and output (if applicable)

Reinforce need for rest, sleep

Encourage gradual progression of activity and participation in ADLs as tolerated

Advise patient to weigh self daily: same time, clothing, and scale; report changes in weight of 2 lb or more to home health nurse and/or physician

Instruct patient to check BP at same time each day and report changes to physician

Teach symptoms of UTI (i.e., dysuria, foul-smelling urine, fever >101°F [38.5°C]) and encourage patient to report these findings to physician

Advise patient to avoid taking over-the-counter medications without physician approval

Peritoneal Dialysis

Perioneal dialysis (PD) is one form of treatment for acute or chronic renal failure; dialysate fluid is introduced into the abdominal cavity, using the peritoneum as a semipermeable membrane between the dialysate and the blood found in abdominal vessels; fluid may be instilled via manual exchanges (Figures 10-22 and 10-23) or machine

Types of PD include intermittent peritoneal dialysis (IPD), continuous ambulatory peritoneal dialysis (CAPD), and continuous cycling peritoneal dialysis (CCPD); access devices may be temporary or permanent

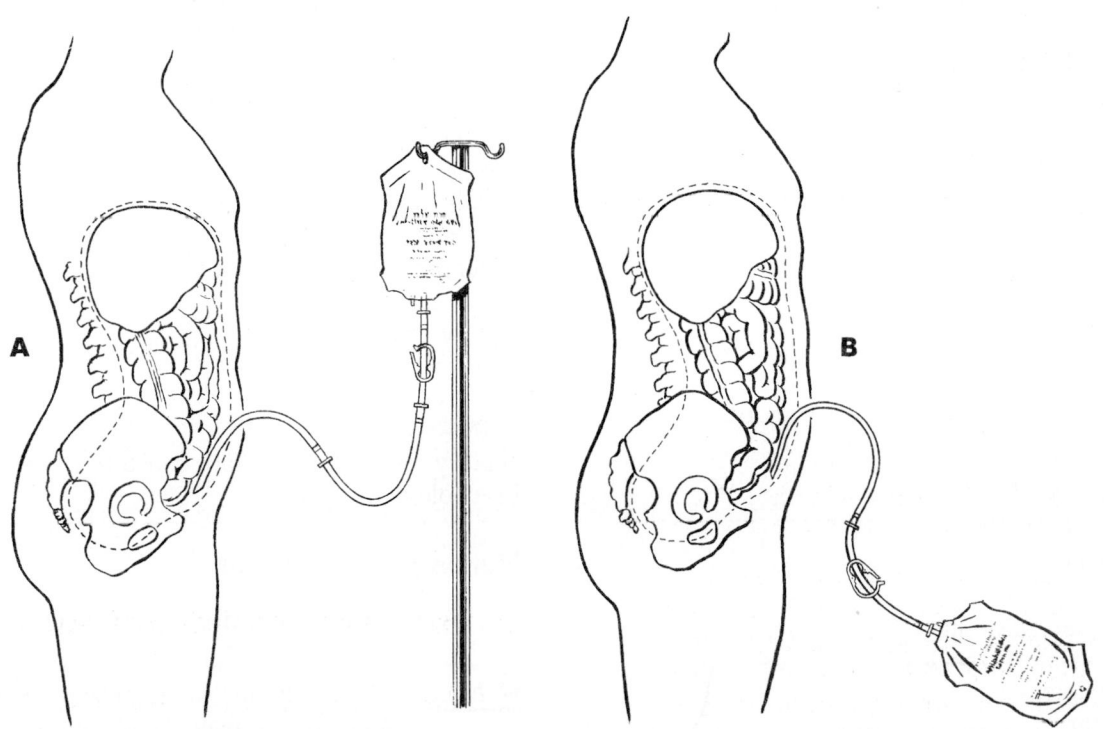

Figure 10-22 Peritoneal dialysis. **A,** Inflow. **B,** Outflow. (From Thompson JM et al: *Mosby's clinical nursing,* ed 3, St Louis, 1993, Mosby.)

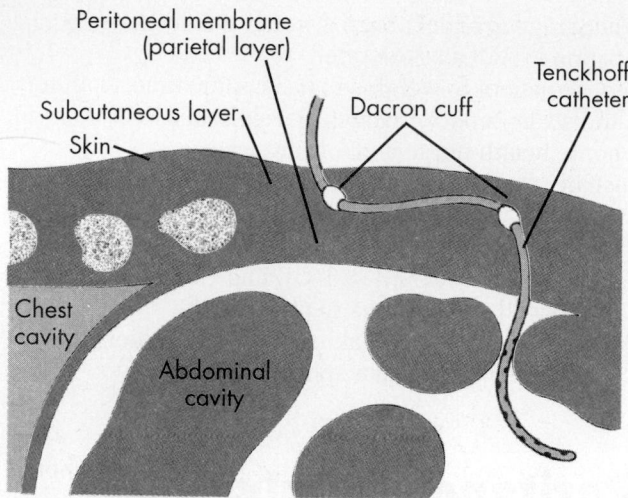

Figure 10-23 Peritoneal catheter. (From Lewis SM, et al: *Medical-surgical nursing: assessment and management of clinical problems,* ed 4, St Louis, 1996, Mosby.)

Assessment

Subjective data

Abdominal pain, tenderness
Thirst
Headache
Fatigue
Nausea
Anxiety

Objective data

Abdominal rigidity
Vomiting
Diarrhea
Decreased/absent bowel sounds
Catheter insertion site
  Redness
  Swelling
  Drainage
Dialysate
  Cloudy
  Red
  Fecal colored
  Foul smelling
Hypervolemia
  Hypertension
  Tachycardia
  Jugular venous distention
  Tachypnea, rales, crackles
  Postural edema
  Weight gain
Hypovolemia

Hypotension
Bradycardia
Flat neck veins
Weight loss
Dry mucous membranes
Confusion
Elevated temperature

Diagnostic tests

Serum electrolytes: abnormal levels
Serum BUN/creatinine: levels elevated above patient's
  normal range
Glucose
Protein
See Renal failure (p. 685)

Potential complications

Leakage/extravasation of dialysate
Hyperglycemia
Peritonitis
Bowel adhesions
Hyperosmolar coma
Perforated bladder/bowel
Hemorrhage
Respiratory conditions

Collaborative management

Therapeutic management

Medications
  Analgesics
  Antacids
  Anticoagulants (history of thrombophlebitis only)
  Antiemetics
  Antihypertensives
  Antimicrobials
  Vitamins
  Ferrous sulfate
  Diuretics
  Calcium
Fluid restriction
Daily weight
Dietary restrictions (dietary consult)
Psychological consult

Nursing management

PATIENT PROBLEMS/NURSING DIAGNOSES

● **NDX:** Fluid volume excess related to fluid accumulation or inability of kidneys to excrete water

Monitor intake and output frequently *so abnormalities will be identified and treated*

Restrict fluid as ordered

Monitor for signs and symptoms of fluid accumulation

  Weight gain (check daily: same time, clothing, and scale when peritoneal cavity is drained)

  Elevated BP

  Dyspnea

  Increased abdominal girth

Monitor serum blood work for abnormalities associated with the following:

  Fluid volume excess: elevated sodium/potassium/pH (electrolyte accumulation)

  Inadequate dialyzing: elevated BUN/creatinine (nitrogenous waste build-up)

  Failure of kidney to produce erythropoetin: decreased Hct (anemia may be associated with uremia)

Ensure tubing is patent *to allow fluid to drain without obstruction*

Implement and maintain accurate dialysis record *so that treatments may be evaluated/amended as needed*

  Strength of solution: 1.5%, 2.5%, or 4.25% dextrose

  Amount of solution instilled/returned

  Time dialysis cycle begins/ends

  Number of exchanges

  Medication used in dialyzing solution

  Weight before and after treatment

Assess bowel status daily; constipation may cause problem with dialysate inflow or outflow

EXPECTED OUTCOMES

Weight remains stable

Abdominal girth is unchanged

BP, P, and breath sounds are within patients normal range

● **NDX:** Fluid volume deficit related to dialysate with high glucose concentration over long periods

Monitor intake and output frequently *so that abnormalities with fluid balance will be identified and treated*

Replace fluid as ordered

Monitor for signs and symptoms of fluid deficit

  Weight loss (check daily same time, scale, and clothing)

  Lowered BP

  Nausea

  Muscle cramps

Implement and maintain accurate dialysis record *so that treatments may be evaluated/amended as needed*

  Strength of solution: 1.5%, 2.5%, or 4.25% dextrose

  Amount of solution instilled/returned

Time dialysis cycle begins/ends

Number of exchanges

Medication used in dialyzing solution

Weight before and after treatment

EXPECTED OUTCOMES

Intake and output are balanced

Weight is stable

Skin turgor is good

● **NDX:** Risk for infection related to peritoneal dialysis catheter (peritonitis and/or infection at catheter insertion site)

Report any temperature elevation above patient's normal range to physician *for evaluation/treatment*

Monitor WBCs for elevation *(may indicate infection)*

Maintain sterile technique and institutional policy when performing dialysis exchanges and dressing changes

Collect samples of dialysate for culture and sensitivity tests if solution is turbid, bloody, or malodorous per policy

Monitor catheter insertion site for signs and symptoms of infection (e.g., erythema, edema, pain, drainage) and report to physician for evaluation/treatment

EXPECTED OUTCOMES

Insertion site is clean and dry

T remains within patient's normal range

Outflow dialysate is clear and without odor

● **NDX:** Body image disturbance related to presence of peritoneal catheter

Provide an accepting and supportive atmosphere *to maintain patient's self-esteem and promote verbalization of feelings, fears, concerns, and questions*

Explore how having peritoneal catheter has affected daily life, activities *to provide emotional support and suggest methods of problem management*

Identify positive features of patient's life *to promote feelings of self-worth*

Offer assistance from other professionals (psychologist, sexual counselor) *to assist in management of emotional changes*

Encourage communication with significant other(s) and/or members of support group *to decrease feelings of isolation*

Explain that tight pants can cause irritation at exit site and bikinis or girdles may disrupt catheter and should not be worn

Explain that there are no social limitations; patient may participate in sports not requiring direct body contact

EXPECTED OUTCOMES

Seeks psychosocial support when needed
Comfortably verbalizes fears, feelings, and concerns

ADDITIONAL NURSING DIAGNOSES
TO CONSIDER

Pain/discomfort related to dialysis process
Ineffective individual/family coping related to diagnosis of chronic illness
Noncompliance to prescribed treatment regimen related to denial of chronic disease

Patient/family teaching

Explain surgical procedure for catheter placement and peritoneal dialysis procedure; encourage questions, verbalization of concerns and feelings
Explain purpose of prescribed medication regimen
Explain reasons for dietary/fluid restrictions
Teach about ordered medications: names, dosages, schedules, purposes, and side effects

Home care considerations

Emphasize importance of ongoing outpatient care
Reinforce importance of good handwashing technique for patient and others with whom patient comes in contact; maintain aseptic technique when performing dialysis exchanges
Reinforce actions aimed at decreasing infection
Protect catheter from damage
Keep sterile cap/dressing in place
Wash catheter insertion site gently with soap and water, rinse well, and pat dry
Advise patient to avoid interacting with persons who have infections (e.g., colds/flu)
Encourage patient to report any T increase to physician
Encourage patient to report turbid, cloudy, malodorous, bloody, or feces-stained dialysate to physician immediately
Encourage patient to report redness, pain, swelling, or drainage from catheter insertion site to physician
Reinforce importance of adhering to dietary/fluid restrictions (e.g., adequate protein, sodium restriction)
Reinforce need for rest, sleep
Encourage gradual progression of activity and participation in ADLs as tolerated
Advise patient to weigh self daily: same time, clothing, and scale; report changes in weight of 2 lb or more to home health nurse and/or physician
Instruct patient to check BP at same time each day and report changes to physician
Teach symptoms of UTI (i.e., dysuria, foul-smelling urine, T elevation) and encourage patient to report to physician

Advise patient to avoid taking over-the-counter medications without physician approval
Advise patient to avoid straining during bowel movements and ask physician for stool softeners/laxatives as needed

Nephrectomy: Total/Partial

Total or partial surgical removal of a kidney via a flank, transabdominal, or thoracoabdominal incision; indicated in the treatment of renal malignancy, chronic pyelonephritis, trauma, polycystic kidney disease, renal vascular disease, congenital deformity, or renal calculi, or for the purpose of donation

Assessment

Subjective data (postoperative)

Pain

Objective data (postoperative)

Urine output: character, amount, color
Patent drainage systems
Ureteral catheter
Nephrostomy tube stents
Site of incision: redness, swelling, drainage
Fever
Anxiety

Diagnostic tests

Blood typing, cross matching, tissue compatibility testing (done preoperatively)
Serum electrolytes: abnormal results
BUN/creatinine: elevated
Coagulation studies: abnormal clotting patterns
CBC: decreased Hct/Hgb, elevated WBC
Chest x-ray: abnormalities in lung(s): pneumonia/atelectasis
Urinalysis: WBC, RBC, sediment, bacteria
Urine culture and sensitivity
Urine creatinine clearance (24 hr): inadequate processing of waste by kidney(s)
IVP: abnormalities in kidney(s), ureter(s), bladder
Renal arteriogram: inadequate blood supply to kidney(s)
Renal venogram: inadequate venous drainage system of kidney(s)
Renal ultrasound: abnormalities in kidney(s), ureter(s), bladder

Potential complications

Pneumonia
Pneumothorax
Hemorrhage/shock
Paralytic ileus
Infection

Collaborative management

Therapeutic management

Medications
  Analgesics
  Antiemetics
  Antibiotics
  Stool softeners/laxatives
  IV fluids
Nasogastric tube
NPO until bowel sounds return
Incentive spirometer
Wound/drain management
Psychological consult

Nursing management

PATIENT PROBLEMS/NURSING DIAGNOSES

● **NDX:** Risk for fluid volume deficit related to hypovolemia or hemorrhage

Monitor intake and output frequently *so that abnormalities with fluid balance will be identified and reported*
Assess surgical dressing, tubes, stents, and catheters for patency and bleeding qh and report to physician
Monitor urinary output for evidence of excessive hematuria (urine is expected to be pink tinged not bright red)

EXPECTED OUTCOMES

Patient's intake and output are in balance
Stents, catheters are patent
Urine is pink to yellow

● **NDX:** Pain related to nephrectomy

Assess type, intensity, location, and duration of pain and document *so that changes may be noted*
Identify verbal and nonverbal responses to pain
Ensure that catheters/tubes are patent *to promote optimal drainage/prevent pressure from backflow*
Secure catheters/tubes *to prevent pulling sensation or dislodgement*
Offer analgesics, document effectiveness and tolerance *so that pharmacologic changes may be made as needed*

Institute nonpharmacologic comfort measures
  Optimal positioning
  Relaxation techniques/guided imagery
  Restful environment
  Diversional activity
  Splint incision when turning, coughing, and deep breathing

EXPECTED OUTCOME

Patient assumes relaxed posture and verbalizes increasing comfort

● **NDX:** Altered urinary elimination related to nephrostomy tube, ureteral catheter, and surgical intervention

Assess patient's previous voiding pattern and begin voiding diary *to document changes*
Monitor for signs and symptoms of UTI (e.g., dysuria, frequency, urgency) and report to physician for evaluation and treatment
Maintain patency of catheters *to promote optimal flow of urine*
  Tubing below level of bladder to allow for gravity flow
  Assess for clamping/kinks in tubing
  Secure catheters while still allowing for patient movement
  Irrigate tubes cautiously, using small volume and only when ordered *to prevent damage*
  Label each tube clearly and record drainage from each tube separately *to allow for accurate assessment of output from each system*
If nephrostomy tube is in place
  Tape to flank
  Do not clamp
  Irrigate only with physician's order (may be continuous or intermittent)
  Have extra tube available at bedside *for emergency use if tube is dislodged*
  Notify physician immediately if nephrostomy tube becomes dislodged
After urinary bladder catheter is removed, institute measures to facilitate voiding
  Privacy
  Comfortable positioning
  Running tap water
  Placing patient's hand in warm water
  Applying heat to suprapubic area (if ordered)
  Pouring warm water over perineum
  Relaxation techniques
  Applying oil of peppermint (a few drops in bedpan/urinal or on cotton ball in front of urinary meatus)
  Stroking inner aspect of thigh gently with ice
  Offering analgesic

Voiding 1 to 2 hr after fluid intake
Double voiding (to empty bladder more completely)
Encourage patient to drink at least 2500 ml/day (unless contraindicated) to promote adequate output

EXPECTED OUTCOMES

Patient's intake balances output
Regular voiding pattern is established

● **NDX:** Risk for infection related to surgical incision/presence of tubes, catheters

Assess incision q4h for presence of erythema, edema, tenderness, and drainage; document findings *so that changes may be identified and treated*
Report signs and symptoms of infection (fever/chills) to physician *so that appropriate interventions may be implemented*
Obtain wound culture as ordered *to identify bacteria*
Monitor for elevation of WBC, *indicates presence of infection*
Administer and monitor tolerance of ordered antibiotics

EXPECTED OUTCOME

Incision is intact and dry

● **NDX:** Dysfunctional grieving related to loss of body organ

Provide an accepting and supportive atmosphere *to maintain patient's self-esteem and promote verbalization of feelings, fears, concerns, and questions*
Explore how losing a kidney (or part) and/or donating kidney for transplantation has affected patient and and patient's family
Identify positive features of patient's life *to promote feelings of self-worth*
Offer assistance from other professionals (psychologist, clergy, sexual counselor) *to assist with management of emotional changes*
Encourage communication with significant other(s) and/or members of support group *to decrease feelings of isolation*

EXPECTED OUTCOMES

Seeks psychosocial support when needed
Comfortably verbalizes fears, feelings, and concerns and uses effective coping measures

ADDITIONAL NURSING DIAGNOSES TO CONSIDER

Ineffective breathing patterns (postoperatively) related to effects of anesthesia
Altered tissue perfusion: peripheral, cardiopulmonary, and GI related to postoperative complications
Ineffective individual/family coping related to surgical removal of major body organ

Patient/family teaching

Explain surgical procedure; encourage questions, verbalization of concerns and feelings
Explain purpose of prescribed medical/surgical regimen
Explain reasons for dietary/fluid restrictions
Explain importance of turning, coughing, and deep breathing q2h; instruct in use of incentive spirometer and splinting postoperatively
Teach about ordered medications: names, dosages, schedules, purposes, and side effects

Home care considerations

Emphasize importance of ongoing outpatient care
Reinforce importance of good handwashing technique for patient and others with whom patient comes in contact
Advise patient to avoid interacting with persons who have infections (e.g., colds/influenza)
Reinforce need for rest, sleep
Encourage gradual progression of activity and participation in ADLs as tolerated; no heavy lifting until approved by physician
Advise patient to avoid activities (e.g., contact sports) that may endanger remaining kidney
Advise patient to alert other health professionals of presence of nephrostomy or ureteral catheter and history of nephrectomy
Encourage patient to report fever >101°F (38.5°C) to physician
Reinforce method of caring for incision, dressing, tubes, and drains (refer to home health agency as needed)
Encourage patient to report to physician redness, pain, swelling, or drainage from incisional site
Instruct patient to institute measures to prevent UTI (see p. 648)
Teach symptoms of UTI (dysuria, foul-smelling urine, fever >101°F [38.5°C]) and encourage patient to report to physician
Advise patient to avoid taking over-the-counter medications without physician approval
Advise patient to avoid straining during bowel movements and ask physician for stool softeners/laxatives as needed

Renal Transplantation*

A functioning kidney is removed from a living donor or a human cadaver and is transplanted into the right or left iliac fossa of the recipient; the renal blood vessels of the donor organ are anastomosed to the recipient's iliac artery and vein, and the ureter is transplanted into the bladder or anastomosed to the recipient's ureter to establish urinary tract continuity (Figure 10-24)

Assessment

Subjective data (postoperative)

Pain
Anxiety
Depression

Objective data (postoperative)

Rejection of kidney (Table 10-10)
Decreased urinary output
Hematuria
Decreased/diminished breath sounds
Tachypnea
Tachycardia
Hemorrhage

*See Nephrectomy (p. 696) for care of donor

Diagnostic tests

See Renal Failure, p. 685
Blood typing/cross matching/tissue compatibility testing (done preoperatively)
Chest x-ray: abnormalities in lung(s); pneumonia/ atelectasis
ECG: dysrhythmias

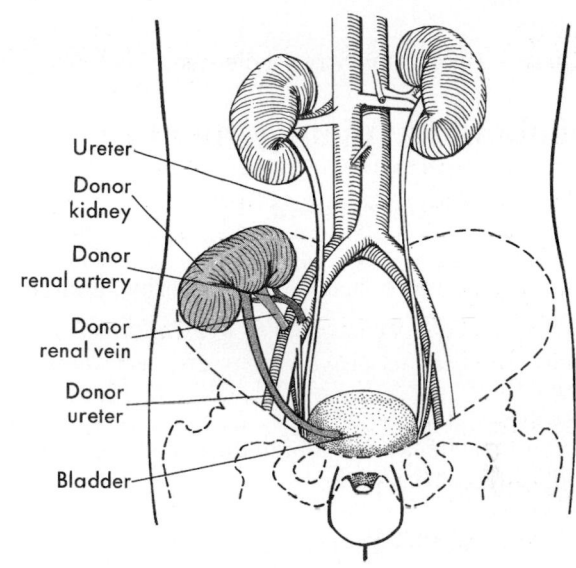

Ureter
Donor kidney
Donor renal artery
Donor renal vein
Donor ureter
Bladder

Figure 10-24 Location of transplanted kidney showing anastomosis of renal artery, renal vein, and ureter. (From Phipps WJ et al: *Medical-surgical nursing: concepts and clinical practice*, ed 5, St Louis, 1995, Mosby.)

Table 10-10 Classification of Rejection

Hyperacute	Acute	Chronic
Rejection occurs as soon as new kidney is implanted	Rejection occurs 1 wk to 3 months after kidney has been implanted	Rejection occurs at any time after surgery
Rejection is caused by presence of antibodies in recipient that cause polymorphonuclear leukocytes to clot, thus blocking glomerular and peritubular capillaries	Immune response leukocytes and RBCs invade vascular endothelium and intertubular vasculature; renal blood flow is decreased; therefore necrosis of renal tubules occurs	There is gradual decline in kidney function; glomerular filtration is decreased, and serum creatinine and serum urea nitrogen are elevated; proteinuria occurs, and sodium is decreased in urine
Rejection is usually irreversible	Rejection may be reversible	Early detection and treatment may decrease decline in kidney function
Transplanted kidney is removed immediately	Attempt is made to save new kidney	Attempt is made to save kidney
Patient resumes hemodialysis	Patient may need to resume dialysis treatments	Patient may need to resume dialysis treatments

Potential complications

Rejection
Ureteral fistula/obstruction
Renal artery stenosis
Shock
Paralytic ileus
Diabetes
Cushing's syndrome
GI bleeding
Glaucoma
Reappearance of primary renal disease

Collaborative management

Therapeutic management

Medications
  Immunosuppressive agents (Cyclosporine, Imuran)
  Analgesics
  Antacids
  Antiemetics
  Antibiotics
  Insulin (may be needed if high-dosage steroids used)
  Stool softeners/laxatives
  IV fluids
NPO until bowel sounds return
Incentive spirometer
Wound/drain management
Hemodialysis
Psychological consult

Nursing management

PATIENT PROBLEMS/NURSING DIAGNOSES

● **NDX:**   Risk for fluid volume excess or deficit related to postoperative diuresis, changes in renal perfusion

Monitor intake and output frequently *so that abnormalities with fluid balance will be identified and reported*
Weigh patient daily: same time, clothing, and scale *to ensure accurate and reliable results*
Monitor for signs and symptoms related to fluid balance changes
  Change in skin turgor, mucous membranes
  Change in CVP
  Abnormal serum electrolytes
Restrict/administer fluids as ordered; monitor and document patient response to therapy

EXPECTED OUTCOMES

Vital signs and weight are stable and within patient's normal range
Skin turgor is good

● **NDX:**   Pain related to renal transplantation surgery

Assess type, intensity, location, and duration of pain and document *so that changes may be noted*
Identify verbal and nonverbal responses to pain
Ensure that catheters/tubes are patent *to promote optimal drainage, prevent pressure from backflow*
Secure catheters/tubes *to prevent pulling sensation*
Offer analgesics, documenting effectiveness and tolerance *so that pharmacologic changes may be made as needed*
Institute nonpharmacologic comfort measures
  Optimal positioning
  Relaxation techniques/guided imagery
  Restful environment
  Diversional activity
  Splint incision when turning, coughing, and deep breathing

EXPECTED OUTCOME

Patient assumes relaxed posture and verbalizes increasing comfort

● **NDX:**   Risk for infection related to immunosuppression, incision, or presence of drains and catheters

Assess incision (transplant site) for presence of erythema, edema, tenderness, and drainage; document findings *so that changes may be identified and treated*
Report signs and symptoms of infection (e.g., fever/chills) to physician *so that appropriate interventions may be implemented*
Obtain wound culture, as ordered, *to identify bacteria*
Obtain urine culture if urine is cloudy or malodorous *to identify bacteria*
Monitor for elevation of WBC, *which indicates presence of infection*
Monitor for decrease in WBC, *which indicates immunosuppressive response*
Administer and monitor tolerance of ordered antibiotics

EXPECTED OUTCOMES

Patient is afebrile
Incision is clean and dry
WBCs are within normal range for patient

● **NDX:**   Altered urinary elimination related to renal transplantation

Assess patient's previous voiding pattern and begin voiding diary *to note changes*
Urine may be blood tinged in immediate postoperative period; determine whether irrigation may be performed if needed *to dislodge clots*

Monitor for signs and symptoms of UTI (dysuria, frequency, urgency) and report to physician *for evaluation and treatment*

Maintain patency of catheters *to promote optimal flow of urine*

Tubing below level of bladder to allow for gravity flow

Assess for clamping/kinks in tubing

Secure catheters while still allowing for patient movement

Irrigate tubes as ordered

Label each tube or catheter clearly and record drainage from each tube separately *to accurately assess output from each system*

Monitor for and report abdominal/bladder distention *to prevent tension on anastomosis*

After urinary catheter is removed, encourage patient to void q1h to 2h *to decrease bladder distention and tension on anastomosis*

Institute measures to facilitate voiding

Privacy

Comfortable positioning

Running tap water

Placing patient's hand in warm water

Applying heat to suprapubic area (if ordered)

Pouring warm water over perineum

Relaxation techniques

Applying oil of peppermint (a few drops in bedpan/urinal or on cotton ball in front of urinary meatus)

Stroking inner aspect of thigh gently with ice

Offering analgesic

Voiding 1 to 2 hr after fluid intake

Double voiding (to empty bladder more completely)

Encourage patient to drink up to 2500 ml/day (unless contraindicated) *to promote adequate output*

EXPECTED OUTCOMES

Patient's intake balances output

Regular voiding pattern is established

● **NDX:** Body image disturbance related to new organ

Provide an accepting and supportive atmosphere *to maintain patient's self-esteem and promote verbalization of feelings, fears, concerns, and questions*

Explore how receiving a new kidney and concern for donor have affected patient and patient's family

Explain side effects of immunosupressants that may cause appearance changes

Identify positive features of patient's life *to promote feelings of self-worth*

Offer assistance from other professionals (psychologist, clergy, sexual counselor) and kidney recipients *to assist in management of emotional changes*

Encourage communication with significant other(s) and/or members of support group *to decrease feelings of isolation*

EXPECTED OUTCOMES

Seeks psychosocial support as needed

Comfortably verbalizes fears, feelings, and concerns

ADDITIONAL NURSING DIAGNOSES
TO CONSIDER

Ineffective breathing patterns (postoperatively) related to anesthesia

Noncompliance to prescribed treatment plan related to change in condition

Ineffective individual/family coping related to surgical placement of major body organ

Patient/family teaching

Explain surgical procedure; encourage questions, verbalization of concerns and feelings

Demonstrate appropriate handwashing technique

Explain reasons for dietary/fluid restrictions

Explain importance of turning, coughing, and deep breathing regularly; instruct in use of incentive spirometer and splinting

Explain importance of early ambulation/activity

Teach about ordered medications: names, dosages, schedules, purposes, and side effects

Home care considerations

Emphasize importance of ongoing outpatient care

Reinforce importance of good handwashing technique for patient and others with whom patient comes in contact

Advise patient to avoid interacting with persons who have infections (e.g., colds/flu)

Reinforce need for rest, sleep

Encourage patient to report signs and symptoms of rejection to physician

Redness, swelling, tenderness over transplant site

Fever

Decreased urinary output

Edema

Emotional/mental status changes

Provide written information about potential side effects of immunosuppressive medications and encourage patient to report to physician difficulties in tolerating medication

Encourage patient to wear medical alert/identification bracelet

Advise patient to check BP at same time each day and report changes to physician

Advise patient to weigh self daily: same time, clothing,

and scale; report change of 2 lb or more to physician

Encourage gradual progression of activity and participation in ADLs as tolerated; restrict lifting and driving as advised by physician

Advise patient to avoid activities (e.g., contact sports) that may endanger new and remaining kidney

Advise patient to alert other health professionals (e.g., dentist) of presence of new kidney

Reinforce need to comply with dietary/fluid restrictions (e.g., avoiding alcoholic beverages unless approved by physician)

Advise patient to consult with physician regarding resumption of sexual activity, contraception methods

Encourage patient to report fever >101°F (38.5°C) to physician

Reinforce method of caring for incision, dressing, catheters, and drains (refer to home health agency as needed)

Encourage patient to report to physician redness, pain, swelling, or drainage from incisional site

Instruct patient to institute measures to prevent UTI (see p. 648)

Explain reasons for and importance of having blood drawn as ordered

Encourage eye examinations every 6 months to assess for visual changes; routine physical examination and laboratory follow-up

Teach symptoms of UTI (dysuria, foul-smelling urine, fever >101°F [38.5°C]) and encourage patient to report to physician

Advise patient to avoid taking over-the-counter medications without physician approval

Advise patient to avoid straining during bowel movements and ask physician for stool softeners/laxatives as needed

BIBLIOGRAPHY

Ackley BJ, Ladwig GB: *Nursing diagnosis handbook: a guide to planning care,* ed 2, St Louis, 1995, Mosby.

Beare PG, Myers JL: *Principles and practice of adult health nursing,* ed 2, St Louis, 1994, Mosby.

Brundage DJ: *Mosby's clinical nursing series: renal disorders,* St Louis, 1992, Mosby.

Dunn SA: How to care for the dialysis patient, *Am J Nurs* June, 26, 1993.

Gray M: *Mosby's clinical nursing series: genitourinary disorders,* St Louis, 1992, Mosby.

Helberg JL: Patients' status at home care discharge, *IMAGE J Nurs Sch* 25(2):9, 1993.

Jones KR: Risk of hospitalization for chronic hemodialysis patients, *IMAGE J Nurs Sch* 24(2):88, 1992.

Kim MJ et al: *Pocket guide to nursing diagnoses,* ed 6, St Louis, 1995, Mosby.

LeMone P: Analysis of a human phenomenon: self-concept, *Nurs Diagn* 2(3):126, 1991.

McCance KL, Huether SE: *Pathophysiology: the biological basis for disease in adults and children,* ed 2, St Louis, 1994, Mosby.

McClosky B: The NIC taxonomy structure, *IMAGE J Nurs Sch* 25(3):187, 1993.

McCormick KA et al: Urinary incontinence in adults, *Am J Nurs* 92(10):75, 1992.

McFarland GK, McFarlane EA: *Nursing diagnosis and intervention planning for patient care,* ed 2, St Louis, 1993, Mosby.

Mehmert PPA, Delaney CW: Validating impaired physical mobility, *Nurs Diagn* 2(4):14, 1991.

Melman A: Urinary tract infection: specific concerns in elderly patients, *Consultant* July, 115, 1992.

Moore S et al: Nerve sparing prostatectomy, *Am J Nurs* April, 59, 1992.

Moore S, Newton M, Yancey R: How to irrigate a nephrostomy tube, *Am J Nurs* July, 6, 1993.

Norris J: Nursing intervention for self-esteem disturbances, *Nurs Diagn* (2):48, 1992.

Ouellet LL, Rush KL: A synthesis of selected literature on mobility: a basis for studying impaired mobility, *Nurs Diagn* (2):72, 1992.

Pagana KD, Pagana TJ: *Mosby's diagnostic and laboratory test reference,* ed 2, St Louis, 1995, Mosby.

Pearson: Liquidate a myth . . . , *Urol Nurs* 13(3):86, 1993.

Peterson KJ, Solie CJ: Interpreting lab values in chronic renal insufficiency, *Am J Nurs* May, 56B, 1994.

Radziewicz RM, Schneider SM: Using diversional activity to enhance coping, *Cancer Nurs* 15(4):29, 1992.

Resnick B: Retraining the bladder after catheterization, *Am J Nurs* November, 46, 1993.

Rogers J: Pass the cranberry juice, *Nurs Times* 87(48):6, 1991.

Scheck DN, Pappas PG: Lower urinary tract infections in women: a pragmatic approach, *Hosp Med* May: 48, 1993.

Sparks SM: Exploring electronic support groups, *Am J Nurs* December: 62, 1992.

Thayer D: How to assess and control urinary incontinence, *Am J Nurs* October: 42, 1994.

US Department of Health and Human Services: Benign prostatic hyperplasia: diagnosis and treatment, Pub No 94-0582, Rockville, Md, 1994, US Government Printing Office.

US Department of Health and Human Services: Urinary incontinence in adults, Pub No 92-0040, Rockville, Md, 1992, US Government Printing Office.

Willis D: Taming the overgrown prostate, *Am J Nurs* February 4, 1992.

BARNES

CARE PATH
750 CYSTECTOMY WITH NEOPLASM

SERVICE		PHYSICIAN		
PRIMARY NURSE		PRIMARY NURSE		
DC DATE	ADM DATE	DATE OF SURGERY	A-8	

PROBLEM NUMBER	PATIENT PROBLEMS / NURSING DIAGNOSES
#1	ALT. IN URINARY ELIMINATION R/T
#2	LACK OF KNOWLEDGE R/T
#3	ALT. IN COMFORT R/T

PROB.NO.		ADM. DAY 1	DAY 2 DOS	DAY 3 POD 1 OU	DAY 4 POD 2 OU	DAY 5 POD 3 OU	DAY 6 POD 4 OU	DAY 7 POD 5
#1 #2	ASSESSMENT/MONITORING	Adm. work-up	Freq Postop VS;	VS q̄ 4 ×1 ×2 ×3 ×4 ×5 ×6 drsg; NG Stoma viability Stent position Urine output ≥30 cc/hr Monitor labs Pain control Lung sounds Bowel sounds	VS q̄ 4 ×1 ×2 ×3 ×4 ×5 ×6 Stoma viability Stent position Urine output ≥30 cc/hr Monitor labs Pain control Lung sounds Bowel sounds	VS q̄ 4 ×1 ×2 ×3 ×4 ×5 ×6 Stoma viability Stent position Urine output ≥30 cc/hr Monitor labs Pain control Lung sounds Bowel sounds	VS q̄ 4 ×1 ×2 ×3 ×4 ×5 ×6 Stoma viability Stent position Urine output ≥30 cc/hr Monitor labs Pain control Lung sounds Bowel sounds **Hemodynamically stable**	VS q̄ shift ×1 ×2 ×3 Wound open to air Staples intact Stoma viability Stent position Urine output ≥30 cc/hr Monitor labs Pain control Lung sounds Bowel sounds
#2	CONSULTS	Surg. CNS	Social Work	Home Health				
#1 #3	PROCEDURE/TEST	Adm. Labs UA with Micro Urine C & S CXR ECG Mark stoma placement Type & Cross 4 units PRBC	Irrigate NG tube q̄ 4° ×1 ×2 ×3 ×4 ×5 ×6 Check pH CBC, 6 in PAR Check NG pH q̄ 4° ×1 ×2 ×3 ×4 ×5 ×6	CBC, 6 Pulse Oximetry ×1			DC NG tube	IVP Prep
#1 #3	TREATMENT	Weight TWE till clear. Betadine scrub Measure/order TEDS	TEDS sequential stocking IS / TCDB q̄ 2 ° ×1 ×2 ×3 ×4 ×5 ×6 ×7 ×8 ×9 ×10 ×11 ×12 O₂	D/C sequential TEDS IS/TCDB q̄ 2 ° ×1 ×2 ×3 ×4 ×5 ×6 ×7 ×8 ×9 ×10 ×11 ×12 Weight D/C O₂ Ted Hose	IS / TCDB q̄ 2 ° ×1 ×2 ×3 ×4 ×5 ×6 ×7 ×8 ×9 ×10 ×11 ×12 Weight Ted Hose	**No atelectasis** Using IS independently Ted Hose	Using IS independently Ted Hose	Using IS independently Ted Hose
#3	ACTIVITY	UP AD LIB	Bed rest	Up with assist Chair/amb TID ×1 ×2 ×3 Bed bath	Up with assist Chair/amb TID ×1 ×2 ×3 Assist bed bath	Increase amb QID ×1 ×2 ×3 ×4 Assist bath	Amb QID ×1 ×2 ×3 ×4 Assist bath	Amb QID ×1 ×2 ×3 ×4 Assist bath

Used by permission of Barnes Hospital, St. Louis, Missouri.

Continued.

BARNES

CARE PATH
750 CYSTECTOMY WITH NEOPLASM

CNS	DIETARY	RT
HOME HEALTH	OT	OTHER
PT	SW	OTHER

A-8

PROBLEM NUMBER	PATIENT PROBLEMS / NURSING DIAGNOSES

DAY 8 POD 6	DAY 9 POD 7	DAY 10 POD 8	DAY 11 POD 9	POST DC	DC OUTCOMES
VS q̄ shift ×1 ×2 ×3 Wound open to air Staples intact Stoma viability Stent position Urine output ≥30 cc/hr Monitor labs Pain control Lung sounds Bowel sounds	VS q̄ shift ×1 ×2 ×3 Wound open to air Staples intact Stoma viability Stent position Urine output ≥30 cc/hr Monitor labs Pain control Lung sounds Bowel sounds	VS q̄ shift ×1 ×2 ×3 Wound open to air Staples intact Stoma viability Stent position Urine output ≥30 cc/hr Monitor labs Pain control Lung sounds Bowel sounds **No leaking, skin problems with ostomy equipment U.O. = ³ prior to stent removal**	VS q̄ shift ×1 ×2 ×3 Wound open to air Staples intact Stoma viability Stent position Urine output ≥30 cc/hr Monitor labs Pain control Lung sounds Bowel sounds		**Afebrile: VSS** **Stoma Viable** **U. O. = ³ than before stent removal** **Wound intact** **Lungs clear** **Labs WNL** **Hemodynamically stable**
					DC with MD/clinic/f/u in 2 weeks home health ref. form completed
DC Urinary stent Modified IVP					
Using IS independently	**Using IS at 90 - 100% of preop level**				**No pulmonary complications** **Loop functioning** **Weight stable** **No thrombophlebitis**
Ted Hose	Ted Hose	Ted Hose	Ted Hose	Ted Hose	
Amb QID ×1 ×2 ×3 ×4 Independent personal hygiene	UP AD LIB	UP AD LIB	**Amb independently**		**As before adm with restrictions involving limited exertional activity**

		ADM. DAY 1	DAY 2	DAY 3	DAY 4	DAY 5	DAY 6	DAY 7
#1	MEDS/IVS	IVF Bowel Prep	IVF IV Antibiotics H_2 antagonist IV PCA IV Antacid per NG tube	IVF IV Antibiotics H_2 antagonist IV PCA IV Antacid per NG tube	IVF IV Antibiotics H_2 antagonist IV PCA IV Antacid per NG tube	IVF IV Antibiotics H_2 antagonist IV PCA IV Antacid per NG tube	IVF IV Antibiotics H_2 antagonist IV DC PCA; oral analgesic DC antacid	IVF IV Antibiotics DC H_2 antagonist PO analgesia
#1	NUTRITION	Clear liquid NPO after MN	NPO	NPO	NPO	NPO	Clear liq.	Clear liq.
#1 #2	PATIENT/FAMILY EDUCATION	Preop: IS, Activity Postop goals Intro Ostomy booklet Plan of Care Primary Nsg.	Postop orders, plan of care, pain control Explain ostomy teaching plan	Ostomy Teaching booklet	Demonstrate pouch/valve & connector		Review pouch chg. with pt. Assist pt with flange & pouch chg. Review teaching booklet	Review teaching booklet. Review ostomy/skin care, pouch, flange change. Instruct pt on IVP procedure
#1 #2	DISCHARGE PLANNING	**Pt / family verbalizes understanding of care path.** **Plan of care has been mutually set with pt/family.**			SW: initial interview regarding: living situation, support systems, resource needs		CNS, SW, HH review DC plan	
#1 #2	PSYCHOSOCIAL / EMOTIONAL NEEDS	Nursing: initial assessment Identify support person(s)	Nursing: Therapeutic emotional care	Nursing: Therapeutic emotional care	SW: initiate support. Assess counseling needs. Provide emotional support	Nursing/SW: Provide emotional support	Nursing / SW: Provide emotional support	Nursing / SW: Provide emotional support
	SIGNATURES							

3100-51

Continued.

	DAY 8	DAY 9	DAY 10	DAY 11	POST DC	DC OUTCOMES
4	Heplock IVF	Heplock IVF	Heplock IVF	DC Heplock		**Pain controlled with oral analgesics** **No gastric distress** **No UTI**
	PO antibiotics PO analgesia	PO antibiotics PO analgesia	PO antibiotics PO analgesia	PO antibiotics PO analgesia	PO antibiotics PO analgesia	
	Full liq.	Soft	Reg prior	Reg as before adm.	Reg as before adm.	**Tolerating diet as before adm.**
	Review night drainage system	Reinforce ostomy education Encourage independence with ostomy care	Pt assist with flange, pouch change. Review home needs. Review community resources available. Instruct on wound care Instruct S/S VTI.	Review disch. needs, Review ostomy care, Review how to order supplies.		**Able to verbalize/demonstrate:** **Use of valve, Application/ removal of pouch/flange.** **Night drainage system** **stoma skin care** **S/S wound infection** **S/S UTI**
	HH: Assess home needs (Barnes) outside home health referral initiated by SW		SW/HH/nursing Finalize DC plans outside home health referral initiated by SW	HH: visit pt to explain services (Barnes) Nursing: inventory ostomy supplies with pt SW/HH/Nursing/MD: plans finalized pt discharged		**Home with appropriate level of care** **HH visit scheduled for next day**
	Nursing/SW: Provide emotional support	Pt able to verbalize, identify lifestyle changes				**Identifies support systems & resources.** **Is able to look at stoma**

3100-51

Female Reproductive System/ Women's Health

Female Reproductive System Assessment

● Subjective Data

Lower abdominal pain
Cramps
Vaginal bleeding: color and amount
Vaginal discharge
  Mucoid
  Thick, white
  Frothy, watery, yellow-green
  Thick, yellow-green or brown, and bloody
  Yellow
  Gray or green
  Odoriferous
  Duration
Itching
Swelling
Redness
Painful intercourse
Urination
  Stress incontinence
  Burning on urination
  Pain, urgency, or frequency

Breasts
  Tenderness
  Pain
  Stinging sensation
  Burning

● Objective Data

General appearance (Figures 11-1 and 11-2)
Vital signs (VS), weight
Breasts
  Size
  Symmetry
  Contour
  Lesions
  Lumps, bumps
  "Orange peel" texture
  Venous pattern
  Moles, nevi
  Dimpling or skin retraction

Fixation, nonmobile
  Erythema
Nipples
  Color
  Discharge (serous, bloody, purulent)
  Inversion
Abdomen
  Contour
  Lesions
  Scars
  Stretch marks
  Symmetry
  Visible pulsations
  Visible peristaltic waves
  Presence of bowel sounds in each quadrant
External genitalia
  Labia majora/minora
    Edema
    Redness
    Leukoplakia
    Lumps

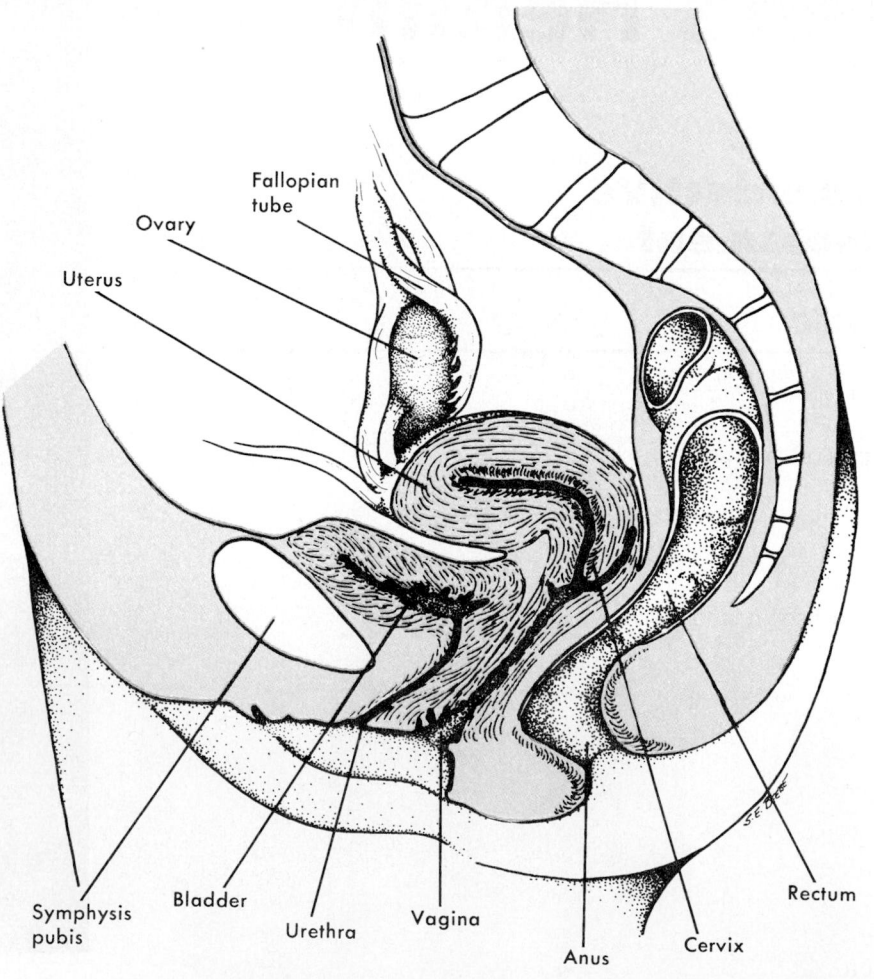

Figure 11-1 Female reproductive system.

Lesions, lacerations
Symmetry
Pigmentation (nevi)
Clitoris
Edema
Redness
Adhesions, lesions
Urethral orifice
Size
Redness
Discharge
Discharge
Bloody
Purulent
Odoriferous
Introitus
Presence or absence of hymenal ring
Hymenal tags
Cystocele, rectocele, enterocele
Uterine prolapse
Edema
Redness
Drainage
Mucoid (normal)

Thick, white, cheesy (typical of moniliasis)
Purulent
Frothy, watery, yellow-green (typical of trichomoniasis)
Thick, yellow-green or brown, and bloody (typical of upper genital tract infection)
Bloody
Yellow: thin with odor
Gray or green
Perineum
Scars
Redness
Edema
Excoriation

● Pertinent Background Information

Concurrent diseases or conditions

Menstrual cycle
Age at onset
Length of cycles (duration)
Interval between cycles

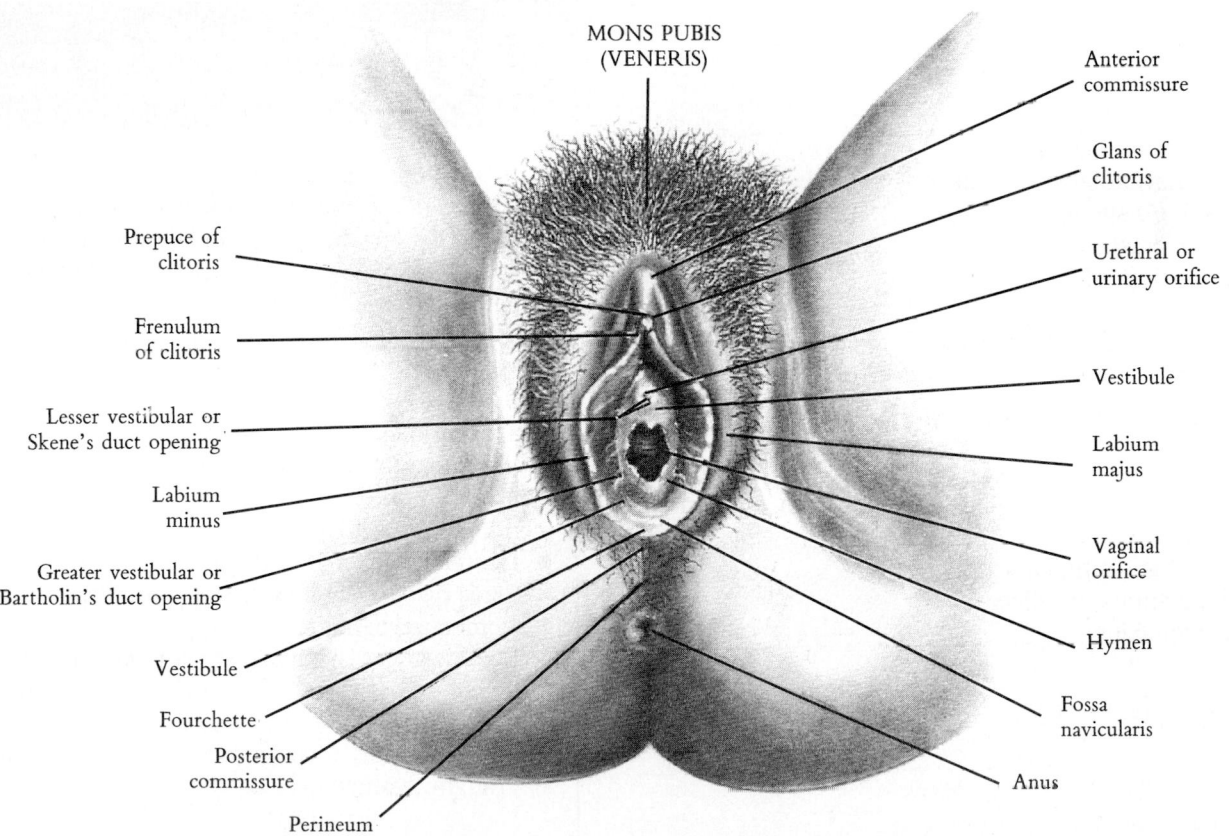

MONS PUBIS
(VENERIS)

Anterior
commissure

Glans of
clitoris

Urethral or
urinary orifice

Vestibule

Labium
majus

Vaginal
orifice

Hymen

Fossa
navicularis

Anus

Prepuce of
clitoris

Frenulum
of clitoris

Lesser vestibular or
Skene's duct opening

Labium
minus

Greater vestibular or
Bartholin's duct opening

Vestibule

Fourchette

Posterior
commissure

Perineum

Figure 11-2 External female genitalia. (From Seidel HM et al: *Mosby's guide to physical examination,* ed 3, St Louis, 1995, Mosby; originally from Bobak, Jensen, and Zalar, 1989.)

Regularity of cycles
Duration, amount, type of flow
Number of tampons or napkins used
Date of most recent douching
Date of last menstrual period (LMP)
Associated symptoms (pain, menorrhagia, metrorrhagia, breast symptoms)
Pregnancy
Number of pregnancies and outcome of each
Complications of pregnancy and delivery and/or abortion
Lactation history
Number of infants breast fed
Duration of breast feeding
Lactation suppressant medications
Contraceptive history
Type of method used
Duration
Effectiveness
Side effects
Menopause
When occurred
Related symptoms
Hot flashes; night sweats
Dry vaginal mucosa
Insomnia
Gastrointestinal (GI) system
Constipation
Hemorrhoids
Endocrine system
Hypothyroidism
Hyperthyroidism
Stein-Leventhal syndrome
Cushing's syndrome
Blood dyscrasia
Hypertension
AIDS
Sexually transmitted diseases

Previous surgery or illness

Gynecologic surgery
Other major surgery or illness (of abdomen, endocrine system)
Sexually transmitted diseases
Pelvic inflammatory disease
Vaginal infections

Family history

Cancer (ovarian, breast)
Sickle cell disease
Thyroid disorder
Diabetes
Multiple pregnancies

Congenital anomalies
Death resulting from gynecologic-related conditions
Maternal diethylstilbestrol (DES) usage

Social history

Sexual activity: abnormal lesions or discharge in sexual partner, condom use
Contraception
Douching habits
Clothing habits (cotton or nonventilated underwear)
Patterns of tobacco, alcohol, and prescription/nonprescription drug use
Occupational hazards, radiation, toxins

Medication history

Oral contraceptives
Estrogen replacement therapy
Phenothiazines
Digitalis
Diuretics

Gerontologic Considerations

● Many older women are reluctant to seek medical care for problems of the reproductive system. This may be related to cultural factors, embarrassment, or lack of knowledge. Routine gynecologic examination should continue as part of the physical examination even after menopause.
● Certain forms of cancer of the reproductive tract are more common with aging. Any vaginal bleeding should be reported to the physician promptly, as should pelvic pain, pruritus, or skin lesions in the genital region.
● Decreased level of estrogen with aging and systemic disease such as diabetes predispose older women to vaginitis.
● Breast cancer risk increases for women older than 40 years of age. Breast examination should continue throughout the lifespan. The American Cancer Society recommends an annual mammogram for women over age 50.

Modified from Christensen BL, Kockrow EO: *Foundations of nursing,* ed 2, St Louis, 1995; Mosby.

● Diagnostic tests

Bimanual examination
Basal body temperature (T)
Cervical mucus testing (Billing's method)
Papanicolaou (Pap) test
Wet mount
Culture
Computed tomography (CT) scan
Magnetic resonance imaging (MRI)
Breast biopsy and aspiration
Cervical biopsy
Endobiopsy
Dilation and curettage (D & C)
Cervical conization (cone biopsy)
Colposcopy
Hysteroscopy
Culdoscopy
Culpotomy
Endoscopy
Laparoscopy
Ultrasound
Insufflation
Mammography
Thermography
Radionuclide imaging
Galactography
Hysterography
Hysterosalpingography
Bone densitometry
Bone scan

Laboratory studies

Human chorionic gonadotropin (HCG) level
Serum testosterone/dehydroepiandrosterone sulfate
  (DHEAS)

Estradiol
Progesterone
Serum luteinizing hormone (LH) and follicle-
  stimulating hormone level (FSH)
Thyroid function studies
  Thyroid stimulating hormone (TSH)
  Basal metabolic rate (BMR)
  Protein-bound iodine (PBI) level
  T_3 and T_4
Adrenal function
  17-ketosteroids
  Corticosteroids
Venereal disease research laboratory (VDRL) test

Pelvic Inflammatory Disease

An infectious process of the pelvic cavity that may include the fallopian tubes, ovaries, pelvic peritoneum, veins, and pelvic connective tissue (Figures 11-3 and 11-4)

Assessment

Subjective data

Abdominal and pelvic pain
Low back pain
Dyspareunia (painful intercourse)
Malodorous, purulent vaginal discharge
Malaise, general aching

Objective data

Fever
Nausea, vomiting

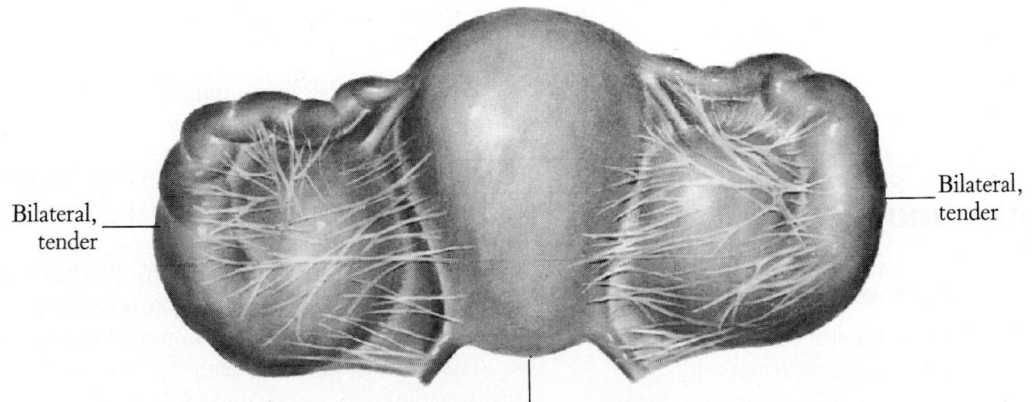

Bilateral, tender

Bilateral, tender

Movement of cervix painful

Figure 11-3   Pelvic inflammatory disease. (From Seidel HM et al: *Mosby's guide to physical examination,* ed 3, St Louis, 1995, Mosby.)

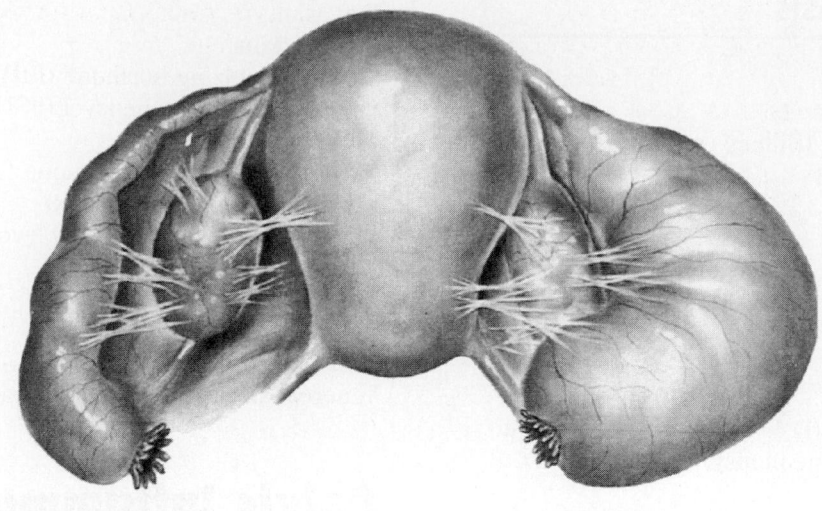

Advanced   Pyosalpinx

Figure 11-4 Salpingitis. (From Seidel HM et al: *Mosby's guide to physical examination,* ed 3, St Louis, 1995, Mosby.)

Pruritus or maceration of vulva
Diarrhea
Bloating

Diagnostic tests

Elevated white blood cell count (WBC)
Elevated erythrocyte sedimentation rate
Culture of purulent secretions positive for
  organisms
Laparoscopic visualization of pelvic inflammation
Ultrasound of tubo-ovarian abscess, if present
Needle culdocentesis for WBCs or nonclotting
  blood

Potential complications

Urinary tract infection (UTI)
Peritonitis
Tubo-ovarian abscess
Infertility
Paralytic ileus

Collaborative management

Therapeutic management

Antibiotics as determined by sensitivity
Bed rest in semi-Fowler's position or position of
  comfort
Parenteral fluids
Nasogastric suctioning if ileus is present
Removal of intrauterine device if present

Removal of tampon if present
Analgesics

Nursing management

PATIENT PROBLEMS/NURSING DIAGNOSES

● **NDX:** Pain related to pelvic inflammation and pro-
            tective guarding

Maintain complete bed rest in semi-Fowler's position or
  position of comfort *to reduce movement, which can increase the sensation of pain*
Administer analgesics as needed
Increase activity as tolerated

EXPECTED OUTCOME
Patient states that pain is relieved

● **NDX:** Risk for impaired skin integrity secondary to
            vaginal drainage

Assist and teach patient to perform gentle perineal care
  q3h to 4h and prn; blot skin dry (avoid rubbing) *to
  prevent excoriation*
Teach patient to wipe from front to back after elimination *to prevent urethral contamination*
Ensure that bed covers do not result in excessive
  warmth of perineal area

EXPECTED OUTCOME
Patient's skin integrity is maintained as evidenced by
  absence of excoriation of perineal area

Patient/family teaching

Explain importance of handwashing both before and after contact with perineum

Explain need to use perineal pads, change them as needed, and wrap and properly dispose of them; avoid use of tampons

Explain that a shower is preferred to a tub bath

Promote good nutrition with diet as tolerated

Teach measures to prevent disease if condition is caused by gonococcus or chlamydia

Home care considerations

Emphasize need for sexual partner to be examined or treated

Discuss condom use

Discuss alternate methods of conception control if condition is related to an intrauterine device (IUD)

Explain importance of avoiding douching, intercourse, or use of tampons for 1 wk after antibiotic therapy or as directed by physician

Discuss symptoms of recurrence that should be reported to physician

Toxic Shock Syndrome

An acute bacterial infection caused by penicillinase-resistant Staphylococcus aureus; *may lead to septic shock and release of exotoxins; most often associated with continuous use of super-absorbent tampons during menses*

Assessment

Subjective data

Myalgia
Sore throat
Headache
Profound fatigue

Objective data

Sudden onset of high fever

Vomiting

Watery diarrhea

Macular erythematous rash (sunburnlike) on palms and soles

Eventual desquamation within 1 to 2 wk after rash appears

Impaired joint mobility

Decreased circulation of fingers and toes

Alterations in level of consciousness (LOC): disorientation, confusion

Vaginal, oropharyngeal, or conjunctival hyperemia

Severe peripheral edema

Diminished urine output

Hypotension

Diagnostic tests

Elevated
  WBC and differential
  Blood urea nitrogen (BUN)
  Creatinine
  Bilirubin
  Aspartate aminotransferase (AST)
  Creatinine phosphokinase (CPK)
Decreased: platelets

Potential complications

Pulmonary edema

Adult respiratory distress syndrome (ARDS)

Sudden hypotension progressing to shock

Disseminated intravascular coagulation (DIC)

Collaborative management

Therapeutic management

Antibiotics

VS monitoring

Parenteral fluids to 3000 ml/day unless contraindicated

Septic shock management as indicated

Nursing management

PATIENT PROBLEM/NURSING DIAGNOSIS

● **NDX:** Altered: tissue perfusion related to exchange problems associated with septic shock and/or ARDS

For specific desired outcome and interventions, see Shock syndrome (p. 150) and Adult respiratory distress syndrome (p. 311)

Patient/family teaching and home care considerations

Explain need to avoid use of tampons until vaginal cultures are negative

Instruct patient to thoroughly wash hands before tampon insertion

Instruct patient to use tampons made of cotton, avoiding the super-absorbent, noncotton type

Explain need to change tampons frequently and rotate using tampons and sanitary napkins (consider wearing napkins at night)

Emphasize importance of avoiding tampons altogether if there is a concurrent skin infection such as a boil caused by *Staphylococcus aureus*

If the following symptoms occur, instruct patient to discontinue use of tampons immediately and report symptoms to physician

Nausea

Vomiting

Diarrhea

Fever

Hydatidiform Mole

Tumor mass of chorionic cells in the uterus that mimics pregnancy; approximately 10% become malignant

Assessment

Subjective data

Uterine cramping

Objective data

Vaginal bleeding (dark brown or bright red; scant or profuse)

Enlarged uterus (larger than pregnant uterus for same date)

Absence of fetal heart tones

Absence of fetal movement

Vaginal expulsion of vesicular tissue

Hypertension

Hyperthyroidism

Nausea, vomiting

Excessive weight loss

Anemia

Diagnostic tests

Ultrasonography

Elevated HCG titer

Collaborative management

Therapeutic management

Evacuation of mole by suction curettage

Routine preprocedural and postprocedural care

Ongoing ambulatory care

Nursing management

PATIENT PROBLEM/NURSING DIAGNOSIS

● **NDX:** Anxiety related to situational crisis associated with pseudocyesis

Encourage verbalization about outcome of diagnosis and treatment

Use active listening skills and assist patient and family with use of adaptive coping strategies *to reduce anxiety about pseudocyesis*

Involve bereavement counselor as appropriate

Involve spouse/significant other in dealing with loss/grief

EXPECTED OUTCOME

Patient demonstrates a reduction in anxiety and exhibits appropriate coping behaviors

Patient/family education

Explain condition and related physiology

Provide information about preprocedural and postprocedural care

Explain preoperative and postoperative vital signs and care routines

Home care considerations

Reinforce physician's explanation of current condition, risk factors, avoidance of pregnancy (usually for 1 year), need for periodic HCG titers, chest x-ray examinations, and follow-up outpatient care

Dilation and Curettage

Expansion of the cervix and scraping of the endometrial lining of the uterus for diagnostic and/or therapeutic purposes; may detect uterine malignancy, evaluate fertility or dysfunctional uterine bleeding, or treat incomplete abortion, dysmenorrhea, or heavy bleeding

Assessment

Subjective data

Pelvic and low back pain

Objective data

Excessive vaginal bleeding

Hematuria

Foul odor of vaginal drainage
Elevated temperature

Potential complications

Endometritis
Sepsis
Uterine rupture
Hemorrhage

Collaborative management

Therapeutic management

Vital signs
Parenteral fluids
Pad count as indicated
Intake and output for 2 to 4 hr; notation of amount and color of first-voided urine after procedure
Analgesics as indicated

Nursing management

PATIENT PROBLEMS/NURSING DIAGNOSES

● **NDX:** Pain related to uterine cramping

Administer analgesics as ordered to reduce sensation of pain and cramping
Maintain bed rest immediately after procedure, progressing to activity as tolerated

EXPECTED OUTCOME

Patient experiences minimal discomfort

● **NDX:** Risk for infection related to traumatized intrauterine tissue secondary to intrauterine curettage

Administer perineal care after elimination as necessary
Monitor temperature and pulse *to identify presence of fever or tachycardia related to infection*
Explain importance of wiping from front to back after elimination *to prevent contamination of urethra with fecal bacteria/matter*
Explain that shower is preferred to tub bath for 3 to 4 days
Note amount, color, and odor of vaginal drainage and change perineal pads as necessary
Understand that vaginal packing, if used, is usually removed by physician because there is a potential for bleeding

EXPECTED OUTCOME

Patient does not develop endometritis or vaginitis as evidenced by euthermia and normal drainage

Patient/family teaching and home care considerations

Explain that vaginal bleeding or spotting may continue for a week and that mild cramps may continue for 2 to 3 days
Explain that minimal activity is recommended for 2 to 3 days based on personal comfort level
Explain that coitus, douching, and use of tampons should be delayed for 1 to 2 wk or as indicated by physician *to prevent infection*
Discuss symptoms that should be reported to physician
Excessive bleeding, heavier than a menstrual period
Foul odor of vaginal drainage
Temperature >100°F (37.8°C)
Severe lower abdominal cramps or pain

Tubal Pregnancy and Salpingectomy

tubal pregnancy: Implantation of the fertilized ovum in the fallopian tube is the most common type of ectopic pregnancy; often related to pelvic inflammatory disease resulting in tubal stricture after salpingitis
salpingectomy: Removal of the fallopian tube

Assessment

Preoperative observations/findings

UNRUPTURED TUBE

Low abdominal pain and tenderness: unilateral or generalized
Vaginal bleeding: usually scanty and dark brown; intermittent or continuous
Signs of pregnancy
Amenorrhea
Nausea, vomiting
Urinary frequency
Breast changes

RUPTURED TUBE (Figure 11-5)

Severe lower abdominal pain: may be sudden and stabbing
Vaginal bleeding may or may not be present
Dizziness
Fainting
Pallor

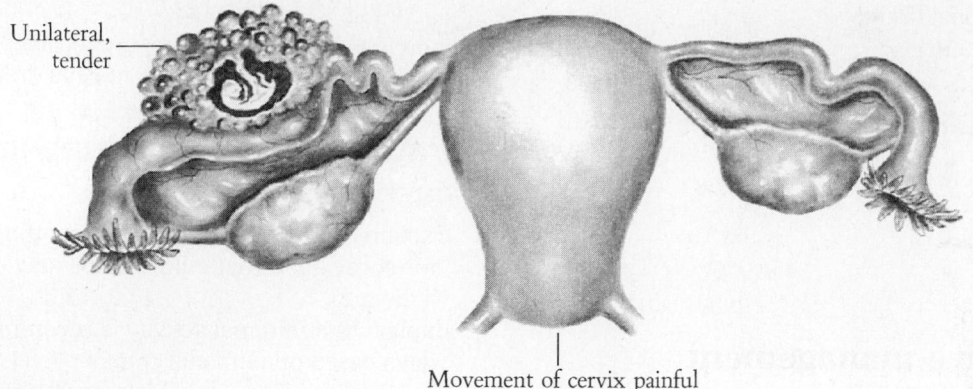

Unilateral, tender

Movement of cervix painful

Figure 11-5 Ruptured tubal pregnancy. (From Seidel HM et al: *Mosby's guide to physical examination,* ed 3, St Louis, 1995, Mosby.)

Progressive supine hypotension
Referred supraclavicular pain

Diagnostic tests

Ultrasonography
Culdocentesis (positive for free blood)
Laparoscopy
Complete blood cell count (CBC), electrolytes, type and screen/cross
Urinalysis
Pregnancy test

Postoperative observations/findings

Site of incision
  Redness
  Pain
  Swelling
  Drainage
Elevated temperature
Feelings of loss and grief

Potential complications

Incisional infection
Paralytic ileus
Pneumonia
Hemorrhage, anemia
Shock

Collaborative management

Therapeutic management

Parenteral fluids
Analgesics

Antiflatulent medications
Indwelling catheter to closed gravity drainage
Vital signs
Intake and output
Anti-Rh globulin as indicated
Progression of postoperative diet from clear liquids to full meal after return of bowel sounds

Nursing management

PATIENT PROBLEMS/NURSING DIAGNOSES

● **NDX:** Pain related to incision and abdominal distention

Assist patient with assuming position of comfort *to minimize sensation of pain*
Administer analgesics as ordered
Auscultate abdomen for bowel sounds; insert rectal tube and/or give Harris flush as ordered *to decrease abdominal distention*

EXPECTED OUTCOME
Patient reports that discomfort is minimal

● **NDX:** Anticipatory grieving related to loss of pregnancy

Encourage verbalization of feelings
Assist patient with working through grieving process by using supportive statements *to enable patient to articulate and address feelings*
Involve grief/bereavement counselor as appropriate
Involve spouse or significant other with loss and grief

EXPECTED OUTCOME

Patient demonstrates successful progress through grieving process with absence of characteristics of dysfunctional grieving

● **NDX:** Impaired physical mobility, related to discomfort in the immediate postoperative period

Observe site of incision and reinforce and change dressing as necessary; ensure that patient *understands that incision is secure and to increase activity based on comfort*

Encourage and assist patient as needed with ambulation; increase activity to tolerance

Involve social service worker regarding placement of other children at home if necessary *because mother's emergency surgery prohibits preoperative planning for their care, and temporary limitations in physical mobility may limit mother's ability/responsiveness to manage care of other children*

EXPECTED OUTCOMES

Patient is fully ambulatory before discharge
Performs self-care activities

Patient/family teaching

Discuss symptoms of wound infection to report to physician
Explain need for activity to tolerance
Explain importance of planned rest periods

Home care considerations

Emphasize importance of prevention of pregnancy for 2 to 4 months or as indicated by physician
Explain that childbearing ability can be diminished, especially if tubal pregnancy was a result of PID or anomaly of the tube resulting in bilateral obstruction

Total Abdominal Hysterectomy and Bilateral Salpingo-Oophorectomy

Surgical removal of the uterus, cervix, both fallopian tubes, and ovaries through an abdominal incision or laparoscopic procedure to treat malignant neoplastic

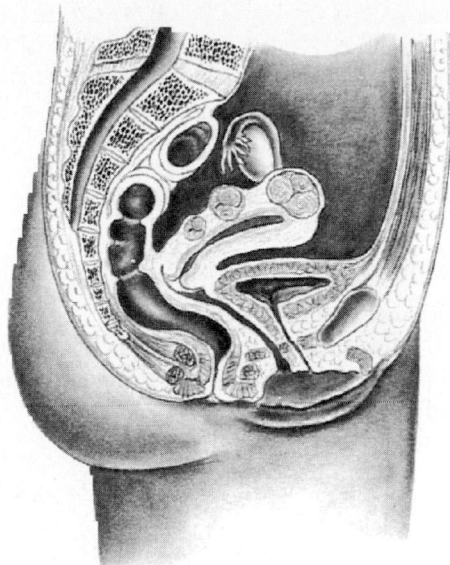

Figure 11-6 Myomas of the uterus (fibroids). (From Seidel HM et al: *Mosby's guide to physical examination*, ed 3, St Louis, 1995, Mosby.)

disease, leiomyomas (Figure 11-6), and chronic endometriosis

Assessment

Subjective data

Difficulty in voiding
Maladaptive comments related to self-concept

Objective data

Vaginal discharge other than serosanguineous and/or with foul odor
Redness, pain, swelling, or drainage at incision site
Fever
Diminished or absent bowel sounds

Diagnostic tests

Urine culture and sensitivity after catheter removal
Hgb and Hct postsurgically

Potential complications

Infection: intraabdominal or incisional
Urinary tract infection
Paralytic ileus

Pneumonia
Hemorrhage
Thrombophlebitis
Pulmonary embolus

Collaborative management

Therapeutic management

NPO until bowel sounds are audible
Parenteral fluids until liquids or diet is tolerated
Indwelling catheter to low-gravity drainage system
Intake and output
BP, T, P, and R per postoperative procedure
Analgesics and stool softeners
Hormone replacement as indicated

Nursing management

PATIENT PROBLEMS/NURSING DIAGNOSES

● **NDX:** Altered tissue perfusion: peripheral related to interruption in arterial and venous flow secondary to surgical intervention

Monitor vital signs as ordered
Avoid sitting with knees bent and/or crossing legs *to prevent peripheral pooling of blood*
Apply antiembolic stockings as ordered
Auscultate bowel sounds; maintain NPO status until bowel sounds are active *to prevent abdominal distention*
Assist with ambulation as needed
Encourage ambulation and/or leg exercises *to increase peripheral tissue perfusion*

EXPECTED OUTCOMES

Patient's vital signs remain within normal presurgical limits
Circulation remains normal without evidence of pelvic stasis or peripheral thrombophlebitis
Bowel function is resuming

● **NDX:** Pain related to surgical incision(s)

Administer analgesics as ordered
Assist patient in assuming a position of comfort
Place pillow on abdomen *for support when patient is coughing to reduce sensation of pain*
Assist with personal hygiene as necessary

EXPECTED OUTCOME

Patient reports that she is comfortable and pain is reduced

● **NDX:** Ineffective breathing pattern related to discomfort and postsurgical status

Assist with turning, coughing, and deep breathing, decreasing frequency as patient becomes more active
Assist and teach patient to use incentive spirometer as indicated *to promote adequate ventilation/prevent pooling of secretions*
Auscultate chest for breath sounds

EXPECTED OUTCOME

Patient has normal breath sounds on auscultation, and inhalation/exhalation pattern enables adequate ventilation

● **NDX:** Impaired skin integrity related to surgical incision(s)

Observe incision for condition
Cleanse incision area as indicated; keep clean and dry
Report signs of infection to physician: redness, swelling, or discharge
Change or reinforce dressing as necessary
Explain to patient importance of avoiding lifting or placing strain on abdominal muscles (avoid straining at stool) *to ensure that incisional skin integrity is maintained*

EXPECTED OUTCOME

Patient's incision remains clean, dry, and intact without signs of infection

● **NDX:** Colonic constipation related to NPO status and manipulation of pelvic and abdominal structures during surgery

Progress to high-protein or high-residue diet as ordered
Encourage adequate fluid intake *to prevent constipation*
Give Harris flush or insert rectal tube *to expel gas as indicated*
Assist patient with assuming lateral Sims position *if it promotes expulsion of flatus*
Encourage ambulation *to promote muscle activity and bowel motility*
Give stool softeners or mild laxatives as ordered *to prevent constipation*

EXPECTED OUTCOME

Patient has expelled flatus and defecated before discharge

● **NDX:** Altered urinary elimination related to post-surgical sensory motor impairment

Maintain closed gravity drainage system if patient has indwelling catheter *to prevent infection*

Promote micturition at regular intervals when catheter is removed *and monitor/report difficulty in voiding*

Monitor intake and output; encourage fluids

EXPECTED OUTCOME

Patient voids q.s. without difficulty

● **NDX:** Self-esteem disturbance related to body image change and value of reproductive organs

Encourage patient's comments and questions about surgery, progress, and prognosis *to prevent internalization of negative thoughts*

Reinforce correct information and provide factual information *to correct any misconceptions;* common misconceptions are that after a hysterectomy a woman grows fat and flabby; develops facial hair; becomes wrinkled, old, and masculine; loses her mind; or becomes depressed and nervous; normal concerns to address are fear of death, disfigurement, cancer, loss of femininity, pain, loss of childbearing ability, and changes in sexuality

Encourage verbalization of feelings with significant other *to address and resolve body image and self-esteem issues*

Discuss hormone replacement therapy if appropriate

EXPECTED OUTCOMES

Demonstrates adaptive responses related to self-concept

Asks appropriate questions

Gives correct information related to procedures and prognosis

Indicates that she has discussed concerns with significant other

Patient/family teaching

Instruct patient to ambulate at regular intervals and to avoid sitting for prolonged periods at home or when travelling

Instruct patient to care for incision with general cleanliness and daily bathing; to report signs of infection to physician, including redness, swelling, pain, discharge, increase in vaginal drainage, and foul odor

Explain need to avoid constipation and straining at stool

Home care considerations

Explain need to avoid coitus, douching, tampons, or anything in vagina for 4 to 6 wk or as indicated by physician

Explain need to avoid heavy lifting and vigorous activity for 6 wk after surgery

Emphasize importance of maintaining regular outpatient gynecologic examinations

Explain need to take estrogen-progesterone hormones as ordered (if surgical menopause is caused by removal of all ovarian tissue)

Perinatal

Assessment

Observations/findings

Age
Height
Prepregnancy weight
Current weight
History of infertility
Menstrual history
  Age at onset, length of, interval between, and regularity of cycles
  Last menstrual period (LMP)
  Expected date of delivery (EDD)
Pregnancy history
  Gravida
  Term births
  Preterm births
  Spontaneous abortions (miscarriages)
  Induced abortions
  Stillbirths
  Date of each birth (month and year)
    Weeks of gestation
    Duration of labor in hours
    Spontaneous or induced labor
    Type of birth (vaginal or cesarean)
    Children living (ages, any developmental problems)
    Multiple births
    Maternal, fetal, or neonatal complications
Blood pressure, temperature, pulse, and respirations
Fetal heart rate (FHR)
Blood type and Rh factor
Rubella titer
Urine protein and glucose
Date and results of last Papanicolaou (Pap) test
Previous major illnesses and surgeries
Current health problems
Breast changes
  Fullness

Tingling
Heaviness
Darkening of areola
Presence of colostrum
Turgid nipples and engorged areolas with sexual stimulation
Nipples: extraverted or inverted

Cardiovascular changes
Increase in heart rate of 10 to 15 beats/min from baseline from 14 to 30 wk of pregnancy
Slight decrease in BP during second trimester with return to previous baseline BP in third trimester <15 mm Hg in either systolic or diastolic
Tendency toward dependent edema

Hematologic changes during pregnancy
Blood volume increases and peaks by 30 to 34 wk
Red blood cell (RBC) production accelerates
Hgb declines because of hemodilution (physiologic anemia)
Reticulocyte count increases because of hematopoiesis
White blood cell count (WBC) increases up to 25,000 mm^3: normal range 5000 to 15,000 mm^3
Total plasma proteins decrease to 3 to 3.5 g/dl (normal range 4 to 4.5 g/dl) because of fall in albumin level
Sedimentation rate increases because of decrease in total plasma proteins

Respiratory changes
Nasal stuffiness because of estrogen-initiated hyperemia
Sinus stuffiness
Prone to nose bleeds
Increased oxygen consumption
Decreased functional residual capacity and residual volume of air
Increased tidal volume, minute ventilatory volume, and minute oxygen uptake
Increased respiratory rate
Compensated respiratory alkalosis

Basal metabolism
Increases by 15% to 20% at term
Lassitude and fatigability in early pregnancy
Heat intolerance in late pregnancy

Urinary changes
Frequency of urination
Increased bladder capacity
Increased glomerular filtration rate
Mild proteinuria
Mild glycosuria

Gastrointestinal (GI) changes
Tender gums
Excessive salivation
Transitory nausea and vomiting in first trimester
Heartburn and acid indigestion (esophageal regurgitation and decreased emptying time)

Unusual food preferences
Constipation
Hypercholesterolemia
Decreased gallbladder emptying time

Neurologic changes
Lightheadedness or faintness in early pregnancy
Headache associated with pregnancy-induced hypertension
Sensory changes in legs with compression of pelvic nerves

Musculoskeletal changes
Decreased abdominal muscle tone
Increase in lumbosacral curve
Hypermobility of pelvic joints
Waddling gait near term
Prone to carpal tunnel syndrome
Acroesthesia (numbness and tingling of hands)

Integumentary changes
Thickened skin
Increased subdermal fat
Hyperpigmentation
Chloasma (mask of pregnancy)
Linea nigra
Increased hair and nail growth
Accelerated sebaceous and sweat gland activity
Increased fragility of cutaneous elastic tissues resulting in striae gravidarum (stretch marks)
Acne vulgaris (preexisting)
Aggravated in first trimester
Improved in third trimester
Angiomas (vascular spiders) on neck, thorax, face, and arms
Thinning and softening of fingernails and toenails
Patterns of tobacco, alcohol, and prescription/nonprescription drug use
Chemical dependency/substance abuse
Patterns of nutrient intake
Planned method of feeding infant
Self-esteem and perceived ability to cope with life situations
Body image resulting from physiological changes of pregnancy
Desire for participation in prepared childbirth classes
Plans for postdischarge newborn care at home
Concurrent conditions
Diabetes
Cardiovascular conditions
Severe anemia
Epilepsy
Asthma or other pulmonary conditions
Drug sensitivities
Renal disorders
Sexually transmitted disease
Patterns of work or employment
Activity/exercise patterns

Diagnostic tests

Pregnancy test confirmation
Blood typing and Rh factor identification
  Hemoglobin (Hgb) and hematocrit (Hct)
  VDRL (Veneral disease research laboratories) test
  Pap test (cervical cytology test)
  Urinalysis
  Irregular antibody screen
  Rubella antibody titer
  TORCH screen as indicated
  SMA
  Sickle cell test
  GC culture at 36 wk
  Alpha fetoprotein between 10 and 16 wk
  Hepatitis BsAg
  Tb, HIV as indicated
  Fasting blood sugar (FBS) screening (at 26 weeks' gestation if no high-risk factors for diabetes are present)
  Glucose tolerance tests for diabetes as indicated and per facility protocol; 1 hr glucola at 26 wk as indicated
  Chorionic villus sampling as indicated
  Amniocentesis before or at 16 wk for genetic screening
  Ultrasound as indicated
  Biophysical profile (as indicated): fetal breathing movements, gross body movements, fetal tone, amniotic fluid index, nonstress test

Collaborative management

Therapeutic management

See Figure 11-7
Uncomplicated pregnancy visit schedule

  Every 4 wk during first 28 wk
  Every 2 to 3 wk until 36 wk
  Weekly until birth
Nonstress testing (NST)
Contraction stress testing (CST)
Antibiotics for treatment as indicated
Prenatal vitamins and iron supplements
Counseling and other referrals as indicated for high-risk pregnancy
Genetic counseling as indicated

Patient/family teaching

Discuss danger signals to report immediately to primary health care provider
  Any vaginal bleeding
  Swelling of face or fingers
  Severe or continuous headache
  Dimness or blurring of vision
  Muscular irritability (or convulsions)
  Abdominal pain or epigastric pain
  Persistent vomiting
  Chills or fever
  Dysuria
  Diarrhea
  Cramping
  Change in character of vaginal discharge
  Pelvic heaviness or pressure
  Contractions
  Escape of fluid from vagina
  Abrupt decrease in fetal movements during last trimester
Emphasize importance of avoiding smoking, alcohol, and illicit drugs including opium derivatives, barbiturates, amphetamines, PCP, cocaine, marijuana, benzodiazepines

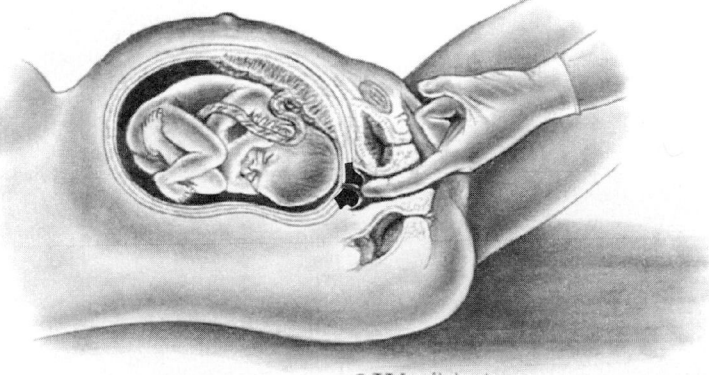

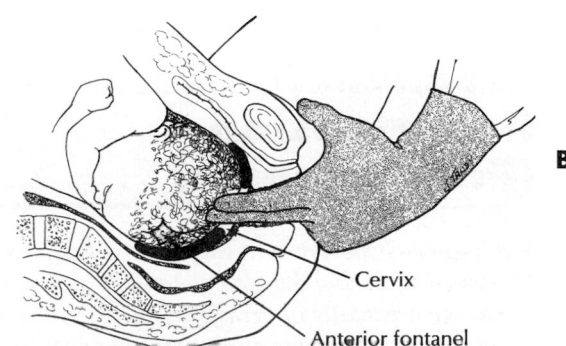

Cervix

Anterior fontanel

Figure 11-7   Vaginal examination. **A,** Undilated, unaffected cervix. Membranes intact. **B,** Palpation of sagittal suture line. Cervix effaced and partially dilated. (From Bobak IM et al: *Maternity nursing,* ed 4, St Louis, 1995, Mosby.)

Emphasize importance of avoiding any nonprescription drugs including aspirin and nose drops without consulting physician and prescription drugs that can be abused

Explain need to check with primary health care provider before traveling

Discuss methods to alleviate nausea, hemorrhoids, and/or varicose veins

Explain importance of toxoplasmosis precautions (e.g., avoiding cat litter)

Emphasize importance of ongoing outpatient care

Explain need to avoid excessive fatigue when exercising

Explain need to maintain good body mechanics when bending, lifting, or walking

Explain need to rest periodically with legs elevated

Encourage rest when feeling fatigued

Explain need to avoid use of constricting garments, especially on lower extremities

Explain need to drink adequate amounts of fluid to 3000 ml/day unless contraindicated

Emphasize importance of well-balanced diet

Explain need to wear well-fitting, supportive brassiere

Explain need to wear only low-heeled shoes if backache or unstable balance occurs with higher-heeled shoes

Emphasize importance of maintaining normal bowel habits with adequate fluid intake, reasonable exercise, and diet high in fiber

Mild laxatives such as prune juice, milk of magnesia, bulk-producing substances, or stool softeners may be taken when necessary

Avoid use of nonabsorbable oil preparations and any other nonprescription medications without consulting physician

Emphasize importance of avoiding intercourse when there is a risk of spontaneous abortion or preterm labor

Discuss pros and cons of breast-feeding vs. formula feeding

Discuss special caretaking considerations for working mothers

Pregnancy-Induced Hypertension (Preeclampsia)

Syndrome of hypertension, edema, and proteinuria occurring during the second half of pregnancy, characteristically in primigravidas; resolves within 10 days postpartum; the etiology is unknown but could be caused by increased vasoconstrictor tone, abnormal prostaglandin action, or immunological factors (Figure 11-8)

Assessment

Subjective data

Edema (Figure 11-9)
  Face
  Fingers
Irritability, emotional tension
Nervousness
Nausea, vomiting
Visual disturbances (scotomata, blurred vision)
Severe generalized headache
Epigastric pain or right upper quadrant pain

Objective data

Elevated BP
Proteinuria
Pretibial pitting edema
Hyperreflexia
Altered level of consciousness
Oliguria
Pulmonary edema
Cyanosis
Onset of labor
Magnesium blood level >7.5 mEq/L

Pregnancy-induced hypertension

BP >140/90 mm Hg or rise in systolic pressure of 30 mm Hg above normal and diastolic pressure 15 mm

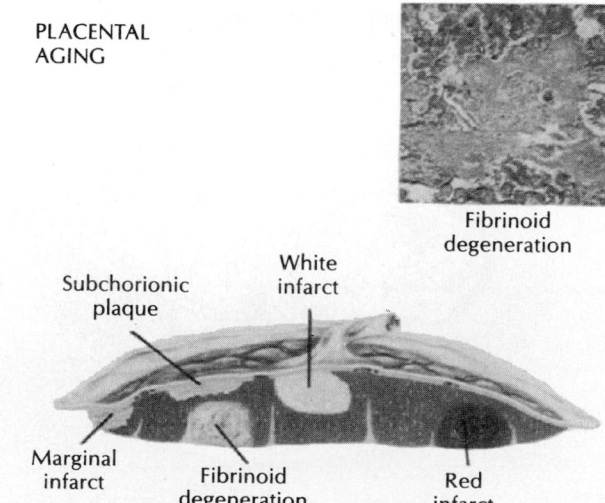

Figure 11-8   Effects of severe PIH on placenta with resultant placental insufficiency. (From Bobak IM: *Maternity and gynecologic care: the nurse and the family,* ed 5, St Louis, 1993, Mosby.)

Hg above normal on two occasions at least 6 hr apart

Mild preeclampsia

Mild preeclampsia is disease progression; includes the following:

Proteinuria >0.3 g/L per 24 hr or 1 g/L in two random specimens collected at least 6 hr apart

Dependent edema

Severe preeclampsia

BP >160/110 mm Hg or systolic pressure of 50 mm Hg above normal, diastolic pressure of 35 mm Hg above normal

Proteinuria: >5 g daily (or 3+ to 4+ based on semiquantitative assay)

Massive generalized edema

Cerebral or visual disturbances

Oliguria: 400 ml or less in 24 hr

Rising plasma creatinine

Diagnostic tests

CBC, differential and platelet count

Liver enzyme

  Serum AST aspartate aminotransferase (previously known as SGOT)

  Serum ALT alanine aminotransferase (previously known as SGPT)

  Lactate dehydrogenase (LDH)

  Creatine phosphokinase (CPK)

  Alkaline phosphatase

Mg^+, Ca^+ levels

BUN, uric acid, creatinine

Serum electrolytes as indicated

Urine (24 hr) for total protein and creatinine

NST and CST as indicated

Coagulation profile: fibrinogen, fibrin degradation products (fibrin split products), prothrombin time (PT), partial thromboplastin time (PTT)

Blood type and crossmatch

Lecithin/sphingomyelin (L/S) ratio and PG (phosphatidylglycerol) as indicated

Fetoscope/Doppler for fetal heart tones by 20 weeks' gestation

Ultrasound for size and dates as indicated; biparietal diameter (BPD) at 16 to 18 weeks' gestation

Amniocentesis (p. 729)

Biophysical profile

Potential complications

HELLP syndrome (*H,* hemolytic anemia; *EL,* elevated liver enzymes; *LP,* low platelets)

Acute fatty liver of pregnancy

Hypertensive crisis

Vascular overload, congestive heart failure (CHF)

Uteroplacental insufficiency (UPI)

Intrauterine growth retardation (IUGR)

Central nervous system (CNS) disturbances

Cerebrovascular accident (CVA)

Seizures

Fetal loss

Prematurity

Magnesium sulfate toxicity

  Respiratory arrest

  Flushing

  Thirst

  Diaphoresis

  Anxiety

  Drowsiness

  Lethargy

  Slight slurring of speech

  Ataxia

  Flaccidity

  Hypotension

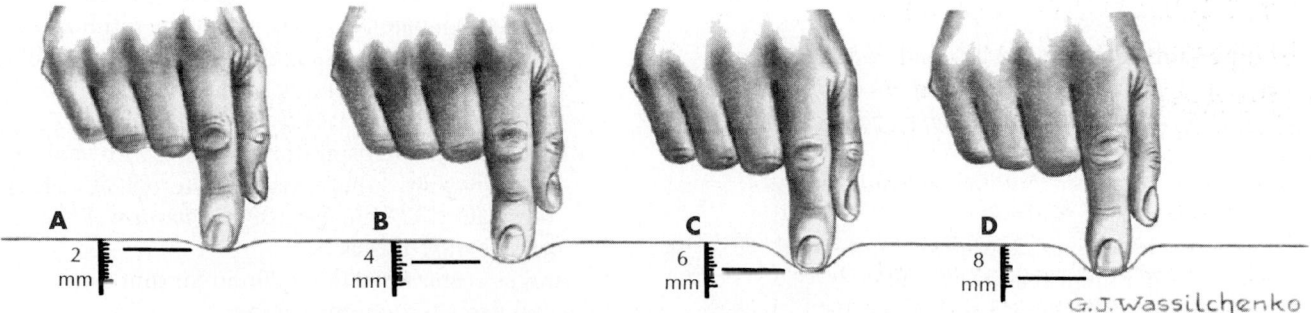

Figure 11-9 Assessment of pitting edema: **A,** +1; **B,** +2; **C,** +3; **D,** +4. (From Bobak IM: *Maternity and gynecologic care: the nurse and the family,* ed 5, St Louis, 1993, Mosby.)

Hyporeflexia; disappearance of patellar reflex
Essential hypertension
Disseminated intravascular coagulation (DIC)
Abruptio placentae

Collaborative management

Therapeutic management

Diagnostic tests as indicated
Bed rest in semi-Fowler's position or lateral position
Weigh patient daily: same time, clothing, and scale
VS with BP
Seizure precautions
Electronic fetal monitoring as indicated
IV fluids as indicated
Antihypertensives as indicated: hydralazine; if ineffective physician may progress to labetalol (Trandate), diazoxide (Hyperstat), sodium nitroprusside, nifedipine
Anticonvulsives as indicated: magnesium sulfate
Oxytocin infusion for birth induction as indicated
Respiratory services as indicated
Invasive hemodynamic monitoring as indicated
Social services support as indicated

Nursing management

PATIENT PROBLEMS/NURSING DIAGNOSES

● **NDX:** Risk for injury and altered tissue perfusion: uteroplacental, renal, related to biochemical regulatory dysfunction

Mild preeclampsia
Encourage rest with legs elevated *to promote tissue perfusion*
If bed rest is prescribed, lateral position is preferred
Monitor VS per hospital protocol
Assess BP q4h while awake with patient in same position with BP cuff at level of the heart
Assist with daily hygiene
Check urine for pH, protein, blood, glucose, and acetone more frequently as condition becomes more acute
Limit visitors as indicated by condition; encourage brief but frequent visits by toddlers or other children, because they help *to reduce patient's anxiety about his or her welfare*
Maintain seizure precautions *to avoid injury*
Oral airway at bedside
Padded siderails; crib bumpers can be used
Suction equipment readily available
Oxygen ready to use
Call light within easy reach

Magnesium sulfate, calcium antidote, and hydralazine readily available
Auscultate FHR for a full min q8h and prn or use electronic fetal monitor for 20 or more min q8h
Report nonreassuring fetal heart rate pattern to physician
Provide diversionary activities
Television
Painting
Reading, books on tape
Needlework

Severe preeclampsia
Continue with ongoing care of mild preeclampsia and *increase* frequency of nursing functions as condition progresses
Place patient in quiet, darkened room
Keep padded siderails up at all times
Maintain complete bed rest in lateral position *to promote tissue perfusion*
Limit visitors
Assess BP, P, and R qh and prn
Auscultate chest for breath sounds prn: report any evidence of pulmonary congestion as a result of limited mobility to physician *because impaired respiratory efficiency could adversely impact quality of tissue perfusion caused by hypoxemia*
Maintain closed gravity drainage system as ordered
Have emergency delivery pack available
Measure intake and output q4h and prn; report output <30 ml/hr
Check urine protein q4h as ordered
Invasive hemodynamic monitoring as ordered
Administer parenteral fluids as ordered based on hemodynamic value or other order *to ensure appropriate volume of circulating fluids, which enhances tissue perfusion*
Administer magnesium sulfate as ordered
Observe patient for progressing signs of magnesium sulfate toxicity
Assess deep tendon reflexes (DTRs) q4h to 8h and before each dose of magnesium sulfate or qh if patient is receiving continuous magnesium sulfate infusion; if patellar reflex is absent, withhold next dose of magnesium sulfate until magnesium blood level is drawn and notify primary health care provider
Assess need for respiratory support with vital signs if magnesium sulfate is administered with a respiratory rate <12/min *because magnesium sulfate depresses respirations*
Assess respiratory rate q30min for four times and prn after administration
Keep calcium antidote at bedside

Administer hydralazine 5 mg IV bolus when diastolic BP reaches 110 mm Hg as ordered *to reduce blood pressure*

If diastolic pressure is not lowered to 90 to 100 mm Hg in 20 minutes, increase the dose in 5 mg increments (10, 15, 20 mg) q20 min to 30 min as ordered (maximal effect is seen 20 to 30 min after administration)

Assess BP q5 min and report to physician

Do not leave patient unattended at any time during administration of hydralazine *because a rapid decrease in blood pressure could result in shock, with subsequent lack of perfusion*

Never leave patient alone when convulsion is pending

Note and report symptoms of *impending seizure activity*

Extremely high BP

Severe headache

Extreme irritability

Acute anxiety

Visual disturbances

Intrapartum care

See Oxytocin infusion: augmentation or induction of labor if labor is induced

Maintain separate IV lines for concurrent administration of oxytocin and magnesium sulfate *to ensure that there is not potential for a bolus dose of either drug*

Ensure that cross-matched blood is immediately available from blood bank if cesarean birth is performed

Prepare for neonatal stimulation and resuscitation

Notify pediatrician to be present at time of birth *to manage infant who may have CNS depression as a result of maternal medications*

Notify admitting nursery that mother had magnesium sulfate

Immediate Postpartum Care

Continue with ongoing care of severe preeclampsia and decrease frequency of nursing functions as patient's condition improves

NOTE: Birth is considered the "treatment" for PIH; however, symptoms may not subside for 2 to 7 days, and an eclamptic seizure is possible during that time

EXPECTED OUTCOMES

Patient's level of consciousness does not change and patient does not have seizures

Fetus does not show signs of compromise

Physiologic metabolic needs are minimized

Tissue perfusion is maximized

BP readings are maintained or lowered

● **NDX:** Fluid volume excess related to increased fluid retention and edema associated with pregnancy-induced hypertension

Weigh patient daily: same time, clothing, and scale to reduce variables that may not indicate a true weight

Assess BP and P q4h and prn; same arm in same position; report tachycardia of ≥120 beats/min and tachypnea to primary health care provider

Report significant hemodynamic values, neck vein distention, pulmonary rales, dyspnea, shortness of breath (SOB), cyanosis, or pallor to physician *because these signs are indicative of fluid volume excess*

Measure intake and output

Check urine protein as ordered

Maintain diet as ordered

Maintain availability of blood products for immediate use if necessary

Maintain separate IV lines for concurrent administration of magnesium sulfate and oxytocin *to limit the potential of a bolus dose of either drug*

Document use of pump and infusion rates per hospital policy

EXPECTED OUTCOMES

Patient's signs and symptoms do not indicate CHF

Edema is minimal

Circulating fluid volume is adequate

Patient/family teaching

Undelivered patient

Discuss symptoms of recurrence or progression to report to primary health care provider

Discuss procedure for urine collection and appropriate storage based on type of laboratory tests if ordered

Delivered patient

See appropriate standard, depending on method of birth: Cesarean birth (p. 753) or Postpartum care (p. 749)

Emphasize importance of physician's appointment during sixth postnatal wk to rule out chronic hypertension

Discuss conception control methods to use until no longer indicated by physician

Home care considerations

Emphasize importance of planned rest periods

Emphasize importance of keeping physician's appointments

Teach name of medication, dosage, time of administration, purpose, and side effects

Explain need to avoid taking over-the-counter medications without physician approval

Explain need for modified activity or activity restriction as indicated

Teach patient how to use BP monitoring device if ordered

Teach patient how to check urine for protein if ordered

Teach patient how to do fetal movement counting (fetal kick counts)

Discuss symptoms that may indicate progression of preeclampsia such as blurred vision, epigastric pain, increased edema, decreased fetal movement

Assess need and plan for assistance at home (meal preparation, housekeeping, child care)

Explain signs of labor and when to call primary health care provider/report to hospital

Assess plan for transport to hospital if necessary including transport availability, child care arrangements

Eclampsia

Progression of preeclampsia characterized by tonic and clonic convulsions

Assessment

Observations/findings

Seizure
  Twitching and blinking of eyes
  Crying or screaming
  Loss of consciousness
  Tachypnea
  Description
    Tonic
      Rigid body
      Jaws fixed
      Hands clenched
      Legs inverted
      Cyanosis
      Breath-holding
      Length of seizure activity
    Clonic
      Twitching of facial muscles
      Frothing at mouth; may be tinged with blood
      Biting of tongue
      Urinary or fecal incontinence

Postseizure assessment

Subjective data

Headache
Amnesia
Nausea/vomiting
Muscle soreness; backache

Objective data

Oliguria
Altered level of consciousness
Aspiration; choking
Vital signs: blood pressure, pulse, respirations

Diagnostic tests

Magnesium sulfate levels
Blood chemistries as indicated
Ultrasound/x-ray examination as indicated
Electronic fetal monitoring
Cardiac monitoring
See Pregnancy-induced hypertension (PIH) (p. 722)

Potential complications

Respiratory distress
  Difficulty in breathing
  Diminished breath sounds
  Cyanosis
  Tachycardia, tachypnea
Fetal compromise
Signs of onset of labor
See Pregnancy-induced hypertension (PIH) (p. 722)

Collaborative management

Therapeutic management

Anticonvulsives as indicated
Magnesium sulfate therapy as indicated (for 24 hr after birth)
Neurologic checks with vital signs
Sedatives as indicated
Antihypertensives
IV fluids as indicated
NPO
Delivery of newborn when stabilized
Oxygen therapy

Nursing management

PATIENT PROBLEM/NURSING DIAGNOSIS

● **NDX:** Risk for injury related to physiologic processes and effects of seizure

Prevent injury by doing the following:
  Removing surrounding furniture if on floor
  Supporting and protecting head; turning head to side
    if possible
  Gently restraining limbs
  Never leaving patient unattended
Insert oral airway when able; *never attempt to force jaws
  open*
Loosen constrictive clothing
Suction oropharynx and nasopharynx prn
Administer oxygen per nasal cannula or face mask at 10
  to 12 L/min for 10 min as ordered
Maintain NPO
Give mouth care when reactive and inspect for damage
  caused by biting soft tissue or tongue
Auscultate FHR q1h to 2h and prn or monitor FHR
  with electronic monitor *to assess fetal status*
Maintain closed gravity drainage system
  Measure urinary output qh
  Report output <30 ml/hr to primary health care
    provider
Maintain parenteral fluids as ordered
Invasive hemodynamic monitoring as indicated
Measure intake and output
Assess neurologic status immediately after seizure and
  prn
  Pupillary size and reaction to light
  LOC
Assess BP and pulse q15min for six times and prn;
  leave BP cuff on arm continuously *to reduce stimuli
  (of attaching/removing cuff) that could precipitate
  another seizure*
Do not take temperature unless necessary; take axil-
  lary temperature *to reduce seizure stimuli*
Do not move patient unnecessarily *to reduce seizure
  stimuli*
Reorient patient to environment when conscious
Provide emotional support
Administer medication as ordered: anticonvulsives,
  sedatives, hypotensives
Protect from extraneous stimuli
  Keep room darkened; light only enough to make
    observations and provide care
  Avoid sudden noises
  Avoid jarring bed
  Converse only if absolutely necessary
Observe for onset of labor
Reinforce primary health care provider's explanation of

what has happened and maternal and fetal prognosis
  to both patient and spouse or significant other
See interventions for Severe preeclampsia (p. 724)
See Pregnancy-induced hypertension (PIH) (p. 722)

EXPECTED OUTCOME
Patient is protected from injury to self and fetus

Hyperemesis Gravidarum

*Excessive or pernicious vomiting during pregnancy,
  potentially leading to dehydration and/or starvation*

Assessment

Observations/findings

Nausea and vomiting usually in morning and/or after
  meals
Epigastric pain
Hiccups
Heartburn
Thirst: may be severe
Weight loss
Oliguria
Concentrated urine
Dry skin
Poor skin turgor
Emesis of food, mucus, and/or bile
Metabolic acidosis evidenced by headache, mental dull-
  ness, disorientation

Diagnostic tests

Blood chemistries/electrolytes
Hgb/Hct
Coagulation profile
Hemodynamic monitoring as indicated
Cardiac monitoring

Potential complications

Dehydration
Jaundice
Tachycardia
Elevated temperature
Alkalosis
Malnutrition, starvation
Emotional disturbances regarding pregnancy and fam-
  ily relationships
Withdrawal
Depression

Collaborative management

Therapeutic management

IV fluids as indicated

Total parenteral nutrition (TPN)/intralipids as indicated

Central venous catheter as indicated or PICC line as indicated

Frequent, small meals or continuous nasogastric tube feedings as indicated

Nursing management

PATIENT PROBLEMS/NURSING DIAGNOSES

● **NDX:** Fluid volume deficit related to vomiting and altered nutrition related to dehydration and hyperemesis

ACUTE CARE

Activity as tolerated

Maintain NPO status for 24 to 48 hr

Administer parenteral fluids with B complex vitamins and vitamin C as ordered *to replace/maintain fluid volume*

Administer electrolyte replacement or TPN as ordered

Dipstick urine for pH, protein, blood, glucose, acetone, and specific gravity q 8h to 12h *to assess uroconcentration*

Maintain feeding/parenteral nutrition as ordered

Maintain patent IV access *to ensure open line for fluids*

Measure intake and output q2h to 4h

Administer medications as ordered; may include antihistaminics, antiemetics, anticholinergics, and sedatives

Administer oral hygiene q2h and prn, especially after episodes of vomiting

Assess BP, T, P, and R q4h and prn

Hemodynamic monitoring as ordered

CONVALESCENT CARE

Continue with acute care and decrease frequency of nursing functions as patient's condition improves

Serve small, frequent meals of solid foods high in carbohydrates such as crackers, dry toast, and cereal five to six times each day *to prevent gastric distension with potential for nausea/vomiting and fluid loss*

Serve small amounts of liquids such as hot tea, crushed ice, carbonated beverages, and cold fruit juices an hour after each meal *to ensure consumed solids don't mix with liquids at the same time, which could precipitate nausea*

Increase amounts of solid food and fluids slowly according to tolerance

Serve food attractively and at proper temperature *to prevent nausea*

Provide foods patient craves; avoid foods and fluids high in fat, *which might contribute to nausea, vomiting, and subsequent fluid loss*

Remove meal tray from bedside as soon as patient has finished

Avoid exposing patient to odors that are nauseating; ask patient which odors she finds nauseating

Certain foods

Room deodorizers

Colognes and perfumes

Mouthwash solutions

EXPECTED OUTCOME

Patient does not lose weight and is <10% dehydrated

● **NDX:** Anxiety related to change in health status and situational crisis

Provide private room if possible

If possible, have the same person care for patient each shift

If requested, facilitate supportive family member or friend visitation

Maintain calm and safe environment *to decrease anxiety*

Decrease stimuli

Talk with and reassure patient

Explore coping mechanisms

Encourage verbalization *to express feelings of anxiety and deal with them*

Request psychiatric evaluation if indicated

Talk to patient in a soothing voice

EXPECTED OUTCOMES

Patient verbalizes feeling less anxious

Exhibits relaxed facial expression

Responds to staff in an appropriate manner

Asks questions about care and prognosis

Patient/family teaching

Explain that termination of pregnancy may be indicated for unwanted pregnancy

Explain that therapeutic abortion may be indicated for deteriorating physical and/or mental condition such as that caused by persistent elevated temperature despite adequate hydration, tachycardia, jaundice, retinal hemorrhage, profound depression, or delirium

Refer to home health agency as indicated

Home care considerations

Explain need for well-balanced diet with adequate fluid intake at scheduled times

Discuss symptoms of recurrence to report to physician

Emphasize importance of planned rest periods

Reinforce physician's explanation of effect of condition on fetus

Explain that symptoms nearly always disappear by fourth month of pregnancy

Teach name of medication, dosage, time of administration, purpose, and side effects

Explain need to avoid taking over-the-counter medications without physician approval

Emphasize importance of ongoing outpatient care

Amniocentesis

Withdrawal of amniotic fluid through a needle inserted through the maternal abdominal and uterine wall to assess fetal health, maturity, genetic karyotype, and/or sex

Assessment

Potential complications

Fainting

Abdominal pain

Nausea

Preterm labor

Fetal hyperactivity or hypoactivity

Fetal tachycardia: >160 beats/min

Fetal bradycardia: <120 beats/min

Maternal hemorrhage

Fetal hemorrhage

Intraamniotic infection
  Tachycardia
  Elevated temperature
  Foul odor of amniotic fluid

Collaborative management

Therapeutic management

Obtain consent

Laboratory tests as indicated

Ultrasound just before or during procedure

Nursing management

PATIENT PROBLEM/NURSING DIAGNOSIS

● **NDX:** Risk for injury related to invasive procedure; transabdominal access to intrauterine cavity

Auscultate FHR *to validate fetal well-being*

Explain that procedure is usually not harmful to mother or fetus

Explain that procedure is virtually painless

POSTPROCEDURE CARE

Apply adhesive bandage to site of injection

Palpate fundus for fetal activity

Monitor FHR with electronic monitor if possible or auscultate FHR q15min twice

Assess BP, P, and R

Position on side if patient experiences profuse diaphoresis, fainting, or nausea

Reinforce primary health care provider's explanation of reason for procedure
  Assessment of fetal maturity and health
  Diagnosis of genetic defects
  Sex determination

Discuss symptoms to report to primary health care provider
  Any vaginal drainage, discharge, spotting, or bleeding
  Fetal hyperactivity, diminished activity, or absence of fetal movement
  Any signs of infection
    Elevated temperature
    Chills
  Abdominal pain
  Cramps
  Contractions

EXPECTED OUTCOME

Patient does not experience injury (complications) to self or fetus

Care of Woman With Diabetes During Last Trimester of Pregnancy

Women with diabetes are frequently hospitalized during the last trimester of pregnancy to monitor insulin needs, which are usually higher than during the previous two trimesters, and to monitor fetal well-being because of the increased fetal and neonatal morbidity and mortality associated with maternal diabetes

Assessment

Objective data

Large weight gain

Presence of risk factors
  Previously diagnosed glycosuria
  Insulin dependent
  Positive family history
  Obesity >200 lb
  Previous large-for-gestational-age (LGA) baby
  Previous stillbirth
  Previous congenital anomalies

Habitual abortion
Maternal age ≥25 years

Diagnostic tests

Blood glucose screening
Glucose loading test, oral glucose tolerance test (OGTT)
Urine glucose/acetone
NST/CST
Blood chemistries as ordered

Potential complications

Hypoglycemia (p. 482)
Diabetic ketoacidosis
PIH (p. 722)
  Hypertension
  Edema (especially of face and hands)
  Proteinuria
Anxiety
Spontaneous abortion
Third trimester intrauterine fetal demise
Hydramnios
Worsening diabetes: increasing insulin requirements
Pyelonephritis
Increased congenital anomalies in newborn
  Cardiac defects
  Neural tube defects
  Caudal regression syndrome
  See Infant of diabetic mother (IDM)
Newborn respiratory distress
Newborn macrosomia
Newborn hypocalcemia
Newborn hypoglycemia

Collaborative management

Therapeutic management

Glucose screening tests as indicated
Insulin as indicated on sliding scale; continuous insulin infusion pump may be preferred
IV fluids as indicated
American Dietetic Association (ADA) diet as indicated
Monitored weight gain
Urine testing as indicated for blood, glucose, ketones, protein, bilirubin, and pH
Nonstress tests, biophysical profile

Nursing management

PATIENT PROBLEM/NURSING DIAGNOSIS

● **NDX:** Risk for injury to mother and fetus related to hypoglycemia/hyperglycemia

Maintain patient on NPH or other long-acting insulin as ordered; as EDC approaches, patient's insulin may be regulated by home monitoring of blood glucose and regular insulin on a sliding scale
Monitor blood glucose as ordered
Replace foods not eaten with appropriate exchanges *to ensure euglycemia;* see Diabetic food replacement in ADA publication
Auscultate FHR tid and prn
Weigh patient daily: same time, clothing, and scale *to ensure consistency*
Measure intake and output as indicated
Encourage verbalization about concerns for fetus and self as a result of diabetes
Reinforce primary health care provider's explanation of status of fetus and reasons for laboratory studies
Explain procedure for implications of nonstress testing or contraction stress test as a method of evaluating fetal status in the presence of maternal diabetes

ADDITIONAL NURSING DIAGNOSES
TO CONSIDER
Anxiety
Altered nutrition: less or more than body requirements
Situational low self-esteem

EXPECTED OUTCOMES
Achieves and maintains euglycemia
Has no injuries (complications to self or fetus)

Patient/family teaching

Explain need for antepartum surveillance
Explain potential need for planning birth if cesarean
Discuss referral to home health care agency if ordered

Home care considerations

Discuss need for following diabetic regimen
Discuss maternal perception of fetal movement
Discuss symptoms of hypoglycemia and appropriate treatment
Discuss symptoms of diabetic ketoacidosis and appropriate treatment (p. 488)
Discuss symptoms to report to primary health care provider
  Diminished fetal activity
  Signs of PIH
  Signs of labor
  Signs of uncontrolled diabetes
Demonstrate and have patient and/or significant other return demonstrate
  Home glucose monitoring
  Use of sliding scale insulin dosing for injection
  See Insulin therapy teaching guide (p. 476)

Intrapartum Care of Woman With Diabetes

Insulin needs vary during labor and delivery, necessitating careful patient observation and monitoring of glucose levels

Assessment for hypoglycemia

Subjective data

Hunger
Palpitation
Weakness, fatigue
Dizziness
Headache

Objective data

Perspiration
Tachycardia
Tremor
Pallor
Blurred or double vision
See Care of mother in first stage of labor (p. 738)
See Care of mother during birth

Diagnostic tests

Blood glucose monitoring
Electrolytes as ordered
Electronic fetal monitoring
Real-time ultrasound

Potential complications

See Care of woman with diabetes during last trimester of pregnancy (p. 729)
Hypoglycemia of mother and infant after birth

Collaborative management

Therapeutic management

Decreased insulin requirements
Continuous IV infusion of insulin if blood glucose is >4 mg/dl
Capillary blood glucose monitoring q1h to 2h
IV fluids as indicated
NPO as indicated
For elective cesarean birth
  No insulin in morning
  Early morning birth (8 to 9 A.M. preferred because of glucose levels)
Monitoring of glucose after birth

Observation for insulin reaction
Family planning counseling and implications for future pregnancies, especially preconceptual counselling

Nursing management

PATIENT PROBLEM/NURSING DIAGNOSIS

● **NDX:** Risk for injury to mother and fetus related to hypoglycemia/hyperglycemia and possible uteroplacental insufficiency during labor

INTRAPARTUM CARE

Administer parenteral fluids; electrolyte solutions may be ordered
Monitor fetus via internal electronic fetal monitoring if possible
Check blood glucose as ordered q1h to 3h
Be aware that regular insulin is preferred to long-lasting insulin *because of fluctuations in use of insulin during active labor*
See Care of mother in first stage of labor (p. 738)
See Care of mother during birth
See Fetal compromise (p. 745)
See Care of mother monitored via EFM (p. 746)

IMMEDIATE POSTPARTUM CARE

See Postpartum care
Observe for symptoms of hypoglycemia
Be aware that insulin dosage will be adjusted to prepregnant state needs *because demand for insulin will decrease*
Use regular insulin based on blood glucose tests for first 24 to 48 hr as ordered *to maintain better short-term control of glucose level*
Progress to NPH or other long-acting insulin after first 24 to 48 hr as ordered, when patient is maintaining stable diet
Check blood glucose levels periodically if ordered

EXPECTED OUTCOME

Mother maintains euglycemia, and fetal heart rate pattern is reassuring

Patient/family teaching

Explain need for NPO status during labor
Explain need for changes in insulin requirements
Explain that insulin and dietary needs may vary because of lactation postpartum
Discuss changes in administration of insulin
Explain need for more frequent capillary glucose monitoring

Home care considerations

Explain need to avoid persons with infections, especially upper respiratory infections (URIs), during puerperium

See Care of women with diabetes during last trimester of pregnancy (p. 729)

The patient and significant other should demonstrate knowledge of diabetic regimen changes and intent to follow plan of care

Premature Rupture of Membranes

Rupture of the bag of waters 12 hr or more before the onset of labor; the etiology is unknown, but it is associated with hydramnios, multiple gestation, preterm labor, cervical incompetence, trauma, and amnionitis

Assessment

Objective data

Fluid leaking from vagina
Positive nitrazine paper test (alkaline amniotic fluid)

Diagnostic tests

Nitrazine paper test (positive); false positives may occur with contact with cervical mucus, blood, semen, antiseptics, and alkaline urine
"Fern" pattern on dried microscope slide
Fluid cultures as indicated
Presence of amniotic fluid pool in vagina

Potential complications

Bleeding
Intraamniotic infection
  Foul odor of vaginal discharge
  Maternal elevated temperature
  Maternal tachycardia
  Maternal leukocytosis
Meconium-stained amniotic fluid
Umbilical cord protruding from introitus
Compression of the umbilical cord
Fetal compromise
  Fetal tachycardia: >160 beats/min
  Fetal bradycardia: <120 beats/min
  Variable decelerations on electronically monitored fetus
Preterm birth of premature infant
See Care of Mother in First Stage of Labor (p. 738)

Collaborative management

Therapeutic management

Oxytocin induction of labor as indicated based on gestational age
Fetal heart rate monitoring
Introital and rectal culture for group B streptococcus
Fetal maturity testing
IUPC (intrauterine pressure catheter) as indicated
CBC and differential

Nursing management

PATIENT PROBLEM/NURSING DIAGNOSIS

● **NDX:** Risk for infection related to premature rupture of membranes

Assess T, P, and R q4h
Auscultate FHR or use electronic FHR monitor q1h to 4hr and prn
Avoid vaginal examinations *to limit opportunity for introduction of opportunistic infection-producing organisms*
Observe drainage of amniotic fluid for color, amount, and odor q2h to 4h and prn
Administer perineal care with antiseptic solution after each elimination, q2h to 4h and prn *to reduce potential for infection*
Keep patient clean and dry: change pad under buttocks q2h to 4h and prn *to prevent pooling of secretions*
Palpate fundus for uterine activity q1h to 2h and prn; report onset of contractions to physician
Administer antibiotics if ordered
Prepare oxytocin induction as ordered if labor does not begin within 24 hr of premature rupture of membranes (PROM) and patient is near EDC *to avoid prolonged period of membrane rupture with increasing potential for infection*
Decrease frequency of nursing functions as patient's condition stabilizes
Carefully clean perineal region; wipe from front to back after elimination *to prevent urethral/bladder infection*
Make note of PROM on newborn's chart so that nursery will observe for possible respiratory distress, meconium aspiration, and pneumonia at and after delivery

EXPECTED OUTCOMES

Patient is treated for infection or does not have symptoms of infection
Fetus/newborn does not have undesirable sequelae, or infection is treated

Patient/family teaching

Discuss with patient that because amniotic fluid is continually produced, she will not experience a "dry" labor

Report any signs of onset of labor; labor usually begins within 24 hr after rupture of membranes

Placenta Previa

Total, partial, or low implantation of the placenta over the internal cervical os (Figure 11-10); occurs most often in multiparas; total and partial placenta previa prohibits vaginal delivery (the fetus is delivered cesarean); with low implantation the fetus can sometimes be delivered vaginally with the presenting part acting as a tamponade against the placenta

Assessment

Objective data

Painless vaginal bleeding: intermittent to constant flow
Soft, relaxed uterus

Diagnostic tests

Ultrasound to identify position of placenta
Amniography
Speculum vaginal examination
Hgb/Hct; CBC
Amniocentesis for fetal maturity as indicated
Clotting studies
Electronic fetal monitoring: continuous

Potential complications

Fetal bradycardia: <120 beats/min
Monitored fetus: late decelerations

Absence of fetal heart tones
Maternal shock
Fetal hyperactivity, hypoxia
Neonatal anemia, shock (hypovolemic)
Cesarean birth

Collaborative management

Therapeutic management

Cesarean birth for nonreassuring FHR pattern or to control hemorrhage
Tocolytic agents as indicated if infant is preterm
IV fluids as indicated
Type and cross match 2 to 4 units of fresh whole blood and/or other blood products as available

Nursing management

PATIENT PROBLEMS/NURSING DIAGNOSES

● **NDX:** Altered tissue perfusion (fetal) related to malaligned placenta and hypovolemia associated with bleeding

NOTE: Amount of bleeding and position of placenta determine care and the frequency of monitoring vital signs
Maintain complete bed rest
Never do a manual vaginal or rectal examination, which could stimulate bleeding
Avoid rectal stimulation; no enemas, which could stimulate a bleeding episode
Monitor intake and output
Initiate parenteral fluids as ordered *to ensure fluid balance;* monitor IV site and flow *to ensure patency*
Place patient in high-Fowler's or lateral position if membranes are ruptured; avoid supine position
Place patient in position of comfort if membranes are not ruptured

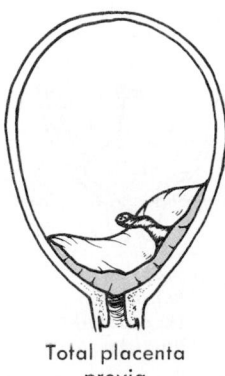
Total placenta previa

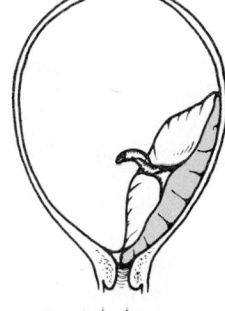
Partial placenta previa

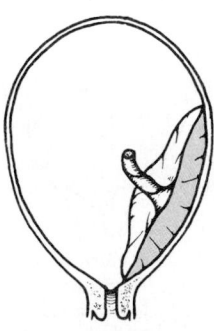
Low implantation

Figure 11-10 Placenta previa (abnormal implantation).

Assess BP, P, and FHR q15min to 2h and prn

Assess pulse oximeter oxygen saturation if respiratory complications are present or impending

Observe amount, color, and character of vaginal drainage q15min to 2h and prn depending on amount of bleeding

Administer perineal care with antiseptic solution after every elimination and prn

Report saturation of more than one perineal pad q30 min

Weigh pads and linen to estimate blood loss as ordered

Administer transfusions and volume expanders as ordered

Immediately report any sign of onset of labor to physician

Monitor FHR electronically as indicated

Prepare for double setup for potential cesarean delivery and/or vaginal delivery as indicated

Administer oxygen by mask or nasal cannula as indicated *to ensure oxygen saturation of maternal Hgb, which enhances appropriate fetal tissue perfusion*

Continue with care and decrease frequency of nursing functions as patient's condition stabilizes

Explain and prepare for diagnostic tests if ordered
Ultrasonography
Amniography
Placenta scan

Prepare for delivery as ordered

See Cesarean birth (p. 753) or Postpartum care (p. 749)

EXPECTED OUTCOMES

Patient does not hemorrhage, and FHR is reassuring

● **NDX:** Anticipatory grieving related to potential loss of fetus

Correct any misconceptions that patient and significant other(s) have about prognosis, procedures, and plan of care

Provide ongoing information about status and plan of care *to ensure understanding by patient and significant other(s)*

Facilitate discussion between patient and significant other(s) about anxieties, fears, and potential fetal loss

EXPECTED OUTCOME

Patient expresses feelings and concerns and maintains constructive interpersonal relationships with family and health care providers

Abruptio Placentae

Premature separation of the placenta occurring before the third stage of labor (Figure 11-11); may be associated with cocaine use, elevated BP, maternal trauma

Assessment

Subjective data

Uterus
Extreme tenderness
General or localized pain
Pain: may be absent to severe
Low back pain
Extreme anxiety

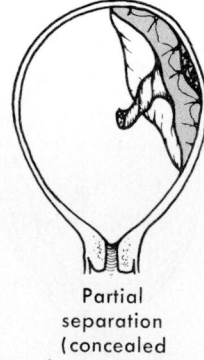 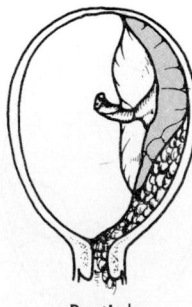 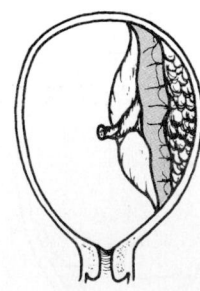

Partial separation (concealed hemorrhage)

Partial separation (apparent hemorrhage)

Complete separation (concealed hemorrhage)

Figure 11-11 Abruptio placentae (premature separation).

Objective data

Uterus
  Sudden enlargement: symmetrical or asymmetrical
  Progressive decrease of relaxation between contrac-
    tions developing into continuous boardlike
    rigidity
  Uterine tachysystole and hypertonus on monitored
    patient
  Hyperactive fetus
Vaginal bleeding may or may not be present
Hemorrhage: usually concealed
Port wine-colored amniotic fluid may be
  present
Rising uterine fundus
FHR
  Bradycardia: <120 beats/min
  Heart tones: may be absent
  Monitored fetus may have late decelerations
Hypovolemia
Hypotension
Tachycardia

Diagnostic tests

CBC, coagulation profile (platelets, fibrinogen,
  PT/INR, APTT, fibrin degradation products [fibrin
  split products])
Continuous external fetal monitoring

Potential complications

Fetal compromise (p. 745)
DIC (p. 252)
Hypofibrinogenemia
Hypoprothrombinemia
Bleeding from mucous membranes
Bruising; ecchymosis
Oliguria progressing to anuria
Maternal hypovolemic shock (p. 151)
Renal failure

Collaborative management

Therapeutic management

Cesarean birth for compromised fetus, maternal
  hemorrhage, or unstable maternal condition
IV fluids as indicated
NPO (if near or in shock or delivery imminent)
Volume expander or blood transfusion as
  indicated
Oxygen 8 to 10 L/min as indicated
Analgesics

Nursing management

PATIENT PROBLEMS/NURSING DIAGNOSES

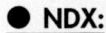 **NDX:** Altered tissue perfusion: placental related to
hypovolemia associated with hemorrhage of
abrupted placenta

IMMEDIATE CARE

Administer oxygen as ordered
Remain with patient at all times
Maintain complete bed rest in position of comfort
Palpate fundus for presence of uterine contractions and
  relaxation
    Report increasing uterine intensity or sustained uter-
      ine contraction to primary health care provider
    Instruct patient to report any sudden increase in pain
Prepare for immediate birth and neonatal resuscitation
Obtain type and cross match of 2 to 4 units of packed
  cells if ordered by physician
Assist with amniotomy if done by physician
Monitor fetus internally with spiral electrode if possible
Assess BP, P, and FHR q5min to 15min
Perform tilt test prn
Administer transfusions or volume expanders as
  ordered

STABILIZATION CARE

Control pain carefully as ordered; small doses of anal-
  gesics are preferred
Weigh pads and linens to estimate blood loss as
  ordered
Allay anxiety as much as possible
Explain all actions taken
Ask patient to verbalize any changes in feeling and sen-
  sorium
Reinforce primary health care provider's explanation
  for cesarean birth if necessary
Notify postpartum nurses to observe patient for the
  following:
  Incisional hematoma
  Disparate intake and output
See Cesarean birth (p. 753) or Postpartum care
  (p. 749)

EXPECTED OUTCOMES

Patient's condition does not develop into hypovolemic
  shock, and fetus's hydration is maintained
Fetus does not experience a negative sequelae

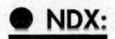 **NDX:** Fluid volume deficit related to active loss
of blood from abrupted placenta before
delivery

Initiate and maintain parenteral fluids as ordered
Hemodynamic monitoring as ordered
Maintain patent IV line
Measure intake and output qh
Connect indwelling catheter (Foley) to closed gravity
system as indicated

EXPECTED OUTCOMES

Hgb/Hct are restored to or maintained at previous
levels
Skin turgor is adequate

Patient/family teaching

Explain aspects of care to patient/significant other(s)
Reinforce primary health care provider's explanation of
plan of treatment and expected prognosis
Attempt to maintain a calm, reassuring demeanor and
environment
Assist with rhythmic breathing and relaxation techniques during episodes of pain associated with uterine
hypertonus

Prolapsed Umbilical Cord

*Protrusion of the umbilical cord in advance of the
presenting part; it should be suspected after
amniotomy or spontaneous gross rupture of
membranes and should be ruled out by vaginal
examination (Figures 11-12 and 11-13)*

Assessment

Observations/findings

Umbilical cord: may or may not be visible at introitus
Meconium-stained amniotic fluid
Fetal bradycardia: <120 beats/min
Slowing pulsations of visible cord
Severe, variable decelerations of FHR

Diagnostic test

Vaginal examination for prolapse verification

Potential complications

Fetal compromise (p. 745)
Fetal hypoxia
Fetal hypoxemia
Fetal acidemia
Fetal acidosis
Fetal asphyxia
Fetal death, stillborn

Collaborative management

Therapeutic management

Bed rest (knee-chest position for acute episode)
Cesarean birth
Oxygen therapy as indicated
IV therapy as indicated

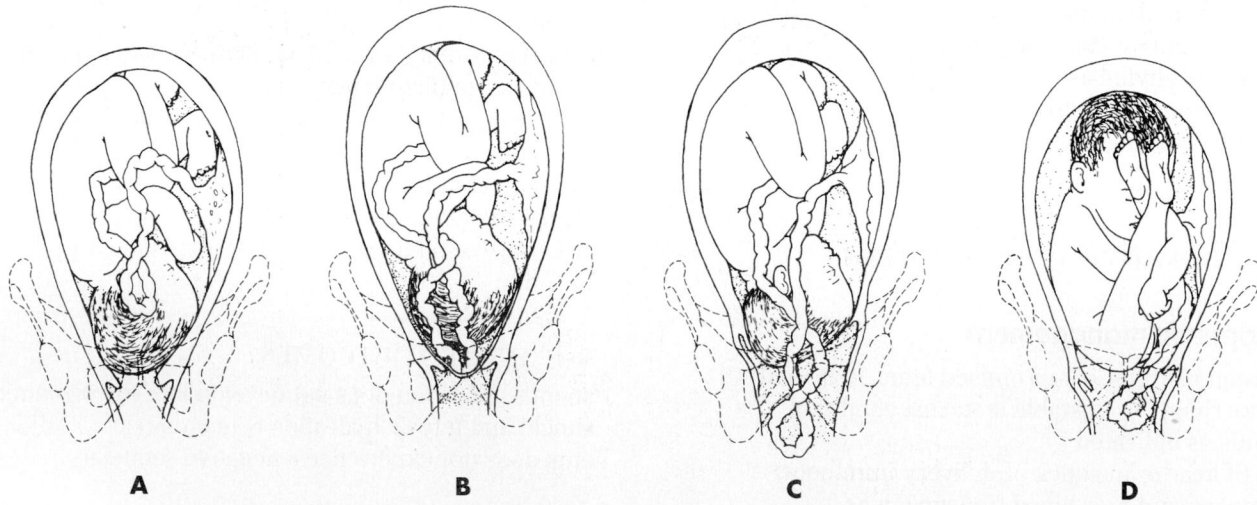

A	**B**	**C**	**D**

Figure 11-12   Prolapse of umbilical cord. Note pressure of presenting part on umbilical cord, which endangers fetal circulation. **A,** Occult (hidden) prolapse of cord. **B,** Complete prolapse of cord. Note membranes are intact. **C,** Cord presenting in front of fetal head and may be seen within vagina. **D,** Frank breech presentation with prolapsed cord. (From Bobak IM et al: *Maternity nursing,* ed 4, St Louis, 1995, Mosby.)

Nursing management

PATIENT PROBLEM/NURSING DIAGNOSIS

● **NDX:** Risk for injury (fetal) related to potential cord compression associated with prolapse of umbilical cord

Prepare for immediate birth; cesarean is usually done
Notify OR and neonatal resuscitation team to attend birth
Maintain absolute bed rest
Never attempt to replace a prolapsed cord into vagina, *which could compress the cord and impede circulation to/from the fetus*
Prevent cord compression
  Elevate presenting part sufficiently *to relieve pressure on the umbilical cord until delivery*
  Pressure of examiner's sterile gloved hand (cord between two spread fingers) *to elevate the presenting part*
  Knee-chest or exaggerated Trendelenburg's position
  Do not manipulate cord
  Rapid filling of urinary bladder with 500 to 700 ml of normal saline through indwelling catheter may help *to elevate the presenting part and reduce compression of the fetal head on the cord*

Assess FHR q2min to 5min, preferably with an electronic fetal monitor
Administer oxygen (10 to 12 L/min) by face mask as ordered; *increased saturation of maternal oxygenation may be of some benefit to the fetus*
Gently cover exposed cord with sterile saline compresses
Stay with patient at all times

EXPECTED OUTCOMES

Circulation is maintained through umbilical cord as evidenced by absence of fetal compromise
Fetal heart rate is in the normal range, and there is absence of severe variable decelerations on an electronically monitored fetus

ADDITIONAL NURSING DIAGNOSES TO CONSIDER

Altered tissue perfusion: fetal
Maternal fear

Patient/family teaching

Allay anxiety as much as possible by explanation to patient about importance of maintaining special position and not bearing down or pushing with contractions

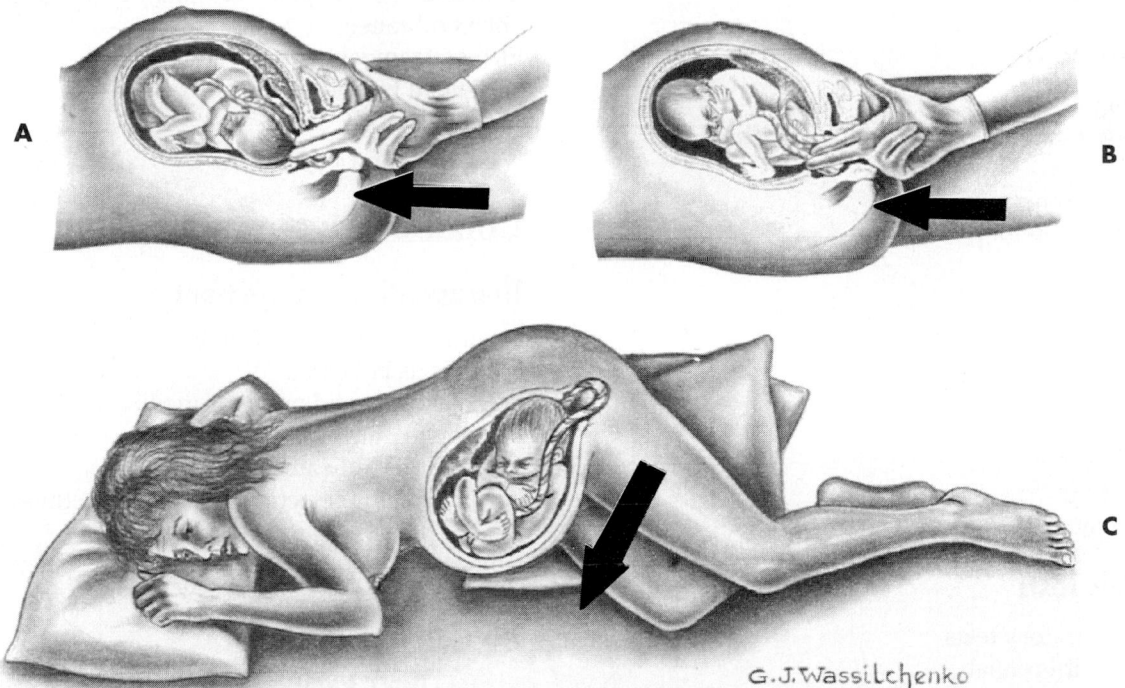

Figure 11-13 Arrows indicate direction of pressure against presenting part to relieve compression of prolapsed umbilical cord. Pressure exerted by examiner's fingers in **A,** vertex presentation, and **B,** in breech position. **C,** Gravity relieves pressure with woman in modified Sims position with hips elevated as high as possible with pillows. (From Bobak IM et al: *Maternity nursing,* ed 4, St Louis, 1995, Mosby.)

Teach patient panting and blowing techniques for use during uterine contractions *to prevent pushing and additional pressure on the prolapsed cord*

Reinforce primary health care provider's explanation of need for immediate delivery

See Postpartum care (p. 749) or Cesarean birth (p. 753)

Care of Mother in First Stage of Labor

Physiologic process by which the fetus is expelled from the uterus

early labor: *Dilation of 0 to 4 cm with mild to moderate irregular contractions*

active labor: *Dilation of 4 to 8 cm with moderate to strong regular contractions every 2 to 5 min*

transitional labor: *Dilation of 8 cm to complete dilation with strong contractions*

Assessment

Subjective data

Behavior
  Surge of energy and activity
  Talking frequently
  Anxious
  Fear of isolation

Objective data

Rupture of membranes
Uterine contractions: regular with increasing intensity and frequency
Transitional labor
  Nausea and vomiting
  Irritability
  Loss of coping mechanisms
  Hiccups and/or belching
  Trembling and/or shaking of legs
  Chilling
  Perspiration
  Rectal pressure
  Urge to push
  Hypersensitive abdomen

Diagnostic tests

Baseline laboratory tests
  CBC with differential
  Hgb/Hct
  VDRL serology
  Chemistries
Urinalysis

Cultures as indicated by history of signs and symptoms
Ultrasound examination as indicated
Electronic fetal monitoring
Fetal scalp pH testing
Vibroacoustic stimulation
Score of Biophysical Profile (if done before onset of labor (Table 11-1)

Potential complications

Nonreassuring findings
  Fetal tachycardia: >160 beats/min
  Fetal bradycardia: <120 beats/min
  Meconium-stained amniotic fluid
  Foul-smelling amniotic fluid
Fetal hyperactivity
Monitored labor (p. 746)
  Severe variable decelerations: <70 beats/min for more than 30 sec
  Uncorrectable, repetitive late decelerations of any magnitude
  Absence of variability
  Prolonged deceleration
  Unstable FHR; sinusoidal pattern
Supine hypotension syndrome
Inadequate uterine relaxation
  Contractions lasting longer than 90 sec
  Relaxation between contractions less than 30 sec
Arrest of labor
Intraamniotic infection secondary to prolonged rupture of membranes
Elevated temperature
Distended bladder
Dehydration
Hemorrhage

Collaborative management

Therapeutic management

Laboratory tests as indicated
IV fluids as indicated
Prenatal chart and previous medical chart ordered to labor and delivery unit
Analgesia as indicated
Preparation for selected/indicated anesthesia by anesthesiologist/nurse anesthetist
Supportive care to patient and family

Nursing management

PATIENT PROBLEMS/NURSING DIAGNOSES

● **NDX:** Risk for injury to mother related to physiologic processes of labor

Table 11-1 Biophysical Profile

A. Description: A Physical Examination of the Fetus with Realtime Ultrasound Measurements

Fetal breathing movements (FBM)
Fetal movement (FM)
Fetal tone (TON)
Amniotic fluid index (AFI)
Nonstress test (NST)

B. Interpretation

Biophysical Variable	Normal (score = 2)	Abnormal (score = 0)
Fetal breathing movements (FBM)	At least one episode of FBM of at least 30 sec duration in 30 min observation	Absent FBM or no episode of ≥30 sec in 30 min
Gross body movements (FM)	At least three discrete body/limb movements in 30 min (episodes of active continuous movement considered as a single movement)	Two or fewer episodes of body/limb movements in 30 min
Fetal tone (TON)	At least one episode of active extension with return to flexion of fetal limb(s) or trunk; opening and closing of hand considered normal tone	Slow extension with return to partial flexion, or movement of limb in full extension, or absence of fetal movement
Amniotic fluid index (AFI)*	AFI ≤1 cm	AFI <1 cm
Nonstress test (NST)	Reactive	Nonreactive

C. Record Biophysical Profile

Parameter	Score
FBM	_____
FM	_____
TON	_____
AFI	_____
NST	_____
TOTAL:	_____

D. Management Based on Interpretation and Score

Score	Action
8-10	Equivalent to reactive NST; manage per protocol
4-6	If pulmonary maturity is favorable, deliver; if not, repeat test in 24 hr; if score persists, deliver if maturity is certain; otherwise, treat with steroids and deliver in 48 hr
0-2	Evaluate for delivery

*Amniotic fluid index: The summation of deepest vertical pocket of amniotic fluid in each of the four quadrants of the amniotic sac. Measurements are done in centimeters and perpendicular to the floor.

Assess temperature q2h after rupture of membranes
Consider plotting cervical dilation and fetal descent over time on square-ruled graph paper (Friedman curve)
Administer clear liquids as ordered
Measure intake and output
Have patient void q2h and prn
Check urine for glucose and protein

Maintain complete bed rest in position of comfort if membranes are ruptured, especially if presenting part is not yet engaged; otherwise, encourage ambulation as tolerated
Assist patient to bathroom if presenting part is well applied to cervix as ordered
Initiate lactated Ringer's solution or other IV solution as ordered

Prehydrate with 500 to 1000 ml of fluid before anesthetic procedure as ordered

Maintain dosing of prelabor medications or drugs as ordered (e.g., anticonvulsants, antihypertensives, or methadone)

See ASPO (Lamaze) review sheet (Figure 11-14)

EXPECTED OUTCOMES

Patient does not experience any injury related to labor as evidenced by adequate hydration, skin turgor, void-

THE PROCESS	WOMAN	BREATHING	LABOR COACH

Beginning
Loss of mucus plug
Rupture of membranes
Contractions
    Regular or irregular
    Closer together
    More intense
	Rest
	Relax
	Sugar foods
			Time contractions
			Inform doctor
			Rest
			Eat

Progress
Effacement
Dilatation
Contractions
    Closer together
    Stronger
	Relax and focus
	Slow chest breathing as needed
		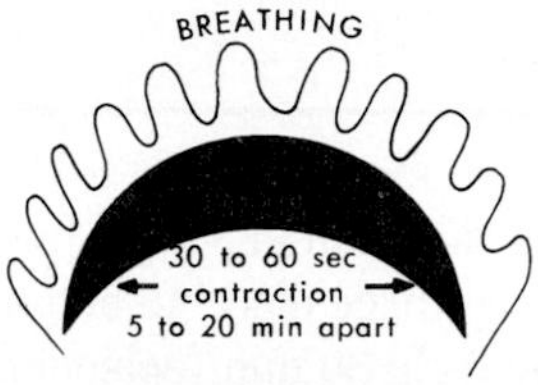 BREATHING
		30 to 60 sec contraction 5 to 20 min apart
		Cleansing breath
		6-9 breaths per min, in through nose, out through mouth
		Effleurage
		Cleansing breath
			Prep room time
			  45 min to 1 hr
			
			Check for comfort
			  Positioning
			    Side position—top leg bent, supported with pillow—either side
			    Tailor sit—head supported
			    Reclining chair—head of bed up, knees bent—pillow under each arm
			    Head up 90 degrees—lean on overbed table with pillow
			    All fours—on hands and knees during contractions—relax to side between
			    Effleurage
			    Counter pressure in back or groin

Labor more active—increasing dilatation	Accelerated, decelerated breathing as needed	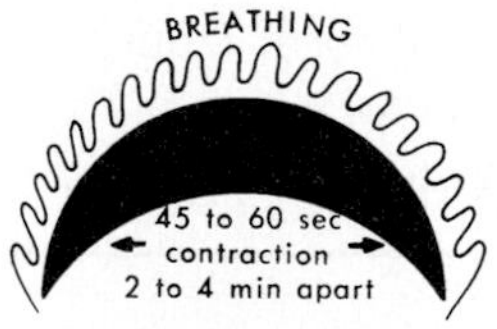 BREATHING
		45 to 60 sec contraction 2 to 4 min apart
		Cleansing breath
		Accelerating short, shallow pants through nose or mouth, decelerating as contraction fades
		Effleurage
		Cleansing breath
			Release tension
			Time contractions
			  Begins
			  Half over
			  Ends
			Breathe with her if needed
			Give verbal support
			Between contractions
			  Ice chips
			  Water
			  Lollipops
			  Washcloth
			
			Back labor 25% to 30%
			Off back use position numbers 1, 2, 4, and 5
			Counter measure
			  Fists, tennis balls, rolling pin, massage, pelvis rock

Transition
Dilatation going to completion
Possible signs
  Irritability
  Hiccups
Belching
Trembling
Nausea
Perspiration or chills
Contractions
  Longest
  Strongest
  2-3 peaks
Rectal pressure
Urge to push
	Transition breathing as needed
	Blow with urge to push
		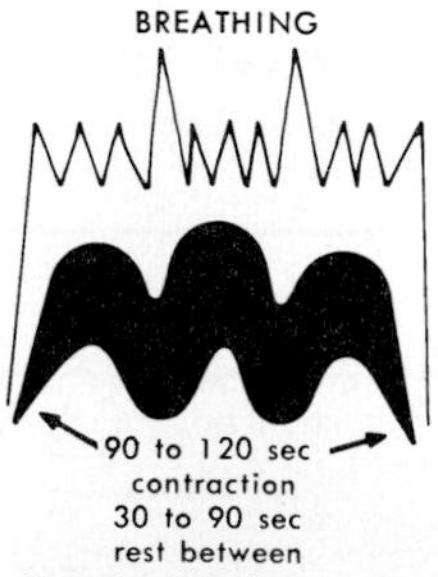 BREATHING
		90 to 120 sec contraction 30 to 90 sec rest between
		Cleansing breath
		8 or 6 or 4 or 2 fast, shallow pants, blow. Repeat. Blow if urge to push occurs
		Cleansing breath
			Great need for firmness, direction, and support
			Take one contraction at a time
			Keep blowing in control
			Call nurse when first feels like pushing
			Check for hyperventilation

Figure 11-14 ASPO (Lamaze) review sheet. (Prepared by the teachers of the American Society of Psychoprophylaxis in Obstetrics of Los Angeles, Inc., with permission of the Board of Directors of ASPO of Los Angeles, Inc.)

THE PROCESS	WOMAN	BREATHING	LABOR COACH

Birth
  Good pushing routine may take
    several contractions
  Pushing may not feel good for
    3 or 4 contractions
	Push with contractions
	Stop pushing as directed by
	  doctor or nurse
			Labor room
			  Elevate bed as desired
			  Remind her of technique
			    Pushing position after
			    2 cleansing breaths,
			    elbows into bed, push
			    gently during contrac-
			    tion, think vagina,
			    forceful pushing will
			    alleviate discomfort,
			    2 cleansing breaths
			    after contraction
			  Coach dress for delivery now

First baby—push in
  labor room until
  baby's head shows
Second baby—to delivery
  room as soon as completely
  dilated
		2 cleansing breaths
		Perform gentle pushing
		2 cleansing breaths
		Stop pushing
		Be sure to follow doctor's
		  directions, stop pushing when
		  directed—blow, then pant,
		  pant blow.
			Delivery room
			  Take 2 pillows
			  Encourage
			  Push as before, support
			    her head and shoulders
			    as she pulls herself up
			
			  Push as before, support
			    her head and shoulders
			    as she pulls herself up
			  Be sure she follows
			    doctor's directions
			  Listen for doctor's command
			    —stop pushing, etc.,
			    and repeat to her

As head comes to outlet may
  experience burning or stinging
  sensation on perineum, extreme
  pressure on anus—may feel
  as if it's "turning inside out"			

Expulsion of the placenta—placenta,
  membranes, umbilical cord are
  delivered
	Enjoy baby!	Push as directed.	Enjoy baby!

CONGRATULATIONS

Figure 11-14, cont'd. For legend see p. 740.

ing pattern (absence of distended bladder); has absence of fever

● **NDX:** Pain and anxiety related to physiologic process of labor

ACTIVE LABOR

Give back rub qh and prn between contractions

Apply pressure to sacrum as needed during contractions

Apply cool compress to forehead prn

Change pad under buttocks when moist, q30min to 60 min and prn

Assist with breathing techniques and teach to significant other who can assist patient

Change gown and linen as necessary

Turn off bright overhead lights when not needed

Clip call bell to bottom sheet within easy reach to ensure that staff is promptly notified of patient's needs

Relieve discomfort with medication as ordered

Assist physician with local or regional anesthetic; take BP and P q10min for three times after anesthetic is administered and until stabilized

Avoid talking to patient during contractions

Reposition patient q30min and prn; lateral position is preferred

TRANSITIONAL PHASE OF LABOR

Encourage deep ventilation before and after each contraction when patient is in active labor and during transition period

Avoid urge to push by panting and/or blowing in rapid sequence with contractions until completely dilated

Have emesis basin readily available

Have patient void to ensure empty bladder

Cover feet with blanket or have patient wear socks if chilling occurs

Tell patient that the transition stage usually lasts no more than 1 to 2 hr and then she will be allowed to push and deliver infant

Maternal-Fetal Assessment Frequencies

LOW-RISK PATIENTS

Temperature and pulse q4h (if ROM, then qh)
Blood pressure qh
Evaluate and record the FHR and UC q30min in the active phase of the first stage of labor and q15min during the second stage

HIGH-RISK PATIENTS

Temperature, pulse, and blood pressure qh or more frequently if situation necessitates
Evaluate and record the FHR and UC every 15 minutes in the active phase of the first stage of labor and every 5 minutes during the second stage

Palpate abdomen very lightly and only as often as necessary if abdomen is hypersensitive
Avoid having persons in labor room who are not directly caring for patient or providing support
Accept aggression or other coping behaviors; avoid negative comments
Avoid unnecessary talking or expression of feelings to meet own needs
Focus on patient and support her
  Calm voice
  Touch
  Positive reinforcement after contractions

EXPECTED OUTCOMES

Experiences manageable pain and minimal anxiety as evidenced by verbalization of same
Complies with assistive directions by staff
Has continuing interaction with significant other/ family

● **NDX:** Altered oral mucous membrane related to mouth breathing

Administer oral hygiene qh and prn between contractions
  Suck on ice chips, wet washcloths, or sour lollipops unless contraindicated
  Rinse mouth with water and/or mouthwash
  Apply petroleum jelly or antichapping lipsticks to dry lips prn

EXPECTED OUTCOME

Patient does not experience disruption in tissue layers of oral cavity

● **NDX:** Risk for injury (fetal) related to uterine contractions of labor and/or uteroplacental insufficiency

Note frequency, duration, and strength of contractions q30min to 60min and prn in early labor; increase to q15min to 30min in active labor
Auscultate FHR immediately after uterine contractions, preferably for 1min if not electronically monitored during labor (q15min to 30min and prn)
Assess BP and P qh and prn
Assess T, P, and R q2h to 4h and prn
Auscultate FHR immediately after membranes rupture or amniotomy is done
Turn mother to lateral position, increase rate of plain IV, administer 100% oxygen by face mask, and notify physician immediately if fetal stress is evident by auscultation or electronic fetal monitoring

EXPECTED OUTCOME

Patient gives birth to newborn in good condition with Apgar score ≥8 at 5 min of age

Patient/family teaching

Allay anxiety as much as possible by doing the following:
  Explain reasons for performing all procedures
  Encourage spouse or significant other to remain with patient to provide support during labor
  Assist spouse or significant other to listen to fetal heart tones with stethoscope, fetoscope, or ultrasound stethoscope
  Provide supportive care based on patient's knowledge of labor process
  Ask patient if she wants additional support persons present for labor and birth
  Inform waiting family members and friends of patient's progress and let patient know that they are interested in her
  Reduce environmental stimuli that may contribute to anxiety and tension; provide relaxed, restful atmosphere
  At appropriate intervals reassure patient that labor is progressing and that both patient and fetus are doing fine

EXPECTED OUTCOMES

Patient understands process of labor and rationale for procedures and is supported by significant other in coping with anxiety

Procedural Care of Mother During Delivery: Second and Third Stages of Labor

The stage of expulsion of the fetus, placenta, and membranes from the mother at birth after complete dilatation of the cervix

Assessment

Subjective data

Extreme anxiety
Patient stating, "Baby is coming"
Desire to defecate, fear of losing control

Objective data

Involuntary bearing down
Pushing
Grunting sounds
Vomiting episode
Involuntary shaking of legs
Perspiration between nose and upper lip
Increase in bloody show
Prolonged second stage
  More than 1 hr for multigravidas
  More than 2 hr for primigravidas

Diagnostic tests

Electronic fetal monitoring
Cord blood: gases, pH, and other tests as ordered

Potential complications

High-risk birth
Birth asphyxia
Difficult birth
  Shoulder dystocia
  Breech presentation
  Cephalopelvic disproportion
Forceps delivery
Vacuum extraction
Cesarean birth
Infant bruising, fractures

Nursing management

CARE DURING DELIVERY

Auscultate FHR q5min and/or after each push if electronic monitor is not used (if electronic monitor was used continuously during labor, then it should be continued in the delivery room until the time of delivery)
Check BP and P q5min to 10min
Pad stirrups if used
Administer oxygen mask at 10 to 12 L/min as ordered
Understand that low- to semi-Fowler's position with lateral tilt is preferred while pushing
Assist with breathing techniques
  Deep ventilation before and after each contraction
  Breathing technique and pushing with contractions
Observe perineum while pushing
Notify physician if second stage is prolonged
Prepare perineum according to hospital procedure
Place nurse, spouse, and/or labor coach at head of delivery table to encourage patient during delivery process
Encourage long, sustained pushing rather than frequent short pushes
Encourage patient to push when she feels urge to push
Encourage complete relaxation between contractions
Reassure patient that she is doing well and is advancing fetus with each push
Apply cool, moist cloth to forehead as needed
Keep DeLee suction catheter available and ready to use if meconium-stained amniotic fluid is present
Plan for suctioning of naso-oropharynx after delivery of fetal head and before delivery of thorax to prevent meconium aspiration
Assist physician or nurse-midwife as needed

IMMEDIATE POSTPARTUM CARE
(FOURTH-STAGE CARE)

Encourage mother to inspect infant as soon as possible
Place infant on maternal abdomen to provide skin-to-skin contact if delivery room is warm
See Care of newborn (p. 761)
Defer neonatal eye therapy for 1 to 2 hr after birth to promote eye contact with mother
Assess BP and P q10min to 15min for four times and prn
Add oxytocic drug as ordered to parenteral fluids
Palpate fundus, noting location and tonus q5min to 10 min for four times
Administer perineal care before removing legs from stirrups *to cleanse and inspect perineum*
Place sterile perineal pad under buttocks before transporting patient to recovery area
Place ice pack on episiotomy unless otherwise ordered *to reduce swelling*
Assist with infant's warm water bath if newborn's temperature is stable as indicated
Maintain mother's warmth with blankets as needed
Place radiant heat warmer over upper part of mother's bed or place dry, warmly blanketed newborn next to mother *so that she can visually inspect, touch, and/or*

breast-feed nude infant while preventing neonatal heat loss

Encourage mother and spouse and/or labor coach to be with infant in delivery area, providing them with as much privacy as feasible unless this is contraindicated by maternal or neonatal pathologic condition

Encourage mother to freely express her feelings about herself and her infant

Explain that behaviors manifested in labor are normal and there is no reason to be embarrassed if mother is apologetic for behavior

See Postpartum care (p. 749)

Oxytocin Infusion: Augmentation or Induction of Labor

Oxytocin infusion may be used to either begin the labor process or to augment a labor that is progressing slowly because of inadequate uterine activity

Diagnostic tests

FHR-UC monitoring
Cephalopelvic disproportion (CPD) measurements
Ultrasound as ordered

Assessment

Observations/findings

Dysfunctional labor pattern (Table 11-2)
Absence of cephalopelvic disproportion
Bishop score (Table 11-3)

Potential complications

Fetal compromise
 Hyperactive fetus
 Fetal tachycardia: >160 beats/min

Fetal bradycardia: <120 beats/min
Late decelerations
Prolonged deceleration
Severe variable decelerations
Uterine hyperstimulation
 Contractions longer than 90 sec
 Contractions occurring more frequently than q2min
 Peak pressure of contraction >90 mm Hg pressure
 Inadequate uterine relaxation: less than 30 sec between contractions
 Intrauterine resting tone >15 mm Hg pressure between contractions
 Sustained tetanic uterine contraction
Meconium-stained amniotic fluid
Maternal hypertension
Water intoxication
 Rising BP
 Edema of face, fingers, and around eyes
 Shortness of breath
 Difficulty in breathing
 Urinary output <30 to 50 ml/hr
Abruptio placentae: sudden, severe uterine pain (p. 734)

Table 11-2 Dysfunctional Labor Patterns

	Nulliparas	Multiparas
Prolonged latent phase	>21 hr	>14 hr
Protracted active phase	<1.2 cm hr	<1.5 cm hr
Secondary arrest: *no change*	>2 hr	>2 hr
Prolonged deceleration phase	>3 hr	>1 hr
Protracted descent	<1 cm hr	<2 cm hr
Arrest of descent	>1 hr	>½ hr

Table 11-3 Bishop Scoring System

Score	0	1	2	3
Station of presenting part	−3	−2	−1/0	+1/+2
Dilatation in cm	0	1-2	3-4	>5
Effacement in cm	>2.5	2	1	<0.5
Consistency	Firm	Medium	Soft	—
Position of os	Posterior	Central	Anterior	—

Precipitate delivery
Hemorrhage
Shock
Uterine rupture

Collaborative management

Therapeutic management

Baseline FHR-UC recording
Oxytocin infusion at a rate of 0.5 mU/min and increasing for desired results at 15- to 20-min intervals in increments of 1 to 2 mU/min not to exceed 20 mU/min or per institutional protocol
Continuous FHR-UC monitoring
Analgesia
Tocolytic agents for excessive uterine activity that persists following oxytocin discontinuation, after supportive treatment is provided (lateral position and oxygen by mask), and fetal distress is present; terbutaline 0.25 mg IV push or magnesium sulfate 4 g, 10% solution IV over 15 to 20 min, or nifedipine per protocol

Nursing management

PATIENT PROBLEM/NURSING DIAGNOSIS

● **NDX:** Risk for injury related to augmentation of labor and potential uterine hyperstimulation

See Care of mother in first stage of labor (p. 738)
Encourage ambulation as tolerated with maternal-fetal assessments at prescribed frequencies
Ensure that physician is immediately available
Apply fetal monitoring; obtain baseline strip before start of IV oxytocin
Place patient in position of comfort; lateral position is preferred *to prevent supine hypotension syndrome*
Always piggyback oxytocin solution into main IV line (10 U oxytocin in 1000 ml IV fluid = 10 mU/ml) or as per institutional protocol
Administer oxytocin via controlled infusion device as ordered
Monitor dose in mU/min q15min to 30min and before each increase
Increase rate of oxytocic solution as ordered to produce contractions every 2 to 3 minutes of 30- to 60-second duration
Assess BP, P, and FHR q15min to 30min or as ordered
Observe contractions for frequency, duration, strength, and relaxation before every dosage increase
Administer analgesics as ordered
Assist in breathing and relaxation techniques (p. 740)
Measure intake and output q2h
Prepare for birth as indicated

Reinforce physician's explanation of reason for augmentation or induction of labor

EXPECTED OUTCOME
Patient and fetus are not compromised as a result of oxytocin infusion

Patient/family teaching

Reinforce physician's explanations
Discuss indications for procedure
Explain administration procedure
Discuss expected effects of oxytocin induction/augmentation of labor
Explain differences between induction/augmentation and normal, spontaneous contractions

Fetal Compromise

A symptom complex indicative of a critical response to stress; may include hypoxemia/hypoxia and/or acidemia/acidosis

Assessment

Observations/findings

Fetal tachycardia: >160 beats/min
Fetal bradycardia: <120 beats/min
Meconium-stained amniotic fluid
Fetal hyperactivity or hypoactivity
Monitored fetus
  Nonreassuring FHR patterns
    Progressive increase or decrease in baseline FHR
    Tachycardia: 160 beats/min or greater; progressive decrease in baseline variability
    Severe variable deceleration; FHR <70 beats/min for longer than 30 sec with the following:
    Rising baseline FHR
    Decreasing variability
    Slow return to baseline (may be with overshoot)
    Late decelerations of any magnitude that are uncorrectable
    Absence of variability
    Prolonged deceleration
    Severe bradycardia
    Unstable FHR; sinusoidal pattern

Diagnostic tests

Electronic fetal monitoring
Amniocentesis
Cord blood studies
Fetal scalp sampling: pH <7.0

Potential complications

Fetal death
Neonatal death
CNS disorders
Meconium aspiration syndrome
Intracranial hemorrhage
Hypoxemia
Hypoxia
Acidemia
Acidosis
Asphyxia
Hypoglycemia

Collaborative management

Therapeutic management

Discontinue tocolytic therapy as applicable
Administer oxygen to patient: 10 to 12 L/min with face mask
Deliver infant as indicated
Fetal blood sampling as indicated
IV fluids as indicated
Laboratory tests as indicated
Continuous fetal evaluation until time of birth
Neonatal resuscitation required at birth

Nursing management

PATIENT PROBLEMS/NURSING DIAGNOSES

● **NDX:** Risk for injury (fetal) related to episode(s) of fetal distress

Intervene methodically; it is not necessary to proceed with subsequent steps if intervention corrects FHR pattern
Change maternal position to where FHR pattern is most improved
Correct maternal hypotension: elevate legs; increase rate of maintenance IV infusion
Discontinue oxytocin if infusing
Administer oxygen by face mask at rate of 10 to 12 L/min or as ordered
Fetal scalp or acoustic stimulation may be done *to assess FHR variability* if patient is making good progress toward vaginal delivery
Perform vaginal and/or speculum examination *to check for prolapsed cord*
Assist physician with fetal blood sampling as indicated
Prepare for birth as indicated
Explain briefly to patient the reasons for actions taken

EXPECTED OUTCOMES

Fetus has minimal compromise
Fetus/infant is delivered in good condition

● **NDX:** Anxiety/fear related to uncertain fetal outcome and unfamiliarity with care required to treat fetal compromise

Explain all interventions to mother and significant other such as the following:
　Reasons for procedure
　How procedures are to be done
　Available options
　Results expected from procedure
Simplify explanations and repeat as necessary
Provide realistic, factual information regarding fetal status
Provide information regarding availability of neonatal intensive care unit should infant require this type of care
Reassure patient that emergency equipment and experienced personnel are available for birth
Encourage patient to express concerns
Offer choices where feasible
Provide information regarding the following:
　Known possible causes of fetal compromise
　Misconceptions
Postdelivery
　Ensure that parents see newborn before transport to nursery
　Allow mother to hold and/or stroke newborn if possible

EXPECTED OUTCOME

Patient and significant other verbalize understanding of required care and are able to verbalize fears and concerns regarding newborn

Care of Mother Monitored via Electronic Fetal Monitor

Refer to Care of the mother during labor (p. 738)
The following guidelines relate to patient teaching and functioning of the monitor:
Explain that fetal status via FHR can be continuously assessed even during contractions
Explain that lower activity on strip chart shows uterine activity; upper panel shows FHR
Reassure patient and significant other that prepared childbirth techniques can be implemented without difficulty

Explain that effleurage performed during external monitoring can be done on sides of abdomen or upper thighs

Relate that breathing patterns based on timing and intensity of contractions can be enhanced by observation of uterine activity panel of strip chart for onset of contractions

Note peak of contraction; knowing that contraction will not get stronger and is half over is usually helpful

Note diminishing intensity

Coordinate with appropriate breathing and relaxation techniques

Reassure patient/significant other that use of internal mode of monitoring does not restrict patient movement

Explain that use of external mode of monitoring usually requires patient cooperation in positioning and movement

Reassure patient and significant other that use of monitor does not imply fetal jeopardy

● External Monitoring

Ultrasound transducer

Monitors FHR with high-frequency sound waves

Perform Leopold maneuvers to assess best position for transducer

Tap transducer before use to ensure sound transmission

Apply ultrasound transmission gel to maternal abdomen; clean abdomen and transducer and reapply gel q2h and prn

Massage reddened skin areas and reposition belt or adhesive device q2h and prn

Auscultate FHR with stethoscope or fetoscope if in doubt as to validity of tracing

Position and reposition transducer prn to ensure clear, interpretable FHR data

Tocotransducer

Monitors uterine activity via pressure-sensing device placed on the maternal abdomen

Position and reposition qh and prn on the fundus where least maternal tissue is in evidence

Maintain abdominal strap snugly

Adjust penset *between* contractions to print between 15 and 20 mm Hg on strip chart

Palpate fundus q30min to 60min to gauge strength of contraction; only frequency and duration of contractions can be assessed with tocotransducer

Do not assess patient's need for analgesic based on uterine activity displayed on strip chart

Massage reddened areas under transducer and belt qh and prn

● Internal Monitoring

Spiral electrode

Obtains fetal ECG from presenting part and converts it to FHR

Ensure that color-coded wires are appropriately attached to push post on leg plate

Apply electrode paste to leg plate q2h and prn

Observe FHR panel of strip chart for long- and short-term variability

Turn electrode counterclockwise to remove; never pull straight out from presenting part

Intrauterine pressure catheter

Catheter (may be fluid-filled) that internally monitors intrauterine pressure

Flush open system catheter with sterile water before insertion and prn

Ensure that black mark on catheter is visible at introitus

Maintain height of strain gauge at miduterine level

For open system catheters: turn stopcock off to patient, then with pressure valve of strain gauge released, flush strain gauge, remove syringe, and set stylus to 0 line of chart paper; test further according to manufacturer's instructions q3h to 4h and prn

For closed system catheters: set baseline rate between uterine contractions when uterus is relaxed

Assess proper functioning by tapping catheter, asking patient to cough, or applying fundal pressure; observe appropriate inflection on strip chart

Maintain catheter taped to patient's leg to prevent dislodgement

Nonstress Test

Basis for Nonstress Test (NST) is that the healthy fetus will exhibit acceleration of FHR and average FHR variability with fetal movement or in response to vibroacoustic stimulation

Assessment

Observations/findings

Accelerations of FHR

Other periodic changes in FHR

Baseline changes in FHR
Evidence of fetal movement on strip chart
  Blips
  Spikes
  Momentary increases in uterine pressure

Diagnostic tests

INTERPRETATION OF RESULTS OF NST

Reactive: two or more accelerations of FHR with an amplitude of 15 beats/min lasting 15 sec or more associated with fetal movement in a 10 min period *or* five or more FHR accelerations in a 20 min period

Nonreactive: either less than two accelerations of FHR with an amplitude below 15 beats/min or lasting less than 15 sec, *or* absence of accelerations associated with fetal movement in a 10 min period, *or* less than five FHR accelerations in a 20 min period

Suspicious: definite accelerations of FHR associated with fetal movement; however, number of accelerations or amplitude and duration do not meet criteria of reactive or nonreactive test

Unsatisfactory: quality of FHR recording is not adequate for interpretation

Potential complications

Identification of fetal compromise
Detection of uteroplacental insufficiency

Collaborative management

Therapeutic management

Begun at 32 to 34 weeks in high-risk patients
If nonreactive, proceed to VST and/or CST
If reactive, repeat 1 to 2 times per week until delivery or until nonreactive

Nursing management

Explain general use of equipment and procedure to patient and significant other
Give full liquid meal (if not taken before test) to reduce bowel sounds if ordered
Request patient to void
Assist patient with assuming semi-Fowler's position with lateral uterine tilt
Monitor FHR and uterine activity externally until test can be interpreted
Confirm fetal movement by palpation or patient confirmation
Reinforce implications of reactive and nonreactive tests

VIBROACOUSTIC STIMULATION TEST (VST)

Monitor FHR and UA until at least 10 to 15 min of interpretable data is obtained
Apply artificial larynx firmly to the maternal abdomen over the fetal head
Depress the button on the artificial larynx from 1 to 10 sec according to facility procedure
Observe the FHR strip
  Reactive test: increase in FHR of at least 15 beats/min from baseline in response to vibroacoustic stimulation
  Nonreactive test: no response of FHR to vibroacoustic stimulation; consider proceeding to contraction stress test

Contraction Stress Test

Assessment of uteroplacental reserve by means of "stressing" the fetus with contractions and observing the resultant FHR pattern

Assessment

Observations/findings

Periodic changes in FHR
  Accelerations
  Decelerations: early, late, variable
Baseline changes in FHR
  Tachycardia
  Bradycardia
  Absent or minimal variability
  Sinusoidal pattern

Interpretation of results

Negative: three contractions >40 sec duration in a 10 min period without late decelerations; there is usually a good baseline variability and acceleration of FHR with fetal movement
Positive: persistent and consistent late decelerations occurring with more than half the contractions
Hyperstimulation: contractions occurring more often than q2 min and/or lasting longer than 90 sec
  Uterine hypertonus: rise of baseline uterine tone
  Late decelerations occurring during or after excessive uterine activity
Suspicious: late decelerations occurring with less than half the uterine contractions once an adequate contraction pattern has been established
Unsatisfactory: inadequate contraction pattern or tracing too poor to interpret; test is not interpretable and cannot be used for clinical management

Potential complications

Uterine hyperstimulation
Elevated BP
Onset of labor
Supine hypotension syndrome
Clarity of strip chart tracing
Fetal compromise
Emergency birth

Collaborative management

Therapeutic management

AFTER NONREACTIVE NST

If positive CST, imminent birth
If negative CST, repeated per hospital protocol until
  birth or until CST becomes positive

PREPROCEDURAL CARE AND TEACHING

Explain general use of equipment and procedure to patient and significant other
Give full liquid meal (if not taken before test) to reduce
  bowel sounds if ordered
Request patient to void
Assist patient with assuming semi-Fowler's or lateral tilt
  position
Understand that contractions can be stimulated by dilute IV oxytocin or nipple stimulation

NIPPLE-STIMULATED CONTRACTIONS

Monitor FHR and uterine activity externally to determine baseline until at least 10 min of interpretable
  data are obtained
Assess BP and P q15min
Defer nipple stimulation if three unstimulated contractions of greater than 40 sec duration occur within a
  10 min period
Apply warm, moist washcloth to both breasts for several minutes
Instruct patient to massage and/or roll nipple of one
  breast for 10 min; if uterine contractions do not occur, stimulate both breasts for 10 min
Restimulate breasts intermittently as needed to maintain uterine contractions
If nipple stimulation does not produce desired uterine
  activity, proceed to oxytocin-stimulated contraction
  stress test

OXYTOCIN-STIMULATED CONTRACTIONS (OXYTOCIN CHALLENGE TEST; OCT)

Administer parenteral fluids with oxytocin piggybacked
  into main IV line; deliver with infusion pump in
  mU/min
Assess BP and P q15min

Monitor FHR and uterine contractions externally to determine baseline uterine activity until 10 min of interpretable data are obtained before administration of
  oxytocin
Defer oxytocin infusion if three unstimulated contractions of greater than 40 sec duration occur within a
  10 min period; interpret the results
Increase dosage of oxytocin q15min to 20min as
  ordered
Discontinue oxytocin when three uterine contractions
  of greater than 40 sec duration have occurred within a
  10 min period

POSTPROCEDURE CARE

Continue to monitor FHR and uterine contractions until
  uterine activity is diminished to pretest baseline
Interpret results of test
Teach patient signs of onset of labor; labor almost
  never begins within 48 hr if fetus is less than
  38 weeks' gestational age

EXPECTED OUTCOMES

Complications are absent or minimized
Patient complies with procedure instructions

Postpartum Care

*Care after birth of a fetus through the vaginal canal
throughout the maternal recovery period to 6 wk
after birth*

Assessment

Observations/desirable findings

Skin
  Mask of pregnancy
  Striae
Breasts
  Colostrum
  Breast milk
Abdomen
  Uterine involution
    Firm (Figure 11-15)
    Midline
    1 to 2 finger breadths (cm) below umbilicus and de-
      creasing
  Relaxed abdominal muscles
Lochia
  Color: rubra, serosa, or alba
  Flow: heavy, moderate, light, or scant
Perineum: episiotomy clean and intact (Figure 11-16)
Appropriate psychoemotional responses to child-
  birth

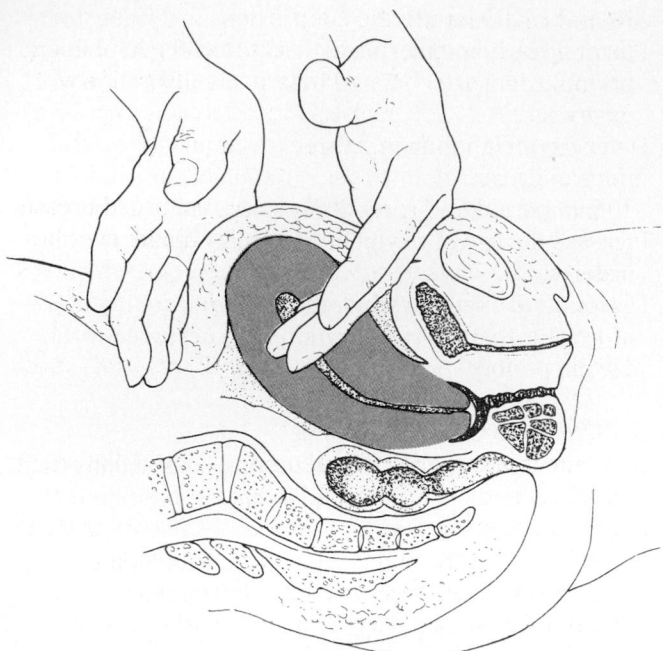

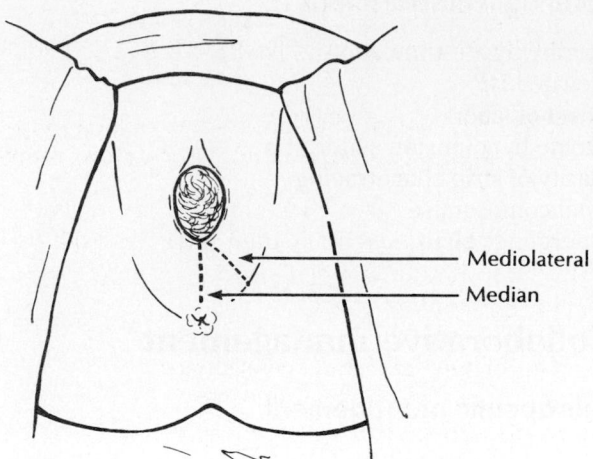

Figure 11-16 Types of episiotomies. (From Bobak IM et al: *Maternity nursing,* ed 4, St Louis, 1995, Mosby.)

Figure 11-15 Palpating fundus of uterus during first hour after delivery. Note that upper hand is cupped over fundus; lower hand dips in above symphysis pubis and supports uterus while it is massaged gently. (From Bobak IM et al: *Maternity nursing,* ed 4, St Louis, 1995, Mosby.)

Diagnostic tests

Hgb/Hct
CBC with differential if indicated
Electrolytes if indicated

Potential complications

Hemorrhage; soft, relaxed fundus
  Retained placental fragments
  Hematoma of episiotomy site
Infection
  Elevated temperature
  Diaphoresis
  Chilling
  Nausea, vomiting
  Tachycardia
  Foul odor of lochia
  After pains
  Drainage from episiotomy
  Edema, redness, or discoloration at incisions or
    lacerations
  Gaping sutures at incisions or lacerations
Bladder distention and/or inability to void
Painful hemorrhoids
Constipation
Thrombophlebitis

Pulmonary embolus
Engorged breasts; sore nipples
Behavioral changes
  Depression
  Withdrawal
  Lack of contact with, or care of, newborn
  Newborn abuse
  Newborn neglect

Collaborative management

Therapeutic management

Postpartum assessment with vital signs
Neurologic checks and spinal dermatomes check,
  along with vital signs, if regional anesthesia is
  received
IV fluids
Oxytocics as indicated
Pain medications, stool softeners, antiflatulents as indi-
  cated
Breast binder if indicated
Lactation suppression drugs
Ice bag to perineum as indicated
Topical anesthetic to episiotomy as needed
Anesthetic ointment for hemorrhoids
Foley catheter if indicated
Progressive ambulation as tolerated
Laboratory tests as indicated
Regular diet as tolerated; encourage oral fluid and
  snacks
Intake and output as indicated
Anti-Rh globulin as indicated
Rubella vaccine as indicated

Nursing management

PATIENT PROBLEMS/NURSING DIAGNOSES

● **NDX:** Risk for fluid volume deficit related to active loss associated with postpartum hemorrhage

Assess the following q15min until stable then q4h to 8 hr per institution policy
  Fundus location and tone
  Episiotomy condition
  Lochia amount, color, and consistency
  Temperature, pulse, blood pressure
  Level of consciousness
If fundus is soft and/or relaxed, massage until firm *to prevent excessive blood loss*
Teach mother normal parameters of lochia and instruct her to call provider if there is abnormally heavy flow
Change perineal pads q30min to 60min and/or as needed; report excessive bleeding to provider
Avoid unnecessary massage of fundus, *which can cause uterine relaxation and hemorrhage*
Maintain parenteral fluids with oxytocics *to contract uterus,* as ordered
Encourage fluids po unless contraindicated
Measure intake and output for 24 hr or as ordered
Remain with patient during the first time out of bed *in case hemodynamic changes or orthostatic hypotension results in dizziness/faintness*

EXPECTED OUTCOME

Patient does not become hypovolemic as a result of excessive blood loss; has vital signs that are within normal limits

● **NDX:** Pain related to episiotomy, afterbirth pains, and/or breast discomfort

Note time when sensation has returned to lower extremities after spinal anesthetic
Manage pain; administer medication as ordered
Apply ice bag to perineum as ordered *to reduce swelling and sensation of pain*
Maintain warmth with blankets; avoid drafts in patient care unit
Use sitz bath tid and prn if ordered
Administer anesthetic spray to episiotomy and hemorrhoids prn *to reduce discomfort*
Apply anesthetic ointment to hemorrhoids prn
Shower or bathe daily; avoid washing nipples of breast-feeding mothers at any other time *because it removes natural oils and contributes to skin irritation and discomfort*
Have mother wear supportive bra at all times *to reduce discomfort of heavy breasts*

Assess breasts q4h to 8h and prn
If breast-feeding, place warm, moist towel packs on engorged breasts for 15 to 30 min q1h to 3h *to stimulate let-down reflex,* then massage and manually express breasts or have infant nurse
If formula feeding
  Never massage or manually express engorged breasts
  Have mother wear snug-fitting breast binder over bra and use ice bags q1h to 3h for 15 min on each side if breasts are engorged *to reduce circulation and subsequent engorgement*
  Stand with back toward water in shower *to avoid stimulation of breasts*
Anticipate need for pain relief
Administer pain medication as ordered and document effectiveness
Instruct mother to squeeze buttocks together when sitting down if episiotomy is painful with ambulation
Encourage mother to use relaxation techniques learned in labor for afterbirth pains during breast-feeding

EXPECTED OUTCOMES

Pain is relieved or minimized
Uterine fundus is firm and pain free
Patient is able to demonstrate proper breast care

● **NDX:** Risk for infection related to incision and/or lacerations

Instruct patient on perineal care per hospital policy
Change perineal pad from front to back after each elimination *to prevent urethral contamination*
Observe condition of episiotomy and document same q8h to 12h
Watch for elevated temperature or other changes in vital sign parameters
Note and report any abnormal, foul-smelling drainage or discharge, *which is indicative of an infectious process*
Administer antibiotics as ordered

EXPECTED OUTCOME

Patient's episiotomy and/or lacerations heal without infection as evidenced by absence of edema and drainage

● **NDX:** Urinary retention (potential) related to trauma and subsequent edema associated with childbirth process

Avoid distention of bladder; encourage voiding within 6 to 8 hr after delivery or catheterize as ordered
Encourage daily fluids to 3000 ml unless contraindicated

Encourage patient to void q4h to 6h as able

Employ techniques *to assist voiding as needed,* including voiding in sitz bath if this is the only way the patient can comfortably void

EXPECTED OUTCOMES

Patient does not experience bladder distention; voids q.s. following birth

● **NDX:** Constipation related to pain of episiotomy and hemorrhoids secondary to childbirth process

Ensure adequate fluid intake

Sitz bath may help *to relax perianal muscles before bowel movement*

Give stool softeners or laxative as ordered

Encourage patient to ambulate as tolerated, increasing progressively

Maintain regular diet with between-meal snacks; increase amount of fruit and roughage

Anesthetic spray/ointment applied to perianal area and episiotomy site may *provide pain relief and subsequently permit bowel movement*

EXPECTED OUTCOME

Patient has bowel movement with minimal discomfort

● **NDX:** Risk for altered parenting related to transition to parenthood and role change

Recover mother and newborn in same bed under radiant heat warmer if possible *to promote visual inspection, skin to skin contact, and attachment*

Assist with holding and inspecting newborn as soon as possible and before 6 hr after birth and prn until mother is able to become actively involved in newborn care

Encourage mother to have newborn at bedside as much as she desires *to promote attachment behaviors*

Meet mother's dependency needs during "taking in" phase

Encourage verbalization; mothers are usually extremely talkative, repeatedly relating experience of labor and birth

Understand that enthusiastic listening by nurse helps experience become more meaningful to parents

Meet mother's needs during "taking hold" phase

Reassure mother that she is performing well in all aspects of self-care and newborn care

Avoid intervening between mother and newborn regardless of how awkward her skills seem

Positively reinforce all tasks done well

Avoid negative criticism at all times, unless solicited by parent

Assist and teach mother to perform all newborn care tasks: (e.g., bathing, feeding, diapering, cord care, cuddling)

Teach mother and visitors proper handwashing technique

Involve spouse or significant other in newborn care and teaching

Observe mother-newborn interaction; report to physician

Mother not holding newborn while feeding

Lack of eye contact between mother and newborn

Absence of verbalization of mother to newborn

Lack of physical contact with newborn

Encourage verbalization about role of mothering, effect of new family member, and sibling rivalry, if applicable

Encourage visits by healthy siblings unless contraindicated

See Care of newborn (p. 761)

EXPECTED OUTCOMES

Demonstrates adequate newborn caretaking skills

Provides an optimal environment for newborn growth and development

● **NDX:** Situational low self-esteem in response to feelings of inadequacy associated with responsibilities of parenthood related to birth experience

Encourage discussion of real and perceived problems

Help mother validate the reality of her labor and birth experience

Give reassurance concerning her ability *to promote self-perception of adequacy and competency as a mother*

Help patient accept emotional ups and downs of postpartum period and explain that these feelings and changes are common during this time

Encourage rest periods throughout the day *to prevent sleep deprivation*

Provide opportunity for parent/infant interactions and involve father or significant other as possible

Support and encourage parents and/or significant other in interactions and caring for newborn

EXPECTED OUTCOME

Mother demonstrates effective emotional adjustment and healthy self-esteem as evidenced by positive statements about self and abilities to care for infant

Patient/family teaching

Caution patient to avoid coitus or douching for 4 to 6 wk or as indicated

Demonstrate breast care and manual expression if mother is breast-feeding

Emphasize importance of nutritious diet
Explain need to carefully clean perineal region
  Wipe from front to back after urinating
  Administer perineal self-care
  Apply perineal pad from front to back
  Wash vulva and perineum, including sutures, before
    washing anal area when showering
Relate that absorbable sutures do not need to be
  removed
Instruct patient to use anesthetic spray and/or oint-
  ment to treat perineal area and/or hemorrhoids
Caution patient to avoid constipation; stool softeners or
  mild laxatives may be necessary
Discuss symptoms to report to provider
  T >100°F (37.8°C)
  Foul odor of lochia
Relate that shower or tub bath may be taken
Explain that lochia may continue for 3 to 4 wk, chang-
  ing from red to brown to white
Relate that menses will return 6 to 8 wk after birth
  often despite breast-feeding
  Explain that some nursing mothers do not menstruate
    until they wean infant from breast, whereas others
    resume menstruation at various times while nursing
  Emphasize that pregnancy is possible 4 to 6 wk after
    birth, whether mother is breast-feeding or not;
    discuss availability of nonprescription methods of
    contraception

Home care considerations

Caution patient to avoid lifting anything heavier than
  the infant for 2 to 3 wk
Explain need for planned rest periods
Relate that sitz bath and perineal light may be used at
  home prn
Explain need for mild exercise initially
  Do not start vigorous exercise until approved by
    provider
  Explain that Kegel exercises can be begun during
    early puerperium
Discuss normalcy of postpartum depression
Discuss need to plan for care of other children at home
  and discuss possible behavioral changes necessary
  because of new family member
Teach name of medication, dosage, time of administra-
  tion, purpose, and side effects
Emphasize importance of ongoing outpatient care in-
  cluding postpartum checkup
Emphasize the normalcy of feelings that may be
  disturbing
  Initial lack of feeling of love for infant
  Variations from prenatal expectations of what infant
    would look like; disappointment in sex, weight, or
    appearance

Frustration caused by increased demands on
  time
Feelings of being trapped
Unsettled feelings about being a mother and
  parent
Feelings of tension, nervousness, and fatigue
Discuss how to contact available community
  resources
  Housekeeping agencies
  Nursing care agencies
  Diaper services
  Family planning organizations
  Breast-feeding organizations: La Leche League*
  Parenting groups
  Publications on infant care
    Growth and development
    Parenting
    Health care
    Infant stimulation
Discuss proper principles and practice of infant care

Cesarean Birth

*Birth of a fetus through a uterine incision; most com-
mon is the transverse lower segment incision, with
the classic vertical cesarean incision done less
frequently*

Assessment

Observations/findings

  INDICATIONS
CPD in current pregnancy
Fetal compromise
Failure to progress in labor/dystocia
Malposition of fetus
  Breech presentation
  Transverse lie
  Abnormal vertex presentation
Umbilical cord prolapse
Abruptio placentae
Placenta previa

Preoperative/diagnostic tests

Fetal monitoring for fetal well-being
ECG monitoring
CBC with differential
Electrolytes

*La Leche League International, 9616 Minneapolis Ave, Franklin
Park, IL 60131.

Hgb/Hct
Type and cross match for blood
Urinalysis
Amniocentesis for fetal lung maturity as indicated
X-ray examination as indicated
Ultrasound as ordered

Potential complications

Hemorrhage; soft, relaxed uterine fundus
Shock
Anemia
DIC
Infection
  Elevated temperature
  Tachycardia
  Foul odor of lochia
Site of incision
  Redness
  Pain
  Swelling
  Drainage
Cystitis
Engorged breasts
Pneumonia
Paralytic ileus
Thrombophlebitis
Pulmonary embolus
Behavioral changes
  Guilt
  Depression
  Withdrawal
  Lack of contact with or care of newborn
Anesthesia reaction: malignant hyperthermia
Fetal injury during surgery
Fetal blood loss during surgery
Neonatal depression/resuscitation at birth

Collaborative management

Therapeutic management

IV fluids as indicated
Anesthesia: regional or general
Agreement of significant other to attend cesarean
  birth
Diagnostic tests as indicated
Oxytocic administration as indicated after birth
Vital signs per recovery room protocol
Abdominal surgery skin preparation
Foley catheter insertion
See Postpartum care (p. 749) for routine medical man-
  agement

Nursing management

PATIENT PROBLEMS/NURSING DIAGNOSES

● **NDX:** Knowledge deficit related to lack of information about procedure and precesarean delivery care

Discuss with mother and significant other the reason
  for cesarean birth
Explain "normal" preoperative procedures and potential
  variations for current situation
Witness consent form and obtain baseline vital signs
Draw blood for CBC, electrolytes, type, and screen
Obtain urine for urinalysis
Insert Foley catheter
Maintain NPO status
Perform abdominal surgery preparation per hospital
  policy and aseptic technique principles and explain to
  patient/family
Administer IV fluids as ordered
Remove contact lenses and jewelry
Discuss presence of significant other in operating room
  as appropriate
Encourage parents to attend preparatory classes
  specifically for cesarean birth if cesarean is
  elective
Inform father that immediately postdelivery, he may
  hold infant close to mother's face and arms unless
  contraindicated

EXPECTED OUTCOME

Patient verbalizes rationale for cesarean birth and cooperates with presurgical preparations

● **NDX:** Pain related to postoperative condition

Anticipate need for pain medications and/or additional
  methods of pain relief
Note, document, and identify the following:
  Reports of pain at incisional site: abdomen
  Facial grimace of pain
  Decreasing mobility
  Relief/distraction behavior
  Pain scale score
Administer pain medication as ordered, preferably via
  patient controlled analgesia pump, and evaluate its ef-
  fectiveness
Monitor effectiveness of epidural if used
Provide other comfort measures that may be
  helpful such as repositioning or supporting with
  pillows

EXPECTED OUTCOME

Pain is minimized/controlled and patient verbalizes
  that she is comfortable

● **NDX:** Altered tissue perfusion: cardiopulmonary, peripheral related to interruption of flow secondary to postoperative immobility

Assess respiratory status with vital signs
Document and report increased respiratory rate, nonproductive cough, audible rhonchi, rales, or upper airway congestion
Note symptoms of pulmonary embolus
  Restlessness
  Chest pain
  Diaphoresis
  Dyspnea
  Tachycardia
  Change in BP
  Abnormal breath sounds
Encourage patient to cough, turn, and deep breathe q2h during first postoperative day, then prn
Demonstrate splinting *to support incision*
Encourage use of incentive spirometer
Encourage early ambulation *to promote peripheral circulation*
Discuss elevating feet prn and not crossing legs *to avoid constricting circulation*
Check Homan's sign with vital signs: *pain in calf associated with dorsiflexion is indicative of thrombophlebitis*
Note symptoms of deep vein thrombosis formation
  Localized tenderness
  Calf pain
  Redness
  Swelling
  Elevated temperature
  Positive Homan's sign

   EXPECTED OUTCOMES
Patient does not have respiratory congestion
Shows no signs or symptoms of pulmonary embolism or deep vein thrombosis during hospitalization

● **NDX:** Altered urinary elimination (postremoval of Foley catheter) and/or constipation related to manipulation or trauma secondary to cesarean birth

Encourage voiding q4h to 6h if possible
Employ techniques to encourage voiding as needed
Explain perineal care procedures per hospital policy
Palpate lower abdomen if patient reports bladder distention and inability to void *to assess for urinary retention*
Encourage mother to do the following:
  Ambulate as tolerated
  Increase intake of fluids (2000 to 3000 ml/day)
  Increase fruit and roughage in diet
Give stool softener/laxative as ordered *to prevent constipation*

Administer antiflatulents as ordered *to reduce discomfort associated with flatus*
Monitor intake and output until eliminating adequately

   EXPECTED OUTCOMES
Voids spontaneously without discomfort
Has a bowel movement within 3 to 4 days after surgery

● **NDX:** Situational low self-esteem in response to feelings of inadequacy associated with unanticipated cesarean birth and interruption of anticipated childbirth experience

Encourage mother to verbalize fears and feelings of guilt and/or blame
  Sense of failure at not giving birth "normally"
  Feelings of being cheated or disappointed
  Feelings of intrusion caused by surgical procedure
Provide support through reassurance and open communication *to promote feelings of adequacy and competence in self-care and newborn care*
Include significant other in discussions
Provide positive feedback to mother and significant other

   EXPECTED OUTCOMES
Verbalizes feelings of self-worth
Demonstrates appropriate coping skills

● **NDX:** Risk for infection or injury related to surgical procedure

Monitor for elevated temperature or tachycardia as signs of infection
Observe incision *to identify signs of infection*
  Redness
  Tenderness
  Swelling at incision site
  Reports of pain
  Unusual discharge
  Elevated temperature
Change dressing prn or ordered *to inspect incision and observe for symptoms of infection*
Assess fundus, lochia, and bladder and vital signs as ordered
Evaluate vital signs for symptoms of infection (fever and tachycardia) or hemorrhage q4h and prn
Massage fundus if boggy or does not remain firm
Notify provider of deviations from normal parameters
  Boggy, displaced uterus
  Uterine tenderness at palpation
  Persistent discharge of lochia rubra
  Profuse bleeding
  Foul-smelling lochia

EXPECTED OUTCOMES

Patient's incision is clean and dry, without any signs or symptoms of infection

Uterine involution progresses normally

Patient/family teaching

Discuss the following with mother and significant other during the postpartum period

Need to avoid coitus or douching for 4 to 6 wk or as indicated by physician

Breast care and manual expression if breast-feeding

Need to avoid sitting with knees bent for long periods

Care of incision

Symptoms of wound infection to report to provider

Importance of nutritious diet

Need to avoid constipation; stool softeners or mild laxatives may be necessary

Lochia may continue for 3 to 4 wk, changing from red to brown to white

Menses will return 6 to 8 wk after birth unless breast-feeding

Explain that some nursing mothers do not menstruate until weaning infant from breast

Explain that others resume menstruation at various times while nursing

Explain that pregnancy is possible whether mother is breast-feeding or not, 4 to 6 wk after birth

Discuss availability of nonprescription methods of contraception

Name of medication, dosage, time of administration, purpose, and side effects

Importance of follow-up outpatient care including postpartum checkup

Home care considerations

Advise patient to avoid lifting anything heavier than infant for 4 to 6 wk

Encourage planned rest periods

Advise patient that showers may be taken

Explain importance of exercise, need to avoid vigorous exercise until approved by provider

Discuss normalcy of postpartum depression

Advise about need to plan for care of other children at home and discuss possible behavioral changes necessary as a result of new family member

Discuss normalcy of feelings that may be disturbing to mother

Initial lack of feeling of love for newborn

Variations from prenatal expectations of what newborn would look like: disappointment in sex, weight, or appearance

Frustration resulting from increased demands on time

Feelings of being trapped

Unsettled feelings about being a mother and parent

Feelings of tension, nervousness, and fatigue

Instruct patient on how to contact available community resources

Housekeeping agencies

Nursing care agencies

Diaper services

Family planning organizations

Breast-feeding organizations: La Leche League, lactation institutes

Cesarean birth groups (such as C/Sec. Inc.)

Parenting groups

Publications on infant care

Growth and development

Parenting

Health care

Infant stimulation

See Care of newborn (p. 761)

Home care considerations for breast-feeding

Discuss, demonstrate, and return-demonstrate breast-feeding principles related to cesarean birth as follows

If desired, breast-feeding is possible

Feed only breast milk to newborn

Do not supplement with formula or water routinely (see Breast-feeding below)

Take pain medication 20 to 30 min before nursing

Proper positioning prevents and relieves discomfort (Figure 11-17)

Instruct mother to do the following:

When lying on either side

Put newborn on side facing you

Pull newborn's buttocks toward abdomen

Use pillows to support the back and protect abdomen

When sitting up in bed

Use pillows under both knees to support them

Place a pillow under each arm and another over abdomen

Put newborn on side toward you in "crook" of your arm, with newborn's face and belly facing toward the mother

Breast-Feeding

Assessment

Observations/findings

Breasts

Hardness

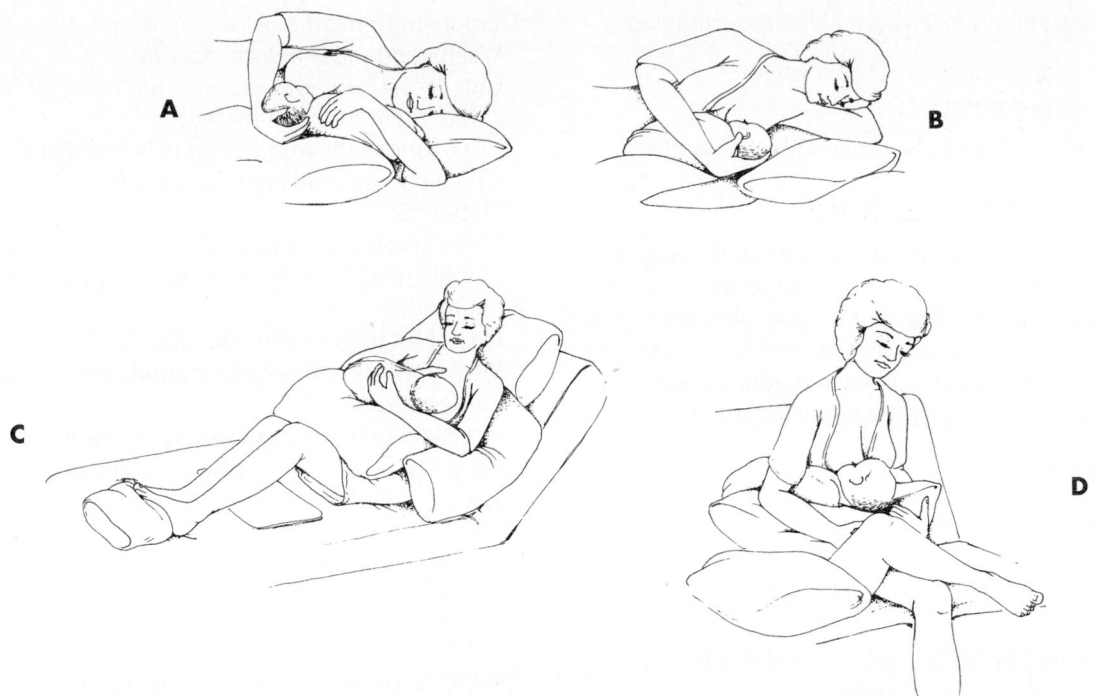

Figure 11-17 Comfortable breast-feeding positions after cesarean delivery. **A** and **B,** Side-lying position. **C,** Sitting in bed. **D,** "Football" hold.

Tenderness
Pain
Redness
Condition of nipples
Dehydration
Newborn
  Nursing more frequently than q2h
  Voiding less than six times daily

Potential complications

Engorgement
Nipple problems
  Blistered, cracked nipples
  Inverted nipples
  Sore nipples
Mastitis
Nipple confusion of newborn

Collaborative management

Therapeutic management

Antibiotics for mastitis as indicated
Referral to lactation specialist/consultant
Increase of caloric intake by 500 calories/day
Increase of fluid intake to 3000 ml/day unless contraindicated
Contraception counseling
Family planning counseling referrals as indicated

Nursing management

PATIENT PROBLEMS/NURSING DIAGNOSES

● **NDX:** Risk for fluid volume deficit in newborn related to inadequate breast-feeding

Instruct mother to do the following:
  Feed newborn when hungry
  Begin feeding newborn on one side for 10 to 30 min or until newborn begins to slow down
  Break suction of newborn's mouth on nipple by placing finger inside mouth between gums
  Avoid pulling newborn off breast without releasing suction
  Burp newborn in a sitting position after nursing at each breast
  Place newborn on opposite breast for 10 to 30 min or until newborn begins to slow down
  Change back to other breast again until newborn seems satisfied and falls asleep
  Replace nursing bra after nursing is completed *to support breasts*
Remind mother that during newborn period total feeding time can range from 20 to 60 min each
Remind mother that best way to tell if newborn is getting enough milk is to listen for swallowing while sucking
Explain that adequate intake and nutrition is judged by six to eight wet diapers per day, newborn sleeping 1 to 2 hr between feedings, and newborn gaining weight

by time of examination with first visit to health care provider

EXPECTED OUTCOME

Newborn receives adequate intake for appropriate weight gain

● **NDX:** Ineffective breast-feeding related to any one of multiple factors including previous history of breast-feeding failure, poor newborn suck reflex, nonsupportive partner, interruption in breast-feeding, and lack of information about appropriate breast-feeding technique

Initiate breast-feeding as soon as mother and newborn are in good condition (may be on delivery table); manually express both breasts q4h until infant can be nursed

See Figures 11-18 and 11-19 for proper body and nipple positioning

Remain with mother for at least her first two breast-feeding experiences if necessary

Have mother assume most comfortable position for her; may be sitting or lying on side

Alternate breast that is used first at each feeding: place safety pin on bra as reminder

Apply small amount of hydrous lanolin to nipples *to prevent dryness and cracking as ordered;* it does not need to be washed off before next feeding

Have mother shower daily for breast and general cleanliness

Do not wash breasts with any solution except water *to avoid removing protective oils from breasts before each feeding*

Avoid using nipple shield; if necessary, use only long enough to draw nipple out *so that infant may grasp and suckle*

Demonstrate hand expression of milk (Figure 11-20)

Wash hands well before starting

Cup breast with either hand (left hand for left breast, right hand for right breast)

Place thumb above and fingers below nipple, 1 to 1½ inches behind nipple on areola (forming the letter "C")

Press in toward back, then roll fingers down toward nipple, while gently pressing thumb and finger together

Do not let fingers slide on skin

Move fingers completely around areola *to reach all milk sinuses*

Alternate between breasts every few minutes

Instruct patient in appropriate techniques and relate information *to promote a successful breast-feeding experience*

Refer to specific instructions in next section

EXPECTED OUTCOMES

Patient demonstrates appropriate breast-feeding skills with minimal discomfort

Expresses satisfaction with the breast-feeding experience

Patient/family teaching

Discuss and assist mother with the following:

Breast-feeding reflex: "let-down" reflex

Handwashing before breast-feeding

Body position (see Figure 11-18)

Nipple position (see Figure 11-19)

Inversion of nipples as indicated

Explain that supply of milk is related to demand

Giving formula only decreases milk supply

No need to supplement

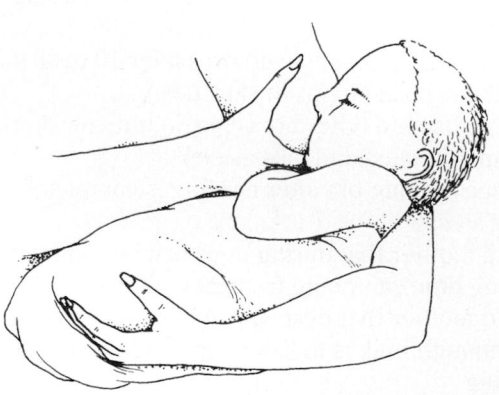

Figure 11-18   Correct body position for breast-feeding. Head of infant is in crook of mother's arm with front of infant facing front of mother.

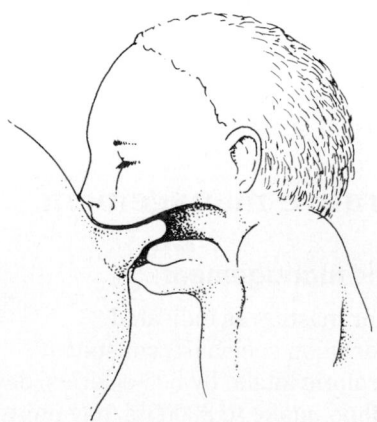

Figure 11-19   Correct latch-on position. Infant's mouth compresses milk-collecting sinuses in areola.

Need for feeding often is on demand (often up to q1½h to 2h; later about q3h; breast-fed newborns usually eat q3h)

Emphasize importance of drinking at least six to eight glasses of liquid each day (water, juice, and milk) and eating a balanced diet including meat, milk, vegetables and fruits, grains and cereals

Relate that milk can be expressed into clean glass containers or into plastic disposable bottle liners

Explain that mother's fluid intake should be a minimum of 3000 ml/day unless contraindicated; a full 8 oz glass of fluid before each nursing session will help ensure adequate maternal hydration

Discuss adjustment of dietary intake to meet infant's needs

Eat well-balanced, high-protein diet

Avoid foods that cause newborn distress (colicky, crying, wakeful); do not arbitrarily omit foods usually eaten

Explain that breast milk normally has a thin, watery appearance

Explain that milk supply will be adequate if newborn nurses regularly; the more nurses, the more milk is produced

Explain that six wet diapers daily of pale-colored urine is indicative that newborn is properly hydrated

Explain that four to six bowel movements daily is normal in breast-fed newborn

Explain that it may be necessary to keep newborn awake during feedings by unwrapping blanket and gently rubbing back or feet

Tell patient not to give prepared formula routinely

Explain that for several days after birth it is normal to experience uterine cramping while nursing

Explain that milk flowing from opposite breast while nursing is normal

Caution patient to avoid plastic-coated breast shields in bra between feedings; a clean, ironed handker-chief or Woolwich shield from La Leche League is preferred

Discuss treatment for engorged breasts

Place very warm towel packs on breasts for 15 min

Massage from outer breast to areola

Manually express milk or nurse newborn

Caution patient that a breast-feeding woman can become pregnant and should be aware of contraceptive methods other than oral contraceptives, which are usually contraindicated for at least the first 3 months after giving birth

Relate that breast milk normally leaks during coitus

Discuss symptoms of complications to be reported to health care provider

Home care considerations

Advise patient to limit visitors and household duties for the first month postpartum

Suggest that patient have relatives or friends assist with household chores, shopping, and meals prn

Explain need for planned rest periods and napping when able

Discuss how to contact local breast-feeding organizations for further information while at home

La Leche League

Lactation Institute

Lactation specialists/consultants in private practice

Breast-feeding clinics

Postpartum Hemorrhage

Maternal postdelivery blood loss resulting from uterine atony, lacerations, and/or retained products of

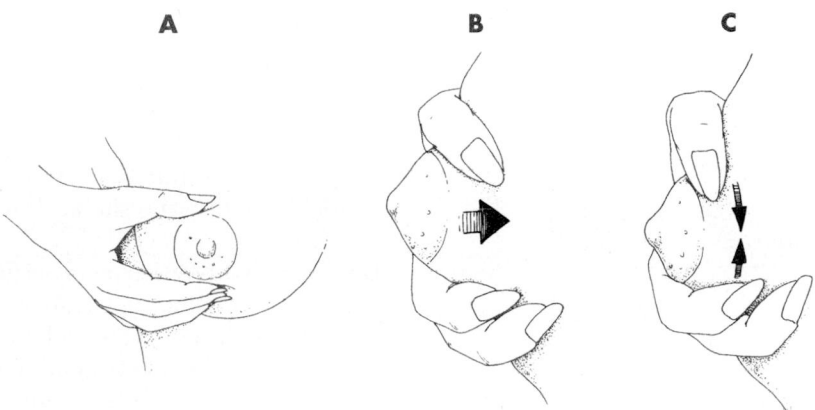

A   **B**   **C**

Figure 11-20   Hand expression of breast milk. **A,** Place thumb and fingers about 1 to 1½ inches behind nipple, forming *C* shape. **B,** Press in toward body. **C,** Firmly press fingers together on lacteal sinuses to express milk.

conception; predisposing factors include overdistended uterus (macrosomic baby, multiple gestation, hydramnios), unusually short (≤4 hours) or prolonged labor, preeclampsia (PIH) treated with magnesium sulfate, chorioamnionitis

Assessment

Observations/findings

Uterine atony
  Relaxed fundus
  Dark bleeding
  Boggy, distended uterus
  Expulsion of clots
Genital lacerations
  Constant trickle of bright red blood
  Firm fundus
Retained placental tissue
  Dark bleeding
  Boggy, distended uterus
  Abdominal pain
Hematoma
  Bruising
  Edema
  Pain
Tachycardia
Progressive hypotension

Diagnostic tests

Vaginal examination
Clotting studies
Hgb and Hct
CVP monitoring

Potential complications

Shock
  Pallor
  Restlessness
  Weak, rapid pulse
  Decreased BP
  Chills
  Difficulty in breathing
  Air hunger
See Hypovolemic shock (p. 151)
DIC
Postpartum infection
Anemia
Transfusion hepatitis
Hysterectomy (for placenta accreta)

Collaborative management

Therapeutic management

Dilation and curettage (D & C) as indicated
Repair of lacerations
Manual removal of placental fragments
Insertion of uterine packing as indicated
IV fluids, volume expanders, or blood products
NPO
Strict intake and output
VS as indicated
Antiembolic stockings as indicated
Oxygen therapy as indicated
Medications as indicated (prostaglandin, iron
  therapy)
Oxytocin infusion as indicated
Prostin E2 (PG E2) vaginal suppository as indicated
Vaginal packing as indicated

Nursing management

PATIENT PROBLEMS/NURSING DIAGNOSES

● **NDX:** Fluid volume deficit related to hypovolemia associated with postpartum hemorrhage

Never leave patient unattended during active bleeding
Massage relaxed, boggy fundus until firm; *do not over-massage or push hard on a relaxed fundus*
Administer oxygen at 10 to 12 L/min if ordered
Administer parenteral fluids with oxytocics as ordered
  Example: oxytocin 20 to 30 units in 1 L solution infused at rate of 200 ml/hr (DO NOT administer an undiluted IV bolus of oxytocin)
Administer volume expanders or blood as ordered
Assess BP, P, and R q15min until stable, then as ordered
Palpate fundus and observe amount of vaginal bleeding q15min until stable
Measure intake and output
Weigh pads and linens *to estimate blood loss* (1 ml = 1 g)
Apply antiembolic stockings to legs *to enhance venous return*
Maintain warmth with blankets
Allay anxiety as much as possible by remaining with patient and offering simple, brief explanations of care
Be aware that physician may order prostaglandin IM (or PG E2 vaginal suppository) *to control atony*
Continue with acute care and decrease frequency of nursing functions as patient's condition improves
Observe for side effects of iron therapy if ordered

Reinforce primary health care provider's explanation of
the following, if done
Vaginal examination
Insertion of uterine packing
D & C

EXPECTED OUTCOMES

Patient receives adequate fluid replacement with no untoward effects
Does not have symptoms of hemorrhagic/hypovolemic
shock

● **NDX:** Pain and discomfort related to uterine massage and uterine contraction

Explain purpose of frequent postpartum assessments
Palpation of fundus for height, position, and tone
Uterine massage if necessary
Lochia flow
Encourage patient to palpate fundus and learn what
firm uterine tone feels like
Encourage patient to check fundus periodically and
massage prn
Apply ice pack to perineum as needed *to reduce pain,
swelling*
Promote comfort by position changes
Provide emotional support, especially if pain medica-
tion is contraindicated
Administer medications as ordered by primary health
care provider and check for any reactions
Minimize other factors that could be contributing to
discomfort such as distended bladder, episiotomy
pain, or "afterbirth" pain

EXPECTED OUTCOMES

Verbalizes symptoms to report
Demonstrates self-care as taught

Patient/family teaching

Discuss symptoms to report to primary health care
provider
Passage of large or several clots
Large amount of bleeding: more than a menstrual
period
Pain
Foul odor of vaginal drainage
See Postpartum care (p. 749)
Teach name of medication, dosage, time of administra-
tion, purpose, and side effects

Newborn

● Care of Newborn

Assessment
Observations/findings

GENERAL

Apgar scores
Quality of cry and respirations
Skin color
Apical P and heart rate
Respiratory rate
Muscle tone
Reflexes
Thermal control
Cord condition
Feeding and sucking pattern
Stool pattern
Voiding pattern
Congenital defects

SPECIFIC

Apgar scores
Heart rate; presence of murmur
Respiratory effort
Muscle tone
Reflex irritability
Color
Abnormalities or malformations
Head circumference: normal 33 to 35 cm
Chest circumference: normal 30 to 33 cm
Birth-related trauma: presence of caput, cephalo-
hematoma, and forceps marks
Amount of subcutaneous fat
Cry
Lusty
Feeble
High pitched
Absent
Asymmetrical facies
Umbilical cord
Drainage
Bleeding
Number and type of vessels
Presence or absence of Wharton's jelly
Unusually high or low temperature: normal, 97.7°F
(36.5°C) axillary
Edema (except for presenting part)
Color
Pink
Jaundice
Pallor

Gray, dusky
Cyanosis
Plethora
GI system
  Hard and soft palate intact
  Refusal to feed
  Excessive mucus
  Regurgitation; vomiting
  Abdominal distention
  Imperforate anus
  Stools
    Meconium
    Bloody
    Diarrhea
    Absent
Neurologic system
  Moro's reflex: present, absent, asymmetrical, or
    hyperactive
  Sucking reflex: strong or weak
  Rooting reflex: good or poor
  Reflexes: grasp (palmar and plantar), tonic neck, step-
    ping and Babinski
  Suck/swallow coordination
  Tremors
  Twitching
  Seizure activity
  Loss of motion of an extremity
State of consciousness
  Deep sleep
  Active REM sleep
  Drowsy
  Wide awake (quiet alert)
  Active awake (active alert)
  Crying
Respiratory rate: normal 40 to 60/min
  Tachypnea
  Shallow or periodic breathing
  Nasal flaring
  Retractions
  Expiratory grunt
Cardiovascular rate: normal 120 to 160 beats/min
  Tachycardia
  Bradycardia
  BP: normal 60/30 to 90/50 mm Hg
Musculoskeletal system
  Muscle tone
  Muscle strength
  Limpness
  Weakness
  Rigidity
  Asymmetry
  Swelling of skull or spine
  Abnormal position or posture of extremity
Skin
  Milia

Birthmarks
Pustules
Abrasions
Rash
Petechiae
Ecchymosis
Condition of circumcision
Genitourinary system
  Hypospadias
  Epispadias
  Undescended testicles
  Indeterminate sex
  Failure to void

Diagnostic tests

Cord blood samples
Phenylketonuria (PKU; newborn screening examination)
Hct; thyroid studies (T_3, T_4)
Bilirubin

Potential complications

Altered thermoregulation
Birth injuries
Hyperbilirubinemia
Congenital defects
Need for resuscitation at birth

Collaborative management

Therapeutic management

Vitamin K IM injection
Newborn screening examination (PKU, thyroid)
Hepatitis B vaccine
Eye prophylaxis
Feeding schedule
Cord care protocol
Circumcision care
Chemstrip as indicated
Hct
Daily weights
Rectal temperature once, then axillary temperature per
  protocol

Nursing management

POSTBIRTH NURSING PROCEDURES
Perform stabilization procedures (Figure 11-21)
Take Apgar scores at 1, 5, and 10 min after birth
Apply clamp to umbilical cord
Identify newborn according to facility policy: bracelet,
  necklace, and/or footprints
Perform screening examination for congenital defects

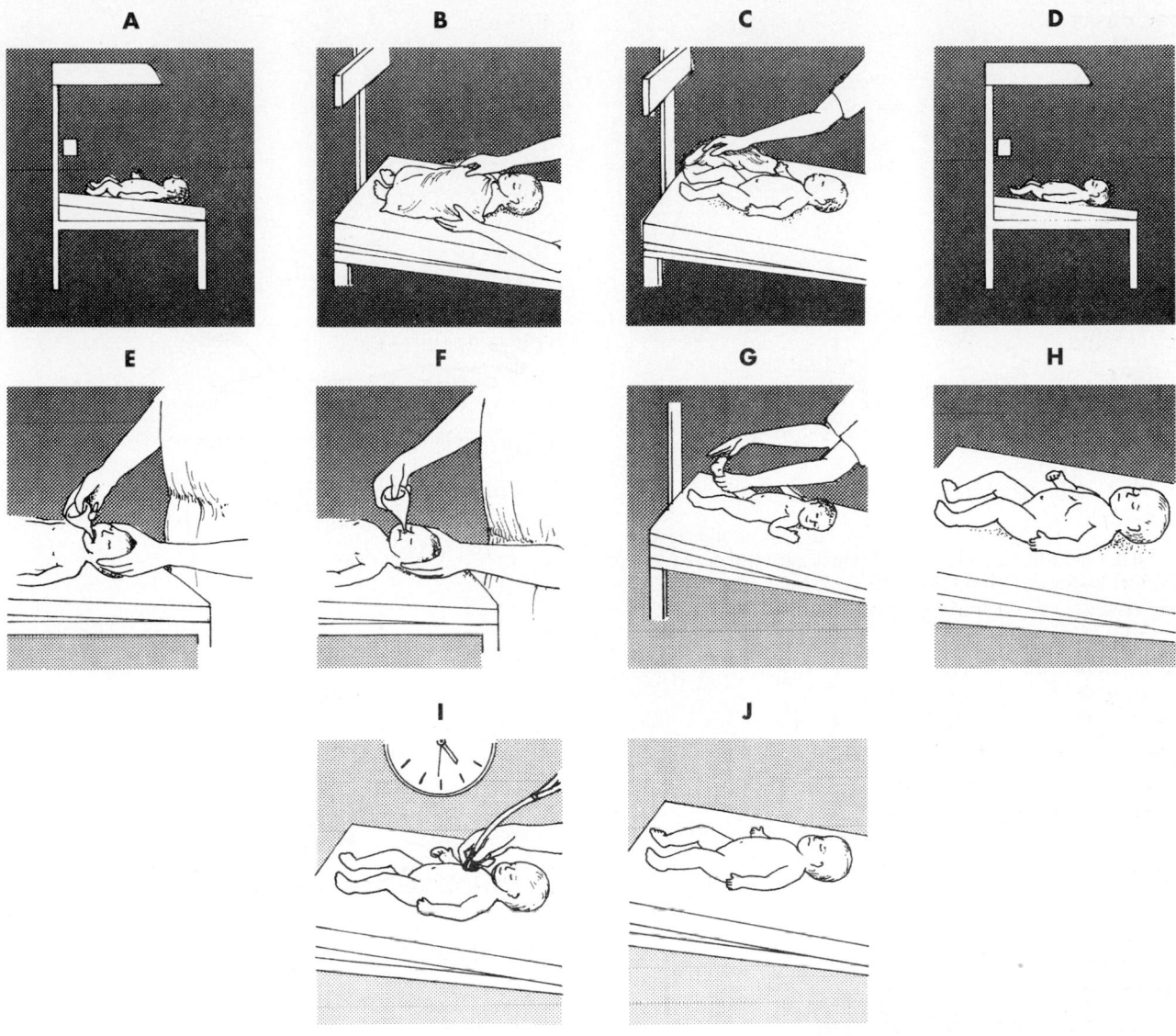

Figure 11-21 Immediate stabilization of newborn at delivery—sequence of interventions for assessment at birth. **A,** Place newborn under radiant heat warmer in slight Trendelenburg position. **B,** Dry immediately. **C,** Remove wet linens. **D,** Position newborn with head and neck in "sniffing" position. **E** and **F,** Suction oropharynx, then nasopharynx with bulb syringe *as needed. Not shown:* Suction oropharynx, trachea, and stomach as necessary with 10-French catheter connected to wall suction of 80 to 100 mm Hg per gauge. **G,** Tactile stimulate by slapping twice on sole of foot. **H,** Assess respirations. **I,** Assess heart rate by apical pulse. **J,** Assess color. Resuscitate as indicated by assessment.

Assist with newborn's warm water bath as indicated (LeBoyer deliveries)

Show warmed newborn to parents; identify sex and check identification bracelets initially and at each visit to mother and at discharge

Encourage parents to hold newborn as condition of newborn and parents permits to promote attachment and family-centered care

Perform the following according to facility policy
Weigh newborn
Measure length and head circumference
Administer medication as ordered

Eye prophylaxis
Vitamin K therapy
Do resuscitation documentation
Do newborn admitting assessment
Perform cord care

Perform neuromuscular maturity and physical maturity assessment (Ballard rating) (Figures 11-22, 11-23, and 11-24)

Give sponge bath daily until umbilical cord falls off, then bathe daily, washing hair two to three times per wk

Perform neonatal behavioral assessment and share infant responses with parents

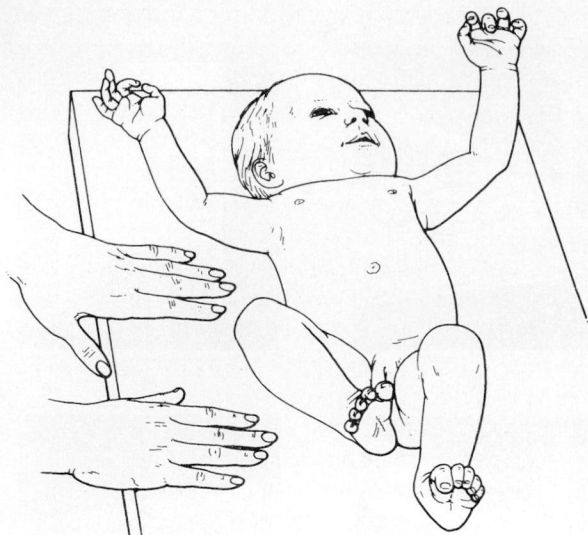

Figure 11-22 The Moro or startle reflex. Note the position of the arms and the index finger and thumb. (From Scipien GM et al: *Pediatric nursing care,* St Louis, 1990, Mosby.)

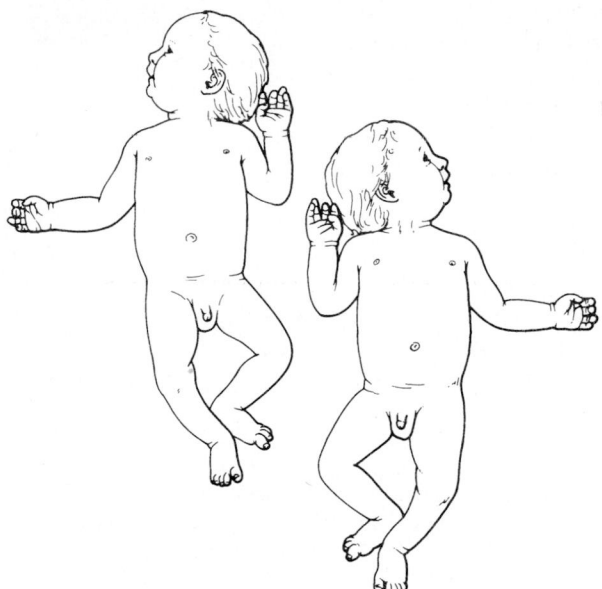

Figure 11-23 The tonic neck reflex demonstrating the typical asymmetrical fencer position. (From Scipien GM et al: *Pediatric nursing care,* St Louis, 1990, Mosby.)

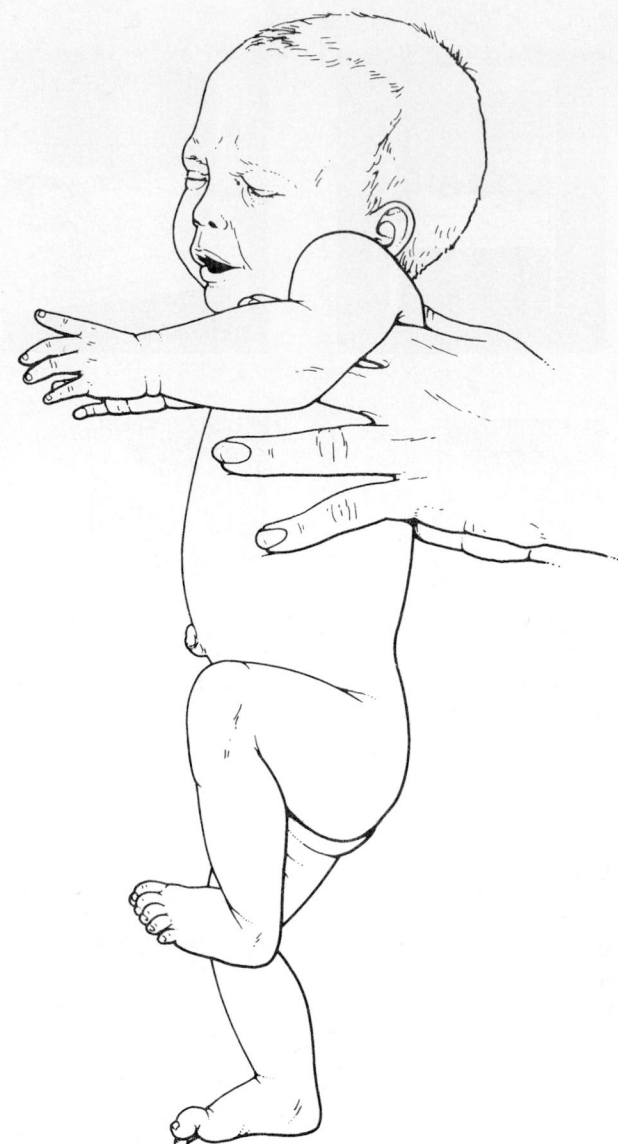

Figure 11-24 The stepping reflex. (From Scipien GM et al: *Pediatric nursing care,* St Louis, 1990, Mosby.)

Administer circumcision care; apply petrolatum gauze to penis as appropriate

Perform newborn assessments as required by policy and/or newborn condition; particularly note the following:

Note time of first voiding and meconium stool

Auscultate heart rate hourly twice and prn

Report rate above 180 or below 100 beats/min to primary health care provider

Report heart sounds heard on right side of chest

Report murmur

Assess respiratory rate q30min for four times and prn

Assess quality of respirations and report if abnormal

Perform heel puncture for blood glucose testing if newborn is at risk for hypoglycemia or hypothermia

Provide for sucking needs with pacifier as indicated (be aware that homemade pacifiers are unsafe)

Check rectal temperature one time to determine patency of anus

Administer eye prophylaxis and vitamin K therapy as ordered

Administer sterile water to establish adequate sucking/swallowing if this has not been established by infant breast-feeding in the delivery room, followed a few minutes later by 5% glucose water, breast-feeding, or formula per facility policy or as ordered

Administer feedings as ordered

Apply alcohol or triple dye to cord according to facility policy; remove cord clamp when cord is dry (usually about 24 hr after birth)

● **NDX:** Ineffective thermoregulation related to cold stress, hypoglycemia, hypoxemia, or immature thermoregulation mechanism

Recover mother and baby together under radiant heat warmer if possible (e.g., provide neutral thermal environment for infant with warmed blankets)

Observe newborn nude, if possible, for 1 to 2 hr postbirth while maintaining neutral thermal environment

Maintain axillary T at 97.7°F (36.5°C); check q30min/2 hr and until stable

Avoid bathing for first hour and until axillary T is stable at 97.7°F (36.5°C) and other VS are stable *to prevent cold stress*

Return to radiant warmer after bath until axillary T restabilizes to 97.7°F (36.5°C)

EXPECTED OUTCOME

Newborn maintains normal axillary T of 97.7° to 98.6°F (36.5° to 37°C)

● **NDX:** Ineffective airway clearance related to coordination of suck-swallow-gag reflexes

Keep bulb syringe in crib at all times; suction as needed

Hold newborn for feedings: *never prop bottles* (be aware that although demand feedings are preferred, newborn may need to be awakened if longer than 4 to 5 hr intervals occur between feedings)

Reposition q2h and prn; place on right side or abdomen after feedings for at least 30 min

Periodically reassess respiratory rate and rhythm

Perform "football hold" and use obstructed airway maneuvers recommended by American Heart Association as needed for choking

EXPECTED OUTCOME

Newborn maintains patent airway as evidenced by normal respiratory rate, depth, and rhythm and clear breath sounds

Patient/family teaching

Teach principles of, demonstrate and have parents return-demonstrate, and document inpatient teaching plan

Newborn care: bathing, feeding and burping, changing diaper, caring for cord and/or circumcision, taking temperature (rectal and axillary)

Instructions for formula preparation or pumping and storage of breast milk

Breast-feeding or formula feeding

Discuss issues related to use of disposable and recyclable cotton diapers

Review

Importance of dressing newborn according to temperature of day; avoid overheating

Importance of natural home environment; avoid unnatural quietness and overheating of home

How to seek assistance for newborn problems and concerns of parenthood (e.g., pediatrician's phone number, support groups)

Discuss conflicts of parental roles

Idealized versus realistic role of parenting

Love, resentment, or indifference toward newborn

Personal needs and demands of parenting

Describe how to obtain emergency care if required

Identify abnormal signs and symptoms to report to provider

Jaundice

Fever lasting longer than 24 hr

Newborn pulling on ears

Productive cough

Vomiting

Refusal to eat

Diarrhea

Lethargy

BIBLIOGRAPHY

Affonso D: Assessment of maternal postpartum adaptation, *Public Health Nurs* 4(1):9-20, 1987.

Avery M, Rossi M: Gestational diabetes, *J Nurse Midwifery* 39(2) supp., 9-19, 1994.

Akins S: Postpartum hemorrhage: a 90s approach to an age-old problem, *J Nurse Midwifery* 39(2) supp., 123-134.

AWHONN: Cervical ripening and induction and augmentation of labor, *Practice Resource.* Washington, DC, 1993, AWHONN.

Baurmann P, McFarlin B: Prenatal diagnosis, *J Nurse Midwifery* 39(2) supp., 35-51, 1994.

Chute G: Promoting breastfeeding success: an overview of basic management, *NAACOG's Clinical Issues in Perinatal and Women's Health Nursing* 3(4):570-582, 1992.

Combs CA, Murphy EL, Laros RK: Factors associated with postpartum hemorrhage with vaginal birth, *Obstet Gynecol* 77-76, 1991.

Dildy G, Clark S: Umbilical cord prolapse, *Contemp OB/GYN* 38(11):75-80, 1993.

Edge V, Miller M: *Women's health care,* St Louis, 1994, Mosby.

Flagler S, Nicoll L: A framework for the psychological aspects of pregnancy, *NAACOG's Clinical Issues in Perinatal and Women's Health Nursing* 1(3):267-278, 1990.

Gilbert E, Harmon J: *High-risk pregnancy and delivery,* St Louis, 1993, Mosby.

Hansen C: Baby blues: identification and intervention, *NAACOG's Clinical Issues in Perinatal and Women's Health Nursing* 1(3):369-374, 1990.

King T: Clinical management of premature rupture of membranes, *J Nurse Midwifery* 39(2) supp., 81-90, 1994.

Lawrence R: *Breastfeeding: a guide for the medical profession,* ed 4, St Louis, 1994, Mosby.

Mandeville L, Troiano N: *High-risk intrapartum nursing,* Philadelphia, 1992, JB Lippincott.

Martin J, Troiano N: Principles in hemodynamic assessment, *NAACOG's Clinical Issues in Perinatal and Women's Health Nursing* 3(3):377-384, 1992.

Miles J et al: Postpartum eclampsia: a recurring perinatal dilemma, *Obstet Gynecol* 76:328-331, 1990.

Phillips C: *Family-centered maternity and newborn care,* ed 4, St Louis, 1996, Mosby.

Rhode MA, Barger M: Perineal care, *J Nurse Midwifery* 35(4):195-205, 1990.

Roberts J: Current perspectives on preeclampsia, *J Nurse Midwifery* 39(2):70-90, 1994.

Romero R, Ghidini A: Premature rupture of membranes: amniotic fluid infection, *Contemp OB/GYN* 38(11):75-80, 1993.

Sauer T, Harvey C: Pregnancy-induced hypertension, *Crit Care Nurs Clin North Am* 4(4):703-710, 1992.

Tappero EP, Honeyfield ME: *Physical assessment of the newborn,* Petaluma, Calif, 1993, NICU INK Book Publishers.

Zerbe M, Bashore R: Critical hemorrhage during pregnancy, *Crit Care Nurs Clin North Am* 4(4):729-736, 1992.

CATHERINE MCAULEY HEALTH SYSTEM
Ann Arbor, Michigan 48106

Critical Path for: Gynecologic Malignancies
NMP(s): N-K-024: Gynecologic Surgery   Variance Yes_____ No_____
C-P-090: Postoperative Gynecology Patient   DRG/ICD9 Code: DRG - 353, 354, 355, 357
Primary Nurse(s): _____
Case Manager: _____

	Date_____ PPT Appointment	Date_____ ☐ Inpatient Admission (SDA N/A)	Date_____ Surgery ☐ Admission
ACTIVITY	☐ Ambulate as tolerated	☐ Ambulate as tolerated	• Reposition with encouragement q 2-4 hr x 12 hr ☐ Evening: dangle and take steps at bedside ☐ Braden Scale = _____
ASSESSMENT	• History and physical by MD or PA in PPT ☐ Nursing data base by unit RN in PPT (Include assessment psych/social/spiritual needs/feeling r/t sexuality) ☐ Special needs_____ _____ • Describes procedure R/T changes in body function • Opportunity to discuss feeling R/T surgery and recovery • Mutual goal setting initiated	• Complete nursing data base and admission profile • VS q shift • Assess response to bowel prep	• Implement NMP for postop Gyn pt. • Complete nursing data base and admission profile • Assess surgical drsg/incision with VS checks and prn • Assess characteristics of urine and voiding while on I & O • VS q 2 hr x 2, q 4 hr x 4 • LOC c/VS checks x 12 hr • Breath sounds q 8 hr • Bowel sounds q 8 hr until passing gas then BID until first BM • Assess patency tubes/drains
CONSULTS REFERRAL	☐ Cardiology Other:_____ ☐ Anesthesia _____ ☐ Social work ☐ Pastoral care ☐ Home Care	• Follow-up preop referrals • Notify HO with values outside of parameters	☐ Notify HO with values outside of parameters
TREATMENTS (Meds, Diet, etc.)	• Explanation of perioperative procedures • Instruct medications to take day of surgery per anesthesia guidelines • Iron po if donating blood • Stop ASA 10 days or NSAIDS 3 days before OR	• NPO x water, bowel prep, and medications • Start IV per MD order • I & O q shift • Bowel prep per MD order • Measure and order SCD • Medications as ordered	• Strict NPO • IV per MD order ☐ Foley cath to DD ☐ Suprapubic to DD ☐ NG to SX • Other drains_____ or ostomy: _____ • I & O q 4 hr or as ordered ☐ Instruct use of incentive spirometer ☐ C & DB with use IS • SCD • Pain management • Meds as ordered
DC PLANNING	• Assess home; D/C plans/needs	• Continue	• Continue
PATIENT EDUCATION	• MD office/PPT provides Gyn class flier ☐ Attends Preop Gyn class • Implement NMP: K/D R/T Gyn surgery • Initiate PER	• Instruct use of incentive spirometer, leg exercises, C & DB • Reinforce preop education	• Refer to PER, PCIS
DIAGNOSTICS	• Anesthesia guidelines ☐ Autologus or directed donor blood donations		• Labs R/T surgery • CBC
SIGNATURES			
SHIFT/INITIALS			

6111-017 4/94

Used by permission of St. Joseph Mercy Hospital, Ann Arbor, Michigan.

Continued.

CATHERINE MCAULEY HEALTH SYSTEM
Ann Arbor, Michigan 48106
Critical Path for: Gynecologic Malignancies
NMP(s): N-K-024: Gynecologic Surgery   Variance   Yes____   No____
C-G-066: Postoperative Gynecology Patient   DRG/ICD9 Code: DRG - 353, 354, 355, 357
Primary Nurse(s): _____
Case Manager: _____

	Date_____ POD 1	Date_____ POD 2	Date_____ POD 3	Date_____ POD 4	Date_____ POD 5	Date_____ POD 6
ACTIVITY	☐ Ambulate BID, progress as tolerated • Assess with AM Care	• Ambulate TID to QID in hallway, progress as tolerated				
ASSESSMENT	• Assess integrity of surgical drsg(s) • Continue to assess characteristics of urine and voiding while on I & O • VS q 4 hr • Breath sounds q 8 hr W/A • Bowel sounds q 8 hr W/A • Assess tubes/ drains prn • Weight qd	• Drsg removed per MD; assess incision q 8 hr W/A. Assist with care • VS q 4 hr	• VS q 4 hr to q shift			
CONSULTS REFERRALS	• Continue as applicable					
TREATMENTS (Meds, Diet, etc.)	• Strict NPO • IV per MD order • Foley catheter to DD • NG to sx • Continue drains • Other_____ • I & O q 4° or as ordered • Assist with use IS, C & DB • SCD • Pain management • Other meds	Diet_____ IV: Yes☐ No☐ Foley: Yes☐ No☐ NG: Yes☐ No☐ ____ Yes☐ No☐	Diet_____ IV: Yes☐ No☐ Foley: Yes☐ No☐ NG: Yes☐ No☐ ____ Yes☐ No☐	Diet_____ IV: Yes☐ No☐ Foley: Yes☐ No☐ NG: Yes☐ No☐ ____ Yes☐ No☐	Diet_____ IV: Yes☐ No☐ Foley: Yes☐ No☐ NG: Yes☐ No☐ ____ Yes☐ No☐	Diet_____ IV: Yes☐ No☐ Foley: Yes☐ No☐ NG: Yes☐ No☐ ____ Yes☐ No☐
DC PLANNING	• Continue	• D/C info sheet given to pt. per RN assessment				
PATIENT EDUCATION	• Refer to PER	☐ Pt. instructed in incision care	☐ Pt. participates in incision care • D/C education with pt and/or SO per RN assessment			• Discharge prescriptions per MD
DIAGNOSTICS	• CBC, platelets, BUN, CR, Lytes in AM		• CBC, platelets, BUN, CR, Lytes in AM			
SIGNATURES						
SHIFT/INITIALS						

6111-017 4/94

CATHERINE MCAULEY HEALTH SYSTEM
Ann Arbor, Michigan 48106
Critical Path for: Gynecologic Malignancies
NMP(s): N-K-024: Gynecologic Surgery   Variance Yes_____ No_____
C-G-066: Postoperative Gynecology Patient   DRG/ICD9 Code: DRG - 353, 354, 355, 357_____
Primary Nurse(s): _____
Case Manager: _____

	Date_____ POD 7	Date_____ POD 8	Date_____ POD 9	Initial box if PATIENT OUTCOMES met. If not, document variance. NA = not applicable
ACTIVITY	☐ Ambulate ad lib			☐ Ambulated as tolerated Date_____
ASSESSMENT	• Assess incision BID prn • Assess characteristics urine voiding pattern prn • VS q shift • Breath sounds BID prn • Bowel sounds BID prn			☐ Collaborative NMP completed Date_____ ☐ Incision clean, dry, & intact Date_____ ☐ Urinating without difficulty Date_____ ☐ BP, HR, & temp at baseline Date_____ ☐ Lungs CTA/baseline Date_____ ☐ Passing flatus Date_____ ☐ Goal setting completed Date_____
CONSULTS REFERRALS	• Continue as applicable _____			Consults completed: ☐ Social service Date_____ ☐ Pastoral care Date_____ ☐ Home care Date_____ ☐ APS Date_____ ☐ Other_____ Date_____
TREATMENTS (Meds, Diet, etc.)	Diet_____ ☐ Foley cath ☐ Suprapubic tube ☐ Other_____ • I & O prn • Pain management • Other meds			☐ General diet Date_____ ☐ Performs ISC Date_____ ☐ D/C'd with Foley-dd; care instructed with demonstration Date_____ ☐ Leg bag use instructed with demonstration Date_____ ☐ Suprapubic tube care Date_____ ☐ Ostomy care: type Date_____
DC PLANNING	• Continue			☐ Discharged Date_____
PATIENT EDUCATION	• Continue prn			☐ Chemotherapy information Date_____ ☐ Radiation therapy information Date_____ ☐ KD NMP completed Date_____ ☐ D/C Education completed (see PER) Date_____ ☐ BSE video viewed Date_____ ☐ Other_____ Date_____
DIAGNOSTICS				
SIGNATURES				
SHIFT/INITIALS				

6111-017 4/94

BARNES

**CARE PATH®
702
VAGINAL HYSTERECTOMY**

SERVICE		PHYSICIAN			
PRIMARY NURSE		PRIMARY NURSE			
DC DATE	ADM DATE	DATE OF SURGERY		**A-8**	

PATIENT PROBLEMS/NURSING DIAGNOSES

Problem Number	
#1	LACK OF KNOWLEDGE
#2	ALTERATION IN COMFORT
#3	POTENTIAL ALTERATION IN URINARY ELIMINATION
#4	POTENTIAL FOR INFECTION
#5	POTENTIAL ALTERATION IN BOWEL ELIMINATION
#6	POTENTIAL ALTERATION IN BODY IMAGE * IF APPROPRIATE

#	2, 3, 4, 5, 6			3	3, 4, 5
	ASSESSMENT/MONITORING	**CONSULTS**	**PROCEDURES/TEST**	**TREATMENT**	**ACTIVITY**
PRE ADMIT	Risk factors for surgery Emotional response Comprehension of preop instructions		Type & X Autologous Donation CBC *CXR *ECG		
DAY 1 OP DAY	Pain control I & O S & Ss of shock Vaginal drainage, vaginal packing Bowel sounds Lung sounds Activity level Tolerance of PO fluids N/V VS Fall prevention **VS stable** **Pain controlled w/PCA**	Anesthesia		Foley	TCDB q 2 hr ×1 ×2 ×3 ×4 ×5 ×6 ×7 ×8 ×9 ×10 ×11 ×12 Dangle 6 hr postop Tolerates dangling at bedside

SIGNATURE	INIT.	SIGNATURE	INIT.	SIGNATURE	INIT.

BARNES

CARE PATH®
702
VAGINAL HYSTERECTOMY

CNS	DIETARY	RT
HOME HEALTH	OT	OTHER
PT	SW	OTHER

A-8

Problem Number	PATIENT PROBLEMS/NURSING DIAGNOSES

2, 4, 5	4	1	1, 2, 3, 4, 5, 6	1	INITIALS (SEE KEY AT BOTTOM)		
MEDS / IVS	NUTRITION	PATIENT/FAMILY EDUCATION	DISCHARGE PLANNING	PSYCHOSOCIAL/ EMOTIONAL/ SPIRITUAL NEEDS			
		Reason & implications of surgery (Loss of fertility) Preop teaching: Tests Procedure NPO after MN Activities before surgery IV Foley Immediate postop activities: TCDB Activity PO intake Pain control **States reason surgery is necessary.** **States organ(s) removed during surgery** **Defines term "sterilization"**		*Social Work for: Needs expressed by pt. High risk for problems with coping (no children, childcare problems during hospitalization)			
IV PCA *ATDs	Clear liquids after surgery Advance Diet as tolerated **Tolerates PO fluids w/o nausea**	Function of PCA Importance of early ambulation, PO intake, and return of bowel and bladder function	*Social Work if advanced age, ≥70 living alone, and/or financial concerns **Pt./family verbalizes understanding of Care Path.** **Estimated length of stay and plan of care mutually set with pt./family**				
SIGNATURE	INIT.	SIGNATURE	INIT.	SIGNATURE			INIT.

Continued.

#	2, 3, 4, 5, 6				3	3, 4, 5
	ASSESSMENT/MONITORING	**CONSULTS**		**PROCEDURES/TEST**	**TREATMENT**	**ACTIVITY**
DAY 2 POD 1	Pain control I & O S & Ss of shock Vaginal drainage, vaginal packing Bowel sounds Voiding Tolerance of diet VS Emotional response **Pain controlled with PO meds**			*CBC	d/c foley in AM **Voiding w/o pain, frequency, urgency, or retention**	Up with assistance **Ambulates with assistance**
DAY 3 POD 2	DC Day					Up ad lib Independent in ambulation
DISCHARGE	**Vital signs stable** **H & H WNL** **Vaginal drainage similar to menstrual bleeding in amount and character** **Absence of dysuria, hematuria, burning, frequency, or urgency**				**Voiding w/o pain, frequency, or urgency**	**Able to ambulate and perform self- care as before surgery.**
	SIGNATURE	**INIT.**	**SIGNATURE**		**INIT.**	**SIGNATURE**	**INIT.**

2, 4, 5	4	1	1, 2, 3, 4, 5, 6	1	INITIALS		
MEDS/IVS	**NUTRITION**	**PATIENT/FAMILY EDUCATIONS**	**DISCHARGE PLANNING**	**PSYCHOSOCIAL/ EMOTIONAL/ SPIRITUAL NEEDS**	(SEE KEY AT BOTTOM)		
IV: Hep lock/KVO in PM PO analgesic d/c PCA in PM if tolerates PO fluids *ATBs *Stool softeners	Regular Diet Tolerates PO intake w/o nausea & vomiting	PO pain meds Begin DC teaching: (S & Ss to report to MD) Increased vaginal discharge Temp ≥101°F (38.5°C) Urinary incontinence, dysuria, painful urination Activity: Up ad lib, no driving for 2 weeks, no heavy lifting for 6 weeks, no douching, intercourse, or tampons until directed by MD Diet: regular as permitted d/c meds: purpose, dosage, route, schedule, side effects of analgesics and laxatives, stool softeners, and other prn.		Provide opportunity to discuss physical, psychosocial, and sexual impact of surgery			
	Regular Diet	Reinforce DC teaching		Provide opportunity to discuss physical, psychosocial, and sexual impact of surgery			
Pain control with PO medication	**Able to tolerate PO intake w/o nausea and vomiting**	**Verbalizes understanding of signs to report to MD, activity limitations, diet, personal hygiene, and medications**	**Able to perform ADLs independently or with assistance of appropriate community resources**	**Able to verbalize concerns about impact of surgery**			
SIGNATURE	**INIT.**	**SIGNATURE**	**INIT.**	**SIGNATURE**			**INIT.**

Integumentary System

Integumentary System Assessment

● Subjective Data

Skin
  Itching
  Painful
  Rash
  Oily
  Dry
  Rough
  Bumpy
  Thin
  Peeling
  Puffy
  Blisters
  Hot
  Cold
  Changes in skin color
  Liver spots: aging spots
  Boils
  Use of Retin-A, antibiotics

● Objective Data

Skin
  Color
    Cyanosis
      Lips
      Circumoral area

Mucous membranes
Earlobes
Nail beds
Jaundice: sclera, skin
Pallor: conjunctiva, nail beds
Pigmentation distribution; freckling, moles
Turgor
Elasticity
Intactness
Rashes
Moisture
Temperature (T)
Cleanliness
Odor
Edema
Needle marks
Insect bites
Scabies
Acne, calluses, corns
Exudate
Uremic frost: beard, eyebrows
Sclerema
Striae
Pressure areas over bony prominences
Decubitus ulcers
Nails
Cleanliness
Brittleness
Condition of surrounding tissue
Clubbing of fingers and toes
Lines, pitting
Ram's horn shape: turning under fingertip
Spoon shape: concave
Hair
Distribution and configuration
Texture
Color
Quantity
Parasites
Alopecia
Lesions
Macula (<5 mm) (freckles, moles)
Flat
Discolored
Papule (<5 mm) (warts, eczema)
Elevated
Discolored
Patch (>5 mm) (port wine marks)
Flat
Discolored
Scaly
Vesicle (blister, varicella)
Elevated
Superficial
Serous exudate
Pustule (acne, impetigo)

Elevated
Purulent exudate
Bulla (large blister, pemphigus)
Flaccid
Tense
Plaque (psoriasis, keratosis)
Thickened
Coalesced papules
Elevated
Tumor (>5 cm) (neoplasm)
Solid
Elevated
Cyst (sebaceous cyst)
Semisolid
Palpable
Encapsulated
Serous or purulent exudate
Crust (scab, eczema)
Dried exudate
Elevated
Wheal (urticaria, bites)
Solid
Irregular shape
Elevated
Itchy
Transient
Scale (psoriasis, dermatitis)
Elevated
Flaky
Irregular
Nodule (lipoma)
Elevated
Firm
Palpable
Deep
Comedo: blackhead/whitehead
Chancre
Small
Hard or ulcerated
Excoriation (abrasion)
Loss of epidermis
Linear
Ulcer (decubiti)
Loss of epidermis, dermis
Concave
Exudate
Cicatrix: scar
Whealed dermis
Occasionally raised
Keloid: excessive collagen formation around lesion or scar
Irregular shape
Elevated
Beyond scar border
Petechia
Small

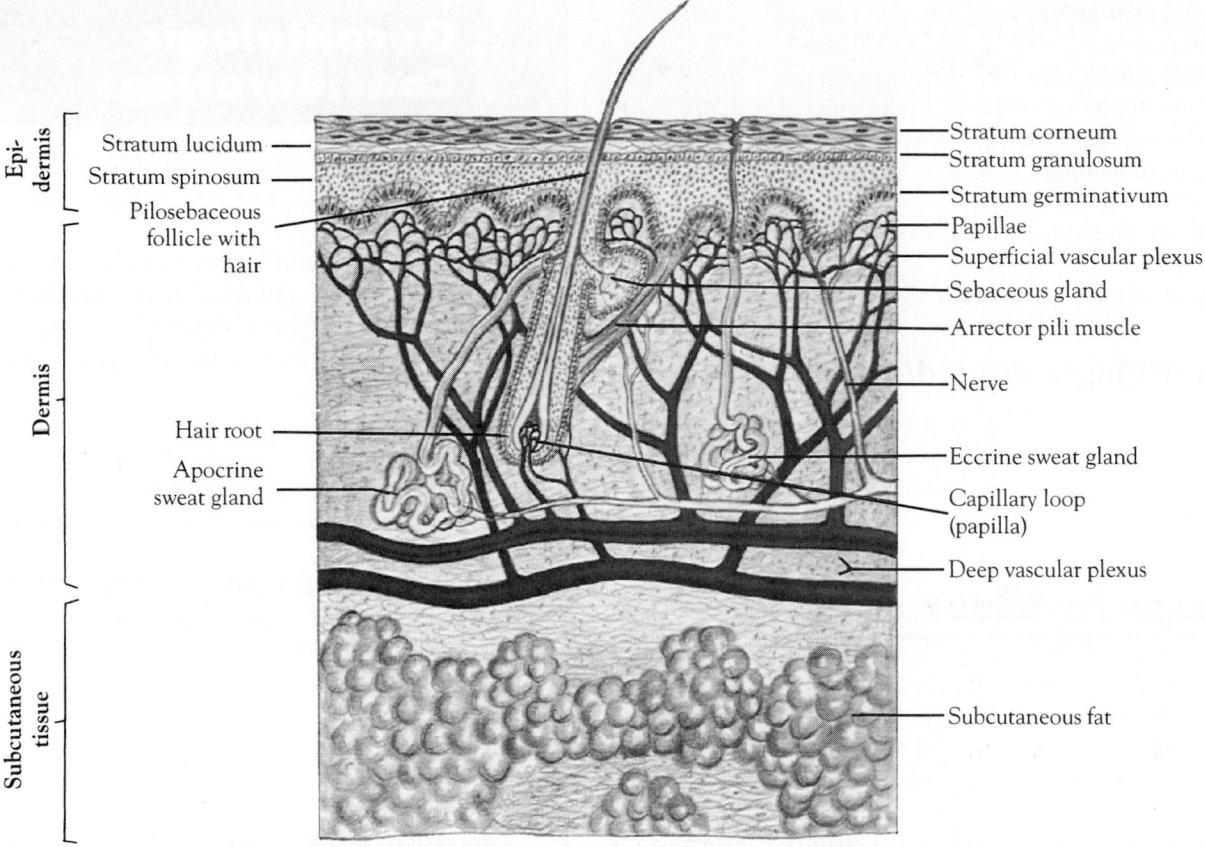

Figure 12-1 Structures of skin. (From Thompson et al: *Mosby's clinical nursing,* ed 3, St Louis, 1993, Mosby.)

Bright red
Flat
Fissure (athlete's foot)
  Small
  Deep
  Red
  Linear
Telangiectasia (rosacea)
  Fine red line
  Irregular
Erosion (varicella)
  Moist
  Depressed
  Shiny
Lichenification (chronic dermatitis): thick, rough
  epidermis

● Pertinent Background Information

Family history and concurrent diseases

Allergies
Exposures to external allergens
  Cosmetics

Soaps
Medication
Plants
Chemicals
Exposures to internal allergens
  Drugs
  Food
Travel history
Exposure to parasites
Response to sun

Medication presently being taken

Injectable medication
Prescription medication
Over-the-counter medication
Creams, lotions, ointments
Hygienic practices
Sexual practices

● Diagnostic Tests

Diagnosis of causative disease
Skin and lesion cultures
Gram stain for organism identification

Electron microscopy
Diascopy
Immunofluorescence (IF)
Lupus erythematosus preparation
Punch biopsies, cytology
Allergy skin testing
Blood culture
Skin scraping: potassium hydroxide (KOH) testing for
  fungus
Complete blood count (CBC)

Gerontologic considerations

The aging process elicits many alterations in the integumentary system that can cause physical and emotional changes in the individual (see Gerontologic
  Considerations box)

Pressure Ulcer

*An area of cellular necrosis usually over a bony
  prominence that results from tissue hypoxia attributed
  to pressure, shearing, friction, moisture, poor
  nutrition, fever, altered circulation; these alone or in
  combination can contribute to skin frailness and
  reduce its ability to withstand the irritating factors
  (Table 12-1)*

Assessment

Subjective data

Pain, numbness

Objective data

Location of pressure area; risk score assessment
  Back of head
  Ear rims, cheeks
  Shoulder blades, acromion process
  Elbows, heels, toes
  Sacrum, buttocks, coccyx
  Hips, greater trochanter, ischial tuberosities
  Inner knee; medial, lateral malleolus
  Medial, lateral condyles
  Breast (women), genitalia (men)
  Assess stage of necrosis (see box on p. 780)
Immobility
Elevated temperature
Medical history (diabetes, carcinoma, anemia)
Nutritional status
Age, weight, mental acuity
Moisture, incontinence, perspiration
Hydration

Gerontologic Considerations

- Physiologic changes make the skin of the older
  person more fragile and susceptible to impairment.
- Aging changes include decreases in tissue fluid,
  subcutaneous fat, and sebaceous secretions.
  This results in dryness, flaking, pruritus, loss of
  elasticity, altered turgor, and a wrinkled appearance.
- Hyperkeratotic changes are typically seen in the
  nails, making them thick and difficult to care
  for. Podiatric care is recommended for older
  adults, particularly those with circulatory impairment.
- Circulatory changes and decreased mobility increase the risk of senile purpura and decubitus
  ulcers.
- Significant hair and scalp changes can manifest
  with aging:
  - Loss of pigmentation leading to graying
  - Decreased thickness and increased incidence
    of balding
  - Increased incidence of seborrheic dermatitis
    of the scalp requiring special care
  - growth of facial hair on women, which can be
    damaging to self-image
  - Localized clusters of melanocytes surrounded
    by areas of decreased pigmentation result in
    "age spots."
- The incidence of basal and squamous cell carci-
  noma increases with age, particularly in individ-
  uals who have had a high level of sun exposure.
  Aging skin should be closely inspected for
  changes in the appearance of moles or warts.

From Christensen BL, Kockrow EO: *Foundations of nursing,* ed 2, St
Louis, 1995, Mosby.

Diagnostic tests

Lesion culture
CBC, electrolytes
Serum albumin
Fasting blood sugar, (FBS)

Potential complications

Infection
Further necrosis

Table 12-1 Pressure Ulcer Prevention

Contributing Factor	Interventions
Inactivity	Perform range of motion (ROM) exercises to all extremities Promote self-care activities Provide assistive devices: cane, walker, wheelchair
Immobility	Assess care givers' ability to provide care Maintain turning schedule Avoid friction, shearing, sliding Institute small, frequent position changes Prop with pillows for comfort Initiate use of pressure-reducing devices: foam, gel, water, air mattress
Incontinence	Assess need for fecal management device Provide perineal, perianal care after each voiding or bowel movement Assess for possible urinary management device: internal, external catheter Offer bedpan or use of commode at scheduled times
Malnutrition	Provide diet high in protein, carbohydrate, vitamins C and E Offer between-meal snacks; Ensure; Carnation instant breakfast Offer small, frequent meals (6/day)
Decreased sensation/mental acuity	Assess neuromuscular function; avoid overexposure to heat, cold Assess care givers' ability to provide care if needed Maintain warmth without added weight

Change	Patient Problem	Interventions
Reduced body temperature/ circulation	Cold extremities, pressure ulcers	• Maintain warmth with use of warm stockings, knee and ankle warmers, bed socks, and blankets that provide heat but not extra weight • Encourage use of fleece-lined slippers, mittens, boots, hats • Encourage ambulation, exercises • Provide pressure-reducing devices: air, foam mattress, circulating air mattress • Avoid massaging skin
Decreased moisture retention	Dry, rough, flaky skin	• Encourage use of creams and mild soaps; avoid antibacterial types, which tend to be drying • Maintain and protect skin with emollient application to entire body to prevent dryness • Avoid direct sunlight and wear a sunscreen cream • Encourage fluid intake of 3000 ml/day if allowed • Maintain adequate humidity
Inadequate nutrition/ hydration		• Evaluate knowledge of good nutrition • Maintain diet high in protein, carbohydrates, and vitamins; encourage small, frequent meals • Evaluate ability to chew, encourage to take small bites and chew food well • Provide alternate methods of preparing food to enhance intake: soft, puréed • Refer to community agencies for meals: Meals-on-Wheels

Stages of Necrosis

I. Erythema only, no break in skin
II. Partial thickness; loss of skin involving epidermis, often into dermis
III. Full thickness; involves epidermis, dermis into or exposing subcutaneous tissue
IV. Deep tissue loss through subcutaneous tissue into fascia, muscle, bone

Collaborative management

Therapeutic management

Diet, vitamin, mineral supplements
Surgical and chemical debridement
Systemic and topical antibiotics
Enterostomal nurse/clinical nurse specialist
  Stage assessment assistance
  Treatment suggestions
  Resources

Nursing management

PATIENT PROBLEMS/NURSING DIAGNOSES

● **NDX:** Impaired skin integrity related to immobility

Preventive measures
  Elevate head of bed only enough to maintain comfort *to prevent sliding and possible shearing*
  Maintain skin integrity by keeping skin clean and dry
  Perform skin care daily and prn
  Bathe with mild soap and warm water; remove powder and ointments
  Rinse skin and pat dry thoroughly
  Apply lotion to feet, elbows, and back and massage very gently; remove excess
  Administer perineal care after elimination
Turn patient q2h: side, back, side *to relieve pressure;* lift patient when turning *to prevent friction;* avoid positioning directly on trochanter when lying on side
Assess and monitor pressure points qid and prn
Assist and teach patient to change position slightly q15min to 30min *to avoid pressure and fatigue*
Maintain clean, comfortable bed with wrinkle-free sheets
Administer back rubs with bland emollient; avoid alcohol

Prevent and eliminate pressure and friction by placing pillows between pressure areas (knees, ankles)
Prevent pressure with the following devices
  Alternating pressure mattress
  Foam or static air mattress overlay
  Pressure reduction replacement mattress
  Flotation mattress
  Silicone pads
  Heel and elbow guards *to reduce friction*
Assist with and teach active or perform passive ROM exercises to all extremities q4h
Increase activity as allowed: assist patient out of bed and into chair; avoid sitting for more than 30 min; provide pressure relief while in chair; avoid donut-type devices

EXPECTED OUTCOMES
Verbalizes understanding of procedures needed to prevent tissue breakdown
Participates in treatment/activities
Expresses sense of well-being

● **NDX:** Impaired skin integrity related to mechanical factors

Assess skin and identify stage of ulcer development
Involve enterostomal therapist/clinical nurse specialist if available
Eliminate causative factors
Initiate appropriate ulcer care for stages I and II
  Cleanse skin at least q8h with mild soap and water and pat dry
  Massage skin gently *to increase circulation;* avoid vigorous rubbing; bathe only as necessary
  Do not massage reddened areas *because it may cause deep tissue trauma*
  Turn q1h to 2h; use turn sheet or lift patient; avoid sliding *to prevent friction*
  Maintain wrinkle-free sheets
  Provide special pads, mattresses, beds as indicated
  Position patient on unaffected areas
  Protect skin surface and affected area with one or combination of the following
    Apply Skin Prep/gel around area to prepare skin for dressing
    Cover area with transparent dressing (Opsite) or hydrocolloid wafer barrier (Duoderm); bruised skin should not be covered
    Continue one type of application, or a combination, for 48 to 72 hr; if improvement is apparent, continue applications; if no improvement is noted, begin another type of treatment
Initiate appropriate ulcer care for stages III and IV
  Assess ulcer for size, location, color, odor, and amount and type of drainage

Monitor temperature for elevation

Evaluate ulcer for infection and culture as needed

Administer wound care according to hospital standard of care

If healing is not evident, prepare for debridement as ordered

After debridement, change dressings as ordered; may range from gauze to hydrocolloids to absorbent gel-type dressing

EXPECTED OUTCOMES

Exhibits skin/tissue color, integrity, and temperature returning to normal

Demonstrates ability to perform exercises/activities to prevent further tissue damage

● **NDX:** Impaired skin integrity related to malnutrition

Assess patient's ability to chew and swallow food, determine dietary preferences, and provide appropriate type of diet; assist with feeding as needed

Explain diet rationale to patient and the need for high-protein, high-carbohydrate foods to promote healing; involve nutritionist/registered dietitian and perform calorie count

Offer frequent, small feedings on attractive trays; provide supplemental feedings

Promote involvement of significant other(s) *to provide support*

Encourage involvement in food selection

Increase fluid intake to 2500 ml/day if not contraindicated

Weigh patient daily: same time, clothing, and scale; report 0.5 kg loss to physician

Monitor CBC, electrolytes, and serum albumin

Measure intake and output q8h; ensure intake equals output

EXPECTED OUTCOMES

Regains/maintains weight consistent with age/height

Participates in meal planning

Presents normal laboratory values

Patient/family teaching

Provide written instructions for pressure ulcer care

Demonstrate cleansing procedure and application of medication and dressings as ordered; observe return demonstrations

Explain dietary regimen and provide written instructions

Stress importance of daily weights

Discuss signs and symptoms to report to physician
  Weight loss; elevated temperature

Increased drainage from ulcer

Foul odor from ulcer

Further necrosis around ulcer

Reddened areas at other pressure points

Explain importance of increasing activity as tolerated, changing positions frequently while in bed, and avoiding pressure on affected area

Promote follow-up visits with physician

Home care considerations

Assess and continue with patient/family education and evaluate/discuss

Pressure ulcer prevention (see Table 12-1)

Nutrition and dietary intake

Intake and output

Care of pressure ulcer, use of sterile technique; adequate dressings, medications, correct procedure

Knowledge of where and what items to purchase as needed

Importance of changing position, increasing activity

Cellulitis

An acute streptococcal, staphylococcal infection of all layers of the skin and subcutaneous tissue, usually caused by bacterial invasion through a broken area in the skin such as skin trauma or ulceration; however, it may occur with no site of entry evident such as in lymphedema; it occurs as a result of a breakdown of tissues by enzymes produced by the invading bacteria

Assessment

Subjective data

Localized pain, redness, swelling, tenderness of skin

Headache

Objective data

Lymphangitic streaks

Skin resembling skin of orange (peau d'orange)

Presence of open wound

Amount, color, odor of drainage

Fever, chills, malaise

Tachycardia

Hypotension

Diagnostic tests

CBC: increased white blood cell count (WBC), eosinophils

Erythrocyte sedimentation rate (ESR) increased
Cultures: lesion and blood

Potential complications

Systemic infection
Ulceration

Collaborative management

Therapeutic management

Antibiotics, analgesics, antipyretics
Position and immobilization of extremity
Alternate cool/warm compresses
Diet, activity

Nursing management

PATIENT PROBLEMS/NURSING DIAGNOSES

● **NDX:** Impaired skin integrity related to altered turgor, circulation, and edema

Assess impairment: size, depth, color, drainage q4h *to form basis for treatment*
Maintain bed rest with extremity elevated and immobilized for 2 or 3 days *to decrease edema and promote circulation*
Change dressings prn *to promote comfort*
Maintain aseptic techniques *to prevent spread of infection*
Apply compresses, alternating cold *to reduce discomfort* and warm *to increase circulation*
Monitor temperature q4h; report elevation to physician
Administer antibiotics *to reduce infection*

EXPECTED OUTCOMES

Lesion begins to heal, and area is free of further infection
Skin is clean and dry, and surrounding area is free of swelling
Temperature returns to normal

● **NDX:** Impaired physical mobility related to pain, discomfort

Maintain elevation of each extremity *to reduce swelling and pain*
Assist with use of cane, crutches, walker *to aid in ambulation*
Explain importance of maintaining elevation to just above heart level *to increase circulation*

EXPECTED OUTCOMES

Begins to engage in usual activities
Uses appropriate mobilization device correctly

● **NDX:** Pain related to tissue inflammation

Assess pain for intensity using pain rating scale
Maintain affected extremity in prescribed position *to promote comfort*
Explain need for immobilization for 48 to 72 hr *because it reduces inflammation*
Administer analgesic as appropriate; assess effectiveness
Change position frequently, maintaining alignment, *to prevent pressure and fatigue*
Assist with and teach alternate pain relief measures: imagery, relaxation *to lessen preoccupation with pain*
Promote diversional activities *to decrease attention on pain*

EXPECTED OUTCOMES

Reports a reduction in pain and discomfort that is at a tolerable level
Appears calm; has relaxed facial expression
Alternates sleep with activity appropriately

Patient/family teaching

Demonstrate wound care and dressing-change procedure; stress importance of clean technique
Discuss maintaining prescribed elevation and immobilization of extremity
Encourage activity to tolerance using supportive devices: sling, crutches
Explain signs and symptoms to report to physician
  Wound pain or increased drainage
  Fever, chills, headache
  Odor from dressings and wound
Discuss medication schedule including name, purpose, dosage, and side effects
Stress importance of balanced diet to promote wound healing
Promote follow-up visits with physician

Home care considerations

Assess and continue with patient/family teaching and evaluate/discuss understanding of the following:
  Pressure ulcer prevention (see Table 12-1)
  Nutrition and dietary intake
  Intake and output
  Care of wound; use of clean technique; adequate dressings, medications, correct procedure

Knowledge of where and what items to purchase as needed

Importance of changing position, increasing activity

Pruritus

A sensation that evokes the desire to scratch, which can be a symptom of localized primary skin disorders (eczema, irritation, allergic reactions) or a systemic disease (renal failure, liver or thyroid disease, opiate drugs, psychological problems); the sensory nerve endings promote the itching sensation, but exactly how and why are unknown; there are four main areas affected: pruritus ani, occurring usually in men; pruritus vulvae, found in women; otitis externa occurs in the external ear canal; and generalized pruritus may signify a systemic disease

Assessment

Subjective data

Itchiness, discomfort
Level of stress, tension
History of liver, renal disease
Pattern of itching: at all times, occasional, seasonal

Objective data

Location, distribution of pruritus
Erythema, scaling of area
Signs of scratching
Signs of ascites, urine retention

Diagnostic tests

Culture of area
Biopsy
CBC, BUN
FBS
Serum bilirubin, iron
Stool for hemocult, parasites
Urinalysis
Sulfobromophthalein retention test

Potential complications

Increased excoriation
Fissures
Secondary infection

Collaborative management

Therapeutic management

Topical preparations, steroid cream
Antihistamines: diphenhydramine (Benadryl), terfenadine (Seldane)
Antianxiety agents: hydroxyzine (Atarax, Vistaril)
Psychotherapeutic agents (for antipruritic effect); chlorpromozine (Thorazine)
Cool compresses
Sitz baths
Emollients
Psychological counseling as needed

Nursing management

PATIENT PROBLEMS/NURSING DIAGNOSES

● **NDX:** Impaired skin integrity related to scratching of affected areas

Encourage patient to maintain excellent hygiene *to prevent infection and further impairment*
Apply topical lotions and creams if not contraindicated *to reduce sensation to scratch*
Administer cooling compresses or baths *to soothe the area*
Advise and discuss importance of keeping nails short *to prevent further tissue damage*
Encourage patient to use tepid water and pat skin dry *to avoid irritating tissues*
Apply mittens if urge to scratch is uncontrollable
Administer antibiotics if skin is infected
Monitor laboratory results *to assist in identifying underlying systemic disease*

EXPECTED OUTCOMES

Expresses a decreased desire to scratch affected areas
Exhibits no signs of infection
Maintains short fingernails

● **NDX:** Pain related to itching caused by irritation, inflammation, or a systemic condition

Maintain patient in a position of comfort
Administer antianxietics, antihistamines, psychotherapeutics *to reduce discomfort*
Apply soothing emollients *to decrease itching sensation and increase moisture in the skin*
Provide diversional activities *to decrease attention on discomfort*
Change position frequently in small ways *to prevent fatigue*

Offer back rubs *to soothe and promote comfort*
Encourage verbalization of concerns, fears, and
stress factors *to prevent further aggravation of
pruritus*

EXPECTED OUTCOMES
Exhibits less discomfort and decreased scratching
Utilizes discomfort-reducing methods successfully

Patient/family teaching and home care considerations

Explain and discuss the importance of avoiding the
following:
Excess heat/dryness in the home
Clothing that is tight fitting and/or made from rough
fabrics
Polyester fabrics that do not allow for ventilation
Irritating soaps, laundry detergents
Explain importance of keeping nails short
Discuss medications schedule and possible side
effects
Evaluate procedure for compress application
Explain signs of infection: redness, pain, drainage,
fever; need to promptly report these symptoms to
physician
Discuss importance of physician follow-up visits

Burn Management

● Causative Factors of Burns

thermal: Caused by exposure to flame, hot liquids,
radiation
chemical: Caused by contact, inhalation, ingestion of
acids, alkalies, vesicants
electrical: Caused by electrical current passing through
the body and into the ground

Assessment: full-thickness burns (Table 12-2)

Observations/findings

Percentage of body surface involved (Figure 12-2)
Classification (Table 12-3)
Anatomical location
Age of patient
Causative agent
History of preexisting illness
Other body trauma
Fractures
Deep tissue destruction
Respiratory tract trauma
Respiratory distress caused by toxic inhalation
Hypotension, tachycardia, shock
Presence of pain

Diagnostic tests

CBC, electrolytes, serum albumin, oxyhemoglobin,
BUN, creatinine, bilirubin, alkaline phosphatase
Arterial blood gases (ABGs), glucose, carbooxyhemo-
globin
Urinalysis for Hgb, myoglobin, albumin, glucose, ace-
tone, specific gravity
Chest and body radiology, bronchoscopy, lung scan
Electrocardiogram (ECG)

Potential complications

Hyponatremia (first 48 hr)
Hypernatremia (after 48 hr)
Hyperkalemia (first 48 hr)
Hypokalemia (after 48 hr)
Hypoproteinemia
Dehydration
Hypoxia
Circulatory collapse

Table 12-2 Assessment of Burn Injury

Degree	Depth	Characteristics
Superficial (first degree)	Epidermis only; devitalization of epidermis and dilation of intradermal vessels	Pain; erythema; blanching with pressure; normal texture
Partial-thickness (second degree)	Destruction of epidermis and part of dermis	Erythema; blisters; pain; blanching with pressure; firm texture
Full-thickness (third and fourth degree)	Destruction of all layers of skin extending into subcutaneous tissue, muscle, nerves, and bone	Dryness; pale, white, brown, or red color; charring; no capillary refill; no pain; firm and leathery texture

Hematuria, oliguria
Anemia
Adult respiratory distress syndrome (ARDS)
Gastric atony
Septic shock
Curling ulcer (as early as first week, as late as ninth
week)
Fecal impaction
Emotional shock
Disseminated intravascular coagulation (DIC)

Collaborative management

Therapeutic management

Narcotics, sedatives, analgesics, insulin, tetanus
Broncholytic agents, steroids, diuretics, antacids

Antibiotics, vasodilators
Mechanical ventilation, endotracheal tube
Tetanus vaccine
Parenteral fluids with electrolytes and vitamins
Hemodynamic monitoring, Swan-Ganz catheter
Transfusion/plasma
Nasogastric suction/indwelling urinary catheter
Diet, NPO, total parenteral nutrition (TPN), fluid re-
placement formula, tube feedings
Burn care
Escharotomy, fasciotomy
Skin graft
Oxygen therapy, IPPB
Chest physiotherapy
Mechanical ventilation
Social worker
Assist with body image disturbance

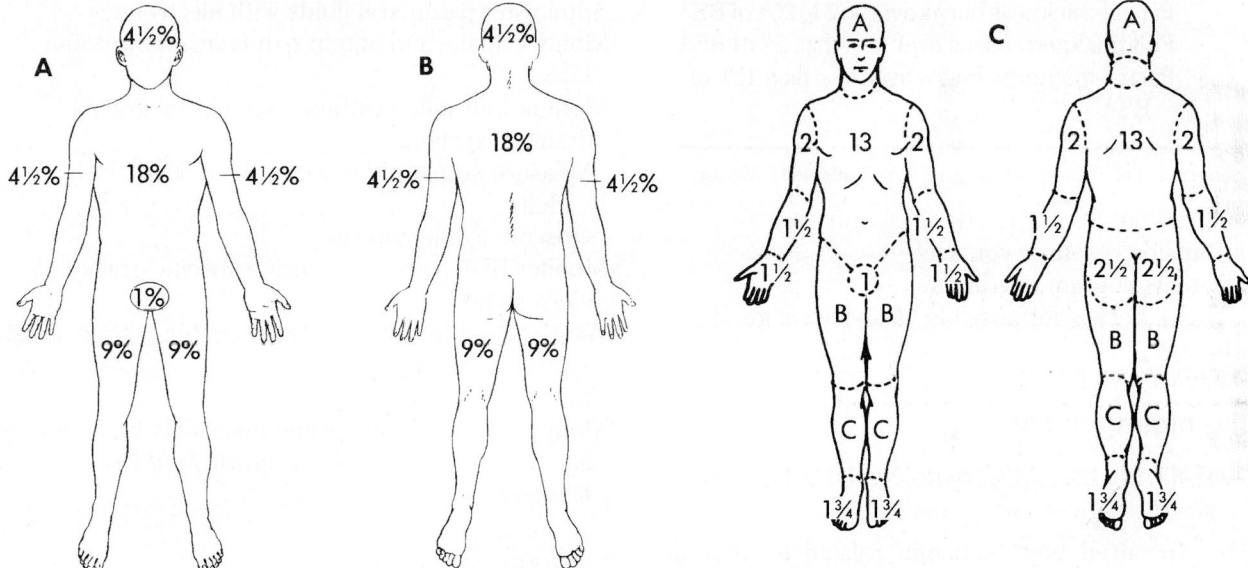

Relative percentages of areas affected by growth
(age in years)

	0	1	5	10	15	Adult
A: half of head	9½	8½	6½	5½	4½	3½
B: half of thigh	2¾	3¼	4	4¼	4½	4¾
C: half of leg	2½	2½	2¾	3	3¼	3½

Second degree _____ and
Third degree _____ =
Total percent burned ___

Figure 12-2   Estimation of adult burn injury: rule of nines. **A,** Anterior view. **B,** Posterior view.
C, Estimation of burn injury: Lund and Browder chart. Areas designated by letters *(A, B,* and *C)*
represent percentages of body surface area that vary according to age. The accompanying table
indicates the relative percentages of these areas at various stages in life. (From Sabiston DC Jr, editor:
Textbook of surgery: the biological basis of modern surgical practice, ed 11, Philadelphia, 1977, WB
Saunders Co.)

Table 12-3 American Burn Association Classification of Burn Injury

Class	Description
Major	Full-thickness burns over 10% or more of body surface area (BSA)
	Partial-thickness burns over 25% of BSA
	All burns on face, hands, eyes, ears, feet, or perineum
	All inhalation and electrical burns
	All burns complicated by trauma
	All burns in poor-risk patients
Moderate	Full-thickness burns over 2% to 10% of BSA
	Partial-thickness burns over 15% to 25% of BSA
Minor	Full-thickness burns over less than 2% of BSA
	Partial-thickness burns over less than 15% of BSA

From Thompson et al: *Clinical nursing*, ed 3, St Louis, 1993, Mosby.

Supply outside resource contacts
Rehabilitation program exercises
Occupational therapy for possible lifestyle change
Hydrotherapy

Nursing management

PATIENT PROBLEMS/NURSING DIAGNOSES

● **NDX:** Impaired gas exchange related to altered alveolar-capillary membrane and/or hypovolemia

Assess respiratory status
Monitor breath sounds qh; observe for decreased breath sounds, tachypnea, dyspnea, cough, pallor, and cyanosis
Monitor ABGs and vital signs *to assess hypoxic status*
Assess for signs of hypoxia: tachycardia, altered mental acuity
Maintain patent airway; perform orotracheal suction as needed; position patient for optimal ventilation *to prevent airway obstruction*
Monitor mechanical ventilation and endotracheal tube for correct settings and function *to assist in airway management*
Assist patient with turning q2h and deep breathing qh *to prevent hypostatic pneumonia*

Provide rest periods; avoid overexertion and assist with ADLs as needed *to reduce overtaxation of respiratory system*
Administer oxygen therapy *to reduce hypoxic state*
Administer broncholytic agents *to open alveoli and increase respiratory competency*
Assist/perform chest physiotherapy and incentive spirometer *to drain and expand the lungs*

EXPECTED OUTCOMES

Respirations are slow, regular
Breath sounds are clear
ABGs are within normal limits

● **NDX:** Fluid volume deficit related to burns

Monitor for dehydration, reduced skin turgor, dry mucous membranes, decreased mental acuity
Maintain NPO
Administer parenteral fluids with electrolytes
Monitor intake and output q4h *to assess hydration status*
Monitor indwelling catheter and closed gravity drainage system
Measure output qh; report <30 to 50 ml/hr in adults
Observe for hematuria
Monitor BUN, creatinine, urine specific gravity, electrolytes
Weigh patient daily: same time, clothing, scale, *to assess hydration status*
Monitor mental acuity q8h
Monitor wound drainage and insensible fluid loss and add to output *to establish accurate fluid loss measurement*

EXPECTED OUTCOMES

Intake is balanced with output
Skin turgor is normal
Mucous membranes are moist
Electrolytes are within normal limits

● **NDX:** Altered tissue perfusion: cardiopulmonary, gastrointestinal (GI), peripheral, renal, cerebral related to hypovolemia/edema

Cardiopulmonary system
  Assess for signs of dehydration
    Skin turgor if able
    Mucous membranes
    Decreased urine output
  Monitor vital signs q1h to 2h (48 hr)
  Monitor CVP, Swan-Ganz lines
  Monitor for dysrhythmias

Administer blood replacement as prescribed

Monitor CBC, electrolytes, arterial gases

Encourage leg movement if able *to promote venous return*

Assess respiratory status q2h to 4h: depth, rate, quality

GI system

Assess bowel sounds q4h; measure girth if sounds are absent *to monitor for ileus,* a possible complication in first 24 hr

Observe for nausea/vomiting, gastric distention

Monitor nasogastric tube functioning

Measure output q4h

Maintain patency

Observe for signs of bleeding; *may indicate stress ulcer*

Maintain bowel function

Provide softeners, natural laxatives

Observe for diarrhea, constipation

Monitor for signs of bleeding, tarry stools

Peripheral system

Monitor extremities for color, temperature, mobility, sensation, edema

Assess pedal pulses q4h

Monitor antiembolic stockings if applicable; remove daily and observe skin for redness

Encourage ROM exercises to unaffected extremities *to promote circulation*

Provide warmth to extremities

Elevate affected extremity *to reduce edema and encourage circulation*

Assess for compartment syndrome: unrelenting calf, thigh, arm pain, edema

Renal system

Maintain NPO

Administer parenteral fluids

Monitor intake and output q4h

Monitor indwelling catheter and closed gravity drainage system

Measure output qh; report <30 to 50 ml/hr in adults; 1 to 1.5 ml/kg/hr in children

Observe for hematuria; monitor with Hemastix; monitor specific gravity

Assess skin turgor for dehydration

Monitor BUN, creatinine, urine specific gravity *to assess renal function*

Weigh patient daily: same time, clothing, scale *to prevent possible fluid overload*

Cerebral system

Assess mental acuity and level of consciousness (LOC) q8h

Assess neurologic status; document baseline assessment

Monitor blood gases; report decrease in Po_2 to physician

EXPECTED OUTCOMES

Tissue perfusion is adequate as evidenced by normal vital signs, balanced intake and output, normal laboratory results and ABGs

Respirations are slow, regular

Peripheral pulses are present

Available skin turgor, mucous membranes are normal

Mental acuity is normal

● **NDX:** Risk for infection related to inadequate primary defenses, trauma

Maintain isolation precautions, scrupulous handwashing, and aseptic technique; wear gown, mask, gloves as indicated *to prevent further infection*

Monitor vital signs q2h to 4h to assess for signs of infection: fever and tachycardia

Monitor for other signs of infection: increased redness and pain, purulent drainage, odor

Monitor invasive hemodynamic monitoring lines and indwelling urethral catheter for infection; culture as indicated

Assess laboratory values: WBC, urinalysis, leukocytosis

Limit visitors to patient's *significant* others, especially exclude people with upper respiratory infections (URIs)

Administer tetanus toxoid as indicated

Administer topical/systemic antibiotics as indicated; assess effectiveness, side effects

Monitor for sepsis: fever, tachypnea, altered sensorium, decreased platelets, hyperglycemia

Initiate local burn therapy using the following principles, which are general considerations

Obtain culture for burn areas as needed

Cleanse burn and remove all pieces of detached epithelium; cleanse with saline or mild soap and tap water (hexachlorophene is not recommended)

Debride, using sterile equipment

Remove dirt and blood

Shave surrounding area

Prevent destruction of viable epithelium; prevent burned surfaces from touching viable skin or other burned surfaces

Produce environment unfavorable to bacterial growth

Aid separation of burn slough

Apply skin coverage as soon as possible

Initiate one of the following topical burn agents as ordered

Silver nitrate: antiinfective agent; penetrates burn slowly, is very painful; burn/dressings must be kept saturated; causes electrolyte imbalance and turns all surfaces black

Povidone-iodine (Betadine): broad-spectrum antiinfective; is very painful and may cause increased iodine absorption

Silver sulfadiazine 1% (Silvadene)
    Broad-spectrum antibiotic; is slow to absorb but relatively painless; may decrease WBC
    Monitor serum chloride and pH; WBC
    Mafenide acetate (Sulfamylon): antiinfective agent; penetrates burn well but is painful; may cause rash, decreased $Paco_2$
Examine wounds daily and prn to assess change in odor, appearance, amount of drainage
Apply dressings to prevent skin-to-skin contact: each finger, toe

EXPECTED OUTCOMES

Burned areas begin to heal adequately
Temperature is normal
Laboratory values are within normal limits
Surrounding tissue is clean, dry, and intact

● **NDX:**   Impaired skin integrity related to trauma

Assess skin for signs of trauma, rashes, reddened areas
Maintain in prescribed position or position of comfort
Assess pressure areas; change position and support with pillows, padding as indicated
Provide bathing and oral care as needed
Monitor mucous membranes if nasogastric tube is in place; keep nares moist
Administer lotions to unaffected areas *to promote comfort and prevent breakdown*
Assess size, depth, color of burned area; observe surrounding tissue for redness or necrosis
Maintain isolation procedures as indicated
Monitor burn covering, dressing prn
    Dressings: gauze in layers; fine mesh to cover area, then coarse mesh to absorb drainage, and lastly a pressure dressing; change bid
    Hydrocolloid (DuoDerm) aids in healing; leave on 4 to 5 days
    Polyurethane foam (Epi-Lock) remains 1 wk
Monitor skin graft area
    Homograft: from deceased person
    Autograft: from unburned area of patient

Heterograft: pigskin or synthetic
    Autologous: epithelium cells cultured into sheets
Maintain correct body alignment and elevate affected graft, dressing site if appropriate
Monitor sites for signs of healing
Maintain dressings/grafts as indicated

EXPECTED OUTCOMES

Healing is adequate
Burn sites are regenerating new tissue
Other tissue/skin areas are free from trauma

● **NDX:**   Impaired physical mobility related to decreased strength and endurance

Maintain bed rest in prescribed position *to promote healing*
Monitor neuromuscular status q4h *to prevent contractures*
Maintain body alignment within parameters of treatment
Prevent contractures and/or hypertrophy
    Head and neck: do not use pillows (Figure 12-3)
    Hand (Figure 12-4)
    Upper chest, axilla, and arms (Figure 12-5): maintain arm at 90-degree angle, away from body and slightly above shoulder
    Ankles and feet (Figure 12-6): use footboard with patient in supine position
    Legs: traction/splints may be used
Explain necessity of positions, which can be uncomfortable; position of comfort can be position for forming contractures
Administer analgesics before procedures *to reduce pain and enhance movement*
Apply and maintain pressure dressings on graft partial thickness wounds *to prevent scarring and contractures*
Assist with and teach active or perform passive ROM exercises on unaffected extremities *to maintain muscle strength*
Coordinate care to allow for rest periods *to prevent fatigue*
Encourage patient to perform self-care activities

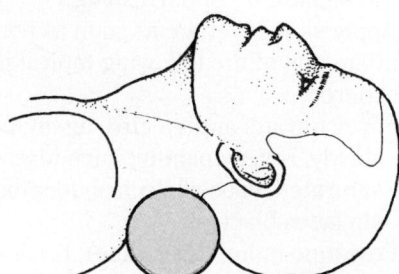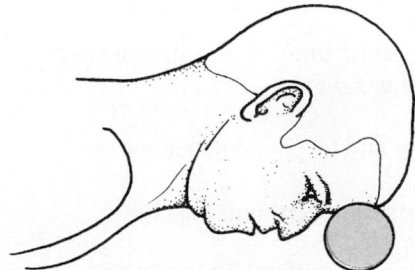

Figure 12-3   Positioning for head and neck burns to prevent contractures.

Change position frequently *to prevent fatigue and pressure;* low-air-loss/air fluidized beds may be required to promote position changes

Refer patient for physiotherapy and/or hydrotherapy as indicated *to provide individualized activity/exercise program*

Ambulate as soon as possible *to prevent respiratory compromise*

EXPECTED OUTCOMES

Participates in prescribed activities and therapy
Maintains correct body alignment
Demonstrates ability to balance rest with activities

● **NDX:** Altered nutrition: less than body requirements related to thermal injury

Maintain adequate hydration, nutrition *to replace lost fluids and promote healing* (Table 12-4)

Provide TPN (p. 64), tube feedings (p. 59) if appropriate *to maintain needed calorie intake*

Monitor serum/finger stick glucose, Clinitest/Acetest *to assess for hyperglycemia*

Provide high-protein, high-calorie diet as ordered and tolerated

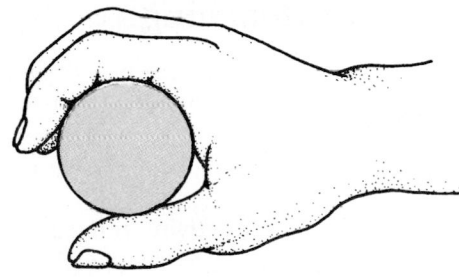

Figure 12-4   Positioning of hand burn to prevent contractures.

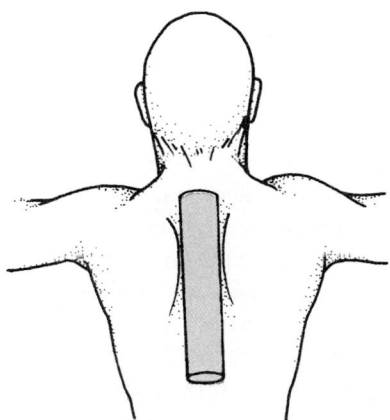

Figure 12-5   Placement of contracture roll for upper chest, axilla, and arm burns.

Protein: 3 g/kg/day
Fat: 20% of calories
Carbohydrate: remainder of calories

Provide small, frequent meals; encourage oral fluids: milk, juice *to assure correct intake and prevent gastric distention*

Perform meticulous calorie count after meals *to evaluate/adjust required intake*

Involve patient in food selection, preferences
Encourage family to provide home-cooked food
Perform oral hygiene before and after meals *to provide comfort and encourage eating*

Assist with feeding as needed; advance position to sitting in chair for meals when tolerated *to prevent aspiration and promote digestion*

Weigh patient daily: same time, clothing, scale *to monitor effectiveness of diet*

EXPECTED OUTCOMES

Regains lost weight to within 2% to 5% of normal
Participates in food selection and calorie count
Selects foods that increase healing potential

PATIENT PROBLEMS/NURSING DIAGNOSES

● **NDX:** Pain related to destruction of tissue

Elevate each extremity periodically *to decrease edema, pain*

Cover burn to decrease discomfort if applicable *because air movement may cause increased pain*

Maintain comfortable temperature/humidity because body temperature regulation may be altered

Assess location, type, and severity of pain; assess intensity with pain rating scale to monitor for increasing intensity, which may indicate complications

Administer analgesics; assess effectiveness of pain relief measures; decrease narcotics as soon as possible *to prevent addiction*

Collaborate with physician and instruct patient in use of patient controlled analgesia (PCA)

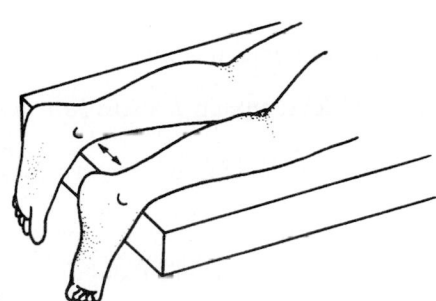

Figure 12-6   Correct foot and ankle positioning to prevent foot and ankle contractures.

Table 12-4 Calculation of Fluid Replacement for Burns: Brooke Formula

NOTE: Many formulas are in use; Brooke formula is moderate and most frequently used

CALCULATION FOR ADULTS

First 24 hr (calculated from time of burn, not admission)

Lactated Ringer's solution: 2 to 4 ml/kg/percentage body surface area (BSA) burned

Five percent dextrose in water: 2000 ml; adjusted to keep urine output at 30 to 50 ml/hr

Half of the solution is to be given in the first 8 hr, and the other half in next 16 hr

Second 24 hr

Colloids (albumin, dextran, or plasma): 0.5 ml/kg/ percentage of body surface area (BSA) burned; half the amount is given in the first 24 hr

Lactated Ringer's solution: half the amount is given in the first 24 hr

Five percent dextrose in water: 2000 ml

Allow time to discuss feelings about pain

Perform dressing changes only after patient is medicated as needed *to provide comfort*

Offer diversional activities *to decrease attention on pain*

Encourage use of alternate pain relief measures: relaxation techniques, imaging, deep breathing

Encourage small shifts in position *to promote comfort*

EXPECTED OUTCOMES

Reports a tolerable pain level

Presents calm, relaxed facial affect

Demonstrates use of alternate pain relief measures

● **NDX:**   Body image disturbance related to possible disfigurement from burns

Assess feelings of loss, anxiety *to assist patient to work through feelings*

Express acceptance of feelings *to prevent feelings of rejection*

Encourage and allow time for verbalization of concerns/feelings; include significant others; provide privacy

Set realistic short-term goals and acknowledge tasks attempted and/or completed *to inspire confidence*

Allow patient to progress through stages of grief at own pace

Maintain nonjudgmental attitude and avoid nonverbal rejection; discourage maladaptive behavior

Assess present coping attitudes and assist patient with identifying successful past behaviors

Promote self-care activities as soon as possible *to foster self-confidence*

Involve patient with unit routine and other burn patients *to increase support base*

Collaborate with social service agencies for financial, family, and educational assistance

EXPECTED OUTCOMES

Begins to acknowledge altered image

Discusses feelings/anxieties with increasing confidence

Undertakes goal setting for future

Participates in self-care activities

ADDITIONAL NURSING DIAGNOSES TO CONSIDER

Constipation related to immobility, medications

Powerlessness related to length of treatment regimen

Fear/anxiety related to risk of disfigurement and/or separation from support groups

Patient/family teaching

Provide written dietary instructions; discuss importance of maintaining normal weight and adequate fluid intake

Explain rehabilitation plan and use of pressure garment if applicable

Discuss maintaining normal activity with planned rest periods; prevent boredom with diversional activities

Demonstrate burn care
  Wash hands
  Cleanse wound with mild soap
  Rinse well
  Pat dry using clean towel
  Apply topical ointment/dressing

Discuss care of healing wound/scars: apply cocoa butter, Nivea cream after washing with mild soap/water and rinsing well bid; may use Silastic gel sheeting to prevent hypertrophic scarring

Wear nonirritating, loose clothing

Explain care of pressure garment
  Wash and rinse well daily with mild soap and water
  Allow to dry flat on towels
  Observe for signs of skin irritation
  Have garment checked for correct fit at follow-up appointments

Promote use of moisturizers, sunscreen to decrease irritation; avoid sunlight, detergents, fabric softeners

Explain symptoms to report to physician
  Fever, malaise
  Bleeding, odor, and drainage from burn area
Discuss medication schedule including name, purpose, dosage, and side effects; caution patient to avoid taking over-the-counter medications unless approved by physician
Avoid contact with persons with infections, especially URIs
Provide names and phone numbers of home health care team
Encourage follow-up visits with physician, physical therapist

Home care considerations

Assess and continue with patient/family teaching and evaluate the following:
  Burn site(s)/skin
    Healing progress
    Signs of infection
    Dressing change procedure; aseptic technique
    Supplies: where and what to purchase
    Pressure garment use if indicated
    Pain control
    Exercise and rehabilitation programs
    ROM exercises to extremities as prescribed
    Diversional activities to prevent boredom and decrease attention on pain
    Rest periods interspersed with activities
  Nutrition/elimination
    Weight

High-carbohydrate, high-protein diet with supplemental vitamins
    Intake of 2500 to 3000 ml/day of fluids
    Bowel function; use of stool softeners, natural laxatives
  Emotional
    Degree of coping with anxiety/body image change
    Knowledge of community resources: homemaker service, counselors, Meals-on-Wheels

BIBLIOGRAPHY

Barnes HR: Alternating transparent and hydrocolloid dressings, *Nursing '93* 23(3):59, 1993.
Beare PG, Myers JL: *Principles and practice of adult health nursing,* ed 2, St Louis, 1994, Mosby.
Bergstrom N et al: How to predict and prevent pressure ulcers, *Am J Nurs* 92(7):52, 1992.
Calistro AM: Burn care basics and beyond, *RN* 56(3):26, 1993.
Doenges ME et al: *Nursing care plans: guidelines for planning and documenting patient care,* ed 3, Philadelphia, 1993, FA Davis.
Flory C: Skin assessment, *RN* 55(6):22, 1992.
Kim MJ et al: *Pocket guide to nursing diagnoses,* ed 6, St Louis, 1995, Mosby.
Maklebust J: Pressure ulcer update, *RN* 54(12):56, 1991.
McCance KL, Huether SE: *Pathophysiology, the biological basis for disease in adults and children,* ed 2, St Louis, 1994, Mosby.
McFarland GK, McFarlane EA: *Nursing diagnosis and intervention: planning for patient care,* ed 2, St Louis, 1993, Mosby.
Motta GJ: How moisture-retentive dressings promote healing, *Nursing '93* 23(12):26, 1993.
Rogers-Seidle FF: *Geriatric nursing care plans,* St Louis, 1991, Mosby.
Schmidtling RE et al: Treating pressure ulcers with a myocutaneous flap, *Nursing '92* 22(7):56, 1992.
Thompson JM et al: *Mosby's clinical nursing,* ed 3, St Louis, 1993, Mosby.

Optic and Auditory Systems

Optic System (Figure 13-1)

Assessment

Subjective Data

Blurred or double vision
Light, flashes, rainbows, or halos seen
Decreased or absent vision
Decreased night or peripheral vision
Objects held too near or far
Needs stronger light to see
Collides with unfamiliar objects
Eye fatigue and strain
Tenderness or pain: sudden or gradual onset
Eyes water and itch
Dryness of eyes
Increased tearing
Trauma to head, face, or eyes
Inability to see in bright light
Headache
Squinting
Frequent falls
Clumsiness

Objective Data

General appearance
Age of patient
Vital signs: elevated blood pressure (BP), temperature (T), pulse (P), or
  respiratory rate (R)

Gerontologic Considerations

- Multiple changes in vision that normally occur with aging include the following:
  - Changes in accommodation, resulting in increased difficulty focusing on close objects (presbyopia), which leads to difficulty reading or doing other close work
  - Decreased color perception and discrimination, particularly with shades of blue, green, and violet
  - Poor adaptation to changes in light, resulting in "night blindness" and increased sensitivity to glare
  - Alterations in depth perception, leading to increased risk of falls
  - Decreased secretion of tears, resulting in complaints of dryness or pruritus, which leads to a high risk for irritation of the cornea
  - Increased incidence of moving particles or "floaters" that interfere with visually based tasks
- Older adults experience an increased incidence of eye disorders including cataracts, retinal detachment, macular degeneration, and glaucoma.

Modified from Christensen BL, Kockrow EO: *Foundations of nursing,* ed 2, St Louis, 1995, Mosby.

Wears glasses, contact lenses, or eye patch
Position of reading material
Conjunctivitis
Drainage
  Amount
  Type
Hemorrhage
Rubbing eyes
Eyelid changes: edema, ptosis, redness, eversion, inversion
Amount of dependence or independence
Visual acuity
Exophthalmos
Ability to close eyelid(s)
Ability to blink
Abnormal eye movement
Opaqueness of eyeball
Increased tearing
Head tilts to improve vision
Squinting
Medication, eyedrops used

Allergies
Strabismus
Nystagmus
Scleral edema, infection, jaundice
Chalazion
Foreign body
Laceration, contusion
Enucleation

● Pertinent Background Information

Concurrent diseases or conditions

Multiple sclerosis
Diabetes mellitus
Hypothyroidism
Hyperthyroidism
Sinus problems
Hypertension
Cerebral-associated diseases, trauma, or tumors
Sexually transmitted diseases
Myasthenia gravis
Glaucoma
Cataract
Retinal detachment
Autoimmune diseases
Arthritis, rheumatism

Previous surgery or illness

Eye surgery or treatments
Head or face trauma
Oxygen therapy as newborn
Coma
Hypertension
Substance abuse
Macular degeneration

Family history

Glaucoma
Diabetes mellitus
Cataracts
Retinitis pigmentosa

Social history

Hazardous job or recreation
Safety precautions taken
Alcohol or drug abuse
Sexually transmitted diseases

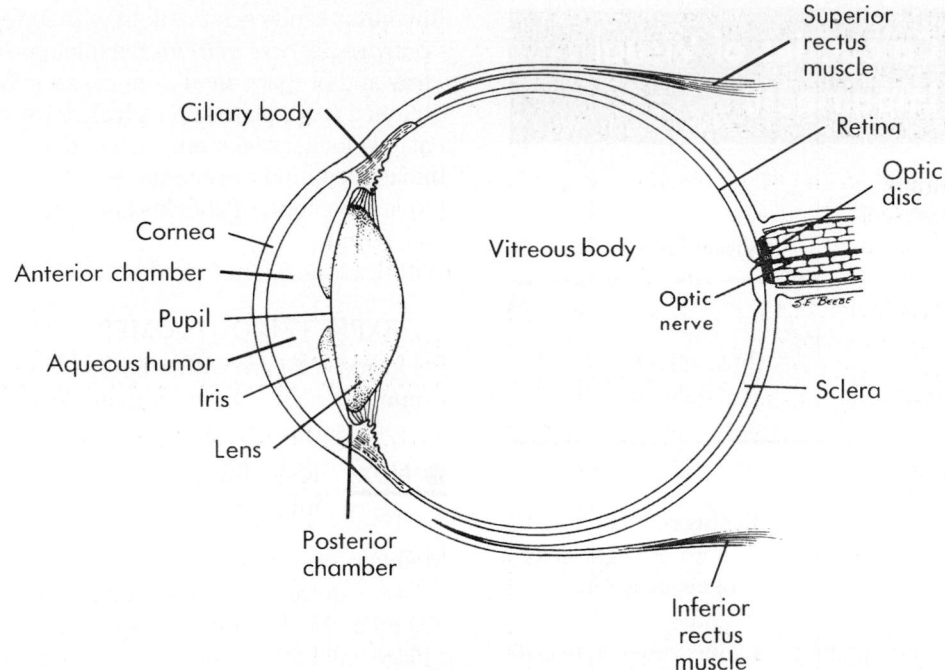

Figure 13-1 The eye.

Medication history

Antibiotics
Antiemetics
Miotics
Acetazolamide
Mydriatics
Beta blockers
Epinephrine derivatives
Steroids (systemic, topical)
Antilipidemic agents
Hydroxychloroquine sulfate (Plaquenil)

Color vision test
Refraction
Microscopic procedures
Conjunctival scrapings

● Diagnostic Tests

Visual fields and acuity
Biopsy and cultures
Magnetic resonance imaging (MRI)
Computed tomography (CT) scan
X-ray studies of orbit and skull
Ophthalmoscopic evaluation: direct, indirect
Slit lamp examination
Tonometry
Fluorescein angiography, stain
Ultrasonography
Gonioscopy
Brain scan
Ultrasound
Electroretinogram (ERG)

Visually Impaired Patient

The loss of visual acuity that encompasses partial or low vision to that of total blindness (Table 13-1)

Assessment

Observations/findings

Status of impairment
  Temporary (eye patch, shield)
  Permanent
Duration of impairment
Degree of visual loss
Degree of acceptance of impairment
Cause of visual impairment: diabetes, stroke, aneurysms, brain tumor, trauma, glaucoma
Condition of eyes: drainage, redness, pain, edema, squinting, abnormal eye movements, rubbing, opacities
Ability to perform activities of daily living (ADLs)

Table 13-1 Categories of Visual Impairment

Category	Visual Acuity (with Optimum Correction)	Visual Field Radius
LOW VISION STATUS		
1	20/70	Not defined
2	20/70 to 20/200	Not defined
BLINDNESS STATUS		
3	Able to count fingers at 3 m; 20/200 to 20/400	Radius reduced to 5-10 degrees regardless of visual acuity status
4	Able to count fingers at 1 m; 20/400 to 20/1200 (5/300)	Radius reduced to 5-10 degrees regardless of visual acuity status
5	No light perception	—

From Thompson JM et al: *Mosby's clinical nursing,* ed 3, St Louis, 1993, Mosby.

Collaborative management

Nursing management

PATIENT PROBLEMS/NURSING DIAGNOSES

● **NDX:** Sensory/perceptual alterations: visual related to impairment

Familiarize patient with surroundings *to promote confidence*

Place all utensils and personal articles within easy reach and maintain consistent placement

Use patient's senses of touch and smell during orientation

Describe location of doors, windows, furniture, bathroom, and other patients

Establish effective lines of communication *to ensure understanding*

Always identify self when approaching or touching patient

Call patient by name

Explain purpose of visit and visit often, especially at night

Use visual aids: magnifying glasses, large print

Encourage and assist patient with independence *to encourage self-care activities:* explain position of food on tray and prepare food as necessary; use clock sequence (e.g., plate at 6 o'clock, fruit at 10 o'clock, milk at 1 o'clock); assist only as needed

Initiate grooming procedures as tolerated

Explain position of articles and place in same position each time

Withdraw assistance gradually

EXPECTED OUTCOMES

Performs self-care within limits of impairment

Communicates effectively using learned skills

● **NDX:** Risk for injury/trauma related to visual impairment

Maintain safe environment *to prevent accidents, injuries*

Place siderails up while patient is in bed

Keep bed in locked, low position

Place call bell and needed articles within easy reach

Maintain environment as described (e.g., furniture, footstools, IV poles, wastebaskets)

Keep doors fully open or closed

Flag chart and bed, indicating degree, type of visual impairment, and eye affected *to provide continuity of care*

Encourage patient to call nurse before ambulating; assist by standing on affected side

Instruct patient to avoid use of sharp items such as razors, scissors, and glass without supervision

EXPECTED OUTCOMES

Demonstrates ability to perform activities in a safe manner

Verbalizes understanding of needed limitations

● **NDX:** Anxiety related to degree of visual impairment

Assess level of anxiety and normal coping mechanisms *to provide a basis for assistance*

Encourage and allow time for verbalization of feelings

Explain daily plan of care and procedures *to reduce anxiety level*

Allow as much independence as safety permits

Provide reassurance by being available and answering all questions

Provide time for use of relaxation measures

Encourage visitors and communication with significant others

Identify and reinforce use of adaptive coping mechanisms *to improve self-esteem*

Present a calm, caring attitude

Provide diversional activities *to reduce attention on anxiety*

EXPECTED OUTCOMES

Identifies causative factors of anxiety

Accepts limitations and seeks ways to use remaining sight

Seeks assistance appropriately

● **NDX:** Body image disturbance related to visual impairment

Discuss with patient and significant others alternatives in managing ADLs: dressing, bathing, grooming

Assess past coping mechanisms that have been successful

Allow time for patient to verbalize feelings *to reduce frustration*

Demonstrate acceptance of these feelings

Provide quiet, encouraging environment

Assist with and teach new skills as needed

Discuss and set small, realistic goals *to increase self-confidence*

Provide praise and encouragement

Promote support by significant other

Encourage involvement with others *to avoid isolation*

Assist patient in discussing and accepting altered visual acuity

Encourage independence as tolerated

Encourage use of other senses: touch, smell, hearing

EXPECTED OUTCOMES

Demonstrates adaptive responses to altered body image

Expresses awareness of change and progresses toward acceptance

ADDITIONAL NURSING DIAGNOSES TO CONSIDER

Self-esteem disturbance related to visual loss

Family coping: potential for growth related to acceptance of visual loss

Risk for injury at home related to loss of vision

Patient/family teaching

Reinforce safety precautions related to furniture placement, sharp objects and corners, scatter rugs, objects on floor

Reinforce physician's explanation of disease, disease process, and need to notify physician of any changes in condition

Assist patient and/or significant other in managing ADLs

Promote self-care within limits of visual impairment

Demonstrate procedure for instillation of eyedrops

Refer to home health care agency and/or organizations for the visually impaired*

Maintain regular outpatient care visits with physician

Home care considerations

See Home care considerations for the visually impaired patient (p. 801)

Acute Glaucoma: Adult Onset

acute (closed-angle) glaucoma: Disease characterized by suddenly impaired vision resulting from intraocular pressure caused by imbalance in production and excretion of aqueous humor; if left untreated may cause optic nerve degeneration, visual field loss, and total blindness

Assessment

Subjective data

Rapid onset of severe pain in eye(s)

Blurred vision

Headache

Rainbows in artificial light

Halos around lights

Nausea

Objective data

Vomiting

Dilated pupil(s)

Diagnostic tests

Tonometry

Gonioscopy

Visual fields

Visual acuity

Ophthalmoscopy

Potential complications

Infection

Increased intraocular pressure (IOP)

---

*American Foundation for the Blind, 15 West 16th St., New York, NY 10011.

Increased visual impairment
Blindness if untreated

Collaborative management

Therapeutic management

Miotic beta blocker eyedrops
Carbonic anhydrase inhibitors
Hyperosmotic agents
Antiemetics
Analgesics
Laser iridotomy
Iridectomy

Nursing management

PATIENT PROBLEMS/NURSING DIAGNOSES

● **NDX:** Pain related to increased IOP

Assess type, intensity, and location of pain; be alert for
  signs of increased IOP
Use pain rating scale to determine analgesia dose
Maintain bed rest in quiet, darkened room with
  head elevated 30 degrees or in position of comfort
Administer analgesics and diuretics: assess for effectiveness, side effects; avoid morphine, which may
  cause nausea and vomiting
Avoid nausea and vomiting, which increase IOP: administer antiemetics as needed
Administer osmotics, carbonic anhydrase inhibitors *to*
  decrease aqueous production
Assess visual acuity
Administer back rubs, position changes *to promote*
  comfort

EXPECTED OUTCOMES

Demonstrates knowledge of pain control measures
Experiences and demonstrates periods of uninter-
  rupted sleep
Exhibits decreased IOP

● **NDX:** Anxiety related to altered health status and
  decreased visual acuity

Assess anxiety level
Discuss previous coping methods *to provide a basis for*
  counseling
Encourage verbalization of anxieties
Maintain calm environment
Provide emotional support
Answer questions honestly
Explain all procedures

Reinforce physician's explanation of disease process
  and surgery if indicated
Visit frequently, especially at night
Explain nursing care plan
Discuss visual limitations as needed
Place all needed articles within reach and strive to keep
  them in same place at all times *to provide continuity of*
  care
Reassure that assistance with ADLs will be available
Assist and teach relaxation techniques: deep breathing,
  meditation, imagery
Provide information and support for possible laser iri-
  dotomy (see Eye surgery, p. 799)

EXPECTED OUTCOMES

Demonstrates adaptive coping measures to reduce
  anxiety
Expresses understanding of disease process

Patient/family teaching

Teach eyedrop instillation procedure to patient and sig-
  nificant other(s)
  Discuss possible side effects
    Interactions of eye medications with those pre-
      scribed for other diseases such as hypertension, di-
      abetes, COPD
    Maleate (Timoptic): depression, bradycardia,
      asthma
    Miotics: blurred vision, diarrhea
    Acetazolamide (Diamox): hyperkalemia, confusion,
      impotence
  Always count drops and do not miss a dose
  Keep extra bottles of drops in case of loss or
    breakage
  Stress that drops will be needed over extended
    period
  Discuss name, dose, and administration times of med-
    ications
  Emphasize need to wear and carry medical alert
    bracelet and card
  Stress importance of never taking medication contain-
    ing atropine or any over-the-counter medications
    without consulting physician
Discuss symptoms of IOP to report to physician
  Severe pain in eye(s)
  Blurred vision
  Headache
  Halos or rainbows
  Nausea, vomiting
Refer to agencies for visually impaired*
Explain importance of follow-up care with physician

---

*Lions Club International, 300 22nd St., Oak Brook, IL 60570.

Home care considerations

See Home care considerations for the visually impaired patient (p. 801)

Eye Surgery

cataract removal with or without intraocular lens transplant: *Surgical removal of a lens that has become opaque because of senile degenerative changes, trauma, or systemic disease (diabetes) or a congenitally opaque lens; an intraocular lens may be implanted simultaneously as an alternative to wearing cataract glasses or contact lenses postoperatively*

corneal transplant: *Surgical procedure to replace a damaged cornea with a healthy, clear donor cornea of equal size*

scleral buckling, retinal cryopexy, photocoagulation: *Surgical repair of a detached retina*

enucleation: *Surgical removal of a blind, painful eye globe while maintaining orbital integrity for insertion of a prosthesis*

iridectomy, iridencleisis, trabeculectomy, sclerotomy: *Surgical incision to release accumulated pressure caused by glaucoma by creating a channel for drainage of the aqueous humor*

NOTE: Patients with retinal detachment may need special positioning in bed, patching of the eye, and restrictions on activity to prevent further or complete detachment

Diagnostic tests

CBC, PT/INR
Ophthalmoscopy
Slit lamp examination
Visual fields

Preoperative assessment and teaching

Reinforce physician's explanation of surgical procedure to ensure patient is informed
Encourage and allow time for verbalization of fears and anxieties
Answer all questions with honesty, empathy, and understanding *to increase patient's confidence and knowledge*
Explain postoperative nursing care plan and availability of staff *to reduce anxiety*
Assess present degree of sight and assist as needed

Provide a safe environment; orient patient to room floor plan, placement of call bell, personal articles
Explain surgical preparation of eye according to hospital policy and physician's order *to involve patient and decrease fear*
Stress importance of wearing eye patch/shield postoperatively
Discuss with patient and teach not to bend, strain, lift heavy objects (more than 5 lb) postoperatively
Discuss importance of trying not to cough, sneeze, or vomit postoperatively
Advise patient not to touch or rub eyes *to prevent trauma or infection*
Explain that all eye make-up is removed before surgery

Postoperative assessment

Subjective data

Nausea
Sudden, severe eye pain

Objective data

Vomiting
Placement of eye bandage(s)
Restlessness
Position to be maintained while in bed

Potential complications

Hemorrhage
Shock
Infection
Decreased visual acuity
Blindness

Collaborative management

Therapeutic management

Medications
  Analgesics
  Antiemetics
  Antibiotics
  Stool softeners
Eye shield or patch
NPO until fully reactive, increase to presurgery diet
Ambulation and activities
Dressing changes/warm or cold sterile compresses
Prescription glasses

Nursing management

PATIENT PROBLEMS/NURSING DIAGNOSES

● **NDX:** Risk for infection related to invasive surgical procedure

Monitor dressing q2h for 4 hr, then q4h if present
Assess for drainage, bleeding, and/or pain: report immediately
Maintain eye shield or patch *to increase protection*
Caution patient not to touch, squeeze, or rub eye
Monitor vital signs q4h until stable

EXPECTED OUTCOMES

Temperature remains normal
Eye remains clean, with no purulent drainage

● **NDX:** Risk for injury/trauma related to altered visual acuity

Assess visual acuity
Keep siderails up at all times
Plan all care with patient; explain daily routines *to increase confidence and reduce anxiety*
Announce yourself when entering room *to avoid startling patient*
Assist with and teach deep-breathing exercises; stress need to avoid coughing, which increases IOP
Keep patient's articles in same place at bedside
Place call bell within easy reach
Enucleation patients have clean, plastic conformer in eye socket *to retain eye shape*
Stress need to avoid vomiting, which increases IOP; administer antiemetics
Increase activities and ambulation when patient demonstrates ability to remain safe
Assist with ambulation as needed; stand on affected side *to provide visual support*
Teach self-care activities and assist as needed

EXPECTED OUTCOMES

Demonstrates understanding of safety precautions
Notifies staff for assistance

● **NDX:** Pain related to surgical procedure

Assess pain intensity using pain rating scale
Administer analgesics; assess pain to ensure that it is not caused by increased IOP or bleeding; monitor for effectiveness
Administer back care and position changes *to relieve discomfort*
Teach and assist with alternate pain relief measures *to decrease attention on discomfort*

EXPECTED OUTCOMES

Reports a reduction of pain
Appears calm and relaxed

● **NDX:** Sensory/perceptual alteration related to impaired vision

Visit frequently *to determine needs and allay anxiety,* especially at night
Encourage patient to express feelings and thoughts
Involve significant others in care and activities *to provide support and assistance*
Reduce noise, traffic in area
Provide balanced rest and activity
Encourage diversional activities *to decrease attention on anxiety*
Allow patient to wear glasses, if allowed, *to increase sensory perception*

EXPECTED OUTCOMES

Accepts and copes appropriately with visual limitations
Uses remaining sight or other senses adequately

Patient/family teaching

General

Instruct patient and/or significant other in care of the eyes
  Dressing changes using aseptic techniques
  Use of eye patch or shield at night
  Method of eyedrop instillation
  Avoid rubbing, squeezing, or touching eye
  Use of eyeglasses as ordered; sunglasses to reduce glare
  Keep an extra bottle of eyedrops in case of loss or breakage and while traveling
Caution patient to avoid constipation, bending, vacuuming, straining, and lifting heavy objects (more than 5 lb)
Provide list of organizations for visually impaired (see p. 802)
Discuss home care with patient and family/significant other(s)
  Arrange furniture for safety and convenience
  Encourage self-care
  Avoid being overprotective
  Provide diversional activities: records, tapes, recorded books; television and reading if able
  Know name of medication, dosage, time of administration, purpose, and side effects
  Avoid using over-the-counter medications, eyedrops, or ointments without physician approval
  Make and keep follow-up appointments with physician

Discuss symptoms to report to physician
  Pain in eye
  Redness
  Drainage
  Decreased visual acuity
  Floaters
  Halos, sparks

Specific

See boxes below

Cataract Removal

Without lens implant, using glasses: explain that
  glasses
  Usually magnify objects 25% to 30%
  Decrease peripheral vision
  Can cause visual disturbance if fit is incorrect
  Allow patient to focus; patient will be unable to
    focus without them
  Are temporary glasses and new ones will be
    prescribed in about 2 to 12 wk
  Sometimes alter distance judgment
Without lens implant, using contact lenses: ex-
  plain that contact lenses
  Will be fitted and worn after 2 to 12 wk
  Allow patient to focus, but patient will need
    glasses for close vision
With intraocular lens implant: explain that lens
  implant
  Aids in focusing, but glasses will be fitted for
    close vision in 8 to 12 wk
  Does not cause depth perception loss

Trabeculectomy, Laser Iridotomy

Discuss signs of increased IOP
  Severe eye pain
  Headache
  Nausea
  Increased tearing
Explain importance of using glaucoma eye drops
  in unoperated eye
Advise to use nonaspirin pain medication to pre-
  vent bleeding

Scleral Buckling, Retinal Cryopexy

Discuss symptoms of further detachment
  Sudden loss of vision
  Severe pain
  Increased floaters
Explain that reading must be avoided for 1 wk

Corneal Transplant

Discuss signs of graft rejection
  Pain
  Inflammation
  Drainage
Explain that sutures will remain in eye up to a
  year

Enucleation

Conformer for eyeball may become dislodged;
  explain that this is of little consequence and it
  need not be reinserted
Discuss use of antibiotic drugs and need to wear
  eye shield until prosthesis is fitted (in about 10
  to 14 days)

Home Care Considerations for the Visually Impaired Patient

Assess and continue with patient/family education and
  monitor the following:
Environmental/safety status
  Evaluate and discuss
    Lighting for ease in movement
    Hand rails, carpet or nonskid treads on stairs
    Carpets and rugs secured to floor
    Presence of telephone and emergency numbers in
      large print
    Presence of Lifeline or Life Dial system for emer-
      gencies

Furniture arrangement adequate to allow a clear
pathway
Presence of smoke detectors, fire extinguishers
Nonslip strips in tub
Medications for easy administration; labeled cor-
rectly and in large enough print for identification
Ability to instill eyedrops correctly (see p. 803)
Presence of medication box that can be filled for
daily use
Presence of clock with large digital numbers or one
that chimes
Use of watch with raised numbers
Use of slippers, shoes in good repair with nonskid
soles
Use and availability of walker, cane
Use of available support groups
Presence of sharp objects, pointed corners
Safe placement of cleaning materials with all poi-
sons clearly marked
Adjusted water temperature to prevent burns
Transportation available for shopping, errands, and
medical appointments
Eye care status
Evaluate and discuss the following:
Dressing change procedure if indicated
Condition of the eye for signs of infections, red-
ness, pain, drainage
Procedure for instilling eyedrops
Medication for correct administration times
Handwashing technique
Personal care and hygiene status
Evaluate and discuss the following:
Availability of a care giver if needed
Ability to bathe self in tub, shower, sponge bath,
with or without assistance
Grooming ability (hair, nails, clothing selection,
shaving, make-up) with or without assistance
Dressing self: able to select and put on clothes with
or without assistance
Height of toilet seat for easy access on and off
Nutritional status
Evaluate and discuss the following:
Ability to prepare meals alone or with assistance
Adequate fluid intake
Selection of food to provide adequate nourishment
Weight to monitor adequate intake
Elimination status
Evaluate and discuss management of bowel elimina-
tion to prevent constipation with natural laxatives
(bran, prunes) or psyllium
Emotional status
Evaluate and discuss the following:
Degree of acceptance attained
Feelings of anxiety, low self-esteem, depression
(see p. 35)

Knowledge of outside support groups available

American Foundation for the Blind
Customer Service Division
15 W. 16th Street
New York, NY 10011
(800) 232-5463

National Eye Institute
National Institute of Health
Bldg. 31, Room 6A25
9000 Rockville Pike
Bethesda, MD 20014
(301) 496-2234

Importance of maintaining social interaction with
family and friends
Availability of communication devices such as
recorded books, telephone, alarm clocks, door-
bell, fire alarm attached to vibrating device
Knowledge of local groups providing braille
instruction

Contact Lens Removal

*Occasionally unconscious, paralyzed, disoriented, or elderly
patients and patients with limited or restricted use of
their arms may be wearing contact lenses; lenses must be
removed to prevent eye damage*

Assessment

Observations/findings

LOC/ability to cooperate
Presence of contact lenses in unconscious patient:
shine flashlight into eye from outer canthus;
lenses will appear around iris or slightly
beyond
Type of lenses
Hard: covers iris, may be tinted
Soft: covers iris, may be tinted
Extended wear (1 wk)
Disposable (1 wk)
Scleral: covers iris and sclera
Small suction cup apparatus for removing contact
lenses is often kept in emergency room

Removal procedure

Wash hands thoroughly before procedure
Removal of hard lenses
Place forefinger at outer canthus of eye
Gently push finger up and then down

Lens will appear from under lid
Store in distilled water, keeping right and left lenses
 separate and containers marked
Removal of soft lenses
 Place thumb and forefinger on lower and upper lid,
  respectively
 Gently open eye
 With other hand gently lift lens off iris, using thumb
  and forefinger
 Store in normal saline solution, keeping right and left
  lenses separate and containers marked, or discard if
  disposable
Removal of scleral lenses
 Place forefinger at edge of and parallel to lower
  lid
 Gently press lid downward until lower edge of lens is
  visible
 Continue gentle pressure, pulling lid toward ear
 Lens will slide out from under lid
 Store in distilled water, keeping right and left lenses
  separate and containers marked
Removal of all types of lenses using suction cup
 apparatus
 Depress bulb between thumb and forefinger
 Position cup over lens
 Slowly release pressure on bulb
 Lens will adhere to cup
 Remove lenses and store in marked containers with
  appropriate solution
If lenses are not visible (eyes rolled back) or difficulty
 is experienced in removal procedure, notify ophthal-
 mologist to remove lenses

Instillation of Eyedrops/Ointments

Preinstillation assessment

Assess patient's ability to hold eyes open and cooperate
Explain purpose of medication, procedure, and side
 effects
Perform medication assessment
 Correct medication, patient, dosage, time, and eye
 Check dropper for defects
 Understand abbreviations
  OD: right eye
  OS: left eye
  OU: both eyes

Instillation procedure (Figure 13-2)

Eyedrops are sterile, and any contamination of the
 dropper or squeeze bottle can cause infection
Always discard when contamination occurs

Position patient in chair with head tilted back or in dorsal recumbent position in bed
Wash hands before procedure
Draw medication into dropper (keep medication from
 going into bulb end) or open squeeze bottle of drops
 or tube of ointment
Gently pull down skin beneath lower lid with thumb
 and place forefinger above upper lid. Put pressure on
 the cheekbone, not on soft tissue of eye
Instruct patient to look upward
Allow time between drops: patient will blink after each
 drop
Instill drops or dab ointment into pocket formation in
 lower lid; do not touch conjunctiva with dropper or
 tube
Instruct patient to close eye gently and not to squeeze
 eye closed or rub it
Wipe off excess medication with tissue
Instruct patient to open and close eye slowly for a few
 minutes to distribute medication evenly

Auditory System (Figure 13-3)

Assessment

Subjective data

Earache (otalgia)
Decreased, absent hearing acuity in one or both ears
Tinnitis
Feeling of fullness in ear
Own voice echoes
Popping noise when yawning or swallowing
Vertigo, dizziness, disequilibrium
Itching in ear
Heart pulsating in ear
Ear drainage
 Dark
 Red

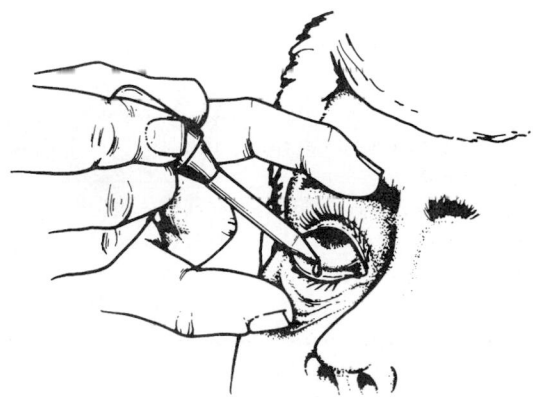

Figure 13-2 Instillation of eyedrops.

Clear
Yellow
Use of oils, cotton swabs, hairpins to clean ears

Objective data

General appearance
Vital signs: elevated BP, T, P, and R
Ability to hear; use of hearing aid
Ability to lip-read or use sign language
Startle reflex
Tolerance of loud sounds
Type, color, and amount of ear drainage
Medication history (streptomycin, salicylates, quinine, gentamycin)
Allergies

● Pertinent Background Information

Concurrent diseases or conditions

Otitis media
Otosclerosis
Acoustic nerve tumor
Labyrinthitis
Ménière's, Graves' disease
Cerebral tumors, contusion, diseases, fractures
Diabetes mellitus
Arteriosclerosis

Hypertension
Hypotension
Mastoiditis
Bleeding disorders

Previous surgery or illness

Stapes mobilization
Syphilis
Otitis media
Head trauma
Mastoidectomy

Social history

Sexually transmitted diseases
Recreational hazards: swimming, diving
Exposure to loud noises
Safety precautions taken
Use of tobacco, coffee, alcohol
Substance abuse

Medication history

Antineoplastics
Diuretics
Narcotics
Narcotic antagonists
Ear drops
Antibiotics

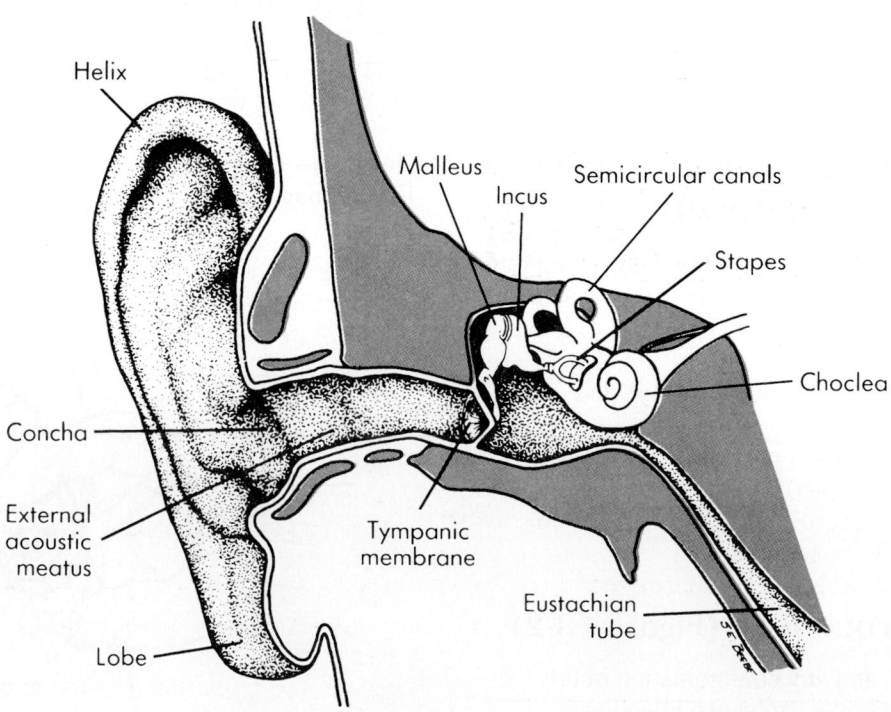

Figure 13-3 The ear.

Salicylates
Quinine

Diagnostic tests

Audiogram, audiometry, whisper test
Mastoid x-ray examination
Tuning fork test (Rinne)
Otological examination to assess for cerumen buildup,
  foreign objects
"Lateralization" tuning fork test (Weber)
Pneumatic otoscopy
Tympanometry, acoustic reflex test
Caloric examination
Electronystagmography (ENG)
Electrocochleography
Tomogram
Cerebral arteriography
CT scan
MRI
Schwabach test
Platform posturography
Culture for pathogens

Hearing-Impaired Patient

*The loss of hearing acuity that encompasses partial
  hearing loss to that of total deafness*
Types of loss
conduction: *An interference of sound waves through
  auditory canal, eardrum, middle ear*
sensorineural: *Injury or disease that affects the inner
  ear and nerve pathways to the brain*

 **Gerontologic Considerations**

- A third of all individuals over the age of 70 have
  significant hearing loss.
- Hearing loss in older adults is most often sensorineural and involves loss of the high frequencies. Hearing loss results in the distortion of
  speech, which can lead to failure to respond to
  directions or inappropriate behaviors often mis-
  interpreted as disorientation.
- Hearing loss can lead to social isolation when
  the older adult is unable to understand and participate in normal conversation.

Modified from Christensen BL Kockrow EO: *Foundations of nursing,*
ed 2, St Louis, 1995, Mosby.

mixed: *Interference with conduction in all three areas:
  external, middle, and inner ear*

Assessment

Observations/findings

Assess hearing acuity and communication skills
Lip-reading or sign language
Hearing aid
Pad and pencil
Flash cards
Determine status and duration of impairment
Assess acceptance of impairment and skills learned
  Well adjusted
  Fear/anxiety
  Anger, hostility
Examine ears for drainage, crusts, cerumen accumula-
  tion, and deformities

Collaborative management

Nursing management

PATIENT PROBLEMS/NURSING DIAGNOSES

● **NDX:** Sensory/perceptual alteration related to
  hearing impairment

Assess level of hearing impairment
Reinforce physician's explanation of hearing impairment
  to increase patient knowledge and feeling of security
Assess and establish means of communication
  Lip-reading (speech reading)
    Speak slowly and enunciate well
    Do not exaggerate sounds
    Have only one person speak at a time
    Stand so patient can see your mouth clearly
    Speak in simple phrases first to determine expertise
      in the skill
    NOTE: Nurses with mustaches may be more difficult
      to understand
    Point to objects of conversation where appropriate
    Avoid chewing gum and shouting
    Rephrase statements if not understood initially
  Sign language
    Determine whether patient can communicate with
      pad and pencil, because most hospital personnel
      are not skilled in sign language
    Enlist cooperation of family/significant other in com-
      munication *to provide support*
  Hearing aid
    Assess patient's ability to use and care for appliance
    Make certain aid is in place and turned on before
      speaking

Establish a pitch that is comfortable for patient
Avoid shouting
Stand so patient can see your face
Pad and pencil
Write messages clearly in short, simple phrases
Develop a checklist of phrases most often used and instruct patient to check appropriate one(s)
Allow time for patient to understand and answer

EXPECTED OUTCOMES

Accepts limitations caused by hearing impairment
Demonstrates positive coping behaviors
Uses learned skills for communicating

● **NDX:**   Risk for injury/trauma related to hearing impairment

Maintain safe environment
Locate bed so door is visible when possible
Orient patient to surroundings; have call bell within reach
Answer call light promptly
Keep siderails up if appropriate
Approach patient carefully if eyes are closed; a gentle touch on patient's arm will arouse but not startle
Explain all procedures *to ensure understanding*
Flag chart and bed indicating type of impairment and ear(s) involved *to provide continuity of care*

EXPECTED OUTCOMES

Understands safety factors associated with hearing impairment
Demonstrates ability to perform activities in safe manner
Notifies staff for assistance

● **NDX:**   Anxiety related to hearing impairment

Maintain quiet, nonstressful environment
Assess level of anxiety *to provide baseline for counseling*
Encourage and allow time for verbalization of feelings
Explain nursing plan of care and involve patient in planning care *to reduce anxiety level*
Display confidence and a caring, nonjudgmental manner
Use pictures when explaining procedures or treatment
Encourage communication with significant other *to provide support*
Avoid using electronic nurse-patient intercommunication system if patient has partial hearing because it can cause frustration
Evaluate patient's ability to use other senses (sight and touch especially) to aid in daily living
Provide diversional activities: puzzles, cards, hobbies *to decrease attention on anxiety*

EXPECTED OUTCOMES

Understands causes of anxiety
Demonstrates positive behaviors in coping with anxiety
Reports a reduction in anxiety level

Patient/family teaching

Reinforce physician's explanation of cause of impairment and prescribed treatment
Explain safety factors important in home environment
Discuss availability of hearing devices: amplifiers, flashing lights on telephones and door bells
Refer to local telephone company and/or hearing institute for assistance
Refer to local schools for classes on lip-reading and/or sign language
Instruct patient in care of hearing aid and to have extra battery available at all times
Demonstrate care of ear dressings and ear drop instillation if applicable
Encourage patient to make and keep follow-up appointments with physician

Home care considerations

See Home care considerations for the hearing-impaired patient (p. 810)

Ménière's Disease

A common disorder of the ear, both auditory and vestibular, that is thought to be caused by an alteration in the metabolism of the labyrinthine fluid of the vestibular system; this in turn causes the membrane of the labyrinth to dilate from the increased production of endolymph; severe attacks can be very disabling

Assessment

Observations/findings

Acute attack
Rapid onset: recurrent deafness
Tinnitus: usually roaring sensation
Incapacitating vertigo
Nausea, vomiting
Disequilibrium: falls toward affected ear
Blurred vision
Photophobia
Nystagmus
History of the following:
Otitis media
Arteriosclerosis
Allergies

Leukemia
Tobacco, alcohol, caffeine abuse
Medication use
Quinine
Salicylates
Streptomycin

Diagnostic tests

Audiologic testing
Audiometry
Electrocochleography
Electrostagmography
Audiogram
Caloric tests
X-ray examination of petrous bone

Potential complications

Dehydration
Increased hearing impairment
Permanent disequilibrium, vertigo
Fractures from falling

Collaborative management

Therapeutic management

Low-sodium or neutral ash diet
Diuretics: hydrochlorothiazide (Diuril), triamterene (Dyazide)
Vestibular depressants: diazepam (Valium), prochloperazine (Compazine), lorazepam (Ativan)
Adrenergic agents: meclizine (Antivert), epinephrine
Surgical interventions: labyrinthectomy, vestibular neurectomy, endolymphatic decompression

Nursing management

PATIENT PROBLEMS/NURSING DIAGNOSES

● **NDX:** Sensory/perceptual alteration related to disequilibrium

Assess audiogram results
Assess patient's hearing acuity, which may be decreased
Flag chart and bed *to indicate impairment and provide continuity of care*
Stand so that patient can see your face
Speak slowly and enunciate carefully
Explain all procedures and nursing care plan *to promote confidence*
Maintain quiet environment *to alleviate confusion*
  Minimize activities in room

Avoid bumping bed
Assist with personal care and activities as needed
Assist and teach patient to deep breathe q2h to 4h and turn on affected side when symptoms subside
Administer antianxiety agents

EXPECTED OUTCOMES
Exhibits a more accepting manner
Appears more aware of surroundings

● **NDX:** Risk for injury/trauma related to disequilibrium, vertigo

Administer vestibular depressant
Maintain bed rest in position of comfort during acute attack *to prevent injury*
Keep siderails of bed up and bed in low position
Discourage smoking
Assess visual acuity because balance depends on it as well as the vestibular system
Instruct patient to call nurse before getting up
Ambulate as ordered
  Observe for vertigo, nausea, and nystagmus
  Provide unobstructed pathway *to prevent accidents*
  Assist with ambulation
  Increase distance as tolerated
Instruct patient to turn head slowly *to prevent vertigo*
Encourage use of walker, cane *to improve equilibrium*

EXPECTED OUTCOMES
Expresses understanding of preventing injury
Uses devices to assist in ambulating

● **NDX:** Risk for fluid volume deficit related to vomiting

Monitor intake and output for severe vomiting to form basis for fluid replacement
  Include emesis, diarrhea, urine
  Administer antiemetics *to reduce vomiting*
Monitor vital signs qid
Provide low-sodium diet as tolerated *to decrease endolymph production*
  Assist with eating
  Avoid caffeine
  Restrict fluid intake as ordered
Assess skin turgor, mucous membranes *to identify dehydration*
Monitor electrolytes *to assess for hypokalemia*

EXPECTED OUTCOMES
Vital signs and electrolytes are within normal limits
Skin turgor is normal
Mucous membranes are moist
Appetite has improved

● **NDX:**   Anxiety related to change in health status

Assess level of anxiety *to assist in planning
    interventions*
Encourage and allow time for discussion of feelings
Explain plan of care and involve patient in care *to re-
    duce anxiety level*
Provide diversional activities *to decrease attention on
    anxiety*
Discuss and teach stress management techniques,
    which may assist in reducing severe vertigo attacks
Reinforce physician's explanation of disease *to decrease
    anxiety and increase knowledge*

EXPECTED OUTCOMES

Exhibits a more relaxed appearance
Discusses and practices relaxation techniques
Understands methods of dealing with vertigo

ADDITIONAL NURSING DIAGNOSES
TO CONSIDER

Body image disturbances related to acute vertigo/
    disequilibrium
Fear related to effects of vertigo

Patient/family teaching

Reinforce physician's explanation of disease process
    and procedures to follow when attacks occur
Explain that vertigo is usually first symptom; patient
    should immediately do the following:
    Take medication as ordered
    Lie or sit down when vertigo appears
    Not walk unassisted
    Notify physician of recurrence
    Stress to patient that progressive hearing loss may oc-
        cur if treatment is not initiated or successful
Explain that tinnitus may always be present; advise pa-
    tient to utilize background music, radio, or TV to over-
    come tinnitus
Discuss importance of leading a normal life when ver-
    tigo is absent
Explain importance of exercise on a daily basis
Discuss importance of not driving when taking medica-
    tion that slows reflexes
Discuss importance of following low-sodium diet or
    neutral ash diet as ordered
Warn patient to avoid ototoxic medications: salicylates,
    quinine, some diuretics, and aminoglycoside antibiotics
Avoid smoking, caffeine, alcohol
Have periodic audiologic examinations

Home care considerations

See Home care considerations for the hearing-impaired
    patient (p. 810)

Ear Surgeries

stapedectomy: *Surgical removal of all or part of the
    stapes footplate and creation of a patent oval window
    and pathway for sound transmission using natural or
    artificial materials, performed for otosclerosis*
myringotomy with tube insertion: *Surgical incision
    into the tympanic membrane to aspirate collected fluid
    and insertion of a ventilating tube to keep the pressure
    equal between the middle and outer ear, performed to
    correct serous otitis media*
tympanoplasty: *Surgical repair of tympanic
    membrane perforated or largely destroyed by infection,
    trauma, otosclerosis, stenosis, or necrosis of the middle
    ear; type performed depends on degree of perforation
    and destruction, as well as ossicular involvement and
    damage*

Preoperative assessment/teaching

Assess hearing acuity in both ears *to provide basis for
    interventions*
Reinforce physician's explanation of procedure
Establish means of communication because hearing
    may be impaired
Encourage and allow time for verbalization of fears and
    anxieties
Explain postoperative patient care plan and availability
    of staff *to reduce anxiety about procedure*
Explain that hearing may not improve immediately

Postoperative assessment

Subjective data

Restlessness resulting from decreased hearing
Location and character of pain
Excessive pain
Hearing acuity
Nausea
Vertigo
Altered taste

Objective data

Vomiting
Character and amount of ear drainage

Potential complications

Infection
Hemorrhage
Decreased hearing acuity
Tinnitus
Facial nerve paralysis
Perforation

Collaborative management

Therapeutic management

Analgesics
Antiemetics
Antihistamines for nasal congestion
Antibiotics
Dressing change schedule

Nursing management

PATIENT PROBLEMS/NURSING DIAGNOSES

● **NDX:** Pain related to surgical procedure and position restriction

Maintain bed rest in quiet environment
Supine position with operative side up for prescribed length of time
  Keep siderails up *to promote slight position changes*
  Do not turn unless ordered
  Provide back rubs prn *to promote comfort and relaxation*
  Elevate head of bed when allowed *to provide comfort*
Assess pain intensity using a pain rating scale of 0 to 5
Administer analgesics and assess effectiveness of pain relief
Report excessive pain to physician; increasing pain may be a sign of bleeding
Avoid nose blowing or sneezing, which increase pain
Avoid vomiting by administering antiemetics

EXPECTED OUTCOMES

Expresses satisfaction with pain relief measures
Appears calm and relaxed in position of comfort

● **NDX:** Risk for infection related to invasive surgical procedure

Monitor vital signs q4h especially temperature
Monitor for signs of infection q4h
  Increased drainage/pain
  Fever
  Headache
  Administer antibiotics as prescribed
Keep outer ear plug clean and dry
Change ear plugs prn
Report excessive bleeding, drainage to physician
Maintain aseptic technique

EXPECTED OUTCOMES

Patient is afebrile
Exhibits no purulent ear drainage

● **NDX:** Sensory/perceptual alteration related to hearing impairment

Assess hearing acuity of affected ear; may be reduced because of ear canal packing
Stand at unaffected side when speaking
Explain that hearing may not improve immediately and that this is not abnormal
  Ear plugs and bleeding decrease hearing acuity
  Hearing usually improves after plugs are removed
Provide and use alternate communicating measures as needed: pen and paper, Magic Slate
Encourage verbalization of thoughts and feelings *to promote feelings of self-confidence*
Involve patient in self-care and assist as needed *to increase independence*

EXPECTED OUTCOMES

Accepts and copes appropriately with hearing impairment
Strives to use remaining hearing or other senses adequately

Patient/family teaching

General

Explain importance of nutritious diet, fluid intake, rest, and activity
Discuss signs and symptoms to report to physician
  Elevated temperature
  Increased pain and/or ear drainage
  Decrease in hearing acuity
Discuss medications: name, dosage, time of administration, purpose, and side effects
Avoid persons with URIs or cold symptoms
Avoid smoking
Encourage follow-up visits with physician

Specific

See boxes below and on p. 810

Stapedectomy

Instruct patient on ear care
  Change only outer ear plug prn
  Keep plug clean and dry
  Avoid nose blowing for 1 wk
  Keep ear covered while outside
  Avoid sneezing; if unavoidable, open mouth wide to sneeze
  Wash hair only after 2 wk
  No air travel or diving for 6 months
Plugs and packing are removed after 1 wk

Tympanoplasty

Discuss precautions and restrictions in ear care
  Wear shower cap when bathing or place lamb's
    wool pledget in ear to protect ear from water
  Avoid blowing nose and sneeze through mouth
  Remove inner ear dressing only if prescribed
    by physician
  May swim or fly after healing has taken place
Explain that meclizine hydrochloride (Antivert)
  may be needed for about 1 month postopera-
  tively to offset vertigo

Myringotomy with Tube Insertion

Discuss special precautions and restrictions
  Keep water out of ear
  Place petroleum jelly–covered cotton or lamb's
    wool pledget in ear before showering or
    shampooing
  Wear well-fitting ear plugs when swimming is
    allowed or wear a cap
  Do not dive because it increases ear pressure
Explain that tube will come out naturally in 2 to 8
  months and there may be bloody drainage; if
  tube is dislodged earlier, instruct patient or par-
  ent(s) to notify physician
Demonstrate ear drop instillation and instruct pa-
  tient or parent(s) to complete prescribed
  course of oral or ear drop antibiotic therapy

Home Care Considerations for the Hearing-Impaired Patient

Assess and continue with patient/family teaching and
  evaluate/discuss the following:
Communication devices
  Hearing aid(s)
  Telephone receivers with amplifiers
  Flashing lights for phones, doorbells, fire alarms, se-
    curity systems
  Vibration attachments for alarm clocks
  Headsets for television, radio, stereo
Care of the ear
  Presence of drainage, pain, tenderness, fever

Use of ear plugs when swimming, showering
Procedure for instilling ear drops
Compliance to medication schedule
Understanding of disease process
  Presence of support group to reduce fear, anxiety,
    and hopelessness
  Knowledge of outside support groups to assist in de-
    creasing feelings of low self-esteem, isolation, and
    depression
  Presence of names, phone numbers of home health
    team
  Knowledge of national support groups such as the
    following:

Self Help for Hard of Hearing
4848 Battery Lane
Bethesda, MD 20814

National Organization for Hearing Research
225 Haverford Ave. #1
Narberth, PA 19072
(610) 664-3135

National Institute on Deafness and Other Commu-
  nication Disorders
National Institute for Health
NIDCD Information Clearing House
P.O. Box 37777
Washington, DC 20013-7777
(800) 241-1044
TDD (800) 241-1055

American Tinnitus Association
P.O. Box 5
Portland, OR 97207
(503) 248-9985

BIBLIOGRAPHY

Beare PG, Myers JL: *Principles and practice of adult health nursing,* ed 2, St Louis, 1994, Mosby.
Brinkmann KL: Why can't your patient hear you? *RN* 54(1):46, 1991.
Cleveland PJ, Morris J: Ménière's disease. *RN* 53(8):28, 1990.
Doenges ME et al: *Nursing care plans: guidelines for planning and documenting patient care,* ed 3, Philadelphia, 1993, FA Davis.
Faucher D et al: Why some eye surgery patients are seeing dots. *Nursing '93* 23(2):41, 1993.
Kim MJ et al: *Pocket guide to nursing diagnoses,* ed 6, St Louis, 1995, Mosby.
McCance KL, Huether SE: *Pathophysiology, the biological basis for disease in adults and children,* ed 2, St Louis, 1994, Mosby.
McFarland GK, McFarlane EA: *Nursing diagnosis and intervention: planning for patient care,* ed 2, St Louis, 1993, Mosby.
Rogers-Seidle FF: *Geriatric nursing care plans,* St Louis, 1991, Mosby.
Seigler BA, Schuring LT: *Ear, nose and throat disorders, Mosby's clinical series,* St Louis, 1993, Mosby.
Smith JF, Graham MD: Exercise helps these postop patients. *RN* 55(2):38, 1992.
Thompson JM et al: *Mosby's clinical nursing,* ed 3, St Louis, 1993, Mosby.
Webber-Jones J: Doomed to deafness? *Am J Nurs* 92(11):37, 1992.

BARNES

CARE PATH
850
SCLERAL BUCKLE PROCEDURE

SERVICE	PHYSICIAN	
PRIMARY NURSE	PRIMARY NURSE	A-8
DC DATE	ADM DATE	DATE OF SURGERY

PROBLEM NUMBER	PATIENT PROBLEMS / NURSING DIAGNOSES
#1	SENSORY ALTERATION
#2	LACK OF KNOWLEDGE
#3	POTENTIAL FOR INJURY
	*AS APPROPRIATE

PROB. NO.		PRE-ADM	DAY 1 DOS PRE-OP	DAY 1 DOS POST-OP
#1 #2 #3	ASSESSMENT/MONITORING	Determine if pt. is diabetic	Preparation for surgery in SDS: **VS stable:** **If SBP > 190** **DBP > 100 notify MD** **If DBP > 110 call Anesthesia** **No arrhythmia** **Pulse 60-100** **No SOB** **Afebrile** Assess if pt. brought meds from home Assess: Normal ECG CXR = NAD **Lab values within Barnes guidelines** Assess NPO status	VS every 30" until at baseline then ×1 ×2 Evaluate degree of visual deficit Evaluate for fall program Evaluate effectiveness of pain control Evaluate symptoms of increased IOP (nausea, vomiting, uncontrolled pain) **Serosanguinous drainage less than half-dollar size**
	CONSULTS	Pvt. MD clearance		Social work as appropriate Diabetes Nurse specialist as appropriate.
#2	PROCEDURE/TEST	In SDS: ECG within 6 months if pt. over 40 yrs. CXR within 1 yr. if pt. over 50 yrs. HCT within 15 days SMA6 within 15 days (see anesthesia guidelines)		
	TREATMENT			
#1 #2 #3	ACTIVITY		Bedrest with BRP	Bedrest with assistance

Used by permission of Barnes Hospital, St Louis, Missouri.

Continued.

BARNES

CARE PATH
850
SCLERAL BUCKLE PROCEDURE

CNS	DIETARY	RT
HOME HEALTH	OT	OTHER
PT	SW	OTHER

A-8

PROBLEM NUMBER	PATIENT PROBLEMS / NURSING DIAGNOSES

DAY 2 POD 1	DAY 3 POD 2	D/C OUTCOMES	RESOURCE INFORMATION
VS ×1 ×2	VS ×1	**VS at baseline**	No bending with head below waist
			No straining
			No lifting over 20 #
Evaluate effectiveness of pain control	**Evaluate minimal or no eye pain**	**Minimal or no eye pain**	May remove patch on arrival home
Evaluate for increased IOP			Wear glasses during the day and eyeshield at bedtime
Evaluate bladder / bowel status	**Voiding without difficulty No constipation Minimal or no drainage**	**Voiding adequately at baseline No straining Minimal or no drainage**	Avoid getting soap in eyes when taking a tub bath or shower
Serous drainage less than size of a dime			Avoid direct sunlight
			Take a cough syrup for persistent coughing
			Do not hold back sneezes
		Discharge to home	If gas / air is injected in the eye, do not fly in an airplane until your doctor gives permission
		MD or clinic follow-up	
		7 - 10 days	Do not drive a car until after F / U appt. with MD
			Call Primary Nurse as needed.
Eye dressing change	Eye dressing change		
AM dilation Eye Exam	AM dilation Eye Exam		
BRP with assistance	Ad lib or as tolerated	**Return to baseline level of ADL**	
Chair ×1 ×2 ×3			

		PRE-ADM	DAY 1 DOS PRE-OP	DAY 1 DOS POST-OP
#1 #2	MEDS/IVS		SDS / OP / OR / Floor Nurse - Initiate dilation x1 x2 x3 x4 IV per Anesthesia	IVFs
#2	NUTRITION	Admitting Nursing: NPO after MN except meds as instructed by MD	NPO except Meds	Clear liquids
#1 #3	PATIENT/FAMILY EDUCATION	Admitting Nursing: Reinforce pt. to bring meds from home as instructed by MD Admitting arrival time	OR Nurses: Review dilating drops, OR procedures, retrobulbar injection	Floor Nurses: Explain call system Positioning per MD order Availability of analgesia / antiemetic Primary Nurse Role **Pt. able to demonstrate use of call system**
#1 #2 #3	DISCHARGE PLANNING		**Pt. / family verbalize understanding of Care Path. Plan of care has been mutually set with pt. / family.**	Nursing: Evaluate home care needs, transportation, support system
#1	PSYCHOSOCIAL / EMOTIONAL / SPIRITUAL NEEDS		Holding area: Give emotional support for surgery, i.e., reassurance - verbal & non-verbal (touch)	Nursing: Give emotional support for decreased vision. Encourage pt. to express feeling about visual loss Assess coping ability. Give reassurance - verbal & non-verbal
	SIGNATURES			

3100-53 (REV. 4/93)

Continued.

850

DAY 2 POD 1	DAY 3 POD 2	D/C OUTCOMES	RESOURCE INFORMATION
D/C IV or change to Heplock Begin post-op eye gtts	D/C Heplock Post-op eye gtts	**Pt. / Care Provider able to administer eye drops**	
Regular diet	Regular diet	**Tolerating regular diet**	
Explain eye meds Teach eye drop instillation	Instruct pt. to wear eye shield or glasses Teach eye drop schedule Reinforce teaching booklet instructions	**Pt. verbalizes Understanding Discharge Instructions**	
Pt. able to instill eye gtts independently Distribute teaching booklet & explain contents Teach cleansing of eye: soft, clean washcloth & tap water. Teach signs of infection: increase in redness, purulent drainage, increase in pain. Teach signs of increased eye pressure (see DOS post-op). Teach observance of any decrease in vision **Pt. able to verbalize eye cleansing, signs of infection, increased eye pressure, and understanding of visual testing.**	**Pt. verbalizes understanding of eye safety and medication schedule.**		
Nursing: Finalize home arrangements and transportation Call Social Worker if needed	D / C pt. with caregiver	**Discharge to home with caregiver to self-care.**	
Nursing: Continue emotional support			

3100-53 (REV. 4/93)

A-8

			VARIANCE	
DATE	TIME	VARIANCE	ACTION PLAN	INITIALS

Immune System

Immune System (Figure 14-1)

Assessment

Subjective data

Cardiopulmonary system
  Shortness of breath (SOB)
  Palpitations, chest pain
Central nervous system (CNS)
  Paresthesia
  Headache
  Photophobia
Gastrointestinal (GI) system
  Loss of appetite, anorexia
  Altered taste sensation
  Nausea, abdominal pain
  Rectal itching
Musculoskeletal system
  Fatigue, malaise
  Joint pain/stiffness, arthralgia
Ophthalmologic: ocular pain

Objective data

Age, race
Gender, ethnic background
Weight loss
Cardiopulmonary system
  Hypertension/hypotension
  Jugular vein distension
  Pericarditis
  Cardiomegaly, dysrhythmia
  Edema

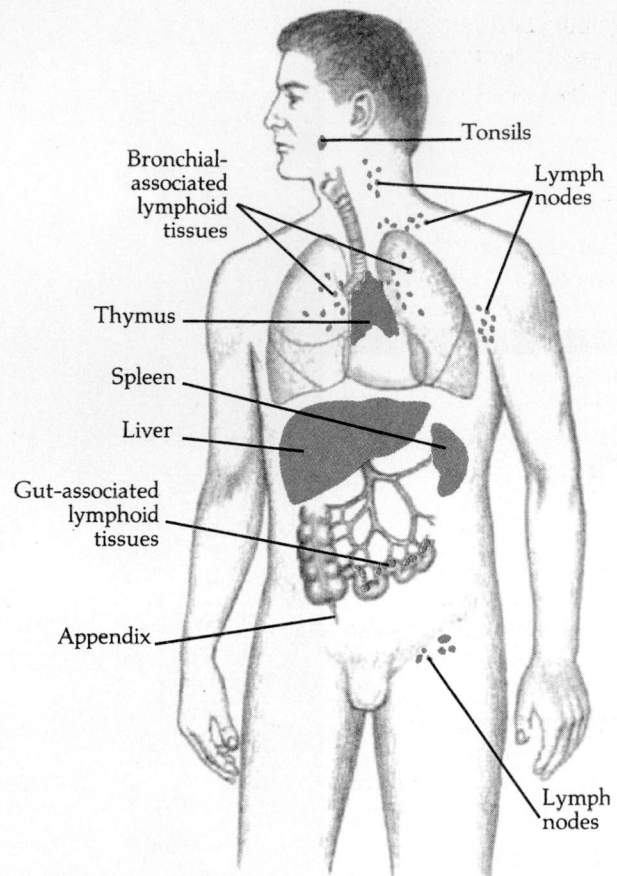

Bronchial-associated lymphoid tissues

Tonsils

Lymph nodes

Thymus

Spleen

Liver

Gut-associated lymphoid tissues

Appendix

Lymph nodes

Figure 14-1 Organization of immune system. Cellular constituents of immune system are derived from bone marrow stem cells. On maturation, these cells are released into peripheral blood and subsequently populate organized tissues of lymphoreticular system. (From Thompson JM et al: *Mosby's clinical nursing,* ed 3, St Louis, 1993, Mosby.)

Cough, dyspnea, wheezing
Tachypnea, intercostal retractions
Cyanosis
Hemoptysis
Lung infiltrates, hemorrhage
Breath sounds; crackles
CNS (Central nervous system)
  Dementia, personality changes, psychosis
  Depression
  Memory impairment
  Poor concentration, slowed thought processes
  Confusion
  Unsteady gait
  Decreased hand coordination
  Raynaud's disease
  Neuritis
  Peripheral nerve vasculitis; foot-drop, wrist-drop
  Tremors
  Seizures

Decreased animation
Withdrawal
Depression
Emotional lability
Psychosis
Nuchal rigidity
Altered level of consciousness (LOS)
Coma
GI system
  Difficulty chewing, swallowing
  Oral/esophageal lesions
  White/gray patches, dried patches may appear hairy
  Red to purple/brown lesions, may appear nodular, macular, plaquelike
  Gingivitis, parotitis
  Perioral/lips: red fissures, crusted, herpetic vesicles
  Vomiting
  Unintentional weight loss
  Abdominal cramping
  Change in bowel habits
  Diarrhea
  Constipation
  Rectal bleeding, fissures
  Peritonitis
Musculoskeletal system
  Weakness of extremities
  Swelling, warmth of joints
  Impaired joint function
  Joint effusions, deformities
  Muscle spasms, atrophy, contracture
  Subcutaneous nodules over pressure points
  Clubbing of fingers
Ophthalmologic system
  Dry eyes, sclera
  Cotton, wool exudate, lacrimation
  Bright subconjunctival masses
  Conjunctival infection
  Blurred vision
  Papilledema
  Diplopia
  Visual field deficits
  Retinal cystoid bodies
  Blindness
Ears/nose/throat status
  Nasal ulcerations
  Sensorineural hearing loss
Integumentary system
  Skin lesions: purple to brown
  Vasculitic skin lesions
  Skin vesicles
  Diaphoresis
  Rashes, hyperpigmentation
  Shiny, taut skin over joints
  Dryness

Sensitivity to the sun
Alopecia
Delayed wound healing
Lymphadenopathy
Hematologic system
Hepatosplenomegaly
Petechiae
Purpura
Easy bruising
Elevated temperature
Renal/genitourinary system
Hematuria, hemorrhagic cystitis
Urine casts
Proteinuria
Comorbidities
Anemia
GI bleeding
Renal calculi
Renal failure
Pericarditis
Myocardial infarction (MI)
Tenosynovitis
Interstitial fibrosis, pneumonitis
Pneumonia
Cerebrovascular accident
Infection, diabetes from steroid use
Graft vs. host disease
Retinopathy

Medical history/risk factors

Hepatitis
Sexually transmitted diseases
Frequent viral illness
Amebiasis
Transfusion of blood products
Chemical exposure
Occupational risks
Chemotherapy
Radiation therapy
Radioactive iodine therapy
Family history

Social history

Exposure to contaminated needles, IV drug use
Multiple sex partners
Sexual preference
Work/productive activities
Stress factors/coping mechanisms
Previous losses/coping mechanisms
Self-concept
Conceptualization of illness
Support network
Living arrangements

Significant other/marriage partner
Ability to perform ADLs
Transportation

Diagnostic tests

Hematologies
Leukocyte count
Lymphocyte count
Complete blood cell count (CBC)
Coagulation profile
Erythrocyte sedimentation rate (ESR)
Blood type and cross/screen
HLA typing
Immunologies
Kveim skin test
Immunofluorescence assay
$T_{4,8}$ cell count
T helper/T suppressor ratio
Serum immunoglobulin
ASO titer, rheumatoid factor
Serum protein levels: IgG, IgA, IgM
C-reactive protein
Antinuclear antibodies
LE prep
Antinuclear antibody
Antidouble-standard DNA antibody
Complement
Viral, serology studies
ELISA for HIV
Western blot test
HBsAg, HBsAb
Herpes zoster (HZ)
Herpes simplex (HS)
Cytomegalovirus (CM)
Epstein-Barr virus (EBV)
VDRL, Fluorescent treponemal antibody absorption (FTA-A)
Toxoplasmosis
Chemistries
LDH
Alkaline phosphatase, AST, ALT
Bilirubin
Serum cholesterol
Serum iron, magnesium
Electrolyte panel, BUN, creatinine
Fasting blood sugar (FBS)
Cultures
Sputum
Spinal fluid
Bone marrow
Mucous membranes
Blood
Stool

Urine
  Urinalysis
  Creatinine clearance
Imaging studies
  X-rays
  Chest
  Joints
Nuclear medicine: Gallium scan
CT scan, MRI
Arthroscopy

Neurophysiology studies
  Stereotactic brain biopsy
  Electromyelography
  Nerve conduction studies
Cardiopulmonary studies
  Arterial blood gases (ABGs)
  Pulmonary function
  Electrocardiogram (ECG), echocardiogram
Biopsies
  Skin
  Kidney
  Lymph nodes
  Bronchial, open lung

Gerontologic Considerations

- Older adults are at increased risk for inflammation and infections resulting from changes in natural defense mechanisms.
  Pathogens are able to enter through breaks in the fragile, dry skin, increasing the risk of skin infections.
  Decreased movement of respiratory secretions increases the risk of respiratory infections.
  Decreased production of saliva and gastric secretions increases the risk of gastrointestinal infections.
  Decreased tear production increases the risk of eye inflammation and infections.
  Structural changes in the urinary system that lead to urinary retention or stasis increase the risk of urinary tract infection.
- Signs and symptoms of infection tend to be more subtle than in younger individuals. Because older persons have decreased body temperature, fever may be more difficult to detect. Changes in behavior such as lethargy, fatigue, disorientation, irritability, and loss of appetite may be early signs of infection.
- Functioning of the immune system appears to decrease somewhat with advanced age. Specific data on this is not conclusive, but research is continuing.
- The older adult's immune system continues to produce antibodies and therefore immunization for diseases such as pneumonia and influenza is recommended.
- Older individuals who have chronic illnesses are generally at increased risk for infection.

From Christensen BL, Kockrow EO: *Foundations of nursing*, ed 2, St Louis, 1995, Mosby.

Acquired Immunodeficiency Syndrome

AIDS includes the final stages of a wide range of health problems caused by the human immunodeficiency virus type I (HIV) (Figure 14-2); this virus attacks the cell-mediated immune system through invasion of CD4 cells, causing a major deficit in the system (see the box on p. 823); the infected person becomes vulnerable to opportunistic infections and cancers (Table 14-1); HIV is transmitted by exposure to infected blood/body fluids; the exposures that put people at risk include sexual contact with an infected partner, receptive anal intercourse, multiple sexual partners, anonymous sexual activity, intravenous drug use, contact with contaminated blood products or tissue through transfusion, transplant, or occupational risk, and infants exposed in utero by infected mothers

Assessment

Subjective data

Cardiopulmonary system: SOB
CNS
  Paresthesia
  Headache
  Photophobia
Ophthalmologic
  Floaters
  Flashing lights in peripheral vision
GI system
  Loss of appetite
  Nausea
  Abdominal pain
  Rectal itching, pain
  Severe fatigue

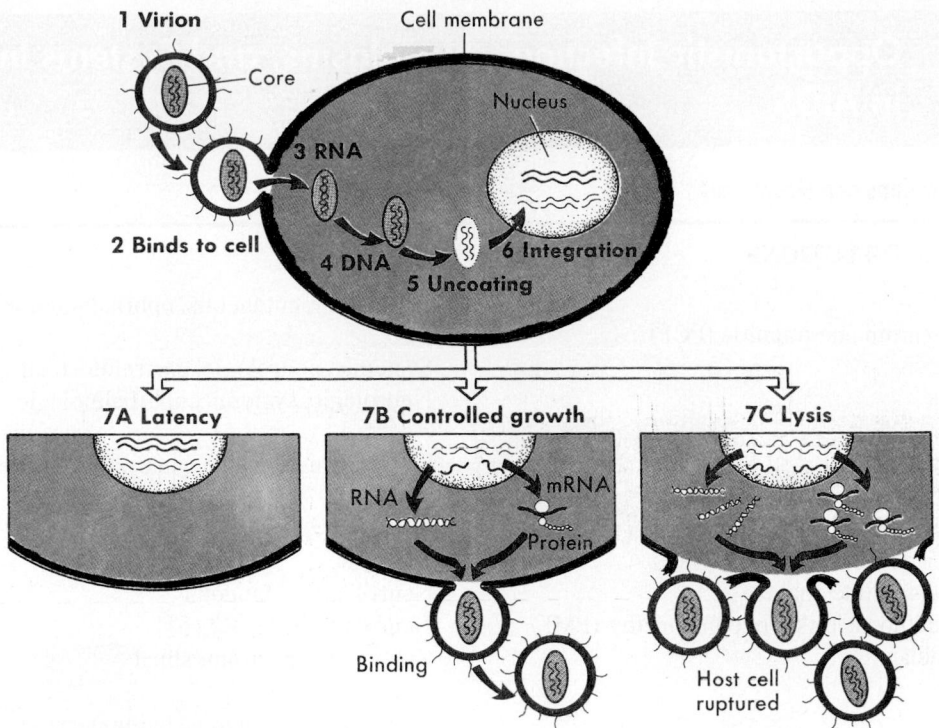

Figure 14-2 Infection and cellular outcomes of the HIV. HIV infection begins *(1)* when a virion, or virus particle, *(2)* binds to the outside of a susceptible cell and fuses with it, *(3)* injecting the core proteins and two strands of viral RNA. Uncoating occurs, during which the core proteins are removed and the viral RNA is released into the infected cell's cytoplasm. *(4)* The double-stranded DNA (provirus) migrates to the nucleus, *(5)* uncoats itself, and *(6)* is integrated into the cell's own DNA. The provirus then can do a couple of things: *(7A)* remain latent or *(7B)* activate cellular mechanisms to copy its genes into RNA, some of which is translated into viral proteins or ribosomes. The proteins and additional RNA then are assembled into new virions that bud from the cell. The process can take place slowly, sparing the host cell *(7B)*, or so rapidly that the cell is lysed or ruptured *(7C)*. (From McCance KL, Huether SE: *Pathophysiology: the biological basis for disease in adults and children,* ed 2, St Louis, 1994, Mosby.)

Objective data

Cardiopulmonary system
  Cough
  Dyspnea
  Wheezing
  Tachypnea
  Cyanosis
  Hemoptysis
  Intercostal retractions
CNS
  AIDS dementia complex
    Memory impairment
    Poor concentration
    Slowed thought processes
    Confusion
    Unsteady gait
    Weakness of extremities, especially lower
      extremities
    Decreased hand coordination
    Tremors

    Seizures
    Decreased animation
    Withdrawal
    Depression
    Emotional lability
    Psychosis
  Nuchal rigidity
  Altered LOC
  Coma
Ophthalmologic system
  Cotton, wool exudate
  Blurred vision
  Papilledema
  Diplopia
  Visual field deficits
  Retinal hemorrhage
  Bright red subconjunctival masses
  Blindness
Ear, nose, throat (ENT) status
  Oral cavity and esophagus lesions

Table 14-1 Opportunistic Infections, Neoplasms, and Systems Involved in AIDS

Opportunistic Infections and Neoplasms	System Involved
OPPORTUNISTIC INFECTIONS	
Protozoal	
Pneumocystis carinii pneumonitis (PCP)	Pulmonary, cutaneous, ophthalmologic
Cryptosporidiosis	Systemic, neurologic, gastrointestinal
Toxoplasmosis	Neurologic, systemic, ophthalmologic
Viruses	
Cytomegalovirus (CMV)	Systemic, neurologic, gastrointestinal, pulmonary, ophthalmologic
Herpes simplex I, II—disseminated	Neurologic, cutaneous
Epstein-Barr virus (EBV)	Systemic
Herpes zoster—multidermal	Neurologic, cutaneous
Progressive multifocal leukoencephalopathy (PML)	Neurologic
Hairy leukoplakia	Cutaneous, gastrointestinal
Fungi	
Candidiasis	Neurologic, cutaneous, pulmonary
Cryptococcosis	Neurologic, systemic
Histoplasmosis	Pulmonary, systemic
Coccidioidomycosis	Pulmonary, cutaneous, systemic
Bacterial	
Mycobacterium avium-intracellular (MAI)	Neurologic, systemic, pulmonary, gastrointestinal
Mycobacterium tuberculosis	Neurologic, pulmonary, systemic
NEOPLASMS	
Kaposi's sarcoma (KS)	Neurologic, cutaneous, ophthalmologic, gastrointestinal
Lymphoma (p. 903)	Neurologic, systemic, gastrointestinal
OTHER ASSOCIATED INFECTIONS, CONDITIONS NOT CONSIDERED OPPORTUNISTIC	
Anemia	Hematologic, systemic
Aspergillosis	Pulmonary, ophthalmologic, systemic
Giardiasis	Gastrointestinal
Klebsiella pneumoniae	Pulmonary
Salmonellosis	Gastrointestinal, cutaneous, skeletal, systemic
Idiopathic thrombocytopenia purpura (ITP) (p. 249)	Hematologic, gastrointestinal, neurologic
Xerostomia	Gastrointestinal

White/gray patches, dried patches may appear
  hairy
Red to purple/brown lesions, may appear macular,
  nodular, or plaque like
Gingivitis, bleeding
Perioral/lips: red fissures, crusted, herpetic vesicles
Integumentary system
  Skin vesicles

Diaphoresis
Rashes
Skin lesions: purple to brown
Dryness
Delayed wound healing
Lymphadenopathy, nodes not fixed or hard
GI system
  Difficulty chewing, swallowing

1993 CDC Classification for HIV Infections in Adults

Category A: Asymptomatic; primary HIV or persistent lymphadenopathy

A1	CD4	T cell count $\geq$500/mm^3
A2	CD4	T cell count 200 to 499/mm^3
A3	CD4	T cell count <200/mm^3

Category B: Symptomatic; examples include candidiasis (oral, vulvovaginal), cervical dysplasia/cancer, diarrhea lasting longer than 1 month, herpes zoster, pelvic inflammatory disease, idiopathic thrombocytopenia

B1	CD4	T cell count $\geq$500/mm^3
B2	CD4	T cell count 200 to 499/mm^3
B3	CD4	T cell count <200/mm^3

Category C: AIDS indicators; examples include candidiasis (trachea, bronchi, lungs), cytomegalovirus (other than liver, spleen, nodes), lymphomas, Kaposi's sarcoma, mycobacterium, pneumocystis carinii, wasting syndrome, encephalopathy

C1	CD4	T cell count $\geq$500/mm^3
C2	CD4	T cell count 200 to 499/mm^3
C3	CD4	T cell count <200/mm^3

Vomiting
Unintentional weight loss, 10% in 1 to 2 months
Abdominal cramping
Intractable diarrhea
Rectal bleeding, fissures
Hematologic system
  Splenomegaly
  Petechiae
  Purpura
  Easy bruising
Night sweats
Elevated temperature

Medical history

Hepatitis
Sexually transmitted diseases
Frequent viral illness
Amebiasis
Exposure to contaminated needles, IV drug use
Transfusion of blood/blood products
Females
  Recurrent vaginal candidiasis
  History of abnormal Pap test

Social history

Multiple sex partners
Sex partner of IV drug user
Bisexual male
Sexual preference
Work/productive activities
Stress factors, coping mechanisms
Previous losses, coping mechanisms
Self-concept
Conceptualization of illness

Diagnostic tests

Leukocytopenia
Lymphocytopenia
RBC, Hct, and Hgb: decreased
Thrombocytopenia
Immunologies
  ELISA: reactive
  Western blot assay or Immunofluorescence assay: positive
  HIV antigen (PCR): positive
  HIV culture: positive
  T$_4$ cells: decreased
  T$_8$ cells: increased
  T helper/T suppressor ratio: inverted
  Serum immunoglobulin: elevated
Chemistries
  LDH: elevated
  Alkaline phosphatase: elevated
  Serum cholesterol: decreased
  Serum iron: decreased
  Electrolytes: imbalanced
Cultures/serologies
  Sputum: pneumocystis carinii, AFB, fungus, MAI
  Spinal fluid: MAI, cryptococcal antigen, HIV, herpes, CMV, viremia, MAI bacteremia
  Bone marrow: disseminated MAI, CMV
  Mucous membranes: candidiasis, herpes
  Blood: cryptococcal antigen, HIV, toxoplasmosis Ag
  Stool: ova and parasites
Imaging studies/nuclear medicine
  Chest radiograph: interstitial infiltrates
  Gallium lung scan: positive
  Bronchoscopy: biopsy positive
  CT scan/MRI: positive for toxoplasmosis lesions, HIV infections

Stereotactic brain biopsy: differentiate intracranial lesions
Neurophysiology studies
    Electromyelography
    Nerve conduction studies: slowed
Cardiopulmonary studies
    ABGs
    Pulmonary function

Collaborative management

Therapeutic management

Oxygen therapy
Chest physiotherapy
Central line catheter
Total parenteral nutrition (TPN)
Appetite stimulants
Parenteral therapy
Chemotherapy
Antiemetics
Antidiarrheals
Antivirals
Antifungals
Biologic modifiers
Sulfonamides
Antipyretics
Analgesics
Radiotherapy

Nursing management

PATIENT PROBLEMS/NURSING DIAGNOSES

● **NDX:**   Impaired gas exchange related to opportunistic pulmonary infections

Assess VS, especially rate, depth, work of breathing and breath sounds q4h and prn *to determine changes from baseline that may indicate infection*
Monitor ABGs, pulse oximetry as ordered; *changes may indicate onset/progression of pulmonary infection*
Administer oxygen therapy as ordered *to maintain optimal oxygen level*
Suction airways prn *to remove secretions if patient is unable to do so*
Obtain sputum specimen for culture *to determine infective agent and appropriate therapy*
Provide chest physiotherapy and postural drainage as needed *to remove secretions, which increase bacterial growth*
Assist patient to turn, cough, and deep breathe q2h and prn *to assist in secretion removal, which promotes better oxygenation*
Position patient in high-Fowler's position, *which provides for optimal respiratory excursion*

Assist patient with relaxation exercises *to decrease rapid, shallow breathing*
Evaluate ADLs in relationship to oxygen demands, assist patient prn *to conserve energy*

EXPECTED OUTCOMES
Patient does not exhibit signs/symptoms of acute respiratory distress, or signs/symptoms are recognized and treated immediately

● **NDX:**   Risk for infection related to suppressed immune system

Screen personnel and visitors for symptoms of infection *to reduce patient's exposure to foreign pathogens*
Use strict sterile technique for all invasive procedures *to prevent pathogen infiltration*
Monitor sites of invasive lines/tubes/drains for signs of infection q8h; *tissue response to pathogen infiltration*
Check body fluids for alteration in color, odor, consistency, *which may indicate infection*
Ensure excellent personal hygiene is maintained, especially after bowel movements *to prevent infection*
Provide uninterrupted periods of sleep and rest *to provide energy to combat invading pathogens*
Ensure required fluid/nutrient intake, supplement with total oral nutrition products prn, institute calorie count as needed *to provide adequate nutrition*
Record intake and output *to ensure balance*
Monitor VS, especially T and breath sounds; *fever is hallmark of infection; increased BP, P may indicate sepsis*
Monitor CBC, WBC results per physician order *so increased WBC, indicative of infection, can be reported and treated promptly*
Maintain skin integrity: *intact skin may prevent entry of microorganisms*
Encourage clearance of pulmonary secretions; turn, cough, deep breathe q2h; perform chest percussion and drainage prn; encourage use of incentive spirometer *to remove secretions, which enhance growth of pathogens*
Maintain intact mucous membranes; scrupulous oral care using soft instruments prn *to prevent a port of entry for pathogens*

EXPECTED OUTCOMES
Patient exhibits improvement, resolution of current infections, and/or new infections do not develop

● **NDX:**   Altered thought processes related to AIDS dementia complex

Assess for disruptions in thinking processes, time management, task orientation, memory, changes in attention span, labile emotions daily: *changes may indicate cerebral involvement*

Assist patient to explore appropriateness of goal setting for the present and future

Assess LOC and orientation q8h and prn *to determine early changes*

Develop a supportive, therapeutic nurse/patient relationship *to promote trust*

Reorient to person, place, time prn

Call patient by name, identify self, and state purpose when entering the room *to prevent distortions of interpretation*

Speak directly to patient, avoid vague comments and conversations not addressing the patient *to decrease multiple stimuli, which may confuse patient*

Be clear and direct when providing instructions, give one direction at a time, break complex tasks into simple steps *to promote feelings of accomplishment*

Redirect misinterpretations of stimuli to reality-centered discussions

Assist patient to clarify thoughts and feelings, learn to recognize reactions to automatic thoughts

Assess environment and attempt to decrease stimuli that the patient may misinterpret

Teach patient how to make more appropriate self-evaluations by examining consistency of thoughts

Adjust lighting to prevent shadows, use night light *to prevent visual distortions*

Make familiar objects, pictures, clock, and correctly dated calendar visible to patient *to assist in maintaining orientation*

Provide radio, TV, newspapers as patient wishes

Develop and maintain with patient a consistent daily schedule; post schedule for patient *to promote routine, reality-based behavior*

Encourage significant others to visit often *to assist in maintaining orientation*

Maintain consistent arrangement of room *to protect patient from injury*

Use soft restraints or jacket restraint only as needed and when patient is alone *to prevent injury*

Encourage acceptance of responsibility for actions

Plan care with patient *to encourage self-control,* encourage patient to make choices as appropriate

Give positive reinforcement for participation in self-care; teach patient to reward self in concrete ways

In collaboration with physician, refer for neuropsychiatric or psychosocial evaluation

EXPECTED OUTCOMES

Actively participates in ADLs to extent possible based on physical limitations

Maintains reality orientation, communicates clearly with others

Participates in developing plan of care, ordering meals, making other choices as appropriate

Expresses delusional thoughts less frequently

● **NDX:** Pain related to involvement of multiple organ systems

Assess nature, intensity, location, duration, and precipitating and alleviating factors; use consistent pain rating scale *to determine baseline and deviations that indicate intervention is needed*

Assess nonverbal signs of pain particular to patient *so that early signs can be noted and treatment started*

Obtain information from patient regarding past pain experiences and methods used for relief

Control environmental factors that may increase perception of pain: temperature, noise, lighting

Assist patient to achieve positions *that promote comfort*

Assist patient to achieve state of minimal physical tension through techniques such as relaxation, music, visualization, diversion *to decrease need for medication*

Provide a restful environment with opportunities to rest during the day and uninterrupted periods of sleep at night

In collaboration with physician, provide analgesic medications as required, observing for therapeutic and side effects

Discuss noninvasive pain relief measures: relaxation, cutaneous stimulation, distraction, hot/cold therapy

EXPECTED OUTCOMES

Verbalizes decrease in or relief of pain

Able to incorporate existing pain while participating in daily activities

● **NDX:** Diarrhea related to GI infection, chemotherapy

Assess usual patterns of elimination: quantity, frequency, color, consistency, presence of overt/occult blood, undigested food

Assess current use of laxatives/antidiarrheals, *which may cause/interfere with current condition*

Evaluate hydration and electrolyte status; maintain record of intake and output, measuring liquid stools *to determine fluid deficit*

Assess abdomen: bowel sounds, distension, softness/firmness

Assess for flatus, cramping

Weigh patient daily: same time, clothing, and scale

Adjust diet to eliminate foods inducing bowel irritation; offer frequent, small meals

Provide protein and electrolyte supplements, total oral or parenteral nutrition

Provide fluids at least in equal amount to output *to maintain balance*

In collaboration with dietitian and patient, maintain calorie count and select nondiarrheic foods

In collaboration with physician, administer antidiarrheals, antiinfective agents

EXPECTED OUTCOMES

Frequency and quantity of abdominal pain, cramping, and diarrheal stools per day are decreased

Weight is maintained or increased if appropriate

Able to identify foods to consume/avoid *to prevent exacerbation*

● **NDX:** Altered nutrition: less than body requirements related to reduced food intake, malabsorption, anorexia, vomiting, diarrhea, stomatitis

Assess nutritional status daily: weight, electrolytes, total protein, serum albumin, Hgb, skin turgor, muscle mass *to determine fluid deficit and weight loss*

Determine amount and types of foods patient likes and is able to tolerate *to increase intake*

Provide for oral hygiene before and after meals *to enhance comfort and sense of taste*

Administer anesthetics to oral mucosa before meals as needed *to promote comfort*

Offer high-calorie, high-protein diet with variation in taste, texture, and presentation of foods *to stimulate appetite*

In collaboration with physician, provide oral and parenteral nutritional supplements *to supply required nutrients and calories*

Serve frequent, light meals and nutritional, high-calorie snacks; *small amounts more easily tolerated*

Assist patient to eat if fatigue is a factor

Present meals in an attractive, pleasing manner

Provide a pleasant atmosphere *to increase desire to eat*: encourage significant others to join patient for meals, remove bedpans/urinals from area, maintain well-ventilated room, serve food as soon as it arrives, remove tray as soon as patient finishes eating

In collaboration with clinical dietitian: calculate number of calories and nutrients *needed to maintain/gain weight and support metabolic needs*

Encourage family to bring favorite foods from home *to enhance patient's appetite*

In collaboration with physician, administer antiemetics before meals as needed

EXPECTED OUTCOME

Weight is maintained within 10% of baseline

● **NDX:** Altered oral mucous membranes related to opportunistic infections

Assess oral mucous membranes q8h to 12h for color, moisture, texture, presence of lesions *to determine baseline and, thereafter, changes indicative of infection*

Assess ease of swallowing *to note any difficulties that may lead to aspiration*

Obtain cultures of lesions per physician order *to determine infective pathogen*

Provide oral hygiene q2h while awake: use instruments appropriate for condition of mucous membranes; avoid abrasives, alcohol-containing mouthwash, and lemon glycerin swabs, *which may cause irritation and a port of entry for infective agents*

Perform oral hygiene as soon as possible after eating *to remove food particles, which enhance growth of pathogens*

Use baking soda, antifungal medications, topical anesthetics per physician order

Apply water-soluble lubricant to lips q2h *to maintain hydration*

Provide foods that are nonirritating to mucous membranes, easily chewed

Avoid very sweet, spicy, acidic foods, *which may cause irritation to membranes*

Provide foods at neutral temperature or per patient tolerance

If patient is unable to assist in oral hygiene: irrigate mouth with soft rubber catheter, use soft utensil to remove debris

Discourage smoking and alcohol use, *which increase dehydration of membranes*

EXPECTED OUTCOMES

Patient is able to take oral nutrition

Oral mucous membranes intact; lesions healing

● **NDX:** Risk for impaired skin integrity related to malnutrition, immobility, opportunistic infection

Assess skin condition q8h; pay close attention to axilla, skin folds, groin and perineal area, heels, scapula, back of head, dependent extremities, sacral area, mucous membranes *for irritation or breaks*

Note condition of skin related to temperature, moisture, color, texture, lesions

Assist with bathing as necessary, use mild soaps, rinse and dry well *to prevent sites of moisture, which enhance skin irritation and bacterial growth*

Do not leave skin moist with lotions; avoid deodorants, cologne

If patient is diaphoretic, rinse and dry skin well, keep clothing and bedding dry

Keep linen wrinkle free, avoid pressure from linen on feet, use foot cradle prn *to prevent areas of pressure*

Lift patient when turning; avoid sliding on sheets, *which may cause shearing of skin*

Prevent pressure on bony prominences using pillows, air therapy beds prn *to promote circulation to all areas*

Encourage small shifts in position q30 min and turn at least q2h *to decrease pressure points*

Increase active mobility *to increase circulation;* encourage walking and sitting in chair, avoid chair sitting in one position for longer than 30 min

Provide for perianal care after each elimination *to prevent irritation and/or promote healing*

Avoid IM injections and multiple venipunctures *to eliminate/decrease sites of invasion*

EXPECTED OUTCOMES
Skin and mucous membranes remain intact
Current skin breakdown is healing

● **NDX:** Bleeding related to thrombocytopenia*

Assess neurologic status q8h: *changes may indicate intracranial bleeding*

Observe urine and stools for obvious blood, test for occult blood per physician order

Assess skin and mucous membranes for extension/new sites of ecchymosis, hematoma q8h

Use smallest gauge needles possible, perform finger sticks (or draw from central line when possible), consolidate blood draws *to decrease number of invasive sites and lower risk of bleeding*

Apply manual pressure for five min to all puncture sites; do not disturb clots/scabs *to prevent fresh, unobserved bleeding*

Avoid rectal T, medications, *which may inadvertently break mucosa, providing a bleeding site*

Use nonabrasive soaps, soft brushes, soft washcloths and towels *to maintain skin integrity*

Assist with ambulation as needed to avoid bumps and falls, *which provide sites of internal bleeding*

Avoid constipation

Transfuse blood products per physician order

EXPECTED OUTCOMES
Skin and mucous membranes remain intact, without bruising/hematoma
Hgb/Hct remain stable

*Not a NANDA-approved diagnosis.

● **NDX:** Fatigue related to chronic disease process

Assess causative/contributing factors; identify activities that are difficult for patient and use excessive energy

Coordinate activities *to provide for undisturbed periods of rest and sleep*

Perform active/passive ROM exercises qid, collaborate with physical therapy to determine most therapeutic exercises *to decrease energy expenditure*

Determine whether patient becomes posturally hypotensive; change positions gradually *to prevent injury*

Monitor for hypotension and tachycardia, *which indicate increased expenditure of energy*

Gauge amount and intensity of activity tolerated by monitoring patient's subjective complaints of fatigue and changes in VS

Assist patient to identify strengths, abilities, interests; assist in development of realistic goals progressing from simple to complex *to conserve energy*

Encourage patient to participate in self-care to tolerance; assist as needed to avoid exhaustion; assist to identify energy patterns and schedule activities appropriately

Teach energy conservation techniques, use of assistive devices

Place patient on falls-prevention protocol

Collaborate with physical therapist to design measures *to maintain activity and independence*

EXPECTED OUTCOMES
Participates in self-care to tolerance
Ability to be active increases; patient states a feeling of increased energy

● **NDX:** Anticipatory grieving related to lifestyle changes, decreased physical abilities, changes in physical appearance, life-threatening prognosis

Be sensitive to changes patient is experiencing; encourage patient to express feelings, frustrations, anger, hopes *to begin work of grieving process*

Provide a therapeutic environment conducive to open discussion; actively listen, perceive nonverbal cues; be patient and empathetic *to facilitate trust*

Encourage questions and provide information freely as patient expresses the desire for knowledge about disease, treatments, and prognosis *to ease fear of the unknown*

Support adaptive behaviors that suggest progression and resolution of the grieving process

Set limits on maladaptive coping behaviors if they interfere with patient's well-being

Provide opportunities for private, uninterrupted time with significant others

Assist in identifying ways to adapt lifestyle as condition changes *to enhance participation and feelings of control*

Provide information regarding support groups, including electronic access groups, for patient and significant others

Collaborate with other professionals (social worker, clergy, psychologist, psychiatrist) *to provide support and facilitate grieving process*

Provide reference for financial assistance, answers to questions regarding medical insurance

Provide information to assist patient in completing advanced directives or similar document *to ensure patient's wishes are known to significant others and care providers*

EXPECTED OUTCOMES

Patient progresses through stages of the grieving process and moves toward acceptance

Demonstrates effective coping mechanisms

Participates in decisions about own future

● **NDX:** Altered sexuality patterns related to limitation imposed by symptoms (fatigue, decreased libido, impotence), fear of rejection by partner, fear of spreading infection to partner

Determine knowledge level about AIDS and attitude about AIDS in relation to sexuality

Clarify uncertainties, misconceptions if present *to ensure relationships are maintained within safe boundaries*

Provide opportunities for expression of concerns, fears *to decrease feelings of isolation*

Be nonjudgmental, aware of how own discomfort level and personal attitude may affect ability to be therapeutic

Provide private time and encourage patient to discuss concerns and feelings with sex partner including imagined responses, fear of rejection *so that unspoken fears do not interfere with relationship*

Provide information about alternate methods for sexual expression while avoiding activities that permit exchange of body fluids, feces, or blood between partners *to prevent transmission of causative agents*

Instruct patient and partner in safer sex guidelines (see box at right)

EXPECTED OUTCOMES

Patient makes informed statements concerning alternate modes of sexual expression

Identifies safer sex practices

Openly discusses concerns and makes plans for safer sexual activities with sex partner

Safer Sex Guidelines

SAFER SEX PRACTICES/PATIENT EDUCATION

Inform previous and present partners (and those with whom you share needles) of their possible exposure to HIV; if partner is female and pregnant, immediate referral for medical evaluation is advised

If female, avoid pregnancy

Selectively choose partners, know partners' sexual histories; limit partners, preferably to one person

Avoid oral-genital contact

Avoid sexual intercourse, especially those practices that may injure tissue such as anal intercourse

Modify practices so that body fluids, blood, and feces are not exchanged

LOW-RISK SEX PRACTICES

Vaginal penetration

Instruct in proper selection and application of latex condoms

Use latex condoms from start to finish to protect from body fluid exchange (natural skin condoms allow the passage of HIV)

Apply spermicide with nonoxol-9 inside and outside of the condom for added protection in the event of condom breakage

Use water-soluble lubricant to decrease friction on mucous membranes (oil-based lubricants may cause the condom to break)

French (wet) kissing

Controversial because HIV is found in saliva, but no instance of transmission via this route is reported; avoid kissing if either partner has mouth sores

Mutual masturbation

Use latex gloves to guard against possible exposure through cuts on hands

UNSAFE SEX PRACTICES

Vaginal, anal, or oral intercourse without a condom or latex barrier (dental dams)

Unprotected penetration of vagina or anus with fingers or hands

Blood contact of any kind

Sharing sex toys or needles

● **NDX:** Social isolation related to social stigma of AIDS and fear of infecting others

Determine patient's support systems, significant others, family, social groups; encourage patient to continue interactions

Encourage expression of feelings of aloneness, rejection, isolation if present

Be nonjudgmental; listen openly and accept feelings being expressed

Reinforce with patient and visitors that AIDS is not communicated through casual contact such as holding hands, hugging *so that touching and usual contacts with others continue*

Assist patient to maintain contact with others via telephone, letters

Encourage visitors to return frequently

Spend time with patient when not required to perform care-giving tasks *to increase feelings of self-worth*

Avoid unnecessary use of barrier techniques that convey fear of care giver contamination

Assist patient in assessing self-worth, achievements positively

Arrange with significant others to bring personal mementos, pictures, favorite videos, books, tapes, surprises such as flowers, balloons

Provide patient and significant others with information about support groups

EXPECTED OUTCOMES

Maintains healthy, supportive interpersonal relationships with significant others

Verbalizes sense of belonging and feelings of being loved and supported

Patient/family teaching

Explain the following:
 Chest physiotherapy and postural drainage
 Importance of turning, coughing, deep breathing
 Pursed lip or diaphragmatic breathing
 Oxygen administration
 Use of walking aids
 Universal precautions and handwashing, especially after using bathroom and before preparing food
 Importance of maintaining clean home environment
 How to handle and store foods to minimize bacterial count
 Disposal of infectious wastes in secured bags
 Washing of soiled linen separately using 1% bleach solution
 Safe disposal of needles in impervious containers
 Not to clean litter boxes, bird cages, fish tanks in order to avoid exposure to toxoplasmosis
 Never to donate blood or semen
 Importance of avoiding persons who may be infectious, persons who have been recently vaccinated, and crowds
 Care of skin and mucous membranes, oral hygiene
 Relaxation techniques, stress management; maintain balance between activity and rest
 Diet choices that increase caloric intake without irritating oral cavity or bowel
 Safer sex practices (see box, p. 828)
 Changes in condition, signs/symptoms of opportunistic infections that need to be reported to physician
 Procedure of taking oral/axillary T and when to notify physician of elevation
 Administration and side effects of medications
 Care of central line, flushing, and medication administration
 Avoid use of alcohol, tobacco, recreational drugs
 Importance of receiving ongoing outpatient care
 Importance of informing all care providers of HIV infection
 Reasons for wearing medical alert ID band; how to obtain band

Home care considerations

Explain that condition/layout of home, safe arrangement of furniture and other household items, and adequate lighting are necessary to prevent accidental injury

Discuss storage of dressing change supplies; oxygen equipment; walking aid; puncture-proof container for needles, gloves, masks; clean linens

Discuss safe disposal and/or cleaning of sharp objects and other blood- or body-fluid contaminated items

Assess assistance available for shopping, cleaning, transportation; arrange providers as needed

Arrange for durable medical equipment as required

Facilitate hospice care if condition requires

Bone Marrow Transplant

A treatment approach that results in the replenishing of depleted bone marrow cell reserves; care is divided into four phases: pretransplant (preparation), conditioning, transplant, and posttransplant (Table 14-2); there are three sources of donor marrow: allogenic is most common and the treatment of choice for patients with aplastic anemia under 50 years of age for which an identical HLA donor can be found; allogenic grafts may also be used for severe immunodeficiency disorders, acute and chronic leukemia, and multiple myeloma. Autologous transplants are being used to treat Hodgkin's and non-Hodgkin's lymphoma; acute leukemia; lymphoma; responsive solid tumors; neuroblastoma; tumors of the breast, ovaries, and testes; small cell lung cancers; in

Explain intake and output measurement; provide measurement tools and list of volumes of various containers; have patient record on bedside record sheet

Explain and demonstrate assessments that will be done and their frequency: inspection of oral cavity, skin, and perineal status; respiratory, cardiac, GI, and neurologic assessments, testing for occult blood in stool and urine

Discuss activity level patient will be expected to maintain: shower and bathroom activities, ambulation and active ROM exercises, use of exercycle

Promote interest in diversionary activities: TV watching, reading, computer/video games, handicrafts, puzzles; consult occupational therapy *to assess patient abilities and interests and provide challenging activities*

Explain all procedures before their occurrence, expected sensations during, patient participation in, and expected duration of procedures

Collaborate with clinical dietitian *to educate patient regarding low-bacteria diet:* only sterile water for drinking/ice cubes, list of permitted foods, not to leave food at bedside, food from home must be approved and cooked the same day it is eaten

Collaborate with clinical pharmacist to explain medication regimen, actions, benefits, and potential side effects

EXPECTED OUTCOME

Patient and significant other verbalize understanding of BMT and related procedures, medication administration, diet, and self-care

● Conditioning Phase

First phase of the clinical course; involves treatment of patient with a pretransplant conditioning regimen; for patients with leukemia, high-dose cytarabine (Ara-C) or cyclophosphamide and total body irradiation (TBI) have become standard; for patients with aplastic anemia, high-dose cyclophosphamide is given with or without TBI; for patients with lymphomas, etoposide and TBI; and for patients with neuroblastoma, cisplatin, etoposide, melphalan, and TBI

Assessment (related to side effects of drugs and TBI)

Subjective data

Nausea
Anorexia

Objective data

Stomatitis/mucositis
Diarrhea
Pancytopenia
Hemorrhagic cystitis
Sensorineural hearing loss
Azotemia, renal tubular dysfunction
Hypocalcemia, hypomagnesia
Hypotension
Fever
Alopecia
Liver toxicity
SIADH
Vomiting
Parotid gland swelling
Erythema
Decreased saliva and tears
Interstitial pneumonia
Hepatic veno-occlusive disease
Comorbidities: pneumonia
Psychosocial
  Response to treatments
  Relationships and support systems
  Coping mechanisms
  Understanding of disease and treatment

Diagnostic tests

CBC, platelet count
RBC, PT/INR, APTT
Electrolytes, calcium, BUN, creatinine, triglycerides
Liver function tests, AST, ALT, bilirubin, alkaline phosphatase
CMV cultures: urine, blood
Urinalysis
Cardiopulmonary tests: ECG (weekly)

Collaborative management

Therapeutic management

Parenteral fluids and nutrition, TPN
Irradiated blood products
High-dose cyclophosphamide
Cyclosporin
Antiemetics
Antipyretics
Antibiotics
Antidiarrheals
Diuretics
Daily weights
Accurate intake and output measurement
Protective environment
Bladder irrigation, three-way foley catheter

TBI (1000 rad over 3 days), or high-dose cytarabine (ARA-C) and fractionated TBI
Cardiac monitoring during TBI and cyclophosphamide

Nursing management

PATIENT PROBLEMS/NURSING DIAGNOSES

● **NDX:** Knowledge deficit regarding sequence of events during TBI procedure

Explain/reinforce physician's information regarding procedure *to decrease fears*
Patient will be alone in room but will be able to communicate with personnel
Patient will be visually monitored and cardiac monitored at all times during procedure
Nurse will remain in radiology department and be available to speak to patient, provide support and comfort prn
Patient must remain positioned without moving during procedure
Patient must wear mask and will be placed in protective isolation following the procedure

EXPECTED OUTCOMES
Patient and significant other verbalize understanding of procedure and degree of patient cooperation required
Patient participates as directed during the procedure

● **NDX:** Potential for hemorrhagic cystitis related to effects of TBI and cyclophosphamide*

Ensure adequate hydration and diuresis 24 hours before, during, and 24 to 48 hours after administration of cyclophosphamide *to prevent/lessen effects of medication on bladder*
Force fluids to 4000 to 5000 ml/day (unless contraindicated); enlist patient to make choices of fluids, offer small amounts frequently *so required volume can be taken*
Administer parenteral fluids per physician order, usually at rapid rates (200 ml/hr) for several hr before, during, and after chemotherapy administration *to decrease concentration of medication*
Insert and maintain indwelling foley catheter (three way for irrigation) *to keep bladder empty thereby decreasing chance of bleeding;* using strict aseptic technique *to prevent introduction of pathogens*
Perform bladder irrigation per physician order; accurately record intake and output *so imbalance can be noted and treated promptly*

---

*Not a NANDA-approved diagnosis.

Test urine for occult blood q2h to 4h *to determine effects of medication on bladder*

EXPECTED OUTCOME
Signs/symptoms of hemorrhagic cystitis do not develop or are recognized and treated without delay

● **NDX:** Altered nutrition: less than body requirements related to nausea/vomiting, anorexia, parotid gland swelling

Assess amount and type of foods and liquids tolerated and desired; sweet and highly seasoned foods usually are not well tolerated
Assess and eliminate predisposing factors when possible: unpleasant odors, perfumes, body positioning, disturbing sights/sounds *to decrease noxious stimuli*
Arrange for quiet rest periods before meals *to conserve energy for eating*
Arrange for visitors to join patient for meals; may bring favorite (approved) foods from home; *food tolerated better in a social setting*
Ensure patient's room is well ventilated and odors controlled; remove trash, bedpans; remove food tray as soon as meal is finished *to prevent delayed responses to negative stimuli*
Provide foods that may be served cold or at room temperature *to assist in odor control*
Encourage patient to control nausea through relaxation, rhythmic breathing, imagery exercises
Have patient remain sitting for 30 min after meals *to prevent fullness and bloating*
Provide clear liquid diet: juices, carbonated beverages, ice pops *to reduce nausea*
Supplement diet with high-protein, total oral nutrition drinks *to reduce volume required to maintain nutrient level*
Remind patient to eat slowly and chew well
Assist patient in or administer oral care before meals; administer topical anesthetics to oral cavity as needed per physician order *to increase comfort*
In collaboration with clinical dietitian, maintain calorie count and develop meal plans *to meet caloric and nutritional needs* while incorporating patient preferences: BMT patients require 33 to 38 kcal/kg and 1.5 g protein/kg
Weigh patient daily: same scale, clothing, and time
Administer total parenteral nutrition per physician order *to provide required nutrients and fluids to support metabolic needs*

EXPECTED OUTCOMES
Maintains body weight within 5% of baseline
Nausea is controlled, allowing patient to take sufficient calories, nutrients, fluids orally

● **NDX:** Risk for infection related to suppressed immune system

Protective environment to be maintained at all times (protocols will vary among centers): care givers and visitors must wash hands with antibacterial scrub and don mask and gloves before entering patient room *to prevent/decrease introduction of organisms*

Doors to patient room to remain closed

No infectious care givers or visitors to enter room

Patient must wear mask if necessary to leave room

All items entering room are to be sterile or cleaned with bactericidal solution

No flowers or plants to be taken to room *(they harbor infective agents)*

Tap water used for bathing only, never drinking

Instruct visitors in use of protective gear, not to use patient's equipment or bathroom *to prevent transmission of microorganisms*

In collaboration with environmental services: ensure all patient equipment, furniture, fixtures are cleaned with bactericidal solution daily; remove trash, soiled linen from room immediately *to decrease exposure to potentially harmful microorganisms*

Maintain low-bacteria diet and caution in handling and preparation of foods: wash hands before and ensure clean utensils used in food preparation; serve foods at proper temperature; wash thick-skinned fruits in alcohol and peel before serving; dispose of uneaten foods outside patient room; sterile water only for drinking and food preparation

Observe for signs/symptoms of infection: redness, swelling, pain, elevated temperature, changes in breath sounds, cough, sputum, reports of sore throat or burning on urination, urinary frequency/character of urine, *which may indicate early onset infection*

Assess skin condition, paying particular attention to skin folds and orifices, *which provide ideal environment for growth of infective microorganisms*

Use central venous catheter for blood draws and medication administration; ensure perianal care is performed after each elimination; prevent constipation/diarrhea; keep patient and linen clean and dry; encourage mobility and position shifts at least q2h *to maintain skin integrity, which provides a barrier to microorganisms*

Pay particular attention to central venous line insertion site for signs of infection; remind physician of catheter schedule change at intervals required by type of catheter; use strict sterile technique whenever manipulating catheter or changing dressing

Perform daily IV tubing changes; do not allow blood to pool and dry in connections or ports *which creates a medium for growth of microorganisms*

Avoid urinary catheterization; if necessary, use strict sterile technique when manipulating catheter and providing catheter care

Encourage pulmonary exercises, use of incentive spirometer q1h while awake

Assess condition of oral mucous membranes q8h; assist patient to provide scrupulous oral hygiene before and after meals and q4h *to maintain integrity*

Ensure adequate intake of calories and nutrients and promote uninterrupted periods of rest and sleep *to provide energy for body defenses*

EXPECTED OUTCOME

Patient does not exhibit signs/symptoms of infection

● **NDX:** Anxiety/fear related to treatment protocols, physical responses to conditioning regimen, and uncertain prognosis

Assess level of anxiety/fear patient possesses; collaborating with social worker, clergy, significant others in assessment process may be helpful

Provide an environment conducive to open discussion; encourage patient to ventilate feelings, worries, fears; *validation of feelings increases self-awareness*

Continue to provide information and clarify misunderstandings regarding disease and course of treatment; be clear and consistent in responses

Visit frequently when not required to perform tasks; reassure patient that he or she will not be alone *to enhance feelings of trust*

Assist patient in using relaxation methods *to cope with new and unsettling situations*

Use touch and positive body language *to decrease anxious feelings*

Encourage continued relationships and frequent visits from significant other(s) *to provide support to patient*

EXPECTED OUTCOMES

Patient verbalizes decreasing anxiety/fears and demonstrates decreasing overt signs of anxiety/fear

● **NDX:** Body image disturbance related to changes in physical appearance and abilities

Discuss with patient perceptions of changes and effects on lifestyle and relationships *to provide an opportunity to begin self-assessment*

Provide an atmosphere of open discussion and allow for genuine expression of feelings regarding changes that are occurring *to facilitate acceptance and trust*

Give correct information about expected positive changes following conclusion of treatment: regrowth of hair, weight gain *to encourage hope*

Assess patient's desire and ability to participate in self-grooming; assist patient as needed

Compliment patient on strengths, successful completion of difficult procedures/tasks, physical appearance, *which assist patient to recognize positive accomplishments*

Assist patient to find ways of improving physical appearance: clothing, hats, scarves, hair pieces, make-up, grooming *to enhance self-concept*

Consult social services, psychiatry services as needed *to assist patient to work through acceptance of changes*

EXPECTED OUTCOMES

Patient verbalizes feelings about losses and effects on lifestyle and relationships and demonstrates positive coping skills and interest in personal appearance

● Transplant Phase

Phase in which histocompatible donor bone marrow is infused to establish a graft and reinstate production of normal blood cellular components; autologous transplant: patient's marrow that was previously harvested, preserved with DMSO, and frozen is thawed and infused; allogenic and syngeneic transplant: marrow is obtained from donor and immediately infused.

Assessment

Subjective data

Chest pain
SOB
Taste of garlic/oyster

Objective data

Reaction to white cells in marrow: chills, fever, hives
Bacterial contamination of marrow: hypotension, fever, shaking chills
Pulmonary overload: tachypnea, dyspnea, crackles, hypertension
Pulmonary emboli: tachycardia, ECG changes
Hematuria: pink or red urine, heme positive (12 to 24 hr postinfusion)
Garlic or oyster smell from patient
Bun/creatinine elevations (lasts for 24 to 48 hr post-infusion)

Collaborative management

Therapeutic management

Administer marrow
  Autologous marrow
    Premedicate patient with diphenhydramine, acetaminophen, and hydrocortisone

Thaw 50 ml bags of marrow one at a time in basin of warm water
Draw contents of bag into syringe and inject quickly into central venous catheter, through running NS IV infusion
Allogenic, synergetic marrow
  Premedicate patient with diphenhydramine, hydrocortisone, and acetaminophen; administer marrow via IV infusion over no more than 4 hr through central venous catheter

Nursing management

POTENTIAL PATIENT PROBLEM

Fluid overload, allergic reaction, pulmonary emboli related to infusion of bone marrow
  Keep epinephrine, diphenhydramine, hydrocortisone at bedside
  Assess patient q5 min during the infusion, then q15 min two times, then q30 min four times *to observe early, subtle changes indicative of overload*
  Have nitroglycerine and oxygen available at bedside in case of chest pain, SOB
  Remain with patient during infusion *to offer support and reassurance*

EXPECTED OUTCOME

Patient exhibits no adverse reactions are prevented or are recognized early and treated promptly

● Posttransplant Phase

The period after infusion of bone marrow is a critical time in which many problems can occur; the degree that the patient is affected may depend on the underlying disease and clinical status before transplant

Assessment

Subjective data

Photophobia, eye pain
Blurred vision
Taste distortion
Nausea, anorexia
Pruritis

Objective data

Skin and mucous membranes
  Petechiae
  Diffuse maculopapular rash; may be first sign of graft vs. host disease
  Bruising
  Breaks, lesions

Hyperpigmentation; onset 2 to 3 weeks after TBI
Jaundice
Perianal erythema, excoriation
Abscess
Oral cavity
  Irritation, swelling
  Erythema, ulcerations
  Leukoplakia
  Secretions: color, amount, consistency
  Herpes infection
  Lymph nodes (cervical, axillary, groin): size, tenderness, pain
GI system
  Vomiting
  Weight loss
  Parotitis: onset 4 to 24 hr posttransplant; resolved in 24 to 72 hr

Graft vs. Host Disease (GVHD)

Acute condition usually appears 2 wk to 3 months after transplant; new bone marrow cells recognize their environment as foreign and try to destroy their new host

Chronic condition appears 3 months to 1 year after transplant; caused by autoreactive T cells and autoantigens

Manifestations
  Skin
    Maculopapular rash
    Erythroderma
    Exfoliative dermatitis
    Bulbous formation
    Desquamation
    Hair loss
    Jaundice
  GI system
    Denuding
    Abdominal pain
    Ileus
  Hepatomegaly/splenomegaly
  Muscle wasting
  Emaciation
  Increased susceptibility to infection
  Pneumonitis
  Hemolytic anemia
  Bone marrow aplasia
  Lymphatic depletion
  Death

Diarrhea: frequency, color, consistency, occult blood, gross bleeding
Urine: color, amount, odor, hematuria, occult blood, presence of sugar
Breath sounds
  Crackles, diminished
  Rate, depth, pattern of respirations
  Cough, character, frequency
  Sputum color, character, frequency
Cardiovascular system
  Apical rate, rhythm
  Dependent edema
Ophthalmologic system: photophobia, abnormal tear secretion
Activity level: fatigue
Comorbidities
  Infections, hemorrhage
  Graft vs. host disease (GVHD) (see box below, left)

Diagnostic tests

Same as conditioning phase, increased frequency of testing (p. 832)

Collaborative management

Therapeutic management

Total parenteral nutrition
IV fluids/electrolytes
Blood products
Pain management
Low-bacteria diet
Daily weights: same scale, time, and clothing
Accurate measurement of intake and output
Maintain protective environment
Incentive spirometer, oxygen therapy, support of respirations
Antibiotics
Antivirals
Antipyretics
Antidiarrheal
Antiemetics
Antifungals

Nursing management

POTENTIAL PATIENT PROBLEM
Bleeding related to thrombocytopenia
  To determine early and/or subtle signs of bleeding:
    Assess neurologic status q8h
    Inspect condition of oral cavity and gums q4h
    Inspect skin q8h for bruising, petechiae, swelling
    Inspect joints q8h for swelling, decreased mobility

Inspect nasal cavity q8h; discourage vigorous nose
blowing

Assess abdomen q8h for distension, firmness, tenderness, *which may indicate GI bleeding*

Test emesis, stool, and urine for occult blood

Use central venous catheter for blood draws and administration of medications *to decrease incidence of
bleeding caused by multiple punctures*

Avoid skin punctures

Avoid use of rough towels and washcloths, razors,
restraints, tight clothing, *which may cause irritation
and subsequent bleeding*

Maintain clutter-free environment; use a night light
to prevent bumping into objects and falling

Administer gentle oral hygiene; to *maintain integrity
of oral mucosa do not use a toothbrush*

Monitor results of CBC, platelet, PT/INR, APTT as
ordered per physician *to note changes indicative of
bleeding*

Administer platelet, other blood products per physician order

Administer H$_2$ blockers and antacids per physician
order

Administer stool softeners prn *to prevent constipation*

EXPECTED OUTCOME

Occult/frank bleeding is prevented or detected and
treated immediately

PATIENT PROBLEMS/NURSING DIAGNOSES

● **NDX:** Altered oral mucous membrane related to infection or conditioning/transplant regimen

Encourage patient to seek needed dental care before
BMT *so oral mucosa and teeth are in optimal condition*

Inspect oral mucous membranes q4h *so therapy can be
started promptly when changes are noted*

Assist patient/provide oral care q4h while awake, as
well as before and after meals and q4h at night to *keep
mouth free of irritating particles and decrease bacteria
count*

Use soft sponge cleaners or gauze

Rinse mouth frequently with nonalcohol mouthwash,
sterile water

If patient wears dentures: assess for proper fit *to prevent irritation;* keep dentures scrupulously clean; remove dentures and rinse mouth often; dental consult
as needed

Keep mouth moist: provide appealing, tepid liquids for
sipping, ice chips, flavored ice pops; use water-soluble
ointment for lips, artificial saliva

Administer topical anesthetic, antihistamine, antacid
mixture as ordered

Administer antifungal medications as ordered

If patient is unable to open mouth for oral care, irrigate
mouth with sterile saline/water solution, allowing to
drain into emesis basin *to remove irritating particles
and enhance healing*

Consult with clinical dietitian *to provide soft foods that
are nonirritating*

Use straws or cups because *hard utensils may be irritating and cause discomfort and breaks in mucosa*

EXPECTED OUTCOMES

Oral mucous membranes remain intact
Healing of disrupted membranes is progressive

● **NDX:** Risk for impaired skin integrity related
to conditioning/treatment regimen and/or
graft vs. host disease (Tables 14-3 and 14-4)

Table 14-3 Proposed Clinical Stage of Graft vs. Host Disease According to Organ System

Stage	Skin	Liver	Intestinal Tract
+	Maculopapular rash over 25% of body surface	Bilirubin 2-3 mg/dl	Greater than 500 ml diarrhea/day
++	Maculopapular rash over 25% to 50% of body surface	Bilirubin 3-6 mg/dl	Greater than 1000 ml diarrhea/day
+++	Generalized erythroderma	Bilirubin 6-15 mg/dl	Greater than 1500 ml diarrhea/day
++++	Generalized erythroderma with bulbous formation and desquamation	Bilirubin >15 mg/dl	Severe abdominal pain with or without ileus

From Thomas ED. Reprinted by permission of *New Engl J Med* 292:896, 1975, Massachusetts Medical Society.

Table 14-4 Overall Clinical Grading of Severity of Graft vs. Host Disease

Grade	Degree of Organ Involvement
I	+ to ++ skin rash; no gut involvement; no liver involvement; no decrease in clinical performance
II	+ to +++ skin rash; + gut involvement or + liver involvement (or both); mild decrease in clinical performance
III	++ to +++ skin rash; ++ to +++ gut involvement or ++ to ++++ liver involvement (or both); marked decrease in clinical performance
IV	Similar to grade III with ++ to ++++ organ involvement and extreme decrease in clinical performance

From Thomas ED. Reprinted by permission of *New Engl J Med* 292:896, 1975, Massachusetts Medical Society.

Assess skin q8h: focus on trunk, palms, soles of feet, ears for maculopapular erythematous rash *so that early changes can be noted and therapy instituted*

Shower/bathe daily and as needed to keep skin clean and dry; pat dry, do not rub *to avoid irritation/ abrasions*

Do not leave skin moist with lotions; avoid perfumes, deodorants, *which may cause allergic reactions*

Keep bed dry and linen wrinkle free *to prevent areas of decreased circulation leading to skin disruption;* use sterile linen and gowns

Use foot cradle, air fluid therapy bed as needed *to maintain circulation to all skin areas*

Turn, sit up in chair, ambulate q2h as tolerated; encourage small shifts in position q30min while in bed

Assist patient to perform perineal care after each elimination *to maintain skin integrity*

Maintain a safe environment and assist patient *to avoid bumps, cuts, scratches*

Instruct patient to avoid scratching

Keep nails short and cut straight across

Protect feet with slippers, shoes when out of bed

Avoid wearing jewelry *because moisture and bacteria can collect underneath, certain metals can irritate, rough edges may scratch*

Assess condition of all invasive sites q8h; maintain strict sterile techniques when changing dressings

EXPECTED OUTCOMES
Skin integrity is maintained
Disrupted skin heals progressively

● **NDX:** Diarrhea related to conditioning/treatment regimen, graft vs. host disease

Observe stools for frequency, amount, consistency, presence of gross/occult blood

Measure liquid stool for inclusion in intake and output calculations

Maintain food diary: eliminate foods that increase/stimulate bowel motility

Cooked foods may be better tolerated than raw fruits and vegetables; omit hot, spicy foods, *which may irritate bowel or enhance peristalsis;* decrease amount of dairy products in diet *to decrease bloated feeling or allergic response*

Encourage foods that decrease bowel motility: rice, bananas

Administer antidiarrheal medications per physician order

EXPECTED OUTCOME
Frequency of stools decreases, consistency becomes more solid

● **NDX:** Impaired gas exchange related to complications of radiation/chemotherapy, BMT

Assess respiratory status q4h to 8h: rhythm, rate, depth, breath sounds, use of accessory muscles, *which indicates decreased function*

Monitor results of ABGs per physician order

Report cough, fever, tachycardia, dyspnea, increased respiratory rate/distress at rest or with activity

Position patient for maximum chest excursion and comfort of respiration: upright supported by pillows or leaning on overbed table

Encourage coughing and deep breathing, use of incentive spirometer q2h while awake *to facilitate movement/removal of secretions*

Suction airways as needed if patient is unable to clear with coughing

Provide oxygen therapy and support ventilation per physician order

Administer medications per physician order

EXPECTED OUTCOME
Patient exhibits breathing patterns that support adequate respiration and gas exchange

● **NDX:** Risk for fluid volume excess related to venoocclusive disease of the liver

Assess volume status

Weigh patient daily: same time, clothing, and scale: *sudden weight gain may indicate liver congestion*

Measure abdominal girth and palpate right upper quadrant q8h to 12h: *increasing girth/tenderness may indicate liver congestion, ascites*

Record accurate intake and output; *positive balance may indicate volume overload*

Assess lung sounds for crackles, wheezes, *which may indicate pulmonary congestion*

Maintain fluid, sodium restrictions as indicated

Monitor results of bilirubin and AST/ALT: *elevated values may indicate compromised liver function*

EXPECTED OUTCOMES

Intake and output remain in balance

Signs/symptoms of volume overload/compromised liver function do not develop or are recognized and treated promptly

● **NDX:** Fatigue related to interrupted sleep patterns, inadequate nutrition, anemia, emotional distress, effects of radiation/chemotherapy

Cluster activities, schedule treatments/tests purposefully *to provide uninterrupted periods of sleep and rest*

Assist patient as needed with meal preparation and consumption, personal hygiene, and daily activities *to conserve energy for required activities*

Assess response to activity; alter sequence or amount of assistance provided if not tolerated

Increase activities slowly and only as tolerated; encourage patient to remain involved in physical activities to tolerance

EXPECTED OUTCOME

Patient is able to participate in daily activities with increasing independence and decreased fatigue

ADDITIONAL NURSING DIAGNOSES TO CONSIDER

Ineffective individual coping related to prolonged disease, uncertain prognosis, multiple life changes, inadequate support systems

Sexuality patterns, altered: impotence, sterility related to disease process, effects of treatment regimen

Pain from oral mucositis related to infection, treatment regimen

Patient/family teaching

Self-care procedures: demonstrate and explain rationale, observe return demonstrations for the following:

Care and flushing of central venous access

Administration of IV medication via central line; use of IV pump

Oral mucous membrane assessment and hygiene

Skin assessment, skin care, perianal care

Handwashing

Use of incentive spirometer

Measurement of intake and output

Occult blood testing of urine and stool

Methods for taking and recording body T

Low-bacteria diet

Instruct in assessment and prevention of the following potential/actual complications

Activity intolerance

Importance of planned rest periods throughout the day and uninterrupted sleep at night

Plan activities for after rest periods

Increase activities to tolerance; seek assistance with ADLs as needed

Importance of changing positions slowly; use of assistive devices as needed

Maintaining a diet high in iron (to combat anemia)

Bleeding

Have emergency telephone numbers on hand; how to reach paramedics, physician

Location of nearest emergency room

Notification of all medical/dental personnel of posttransplant status and medications currently taking

Maintain a safe, clutter-free environment

Avoid over-the-counter medications without consulting physician

Avoid sharp objects; use electric razor

Avoid harsh nose blowing; demonstrate methods for applying pressure for nose bleeding

Infection

Avoid persons who may be infectious, recently vaccinated; avoid crowds

Avoid multiple sex partners

Wash hands before and after eating and toileting

Prevent skin injury, wear protective garments when gardening, cleaning

Avoid overexposure to sun: wear hats, sunscreen

Avoid going barefoot; cut nails straight across

Performing oral hygiene before and after meals and sleep

Avoid drinking fountains

Stomatitis

Explain importance of maintaining oral hygiene routine in morning, before and after meals, and at bedtime

Discuss equipment to use to avoid irritation; avoid alcohol-containing mouthwashes

Teach importance of avoiding irritating foods, controlling temperature and texture to tolerance

Diarrhea
  Discuss importance of maintaining fluid intake at
    least equal to output
  Avoid diet high in fiber, roughage; other foods to
    avoid per individual patient tolerance
  Explain importance of taking prescribed medica-
    tions for diarrhea, avoiding over-the-counter
    medications
Diet
  Explain need to maintain low-bacteria diet
  Discuss need to supplement diet with total par-
    enteral/oral nutrition
  Teach procedures for handling, storing, and cooking
    foods for safe consumption (see box below)
Continuing health care
  Explain importance of keeping appointments for lab-
    oratory, diagnostic work and physician providers
  Provide information regarding community re-
    sources, support groups, home care agencies,
    durable medical equipment suppliers
  Teach names, actions, side effects, potential adverse
    reactions of medications to report to physician

Home care considerations

Explain how to prepare environment to receive patient:
  must be clean and dust free; all surfaces and furniture
  must be washed/vacuumed; environment should be
  clutter free
Remove living flowers and plants
Pets should be boarded elsewhere for the first 100 days
Explain necessity of daily cleaning and damp dusting
  (avoid dry dusting)
Store health care equipment and supplies in clean
  area
Change towels and washcloths at least daily

Temperatures (°F) for Food Safeness	
165° to 195°	This temperature kills most harmful bacteria
140° to 150°	Minimum temperature at which to cook foods to kill bacteria
45° to 140°	Danger zone for food safe-ness; rapid bacterial growth
34° to 45°	Cold or chill food storage; slow bacterial growth
0° to −10°	Frozen food storage

Change bed linens at least twice per week
Clean and dry kitchen utensils immediately after use
Empty trash immediately

Rheumatoid Arthritis

*A chronic, systemic, inflammatory disease of unknown
etiology that is characterized by an inflammatory
reaction in the synovial membrane and leads to
destruction of joint cartilage and subsequent
deformities; the disease may also affect the pulmonary,
cardiac, central nervous, integumentary, and
reticuloendothelial systems; rheumatoid arthritis
occurs more frequently in women and the incidence
increases with advancing age*

Assessment

Subjective data

Fatigue, malaise
Sleep disturbances
Paresthesia of hands and feet
Joint pain and stiffness, especially after periods of rest

Objective data

Weight loss
Dry eyes, sclera
Swelling, warmth, tenderness of involved joints
Impaired joint function
Joint effusions, deformities
Shiny, taut skin over affected joints
Low-grade fever
Muscular weakness, spasms, atrophy, contractions
Subcutaneous nodules over pressure points
Vasculitic skin lesions
Vasculitis of peripheral nerves; wrist-drop and foot-drop
Comorbidities
  Raynaud's phenomenon
  Anemia
  GI bleeding
  Renal calculi
  Pericarditis
  Tenosynovitis
  Interstitial fibrosis, pneumonitis
  Keratoconjunctivitis (Sjögren's syndrome)

Diagnostic tests

CBC, WBC, ESR
ASO titer, rheumatoid factor
C-reactive protein
Antinuclear antibodies

Imaging studies
  Joint radiographs: bone erosion, periarticular
    osteopenia, joint space narrowing
  Arthroscopy with synovial fluid analysis

Collaborative management

Therapeutic management

Physical therapy: paraffin, whirlpool, moist heat,
  cold/heat therapy, ROM exercises
Splints, braces, walking aids
Diet, activity, rest
Antiinflammatories: aspirin, nonsteroidals, ibuprofen,
  naproxen
Corticosteroids
Immunosuppressives: azathioprine
Tranquilizers, antidepressants
Antirheumatic agents: gold, sodium thiomaleate,
  penicillamine
Surgical intervention: total arthroplasty (p. 535), syn-
  ovectomy, arthrodesis
Investigative therapies
  Anti-CD5, anti-CD4 antibody
  DAB$_{488}$ IL-2
  IL-1 receptor antagonist
  TNF alpha inhibitor
  Interferon-gamma
  GMCSF
  Minocycline
  AGM-1470
  Methotrexate
Physical therapy consultation

Nursing management

PATIENT PROBLEMS/NURSING DIAGNOSES

● **NDX:** Pain related to joint inflammation, swelling

Assess location, intensity of pain using consistent pain
  rating scale *to determine tolerance and symptoms for
  which intervention should occur*
Use firm mattress, bedboard, footboard as appropriate
  to provide support
Maintain proper alignment of joints *to increase comfort*
  Extend joints as tolerated
  Avoid external rotation of joints; use supports as
    necessary
  Avoid neck flexion; use thin pillow
Apply splints, braces, traction *to immobilize/support
  joint per physician order*
Handle affected limbs gently, providing support above
  and below joint *to avoid jarring, jerky movements,
  which increase pain*

Monitor effectiveness of treatments: heat/cold, paraffin, whirlpool
Administer skin care and gentle rubs *to enhance feeling
  of comfort*
Use sheepskin, foam, water, air mattress, elbow and
  heel guards
Administer analgesic, antiinflammatory medications
  per physician order
Observe response to medications in terms of pain relief
  and for potential adverse reactions
Discuss and assist patient to use alternate methods of
  pain relief

EXPECTED OUTCOMES
Patient states pain level is tolerable and is able to incorporate existing pain into lifestyle and self-care
  activities

● **NDX:** Self-care deficit: feeding, grooming, toileting,
  bathing, dressing related to limitation of
  physical mobility

Assess current level of functioning; assist patient with
  task analysis of daily activities *to determine priorities*
Administer pain medications before activities
Assist with activities as needed; coach patient through
  daily activities *to simplify task, conserve energy, and increase use of assistive devices*
Consult with physical/occupational therapist *to provide assistive devices: reachers, elevated seats,
  extended shoe horn, large-grip spoons, walking
  aids*
Set goals with patient: encourage short-term, easily
  achieved goals
Be patient; allow sufficient time for patient to complete
  tasks *to enhance compliance and independence*

EXPECTED OUTCOMES
Patient is able to incorporate current level of function-
  ing into performing independent ADLs
Uses assistive devices to increase independence

ADDITIONAL NURSING DIAGNOSES
TO CONSIDER
Body image disturbance related to altered appearance
  and function
Fatigue related to sleep disturbances, chronic illness

Patient/family teaching

Importance of maintaining prescribed exercise, activity,
  rest program
Proper joint alignment and use of supports
Diet management, avoiding undue weight gain
Use of assistive devices and walking aids

Changes in condition that need to be reported to physician

Medication administration and potential side effects, especially means to avoid potential GI effects

Importance of follow-up care with physician and physical therapist

Home care considerations

Assess home for potentially dangerous situations: loose rugs, cluttered furniture, inadequate lighting, many steps, smooth bathtub bottom, dangling cords

Assess assistance available for physical needs, shopping, cleaning, transportation; arrange providers as required

Ensure provision of ADLs and walking aids to take home; contact durable medical equipment provider

Sarcoidosis

A multisystem granulomatous disorder of unknown etiology; any organ system may be involved, but pulmonary manifestations are most common; in most cases the process is benign and self-limiting without residual effects; 10% become chronic conditions, staged according to international standards, based on chest x-ray findings, fatal in 5% of cases; most common in young adults and blacks

Assessment

Subjective data

Anorexia
Arthralgia
Fatigue, malaise
SOB
Palpitations
Mild to severe chest pain (rare)
Ocular pain

Objective data

Fever, night sweats
Weight loss
Arthritis (symmetrical, migratory)
Clubbing of fingers
Respiratory system
  Dyspnea
  Cough: usually nonproductive but may be incapacitating, paroxysms may lead to vomiting
  Hypoxemia
  Diffuse crackles or just at bases

Ophthalmologic system
  Blurred vision, lacrimation
  Conjunctival infection
  Uveitis, iritis
  Blindness (rare)
Cardiovascular system
  Dysrhythmia, conduction defects
  Hypotension
  Jugular vein distension
Integumentary system
  Skin nodules on face, neck, extremities
  Bone cysts in hands, feet
  Nasal mucosa lesions, alopecia
Parotid, cervical lymphadenopathy, splenomegaly

Diagnostic tests

Kveim skin test (intradermal injection of sarcoid tissue suspension): positive in 3 to 6 wk
CBC
Serum protein levels
  C-reactive protein: elevated
  Polyclonal hypergamma globulin: decreased
  IgG: elevated
  IgA, IgM: may be elevated
ESR: elevated
Angiotensin-converting enzyme level: may be elevated
Skin and lymph node biopsy
Cardiopulmonary tests
  Transbronchial biopsy
  Open lung biopsy
  Bronchoalveolar lavage
Imaging/nuclear medicine tests
  Chest radiograph; various hilar lymphadenopathy to diffuse infiltrates and pulmonary fibrosis
  Pulmonary function tests: normal to decreased vital capacity and expiratory flow volumes, decreased compliance
  Gallium-67 scan of lungs
Comorbidities
  Restrictive lung diseases; pulmonary fibrosis
  Complications of steroid therapy; diabetes, infections

Collaborative management

Therapeutic management

Dependent on symptoms, none may be necessary
Serial chest radiographs and pulmonary function testing
Low-calcium, low-sodium, low-potassium diet
Vitamin D supplements
Physical therapy consultation: chest physiotherapy—breathing exercises, percussion, and postural drainage
Oxygen therapy

Supportive/definitive treatment for arthritis

Medications may include: systemic/topical steroids; azathioprine; optic agents; antidysrhythmic agents; calcium chelating agents

Nursing management

PATIENT PROBLEMS/NURSING DIAGNOSES

● **NDX:** Impaired gas exchange related to pulmonary fibrosis or parenchymal lesions

Assess respiratory status: observe for coughing, adventitious sounds, dyspnea, abnormal rate, rhythm *indicative of decreased function*

Obtain sputum specimen for culture *to identify presence of infective agents* as ordered by physician; observe sputum for changes in color, character

Assist patient to use energy conservation techniques

Assist patient to use pursed lip breathing and positioning *to facilitate ease of breathing*

Monitor results of pulmonary function tests, ABGs for changes from baseline

Administer oxygen therapy, breathing treatments per physician order

EXPECTED OUTCOMES

Patient maintains adequate gas exchange and ABGs within baseline

● **NDX:** Pain related to disease-induced arthralgia and ocular discomfort

Assess pain: location, onset, duration, precipitating and alleviating factors *to determine best method to use to enhance comfort*

Use consistent pain rating scale

Assess nonverbal signs of pain

Assist patient to achieve comfortable positions

Assist patient to achieve state of minimal physical tension through relaxation

In collaboration with physician, provide analgesic medications as required, observing for therapeutic results and side effects

EXPECTED OUTCOMES

Patient verbalizes decrease/relief of pain

Incorporates pain into performance of daily activities

Facial expressions and body positioning are relaxed

● **NDX:** Potential for dysrhythmia related to involvement of the cardiac conduction system*

---

*Not a NANDA-approved diagnosis.

Assess VS, including apical and peripheral P q4h

Monitor cardiac rhythm continuously or via daily ECG per physician order

Observe for signs/symptoms of decreased cardiac output: hypotension, chest pain, pallor, cool skin, decreased urine output, tachycardia, fatigue, palpitations

Administer oxygen therapy per physician order

Administer antidysrhythmic medications per physician order

EXPECTED OUTCOMES

Cardiac dysrhythmia is detected and treated promptly

ECG remains within baseline for patient

Patient/family teaching

Explain management of lung disease: administration of oxygen and nebulized medications, chest physiotherapy, positioning, breathing exercises, avoiding persons who smoke

Explain disease process and treatment rationale

Discuss changes in condition that warrant notification of physician: SOB, red/watery eyes, dizziness, chest pain, swollen joints, unusual fatigue, fever

Explain medication administration side effects: need to take steroids with food, antacids; do not take over-the-counter medications without consulting physician

Advise on diet choices to provide balanced nutrition within restrictions

Discuss importance of continued follow-up with physician

Home care considerations

Assess patient support system and ability to provide assistance for physical needs, cooking, cleaning, shopping, and transportation as needed; arrange home care providers as necessary

Assess sufficient, clean space available to store medical equipment and supplies; arrange for durable medical equipment provider as necessary

Systemic Lupus Erythematosus

A chronic autoimmune inflammatory disease of the connective tissues that produces biochemical and structural changes in skin, joints, and muscles, usually with multiple organ involvement; the number of organs involved makes the disease an imitator of many other diseases

Assessment

Subjective data

Malaise
Anorexia
Nausea
Abdominal pain
Headache
Photophobia

Objective data

Fever, weakness
Hemolytic anemia
Thrombocytopenia
GI system
  Vomiting, diarrhea, weight loss
  Hepatosplenomegaly
Genitourinary system
  Hematuria
  Cellular casts*
  Proteinuria*
Cardiovascular system
  Hypertension, cardiomegaly, edema
  Pericarditis, murmurs
  ECG changes, dysrhythmia
Renal system: azotemia, hypoproteinuria
Neurovascular system
  Neuritis, seizures*
  Raynaud's phenomenon
  Vasculitis; necrosis of small arteries
Musculoskeletal system
  Nondeforming arthritis
  Joint warmth and swelling
Integumentary system
  Sensitivity to sun*
  Rash/erythema, "butterfly" over cheeks and bridge of
    nose*
  Partial alopecia*
  Oral/nasal ulcerations*
Respiratory system
  Pleuritis
  Parenchymal lung infiltrates
  Pulmonary hemorrhage
Ophthalmologic system
  Retinal cystoid bodies
  Conjunctivitis
  Diplopia
Personality changes
Depression
Psychosis
Hemolytic anemia*

---

*Four or more of these findings support the diagnosis of SLE

Diagnostic tests

LE prep: positive
Antinuclear antibody (ANA): positive
Anti-DNA antibody: positive
Fluorescent treponemal antibody absorption
  (FTA-ABS): negative
Complement (C3 and C4)
CBC, thrombocytopenia, leukopenia
C-reactive protein
ESR, coagulation profile
Rheumatoid factor
Synovial fluid analysis
Urinalysis
False-positive serology*
Creatinine clearance
Imaging studies: chest radiograph
Skin and kidney biopsy
Comorbidities
  Infection resulting from steroid use
  Renal failure
  MI
  Pneumonia
  Cerebrovascular accident

Collaborative management

Therapeutic management

Medications
  Nonsteroidal antiinflammatory agents
  Corticosteroids
  Antiinfective agents
  Antineoplastic agents
  Antihypertensives
  Analgesics
  Bronchodilators
  Antipyretics
  Antibiotics
Plasmapheresis
Dialysis
Joint arthroplasty
Renal transplant
Diet, activity, rest
Dietary consultation

Nursing management

POTENTIAL PATIENT PROBLEM

Renal, cardiac, and neurologic system dysfunction related to tissue destruction from deposition of immune
  complexes and antibodies
  Assess renal status: monitor for presence of edema,
    nausea, hematuria, hypertension

---

*Four or more of these findings support the diagnosis of SLE

Accurately record intake and output
Monitor results of urinalysis and kidney function
  studies
Assess neurologic status: observe for changes in
  LOC, judgment, mental acuity, speech, personality
  changes
Assess cardiac status: monitor VS, hemodynamic status, cardiac rhythm, presence of edema, jugular vein
  distension

EXPECTED OUTCOME
Changes in renal, cardiac, and/or neurologic function
are detected early, and treatment is initiated

PATIENT PROBLEMS/NURSING DIAGNOSES

● **NDX:**   Impaired gas exchange related to pulmonary
          involvement in SLE

Assess respiratory system: observe for dyspnea,
  cyanosis, diminished breath sounds, coarse/fine
  crackles, tachypnea, bradypnea
Elevate head of bed for ease of respiration
Supply oxygen therapy as ordered by physician
Encourage turning, controlled coughing, deep breathing *to clear lungs and airways*
Administer pulmonary medications as ordered by
  physician: bronchodilators, steroids
Obtain sputum cultures as ordered by physician *to determine presence of infective agents*
Maintain adequate hydration *to facilitate movement of
  secretions*

EXPECTED OUTCOMES
Patient exhibits no signs of respiratory distress

● **NDX:**   Altered nutrition: less than body require-
          ments related to fatigue, nausea, anorexia

Assess nutritional status, maintain calorie count
Consult with dietitian and physician *to develop meal
  plans that incorporate caloric requirements and restrictions based on organ system involvement*
Provide frequent, small meals, *which are more easily
  tolerated*
Provide an environment conducive to pleasant
  eating: provide oral care before meals, remove
  bedpans/urinals, have patient sit up in chair for
  meals
Provide calm, unhurried atmosphere; assist patient to
  eat as necessary
Weigh patient daily: same time, clothing, and scale

EXPECTED OUTCOMES
Patient consumes and retains 80% to 90% of each meal

Weight is maintained within 2% of patient's ideal body
  weight
Intake and output remain balanced

● **NDX:**   Activity intolerance related to poor nutrition,
          painful joints

Coordinate activities *to provide for undisturbed periods
  of rest and sleep*
Assess activity tolerance and range of motion of af-
  fected joints *so plan of care can be altered to meet
  patient needs*
Evaluate pain and effectiveness of current regimen
Administer analgesics as needed before activity *to increase comfort and willingness to participate*
Set goals with patient *to gradually increase activity*
Perform active/passive ROM exercises qid; collaborate
  with physical therapist *to determine most appropriate
  activities*
Provide assistive devices as needed *to ensure safety*
Monitor patient during activity for signs of excess fatigue: changes in VS, dysrhythmia, subjective complaints; discontinue activity based on adverse
  responses
Encourage patient to participate in activities to tolerance; promote a positive attitude; assist as needed *to
  prevent exhaustion*
Consult with clinical dietitian *to plan meals with sufficient calories and nutrients to sustain activity level
  required*
Set activity goals with patient; help patient identify
  progress made

EXPECTED OUTCOMES
Patient participates in care to tolerance
Tolerance for activity gradually increases; patient states
  a feeling of increased energy

● **NDX:**   Risk for infection, related to compromised
          immune system, immunosuppressive med-
          ications, multiple organ system dysfunction

Monitor results of laboratory tests: CBC, WBC differ-
  ential, ESR, C-reactive protein, urinalysis, cultures
Obtain culture of drainage from any site: sputum, urine,
  blood per physician order
Monitor for elevated T
Assist patient to maintain excellent personal hygiene *to
  decrease environment conducive to growth of infective
  microorganisms*
Restrict visitors, care givers who may be infectious
Provide for optimal nutrition and fluid intake *to enhance
  body defense mechanisms*
Avoid multiple injection sites
Use strict sterile technique for all invasive procedures

Administer antibiotics and other antiinfectives per physician order

EXPECTED OUTCOME
Patient exhibits no signs of infection

ADDITIONAL NURSING DIAGNOSES TO CONSIDER

Impaired skin integrity, related to integumentary involvement

Body image disturbance related to change in physical appearance and abilities

Patient/family teaching

Explain natural course of disease process, treatment options

Teach administration and side effects of medications

Discuss need to avoid penicillin, sulfa, phenytoin, oral contraceptives

Advise on significant changes in condition, signs/symptoms of infection that need to be reported to physician

Explain importance of continuing follow-up care

Discuss importance of skin care and protection from the sun (sun block)

Advise avoidance of infected individuals and crowds

Discuss need to wear medical alert ID band, how to obtain the band

Teach importance of notifying all care givers of diagnosis

Explain community resources, Lupus Foundation benefits

Home care considerations

Assess patient's ability to provide for own self-care and daily living needs; arrange for home care providers as needed

BIBLIOGRAPHY

Anastasi JK, Rivera J: Understanding prophylactic therapy for HIV infections, *Am J Nurs* February: 36, 1994.

Anastasi JK, Lee VS: HIV wasting: how to stop the cycle, *Am J Nurs* June: 18, 1994.

Ackley BJ, Ladwig GB: *Nursing diagnosis handbook: a guide to planning care,* St Louis, 1993, Mosby.

Atal M et al: Prevention of gram-positive infections after bone marrow transplantation by systemic vancomycin: a prospective, randomized trial, *J Clin Oncol* 9:865, May 1991.

Beare PG, Myers JL: *Principles and practice of adult health nursing,* ed 2, St Louis, 1994, Mosby.

Belcher A: *Cancer nursing,* St Louis, 1992, Mosby.

Belza et al: Correlates of fatigue in older adults with rheumatoid arthritis, *Nurs Res* 42(2):93, 1993.

Bradley-Springer L: Nutritional support in HIV infection: a multilevel analysis, *IMAGE J Nurs Sch* 23(3):155, 1991.

Carpenito LJ: *Nursing diagnosis application to clinical practice,* ed 5, Philadelphia, 1993, JB Lippincott.

Corless et al: Nursing dependency needs of HIV infected patients part 1: methods and clinical findings, *Nurs Adm Q* 18(2):1, 1994.

Crouch R: Current concepts in autologous bone marrow transplantation, *Semin Oncol Nurs* 10(1):12, 1994.

El-Sadr et al: Evaluation and management of early HIV infection, *Clinical Practice Guideline,* Washington, DC, US Department of Health and Human Resources.

Ezzone et al: Survey of oral hygiene regimens among bone marrow transplant centers, *Oncol Nurs Forum* 20(9):1375, 1993.

Franco, Gould: Allogenic bone marrow transplantation, *Semin Oncol Nurs* 10(1):3, 1994.

Grimes D et al: *Infectious diseases,* St Louis, 1991, Mosby.

Jones et al: *Medical surgical nursing, a conceptual approach,* New York, 1982, McGraw-Hill.

Kelley et al: *Textbook of internal medicine,* Philadelphia, 1989, JB Lippincott.

Keithley JK et al: Nutritional alterations in persons with HIV infection, *IMAGE J Nurs Sch* 24(3):183, 1992.

Kelly PJ, Holman S: The new face of AIDS, *Am J Nurs* 93(3), 1993.

Kim MJ et al: *Pocket guide to nursing diagnoses,* ed 6, St Louis, 1995, Mosby.

Lader: HIV infections of the central nervous system, *Nurs Clin North Am* 28(4):838, 1993.

LeMone P: Analysis of a human phenomenon: self-concept. *Nurs Diagn* 2(3):126, 1991.

Mack CH: Assessment of the autologous bone marrow transplant patient according to Orem's self care model, *Cancer Nurs* 15(6):429, 1992.

McCance KL, Huether SE: *Pathophysiology: the biological basis for disease in adults and children,* ed 2, St Louis, 1994, Mosby.

McClosky G, Bulechek: *Nursing interventions classification,* St Louis, 1992, Mosby.

McFarland GK, McFarlane EA: *Nursing diagnosis and intervention: planning for patient care,* ed 2, St Louis, 1993, Mosby.

Mehmert PPA, Delaney CW: Validating impaired physical mobility, *Nurs Diagn* 2(4):143, 1991.

Miller-Blair, Robbins: Rheumatoid arthritis: new science, new treatment, *Geriatrics* 48(6):28, 1993.

Mudge-Grout C: *Immunologic disorders,* St Louis, 1992, Mosby.

Muma et al: HIV manual for health care professionals, Norwalk, Conn, 1994, Appleton & Lange.

Nokes et al: Development of an HIV assessment tool, *IMAGE J Nurs Sch* 26(2):133, 1994.

Norris J: Nursing intervention for self-esteem disturbances, *Nurs Diagn* 3(2):48, 1992.

Ouellet LL, Rush KL: A synthesis of selected literature on mobility: a basis for studying impaired mobility, *Nurs Diagn* 3(2):72, 1992.

Radziewicz RM, Schneider SM: Using diversional activity to enhance coping, *Cancer Nurs* 15(4):293, 1992.

Roitt IM et al: *Immunology,* ed 3, St Louis, 1993, Mosby.

Singla et al: The role of nutrition support and megesterol therapy in reversing malnutrition in AIDS. *AIDS Patient Care* 7(3):132, 1993.

Sparks SM: Exploring electronic support groups, *Am J Nurs* December: 62, 1992.

Thompson J et al: *Mosby's clinical nursing,* ed 3, St Louis, 1993, Mosby.

Zepp: The "potential for injury" and the risk for falls in patients with HIV disease. *AIDS Patient Care* 7(5):249, 1993.

USC UNIVERSITY HOSPITAL

1500 San Pablo
Los Angeles, CA 90033

MULTIDISCIPLINARY PLAN

DIAGNOSIS HIV with Severe Diarrhea ± Fever	NAME _____
SURGERY _____	ALLERGIES _____
	MR# _____
	ADMIT DATE _____

DISCHARGE OUTCOMES	DRG 490 ALOS 8.4
PHYSIOLOGICAL	Bowel function: diarrhea controlled with treatment of causative organism. Fluid/electrolyte within normal limits. Adequate nutritional intake as evidenced by maintenance of weight and labs within normal limits.
COGNITIVE	Verbalizes medical follow-up plan, and signs and symptoms to report to health care team. Verbalizes modes of transmission of HIV, universal precautions, high and low risk behaviors.
PSYCHOLOGICAL	Anxiety/fear controlled as evidenced by ability to participate in medical decisions/care. Demonstrates methods to manage fear/anxiety. Knowledgeable about available community support.

DISCIPLINE	PRE-OP/ PRE-ADMIT	D.O.S. DATE ___ DAY 1	P.O.#1 DATE ___ DAY 2	P.O.#2 DATE ___ DAY 3	P.O.#3 DATE ___ DAY 4	P.O.#4 DATE ___ DAY 5	P.O.#5 DATE ___ DAY 6
LOCATION		Med/Surg	Med/Surg	Med/Surg	Med/Surg	Med/Surg	Med/Surg
LABS		CBC, Chem 20 Blood culture Stool culture, O & P. AFB, C. difficile	Chem 7 CBC Stool for O & P	Chem 7 Stool for O & P	Chem 7 CBC		CBC
CARDIO-PULMONARY							
IMAGING/ NUCLEAR MEDICINE		CXR Verify with MD any bowel preparations.	Verify with MD any bowel preparations.	Verify with MD any bowel preparations.	Verify with MD any bowel preparations.	Verify with MD any bowel preparations.	Verify with MD any bowel preparations.
SOCIAL SERVICES D/C PLAN REHAB. SERVICES		Assess home situation, and psychological response to illness. Provide support prn.	D/C planning. Home health as indicated.	Continued psychosocial support.		Reassess D/C plan.	
PHARMACY		• K+, electrolyte replacement • IV fluid replacement Antidiarrheals unless salmonellosis. Antibiotic therapy as indicated for identified pathogen.	Electrolyte replacement. IV fluid replacement. Antidiarrheals.				
DIETARY/ NUTRITION		DAT. If n/v clear, advance as tolerated.	NPO status as indicated for testing; otherwise, advance diet. Dietitian/consult.	NPO status as indicated for testing; otherwise, advance diet.	Begin calorie count x3 days	Nutritional supplement as indicated.	

Continued.

USC UNIVERSITY HOSPITAL

1500 San Pablo
Los Angeles, CA 90033

MULTIDISCIPLINARY PLAN

NAME _____
ALLERGIES _____

MR# _____

DIAGNOSIS HIV with Severe Diarrhea ± Fever

SURGERY _____

DISCHARGE OUTCOMES	DRG 490 ALOS 8.4
PHYSIOLOGICAL	Bowel function: diarrhea controlled with treatment of causative organism. Fluid/electrolyte within normal limits. Adequate nutritional intake as evidenced by maintenance of weight and labs within normal limits.
COGNITIVE	Verbalizes medical follow-up plan & signs and symptoms to report to health care team. Verbalizes modes of transmission of HIV, universal precautions, high and low risk behaviors.
PSYCHOLOGICAL	Anxiety/fear controlled as evidenced by ability to participate in medical decisions/care. Demonstrates methods to manage fear/anxiety. Knowledgeable about available community support.

DISCIPLINE	PRE-OP/ PRE-ADMIT	P.O.#6 DATE	DAY 7	P.O.#7 DATE	DAY 8	P.O.#8 DATE	DAY 9	P.O.#9 DATE	DAY 10	P.O.#10 DATE	DAY 11	P.O.#11 DATE	DAY 12
LOCATION													
LABS													
CARDIO-PULMONARY													
IMAGING/ NUCLEAR MEDICINE													
SOCIAL SERVICES D/C PLAN REHAB. SERVICES		Home health plan established as indicated.											
PHARMACY													
DIETARY/ NUTRITION		Diet as tolerated.											

PATIENT NAME: _____

MEDICAL RECORD # _____

MULTIDISCIPLINARY PLAN

DISCIPLINE	PRE-OP/ PRE-ADMIT	D.O.S. DATE	DAY 1 DATE	P.O. #1 DATE	DAY 2 DATE	P.O. #2 DATE	DAY 3 DATE	P.O. #3 DATE	DAY 4 DATE	P.O. #4 DATE	DAY 5 DATE	P.O. #5 DATE	DAY 6
PATIENT ACTIVITY		Up ad lib, as tolerated. Daily wt before breakfast.	Up ad lib, as tolerated. Daily wt before breakfast.	Up ad lib, as tolerated. Daily wt before breakfast.	Daily wt before breakfast.	Daily wt before breakfast.	Daily wt before breakfast.	Daily wt before breakfast.		
EDUCATION		Hospital orientation. Preprocedure instructions.	Preprocedure instructions. Medication education.	Preprocedure instructions.	Preprocedure instructions.	Preprocedure instructions. Nutritional education prn.	Side effects of medication.		

KEY

1. To initiate a problem or intervention, document under corresponding date.

2. Document outcomes under appropriate date for achieving the goal.

3. To discontinue an intervention, or resolve a patient problem, highlight date and initial.

SBFT = small bowel follow through

COLLABORATIVE PROBLEMS

	DATE		DC DATE INIT	DATE		DC DATE INIT

1. Alteration in elimination: diarrhea R/T infection or medication.
2. Skin integrity, impaired, R/T diarrhea, malnutrition, immobility.
3. Potential/actual for infection, R/T immunodeficiency.
4. Alteration in comfort, pain.
5. Fluid/electrolyte imbalance, potential.
6. Anxiety/fear.
7. Potential for injury R/T drug administration (liver/renal toxicities).
8. Alteration in nutrition, < body requirements.
9. Alteration in coping R/T diagnosis/prognosis.
10. Knowledge deficit R/T disease, transmission, medications, &/or follow-up plan.

OUTCOMES

1. Diarrhea diminished.
2. No skin breakdown, or implementation of skin care program.
3. No infection throughout hospitalization, or infection managed with no evidence of systemic infection.
4. Pain controlled at a level ≤3 on 1-10 scale.
5. Fluid/electrolytes improved - approaching normal limits.
6. Verbalizes anxiety/fear.
7. No injury R/T drug administration.

1. Diarrhea controlled.
2. Skin integrity maintained, or improved skin integrity.
4. Continued pain control at level ≤3 on 1-10 scale.
5. Fluids/electrolytes within normal limits.
6. Anxiety diminished. Verbalizes understanding of anxiety & demonstrates methods to manage.
7. Verbalizes signs & symptoms of side effects of meds. Knowledgeable about S/S to report to medical team.
8. Optimal nutritional status is maintained. Albumin/protein within normal limits.
9. Identified appropriate resources to seek prn.

Continued.

PATIENT NAME: _____

MEDICAL RECORD # _____

MULTIDISCIPLINARY PLAN

DISCIPLINE	PRE-OP/ PRE-ADMIT	P.O.#6 DATE ___	DAY 7 DATE ___	P.O.#7 DATE ___	DAY 8 DATE ___	P.O.#8 DATE ___	DAY 9 DATE ___	P.O.#9 DATE ___	DAY 10 DATE ___	P.O.#10 DATE ___	DAY 11 DATE ___	P.O.#11 DATE ___	DAY 12 DATE ___
PATIENT ACTIVITY		Up ad lib.											
EDUCATION		Disease process methods to prevent transmission. Pt risk reduction. Risk factors for infection.											

KEY

1. To initiate a problem or intervention, document under corresponding date.

2. Document outcomes under appropriate date for achieving the goal.

3. To discontinue an intervention, or resolve a patient problem, highlight date and initial.

SBFT = small bowel follow through

COLLABORATIVE PROBLEMS

	DATE				DC DATE INIT	DATE				DC DATE INIT
2. Skin integrity, impaired R/T diarrhea, malnutrition, immobility.										
3. Potential for infection R/T immunodeficiency.										
8. Alteration in nutrition ≤ body requirements.										

OUTCOMES

2. Skin intact, no breakdown.	1. Frequency of stools are within normal limits for patient.			
3. No infection/infection resolving with normal VS & no evidence of systemic infection.	10. Self administration of po meds. Able to verbalize need to maintain treatment/med plan. Verbalizes when to consult medical/health care team.			
8. Nutritional intake supports healing/maintenance of wt.				
10. Verbalizes modes of transmission, precautions, high/low risk behaviors.				

PLAN OF CARE DISCUSSED WITH

	D.O.S. DAY 1	P.O.#1 DAY 2	P.O.#2 DAY 3	P.O.#3 DAY 4	P.O.#4 DAY 5	P.O.#5 DAY 6
DATE INIT SO/P	DATE____	DATE____	DATE____	DATE____	DATE____	DATE____

INTERVENTIONS

Continued assessment/management of elimination, infection, skin integrity, fluid & electrolyte & pain problems.

D.O.S. DAY 1	P.O.#1 DAY 2	P.O.#3 DAY 4	P.O.#4 DAY 5	P.O.#5 DAY 6
Assess risk factors: • recent travel • antibiotic exposure				
• seafood exposure • gay male • common source outbreak, i.e., food poisoning	Encourage participation as much as possible. Monitor for s/sx of adverse effects from meds:	Create private/supportive environment for pt family. Explore pt/family perceptions.	Pace care/rest activities to provide for as much independence as possible.	Explain disease process, methods to prevent transmission.
CASE MANAGER: Assess elimination pattern, quality, quantity, frequency.	• nausea/vomiting, diarrhea, bone marrow suppression	Promote strengths & appropriate coping mechanisms providing	Consult P.T./O.T. prn.	Discuss need to follow safe sex guidelines.
presence of blood. Strict I/O. Monitor VS for hypovolemia.	• renal/liver toxicity • anorexia/rash	support & MSW consult. Assist pt/family to use social network for support, assistance in care.	Education regarding support available in the community.	Discuss pt risk reduction. Maintenance of home environment.
CONSULTING MD: Monitor labs, & s/sx of fluid/electrolyte imbalance.	Assess nutritional status, height, wt, total protein/albumin.	Discuss possible areas of conflict that may arise.	Teach pt about prescribed meds, indications for use, side effects.	Adequate nutritional intake.
SOCIAL SERVICE: Assess skin, monitoring perianal skin condition & provide skin care to prevent breakdown.	Consult Dietary prn. Provide small frequent high caloric meals as tolerated/desired.	When appropriate, encourage pt to document preferences regarding decision		Avoidance of people with infection.
ANOINTING OF THE SICK DATE:____ Monitor for s/sx of septicemia temp>101, <98 wbc/bacteria in urine & blood culture.	Allow for adequate rest & assist with ADLs prn. Monitor tolerance to visitors/phones.	maker/advance directive. Continued nutritional support.		Prevention of injury. Mgmt of activity/rest.
Institute measures to prevent exposure to known sources of infection.				Avoidance of high risk behaviors (i.e., use of ETOH, tobacco, recreational drugs).
Assess pain level, characteristics. Medicate as ordered.				Teach reduction of risk factors for infection:
Enteric precautions. Assess level of anxiety: • provide opportunities to express feeling.				• malnutrition • exposure to infectious sources or invasive procedure
• MSW consult prn.				Avoidance of frequent venipuncture.
Maintain immediate environment to allow for self-control.				

MULTIDISCIPLINARY PLAN UPDATE

DATE	SIGNATURES	DATE	SIGNATURES	DATE	SIGNATURES

Cancer

Assessment

Cancer diagnosis is based on physical and psychosocial assessment, including laboratory data, radiologic studies, biopsies, and surgical procedures. Classifications of tumor, lymph node involvement, and metastasis are used to determine the stage of the malignant condition (see the box on p. 854 and Tables 15-1 and 15-2). The performance ability of the patient is evaluated and may be used to determine the type and length of treatment (Table 15-3).

● Current Condition

General appearance
  Posture
  Body movements
  Hygiene
General survey of mental status
  Orientation
  Attention span
  Speech
Behavior/mannerisms
Chief complaint
Vital signs (VS)
Weight and height
Patient's concerns
Patient's problems or needs
Patient's knowledge of the following:
  Disease process
  Treatment
  Outcome

TNM Classifications*

PRIMARY TUMOR

T_X: Minimal requirements to assess the primary tumor cannot be met

T_0: No evidence of primary tumor

T_{IS}: Carcinoma in situ

T_1, T_2, T_3, T_4: Progressive increase in tumor size or involvement

N: Regional lymph nodes

  N_0: No evidence of regional nodal involvement

  N_1, N_2, N_3, N_4: Increasing degree of demonstrable abnormality of regional lymph nodes

M: Distant metastasis

  M_0: Indicates absence

  M_+: Indicates presence

HISTOPATHOLOGY

G_1: Well-differentiated grade

G_2: Moderately well-differentiated grade

G_3 and G_4: Poorly to very poorly differentiated grade

RESIDUAL TUMOR

R_0: No residual tumor

R_1: Microscopic residual tumor

R_2: Macroscopic residual tumor

STAGING METHOD

cTNM: Staging determined by clinical noninvasive physical examination, laboratory, and radiographic studies

sTNM: Staging information based on surgical procedures, biopsies, and histopathologic analysis

pTNM: Staging determined by correlation of clinical, pathologic, and residual tumor findings

*T, Primary tumor; N, regional lymph nodes; M, metastasis by vascular dissemination.

Table 15-1 Cancer Staging Using TNM* Classifications

Stage	T	N	M	Survival	Comments
I	1	0	0	70%-90%	Mass limited to organ of origin; nodes not involved; operable and resectable
II	2	1	0	50%±	Local spread to surrounding tissue; nodal involvement suspected or proved; operable but without certainty of total resection
III	3	2	0	20%±	Extensive primary tumor with fixation to deeper structures; nodes involved; operable but not resectable
IV	4	3	+	<5%	Distant metastases; inoperable

*T, Primary tumor; N, regional lymph nodes; M, metastasis by vascular dissemination.

● Physical Assessment

Hematologic system

Monitor complete blood cell count (CBC), hemoglobin (Hgb), platelet count

Bleeding/hemorrhage

  Petechiae

  Unexplained bruises or ecchymoses

  Hematomas

  Bleeding from any body orifice

  Prolonged oozing of blood from IM or IV sites

  Change in (VS)

  Change in neurologic status (headache, disorientation)

  Pad count high for menstruating females

Anemia

  Palpitations, chest pain on exertion

  Dyspnea

  Dizziness, syncope

  Fatigue, weakness

  Glossitis, anorexia, indigestion

  Insomnia, hypersensitivity to cold

Table 15-2 Classification of Tumors

Tissue of Origin	Benign	Malignant
Epithelium: surface skin and mucous membranes	Papilloma	Squamous cell or epidermoid carcinoma
	Polyp	Basal cell carcinoma
Glands	Adenoma	Adenocarcinoma
	Cystadenoma	
Connective tissue		
Embryonic fibrous tissue	Myxoma	Myxosarcoma
Fibrous tissue	Fibroma	Fibrosarcoma
Cartilage	Chondroma	Chondrosarcoma
Bone	Osteoma	Osteosarcoma
Fat	Lipoma	Liposarcoma
Synovial membrane	Synovioma	Synovial sarcoma
Blood vessels	Hemangioma	Hemangiosarcoma
Lymph vessels	Lymphangioma	Lymphangiosarcoma
Muscle tissue		
Smooth muscle	Leiomyoma	Leiomyosarcoma
Striated muscle	Rhabdomyoma	Rhabdomyosarcoma
Hematopoietic tissue		
Lymphoid tissue		Malignant lymphoma
		Non-Hodgkin's lymphoma
		Lymphocytic leukemia
Granulocytic tissue		Myelocytic leukemia
Erythrocytic tissue		Erythroleukemia
Plasma cells		Multiple myeloma
Nerve cells		
Glial cells	Glioma	Glioblastoma (astrocytoma)
		Spongioblastoma
Meninges	Meningioma	Meningeal sarcoma
Nerve cells	Neuroma; ganglioneuroma	Neurogenic sarcoma
Neuroectoderm	Nevus	Neuroblastoma
Fibers	Neurofibroma	Neurofibrosarcoma
Retina		Retinoblastoma
Adrenal medulla	Pheochromocytoma	Pheochromocytoma
Nerve sheaths	Neurilemmoma	Neurilemmal sarcoma
Tumors of more than one tissue		
Breast	Fibroadenoma	Cystosarcoma phyllodes
Embryonic kidney		Nephroblastoma (Wilms')
Multipotent cells	Teratoma	
Uterus		Mixed mesodermal
Miscellaneous		
Melanoblasts	Pigmented nevus	Malignant melanoma
		Melanocarcinoma
Placenta	Hydatidiform mole	Choriocarcinoma (chorionepithelioma)
Ovary	Granulosa-theca cell tumor	Carcinoma
Testes	Interstitial cell tumor	Seminoma (spermatocytic)
		Carcinoma (embryonal)
Thymus	Thymoma	Thymoma

Table 15-3 Host Performance Status*

Status	ECOG/Zubrod	Karnofsky (%)
H0: Normal activity	0	90-100
H1: Symptomatic and ambulatory; cares for self	1	70-80
H2: Ambulatory more than 50% of time; occasionally needs assistance	2	50-60
H3: Ambulatory less than 50% of time; requires special nursing and/or medical assistance	3	30-40
H4: Bedridden; may need hospitalization	4	10-20

From American Joint Committee on Cancer, *Manual for staging of cancer,* ed 3, 1988.
*The host performance status is determined at the time of classification; the condition of the patient does not enter into determination of stage but may be a factor in deciding type and time of treatment.

Infection(s), present and past
Temperature, (T)
White blood cell count (WBC), including differential
Skin and mucous membrane integrity
  Skin folds (axillae, buttocks, perineum)
  Body cavities (mouth, vagina, rectum)
  Venous access sites
  Surgical wounds
Respiratory tract
Genitourinary system
Eyes
  Conjunctivitis, iritis
  Infection of eyelid or lacrimal gland
Pain
Type
  Acute
  Chronic
Location, circumstances of onset
Intensity, quality
Activities that increase pain: eating, separation from
  significant other
Effects on patient and family
Relief measures
  Medication
  Distraction, meditation, relaxation, exercises
  Imagery; psychosocial and/or spiritual counseling
  Variables affecting response
    Anxiety/fear
    Ethnic/cultural background
    Past experiences with pain management
    Meaning of pain (recurrence of disease, death)
    Perceptions of pain therapy (fear of addictions)
Skin
Color: pallor, duskiness, jaundice
Integrity
  Breaks, lesions, ulcers
  Petechiae, bruises, erythema, ecchymosis
Temperature
  Local and systemic
  Feeling of warmth and/or cold

Hydration: turgor, edema, perspiration
Hair: distribution, alopecia
Nails: color, texture, clubbing
Eyes, ears, nose, throat
Pupil size and response
Color
Sclera
Cataract formation
Nose: bleeding, drainage, crusting
Mouth, tongue, lips
  Color, moisture; presence of lesions on palate, tongue,
    buccal mucosa, inner surface of lips, and oral
    pharynx
  Color, amount, and consistency of saliva
  Condition of teeth
    Dental caries, rough edges
    Plaque, dental fit
  Mobility of tongue
  Ability to chew and taste
  Breath odor
Parotid gland: size, tenderness, pain
Lymph nodes
  Neck, axilla, groin
  Size, tenderness, pain
  Thyroid size
Gastrointestinal (GI) system
Appetite
Food and fluid intake
  Type, consistency, amount
  Frequency, preferences
Nausea, vomiting
  Frequency, character
  Color, amount
  Factors affecting occurrence
    Anticipation
    Activities, treatments, time of day
    Other associated factors
  Relief measures used; variables affecting response
Abdomen
  Distention

Bowel sounds
  Present: type, frequency, character
  Absent
Rigid, flaccid, tender
Spleen and liver: size, tenderness, pain
Stool
  Normal pattern: frequency (time of last stool),
    amount, color, consistency
  Aids to normal elimination
    Dietary (food and fluid)
    Medications (laxatives)
    Enemas
  Method of elimination: toilet, commode, bedpan
  Artificial orifices: colostomy, ileostomy
  Method of care for excretions from artificial orifices
  Pain related to defecation
  Presence of blood (on surface or mixed throughout)
  Mucus, pus
  Level of mobility/immobility
  Stress
  Diarrhea/constipation
    Frequency, amount
    Consistency, color
    Bleeding, occult bleeding
    Flatulence
    Associated factors
    Medications
    Relief measures, methods of coping

Genitourinary system
  Urine, urination
    Usual pattern
    Frequency, amount
    Color, odor, specific gravity
    Presence of usual constituents
    Character, bleeding
    Any urgency felt
    Effort in starting and stopping
    Pain, burning, itching
    Nocturia
    Incontinence
    Retention
    Method of urine elimination (void, in-and-out
      catheter, Foley, urinary diversion)
    Care measures, methods of coping
  Fluid intake
  Medications (diuretics)
  History of urinary tract infection (UTI)

Respiratory system
  Respiratory rate: depth and character of breathing
  Type of airway
  Patency of airway
  Breath sounds (normal, adventitious, increased,
    decreased)
  Color of skin and mucous membranes
  Chest size and shape
  Chest excursion and symmetry

Position of trachea
Shortness of breath (SOB) on exertion
Use of accessory muscles
Nasal flaring, pursed-lip breathing, clubbing of
  extremities
Cough: ability, frequency, depth, force, productivity
Sputum: color, amount, odor, consistency, time of day
  produced
Audible grunting, snoring, stridor
Frequency of suctioning
Present level and tolerance of activity
History of the following:
  Smoking, pulmonary infection, pulmonary diseases,
    exposure to air pollutants
  Chemotherapy (bleomycin), radiation therapy to
    thorax
Laboratory tests: blood gas, sputum, blood cultures,
  WBC
Diagnostic studies: chest x-ray examination, pul-
  monary function tests

Cardiovascular system
  Heart rate, blood pressure (BP)
  Heart sounds
  Peripheral pulses: rate, rhythm, volume
  Skin color, dryness/moistness
  Decreased cardiac output
    Tachycardia
    Electrocardiogram (ECG) changes
    Dyspnea on exertion, exercise intolerance
    Rales, wheezing, cough
    Edema: location, type

Neurologic system
  Sensorium (awake, alert, lethargic, stuporous,
    comatose)
  Orientation to time, person, place, and situation
  Ability to follow commands
  Memory (recent, remote)
  Attentiveness, distractibility
  Language spoken, clarity, appropriateness
  Ability to read and write
  Motor response
    Voluntary, involuntary
    Gait, balance, paralysis, weakness
  Reflex response: pupil, gag, cough, Babinski sign,
    deep tendon reflex
  Tics, trembling, seizures
  Pain
    Rate pain using pain scale
    Location, onset, duration, type
    Precipitating factors, relief measures
  Sensations: tingling, numbness, leg cramps
  Foot-drop, wrist-drop, hand-grip
  Sensory
    Visual
    Auditory
    Olfactory

Taste
Tactile
Safety measures used

● Pertinent Background Information

Sleep/rest
  Usual pattern; hours of sleep at night
  Difficulties
  Number and duration of daily naps
  Use of sleep aids: name, dosage of drug, frequency of
    use, length of time used
  Symptoms that may affect sleep: pain, anxiety, night
    sweats
  Signs and symptoms of sleep disturbance: irritability,
    anxiety, loss of train of thought
  Care measures
Sexuality
  Sexual history
  Current practices, reproductive history
  Impact of therapies on sexuality/sexual function; reac-
    tion of partner to illness
  Expressions of affection
  Methods of coping
Social
  Support system; most significant other
  Role function
  Housing/living arrangement
  Presence of dependent, independent behaviors
Spirituality (p. 54): beliefs, faith, concerns
Activities of daily living (ADLs)
  Lifestyle (active, sedentary); exercise tolerance
  Degree of immobility
  Household assistance
  Employment, leisure/hobbies
  Other activities and concerns
Home environment
  Care giver, facilities, and equipment available for
    meeting care needs
  Pets
  Concerns
Teaching needs
  During hospitalization
  Self-care
Previous conditions
  Acute or chronic diseases or conditions
  Surgery
  Radiation therapy
  Chemotherapy
  Biologic response modifiers
  Trauma
    Physical
    Emotional

● Psychosocial Assessment

Prediagnostic period (determination of feelings and prior knowledge)

Awareness of signs and symptoms; length of time
  known
Delay in seeking treatment; threats to the following:
  Independence
  Group belongingness
  Influence on others
  Adaptive functioning
  Preexisting stability
  Decision-making ability
  Cherished values
  Desired roles
  Limitless future
  Control over destiny
Information about treatment
  Knowledge deficits
  Level of understanding
  Misconceptions and myths
  Ethnic/cultural beliefs
Knowledge of resources

Diagnostic period

Fears of outcome
Perceptions of threat
Significance of studies
Information about cancer and body functions
  Factual
  Deficits
  Misconceptions
    Myths
    Fantasies
Knowledge and level of understanding
  Diagnostic tests and examinations
  Schedule of tests and examinations
  Reasons for studies and preparation
  Role of patient in studies
  Physical effect of studies; expected symptoms and
    responses
Continuously validate patient's understanding and
  perceptions
Coping methods of patient, significant other, or family
  Daily activities
  Use of work and leisure activities
  Relationships
  Methods of communication
    Ability to disclose: open with family, peers, coun-
      selors, and/or medical and nursing staff
    Inability to communicate; awareness of significance

Behavioral responses
 Anxiety
  Apprehensive expectation
  Fear and worry about negative outcome
 Vigilance and scanning
  Hyperattentiveness
  Distractibility
  Concentration problems
  Impatience
  Feeling "on edge"
 Motor tension
  Jumpiness
  Restlessness
  Inability to relax
  Insomnia
  Strained facies
  Easily startled
Autonomic hyperactivity
 Tachycardia
 Tachypnea
 Dry mouth
 Sweating
 Cold, clammy hands
 Upset stomach
 Nightmares

Confirmation of diagnosis

Knowledge of results and meaning of diagnostic studies
 X-ray examinations
 Imaging
  Computed tomography (CT) scans
  Magnetic resonance imaging (MRI)
 Isotope studies
 Ultrasound examinations
 Endoscopy
 Cytology
 Laboratory data
 Biopsy
Meaning of illness
 Perceived threat to the following:
  Independence
  Job and economic security
  Career goals
  Relationships
  Integrity of body
  Body functions
  Recreational activities
  Sexual attractiveness and functioning
  Intimacy
 Fears of disfigurement and pain
 Secondary gains: alteration in behavior
  Acting out
  Demands for attention
  Controlling behaviors

Methods for handling past crises
Availability of knowledgeable and supportive resources
 Family
 Significant others
 Co-workers
 Social contacts
 Religious counsel
 Community
Behavioral responses
 Shock/denial
  Rejection of reality
  Increased perspiration
  Pallor
  Faintness
  Nausea
  Anorexia
  Insomnia
  Confusion
  Difficulty in concentrating
  Difficulty in working
 Anger
  Impatience
  Bitterness
  Jealousy
  Helplessness
  Increased awareness
  Limited attention span
  Uncooperative behavior
  Attention-seeking behavior
  Loud talking
  Vulgar language
  Multiple complaints
 Guilt/punishment
  Underlying reasons
  Misconceptions about cancer: seen as unclean, contagious
  Diagnosis attributed to something person did or did not do
 Hopelessness (p. 37)
  Quiet
  Withdrawn
  Melancholy
  Older appearance
  Poor posture
  Gait: slow, dragging
  Decreased respiration
 Bargaining
  Depression
  Exhaustion
  Attempts to avoid reality
  Self-questioning
  SOB
  Feelings of weakness
 Panic attack
  Dyspnea

Palpitations
Chest pain
Feelings of choking or smothering
Dizziness
Feelings of unreality
Tingling of hands and/or feet
Hot and cold flashes
Sweating
Faintness
Trembling or shaking
Fear of dying, "going crazy," or doing something un-
  controllable during an attack
Be aware of importance of need to initiate appropri-
  ate interventions rapidly when the following are
  observed:
Agitation
Uncharacteristic, unexplained, extreme behavior
Unrealistic perceptions and expectations
Feelings of the following:
  Worthlessness
  Extreme guilt
  Suicide
Inappropriate resistance to treatment
Use of controversial treatments (e.g., laetrile, mega-
  vitamins, mechanical devices, miracle drugs, psychic
  surgeons, Hoxsey and Krebiozen potions)
Acceptance
  Contemplativeness
  Serenity
  Talks about condition

Treatment phase

Adequate information for informed decision making
  Options for the following:
    Types of surgery
    Radiotherapy
    Chemotherapy
    Biologic response modifiers
  Risks, benefits, and complications for each type of
    treatment
  Results of current research: unpredictable outcome
  Prognosis associated with each therapy
Level of understanding of chosen therapy
  Preparation
  Associated physical changes
  Complications
  Local and systemic effects
Reactions to treatment
  Follows directions
  Alterations in activities of daily living (ADLs)
Expresses needs for the following:
  Hope associated with cure
    Future pleasurable experiences
    Ability to reach some goals

Others being available for support
  Idea that life has meaning
Honesty
  Answers questions
  No protection from the truth
  Not withholding information
Information about the following:
  Treatment; side or toxic effects
  Special procedures or treatments
  Changes in expected outcomes
  Expected patient participation
  Availability and support of resources
  Whether patient can share what he or she has
    learned about care
Expresses feelings or conveys
  Anger
  Fear

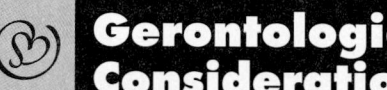

Gerontologic Considerations

- There are more cases of cancer among older
  adults than people of any other age group.
- The incidence of cancer increases with aging,
  possibly as a result of decreased effectiveness of
  the immune system and changes in deoxyri-
  bonucleic acid (DNA).
- The types of cancers seen in older adults are
  prostate, lung, breast, and colon-rectum cancer.
  Cancers of the skin, urinary bladder, vagina,
  and vulva are seen primarily in older adults.
  Chronic lymphocytic leukemia and multiple
  myeloma are seen more frequently in older
  adults than in younger people.
- Many of the early signs and symptoms of cancer
  may be misdiagnosed as normal changes of aging. The importance of routine medical screening and self-examination should be stressed to
  the aging adult.
- Because of fear or past experience, older persons may adopt a fatalistic frame of mind after
  hearing the diagnosis of cancer. Use of the
  terms *tumor* or *growth* may be more acceptable.
- The type of treatment for cancer should be
  based on the older person's wishes and overall
  state of health. Older individuals, their family
  members, and significant others should be presented with all options so that informed decisions regarding treatment can be made.

From Christensen BL, Kockrow EO: *Foundations of nursing,* ed 2, St Louis, 1995, Mosby.

Sadness
Helplessness
Dependency
Powerlessness

Preparation for discharge

Knowledge of continuing care
Methods for dealing with pain (p. 31)
 Increase or decrease in functioning
 Complications of treatment as disease progresses
 Special procedures
 Psychological needs
Daily activity allowances
Signs and symptoms of recurrence or progression
Need for follow-up care
Support groups and counselors: specific information
 and contact person (e.g., wellness community)
Emergency care instructions

Recurrence

Expresses fears of the following:
 Increased dependency
 Increased weakness
 Increased immobility
 Isolation
 Disintegration of relationships
Communicates need for the following:
 Being told death is close
 Information about practical things to do before death
 Discussing pain, pain relief measures, and fear of loss
  of control
 Discussion of beliefs
Ability to continue treatment

Advanced or terminal condition

Knowledge of present diagnosis and prognosis
Symptom-control methods; patient and family
 participation
Responsibilities
 Relationships
 Completion of unfinished business
Ability to discuss fears of the following:
 Inability to continue with life's activities and
  relationships
 Being abandoned
Hospice: alternate methods of care
Meaning of death
 Shameful
 Peaceful
Disengagement
 Life's business finished
 Good-byes said

Psychological withdrawal
Few interactions

Acute Leukemia

*Uncontrolled proliferation of leukocytes and their
 precursors in the bone marrow with infiltration of
 lymph nodes, spleen, liver, and other body organs*
***acute lymphocytic (lymphoblastic) leukemia
 (ALL):*** *Lymphoblasts proliferate in bone marrow and
 lymph nodes and invade other tissues; primarily a
 disease of childhood*
acute myelogenous leukemia (AML): *Proliferation
 of myeloblast (immature polymorphonuclear
 leukocytes); occurs in all age groups but is more
 common in adults*

Assessment

Subjective data

Easily fatigued
Malaise
Irritability
Headache
Abdominal discomfort, nausea
Dysphagia
Anorexia
Palpitations
SOB
Bone/joint pain

Objective data

Elevated temperature
Syncope
Pallor
Petechiae
Easy bruising, ecchymosis
Purpura
Gingival hypertrophy, bleeding, periodontal infections
Oropharyngeal lesions, stomatitis
Epistaxis
Upper respiratory infection (URI)
Urinary infection, uric acid nephropathy
Wound infection: may appear dark red or dark with-
 out pus
Esophagitis
Weight loss
Perirectal abscess
Hepatosplenomegaly
Hypotension
Tachycardia
Cough

Mediastinal mass with tenderness
Enlarged lymph nodes

Medical history

Exposure to ionizing radiation
　Work environment
　Prenatal
　Treatment of preexisting cancer
Genetic factors
　Bloom's syndrome
　Trisomy 21 (Down syndrome; 15 to 20 times the risk)
　Trisomy G (Klinefelter's syndrome)
　Fanconi syndrome
　Philadelphia chromosome present
　Ataxia telangiectasis
　Family history of hematologic disorder
Chemical exposure
　Benzene
　Phenylbutazone
　Arsenic
　Medications
　　Chloramphenicol
　　Alkylating chemotherapeutic agents
Immunodeficiency
Viral exposure

Diagnostic tests

WBC
　Low or elevated, with "left shift"
　Excessively elevated (T cell ALL)
　Blasts
　Lymphocytes (ALL)
　Auer rods (AML)
　Phi bodies (AML)
Reticulocytopenia
　Normochromic (AML)
　Normocytic
CBC: anemia
Platelet count: thrombocytopenia
Chemistries
　Serum uric acid: elevated
　Serum copper: elevated
　Serum zinc: decreased
Urine uric acid: elevated
Hypergammaglobulinemia (AML)
Bone marrow: proliferation of blast cells

Potential complications

Acute infection
Severe anemia
Hemorrhage
Organ failure

Collaborative management

Prevention/detection teaching

Teach importance of limiting exposure time to radiation sources, especially in young children; use proper shields and positioning during necessary x-ray examinations
Explain importance of limiting exposure to toxic chemicals; use proper protective devices during unavoidable exposure
Discuss importance of regular, periodic physical examinations: palpation of lymph nodes, inspection of skin and mucous membranes, palpation of bones and joints, screening laboratory testing
Explain importance of reporting suspect signs and symptoms to physician

Therapeutic management

Chemotherapy
Fluid, parenteral nutritional support
Antibiotics
Radiation therapy (see Transplant preparation, p. 832)
Transfusion of blood components
Bone marrow transplant (see p. 829)
Pain management
Hypnotics

Nursing management

PATIENT PROBLEMS/NURSING DIAGNOSES

● **NDX:** Risk for infection related to suppressed immune system

Screen personnel and visitors for symptoms of infection
Use strict sterile technique for all invasive procedures
Monitor sites of invasive lines/tubes/drains for signs of infection q8h
Check body fluids for alteration in color, odor, consistency
Ensure excellent personal hygiene is maintained, especially after bowel movements
Provide uninterrupted periods of sleep and rest
Avoid chilling; provide socks, extra blankets; keep bed and clothing dry
Ensure required fluid/nutrient intake; supplement with total oral nutrition products prn, institute calorie count prn *to ensure optimum metabolic state to avoid infection*
Record intake and output
Monitor VS, especially T, q4h and prn
Monitor CBC, WBC results per physician order

Administer antibiotics, sulfa-type medications, and other antiinfectives as ordered

Maintain skin integrity *to prevent entry of microorganisms*

Auscultate breath sounds q8h

Encourage clearance of pulmonary secretions: turn, cough, deep breathe q2h; perform chest percussion and drainage as needed; encourage use of incentive spirometer qh

Maintain intact mucous membranes; perform scrupulous oral care using soft instruments q4h and prn

Provide high-calorie, high-protein diet

EXPECTED OUTCOMES

Patient exhibits improvement, resolution of current infections

New infections are not developed

● **NDX:** Altered nutrition: less than body requirements related to reduced food intake, malabsorption, anorexia, vomiting, diarrhea, stomatitis

Assess nutritional status daily: weight, electrolytes, total protein, serum albumin, Hgb, skin turgor, muscle mass

Determine amount and types of foods patient likes and is able to tolerate

Provide oral hygiene before and after meals

Administer anesthetics to oral mucosa before meals prn

Offer high-calorie, high-protein diet with variation in taste, texture, and presentation of foods

In collaboration with physician, provide oral and parenteral nutritional supplements

Serve frequent, light meals and nutritional, high-calorie snacks

Assist patient to eat if fatigue is a factor

Present meals in an attractive, pleasing manner

Provide a pleasant atmosphere *to increase desire to eat:* encourage significant others to join patient for meals, remove bedpans/urinals from area, maintain well-ventilated room, serve food as soon as it arrives, remove tray as soon as patient finishes eating

In collaboration with clinical dietitian: calculate number of calories and nutrients needed *to maintain/gain weight and support metabolic needs*

Maintain calorie count

Encourage family to bring patient's favorite foods from home

In collaboration with physician, administer antiemetics before meals prn

EXPECTED OUTCOME

Weight is maintained within 10% of baseline

● **NDX:** Pain related to involvement of multiple organ systems

Assess nature, intensity, location, duration, and precipitating and alleviating factors

Use consistent pain rating scale *to assess level of pain*

Assess nonverbal signs of pain

Obtain information from patient regarding past pain experiences and methods used for relief

Control environmental factors that may increase perception of pain: temperature, noise, lighting

Assist patient to achieve comfortable positions *to minimize pain*

Assist patient to achieve state of minimal physical tension through techniques such as relaxation, music, visualization, diversion

Provide a restful environment with opportunities to rest during the day and uninterrupted periods of sleep at night *to diminish perception of pain caused by fatigue*

In collaboration with physician, provide analgesic medications as required, observing for therapeutic and side effects

Discuss noninvasive pain relief measures: relaxation, cutaneous stimulation, distraction, hot/cold therapy

EXPECTED OUTCOMES

Verbalizes decrease in/relief of pain

Incorporates existing pain while participating in daily activities

● **NDX:** Fatigue related to chronic disease process

Assess causative/contributing factors; identify activities that are difficult for patient

Coordinate activities to *provide for undisturbed periods of rest and sleep*

Perform active/passive ROM exercises qid; collaborate with physical therapy *to determine most therapeutic exercises*

Determine whether patient becomes posturally hypotensive; change positions gradually; monitor for hypotension and tachycardia

Gauge amount and intensity of activity tolerated by monitoring patient's subjective complaints of fatigue, as well as changes in vital signs

Assist patient to identify strengths, abilities, interests; assist in development of realistic goals to progress from simple to complex

Encourage patient to participate in own care to tolerance; assist as needed *to avoid exhaustion;* assist to identify energy patterns and schedule activities appropriately

Teach energy conservation techniques, use of assistive devices *to minimize fatigue*

Place patient on fall-prevention protocol
Collaborate with physical therapist to design measures *to maintain activity and independence*
Administer filtered, leukocyte-poor red blood cells (RBCs) when ordered

EXPECTED OUTCOMES

Participates in own care to tolerance
Ability to be active increases; states feeling of increased energy

● **NDX:** Potential for bleeding related to thrombocytopenia*

Monitor VS q4h and prn; assess for tachycardia and hypotension
Determine neurologic status q8h to 12h; assess for changing LOC, changing affect, confusion
Assess skin and mucous membranes q8h for increased bruising, bleeding
Observe all urine and stool for gross bleeding; check for occult blood every shift
Maintain integrity of central line; use leur lock connections on all IV tubing
Monitor laboratory results: assess for trends in CBC, platelet count, coagulation studies
Use pull sheet to turn patient *to prevent shearing of tissues and skin trauma*
Use pillows for support of pressure points; avoid excess pressure
Avoid restrictive clothing and bed linen; use bed cradle
Use dental care products appropriate for condition of oral cavity
Use electric razor *to prevent razor cuts*
Avoid vigorous nose blowing
Prevent trauma to decrease risk of bleeding
  Avoid invasive procedures (IM, subcutaneous injections) when possible
  Use smallest gauge needles possible
  Apply manual pressure for 5 to 10 uninterrupted min after any skin puncture *to prevent bruising or hematoma formation*
Provide safe environment: lighting, placement of furniture, well-fitting slippers *to prevent falls*
Prevent constipation; administer stool softeners per physician order
Avoid vomiting; administer antiemetics per physician order
Administer blood components per physician order: platelets are usually ordered at fast rate of infusion and immediately before any invasive procedure for maximal therapeutic effectiveness

---

*Not a NANDA-approved diagnosis.

Administer vasopressors and corticosteroids per physician order

EXPECTED OUTCOME

No signs or symptoms of active bleeding occur

● **NDX:** Anticipatory grieving related to lifestyle changes, decreased physical abilities, changes in physical appearance, life-threatening prognosis

Be sensitive to changes patient is experiencing; encourage patient to express feelings, frustrations, anger, hopes
Provide a therapeutic environment conducive to open discussion: actively listen, tune in to nonverbal cues, be patient and empathetic
Encourage questions and provide information freely as patient expresses the desire for knowledge about the disease, treatments, and prognosis
Set limits on maladaptive coping behaviors if they interfere with patient's well-being
Support adaptive behaviors that suggest progression and resolution of the grieving process
Provide opportunities for private, uninterrupted time with significant others
Assist in identifying ways to adapt lifestyle as condition changes
Provide information regarding support groups for patient and significant others
Collaborate with other professionals (social worker, clergy, psychologist, psychiatrist) *to provide support and facilitate grieving process*
Provide reference for financial assistance, answers to questions regarding medical insurance
Provide information to assist patient in completing advanced directives or similar document to ensure patient wishes are known to significant others and care providers

EXPECTED OUTCOMES

Patient progresses through stages of the grieving process and moves toward acceptance
Demonstrates effective coping mechanisms; participates in decisions about own future

Patient/family teaching

Postdiagnosis

Disease process
  Provide information about disease and treatment
  Discuss symptoms of recurrence or progression of disease to report to physician

Demonstrate how to examine skin and mucous membranes

Emphasize importance of maintaining follow-up appointments for treatment and examinations

Complications

Demonstrate how to check for occult blood in urine and stool

Discuss accident/injury prevention

Avoid restrictive clothing and bed linen

Maintain clutter-free environment

Use assistive devices for ambulation and ADLs as required by condition

Assist patient to select dental hygiene devices and techniques of oral hygiene appropriate for condition of oral mucous membranes and gums

Avoid sports and activities that may result in accidental injury

Handle equipment and sharp objects with care

Discuss prevention of constipation, diet, medications

Infection

Discuss signs and symptoms of infection to report to physician: elevated temperature, sore throat, flu-like symptoms, coughing, burning on urination, infected cuts, lesions that do not heal quickly

Discuss infection-prevention measures: maintain clean environment, avoid handling pets and their equipment, avoid persons with infections and large crowds, practice handwashing techniques (all members of household), routine personal hygiene including perianal care after each elimination

Activity

Discuss importance of maintaining balance between activity and rest

Discuss use of assistive devices as necessary

Discuss importance of assuming activity to tolerance, avoiding fatigue

Nutrition

Consult with clinical dietitian to develop a meal plan, containing necessary calories and fluids, which is consistent with patient's physical condition and considers patient's preferences

Demonstrate administration and management of parenteral nutrition

Anxiety/fear

Explain importance of maintaining open communication with significant others

Teach recognition of early symptoms of depression, maladaptive anxiety/fear

Discuss problem-solving and coping techniques that patient is comfortable practicing

Discuss sources of psychological, financial, spiritual assistance

Medications

Discuss administration, expected therapeutic effects, side effects, and potential adverse reactions of prescribed medication; prepare written instructions

Discuss side/adverse effects that must be reported to physician

Demonstrate use of IV therapy equipment: infusion pump, tubing and connections, storage and handling of medication bags

Need to avoid over-the-counter medications without consulting physician

Home care considerations

Assess ability of patient to provide for physical care needs and ADLs; arrange home care providers as necessary

Evaluate ability of patient to administer own parenteral nutrition and medications; teach significant other(s) to assist or provide care; arrange for home health nurse as needed

Provide sufficient, clean space and refrigeration for storage of supplies and medications

Assess availability of transportation to follow-up appointments; assist with arrangements as needed

Arrange for durable medical equipment: assistive devices, hospital bed, raised commode, IV infusion pump as needed

Assist patient to contact community groups for ongoing psychological/emotional support

Cancer of the Bone (Osteosarcoma)

Rapidly growing malignant bone tumor of unknown etiology occurring most often in the long bones of young people; secondary malignant tumors of the bone metastasize from other primary sites

Assessment

Subjective data

Pain over affected area of extremity, especially at night
Anorexia
Fatigue

Objective data

Limited use of extremity
Weight loss
Localized swelling with or without trauma
Increased skin temperature over affected area

Elevated temperature
Fracture
Spinal cord compression

Diagnostic tests

Serum calcium: decreased
Urine calcium: increased
Alkaline, acid phosphatase: elevated
Imaging/nuclear medicine studies
    Radiographs of affected bones
    Bone scan
    Bone biopsy
    CT scan, MRI

Collaborative management

Therapeutic management

Antineoplastic agents
Radiation therapy
Pain management
Immobilization of limb
Surgical intervention
Potential complications
    Respiratory metastasis
    Pathologic fractures
    Infection at surgical site
Physical therapy consultation

Nursing management

PATIENT PROBLEMS/NURSING DIAGNOSES

● **NDX:**   Pain related to progression of disease process

Assess location, intensity of pain using consistent pain
    rating scale
Use firm mattress, bedboard, footboard as appropriate
Maintain proper alignment of extremities
Extend extremities as tolerated
Avoid external rotation of joints; use supports as
    necessary
Avoid neck flexion; use thin pillow
Apply splints, braces, traction to immobilize/support
    per physician order
Avoid jarring, jerky movements *to prevent potentiation
    of pain*
Handle affected limbs gently, providing support above
    and below joint
Administer skin care
Administer analgesic, antiinflammatory medications
    per physician order
Observe response to medications in terms of pain relief
    and adverse reactions
Discuss alternate methods of pain relief

EXPECTED OUTCOMES
Patient states pain level is tolerable
Incorporates existing pain into lifestyle and self-care
    activities

● **NDX:**   Impaired physical mobility, related to swelling, pain in affected limb, fracture, immobilization device

Provide for bed rest with limb properly aligned, us-
    ing assistive devices as needed: splint, sand bags,
    pillows
Physical therapy consultation to assess activity toler-
    ance, need for assistive devices
Use sheepskin, pressure-reducing mattress, elbow and
    heel guards *to prevent pressure ulcers caused by im-
    paired mobility*
Encourage activity, self-care to tolerance using assistive
    devices as required

EXPECTED OUTCOMES
Participates in activities to tolerance
Demonstrates ability to correctly use assistive
    devices

● **NDX:**   Anticipatory grieving related to lifestyle
changes, decreased physical abilities, changes
in physical appearance, life-threatening
prognosis

Be sensitive to changes patient is experiencing; encour-
    age patient to express feelings, frustrations, anger,
    hopes
Provide a therapeutic environment conducive to open
    discussion: actively listen, perceive nonverbal cues, be
    patient and empathetic *to support grief process*
Encourage questions and provide information freely as
    patient expresses the desire for knowledge about the
    disease, treatments, and prognosis
Set limits on maladaptive coping behaviors if they inter-
    fere with patient's well-being
Support adaptive behaviors that suggest progression
    and resolution of the grieving process
Provide opportunities for private, uninterrupted time
    with significant others
Assist in identifying ways to adapt lifestyle as condition
    changes
Provide information regarding support groups for pa-
    tient and significant others *to deal with grief*
Collaborate with other professionals (social worker,
    clergy, psychologist, psychiatrist) *to provide support
    and facilitate grieving process*
Provide reference for financial assistance, answers to
    questions regarding medical insurance
Provide information to assist patient in completing ad-
    vanced directives or similar document *to ensure pa-*

tient wishes are known to significant others and care providers

EXPECTED OUTCOMES

Patient progresses through stages of the grieving process and moves toward acceptance

Demonstrates effective coping mechanisms; participates in decisions about own future

ADDITIONAL NURSING DIAGNOSIS TO CONSIDER

Altered nutrition: less than body requirements related to anorexia, fatigue

Patient/family teaching

Reinforce physician explanations related to treatment plan, surgical intervention, rehabilitation

Explain chemotherapy/radiation therapy regimen: expected therapeutic effects, side effects, and potential adverse reactions

Explain management of side and adverse effects

Provide information regarding signs and symptoms to report to physician

Discuss importance of following therapy schedule as instructed by physical therapist

Explain importance of taking medication as prescribed

Advise on importance of keeping follow-up appointments with care providers

Home care considerations

Evaluate availability of assistance and ability to provide physical care and home care; arrange home health provider as needed

Assess physical layout: stairs, distance between rooms, arrangement of furniture that may be hazardous; access ability for wheelchair if required

Exhibits ability to provide for durable medical equipment and assistive devices as needed; arranges for provider as needed

Cancer of the Breast/Surgical Intervention

Breast cancer is the leading cancer and the second cause of cancer deaths among women in the United States; the most common form is invasive ductal; the incidence of breast cancer increases with increasing age; surgical intervention may include removal of the entire breast, axillary lymph nodes, and all fat, fascia, and adjacent tissues (modified radical mastectomy); excision and removal of tumor (lumpectomy); excision of tumor and wide margin of healthy tissue (partial mastectomy); removal of one quarter of the breast (quadrantectomy)

Assessment

Subjective data

Postoperative pain
Bone pain caused by metastasis

Objective data

Detection
  Palpable lump: usually painless, upper outer quadrant
  Nipple discharge, retraction
  Dimpling of skin
  Edema (peau d'orange)
  Erythema
  Change in contour of breast
  Axillary adenopathy
  Metastasis: pleural effusions
Postoperative
  Incision site; skin graft site; nipple graft site: redness, edema, drainage
  Wound drains

Risk factors

Female: 99% incidence
Age: more than 40 years of age, increased incidence
Upper socioeconomic status: increased incidence
Nulliparous or first parity after age 30 to 35 years
Family history of breast cancer: mother, sister, maternal aunt, grandmother
Personal history of breast cancer, other cancers
Adverse hormonal milieu
  Early menarche
  Late menopause
  Thyroid disorders
  Diabetes
Lowered immunologic competence
  Thymic atrophy
  Decreased thymus-dependent (T) lymphocytes
  Exposure to excessive radiation
  Use of chemotherapy
  Use of immunosupressives
Obesity, high intake of fat
Chronic psychologic stress

Diagnostic tests

Surgical biopsy
  Estrogen, progestin receptors
  CA 15-3

S-phase index
Ploidy
Needle biopsy
Imaging/nuclear medicine studies: mammography

Potential complications: postoperative

Infection
Hemorrhage, shock
Pneumonia
Brachial plexus damage: contracture, shortening of
  muscles
Metastatic disease

Collaborative management

Prevention/detection teaching

Emphasize that prognosis for most breast cancers is
  more favorable when cancer is detected early
Discuss importance of monthly breast self-
  examinations (most women discover own disease)

Premenopausal: perform 1 wk after menses begin
Postmenopausal: same time each month (for ease of
  remembrance)
Techniques for self-examination
  Visually examine breasts in front of mirror
    (Figure 15-1) (examine with arms at side,
    arms above and behind head, palms of hands
    on hips); notice differences in size, shape, any-
    thing unusual
  While standing: raise one arm over head and exam-
    ine opposite breast, repeating for other breast; re-
    peat examination while lying on back with pillow
    under same shoulder as arm over head, repeating
    for other breast
Methods of examination (all equally effective)
  Wedge method (Figure 15-2): using flat surface of
    three middle fingers, press gently in straight line
    from outer edges toward nipple; repeat in parallel
    lines around breast until all tissue is examined;
    squeeze nipple
  Circular method (Figure 15-3): using flat surface of
    three middle fingers, press gently in small circu-

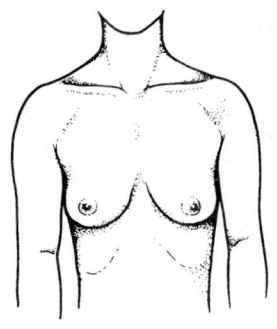
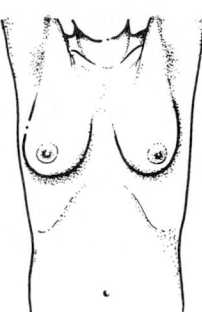
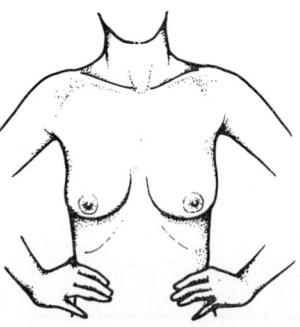
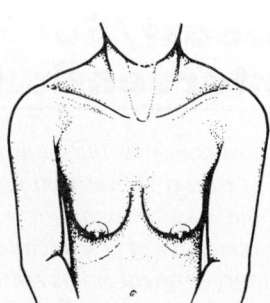

Figure 15-1 Breast self-examination. Visual inspection.

lar motions around the breast, working from outer to inner aspect of breast until all tissue is examined; squeeze nipple

  Vertical strip method (Figure 15-4): using flat surface of three middle fingers, press gently from top outer edge down to the bottom, continuing up and down until you reach the inner aspect of the breast and have examined all tissue; squeeze nipple

Discuss importance of breast examination by professional care giver: every 3 years for women less than 40 years of age, every year for women more than 40 years of age

Explain importance of routine mammography: baseline at age 35 to 40 years; every 1 to 2 years for women age 40 to 49; every year for women more than 49 years of age; earlier/more frequent mammography for women with positive family/personal history

Discuss importance of low-fat, high-fiber diet to reduce endogenous estrogen

Explain need for weight control, reduction

Therapeutic management

Surgical intervention
Postoperative physical therapy
Breast reconstruction
Chemotherapy
Radiation therapy: bradytherapy, teletherapy
Estrogen, androgen, progestin therapy
Reach to recovery program

Nursing management

  PATIENT PROBLEMS/NURSING DIAGNOSES
See perioperative care

● **NDX:** Anticipatory grieving, related to lifestyle changes, decreased physical abilities, changes in physical appearance, life-threatening prognosis

Be sensitive to changes patient is experiencing; encourage patient to express feelings, frustrations, anger, hopes

Provide a therapeutic environment conducive to open discussion: actively listen, perceive nonverbal cues, be patient and empathetic

Encourage questions and provide information freely as patient expresses the desire for knowledge about the disease, treatments, and prognosis

Set limits on maladaptive coping behaviors if they interfere with patient's well-being

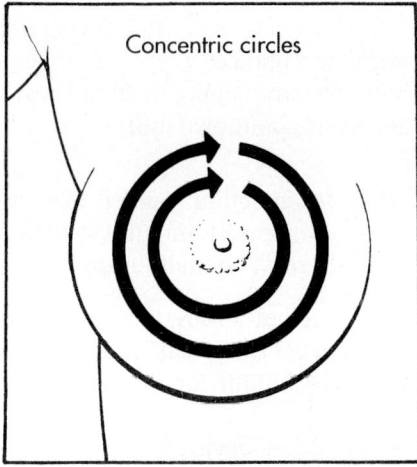

Figure 15-3 Concentric circles. (From Belcher AE: *Mosby's clinical nursing series: cancer nursing,* St Louis, 1992, Mosby.)

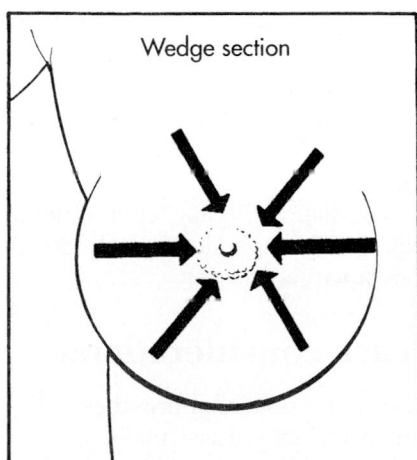

Figure 15-2 Wedge section. (From Belcher AE: *Mosby's clinical nursing series: cancer nursing,* St Louis, 1992, Mosby.)

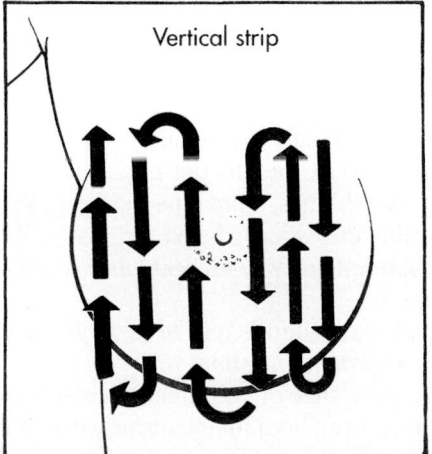

Figure 15-4 Vertical strip. (From Belcher AE: *Mosby's clinical nursing series: cancer nursing,* St Louis, 1992, Mosby.)

Support adaptive behaviors that suggest progression and resolution of the grieving process

Provide opportunities for private, uninterrupted time with significant other(s)

Assist in identifying ways to adapt lifestyle as condition changes

Provide information regarding support groups for patient and significant others *to deal with grief*

Collaborate with other professionals (social worker, clergy, psychologist, psychiatrist) to provide support and facilitate grieving process

Provide reference for financial assistance, answers to questions regarding medical insurance

Provide information to assist patient in completing advanced directive or similar document to ensure patient wishes are known to significant others and care providers

EXPECTED OUTCOMES

Progresses through stages of the grieving process and moves toward acceptance

Demonstrates effective coping mechanisms; participates in decisions about own future

● **NDX:** Risk for infection, related to surgical procedure, depressed immune system from radiation therapy, chemotherapy

During nadir of chemotherapy, limit visitors and crowd exposure *to decrease chances of infection*

Use strict sterile technique for all invasive procedures

Monitor venous access device for signs of infection

Check body fluids for alteration in color, odor, consistency

Ensure excellent personal hygiene is maintained, especially after bowel movements

Provide uninterrupted periods of sleep and rest *to increase resistance to infection*

Ensure required fluid/nutrient intake; supplement with total oral nutrition products prn; institute calorie count prn

Monitor VS, especially T, q4h and prn *to assess for fever*

Monitor CBC, WBC results per physician order

Administer antibiotics, sulfa-type medications, and other antiinfectives as ordered

Maintain skin integrity *to prevent entry of microorganisms*

Auscultate breath sounds q8h *to assess for signs of pulmonary congestion/infection*

Encourage clearance of pulmonary secretions: turn, cough, deep breathe q2h; encourage use of incentive spirometer qh

Provide high CHO, high-protein, low-fat diet *to prevent increased body fat and weight*

Maintain weight within 10% of baseline

EXPECTED OUTCOMES

Patient exhibits no signs of infection

● **NDX:** Potential for lymphedema of affected arm and hand*

Avoid administering parenteral fluids, drawing blood from affected arm

Alternate lying on back and unaffected side

Take BP on unaffected arm only

Check color, sensation, motion in fingers and hand on affected side q1h to 8h as indicated postsurgery

Collaborate with physical therapist to plan exercise regimen and instruct in wrist, hand, elbow, arm exercises

Monitor edema in affected arm: measure upper arm and forearm

EXPECTED OUTCOME

Functioning of affected arm and hand is maintained

Patient/family teaching

Postdiagnosis, postoperative
Instruct patient in precautions for affected arm/breast
Exercise to tolerance; slowly resume housekeeping activities; stop at point of pain
No blood drawing, IV therapy, or injections in affected arm
No BP taken on affected arm
Incision and chest wall may feel numb; avoid accidental injury
Instruct patient to carry handbag on unaffected shoulder or side
Avoid pressure on affected chest wall, arm: sleeping, sexual positions
Report increase in size of arm (sleeves fit tighter)
Gradually increase extent of daily exercise of affected arm and hand; encourage use of affected arm/hand to perform simple care activities; wash face, brush teeth, eating
Discuss types of prostheses, reconstruction (if not performed at time of mastectomy)
Care of incision, signs and symptoms to report to physician
Medication/radiation therapy/chemotherapy regimen: expected therapeutic effects, side effects, potential adverse reactions

Home care considerations

Discuss sources for obtaining prostheses

Teach about availability of assistance for ADLs; arrange home health provider as needed

Discuss availability of transportation to follow-up ap-

---

*Not a NANDA-approved diagnosis.

pointments with care providers; assist with arrangements as necessary
Inform about resources for support groups
Discuss importance of continuing interaction with others

Cancer of the Cervix

Although rates have dramatically decreased over the last 50 years, cancer of the cervix remains the sixth most common cancer among women in the United States; cancer of the cervix is largely influenced by lifestyle factors

Assessment

Subjective data

Pelvic pain (late symptom)
Loss of appetite (late symptom)

Objective data

Unexplained vaginal spotting/bleeding
Postcoital bleeding, postdouche bleeding
Vaginal discharge: watery, purulent, mucoid
Late symptoms
  Irritation
  Vulvitis
  Yellow, foul-smelling vaginal discharge
  Urinary symptoms, leakage of urine or feces from vagina
  Weight loss

Risk factors

Low socioeconomic status: increased incidence
First coitus at early age: within 1 year of menarche
Multiple sex partners
Frequent genital infections; viral exposure
Mismanaged parturition
Nonbarrier contraception
Chronic vaginal douching

Diagnostic tests

CBC
Culposcopy, biopsy
CT scan, MRI
Lymphangiography, needle aspiration

Collaborative management

Prevention/detection teaching

Explain importance of maintaining an accurate menstrual cycle history: frequency, length, amount, color

Maintain good gynecologic hygiene
Avoid frequent douching
Delay beginning sexual activity, especially during teen years
Discuss need for regular, periodic gynecologic examinations including pap test and bimanual examination
  The ACS and ACOG recommend first examination at age 18 or onset of sexual activity, followed by two annual examinations; if these three examinations are normal, the frequency may decrease as determined by the personal physician
Self-visualization examination
  Skin excoriation, ulcers
  Lumps, leukoplakia
  Narrowing of introitus, atrophy

Therapeutic management

Surgical intervention
  Conization
  Cryotherapy, laser ablation
  Hysterectomy (p. 729)
  Loop electrosurgical excision procedure
Radiation therapy
Chemotherapy: advanced disease

Nursing management

See Chapter 11 for surgical interventions (e.g., Hysterectomy, p. 729)

Cancer of the Esophagus

The most common esophageal carcinoma is of the squamous cell or adenocarcinoma type; generally developing in the middle or lower third of the esophagus, this cancer is usually fatal because the condition is advanced before symptoms appear; the highest incidence is in males between the ages of 50 and 70 years

Assessment

Subjective data

Difficulty swallowing
  Early: when swallowing hard, solid food
  Later: constantly when swallowing saliva
Vague epigastric discomfort
Vague feeling of fullness after eating
Loss of appetite
Substernal pain, pyrosis (heartburn)
General malaise

Objective data

Hoarseness, coughing
Glossopharyngeal neuralgia
Foul-smelling breath
Hiccoughs
Esophageal obstruction
  Sialism
  Nocturnal aspiration
  Regurgitation of saliva and food
Weight loss, dehydration
Increased salivation and mucus formation
Eructation
Hepatomegaly
Diaphragmatic paralysis (from phrenic nerve
  involvement)
Cervical/supraclavicular lymphadenopathy

Risk factors

Heavy smoking
Chronic, excessive alcohol intake
Drinking and eating very hot, spicy foods; smoked
  meats
Exposure to foods containing nitrites and nitrates
Nutritional deficiency: riboflavin
Diet high in nitrosamine
History of head and neck tumors, strictures, peptic
  ulcer disease
Family history
  Pernicious anemia
  Gastric polyps
  Gastritis
  Achlorhydria
  Gastric cancer

Diagnostic tests

CBC
Complete chemistry panel
Liver function tests
Imaging/nuclear medicine studies
  Chest radiograph
  Barium studies of the GI tract
  CT scan/MRI
Cardiopulmonary studies
  Bronchoscopy
  Electrocardiogram (ECG)
Endoscopy with biopsy and cytology

Potential complications

Malnutrition, anemia
Fluid and electrolyte imbalance
Aspiration pneumonia
Infection
Metastasis to other organs
Hemorrhage

Collaborative management

Therapeutic management

Pain management
Chemotherapeutic agents
Radiation therapy
Insertion of plastic (Celestin) tubes to maintain
  nutrition
Esophageal surgery (p. 356)
Gastrostomy tube insertion
Speech and occupational therapy

Nursing management

PATIENT PROBLEMS/NURSING DIAGNOSES

● **NDX:** Altered nutrition: less than body requirements related to anorexia, dysphagia,
surgical intervention, radiation therapy,
chemotherapy

Assess nutritional status daily: weight, electrolytes, total protein, serum albumin, Hgb, skin turgor, muscle
  mass *to evaluate response to plan of care and make
  needed changes*
Consult speech therapy *to assess patient's ability to masticate and swallow*
Determine amount and types of foods patient likes and
  is able to tolerate
Provide for oral hygiene before and after meals
Administer anesthetics to oral mucosa before meals prn
Offer high-calorie, high-protein diet with variation in
  taste, texture, and presentation of foods *to enhance
  appetite*
In collaboration with physician, provide oral and parenteral nutritional supplements
Serve frequent, light meals and nutritional, high-calorie
  snacks
Assist patient to eat if fatigue is a factor
Present meals in an attractive, pleasing manner
Provide a pleasant atmosphere *to increase desire to
  eat:* encourage significant others to join patient for
  meals, remove bedpans/urinals from area, maintain
  well-ventilated room, serve food as soon as it arrives,
  remove tray as soon as patient finishes eating
In collaboration with clinical dietitian: calculate number
  of calories and nutrients needed *to maintain/gain
  weight and support metabolic needs*
Maintain calorie count
Encourage family to bring patient's favorite foods from
  home

In collaboration with physician, administer antiemetics before meals prn

EXPECTED OUTCOME

Weight is maintained within 10% of baseline

● **NDX:** Pain related to progressive disease process, surgical intervention

Assess nature, intensity, location, duration, and precipitating and alleviating factors *to establish baseline and evaluate responses to plan of care*
Use consistent pain rating scale
Assess nonverbal signs of pain
Obtain information from patient regarding past pain experiences and methods used for relief
Control environmental factors that may increase perception of pain: temperature, noise, lighting
Assist patient to achieve comfortable positions
Assist patient to reach state of minimal physical tension through techniques such as relaxation, music, visualization, diversion
Provide a restful environment with opportunities to rest during the day and uninterrupted periods of sleep at night
In collaboration with physician, provide analgesic medications as required, observing for therapeutic and side effects
Discuss and institute noninvasive pain relief measures: relaxation, cutaneous stimulation, distraction, hot/cold therapy

EXPECTED OUTCOMES

Patient verbalizes decrease in or relief of pain
Incorporates existing pain while participating in daily activities

● **NDX:** Anticipatory grieving, related to lifestyle changes, decreased physical abilities, changes in physical appearance, life-threatening prognosis

Be sensitive to changes patient is experiencing; encourage patient to express feelings, frustrations, anger, hopes
Provide a therapeutic environment conducive to open discussion: actively listen, perceive nonverbal cues, be patient and empathetic *to support grief process*
Encourage questions and provide information freely as patient expresses the desire for knowledge about the disease, treatments, and prognosis
Set limits on maladaptive coping behaviors if they interfere with patient's well-being
Support adaptive behaviors that suggest progression and resolution of the grieving process

Provide opportunities for private, uninterrupted time with significant other(s)
Assist in identifying ways to adapt lifestyle as condition changes
Provide information regarding support groups for patient and significant other(s)
Collaborate with other professionals (social worker, clergy, psychologist, psychiatrist) *to provide support and facilitate grieving process*
Provide reference for financial assistance, answers to questions regarding medical insurance
Provide information to assist patient in completing advanced directive or similar document to ensure patient wishes are known to significant others and care providers

EXPECTED OUTCOMES

Patient progresses through stages of the grieving process and moves toward acceptance
Demonstrates effective coping mechanisms; participates in decisions about own future

● **NDX:** Ineffective airway clearance, related to esophageal obstruction

Maintain elevated upper body at 30 to 45 degrees *to facilitate respiratory excursion*
Avoid supine positions, gatching knees *to prevent circulatory compromise*
Consult with occupational or speech therapist *to assess swallowing ability and develop plan of care*
Instruct patient in use of tonsil tip suction; have suction available within patient's reach
Suction patient as needed
Provide emesis basin and tissues for expectoration

EXPECTED OUTCOME

Patent airway is maintained

Patient/family teaching

Reinforce physician's explanation of disease and treatment plan
In collaboration with clinical dietitian, speech therapist, and occupational therapist instruct patient regarding diet required, tolerated
Gastrostomy tube management: assessment of placement, tube feedings, flushing, checking for residual
Care of Celestin tube
  Elevating head at all times
  Swallowing only small amounts
  Method for clearing obstruction
Methods for pain management

Discuss importance of maintaining follow-up appointments with care providers, radiation, chemotherapy appointments

Explain medication regimen, side effects, potential adverse reactions

Discuss signs and symptoms to report to physician

Home care considerations

Discuss transportation to care provider visits

Ensure assistance with ADLs: shopping, cooking, cleaning as needed

Teach about durable medical equipment provider for suction equipment and supplies

Discuss importance of clean, sufficient space for storing equipment and supplies, care and maintenance of supplies

Discuss importance of ongoing outpatient care, continued interaction with others who are supportive

Cancer of the Head and Neck

The most common site of head and neck cancer is the larynx; other sites include the oral cavity, pharynx; 90% or more is due to lifestyle or environmental risk factors that are significantly preventable; cancer of the larynx is most commonly caused by squamous cell carcinoma; these cancers are more likely to present with regional lymphatic metastasis at the time of diagnosis

Assessment

Subjective data

Earache
Sore throat lasting longer than 2 wk
Pain

Objective data

Oral cavity: leukoplakia, erythroplasia, other lesions may appear infiltrating, ulcerative, exophytic

Chronic, nonhealing, often painless sores: lips, eyelids, external ear and canal, scalp

Submaxillary, parotid, sublingual glands positive for swelling, adenopathy

Regional lymph nodes may be enlarged, firm, nonmobile, overlying skin may be discolored

Thyroid may be enlarged

Loss of structure/support of external nose, nasal discharge, smell changes, loss of nasal patency

Altered voice tone: hoarseness, cough

Hemoptysis
Glossitis
Dysphagia
Visual changes
Hearing loss
Taste changes

Risk factors

Tobacco use: cigarettes, cigars, snuff, chewing tobacco, pipe

Chronic moderate to heavy use of alcohol

Chronic intake of extremely hot or cold liquids

Exposure to nickel, wood dust, hydrocarbon gases, asbestos, mustard gas, radiation, uranium, syphilis, herpes simplex, Epstein-Barr virus

Chronic inflammatory disease; chronic irritation to oral mucosa from poorly fitting dentures, malocclusion of teeth, poor hygiene

Premalignant lesions: erythroplasia, leukoplakia

Prevention/detection

Explain importance of avoiding tobacco and heavy alcohol use

Discuss importance of proper oral hygiene and routine, preventive dental visits, properly fitting dentures

Teach avoidance of chemical and other carcinogens

Teach about protection from excess exposure to the sun

Discuss maintaining healthy, well-balanced diet

Explain community support groups for quitting smoking and alcohol use counseling

Laryngectomy: Radical Neck Dissection

Removal of larynx and surrounding neck tissue to treat a cancerous condition; a permanent tracheal stoma is created

Assessment

Preoperative

SUBJECTIVE DATA

Pain in "Adam's apple" radiates to ear
Anxiety/fear

OBJECTIVE DATA

Tachypnea
Dysphagia
Hemoptysis
Stridor

Hoarseness
Enlarged cervical nodes
Cough
Behavioral manifestations of fear, anxiety, panic, denial, anger

Postoperative

SUBJECTIVE DATA
Fear of suffocation
Pain at surgical site

OBJECTIVE DATA
Hemorrhage
Airway obstruction: restlessness, tachycardia, use of accessory muscles of respiration, tachypnea, noisy respirations, wheezing, stridor, pallor, cyanosis
Atelectasis
Dehydration
Sputum: amount, character
Incision site: discoloration, swelling, drainage, sloughing of tissue, condition of stoma
Wound drains: amount, character of drainage
Body T elevation
Behavioral manifestations of helplessness, fear, anxiety, anger, frustration

Diagnostic tests

CBC
Type and cross/screen
Electrolytes
Blood chemistries
Epstein-Barr virus antibody titer
Imaging/nuclear medicine studies
  Chest radiograph
  Skull and neck radiographs
  Bone scan
  CT scan, MRI
Cardiopulmonary studies
  ABGs
  Baseline pulmonary function tests
  ECG
Fiberoptic endoscopy studies
Biopsy of suspect lesions

Potential complications

Pneumonia
Respiratory failure
Metastasis
Cardiac erosion
Pneumothorax
Shock
Tracheoesophageal fistula

Collaborative management

Therapeutic management

Radiation therapy
Mechanical support of ventilation, oxygen therapy
Nasogastric tube
Nutritional support, total parenteral nutrition, gastrostomy tube feedings
Parenteral therapy, fluids, medications
Speech therapy

Nursing management

PATIENT PROBLEMS/NURSING DIAGNOSES

● **NDX:** Impaired skin integrity, related to radiation therapy

Assess skin completely q8h
Skin care guidelines
  Avoid bath or shower until ordered by physician
  Do not wash skin in area being irradiated until ordered by physician *to prevent removal of landmarks*
  Do not remove skin markings between treatments
  Avoid use of any products (soap, lotion, deodorants, cosmetics) without checking with physician/nurse
  Avoid tight garments to *prevent rubbing and skin irritation*
  Avoid extremes of temperature
  Dry desquamation: use cornstarch sparingly
  Moist desquamation: use water/saline to keep clean and moist (slow healing)
  Expose skin to air when possible
  Cover broken areas with hydrocolloid dressing; use stretch-type tubular dressing to hold in place

EXPECTED OUTCOME
Patient's skin remains intact and/or impaired skin progressively heals

● **NDX:** Anticipatory grieving, related to lifestyle changes, decreased physical abilities, changes in physical appearance, life-threatening prognosis

Be sensitive to changes patient is experiencing; encourage patient to express feelings, frustrations, anger, hopes *to begin work of grieving process*
Provide a therapeutic environment conducive to open discussion: actively listen, perceive nonverbal cues, be patient and empathetic *to facilitate trust*
Encourage questions and provide information freely as patient expresses the desire for knowledge about the disease, treatments, and prognosis *to ease the fear of the unknown*

Set limits on maladaptive coping behaviors if they interfere with patient's well-being

Support adaptive behaviors that suggest progression and resolution of the grieving process

Provide opportunities for private, uninterrupted time with significant others

Assist in identifying ways to adapt lifestyle as condition changes *to enhance participation and feelings of control*

Provide information regarding support groups for patient and significant other(s)

Collaborate with other professionals (social worker, clergy, psychologist, psychiatrist) *to provide support and facilitate grieving process*

Provide reference for financial assistance, answers to questions regarding medical insurance

Provide information to assist patient in completing advanced directive or similar document to ensure patient wishes are known to significant others and care providers

EXPECTED OUTCOMES

Patient progresses through stages of the grieving process and moves toward acceptance

Demonstrates effective coping mechanisms; participates in decisions about own future

● **NDX:** Altered nutrition: less than body requirements related to dysphagia, radiation therapy, chemotherapy, perceived changes in taste and smell of foods, disinterest in eating

Assess nutritional status daily: weight, electrolytes, total protein, serum albumin, Hgb, skin turgor, muscle mass *to evaluate response to plan of care and make needed changes*

Consult speech therapist to assess patient's ability to masticate and swallow

Determine amount and types of foods patient likes and is able to tolerate

Provide for oral hygiene before and after meals

Administer anesthetics to oral mucosa before meals prn

Offer high-calorie, high-protein diet with variation in taste, texture, and presentation of foods

In collaboration with physician, provide oral and parenteral nutritional supplements

Serve frequent, light meals and nutritional, high-calorie snacks

Assist patient to eat if fatigue is a factor

Provide a pleasant atmosphere *to increase desire to eat:* encourage significant others to join patient for meals, remove bedpans/urinals from area, maintain well-ventilated room, serve food as soon as it arrives, remove tray as soon as patient finishes eating

In collaboration with clinical dietitian: calculate number of calories and nutrients needed *to maintain/gain weight and support metabolic needs*

Maintain calorie count

Encourage family to bring favorite foods from home

In collaboration with physician, administer antiemetics before meals prn

EXPECTED OUTCOME

Weight is maintained within 10% of baseline

● **NDX:** Ineffective airway clearance, related to removal of laryngeal structures, newly created tracheostomy, altered ability to cough and swallow

Assess surgical site around laryngectomy, tracheostomy tube for bleeding and/or excess secretions

Assess respiratory pattern: rate, depth, quality

Auscultate breath sounds for crackles, wheezes

Assess amount of oropharyngeal secretions; have suction readily available within patient's reach

Maintain patient in upright position *to facilitate respiratory excursion*

Apply humidification to tracheostomy per physician order

Suction tracheostomy and mouth prn to keep clear of secretions; use sterile technique

If on ventilator support, hyperoxygenate and/or hyperventilate before suctioning (hospital protocols will vary) *to prevent depletion of oxygen*

Perform tracheostomy care q8h and prn; replace disposable inner cannula with each cleaning *to decrease exposure to pathogens*

Avoid occluding tracheostomy tube when positioning patient or changing bed linens

Maintain manual resuscitator bag at bedside; maintain extra laryngectomy tube of same size and type at bedside *for emergency use*

Assist patient to turn, cough, deep breathe q2h

EXPECTED OUTCOME

Secretions are effectively cleared, and patent airway is maintained

● **NDX:** Risk for impaired skin integrity, related to exposure to tracheostomy secretions

Assess surgical area for signs of wound infection q8h: redness, purulent drainage, edema of tissues, condition of suture lines

Clean skin around stoma q8h and prn *to maintain cleanliness*

Wash with hydrogen peroxide and rinse with saline; pat dry

Place sterile, preslit 4 × 4 gauge around stoma; change prn *to keep stoma clean and dry*

Change laryngectomy tube holder during stoma care and as needed *to keep holder clean and dry*

Ensure laryngectomy holder is snug but not tight around patient's neck *to prevent skin irritation*

Elevate head of bed 45 to 60 degrees *to promote respiratory excursion*

Prevent forward flexion of neck; place small towel under shoulders as needed; remove pillows if necessary

Assess and record output from drains; examine area around drains for signs/symptoms of infection

EXPECTED OUTCOMES

Integrity of surgical incisions and skin around incisions is maintained

Surgical wounds begin to heal without signs or symptoms of infection

● **NDX:** Impaired verbal communication, related to laryngectomy

Provide patient with immediate means of communication; have call light within reach; arrange signs and signals that call for immediate attention

Have paper/pencil, communication board, Magic Slate available for written messages

Read written messages aloud *to confirm meaning with patient*

Avoid asking questions that require *yes* or *no* answers

Be patient; wait for patient to complete message before assuming answer or course of action to take

If call light is answered at nurses' station, ensure patient is not asked questions that cannot be answered simply

Encourage patient to express fears, frustrations related to inability to speak

Encourage and teach visitors to use assistive devices *to communicate with patient*

Collaborate with speech therapy in development of plan of care, assess ability to use artificial larynx

EXPECTED OUTCOMES

Patient/care givers develop an effective communication system

Patient is able to communicate thoughts/ideas, needs, desires to staff and visitors

Patient/family teaching

Preoperative

Reinforce physician's explanation of disease and treatment plan

Demonstrate/explain laryngectomy tube care and suctioning

Explain purpose and location of tubes/drains and their care; gastrostomy tube feedings

Develop a communication system to use postoperatively that incorporates patient's level of ability to read and write and primary language

Schedule visit from speech therapist to explain postoperative course

Provide opportunities for patient to attend support groups or visits from persons who have had similar experiences

Postoperative

Explain importance of maintaining sufficient caloric and fluid intake even though food may not taste or smell appetizing

Review hygiene activities: when showering direct spray under neck, wear shield over stoma, avoid getting soap into stoma, do not use aerosol sprays around stoma

When shaving the face: shield stoma to prevent small hairs from entering; use electric razor to prevent shaving lather from entering stoma site

Explain need to keep stoma lightly covered at all times, avoid tight-fitting necklines, natural fiber scarves, neck jewelry

Discuss importance of covering stoma when coughing

Home care considerations

Teach laryngectomy and stoma care: inner cannula care, removing and replacing outer cannula, suctioning, dressing changes, cleaning stoma, and changing holder

Ensure understanding of medications, diet, administration of tube feedings, signs and symptoms to report to physician

Teach about care of surgical incisions

Refer to community support groups: American Cancer Society; Lost Cord/New Voice Club

Explain importance of clean area to store dressing and suction supplies; care and maintenance of supplies

Establish contact with durable medical equipment agency to supply suction equipment

Make available hand-held mirror

Make available paper and pencil or alternate communication devices

Discuss importance of avoiding persons with URIs smoky environments

Emphasize importance of ongoing outpatient care, continued communication with others who are supportive

Cancer of the Intestine/Colorectal Cancer

Cancer of the small intestine is uncommon; when it occurs it is usually found in the lower duodenum and

Provide opportunities for private, uninterrupted time with significant other(s)

Assist in identifying ways to adapt lifestyle as condition changes *to enhance participation and feelings of control*

Provide information regarding support groups for patient and significant other(s)

Collaborate with other professionals (social worker, clergy, psychologist, psychiatrist) *to provide support and facilitate grieving process*

Provide reference for financial assistance, answers to questions regarding medical insurance

Provide information to assist patient in completing advanced directive or similar document *to ensure patient wishes are known to significant others and care providers*

EXPECTED OUTCOMES

Patient progresses through stages of the grieving process and moves toward acceptance

Demonstrates effective coping mechanisms; participates in decisions about own future

● **NDX:** Diarrhea or constipation related to diseased GI tract, malabsorption, effects of chemotherapy, radiation therapy

Assess usual pattern of elimination and changes experienced

Assess stools for consistency, color, character, presence of occult/gross blood

Auscultate for bowel sounds and measure abdominal girth q8h

Consult with clinical dietitian and physician *to develop nutrition plan consistent with patient condition and tolerance*

Ensure intake is equal to output; include diarrhea in output measurement

Check patient for impaction if no or minimal hard bowel movements

Administer medications: stool softeners, antidiarrheals

EXPECTED OUTCOME

Elimination pattern is maintained within parameters of disease process

Patient/family teaching

Reinforce physician's explanation of disease and treatment plan

Diet management and/or parenteral IV nutrition administration

Advise on activity/rest patterns and their importance

Discuss medications, actions, side effects, potential adverse reactions

Explain radiation, chemotherapy regimen; management of side effects

Discuss importance of follow-up visits with care providers

Home care considerations

Assess patient's ability to care for self and support systems available in the home

Arrange for home care providers as needed to assist with physical and home management needs: shopping, cooking, cleaning

Assess availability of transportation to ensure ability to keep appointments

Ensure adequate, clean storage space for medical supplies; care and maintenance of supplies

Explain importance of ongoing outpatient care, continued interaction with others who are supportive

Cancer of the Kidney and Bladder

Transitional cell carcinomas make up 93% of all bladder cancers; the highest incidence occurs among white men more than 65 years of age; primary renal carcinoma is rare, accounting for 2% of all adult malignancies; most often found in the renal parenchyma, the metastasis rate is high and the prognosis is poor; the incidence of renal carcinoma increases with age

Assessment

Subjective data

Burning, pain on urination
Urgency
Back pain
Fatigue

Objective data

Hypertension
Gross, painless hematuria; may be intermittent
Microhematuria
Frequency of urination
Weight loss
Anemia
Fever, night sweats
Paraneoplastic syndrome associated with renal cancer
  Hypercalcemia
  Hypertension
  Polycythemia

Risk factors

Age: 50 to 70 years
Exposure to carcinogens through skin or vapor
  Aniline dye; rubber and cable industry
  Beta-napthylamine
  4-amino diphenyl
  Tobacco tar
  Benzidine
Exposure to pelvic irradiation
Chronic UTIs
Chronic bacterial cystitis with calculi: strictures, diverticula, paralytic stasis
Chronic intake of analgesics containing phenacetin
Potential risks
  Coffee drinking
  High use of sodium, saccharin, cyclamates
  Urine stasis
  Smoker

Diagnostic tests

Urinalysis
Urine cytology
Complete chemistry panel
Imaging/nuclear medicine studies
  Intravenous pyelogram (IVP)
  Retrograde pyelography
  Nephrotomography
  Ultrasonography
  CT scan
  Renal arteriogram
Cystoscopy

Collaborative management

Therapeutic management

  Nephrectomy, p. 696
  Chemotherapy, p. 922
  Radiotherapy, p. 915

Prevention/detection teaching

Ensure patient and family understand risk factors and the importance of providing detailed occupational history: type and length of exposure, protective measures taken to reduce risk of exposure
Explain need to continue use of protective equipment as needed in work setting
Discuss importance of reporting suspicious signs and symptoms to physician
Explain need for periodic physical examinations: rectal and pelvic examinations, cystoscopy, and cytology

Cancer of the Liver

Malignant tumor most frequently caused by metastatic disease lesions in other organs; primary lesions are rare and may be asymptomatic

Assessment

Subjective data

General weakness
Loss of appetite
Fatigue
Nausea
Abdominal fullness, discomfort
Abdominal pain when coughing or deep breathing
Referred pain to back, scapular, and shoulder area

Objective data

Progressive weight loss
Increased flatulence
Light-colored, bulky stools; stools containing fat
Diarrhea, melena
Low-grade fever
Dehydration
Anemia
Electrolyte imbalance
Jaundice
Edema, ascites

Diagnostic tests

PT/INR: increased
ESR: elevated
Bleeding, clotting times: prolonged
CBC; WBC: leukocytosis
Fasting blood sugar (FBS)
Liver function studies: LDH, ALT, AST
Alkaline phosphatase: elevated
Serum albumin: decreased
Urinalysis
Immunoserologic assay
Serum tumor markers
Stools for steatorrhea
Imaging/nuclear medicine studies
  Chest radiograph
  Abdominal ultrasound
  CT scan, MRI
  Hepatic scintiscan
  Hepatic arteriography
Liver biopsy
Paracentesis cytology

Potential complications

Hypoglycemia
Hepatomegaly/splenomegaly, hepatorenal failure
Hematemesis, GI bleeding
Portal hypertension
Jaundice
Ascites
Peripheral edema
Respiratory distress
Change in mental status, hepatic coma

Collaborative management

Therapeutic management

Pain management
Antiemetics, antacids
Diuretics
Corticosteroids
Therapeutic diet, parenteral nutrition
Parenteral therapy: fluids, electrolytes, vitamins, albumin
Nasogastric aspiration, irrigation if bleeding
Urethral catheter
Percutaneous hepatic arterial catheter for chemotherapy and chemoembolization
Hepatic lobectomy

Nursing management

PATIENT PROBLEMS/NURSING DIAGNOSES

● **NDX:** Pain related to progression of disease process

Assess nature, intensity, location, duration, and precipitating and alleviating factors
Use consistent pain rating scale *to determine baseline and deviations that indicate intervention is needed*
Assess nonverbal signs of pain
Obtain information from patient regarding past pain experiences and methods used for relief
Control environmental factors that may increase perception of pain: temperature, noise, lighting
Assist patient to achieve comfortable positions
Assist patient to achieve state of minimal physical tension through techniques such as relaxation, music, visualization, diversion *to decrease need for medication*
Provide a restful environment with opportunities to rest during the day and uninterrupted periods of sleep at night
In collaboration with physician, provide analgesic medications as required, observing for therapeutic and side effects

Discuss and institute noninvasive pain relief measures: relaxation, cutaneous stimulation, distraction, hot/cold therapy

EXPECTED OUTCOMES

Patient verbalizes decrease in or relief of pain
Incorporates existing pain while participating in daily activities

● **NDX:** Altered nutrition: less than body requirements related to anorexia, malnutrition, fatigue

Assess nutritional status daily: weight, electrolytes, total protein, serum albumin, Hgb, skin turgor, muscle mass
Determine amount and types of foods patient likes and is able to tolerate
Provide for oral hygiene before and after meals
Administer anesthetics to oral mucosa before meals prn
Offer high-calorie, high-carbohydrate diet with variation in taste, texture, and presentation of foods *to enhance appetite*
In collaboration with physician, provide oral and parenteral nutritional supplements
Serve frequent, light meals and nutritional, high-calorie snacks
Assist patient to eat if fatigue is a factor
Present meals in an attractive, pleasing manner
Provide a pleasant atmosphere *to increase desire to eat:* encourage significant other(s) to join patient for meals, remove bedpans/urinals from area, maintain well-ventilated room, serve food as soon as it arrives, remove tray as soon as patient finishes eating
In collaboration with clinical dietitian: calculate number of calories and nutrients needed *to maintain/gain weight and support metabolic needs*
Maintain calorie count
Encourage family to bring patient's favorite foods from home
In collaboration with physician, administer antiemetics before meals prn

EXPECTED OUTCOME

Weight is maintained within 10% of baseline

● **NDX:** Anticipatory grieving related to changes in physical functioning and poor prognosis

Be sensitive to changes patient is experiencing; encourage patient to express feelings, frustrations, anger, hopes *to begin work of grieving process*
Provide a therapeutic environment conducive to open discussion: actively listen, perceive nonverbal cues, be patient and empathetic *to facilitate trust*

Encourage questions and provide information freely as patient expresses the desire for knowledge about the disease, treatments, and prognosis *to ease fear of the unknown*

Set limits on maladaptive coping behaviors if they interfere with patient's well-being

Support adaptive behaviors that suggest progression and resolution of the grieving process

Provide opportunities for private, uninterrupted time with significant other(s)

Assist in identifying ways to adapt lifestyle as condition changes *to enhance participation and feelings of control*

Provide information regarding support groups for patient and significant other(s)

Collaborate with other professionals (social worker, clergy, psychologist, psychiatrist) *to provide support and facilitate grieving process*

Provide reference for financial assistance, answers to questions regarding medical insurance

Provide information to assist patient in completing advanced directive or similar document *to ensure patient wishes are known to significant others and care providers*

EXPECTED OUTCOMES

Patient progresses through stages of the grieving process and moves toward acceptance

Demonstrates effective coping mechanisms; participates in decisions about own future

● **NDX:** Risk for fluid volume deficit related to electrolyte imbalance, poor intake of fluids, NG aspiration

Maintain NPO status per physician order

Administer parenteral fluids with glucose, electrolytes, vitamins

Administer intravenous albumin

Insert NG sump tube to low suction; irrigate with normal saline per physician order, observe aspirate for color, character, and occult/gross blood

Monitor urine output via indwelling bladder catheter: observe color, character, amount

Calculate intake and output q8h

Assess for ankle edema and increasing abdominal girth q8h

Monitor VS and T q4h; provide cooling measures for elevated temperature

Monitor results of blood chemistries and hematologies per physician order

Administer medications per physician order: diuretics, antacids, corticosteroids, chemotherapeutic agents

EXPECTED OUTCOMES

Intake of fluids remains in balance with output

Blood chemistries remain within normal parameters or abnormal results are detected and treated promptly

● **NDX:** Potential for jaundice and GI bleeding related to impaired liver function*

Monitor gastric aspirate and stools for occult/gross bleeding q4h

Observe for bleeding: gums, purpura

Observe for bleeding after injections; avoid needle sticks; use small-gauge needles; hold pressure for 5 uninterrupted min after any skin puncture

Monitor results of coagulation studies per physician order

Monitor skin/sclera for jaundice q8h to 12h

Administer blood products, albumin, vitamin K per physician order

EXPECTED OUTCOME

GI bleeding and jaundice are avoided

● **NDX:** Altered thought processes related to ineffective clearance of metabolites through the liver

Monitor mental acuity q8h: signs of disorientation, lethargy, personality changes, depressed motor ability

Reorient patient as necessary

Provide safe environment: siderails up, call light and needed articles within close reach, walking area free from clutter; provide night light

Provide clear, concise directions; break tasks into small steps and allow time for completion

Maintain continuity of schedule

Monitor serum blood urea nitrogen (BUN) and ammonia levels as ordered by physician

Administer medications including lactulose per physician order

EXPECTED OUTCOMES

Patient remains oriented to self and environment

Blood ammonia levels remain within normal parameters

Patient/family teaching

Reinforce physician's explanation of disease and treatment plan

Discuss importance of maintaining chemotherapy and medication schedules; explain actions, side effects, and potential adverse reactions of medications

Collaborate with clinical dietitian to plan a therapeutic diet consistent with patient's physical condition and preferences

---

*Not a NANDA-approved diagnosis.

Demonstrate care of indwelling catheter if applicable

Discuss signs and symptoms to report to physician: changes in mental acuity, increased abdominal girth, weight gain, jaundice, hematemesis, tarry stools, bleeding from any site, peripheral edema, dyspnea

Emphasize importance of keeping follow-up appointments with care givers

Home care considerations

Assess patient's ability to care for self and assistance available; arrange for home health provider as needed

Assess patient's transportation needs; arrange as necessary

Assess need for assistance with shopping, cooking, cleaning

Ensure clean, adequate area for storage of medical supplies as needed; care and maintenance of supplies

Cancer of the Lung

Epithelial lung cancer is the leading cause of cancer deaths among men and women in the United States; smoking is the single greatest risk factor; the overall survival rate is less than 10% over 5 years

Assessment

Subjective data

Chest pain

Tightness in chest

Shoulder or arm pain: superior vena cava syndrome

Loss of appetite

Pain in right upper quadrant

Bone pain

Objective data

Change in pulmonary habits, change in cough

Respiratory infections

Chronic, productive cough, usually at night

Rust-streaked sputum, hemoptysis

Unilateral wheeze

Dyspnea

Pneumonitis lasting longer than 2 wk with treatment

Lymph node adenopathy

Enlarged liver

Weight loss

Hypercalcemia, anemia

Cushing's disease

Dermatomyositis

Migratory thrombophlebitis

Nonbacterial endocarditis

Disseminated intravascular coagulation (DIC)

Syndrome of inappropriate antidiuretic hormone (SIADH)

Risk factors

Tobacco use: more than 20 pack years—number of packs per day times number of years smoked

Exposure to active or passive tobacco smoke
  Hours per day
  Number of years

Exposure to ionizing radiation

Exposure to carcinogens
  Asbestos
  Aromatic hydrocarbons
  Radioactive ores
  Radon
  Bis ether
  Inorganic arsenic
  Nickel, silver, chromium, cadmium, beryllium, cobalt, selenium, steel

History of lung disease

Low intake of vitamin A

Diagnostic tests

CBC

Complete chemistry panel

Liver function tests

Coagulation panel

Sputum cytology

Cardiopulmonary studies
  Bronchoscopy and bronchial biopsy, brushings and washings
  Fluorescence bronchoscopy

Imaging studies
  Chest radiograph
  Lung, brain, bone scans

Mediastinoscopy, lymph node biopsy

Community support groups for quitting smoking

Collaborative management

Therapeutic management

Pneumonectomy, p. 318

Chemotherapy, p. 922

Radiotherapy, p. 915

Prevention/detection teaching

Importance of avoiding exposure to tobacco smoke, high-risk occupations

Discuss community support groups for quitting smoking

Cancer of the Pancreas

Malignancy in the pancreas is associated with high mortality because of the lack of early symptoms, symptoms similar to those of other diseases, and rapid metastasis to other organs; 50% occurs in the head of the pancreas, and 50% occurs in the body of the pancreas

Assessment

Subjective data

Midepigastric pain, varies in severity; may radiate to lower back and subscapular area; may be related to eating, activity, or the supine position
Loss of appetite
Nausea
Fatigue
Itching skin

Objective data

Signs of biliary obstruction
  Jaundice
  Clay-colored stools
  Dark, concentrated urine
  Rapid weight loss

Diagnostic tests

Serum bilirubin, alkaline phosphatase, amylase, lipase: elevated
Complete chemistry panel, FBS
Liver function tests
Coagulation studies
Imaging/nuclear medicine studies
  Percutaneous transhepatic cholangiography (PTC)
  Endoscopic retrograde cholangiopancreatography (ERCP)
  Arteriography
  Ultrasonography, CT scan
  Upper GI examination
  Abdominal series
  Duodenal secretion cytology
Percutaneous needle aspiration cytology, biopsy

Potential complications

Hyperglycemia, hyperinsulinism; diabetes mellitus
Steatorrhea
Hepatomegaly; bleeding tendencies; vitamin K deficiency; ascites
Thrombophlebitis

Collaborative management

Therapeutic management

Pain management consultation; analgesics
Antiemetics
Vitamin K, pancreatic enzymes, bile salts
Insulin
Clinical dietitian consultation: therapeutic diet
Clinical pharmacist consultation: parenteral nutrition
Parenteral therapy, electrolytes
Nasogastric tube; aspiration
Indwelling urinary catheter
Chemotherapy, radiation therapy
Surgical intervention

Nursing management

PATIENT PROBLEMS/NURSING DIAGNOSES

● **NDX:** Pain related to progression of disease process

Assess nature, intensity, location, duration, and precipitating and alleviating factors
Use consistent pain rating scale *to determine baseline and deviations that indicate intervention is needed*
Assess nonverbal signs of pain particular to patient
Obtain information from patient regarding past pain experiences and methods used for relief
Control environmental factors that may increase perception of pain: temperature, noise, lighting
Assist patient to achieve comfortable positions
Assist patient to achieve state of minimal physical tension through techniques such as relaxation, music, visualization, diversion *to decrease need for medication*
Provide a restful environment with opportunities to rest during the day and uninterrupted periods of sleep at night
In collaboration with physician, provide analgesic medications as required, observing for therapeutic and side effects
Discuss and institute noninvasive pain relief measures; relaxation, cutaneous stimulation, distraction, hot/cold therapy

EXPECTED OUTCOMES

Patient verbalizes decrease in/relief of pain
Patient is able to incorporate existing pain while participating in daily activities

● **NDX:** Altered nutrition: less than body requirements related to anorexia, insulin secretion disorder, nausea, diarrhea, fatigue

Assess nutritional status daily: weight, electrolytes, total protein, serum albumin, Hgb, skin turgor, muscle mass

Determine amount and types of foods patient likes and is able to tolerate

Provide for oral hygiene before and after meals

Administer anesthetics to oral mucosa before meals prn

Offer high-calorie, high-protein diet with variation in taste, texture, and presentation of foods *to enhance appetite*

In collaboration with physician, provide oral and parenteral nutritional supplements

Serve frequent, light meals and nutritional, high-calorie snacks

Assist patient to eat if fatigue is a factor

Present meals in an attractive, pleasing manner

Provide a pleasant atmosphere *to increase desire to eat:* encourage significant other(s) to join patient for meals, remove bedpans/urinals from area, maintain well-ventilated room, serve food as soon as it arrives, remove tray as soon as patient finishes eating

In collaboration with clinical dietitian: calculate number of calories and nutrients needed *to maintain/gain weight, support metabolic needs, and maintain blood glucose within limits*

Maintain calorie count

Encourage family to bring patient's favorite foods from home

In collaboration with physician, administer antiemetics before meals prn

EXPECTED OUTCOME

Patient maintains weight within 10% of baseline

● **NDX:** Anticipatory grieving related to changes in physical functioning and poor prognosis

Be sensitive to changes patient is experiencing; encourage patient to express feelings, frustrations, anger, hopes *to begin work of grieving process*

Provide a therapeutic environment conducive to open discussion: actively listen, perceive nonverbal cues, be patient and empathetic *to facilitate trust*

Encourage questions and provide information freely as patient expresses the desire for knowledge about the disease, treatments, and prognosis *to ease fear of the unknown*

Set limits on maladaptive coping behaviors if they interfere with patient's well-being

Support adaptive behaviors that suggest progression and resolution of the grieving process

Provide opportunities for private, uninterrupted time with significant other(s)

Assist in identifying ways to adapt lifestyle as condition changes *to enhance participation and feelings of control*

Provide information regarding support groups for patient and significant others

Collaborate with other professionals (social worker, clergy, psychologist, psychiatrist) *to provide support and facilitate grieving process;*

Provide reference for financial assistance, answers to questions regarding medical insurance

Provide information to assist patient in completing advanced directive or similar document *to ensure patient wishes are known to significant others and care providers*

EXPECTED OUTCOMES

Patient progresses through stages of the grieving process and moves toward acceptance

Demonstrates effective coping mechanisms; participates in decisions about own future

● **NDX:** Risk for fluid volume deficit related to NPO status, diarrhea, altered glucose metabolism

Administer parenteral fluids, electrolytes, and nutrition per physician order

Calculate intake and output; measure diarrhea and NG aspirate and include in output measurement

Administer insulin per physician order

Monitor VS for signs of dehydration: tachycardia, hypotension, orthostatic hypotension

EXPECTED OUTCOME

Intake remains balanced with output; patient remains hydrated

● **NDX:** Potential for altered glucose metabolism, ascites, bleeding, jaundice related to impaired liver function*

Monitor results of blood glucose, bilirubin, coagulation, CBC, albumin per physician order

Monitor gastric aspirate and stools for gross/occult blood

Perform capillary blood glucose measurements and administer insulin per physician order

Monitor skin and sclera for signs of jaundice

Monitor lower extremities for edema and tenderness

Auscultate abdomen for bowel sounds and measure abdominal girth q8h

Monitor mental status, acuity q8h

Administer medications per physician order

EXPECTED OUTCOME

Potential complications are avoided or are recognized and treated promptly

Patient/family teaching

Provide information about diagnosis and treatment plan

Explain chemotherapy/radiation therapy schedule; ex-

---

*Not a NANDA-approved diagnosis.

pected effects of treatment, side effects, potential adverse reactions

Explain symptomatic care of side and adverse effects

Contact clinical dietitian to assist in planning a therapeutic diet consistent with patient's physical condition and preferences

Contact certified diabetes educator to assist in structuring education related to insulin administration, capillary blood glucose testing, diet, and activity

Discuss medications: administration, therapeutic actions, side effects, potential adverse reactions

Explain importance of reporting changes in condition to physician: weight gain, increase in abdominal girth, jaundice, bleeding from any site, increased pain, hematemesis, tarry/bloody stools, peripheral edema, dyspnea

Discuss importance of follow-up visits with care providers

Home care considerations

Advise where to purchase a capillary blood glucose monitor and supplies for self-testing of capillary blood sugar

Teach importance of refrigerating insulin

Plan for a safe, secure area in which to keep new and used insulin needles/syringes

Discuss patient's and/or family's ability to care for patient and home; obtain home care providers as needed for physical needs: shopping, cooking, cleaning

Plan for transportation to follow-up visits with care providers

Cancer of the Stomach

Carcinoma most frequently occurring in the pyloric segment and along the lesser curvature of the stomach; there are no early, definitive signs of the disease process

Assessment

Subjective data

Feeling of fullness after eating, early satiety
Indigestion
Belching
Epigastric pain or discomfort after eating
Loss of appetite
Malaise, fatigue
General weakness
Dizziness (vertigo, syncope)
Nausea

Objective data

Dysphagia
Weight loss
Pallor
Vomiting
Occult blood in stool

Risk factors

Chronic excessive alcohol intake
Drinking and eating very hot, spicy foods, meats cured with nitrates/nitrites
Exposure to foods containing nitrates, nitrites
Nutritional deficiency: limited intake of vitamins A, C, E, and dairy products
Peptic ulcer disease
Exposure to asbestos, coal, rubber, timber, nickel
Family history
  Pernicious anemia
  Gastric polyps
  Gastritis
  Alchlorhydia
  Gastric cancer

Diagnostic tests

CBC, Hct
Plasma tumor markers
Stool for occult blood
Gastric content analysis
Imaging studies
  Upper GI series
  Endoscopy with biopsy and cytology
  Chest radiography
  Tomography
  Ultrasound

Potential complications

Malnutrition
Fluid and electrolyte imbalance
Hematemesis
Pyloric obstruction
Enlarged axillary, supraclavicular lymph nodes
Epigastric mass
Recurrent phlebitis
Metastasis to the liver

Collaborative management

Therapeutic management

Pain management
Parenteral fluids, total parenteral nutrition
Radiation therapy

Chemotherapy
Surgery: Gastric resection, gastrectomy

Nursing management

PATIENT PROBLEMS/NURSING DIAGNOSES

● **NDX:** Altered nutrition: less than body requirements related to dysphagia, anorexia, nausea, vomiting

Assess nutritional status daily: weight, electrolytes, total protein, serum albumin, Hgb, skin turgor, muscle
mass
Consult occupational therapist *to assess patient's ability
to masticate and swallow*
Determine amount and types of foods patient likes and
is able to tolerate
Provide for oral hygiene before and after meals
Administer anesthetics to oral mucosa before meals
prn
Offer high-calorie, high-protein diet with variation in
taste, texture, and presentation of foods *to enhance
appetite*
In collaboration with physician, provide oral and parenteral nutritional supplements
Serve frequent, light meals and nutritional, high-calorie
snacks
Assist patient to eat if fatigue is a factor
Present meals in an attractive, pleasing manner
Provide a pleasant atmosphere *to increase desire to eat:*
encourage significant other(s) to join patient for
meals, remove bedpans/urinals from area, maintain
well-ventilated room, serve food as soon as it arrives,
remove tray as soon as patient finishes eating
In collaboration with clinical dietitian: calculate number
of calories and nutrients needed *to maintain/gain
weight and support metabolic needs*
Maintain calorie count
Encourage family to bring patient's favorite foods from
home
In collaboration with physician, administer antiemetics
before meals prn

EXPECTED OUTCOME

Patient maintains weight within 10% of baseline

● **NDX:** Pain related to progression of disease
process

Assess nature, intensity, location, duration, and precipitating and alleviating factors
Use consistent pain rating scale *to determine baseline
and deviations that indicate itervention is needed*
Assess nonverbal signs of pain particular to patient *so
that early signs can be noted and treatment started*

Obtain information from patient regarding past pain experiences and methods used for relief
Control environmental factors that may increase perception of pain: temperature, noise, lighting
Assist patient to achieve comfortable positions
Assist patient to achieve state of minimal physical tension through techniques such as relaxation, music, visualization, diversion *to decrease need for medcation*
Provide a restful environment with opportunities to rest
during the day and uninterrupted periods of sleep at
night
In collaboration with physician provide analgesic medications as required, observing for therapeutic and
side effects
Discuss and institute noninvasive pain relief measures:
relaxation, cutaneous stimulation, distraction,
hot/cold therapy

EXPECTED OUTCOMES

Patient verbalizes decrease in or relief of pain
Incorporates existing pain while participating in daily
activities

● **NDX:** Anticipatory grieving, related to lifestyle
changes, decreased physical abilities, changes
in physical appearance, life-threatening
prognosis

Be sensitive to changes patient is experiencing; encourage patient to express feelings, frustrations, anger,
hopes *to begin work of grieving process*
Provide a therapeutic environment conducive to open
discussion: actively listen, perceive nonverbal cues, be
patient and empathetic *to facilitate trust*
Encourage questions and provide information freely as
patient expresses the desire for knowledge about the
disease, treatments, and prognosis *to ease fear of the
unknown*
Set limits on maladaptive coping behaviors if they interfere with patient's well-being
Support adaptive behaviors that suggest progression
and resolution of the grieving process
Provide opportunities for private, uninterrupted time
with significant other(s)
Assist in identifying ways to adapt lifestyle as condition
changes *to enhance participation and feelings of control*
Provide information regarding support groups for patient and significant other(s)
Collaborate with other professionals (social worker,
clergy, psychologist, psychiatrist) *to provide support
and facilitate grieving process*
Provide reference for financial assistance, answers to
questions regarding medical insurance
Provide information to assist patient in completing advanced directive or similar document *to ensure patient
wishes are known to significant others and care providers*

EXPECTED OUTCOMES

Patient progresses through stages of the grieving process and moves toward acceptance

Demonstrates effective coping mechanisms; participates in decisions about own future

Patient/family teaching

Reinforce physician's explanation of disease and treatment plan

In collaboration with clinical dietitian explain nutrition plan consistent with patient's condition, provide written instructions and menu plans

Discuss management of dumping syndrome

Identify with patient support systems, community resources, and support groups

Discuss medication regimen, actions, side effects, and potential adverse reactions to report to physician

Explain importance of keeping follow-up appointments with care providers and diagnostic, therapeutic visits

Home care considerations

Assess patient's ability for self-care; contact home health agency for support as needed

Assess transportation needs to maintain follow-up care

Assess ability to shop, cook, clean; arrange assistance as needed

Discuss importance of ongoing outpatient care, continued interaction with others who are supportive

Cancer of the Testicle/Orchiectomy

Cancer of the testicle occurs most often in males age 15 to 35 years; the incidence is four times greater in whites than blacks; 97% of the cancers are germ cell, which carries a 3 year survival rate of 96% when detected and treated in its early stages

Surgical removal of the testis is most commonly performed in the presence of testicular cancer via an inguinal incision; for more advanced nonseminomatous germ cell cancer, a retroperitoneal lymph node dissection may be necessary

Assessment

Subjective data

Detection
 "Dragging" pain in lower back and abdomen
 Malaise
 Feeling of discomfort in testes

Postoperative
 Pain at operative site
 Anxiety; fear

Objective data

Detection
 Testicular mass, palpable
 Testicular swelling, thickness
 Scrotal edema, discoloration
 Weight loss
 Gynecomastia, nipple pigmentation
 Elevated T
Postoperative
 Hemorrhage
 Swelling at operative site
 Discoloration at operative site
 Condition of suture line
 Wound drains: amount, character of drainage
 Body T elevation
 Pulmonary status
 Hydration status
 Behavioral signs of pain, fear, anxiety, anger, frustration

Risk factors

Age: 15 to 40 years
Cryptorchism (undescended testis)
Previously atrophic testes
Childhood hernia and other genitourinary anomalies
Trauma
Orchitis, especially mumps
Family history of testicular cancer: father, brother
Klinefelter's syndrome
Exposure in utero to diethystilbesterol (DES)

Diagnostic tests

AFP and HCG for tumor markers
Urine for "pregnancy" test
Plasma tumor markers
Imaging/nuclear medicine studies
 Intravenous urography (IVU)
 CT scan
 Radionuclide study
Lymphangiogram

Potential complications

Hemorrhage, shock
Wound infection
Atelectasis, pneumonia
Metastasis; radical lymph node dissection

Collaborative management

Prevention/detection teaching

Instruct regarding time frames for periodic examination by health care provider

Discuss signs and symptoms to report to physician

Explain importance and technique for performing testicular self-examination (beginning at age 15 or before if family history) (Figure 15-5)

Technique: perform after warm shower/bath with relaxed scrotal skin

In standing position

Place middle and index fingers below one testis with thumb on top

Gently roll testis between thumb and finger

Normal findings: rubbery, spongy, smooth, no lumps

Abnormal findings: hard, painless nodule, usually on lateral or anterior surface

Hold one testicle in palm of hand; note weight differences

Therapeutic management

Radiation therapy for seminomatous germ cell tumor

Chemotherapy

Prevention education

Bone marrow transplant

Surgical intervention

Postoperative management (lymph node dissection)

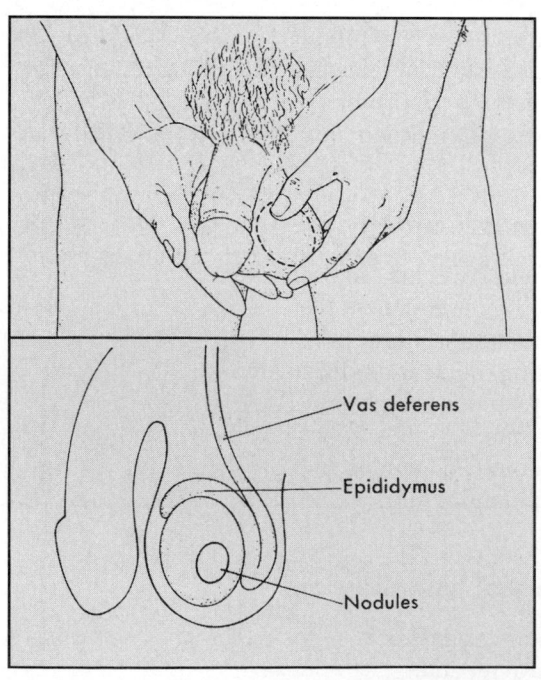

Figure 15-5   Testicular self-examination.

NPO until bowel sounds are active

NG tube: *most patients experience postoperative ileus*

Parenteral fluids until liquids are tolerated

Routine postoperative VS

Analgesics, antibiotics

Scrotal support

Nursing management

PATIENT PROBLEMS/NURSING DIAGNOSES

● **NDX:**   Pain related to scrotal swelling, surgical intervention

Assess nature, intensity, location, duration, and precipitating and alleviating factors

Use consistent pain rating scale *to determine baseline and deviations that indicate intervention is needed*

Assess nonverbal signs of pain particular to patient *so that early signs can be noted and treatment started*

Obtain information from patient regarding past pain experiences and methods used for relief

Control environmental factors that may increase perception of pain: temperature, noise, lighting

Assist patient to achieve comfortable positions

Provide topical cooling and scrotal support measures

Assist patient to achieve state of minimal physical tension through techniques such as relaxation, music, visualization, diversion *to decrease need for medication*

Provide a restful environment with opportunities to rest during the day and uninterrupted periods of sleep at night

In collaboration with physician provide analgesic medications as required, observing for therapeutic and side effects

Discuss and institute noninvasive pain relief measures: relaxation, cutaneous stimulation, distraction

EXPECTED OUTCOMES

Patient verbalizes decrease in or relief of pain

Incorporates existing pain while participating in daily activities

● **NDX:**   Anticipatory grieving related to lifestyle changes, decreased physical abilities, changes in physical appearance, life-threatening prognosis

Be sensitive to changes patient is experiencing; encourage patient to express feelings, frustrations, anger, hopes *to begin work of grieving process*

Provide a therapeutic environment conducive to open discussion: actively listen, perceive nonverbal cues, be patient and empathetic *to facilitate trust*

Encourage questions and provide information freely as patient expresses the desire for knowledge about the disease, treatments, and prognosis *to ease fear of the unknown*

Set limits on maladaptive coping behaviors if they interfere with patient's well-being

Support adaptive behaviors that suggest progression and resolution of the grieving process

Provide opportunities for private, uninterrupted time with significant other(s)

Assist in identifying ways to adapt lifestyle as condition changes *to enhance participation and feelings of control*

Provide information regarding support groups for patient and significant other(s)

Collaborate with other professionals (social worker, clergy, psychologist, psychiatrist) *to provide support and facilitate grieving process*

Provide reference for financial assistance, answers to questions regarding medical insurance

EXPECTED OUTCOMES

Patient progresses through stages of the grieving process and moves toward acceptance

Demonstrates effective coping mechanisms; participates in decisions about own future

● **NDX:** Risk for infection related to suppressed immune system

Screen personnel and visitors for symptoms of infection

Use strict sterile technique for all invasive procedures

Monitor sites of invasive lines/tubes/drains for signs of infection q8h

Check body fluids for alteration in color, odor, consistency

Ensure excellent personal hygiene is maintained, especially after bowel movements

Provide uninterrupted periods of sleep and rest

Ensure required fluid/nutrient intake, supplement with total oral nutrition products prn, institute calorie count prn *to maintain weight within 10% of baseline*

Record intake and output

Monitor VS, especially T, q4h and prn

Monitor CBC, WBC results per physician order

Administer antibiotics, sulfa-type medications, and other antiinfectives as ordered

Maintain skin integrity *to prevent entry of microorganisms*

Auscultate breath sounds q8h

Encourage clearance of pulmonary secretions; turn, cough, deep breathe q2h; use incentive spirometer qh

Maintain intact mucous membranes: scrupulous oral care using soft instruments q4h and prn

EXPECTED OUTCOMES

Improvement, resolution of current infections

New infections do not develop

● **NDX:** Acute urinary retention related to scrotal swelling

Measure urine output every void; assess abdomen for bladder distension

Request patient to inform nurse of bladder fullness and inability to void

Promote measures to facilitate bladder emptying

Ensure privacy, comfortable position for voiding

Run tap water, flush toilet

Place hands in warm water, running water

Pour warm water over penis

Apply heat to suprapubic area

Assist patient to use relaxation techniques

Crede bladder

Stroke inner aspect of thigh with ice

Catheterize patient per physician order

EXPECTED OUTCOMES

Patient is able to empty bladder without use of indwelling catheter

Bladder distension and urinary retention are prevented

Patient/family teaching

Postdiagnosis, postoperative

Avoid constipation

Care of surgical incision

Avoid heavy lifting/straining until cleared by physician

Report signs and symptoms to physician: incision pain, redness, swelling, drainage, elevated T

Medication/chemotherapy/radiation therapy regimen: expected therapeutic effects, side effects, potential adverse reactions; management of side and/or adverse effects

Need to resume usual daily routine as soon as possible

Cancer of the Uterus/Radical Hysterectomy

Assessment

Subjective data

Detection

Lower abdominal and back pain (late disease)

Postoperative
Pain at surgical site

Objective data

Detection
Abnormal vaginal bleeding
Postmenopausal bleeding
Purulent discharge
Endometrial polyps
Enlarged, boggy uterus
Postoperative
Vaginal hemorrhage, drainage (other than serous); foul odor
Incision: redness, edema, drainage
Elevated T
Tachycardia
Amount, color, consistency of contents of surgical drains
Hematuria
Urinary retention
Vaginal leakage of urine
Abdominal distension

Risk factors

Age: over 50 years
Menstrual irregularities
Infertility, anovulation
Nulliparous
Late menopause
Long-term, nonconjugated estrogen use
Obesity, hypertension
Diabetes
Adenomatous hyperplasia

Diagnostic tests

Endometrial biopsy or fractional dilation and curettage (D & C)
Laparotomy with sampling of peritoneal fluid or washings

Potential complications

Hemorrhage
UTI
Constipation, paralytic ileus
Pneumonia
Thrombophlebitis
Pulmonary embolus
Wound infection
Ureteral fistula
Ureter ligation

Metastatic disease: low back pain; decreased urine output
Lymphocyst

Collaborative management

Prevention/detection teaching

Discuss importance of maintaining accurate menstrual cycle history
Frequency, length
Amount, color
Explain importance of routine pelvic examinations

Therapeutic management

Radiation therapy
Chemotherapy
Surgical intervention

Nursing management

PATIENT PROBLEMS/NURSING DIAGNOSES

● **NDX:** Anticipatory grieving related to lifestyle changes, decreased physical abilities, changes in physical appearance, life-threatening prognosis

Be sensitive to changes patient is experiencing; encourage patient to express feelings, frustrations, anger, hopes *to begin work of grieving process*
Provide a therapeutic environment conducive to open discussion: actively listen, perceive nonverbal cues, be patient and empathetic *to facilitate trust*
Encourage questions and provide information freely as patient expresses the desire for knowledge about the disease, treatments, and prognosis *to ease fear of the unknown*
Set limits on maladaptive coping behaviors if they interfere with patient's well-being
Support adaptive behaviors that suggest progression and resolution of the grieving process
Provide opportunities for private, uninterrupted time with significant other(s)
Assist in identifying ways to adapt lifestyle as condition changes *to enhance participation and feelings of control*
Provide information regarding support groups for patient and significant other(s)
Collaborate with other professionals (social worker, clergy, psychologist, psychiatrist) *to provide support and facilitate grieving process*
Provide reference for financial assistance, answers to questions regarding medical insurance

Pat

Preo
Con
tor
de
to
Dis
ma
Dis
va
If pa
re
Post
Tea
co
wo
Disc
an
Exp
Ur
Fr
Ur
El
UI
Disc
ity
Con
hig
co
Adn
Exp
pe
ve
Mar

Hoi

Arrar
teac
tion
Asses
phy
livin
Asses
mer
Plan
sup
Assis
won
cou

Provide information to assist patient in completing advanced directive or similar document *to ensure patient wishes are known to significant others and care providers*

EXPECTED OUTCOMES
Patient progresses through stages of the grieving process and moves toward acceptance
Demonstrates effective coping mechanisms; participates in decisions about own future

● **NDX:** Pain related to progression of disease process, surgical intervention

Assess nature, intensity, location, duration, and precipitating and alleviating factors
Use consistent pain rating scale *to determine baseline and deviations that indicate intervention is needed*
Assess nonverbal signs of pain particular to patient *so that early signs can be noted and treatment started*
Obtain information from patient regarding past pain experiences and methods used for relief
Control environmental factors that may increase perception of pain: temperature, noise, lighting
Assist patient to achieve comfortable positions
Assist patient to achieve state of minimal physical tension through techniques such as relaxation, music, visualization, diversion *to decrease need for medication*
Provide a restful environment with opportunities to rest during the day and uninterrupted periods of sleep at night
In collaboration with physician provide analgesic medications as required, observing for therapeutic and side effects
Discuss and institute noninvasive pain relief measures: relaxation, cutaneous stimulation, distraction, hot/cold therapy

EXPECTED OUTCOMES
Patient verbalizes decrease in or relief of pain
Incorporates existing pain while participating in daily activities

Patient/family teaching
Postoperative
Avoid constipation; use stool softeners, laxatives per physician order
Teach care of suprapubic or indwelling ureteral catheter if patient will be discharged with catheter in place
Teach clean, intermittent, self-catheterization as required
Discuss restrictions: no intercourse, tampons, douching, tub baths for 4 to 6 wk as indicated by physician

---

Avoid prolonged sitting, jarring activities, driving, heavy lifting, vacuuming for 6 wk as indicated by physician
Discuss symptoms to report to physician: elevated T, vaginal bleeding, abdominal cramps, difficulty urinating, change in bowel habits
Discuss that remaining vagina will stretch with sexual intercourse, and normal relations will be possible

Home care considerations
Discuss community resource/support groups for women with cancer/hysterectomy; sexual counseling
Plan for sufficient, clean space to store medical supplies as required
Assess ability to provide for physical and daily living needs: arrange home health provider as needed
Assess transportation availability to follow-up appointments; assist with arrangement as necessary
Reinforce need to continue relationships with supportive people

Cancer of Uterus/Pelvic Exenteration

total exenteration: Removal of all reproductive organs and adjacent tissues; radical hysterectomy, pelvic node dissection, cystectomy with formation of urinary conduit, vaginectomy, and resection of the rectum with colostomy
anterior exenteration: Excludes rectal resection with colostomy
posterior exenteration: Excludes cystectomy with urinary conduit

Postoperative assessment

Subjective data
Pain (may describe level and location)

Objective data
Incision site: redness, edema, drainage
Colostomy, ileostomy, urinary diversion
  Condition of stoma and surrounding skin
  Amount, color, character of output
Elevated temperature
VS: tachycardia, hypotension
Lower extremity edema
Character of popliteal/pedal pulses
Intake and output balance

Ovarian Cancer

Risk factors

Upper socioeconomic status
Hormonal factors
    Nulliparous
    Older at first parity
    Reduced fertility
    Infertility
    Exogenous therapy
Exposure to carcinogens
    Radiation
    Asbestos
History of breast cancer
Family history of breast, colon, or ovarian cancer
History of the following:
    Pentz-Jeghers syndrome
    Mucocutaneous pigmentation
    Intestinal polyps

Subjective data

Dyspepsia
Vague abdominal discomfort
Pelvic pressure
Urinary frequency

Objective data

Change in abdominal girth
Bilateral or unilateral, irregular, immobile ovarian mass
Palpable ovaries after menopause
Adnexal thickening: postmenopausal or nulliparous
    women
Advanced disease
    Weight loss
    Pleural/abdominal effusions
    Bowel obstruction
    Anemia
    Malnutrition

Prevention/detection teaching

Ensure that patient and significant other know and
    understand the following:
    Risk factors
    Importance of maintaining accurate menstrual cycle
        history
        Frequency
        Length of menses
        Amount
        Color
    Need to maintain good gynecologic hygiene
    Need for regular, periodic gynecologic examinations

Importance of cytological Pap examinations
    First smear at onset of sexual activity or age 18
    Second 1 year later, then every 3 years to age 35,
        then every 5 years to age 60
    Annual smears if at high risk
    Signs and symptoms to report to physician
    Early detection is rare (no early symptoms)

EXPECTED OUTCOME

Patient demonstrates knowledge of risk factors associated with ovarian cancer, signs and symptoms requiring health care evaluation, and detection measures for
determining ovarian cancer

Collaborative management

See specific surgery
    Chemotherapy, p. 922
    Table 15-7
    Radiotherapy, p. 915

Cancer of the Vulva/Vulvectomy

*Cancer of the vulva is an uncommon tumor, accounting
    for 5% of all gynecologic tumors; 86% of these
    tumors are squamous cell; surgical intervention may
    include skinning vulvectomy with skin graft (excision
    of the upper layers of the vulva and placement of a skin
    graft from the buttocks or thigh), vulvectomy with
    lymphadenectomy, excision of the vulva (labia
    majora/minora, clitoris, surrounding tissue) and
    pelvic lymph nodes*

Assessment

Subjective data

Itching/skin irritation; pain in the vulvar area

Objective data

Mass, lesion, lump on vulva
Postoperative
    Condition of incision, graft site
    Lower extremities for edema, pulses (pedal, popliteal)
    Constipation or impaction
    Anemia

Risk factors

Age: 70 years and older
Obesity
Hypertension

Smoking
Diabetes
Early menopause
Cervical cancer
Multiple sexual partners or single partner who has had
  multiple partners
Sexually transmitted diseases
Long-term pruritus
Immunosuppression

Diagnostic tests

Biopsy of lesions

Potential complications

Wound breakdown/graft failure
Lymphedema
UTI
Metastatic disease

Collaborative management

Prevention/detection teaching

Need for regular, periodic gynecologic examinations
Importance of maintaining good gynecologic hygiene
Need for periodic self-examination

Therapeutic management

Electrocautery, cryosurgery
Laser treatment
Radiation therapy
  External beam
  Internal implant
Chemotherapy
Surgical intervention
  Wide local incision
  Simple/radical vulvectomy with
    lymphadenectomy
  Skinning vulvectomy
  Psychologic support
  Social services

Nursing management

PATIENT PROBLEMS/NURSING DIAGNOSES

● **NDX:** Pain related to progression of disease process

Assess nature, intensity, location, duration, and precipitating and alleviating factors
Use consistent pain rating scale *to determine baseline
  and deviations that indicate intervention is needed*

Assess nonverbal signs of pain particular to patient *so
  that early signs can be noted and treatment started*
Obtain information from patient regarding past pain experiences and methods used for relief
Control environmental factors that may increase perception of pain: temperature, noise, lighting
Assist patient to achieve comfortable positions
Assist patient to achieve state of minimal physical tension through techniques such as relaxation, music, visualization, diversion *to decrease need for medication*
Provide a restful environment with opportunities to rest
  during the day and uninterrupted periods of sleep at
  night
In collaboration with physician provide analgesic medications as required, observing for therapeutic and
  side effects
Discuss and institute noninvasive pain relief measures:
  relaxation, cutaneous stimulation, distraction,
  hot/cold therapy

EXPECTED OUTCOMES
Patient verbalizes decrease in or relief of pain
Incorporates existing pain while participating in daily
  activities

● **NDX:** Anticipatory grieving related to life-
         style changes, decreased physical abili-
         ties, changes in physical appearance, life-
         threatening prognosis

Be sensitive to changes patient is experiencing; encourage patient to express feelings, frustrations, anger,
  hopes *to begin work of grieving process*
Provide a therapeutic environment conducive to open
  discussion: actively listen, perceive nonverbal cues, be
  patient and empathetic *to facilitate trust*
Encourage questions and provide information freely as
  patient expresses the desire for knowledge about the
  disease, treatments, and prognosis *to ease fear of the
  unknown*
Set limits on maladaptive coping behaviors if they interfere with patient's well-being
Support adaptive behaviors that suggest progression
  and resolution of the grieving process
Provide opportunities for private, uninterrupted time
  with significant other(s)
Assist in identifying ways to adapt lifestyle as condition
  changes *to enhance participation and feelings of control*
Provide information regarding support groups for patient and significant other(s)
Collaborate with other professionals (social worker,
  clergy, psychologist, psychiatrist) *to provide support
  and facilitate grieving process*
Provide reference for financial assistance, answers to
  questions regarding medical insurance

Provide information to assist patient in completing advanced directive or similar document *to ensure patient wishes are known to significant others and care providers*

EXPECTED OUTCOMES

Patient progresses through stages of the grieving process and moves toward acceptance

Demonstrates effective coping mechanisms; participates in decisions about own future

● **NDX:** Risk for impaired tissue integrity (wound breakdown/graft failure) related to stress on operative site

Provide overhead trapeze to *lift and move (do not slide) to prevent shearing of skin*

Maintain bed rest with head of bed elevated 30 to 45 degrees

Provide pressure-relief mattress

Provide bed cradle

Instruct patient not to cross legs

Avoid chair sitting *to prevent ischemic pressure areas on buttocks*

Place pillows between knees while positioned on side

Maintain indwelling urinary catheter

Provide wound care and dressing changes per physician order (dressing may remain in place for several days)

Use sitz bath or whirlpool per physician order *to stimulate circulation and provide comfort*

Avoid straining at stool; provide stool softeners, laxatives per physician order *to prevent development of anal fissures and bleeding associated with constipation*

Assess amount and character of drainage from wound drains; inform physician if amount increases or character changes

Change dressings immediately if soiled with stool/urine

EXPECTED OUTCOME

Wound remains clean and dry; healing begins

Patient/family teaching

Postoperative
  Instruct patient in wound care
    Irrigation and dressing changes
    Sitz baths
  Discuss signs and symptoms to report to care provider
    Unusual odor
    Fresh bleeding
    Perineal pain
    Elevated T
    Increased swelling of operative site/groin
    Frequency, urgency, burning on urination

Instruct patient to elevate legs periodically, avoid prolonged chair sitting, do not cross legs

Avoid constipation; collaborate with clinical dietitian to plan diet high in protein for wound healing that is nonconstipating

Avoid heavy lifting

Resume sexual activity according to physician guidelines
  Discuss options to intercourse
  Explain that fertility is not affected (if no metastasis)

Explain medication/radiation/chemotherapy regimen; expected therapeutic effects, side effects, potential adverse reactions

Discuss management of side effects

Home care considerations

Discuss community resource/support groups for women with cancer; sexual counseling

Assess ability to provide for physical and daily living needs; arrange home health provider as needed

Assess transportation availability to follow-up appointments with care providers; assist with arrangements as necessary

Assess physical space available to store medical supplies

Hodgkin's Disease

Malignant disorder characterized by painless enlargement of lymphoid tissue; usually one lymph node is affected initially, but other nodes and the spleen become involved throughout the lymphatic system (Figure 15-6)

Assessment

Subjective data

Fatigue
Malaise, lethargy
Loss of appetite
Bone pain

Objective data

Enlarged nodes (Table 15-5)
  Initially: supraclavicular and cervical
  Firm, rubbery nodes become hard with sclerosing
  Vary from nontender without skin changes to tender with skin changes
  Cervical node enlargement: venous occlusion, neck edema, airway obstruction

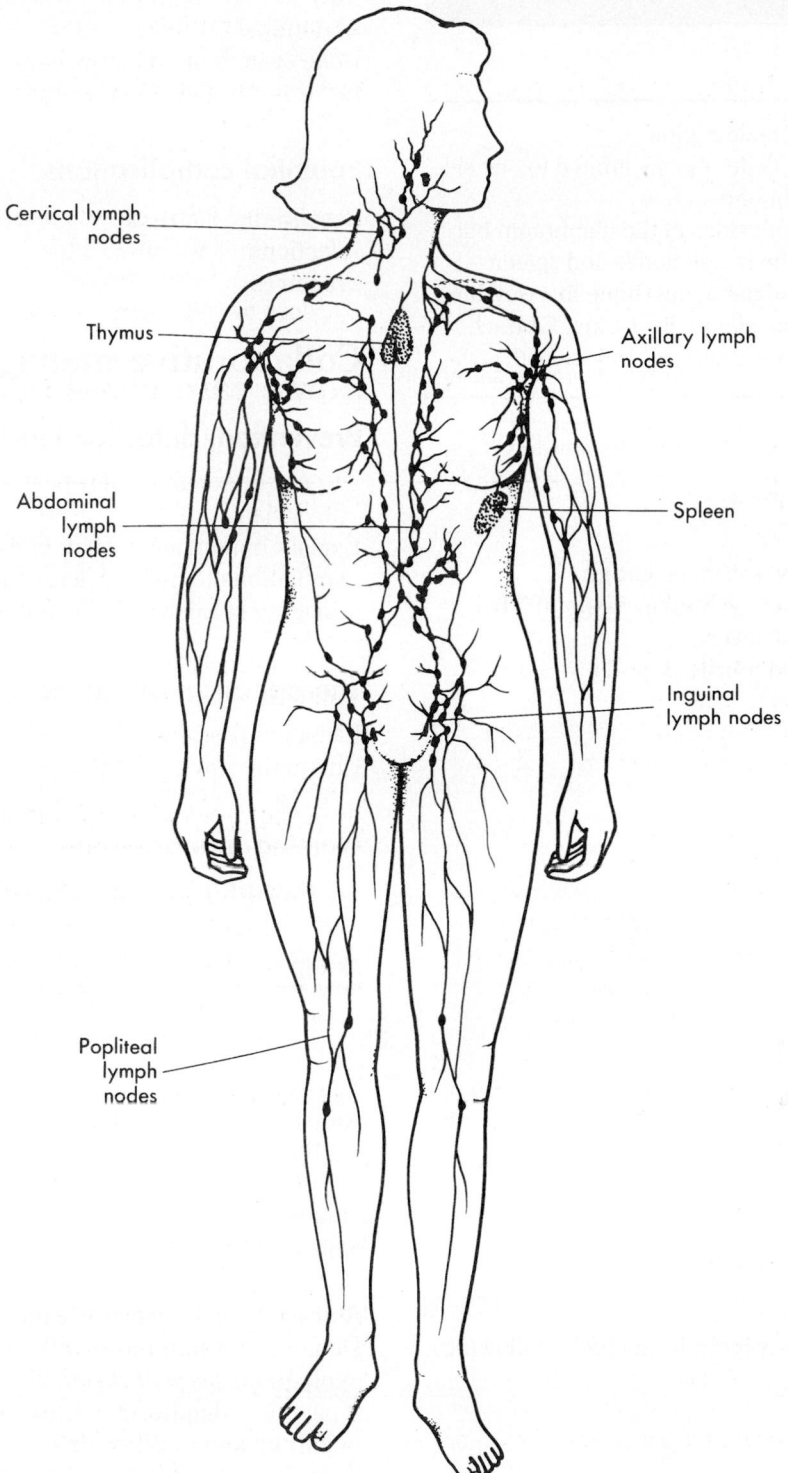

Cervical lymph
nodes

Thymus

Abdominal
lymph
nodes

Axillary lymph
nodes

Spleen

Inguinal
lymph nodes

Popliteal
lymph
nodes

Figure 15-6 Lymphatic system.

Table 15-5 Staging of Hodgkin's Disease

Stage*	Definition
I	Single lymph node region
II	Two or more node regions limited to one side of the diaphragm
III	Disease on both sides of the diaphragm but limited to the lymph nodes and spleen
IV	Involvement of the bones, bone marrow, lung parenchyma, pleura, liver, skin, GI tract, central nervous system, and so forth

From Luckmann J, Sorensen KC: *Medical-surgical nursing: a psychophysiologic approach,* Philadelphia, 1987, WB Saunders.
*All stages are subclassified as A or B to describe the absence (A) or presence (B) of systemic symptoms.

Mediastinal adenopathy: dyspnea, cough
  Inguinal: dysuria, frequency, lumbar discomfort
Pruritus: generalized and severe
T: alternating afebrile and febrile periods
Night sweats
Jaundice
Edema of face and neck
  Weight loss
  Splenomegaly, hepatomegaly

Risk factors

Men: higher incidence
White
Age: under 45, over 70
High socioeconomic status
No or few siblings
History of the following:
  Infectious mononucleosis
  Immunodeficiency syndrome

Diagnostic tests

Normocytic, normochromic anemia
WBC with differential (may include any of the following)
  Neutrophilia
  Monocytosis
  Eosinophilia
  Lymphocytopenia
Abnormal ESR: increased alkaline phosphatase (bone involvement)
Lymph node biopsy
  Reed-Sternberg cells
  Nodular fibrosis

Necrosis
Chest x-rays and CT scan
Gallium scan
MRI
Abdominal CT scan
Bone scan, bone marrow biopsy
Laparotomy, peritoneoscopy

Potential complications

Respiratory distress
Infections
Fractures

Collaborative management

Prevention/detection teaching

Discuss importance of reporting suspect symptoms to physician
Explain importance of scheduling periodic physical examinations to include screening laboratory tests and imaging studies as indicated

Therapeutic management

Radiation therapy
Chemotherapy

Nursing management

PATIENT PROBLEMS/NURSING DIAGNOSES

● **NDX:** Impaired skin integrity related to malnutrition, immobility, opportunistic infection related to cellular immunity (herpes, mumps, varicella, CMV)

Assess skin condition q8h: pay particular attention to axilla, skin folds, groin and perineal area, heels, scapula, back of head, dependent extremities, sacral area, mucous membranes
Note condition of skin related to temperature, moisture, color, texture, lesions
Assist with bathing prn; use mild soaps, rinse and dry well
Do not leave skin moist with lotions; avoid deodorants, cologne *to prevent chemical irritation of skin*
If patient is diaphoretic, rinse and dry skin well; keep clothing and bedding dry
Keep linen wrinkle free; avoid pressure from linen on feet; use foot cradle prn
Lift patient when turning, avoid sliding on sheets *to prevent shearing of skin*
Prevent pressure on bony prominence using pillows, air therapy beds prn

Encourage small shifts in position q30min and turn at least q2h *to promote circulation and prevent pressure ulcers*

Increase active mobility; encourage walking and sitting in chair; avoid chair sitting for longer than 30 min in one position

Provide for perianal care after each elimination

Avoid IM injections and multiple venipuncture

EXPECTED OUTCOMES

Skin and mucous membranes remain intact

Current breakdown is healing

● **NDX:** Fatigue related to chronic disease process

Assess causative/contributing factors; identify activities that are difficult for patient

Coordinate activities *to provide for undisturbed periods of rest and sleep*

Perform active/passive ROM exercises qid; collaborate with physical therapist to determine most therapeutic exercises

Determine whether patient becomes posturally hypotensive; change positions gradually; monitor for hypotension and tachycardia

Gauge amount and intensity of activity tolerated by monitoring patient's subjective complaints of fatigue, as well as changes in VS

Assist patient to identify strengths, abilities, interests; assist in development of realistic goals to progress from simple to complex tasks

Encourage patient to participate in own care to tolerance; assist as needed *to prevent exhaustion;* assist patient to identify energy patterns and schedule activities appropriately

Teach energy conservation techniques, use of assistive devices

Place patient on fall-prevention protocol

Collaborate with physical therapist to design measures *to maintain activity and independence*

EXPECTED OUTCOMES

Patient participates in self-care to tolerance

Ability to be active increases; patient states a feeling of increased energy

● **NDX:** Altered nutrition: less than body requirements related to reduced food intake, malabsorption, anorexia, vomiting, diarrhea, stomatitis

Assess nutritional status daily: weight, electrolytes, total protein, serum albumin, Hgb, skin turgor, muscle mass

In collaboration with physician administer antiemetics, usually on routine schedule *to prevent severe nausea and vomiting caused by medication therapy*

Determine amount and types of foods patient likes and is able to tolerate

Provide for oral hygiene before and after meals

Administer anesthetics to oral mucosa before meals prn

Offer high-calorie, high-protein diet with variation in taste, texture, and presentation of foods

In collaboration with physician, provide oral and parenteral nutritional supplements

Serve frequent, light meals and nutritional, high-calorie snacks

Assist patient to eat if fatigue is a factor

Present meals in an attractive, pleasing manner

Provide a pleasant atmosphere *to increase desire to eat:* encourage significant other(s) to join patient for meals, remove bedpans/urinals from area, maintain well-ventilated room, serve food as soon as it arrives, remove tray as soon as patient finishes eating

In collaboration with clinical dietitian: calculate number of calories and nutrients needed *to maintain/gain weight and support metabolic needs*

Maintain calorie count

Encourage family to bring patient's favorite foods from home

EXPECTED OUTCOME

Patient maintains weight within 10% of baseline

● **NDX:** Pain related to involvement of multiple organ systems

Assess nature, intensity, location, duration, and precipitating and alleviating factors

Use consistent pain rating scale *to determine baseline and deviations that indicate intervention is needed*

Assess nonverbal signs of pain particular to patient *so that early signs can be noted and treatment started*

Obtain information from patient regarding past pain experiences and methods used for relief

Control environmental factors that may increase perception of pain: temperature, noise, lighting

Assist patient to achieve comfortable positions

Assist patient to achieve state of minimal physical tension through techniques such as relaxation, music, visualization, diversion *to decrease need for medication*

Provide a restful environment with opportunities to rest during the day and uninterrupted periods of sleep at night

In collaboration with physician provide analgesic medications as required, observing for therapeutic and side effects

Discuss and initiate noninvasive pain relief measures: relaxation, cutaneous stimulation, distraction, hot/cold therapy

EXPECTED OUTCOMES

Patient verbalizes decrease in and relief of pain

Incorporates existing pain while participating in daily activities

● **NDX:** Risk for infection related to suppressed immune system

Screen personnel and visitors for symptoms of infection
Use strict sterile technique for all invasive procedures *to prevent nosocomial infection*
Monitor sites of invasive lines/tubes/drains for signs of infection q8h
Check body fluids for alteration in color, odor, consistency
Ensure excellent personal hygiene is maintained, especially after bowel movements
Ensure required fluid/nutrient intake; provide high-calorie, high-protein diet; supplement with total oral nutrition products prn, institute calorie count prn
Record intake and output
Monitor VS, especially T, q4h and prn
Monitor CBC, WBC results per physician order
Administer antibiotics, sulfa-type medications, and other antiinfectives as ordered
Maintain skin integrity *to prevent entry of microorganisms*
Auscultate breath sounds q8h
Encourage clearance of pulmonary secretions: turn, cough, deep breathe q2h; perform chest percussion and drainage prn; use incentive spirometer qh
Maintain intact mucous membranes; scrupulous oral care using soft instruments q4h and prn

EXPECTED OUTCOMES
Current infections are improved, resolved
New infections are not developed

● **NDX:** Ineffective airway clearance related to edema and/or enlarged mediastinal lymph nodes

Assess respiratory effort, pattern, breath sounds q4h and prn
Assist patient to achieve comfortable position; sitting position usually decreases work of breathing
Administer oxygen therapy per physician order
Assess patient's response to activity; assist as needed *to prevent respiratory distress*
Position patient *to minimize respiratory effort and maximize quality of ventilation*
Keep emergency airway equipment at bedside

EXPECTED OUTCOME
Effective breathing pattern is sustained

ADDITIONAL NURSING DIAGNOSIS TO CONSIDER
Altered urinary elimination, related to uremia caused by tumor lysis syndrome (p. 910) and increased uric acid

Patient/family teaching

Postdiagnosis
  Discuss symptoms of recurrence/progression to report to physician
  Discuss importance of keeping follow-up appointments with care providers
  Explain medications: therapeutic effects, potential side effects, potential adverse reactions
  Explain management of potential side/adverse effects
Infection
  Discuss importance of reporting signs and symptoms of infection: cold or influenza symptoms, coughing, dysuria, lesions that do not heal quickly, infected cuts
  Explain need to maintain skin integrity: avoid excess scratching, perform careful skin care, observe for skin changes
  Discuss need to maintain clean environment; avoid handling pets; avoid persons with infections and large crowds; perform routine handwashing and personal hygiene
Respiratory distress
  Discuss early signs of respiratory distress to report
    Increasing cough
    Hoarse voice
    Decreased activity tolerance
    Change in breathing pattern
Nutrition
  Collaborate with clinical dietitian to plan meals and instruct patient in selecting foods appropriate to patient's physical condition and considering the patient's preferences
  Instruct patient to weigh weekly and report loss ≥5%
Activities and comfort
  Explain importance of involvement in routine activity as soon as physical condition permits
  Discuss need to balance activity and rest periods
  Explain skin care measures to decrease itching
  Explore pain relief measures acceptable and successful for the patient
Anxiety/fear
  Explain importance of maintaining open communication with significant other
  Teach recognition of early symptoms of depression, maladaptive anxiety/fear
  Discuss problem-solving, coping strategies that patient is comfortable practicing
  Discuss sources of psychologic, financial, spiritual assistance

Home care considerations

Plan for sufficient, clean space to store supplies and medications
Emphasize need to have emergency plans and phone numbers available for periods of acute distress
Explore availability of weighing scale

Assess ability of patient to provide for physical needs
and daily living needs; arrange home health providers
as necessary

Assess availability of transportation to follow-up appointments; assist with arrangements as needed

Assist patient to contact community groups for ongoing
psychological/emotional support

Malignant Lymphoma

*Refers to a grouping of neoplasms originating in lym-
phoid tissue, which are classified by degree and differ-
entiation of cellular content involving either T or B
cell lymphocytes; grouping includes non-Hodgkin's
lymphomas and lymphosarcoma; etiology is unknown,
but a viral source is suspected; it can occur in all age
groups and is more common in men, whites, and
people of Jewish ancestry*

Assessment

Subjective data

Fatigue
Malaise
Pressure symptoms in area of involvement
  GI: difficulty swallowing, loss of appetite, nausea
  Retroperitoneal: abdominal, low back pain
  CNS: numbness, weakness, nerve pain, headache

Objective data

Enlarged lymph nodes
  Cervical and supraclavicular
  Nontender, rubbery, movable, size fluctuations
Enlarged tonsils/adenoids
Oropharyngeal and mediastinal mass
Weight loss
Elevated temperature
Susceptibility to infections related to type of immunity
  affected
Vomiting
Constipation

Diagnostic tests

WBC differential
  Abnormal-appearing lymphocytes (early disease)
  Lymphocytes with monoclonal surface immuno-
    globulin (Ig) (early disease)
Blood chemistries
  Serum calcium: elevated
  Serum copper: elevated
  Lactic dehydrogenase: elevated

Serum albumin: hypoalbuminemia or hypergamma-
  globulinemia (late disease)
Antiglobulin (Coombs): positive
Bone marrow: disease infiltration
Monoclonal Ig spikes

Potential complications

Pleural effusions
Paralysis

Collaborative management

Therapeutic management

Staging procedures
  Biopsies for histologic evaluation
    Lymph nodes
    Tonsils
    Liver
    Bone marrow
    Bowel
    Tissue removed during laparotomy
  Lumbar puncture
  Chest x-ray
  CT scans
    Liver, spleen
    Abdomen
    Bone
    MRI
    Gallium scan
Radiation therapy
Chemotherapy

Nursing management

See Hodgkin's disease (p. 898)

Multiple Myeloma

*Malignant disorder in which immature plasma cells
proliferate in the bone marrow and form osteocyte
tumors of the skeleton; initially, the pelvis, spine, and
ribs are involved; other bones, the lymph nodes, spleen,
liver, and kidneys are affected later; occurs primarily
in males 50 to 70 years of age; diagnosis is often made
in late stages, so prognosis is often poor*

Assessment

Subjective data

Bone pain
  Predominantly severe back pain on movement

Infection

Discuss signs and symptoms of infection to report to physician

Explain importance of avoiding persons with infections or recently vaccinated

Explain importance of avoiding large crowds, common drinking fountains

Discuss importance of maintaining excellent personal hygiene; teach handwashing techniques

Explain importance of avoiding skin disruption; use electric razor, wear gloves when gardening or doing housework

Avoid going barefoot

Instruct on importance of maintaining clean household environment and proper food handling

Anxiety/fear

Explain importance of maintaining open communication with significant other(s)

Teach recognition of early signs of depression, maladaptive anxiety/fear

Discuss problem-solving, coping strategies that patient will be comfortable performing

Discuss sources of psychologic, spiritual, financial assistance

Home care considerations

Plan for sufficient, clean space to store supplies and medications

Emphasize need to have emergency phone numbers available

Discuss availability of weighing scale

Assess availability of transportation to follow-up appointments; assist with arrangements prn

Assess ability of patient to provide for physical and home care needs; arrange home health providers prn

Arrange for durable medical equipment service prn

Assist patient to contact community groups for ongoing psychological/emotional support

Oncologic Emergencies

An oncologic emergency arises from tumor progression or metastasis and can cause irreversible morbidity or death if not promptly recognized and treated

Hematologic Emergencies

Tumor progression may cause hemorrhage via blood vessel erosion or through coagulation abnormalities

such as disseminated intravascular coagulation (DIC)

● Hemorrhage

Observations

Acute hemorrhage, most commonly from the following:

Nose
Bronchus
Stomach
Colon
Carotid artery
Vagina

Associated conditions/factors

Cancer
Stomach
Esophageal
Gynecologic
Head and neck
Colorectal
Leukemia
Lymphoma
Multiple myeloma
Chemotherapy treatment 10 days before
Platelet count <20,000

Interventions

Assess for bleeding; monitor VS and mental status; check mouth, nose, rectum, vagina, and skin; check stools and urine for occult blood

Monitor laboratory data

Notify physician of suspected or frank bleeding

Apply direct pressure for carotid artery hemorrhage

Depending on bleeding site, prepare for the following:
Packing: nose, rectum, or vagina
Occlusion balloon catheter: bronchus
Iced saline lavage: stomach
Iced saline enemas: colon/rectum

Monitor VS q15min; decrease frequency as hemorrhage is controlled

Measure and document amount of blood loss; measure and record intake and output

Maintain calm atmosphere

Support patient and significant other psychologically

Monitor IV fluids and blood products, platelets or fresh-frozen plasma

Prepare patient for surgery or laser surgery when ordered

● Disseminated Intravascular Coagulation (DIC)

Observations

May be hemorrhagic or thrombotic
Clot formation with serous drainage around clot
Increased bleeding from sites of invasive procedures
Ecchymotic extensions
Systemic bleeding to hemorrhage
Thromboemboli in any system
Hypotension
Tachycardia
Cool, pale, clammy skin
SOB
Loss of consciousness

Associated conditions/factors

Cancer
  Lung
  Prostate
Leukemia
Metastases
Sepsis
Infection
Hepatic failure

Interventions

Monitor VS q15min
Assess all body systems for presence of bleeding or thromboemboli and evidence of adequate tissue perfusion
Monitor sites of bleeding; apply pressure
Monitor continuous heparin infusion, IV fluids, and administration of blood products and medications (e.g., vasopressors, antidysrhythmics)
Measure and record intake and output; report deficits
See p. 252 for detailed care

Cardiovascular Emergencies

● Superior Vena Cava Syndrome (SVCS)

Obstructed flow to the right atrium occurs from compression caused by tumor progression or enlarged mediastinal lymph nodes, from intraluminal occlusion caused by some sarcomas, lung cancer, Hodgkin's disease, or lymphomas or from thrombosis caused by central line devices

Observations

Prominent neck and chest veins
Telangiectasia, upper thorax
Facial plethora
Edema of face, neck, upper thorax, upper extremities
Jugular vein distention
Headache, unrelieved
Dizziness
Visual disturbances
Feeling of facial fullness
Dysphagia
Dyspnea
Cough
Hoarseness
Chest pain
Respiratory distress
Altered LOC
Horner syndrome: one-sided drooping of eye with pupil constriction and conjunctivitis with loss of sweating on same side of forehead
Enlarged heart on x-ray examination
CT scan confirmation

Associated conditions/factors

Lung cancer
Hodgkin's disease
Non-Hodgkin's lymphomas
Breast, thymus, testicular, and head and neck carcinomas (metastases)
Chemotherapy via indwelling central line devices
Radiation-induced fibrosis

Interventions

Assess head, neck, upper thorax, and upper extremities for signs of SVCS
Assess mental status, LOC, respiratory status, vision, and voice for changes indicative of SVCS
Report findings indicative of SVCS
Position patient *to reduce edema*
  Semi-Fowler's to high-Fowler's position
  Elevate upper extremities on pillows; overbed table may increase comfort
  Perform passive ROM exercises q4h
Place venous access devices in lower extremities when ordered
Provide skin care for face, eye care to prevent infection and breakdown
Initiate oral hygiene measures
Prevent pressure or trauma to face, thorax, and upper extremities
  Wear loose-fitting bedclothes
  Avoid jewelry

Monitor oxygen administration equipment carefully
Avoid venous punctures for fluid or laboratory studies
Place identification band on lower extremity
Avoid Valsalva maneuver, lifting, or bending
Provide easily chewed foods or full liquid diet
Assist with oral and hygiene measures and diet *to decrease oxygen demand*
Provide information about radiation or chemotherapy as appropriate when scheduled *to reduce anxiety*
Maintain calm, quiet atmosphere
Answer questions and provide information *to reduce anxiety for patient and significant other(s)*
Assess effectiveness of medications administered and observe for toxic or side effects (e.g., chemotherapeutics, anticoagulants, oxygen therapy, steroids)

● Cardiac Tamponade

Cardiac tamponade may be caused by pericardial effusions related to metastatic spread of malignant cells or bleeding from coagulopathies such as DIC; also may result from constrictive pericarditis caused by radiation to mediastinum

Observations

Beck's triad
  Decreased BP with narrow pulse pressure
  Increased central venous pressure (CVP)
  Muffled heart sounds
Pulsus paradoxus: 20 mm Hg or more variation
Kussmaul's sign
Tachycardia
Precordial dullness on percussion
Peripheral constriction; cold, clammy
Tachypnea
Dyspnea, cough
Chest pain
Anxiety, apprehension, feeling of doom
Low-voltage ECG
Enlarged heart on x-ray examination
Effusion on echocardiogram
Jugular vein distention
Ascites
Peripheral edema
Pulmonary congestion
Constriction of pericardial sac
  Audible knock at heart apex
  Friction rub
Shock
Cardiac arrest

Associated conditions/factors

Metastases from the following:
  Lung
  Breast
  Lymphomas
  Leukemias
  Melanomas
Radiation therapy

Interventions

Assess for signs of cardiac tamponade
  Auscultate heart and breath sounds
  Assess carotid, radial, femoral, and pedal pulses
  Assess VS; calculate pulse pressure and presence of pulsus paradoxus
  Monitor respiratory status and continuous ECG
  Assess mental status and LOC
Report signs of cardiac tamponade immediately
Prepare to assist with emergency pericardiocentesis or immediate transfer to ICU or OR
  Observe for dysrhythmias during and after procedure
  Auscultate breath sounds for possible pneumothorax
  Ensure venous access for fluid requirements
  Have airway intubation and suction equipment available
Support patient psychologically
  Explain need for frequent assessment and monitoring
  Provide information about emergency procedures, detailing steps as they are taken
  Remain calm; answer questions clearly
Monitor effect of oxygen therapy
Restrict activities to reduce oxygen demand; assist with positioning, toileting
Position patient to increase venous return
Provide information about further treatments, sclerosing agents, chemotherapy, radiation therapy, or pericardial windows
See p. 146 for further care

Metabolic Emergencies

● Syndrome of Inappropriate Antidiuretic Hormone (SIADH)

Ectopic production of a substance similar to antidiuretic hormone (ADH) by a tumor or stimulation of the posterior pituitary gland to produce ADH by the tumor; or by specific drugs; this causes water intoxication and dilutional hyponatremia, which if unrecognized and treated, may lead to congestive heart failure

Observations

Lethargy
Weakness
Irritability
Confusion
Seizures
Nausea, vomiting
Anorexia
Sudden weight gain, usually without edema
Decreased urine output without change in intake
Congestive heart failure (CHF)
Serum sodium <135 mEq/L
Serum osmolality <280 mOsm/kg H_2O
Urine osmolality >1200 mOsm/kg H_2O
Urine sodium >20 mEq/L
Elevated BUN

Associated conditions/factors

Small cell lung cancer
Lymphoma
Pancreatic cancer
Prostatic cancer
Chemotherapeutic agents
  Vincristine
  Cyclophosphamide
Infections; viral/bacterial pneumonia
Increased intracranial pressure (ICP)

Interventions

Assess for fluid retention and dilutional hypona-
  tremia
Monitor intake and output
Weigh patient daily: same time, scale, and clothing
Assess neurologic and mental status
Evaluate laboratory values for electrolytes
Auscultate lungs for breath sounds
Report adverse signs immediately
In collaboration with physician, restrict fluids to 500 to
  1000 ml/24 hours
Assess effectiveness of parenteral hypertonic saline
  solution and diuretics administered: monitor
  for signs of hypokalemia and hypomagnesemia
  (p. 68)
Provide safety measures (e.g., bed in low position with
  siderails up, call light within reach); assist with am-
  bulation; assist with hygiene and diet *to prevent
  injury*
Maintain seizure precautions
Provide calm, nonstressful environment
Teach patient and significant other signs of SIADH to
  report

● Hypercalcemia

*Elevated calcium levels result from resorption of calcium
  from the bones, which results from bone destruction by
  metastases of the skeleton; prostaglandins, leukocyte
  cytokines, and ectopic production of a substance similar to
  parathyroid stimulates release of calcium from the bones;
  this may result in a gradual or sudden onset of renal failure*

Observations

Polyuria
Nocturia
Polydipsia
Lethargy
Confusion
Disorientation
Bradycardia
Fatigue
Muscle weakness
Hypotonia
Loss of deep tendon reflexes
Dehydration
Nausea, vomiting
Anorexia
Elevated serum calcium
Serum albumin may be decreased with serum calcium
  within normal limits

Associated conditions/factors

Cancer
  Breast
  Lung, squamous cell
  Thyroid
  Kidney
  Ovarian
  Esophageal
  Parotid
  Oral
Ewing's sarcoma
Melanoma
Multiple myeloma
Leukemia
Lymphoma
Immobility
Skeletal metastases
Medications
  Thiazide diuretics
  Lithium

Interventions

Assess for signs and symptoms of hypercalcemia
  LOC and mental status

Pharyngitis
Mucositis, oral infections
GI tract
  Xerostomia
  Esophagitis
  Diarrhea
  Weight loss
Brain irradiation
  Increased intracranial pressure (ICP)
  Sensory perceptual changes
  Hair loss
Genitourinary
  Cystitis
  Hematuria
  Changes in urinary elimination pattern
Cardiorespiratory response
  Tachycardia
  Pericarditis, myocarditis
  Pneumonia

Diagnostic tests

CBC: decreased Hgb
Leukocyte count: decreased to pancytopenia (usually
  receiving chemotherapy also)
Thrombocyte count: decreased
Electrolytes

Potential long-term complications

Lymphedema
Bone marrow suppression
Myelopathy, chronic
Brachial plexopathy
Pulmonary fibrosis
Osteoadinonecrosis
Teleangectasia
Bladder/bowel obstruction
Sterility
Malignancies
Paresthesias

Collaborative management

Therapeutic management

Clinical dietitian for nutrition counseling
Antiemetics, antifungals, antidiarrheals
Viscous lidocaine, topical antacids
Parenteral/nasogastric fluids, nutrition
Urinary anesthesia
Antibiotics
Pain management
Skin care therapist consultation
Blood component administration

Nursing management

PATIENT PROBLEMS/NURSING DIAGNOSES

● **NDX:** Fatigue related to effects of radiation therapy

Assess causative/contributing factors; identify activities
  that are difficult for patient *to plan appropriate assistance*
Coordinate activities to provide for undisturbed periods
  of rest and sleep *to increase energy level*
Perform active/passive ROM exercises qid; collaborate with physical therapist to determine most therapeutic exercises *to maintain muscle tone*
Determine whether patient becomes posturally hypotensive; change positions gradually; monitor for
  hypotension and tachycardia *to prevent accidents and
  decrease fear of movement*
Gauge amount and intensity of activity tolerated by
  monitoring patient's subjective complaints of fatigue,
  as well as changes in vital signs *so activity can be increased as patient's tolerance increases*
Assist patient to identify strengths, abilities, interests;
  assist in development of realistic goals progressing
  from simple to complex *to enhance feelings of accomplishment*
Encourage patient to participate in own care to tolerance; assist as needed *to prevent exhaustion;* assist to
  identify energy patterns and schedule activities when
  energy level is highest
Teach use of assistive devices *to conserve energy*
Place patient on fall-prevention protocol *to prevent
  injury*
Collaborate with physical therapist to design mea-
  sures/activities *to maintain independence*

EXPECTED OUTCOMES

Patient participates in own care to tolerance
Ability to be active increases; patient states a feeling of
  increased energy

● **NDX:** Risk for fluid volume deficit related to nau-
      sea, vomiting, or diarrhea

Monitor intake and output balance q8h to 12h
Inspect skin turgor and mucous membranes for
  hydration
Weigh patient daily: same time, scale, and clothing
Monitor results of electrolytes, blood sugar, Hct as or-
  dered *to determine adequacy of treatment plan*
Maintain oral/parenteral intake of fluids *consistent with
  fluid volume status; push for deficit; restrict for excess*
Offer and assist with oral care *to promote comfort*

EXPECTED OUTCOMES

Fluid intake and output regain or maintain balance

● **NDX:** Impaired skin integrity related to effects of external beam radiotherapy

Assess affected skin areas q8h

Skin care guidelines

  Do not remove skin markings; do not replace if removed, notify radiation oncologist

  Wash skin in area being irradiated with lukewarm water avoiding soaps, which may dry or irritate

  Avoid use of any skin care products (topical medications, lotions, deodorants, cosmetics), especially those containing alcohol or scent *to prevent irritation*

  Avoid tight garments *to prevent rubbing*

  Avoid extremes of temperature

  Dry desquamation: use cornstarch sparingly

  Moist desquamation: use water/saline to keep clean and moist (slow healing, may require days without radiation treatment)

  Expose skin to air *to promote healing* when possible; avoid direct sunlight

  Do not shave affected areas *to avoid cuts or abrasions*

  Cover broken areas with hydrocolloid dressing, using stretch-type tubular dressing to hold in place; avoid bandages, tape, which will irritate skin and cause injury when removed

  EXPECTED OUTCOME

Patient's skin remains intact and/or impaired skin progressively heals

  ADDITIONAL NURSING DIAGNOSES
  TO CONSIDER

Altered urinary/bowel elimination, related to effects of external beam radiation

Altered sexuality patterns, related to fatigue, sterility

Risk for infection, related to suppression of bone marrow

Patient/family teaching

Explain need to avoid persons with infections, especially URIs

Discuss symptoms of infection to report to physician

  Cold, flu, elevated temperature

  Diarrhea and frequency of or burning on urination

  Reddened, painful skin areas

  Mouth redness, swelling, ulceration, bleeding, increased salivation

Emphasize importance of maintaining nutritious diet and fluid intake to 3000 ml/day unless contraindicated

  Take six to eight small meals daily

  Avoid eating immediately before or after treatment

Explain that radiation effects continue for 10 to 14 days after last treatment; tell patient signs of healing will not be seen until 18 to 21 days after last treatment

Explain need for daily oral hygiene—in the morning, after meals, and at bedtime—to keep mouth fresh and clean

Discuss the following symptoms to report to physician

  Mucositis (p. 953)

  Nausea and vomiting (p. 951)

  Inability to eat

  Increasing headache or tiredness

  Severe diarrhea (p. 955)

  Increasing redness, swelling, pain, or pruritus at site of therapy

Emphasize importance of follow-up outpatient care

Teach name of medication, dosage, time of administration, purpose, and side effects

Explain need to avoid taking over-the-counter medications without physician approval

Home care considerations

Assess ability to provide for own physical care and daily living needs; arrange home health providers as needed

Assess availability of transportation to follow-up appointments; assist with arrangements as necessary

Plan for sufficient, clean storage space for medical supplies

● Brachytherapy

Assessment

NOTE: Symptoms will vary depending on isotope used, dosage, and target tissue; intensity of symptoms will also vary.

Head and neck implants (sealed sources of cesium 137, iridium 192) (Figure 15-7)

  SUBJECTIVE DATA

Painful swallowing

Painful speaking

Decreased appetite/anorexia

Fatigue

  OBJECTIVE DATA

Dry mouth/stomatitis

Oral infections

Xerostomia

Thick oral secretions

Erythema/dry desquamation at implant site

Weight loss

Alopecia

Use Voiding measures (p. 656) *to promote voiding when foley catheter is removed*

EXPECTED OUTCOMES

Usual pattern of urinary elimination is maintained; signs of UTI are not present

Patient/family teaching

Explain that patient is not a source of danger from radioactivity to family or others if precautions are followed

Discuss importance of continued activity balanced with periods of rest *to enhance well-being*

Stress importance of continuing follow-up care with physician

Gynecologic implants

Discuss methods *to eliminate constipation prn*

Instruct patient to notify physician of vaginal bleeding (slight spotting is expected)

Discuss signs and symptoms of UTI to report

Instruct patient to use water-soluble lubricant during intercourse (when physician approves resumed sexual activity)

Instruct patient in use of vaginal dilator prn

Prostate implants

Instruct patient to strain all urine for dislodged seeds

Instruct in safe retrieval of seeds with tweezers and foil, need to return to radiation therapy physician

Instruct patient to report changes in urine elimination pattern and/or hematuria

Head and neck implants

Instruct patient to report increased difficulty swallowing or controlling secretions to physician

Home care considerations

Patient is no longer a source of radiation exposure once discharged; however, if seeds are implanted, pregnant women and young children should stay several feet away for first 2 months

Assess patient's ability to provide for own physical and daily living needs; arrange home health providers prn

Assess availability of transportation to follow-up appointments; assist with arrangements as necessary

Chemotherapy

chemotherapy: Systemic cancer treatment using drugs that affect the cell cycle (Figure 15-9) to treat cancer; useful when there is disseminated disease or when there is a high risk of recurrence in the body; can be curative, can prolong life, or can be palliative; is often used as an adjuvant to surgery and/or radiation therapy

Assessment

Observations/findings

Physical response to specific condition

Ability and desire to learn

Barriers to learning: fatigue, denial

Knowledge of plan of care; diagnosis, treatment, expectations of results, patient's perception of his or her role

Attitude related to chemotherapy

Psychosocial response based on patient's coping mechanisms, support system, previous experience with chemotherapy, and amount of information received about disease process

Obtain baseline assessment before beginning chemotherapy and continue throughout treatment period (see assessment, p. 853)

Diagnostic tests

Specific to each medication and expected responses

Potential complications

Side effects and toxicities specific to each medication (see Table 15-7)

Common problems

Bone marrow suppression

Cutaneous manifestations

GI dysfunction

Respiratory dysfunction

Renal dysfunction

Cardiac dysfunction

Sexual and reproductive dysfunction

Electrolyte/chemical imbalance

Musculoskeletal dysfunction

Collaborative management

Therapeutic management

Antineoplastic medications according to protocol or standard regimen

Serial monitoring of results of diagnostic studies

Symptom-specific medications: antiemetics, antidiarrheals, oral anesthetics, antibiotics

Pain management

Parenteral fluids and nutrition

Nursing management

PATIENT PROBLEM/NURSING DIAGNOSIS

See specific condition and/or specific symptomatic care

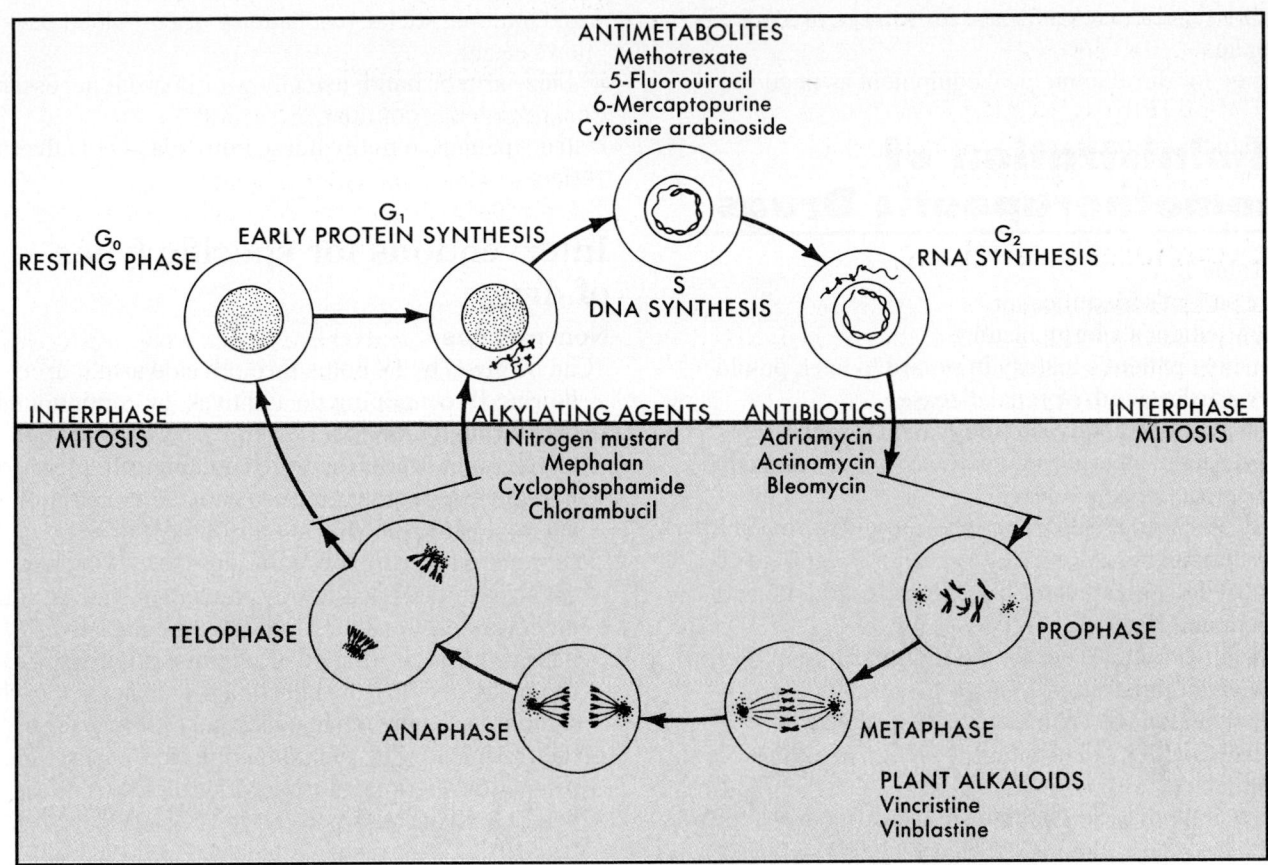

Figure 15-9 The cell cycle. Drugs are identified by where they exert their effect. (From Beare PG, Myers JL: *Principles and practice of adult health nursing*, ed 2, St Louis, 1994, Mosby.)

ADDITIONAL NURSING DIAGNOSES TO CONSIDER

Anxiety/fear related to therapeutic interventions and uncertain outcome

Altered nutrition: less than body requirements related to nausea, vomiting, anorexia, fatigue, stomatitis, decreased food intake

Risk for fluid volume deficit, related to nausea, vomiting, diarrhea

Body image disturbance related to changes in physical appearance and ability to function

Fatigue related to effects of chemotherapy and chronic illness

Patient/family teaching

With help of audiovisual aids, explain how drugs work and expected therapeutic effects of chemotherapy treatment

Provide patient and/or significant other(s) with written material regarding name of drug, action of drug, and potential side effects

Explain method, frequency, and duration of administration of each drug

Provide verbal and written material regarding management of side effects/toxicity

Instruct patient regarding early side effects, such as nausea and vomiting, and side effects that will be delayed such as myelosuppression

Discuss side effects that are reversible

Instruct patient regarding side effects to report to physician

Give written information on how and where to reach health care personnel if necessary

Involve significant other(s) in care planning as much as possible

Home care considerations

Assess patient's ability to provide for own physical and daily living needs; arrange home health providers as needed

Assess availability of transportation to follow-up appointments; assist with arrangements as needed

Facilitate patient joining a community support group for continuing psychosocial and emotional counseling and support

Plan for sufficient, clean space for storage of medical supplies

Arrange for durable medical equipment as needed

Administration of Chemotherapeutic Drugs

See Table 15-7

Verify patient's identification

Review patient's allergy history

Determine patient's history in regard to liver, pulmonary, cardiac, and/or renal disease

Assess patient's ability and motivation to learn

Assess patient's perceived ability to manage and cope with expected side effects

Assess learning needs and concerns; answer questions appropriately

Review educational materials (films, pamphlets) with patient and family

Check physician's order for drug dose, route, rate, and time of administration

Verify that informed consent has been given

Review laboratory data with knowledge of acceptable parameters

Review immediate and long-term side effects of drugs

Calculate dosage, double-check calculation, and ascertain whether dosage is within normal administration range

Know amount and type of diluent to use for reconstitution (mix in biologic safety hood and observe safety precautions [p. 943])

Verify drug dosage with another nurse, pharmacist, or physician

Correctly label drug with patient's name, dose, and route of administration

Administer antiemetic 30 min before administration of chemotherapy if indicated

Have emergency medications and antidote readily available for adverse reaction

Site selection and starting IV

Select site for venipuncture with regard to previous trauma to arm (blood drawing or lymphatic resection) and drug to be given (vesicant vs. nonvesicant); begin at distal portion of extremity

Avoid use of preexisting IV for vesicant drugs

Avoid use of anticubital space, hand, wrist for vesicants and irritants

Avoid use of lower extremities and areas over joints

Wash hands

Start IV, following guidelines of facility's policy and procedures; needle gauge usually No. 23 or No. 25 scalp vein

Avoid multiple sticks; test patency of IV—blood backflows easily

Stabilize arm or hand; use pillow or board if necessary

Ensure patient's comfort

Instruct patient to notify nurse immediately of adverse effects

Interventions for specific types of drugs

Nonvesicants

Can be given by IV bolus through side arm of free-flowing IV containing no additives, by continuous IV drip through a peripheral vein, or by two-syringe technique, with one syringe containing 10 ml of normal saline to test vein before drug administration and to flush vein following injection of drug

When administering through side arm of IV by bolus, check for blood backflow by pinching IV tubing and quickly releasing, before administration of drug, at halfway mark, and at end of administration; before removing needle from injection port, place 4 × 4 with alcohol swab beneath injection port to catch drop

When giving drug by continuous infusion, ensure vein patency throughout infusion period; before removing needle from injection port, place 4 × 4 and alcohol swab beneath infection port to catch drop (prevent spill)

Irritants

Drugs that are capable of producing pain at the IV site or along the vein, with or without inflammatory reaction; never give direct IVP

Can be given by infusion over 30 to 60 min depending on dosage

Check for blood backflow before administration and ensure vein patency throughout infusion period; apply ice pack prophylactically at infusion site to prevent discomfort

Vesicants

Drugs that are capable of causing blister formation and tissue destruction; never give direct IVP

See Extravasation (p. 942)

When given peripherally, avoid sites where damage to underlying tendons or nerves are more likely to occur

Can be safely administered through side arm of newly inserted, free-flowing peripheral IV containing no additives

Check for blood backflow before instillation of each milliliter (as described for nonvesicants)

These drugs are not given as continuous infusions except through a well-established central venous access device

When administering by central venous device, obtain blood backflow before instillation of chemotherapeutic drug (see Care of patient with central venous catheter, p. 67)

Use mechanical or electrical controller for continuous chemotherapy infusion

Keep IV site and as much of limb as possible visible
  Avoid obstructing view of site and vein with tape
  Keep clothing well above site; remove clothing from arm when possible

General interventions

Monitor for allergic reaction: anaphylaxis and extravasation (p. 942) on initiation, continuously during infusion, and then q4h to 8h for 24 hr

Manage pain as indicated and ordered; adjust flow rate of irritating medication to patient tolerance if possible

Know and observe for side or toxic effects and complications during administration, then for 24 to 48 hr; be aware of nadir of drugs ordered

Differentiate between effect of drug and reaction to disease when possible

Infuse parenteral fluids after drug administration to flush tubing, needle, and vein

Apply pressure over site for 3 to 4 min following removal of needle

Document medication, site, and responses or untoward effects of interventions

● Specific Alternate Administration Routes

Intrathecal

Assist physician to perform lumbar puncture (LP)

Observe strict aseptic technique during LP and administration of chemotherapy

Use sterile isotonic diluent without preservatives *to prevent/minimize neurotoxic reactions*

Instruct patient to lie flat for 2 to 4 hr after administration of chemotherapy

Assess for signs of changing neurologic status: sleepiness, headache, changing level of consciousness

Monitor for signs of cerebral spinal fluid leak around insertion site

Intraventricular

Assist physician to insert infusion reservoir

Observe strict aseptic technique during insertion and administration of chemotherapy

Ensure that the volume of CSF removed is equal to the volume of chemotherapy infused

Infusion rate not to exceed 2 ml/min

Assess for signs of changing neurologic status

Assess for signs of infection/bleeding in withdrawn CSF: purulence, color change

Assess for signs of CSF leak around insertion site

Intraarterial

Typically given through implanted pump reservoir into one of several arteries depending on site to be treated

Instruct patient to avoid hot baths/saunas, high altitude, *which may increase rate of pump*

Instruct patient to avoid contact sports/activities

Regional perfusion

Intraarterial infusion into an isolated extremity using tourniquets *to limit systemic absorption*

Performed in the operating room under general anesthesia

Assess for signs and symptoms of deep vein thrombosis, sensorineural changes in affected extremity

Intraperitoneal

Administration directly into the peritoneal cavity

Chemotherapy is mixed in a large volume (1 to 2 L) for maximal distribution

Administration is usually done via Tenckoff catheter or an abdominal implanted port

Warm solution to body temperature before administration

Encourage position changes during dwell time for maximal distribution of solution

Drain solution as ordered

Assess patient for signs of nausea/abdominal pain, peritonitis, respiratory distress

Maintain careful intake and output measurement

Intracavitary

Administration of chemotherapy into a specific body space

Usually excess fluid in the space is removed before administration of chemotherapy

Ensure free flow of solution during administration; aspirate frequently throughout administration

Turn patient side to side q15min for four times; then q2h to 4h to ensure maximum distribution throughout the cavity

Intravesical (urinary bladder)

Avoid fluids 4 hr before administration

Administration via foley catheter; 2 hr dwell time during which patient may not void

Assess for dysuria, hematuria

Text continued on page 942.

Table 15-7 Chemotherapeutic Drugs

Medication	Dosage	Routes of Administration	Side Effects and Toxicities*
ALKYLATING AGENTS			

Busulfan (Myleran)	4-8 mg/day (initially); 1-3 mg/day (maintenance); given according to protocol	po	Myelosuppression
			Low doses
			  Granulocytopenia
			  Platelets, lymphoid elements spared
			Hyperpigmentation
			High doses: leukopenia
			Delayed-refractory: pancytopenia
			Long-term therapy: pulmonary fibrosis (rare)

Chlorambucil (Leukeran)	0.1-0.2 mg/kg; given according to protocol
	2 mg/day maintenance
		po	Myelosuppression: leukopenia
			Nausea and vomiting, mild
			Amenorrhea
			Depressed spermatogenesis
			Long-term therapy
			  Alveolar dysplasia
			  Pulmonary fibrosis
			  Nausea and vomiting
			  Metallic taste
			  Sinus burning

Cyclophosphamide (Cytoxan, Endoxana, CTX)	40-50 mg/kg; given according to protocol
	1-5 mg/kg/day (oral)
		po; IVP
		IVPB
		IVCI
		Intraperitoneal
			Myelosuppression
			  Leukopenia
			  Thrombocytopenia may occur
			Common with high doses
			  Stomatitis
			  Alopecia
			  Hemorrhagic cystitis
			Amenorrhea, dose-limiting
			Testicular atrophy, dose-limiting

Hexamethylmelamine (Atrelamine)	260 mg/m²/day for 14-21 days	po	Nausea/vomiting, abdominal cramps Diarrhea, myelosuppression Peripheral neuropathy, alopecia

Ifosfamide (Ifex)	1000-2000 mg/m²/day for 5 days q4wk	IVP
		IVPB
		IVCI
			Myelosuppression
			  Leukopenia
			  Less thrombocytopenia
			Hematuria—hemorrhagic cystitis
			Alopecia
			CNS toxicity

*See Symptomatic care in Chemotherapy, p. 943.

Nadir	Recovery After Nadir (days)	Indications	Administration and Nursing Implications
10-12 days	42-50	Chronic myelogenous leukemia	Oral tablets may be taken any time of the day
11-30 days 1-10 yr	24-54		
14-28 days	28-42	Chronic lymphocytic leukemia, ovarian cancer, Hodgkin's and non-Hodgkin's lymphoma	Give oral medication as ordered; no specific directions
8-14 days	18-25	Non-Hodgkin's lymphoma, sarcoma, breast, lung, and ovarian cancer; acute and chronic lymphocytic leukemia	Give IV push over 3-5 min through side port of patent IV Give oral doses with or immediately after meals Administer antiemetic before therapy and as indicated Force fluids to 3000 ml/day before administration and 48 hr after
24 hr to several wk			Check output; if falling, notify physician for parenteral therapy orders IV hydration and bladder irrigation usually ordered when high doses given Give within 15 to 30 min after reconstitution
3-4 wk	42	Ovarian cancer Small cell/non–small cell lung cancer	Take 2 hr after meals, at bedtime MAO inhibitor interaction
8-14 days	18-25	Testicular cancer	Give IV over a minimum of 30 min Force fluids to 3000 ml/day before administration and 48 hr after Protector such as MESNA should also be used to prevent hemorrhagic cystitis

Continued.

Table 15-7 Chemotherapeutic Drugs—cont'd

Medication	Dosage	Routes of Administration	Side Effects and Toxicities*

Mechlorethamine (nitrogen mustard, HN$_2$)	IV: 10-16 mg/m²/course
	Intracavity: 0.2-0.4 mg/kg
	Topical: 0.01%
		IVS; intracavitary; intralesional
		Topical
			Myelosuppression, dose-limiting
			  Lymphocytopenia, dose-limiting
			  Thrombocytopenia
			  Granulocytopenia (leukocytopenia)
			Nausea and vomiting, severe onset 1-2 hr, lasting 8 hr
			
			Diarrhea
			Skin rash
			Amenorrhea
			Impaired spermatogenesis
			Vesicant; pain and tissue necrosis if extravasated

Melphalan (Alkeran)	PO: 0.25 mg/kg/day for daily dosage; 0.1-0.15 mg/kg for interval dosage; given according to protocol
	IV: 16 mg/m² at 2 wk intervals for four doses
		po
		Intraperitoneal (Investigational)
		IV
			Myelosuppression
			  Leukopenia
			  Thrombocytopenia
			High-dose therapy: nausea and vomiting
			Long-term therapy
			  Acute leukemia
			  Alopecia
			  Dermatitis
			  Stomatitis

Thio-tepa (triethylene-thiophosphoramide)	IV: 0.3-0.4 mg/kg/day
	Bladder instillation: 60 mg instillations/60 ml
	Given according to protocol; dosage reduced with hepatic or renal dysfunction
		IV, intracavitary, bladder instillation	Myelosuppression
			  Leukopenia
			  Thrombocytopenia
			  Anemia
			Mild
			  Local pain
			  Nausea, vomiting
			  Dizziness
			  Headache

NITROSOUREAS			

Carmustine (BCNU)	IV: 150 mg/m² or up to 200 mg/m²; given according to protocol
	Intraarterial: 100-200 mg/m²
		IV
		Intraarterial
			Myelosuppression, dose-limiting
			  Leukopenia
			  Thrombocytopenia
			Immediate
			  Burning pain at IV site
			  Facial flushing
			  Severe nausea and vomiting onset 2 hr lasting 4-6 hr
			Long-term therapy: pulmonary fibrosis

*See Symptomatic care in Chemotherapy, p. 943.

Nadir	Recovery After Nadir (days)	Indications	Administration and Nursing Implications
7-15 days Within 24 hr	28	Hodgkin's disease, non-Hodgkin's lymphomas, lung cancer, malignant pleural effusions	Give IV push through side port of patent IV; check blood backflow before instilling each ml; flush line with 30 ml IV fluid before each blood check; flush line after administration; monitor for extravasation; give antidote as ordered
6-8 days	10-20		
	Several days		Administer antiemetic before therapy and then as indicated Tell patient a metallic taste may be experienced just after drug injection Inform patient that veins may become discolored Reposition patient q15min for four times after intracavitary instillation
10-12 days	42-50	Breast, ovarian, and testicular cancer, myeloma, melanoma	Give oral doses 2 hr after meals
5-30 days	21-28	Papillary bladder tumors, malignant serous effusions Formerly breast and ovarian cancer and Hodgkin's lymphoma	Give IV push over 2-3 min through side port of patent IV Reposition patient q15min for four times after intracavitary administration Bladder instillation is retained for 2 hr; reposition patient q15min during this period
4-6 wk 3-5 wk	7-14	Multiple myeloma, Hodgkin's disease, non-Hodgkin's lymphoma; brain tumor, colorectal adenocarcinoma; gastric adenocarcinoma, melanoma, hepatoma	Give IV small volume for 15-45 min Apply ice pack at IV site Teach patient to report pain to staff immediately Flush vein before and after administration Administer antiemetics before administration and as ordered after

Continued.

Table 15-7 Chemotherapeutic Drugs—cont'd

Medication	Dosage	Routes of Administration	Side Effects and Toxicities*

Lomustine (CCNU)	100-130 mg/m²; given according to protocol	po	Myelosuppression, dose-limiting
			  Thrombocytopenia
			  Leukopenia
			Nausea, vomiting; onset 2-4 hr
			Anorexia
			Diarrhea

Semustin (investigational) (methyl CCNU)	125-200 mg/m²; given according to protocol; dosage reduced with liver dysfunction and impaired marrow function	po	Myelosuppression, dose-limiting
			  May be cumulative
			  Thrombocytopenia
			  Leukopenia
			  Erythrocytopenia
			Nausea and vomiting; onset 4-6 hr

ANTIMETABOLITES

Medication	Dosage	Routes of Administration	Side Effects and Toxicities*

Cytarabine (Ara-C, Cytosar)	1-3 mg/kg/day given according to protocol; dosage reduced with severe hepatic dysfunction	IV, intrathecal
		IVCI
		SC
			Myelosuppression, dose-limiting
			  Leukopenia
			  Thrombocytopenia
			Nausea and vomiting especially with rapid infusion
			Stomatitis
			High dose: flulike syndrome

5-Fluorouracil (5-FU, fluorouracil)	12 mg/kg/day, not to exceed 800 mg/day; given according to protocol
	Maintenance dosage: 6-15 mg/kg; given according to protocol; dosage adjusted with liver or kidney dysfunction
		Topical
		IVP
		IVPB
		IVCI
			Myelosuppression, dose-limiting
			  Leukopenia (granulocytes)
			  Thrombocytopenia
			Nausea and vomiting
			Alopecia
			Neurotoxicity
			Diarrhea
			Stomatitis

Mercaptopurine (Purinethol, 6-mercaptopurine)	2.5-5 mg/kg/day; given po according to protocol; dosage reduced one third to one fourth with allopurinol	po
		Investigational:
		  IVP
		  IVPB
		  IVCI
		Intrathecal
			Myelosuppression
			  Thrombocytopenia, mild
			  Leukopenia, mild
			Mild nausea and vomiting
			Cumulative hyperbilirubinemia

Methotrexate (MTX, amethopterin)	2.5-5 mg po daily
	50-70 mg/m² IV (low dose)
	100-150 mg/m² IV (high dose)
	IM 15-30 mg daily for 5 day course
	Given according to protocol
		po
		Intrathecal
		Intraarterial
		IVP
		IVCI
		IM
			Myelosuppression
			  Leukopenia
			  Thrombocytopenia
			  Anemia
			    Hgb effect
			    Reticulocytes
			Nausea and vomiting
			Anorexia
			Mucositis
			Hepatoxicity
			Dermatitis

*See Symptomatic care in Chemotherapy, p. 943.

Nadir	Recovery After Nadir (days)	Indications	Administration and Nursing Implications
40-50 days 26-34 days 28-42 days	60 6-10 9-14 24 hr	Palliative: brain tumors, Hodgkin's disease, lung cancer, colorectal adenocarcinoma	Protect oral drug from heat and moisture Teach patient to take on an empty stomach; avoid alcohol after dose
28-63 days 21-35 days 28-42 days	82-89 6-8 hr	GI cancer, brain cancer, Hodgkin's disease, non-Hodgkin's lymphoma	Teach patient to take on an empty stomach (may lessen nausea and vomiting), observe patient preference Absorbed in 30-60 min if stomach is empty
12-14 days	22-24	Acute lymphocytic leukemia, acute granulocytic leukemia	Give IV push over 3-5 min through side port of patent IV; may be given as a continuous infusion Keep patient flat 4-6 hr after intrathecal administration
7-14 days	16-24	Breast cancer, oral lesions, gastric tumors, and colorectal cancer; topically—basal cell carcinomas	Give IV push over 3-5 min through side port of patent IV using two-syringe technique; flush line after therapy Tell patient to expect vein discoloration
7-14 days 12-21 days 11-23 days	14-21	Acute lymphocytic leukemia, chronic granulocytic leukemia	Give oral dose daily
7-14 days 4-7 days 5 days 6-13 days 2-7 days	14-21	Acute lymphoblastic and myeloblastic leukemia, trophoblastic tumors, osteogenic sarcoma, epidermoid cancer of head and neck, multiple myeloma, lung, breast, and ovarian cancer	Ensure that patient knows not to take *any* medication before checking with physician when taking methotrexate po Check patency of IV before administration; flush IV after administration *High-dose* (investigational) Force fluids to 3000-4000 ml/day to ensure high-volume output Check creatinine results with increased dosage, sodium bicarbonate may be ordered to maintain urine pH 7.0

Continued.

Table 15-7 Chemotherapeutic Drugs—cont'd

Medication	Dosage	Routes of Administration	Side Effects and Toxicities*
Methotrexate (MTX, amethopterin)—cont'd			Alopecia Increased ICP Nephrotoxicity
Azacytidine (t-Azacytidine) (investigational)	100-150 mg/m²/day times 5; given according to protocol	IVS IVPB IVCI SC	Myelosuppression: leukopenia Stomatitis Nausea and vomiting; onset 1-3 hr and lasting 3-4 hr Rash Diarrhea Neurotoxicity Hepatotoxicity Hypotension
Thioguanine (6-thioguanine) (investigational)	2-3 mg/kg/day; given according to protocol; dosage reduced with liver or kidney dysfunction	po IVPB	Leukopenia Thrombocytopenia Anemia
VINCA ALKALOIDS			
Vinblastine sulfate (Velban)	0.1-0.4 mg/kg/wk; given according to protocol; dosage decreased with liver disease and neurologic problems	IVP IVS IVCI	Leukopenia, dose-limiting Thrombocytopenia, mild Mild nausea and vomiting Alopecia, mild Mucositis Constipation Ileus Abdominal pain Long-term therapy: neurotoxicity
Vincristine sulfate (Oncovin)	1-2 mg/m²—adult; given according to protocol; dosage decreased with liver disease	IVP IVS IVCI	Myelosuppression, unusual Neurotoxicity, dose-limiting Peripheral neuropathy, dose-limiting Constipation Ileus Alopecia
Vindesine (Eldesine) (investigational)	2-4 mg/m²; given according to protocol; dosage decreased with impaired liver function	IVP IVS IVCI	Neutropenia, dose-limiting Thrombocytopenia Leukopenia Neurotoxicity, dose-limiting at low doses

*See Symptomatic care in Chemotherapy, p. 943.

Nadir	Recovery After Nadir (days)	Indications	Administration and Nursing Implications*
			Administer citrovorum (leucovorin) rescue factor on time as ordered
			After intrathecal administration keep patient flat 4-6 hr
			Never give with salicylates, sulfonamide, phenytoin, ρ-aminobenzoic acid (PABA), alcohol, warfarin, amphotericin B
12-14 days	28	Acute granulocytic leukemia	Give within 8 hr of preparation; usually dilute in Ringer's lactate solution; administer IV push through side port of patent IV; may be ordered as continuous infusion
14-28 days	—	Acute granulocytic and lymphocytic leukemia	Give total oral dose at one time between meals
4-10 days	7-14	Breast and testicular cancer, choriocarcinoma, Hodgkin's disease and lymphoma	Give IV push through side port of freely running IV; check blood backflow before instilling each ml; flush line with 30 ml IV fluid before each blood check; flush line after administration
			Monitor closely for extravasation
			Give antidote as ordered
			Avoid eye contact
			Experimentally given by IV infusion over 24 hr period; monitor site closely
			Administer stool softeners and laxatives as ordered
4-5 days	7	Acute lymphocytic leukemia, breast cancer, sarcomas, Hodgkin's disease, neuroblastoma, non-Hodgkin's lymphoma, small cell lung carcinoma	Ensure patent IV; give IV push over 3-5 min through side port; check blood backflow before instilling each ml; flush line with 30 ml IV fluid before each blood check
			Monitor for extravasation
			Give antidote if extravasation occurs
			Administer stool softeners and laxatives as ordered
5-10 days 5-10 days	15-28	Acute leukemia, lung cancer, esophageal cancer, melanoma	Give IV push over 3-5 min through side port of newly inserted patent IV; flush tubing with 50-100 ml after administration; monitor for extravasation

Continued.

Table 15-7 Chemotherapeutic Drugs—cont'd

Medication	Dosage	Routes of Administration	Side Effects and Toxicities*
Vindesine (Eldesine) (investigational)—cont'd			Alopecia Constipation Paralytic ileus

PODOPHYLLOTOXINS

Medication	Dosage	Routes of Administration	Side Effects and Toxicities*

Etoposide	75-200 mg/m²/day × 3; given according to protocol	IVPB
		PO
			Myelosuppression; dose-limiting
			  Leukopenia
			  Thrombocytopenia
			  Mild nausea and vomiting
			  Alopecia
			  Severe hypotension with rapid infusion

Paclitaxel (Taxol) (investigational)	135-200 mg/m² over 24 hr	IVCI	Cardiotoxicity, dyspnea, urticaria, facial flushing, rash, hypotension, phlebitis, myelosuppression, neurotoxicity, alopecia, stomatitis, diarrhea

VM-26 (Teniposide)	100 mg/m²/wk, 45-50 mg/m²/day; given according to protocol; dosage reduced with prior irradiation/chemotherapy	IVPB
		Intravesicular
			Myelosuppression, dose-limiting
			  Leukopenia
			  Thrombocytopenia
			Hypotension especially with rapid infusion
			Rare anaphylaxis

ANTIBIOTICS

Medication	Dosage	Routes of Administration	Side Effects and Toxicities*
Bleomycin sulfate (Blenoxane, "Bleo")	10-30 units/m² given according to protocol; dosage decreased with renal failure; test dose may be ordered Total cumulative life-time dose not to exceed 400 units	IVPB Intrapleural Intraarterial IVCI IM SC	Anaphylaxis Elevated T with or without chills Hypotension Pulmonary toxicity Mild nausea and vomiting, dose-limiting Cutaneous reactions Alopecia

Dactinomycin (actinomycin D, Cosmegen)	0.5 mg/day for adult; 0.015-0.5 mg/kg for children; both given according to protocol	IVP
		IVS
			Myelosuppression
			  Thrombocytopenia
			  Leukocytopenia
			  Anemia
			Nausea and vomiting, onset 1-2 hr, lasting several days
			Mucositis
			Alopecia
			Skin changes, especially irradiated areas

*See Symptomatic care in Chemotherapy, p. 943.

Nadir	Recovery After Nadir (days)	Indications	Administration and Nursing Implications*
			Administer stool softeners and laxatives as ordered
16 days	20-22	Leukemia, lung cancer, lymphoma, testicular cancer	Give through side port of patent IV over at least 30 min to avoid severe hypotension Take baseline BP before therapy then 15 min into administration and at conclusion
7-10 days	15-21	Ovarian cancer Lung cancer, non–small cell	Cardiac monitor during administration Give via polyethelane tubing Premedicate for allergic reaction Irritant
3-14 days	28	Hodgkin's disease, non-Hodgkin's lymphoma, malignant pleural effusions, bladder cancer; CNS cancer	Give IV infusion in volume five times medication volume; over at least 45 min period through patent IV Take baseline BP before therapy then 15 min into administration and at conclusion Flush line after administration
—	—	Squamous cell carcinoma, Hodgkin's disease, non-Hodgkin's lymphoma, mycosis fungoids, lung cancer, testicular cancer, malignant effusions	Give IV push or IV infusion as ordered after obtaining baseline Be prepared to treat anaphylaxis; have life support equipment and medications available Take T and BP q4h during infusion Assess breath sounds and respiratory function Teach patient to report signs of respiratory difficulty immediately to staff Reposition patient q15min for four times when administering intracavitary doses
14-21 days	22-25	Choriocarcinoma, Wilms' tumor, sarcoma, testicular cancer	Give IV push through side port of patent IV; check blood backflow before instilling each ml, flush line with 30 ml IV fluid before each blood check; flush line after administration Monitor for extravasation; give antidote if extravasation occurs Establish oral and skin hygiene care before therapy Administer antiemetic before administration and as indicated and ordered

Continued.

Table 15-7   Chemotherapeutic Drugs—cont'd

Medication	Dosage	Routes of Administration	Side Effects and Toxicities*
Daunorubicin (Daunomycin, rubidomycin)	30-60 mg/m²; given according to protocol; dosage reduced with impaired renal or liver function	IVP IVS	Myelosuppression; dose-limiting Nausea and vomiting Alopecia
Doxotrubicin (Adriamycin)	60-70 mg/m² single dose; given according to protocol; dosage decreased with hepatic dysfunction Total cumulative lifetime dose not to exceed 450-550 mg/m²	IVP Intraarterial IVS IVCI Intraperitoneal	Myelosuppression: leukopenia, dose-limiting Nausea and vomiting, onset 3-4 hr Stomatitis Marked alopecia Reactivation of irradiated skin areas Cardiotoxicity, dose-limiting
Idamycin (idarubicin HCl)	12 mg/m³/day × 3 (usually with Ara-C); 100 mg/m²/day × 7 or 25 mg/m² IV bolus, then 200 mg/m²/day × 5 continuous IV; dosage reduced with impaired renal or liver function	IV IVCI (investigational)	Severe myelosuppression Nausea, vomiting, abdominal pain Severe diarrhea Mucositis Alopecia Rash: palms, soles of feet Dysrhythmias

Mitomycin (Mutamycin, Mitomycin C)	10-20 mg/m² dose; given according to protocol	IVP
		IVS
		Intraarterial
		Intravesicular
			Myelosuppression cumulative
			  Leukopenia
			    Thrombocytopenia: erythrocytopenia
			Nausea and vomiting, onset 1-2 hr, lasting 6-8 hr
			Stomatitis
			Alopecia
			Purple bands on nails
			Mild nephrotoxicity

Plicamycin† (Mithracin)	0.025-0.050 mg/kg; given according to protocol	IVPB
		IVCI
			Myelosuppression
			  Thrombocytopenia
			  Decreased clotting factors
			  Mild leukopenia

*See Symptomatic care in Chemotherapy, p. 943.
†Used to treat hypercalcemia, not an antitumor agent

Nadir	Recovery After Nadir (days)	Indications	Administration and Nursing Implications
7-14 days	21	Acute lymphocytic leukemia; acute granulocytic leukemia; neuroblastoma	Administer IV push through side port of patent IV Monitor closely for extravasation; give antidote as ordered Tell patient that urine will be colored red
10-14 days	21-24	Acute leukemia, Hodgkin's disease, non-Hodgkin's lymphoma, sarcomas, Wilms' tumor, ovarian, breast, lung, thyroid, and bladder cancer	Give IV push through side port of patent IV; check blood backflow before instilling each ml; flush line with 30 ml IV fluid before each blood check; monitor carefully to prevent extravasation that may cause severe ulceration; flush line after administration with 50-100 ml solution Teach patient to report *any sensation* during administration to staff Give antiemetics before administration and as indicated after Assess cardiac status before administration Institute oral hygiene care before administration
—	—	Leukemia	Give IV push over 10-15 min through side port of free-flowing IV Check blood backflow before instilling each ml; monitor continuous IV closely; flush line Monitor for extravasation; give antidote and follow policy if occurs Assess cardiac status before and during administration
28-42 days	42-56	Cancer of stomach and pancreas	Give IV push over 3-5 min through side port of patent IV; check blood backflow before instilling each ml; flush line with 30 ml IV fluid before each blood check; flush line after administration Monitor closely for extravasation; give antidote if extravasation occurs Administer antiemetics before administration and then as indicated Institute oral hygiene care before therapy Observe for skin changes at IV site or distal to site for 6 wk
14 days	21-28	Hypercalcemia in malignancy	Give in small volume IV over 30-45 min through side port of patent IV; may be ordered as IV infusion given over 4-6 hr for hypercalcemia Observe for extravasation; give antidote as ordered

Continued.

Table 15-7 Chemotherapeutic Drugs—cont'd

Medication	Dosage	Routes of Administration	Side Effects and Toxicities
Plicamycin* (Mithracin) —cont'd			Nausea and vomiting Diarrhea Stomatitis Neurotoxicity Dermatologic reactions Nephrotoxicity Hepatotoxicity
Streptozocin (Zanosar)	1.0-1.5 g/m²/wk; 500 mg-1.0 g/m²/day; given according to protocol	IVS IVPB IVCI Intraarterial	Severe nausea and vomiting Nephrotoxicity, dose-limiting Mild hepatotoxicity Immediate burning pain at IV site; decreases after 15-20 min of infusion
MISCELLANEOUS			
Aminoglutethimide (cytadren)	250 mg bid for 2 weeks then 250 mg qid; given according to protocol	PO	Lethargy, somnolence, malaise Dizziness, fever Adrenal/thyroid insufficiency Myelosuppression
Amsacrine (AMSA)	75 mg/m²/day; 120 mg/m²/wk; given according to protocol; dosage reduced with hepatic dysfunctions	IVCI	Myelosuppression: leukopenia, dose-limiting Neurotoxicity (cerebellar dysfunction, grand mal seizures) Conjunctivitis: nausea and vomiting, mild mucositis Dermatologic toxicity Cardiac dysrhythmias Phlebitis
Asparaginase (Elspar, L-Asparaginase)	10,000-40,000 IU/m²/day, q2-3wk; given according to protocol Skin test may be ordered before administration	IVP IVPB IVSI IM	Anaphylaxis Mild nausea and vomiting Neurotoxicity Hepatotoxicity Pancreatitis Hyperosmolar, nonketotic hyperglycemia

*Used to treat hypercalcemia, not an antitumor agent

Nadir	Recovery After Nadir (days)	Indications	Administration and Nursing Implications
7-14 days	—	Pancreatic islet cell tumors, non–beta cell pancreatic tumors: stomach, carcinoid, colon	Give IV push through side port of patent IV; check blood backflow before instilling each ml; flush line with 30 ml IV fluid before each blood check; flush line after administration; monitor for extravasation (p. 942), give antidote if extravasation occurs Administer antiemetics before therapy and then as indicated Tell patient burning sensation may be experienced; slow infusion to decrease burning Force fluids to 3000 ml/day, unless contraindicated, to ensure adequate urine output Observe for hypoglycemia reactions immediately after administration Have glucose 50% available
4-8 wk	—	Breast cancer	Postural hypotension Given in conjunction with high-dose hydrocortisone to reduce severity to adverse reactions
10 days	21-25	Acute myeloblastic leukemia, lymphoma, sarcoma, lung and breast cancer	Give within 30-60 min of preparation Dilute only in D_5W, never use saline Administer through side port of patent IV Administer corticosteroid eye medication as ordered Tell patient skin may have yellow-orange tinge
—	—	Acute lymphocytic leukemia	Give IV push over 3-5 min through side port of patent IV Take baseline, T, P, R, and BP before administration Be prepared to treat anaphylaxis; have life support equipment readily available

Continued.

Table 15-7 Chemotherapeutic Drugs—cont'd

Medication	Dosage	Routes of Administration	Side Effects and Toxicities*
Cisplatin (Platinol)	80-120 mg/m² ; given according to protocol Higher doses may be mixed in hypertonic saline solution to prevent nephrotoxicity	IVCI Intraarterial Intraperitoneal	Anaphylaxis Nephrotoxicity Ototoxicity Severe nausea and vomiting Hypomagnesemia
Carboplatin (Paraplatin)	360 mg/m² q4wk IV Should not be administered until neutrophils are >2000 and platelets >100,000	IVPB IVCI Intraarterial Intraperitoneal	Myelosuppression Leukopenia Thrombocytopenia Anemia Nausea and vomiting
Dacarbazine (DTIC)	250 mg/m² ; given according to protocol	IVP IVSA Intraarterial	Myelosuppression, dose-limiting Leukopenia Thrombocytopenia Severe nausea and vomiting, onset 1 hr, lasting to 12 hr Immediate burning pain at IV site, decreased with further dilution
Hydroxyurea (Hydrea)	10-30 mg/kg/day; given according to protocol	po	Nausea/vomiting Diarrhea Facial flushing CNS toxicity
Mitotane (Lysodren)	2-6 g/day; given according to protocol	po	Nausea/vomiting, rash Adrenal insufficiency Visual disturbances Myelosuppression Keratoconjunctivitis Prolonged bleeding times
Pentostatin (Covidarabine, DCF)	4 mg/m² every other wk; given according to protocol	IVSP	Hyperuricemia Neurotoxicity Keratoconjunctivitis
Procarbazine (Matulane)	50-200 mg/day; given according to protocol	po	Myelosuppression, dose-limiting Thrombocytopenia Leukopenia Anemia

*See Symptomatic care in Chemotherapy, p. 943.

Nadir	Recovery After Nadir (days)	Indications	Administration and Nursing Implications
18-25 days	39	Testicular and ovarian cancer; squamous cell carcinoma; lung, head and neck cancer	Assess baseline T, P, R, and BP Give by continuous IV infusion Force fluids to 3000 ml/day and give parenteral therapy as ordered 12-24 hr before drug administration Monitor intake and output Mannitol may be ordered with or after administration Ensure output of 100-150 ml/hr before giving medication Give antiemetics as ordered and indicated Be prepared to treat anaphylaxis Have life support equipment and medications available *High-dose*—investigational Parenteral hydration and bladder irrigation may be ordered
21-30 days	28-30	Ovarian cancer	Assess baseline TPR and BP Give by continuous IV infusion Monitor input and output Give antiemetics as ordered and indicated Be prepared to treat anaphylaxis Have life support equipment and medications available
21-28 days	36-50	Malignant melanoma, sarcoma, Hodgkin's disease	Administer small volume IV over 30-60 min through side port of patent IV Flush line after therapy Apply ice pack at IV site Give antiemetics before therapy, then as indicated
24-48 hr	7	Melanoma, chronic Myelocytic leukemia, ovarian cancer, squamous cell cancer of the head and neck	May give with Allopurinal
—	—	Adrenocortical carcinoma	Glucocorticoid, mineral corticoid therapy may be required Avoid use of alcohol
—	—	Hairy cell leukemia	May give with Allopurinal
25-36 days	36-50	Hodgkin's disease and non-Hodgkin's lymphomas, malignant melanoma, lung and brain cancer	Avoid use of alcohol, sympathomimetic drugs, trycyclic antidepressants, CNS depressants, and heavy intake of dark beer, cheese, bananas

Intrapleural

Administration via chest tube; tube clamped for 2 to 6 hr after administration

Discontinue chest tube when drainage is <50 ml/24 hr

Assess respiratory status and onset of chest pain

Intrapericardial

Administered via pericardial catheter with ECG guidance

Assess for ECG changes, onset of chest pain

Extravasation

Escape of agents from a vein into the tissue; escape of certain antineoplastic agents can cause necrosis of local tissue; care must be taken when giving these agents (see Administration of chemotherapeutic drugs, p. 924); vesicant drugs, which can cause tissue necrosis if they infiltrate, include vincristine, vinblastine, doxorubicin (Adriamycin), dactinomycin, daunorubicin, dacarbazine, mitomycin, nitrogen mustard, mithramycin, and streptozocin

Assessment

Observations/findings

Venipuncture site
  During infusion
    Burning
    Pain
    Swelling
    Induration
    Erythema
    Significant change in IV flow rate
    No blood return or questionable blood return (blood return is obtained, but patient questions or complains of pain—drug escape could be above injection site)
  Postinfusion
    Ulceration
    Desquamation
    Necrosis
    Phlebitis
      Pain
      Increased temperature
      Redness
      Swelling
  Predisposing factors
    Sclerotic vascular disease
    Multiple venipunctures

Collaborative management

Therapeutic management

Institute extravasation protocol/standard regimen for specific drug
  Sodium thiosulfate
  Sodium bicarbonate
  Hydrocortisone
  Hyaluronidase
  Warm/cold compresses

Nursing management

PATIENT PROBLEM/NURSING DIAGNOSIS

● **NDX:** Risk for impaired tissue integrity, related to extravasation of chemotherapeutic agents

Take measures to prevent extravasation
  Administer vesicant medication through a freshly inserted IV site with a good blood return
  Select large veins in region with large amount of soft tissue *to avoid possible involvement of tendons should IV infiltrate*
  Check medication dosage and dilution carefully *to avoid error*
  Administer at rate ordered; monitor closely *to decrease immediate side/toxic effects*
  Monitor IV site continuously during infusion *to observe first sign of extravasation*
  Instruct patient to notify staff immediately if burning sensation is felt at site or IV slows or stops
  After infusing medication, infuse neutral solution through IV line as ordered *to remove traces of drug*
  Observe for possible clinical signs of extravasation: pain, burning, swelling, no blood return or questionable blood return
  Observe for possible clinical signs of tissue necrosis: erythema, induration, tenderness, pain, eventual ulceration with tissue breakdown
Initiate protocol/standard regimen for specific drug immediately for any occurrence of extravasation
  Avoid direct pressure to site of extravasation *to prevent spread of drug to surrounding tissue*
  Mechlorethamine (mustargen, nitrogen mustard)
    Aspirate residual drug from existing IV line
    Administer 5 to 6 ml of ⅙ molar solution of sodium thiosulfate through existing IV line and into surrounding subcutaneous tissues *to neutralize drug effects*
    Repeat dosing over next several hours (no dose limit established)
    Apply topical cooling measures for 20 min qh for the next 24 hr
    Elevate and rest extremity

Dactinomycin (actinomycin D, Cosmegen); (Mithramycin, Plicamycin); danorubicin (Daunomycin); doxorubicin (Adriamycin); streptozocin (Zanosar), amsacrine
  Discontinue IV
  Apply topical cooling measures for 24 hr
  Elevate and rest extremity
Vinblastine (Velban); vincristine (Oncovin); vindesine; teniposide; etoposide
  Discontinue IV
  Infiltrate subcutaneous tissues with 1 to 6 ml hyalurondase; repeat over next several hr *to neutralize drug effects*
  Apply topical warming measures for 24 hr *to increase absorption*
  Elevate and rest extremity
Carbustine
  Administer 2 to 6 ml of 1:1 solution of sodium bicarbonate and sterile normal saline into existing IV line and into subcutaneous tissues; may repeat *to neutralize drug effects*
  Total dose not to exceed 10 ml of solution
  Topical cooling measures for next 24 hr
  Elevate and rest extremity

  EXPECTED OUTCOME
Extravasation of chemotherapeutic agents is prevented and/or recognized and treated immediately

Safety in Handling Cancer Chemotherapy Agents

Only pharmacists, physicians, and nurses with special training should prepare chemotherapeutic agents for administration (Table 15-8)
Preparation of cytotoxic agents should be performed in a Class II biologic safety cabinet (hood)
Transport parenteral drugs in plastic cover to prevent spillage and contamination
All equipment and unused drug(s) should be treated as hazardous waste and disposed of according to facility's policy and procedure: place linen in double bag marked "Caution, Chemotherapy"; instruct personnel to observe precautions in handling; wash twice
Personnel who are planning to become or who may be pregnant may request reassignment
Avoid eating, drinking, smoking, and using cosmetics while preparing and/or administering drug
Wash hands thoroughly before putting on gloves and after gloves are removed
Wear disposable cover gowns with closed front and cuffed, long sleeves and latex gloves throughout preparation, administration, and disposal period when handling medication or equipment *to protect against accidental spills*

Wear protective garment and gloves when handling patient excreta during administration and for 48 hr following administration
Syringes and IV sets with Leur-Lok fitting should be used whenever possible *to prevent spillage*
When priming IV line and removing needle from injection port, place alcohol swab and 4 × 4 beneath site *to collect small spills;* discard in hazardous waste container
Occupational Safety and Health Administration (OSHA) recommends drug administration sets should be attached and primed within a hood before the drug is added to the fluid
Wipe up spills immediately; contain spills by gently covering them with disposable absorbent material *to prevent aerosolization* (wear gown, mask, double gloves); place absorbent material in double plastic bag marked "Hazardous Waste" *to prevent accidental spill*

Symptomatic Care in Chemotherapy

● Hematologic Myelosuppression

Inhibition of bone marrow activity resulting in decreased production of blood cells and platelets caused by the effects of chemotherapy, the disease state, or radiation therapy; the majority of chemotherapeutic agents produce some degree of myelosuppression; since the blood count nadirs produced by most chemotherapeutic agents can be predicted, the schedule of drug delivery is designed to coincide with the recovery of the bone marrow; the nurse must be aware of the nadir (the point of lowest drop in blood count) for each chemotherapeutic drug

Leukopenia

Temporary reduction in the total number of circulating WBCs; since the life span of the leukocyte is very brief (6 to 8 hr), leukopenias occur frequently in patients receiving chemotherapy, placing them at risk for infections; a good indication of a patient's ability to fight infection is the absolute granulocyte count (AGC), which is calculated by multiplying the total WBC count by the percentage of neutrophils in the differential:

$$AGC = WBC \times \% \text{ Neutrophils (mm}^3)$$

(Bands + segs = neutrophils)

Table 15-8 Hazards Associated with Chemotherapeutic Drugs

Medication	Route	Hazard	Precaution and Action
ALKYLATING AGENTS			
Cyclophosphamide (Cytoxan)	IV, po	Teratogenic and carcinogenic; skin irritation is rare	Wear protective gloves; flush spills with large amounts of water
Mechlorethamine hydrochloride (Mustargen, nitrogen mustard)	IV, intracavitary, topical, intralesional	Strong vesicant, nasal irritant, highly toxic	Wear protective gloves; protect eyes; wash skin with large amounts of water, sodium carbonate (3%), or isotonic solution of sodium thiosulfate (2.5%); wash eyes with large amounts of water; irrigate with sodium thiosulfate in isotonic solution (contact physician)
Ifosfamide (Ifex)	IV	Teratogenic and carcinogenic; skin irritation is rare	Wear protective gloves; flush spills with large amounts of water
ANTIMETABOLITES			
Cytarabine (Ara-C, cytosar)	IV, SC, IM, intrathecal	Teratogenic; not absorbed through intact skin	Wear protective gloves; wash spills with water
5-Fluorouracil (Fluoroplex, Fluorouracil, Adrucil)	IV, po, topical	Minor inflammatory reaction if skin is broken	Flush spills with large amounts of water
Methotrexate (Mexate, Amethopterin MTX)	IV, IM, intrathecal	Teratogenic, carcinogenic skin irritant	Wear protective gloves; wash spills with water; apply nonmedicated cream for stinging; for systemic absorption of significant quantity notify physician; give folinic acid (leucovorin calcium)
ANTIBIOTICS			
Dactinomycin (Cosmegen, actinomycin D)	IV	Teratogenic; corrosive to soft tissues	Wear protective gloves; protect eyes; rinse spillage in running water for 10 min; rinse with buffered phosphate solution
Bleomycin (Blenoxane)	IV, IM, subcutaneous, intra-arterial, intratumoral, intracavitary	Cytostatic: local, toxic, or allergic reaction	Wear protective gloves; wash spills thoroughly with water
Daunomycin (Cerubidin, Daunorubicin, DNR)	IV	Skin and mucous membrane irritant	Wear protective gloves; wash spills immediately with water or isotonic saline
Doxorubicin (Adriamycin)	IV	Potential teratogenic; suspected carcinogenic skin irritant, but not absorbed into bloodstream	Wear protective gloves; wash spills immediately with large amounts of water

Continued.

Table 15-8   Hazards Associated with Chemotherapeutic Drugs—cont'd

Medication	Route	Hazard	Precaution and Action
ANTIBIOTICS			
Plicamycin (Mithracin)	IV	Rare skin irritation	Wash spills with water
Mitomycin (Mitomycin C, Mutamycin)		Teratogenic; suspected carcinogenic skin irritant	Wear protective gloves; wash spills thoroughly and immediately with large quantities of water; irrigate contaminated eyes with large amounts of water; notify physician
PODOPHYLLOTOXINS			
Etoposide (VP-16)	IV	Suspected teratogenic and carcinogenic irritants	Wear protective gloves; wash spills with large amounts of water
Teniposide (VM-26)			
VINCA ALKALOIDS			
Vinblastine (Velban)	IV	Suspected teratogenic skin irritant	Wear protective gloves; wash spills thoroughly and immediately with large amounts of water
Vincristine (Oncovin)	IV	Suspected teratogenic skin irritant	Wear protective gloves; wash skin with large amounts of water
Vindesine	IV	Suspected teratogenic skin irritant; may produce corneal ulcers	Wear protective gloves; protect eyes; wash areas with large amounts of water
MISCELLANEOUS			
Asparaginase (L-Asparaginase)	IV, IM	Potentially teratogenic	
Azathioprine (Imuran)	IV (investigational)	Potentially teratogenic, suspected carcinogenic skin irritant	Wear protective gloves; protect eyes; wash spills with water immediately
Cisplatin (Platinol)	IV	Suspected teratogen and carcinogen; skin reaction in sensitive patients	Wear protective gloves; rinse spills thoroughly with water
Dacarbazine (DTIC)	IV	Teratogenic, carcinogenic irritant to skin and mucous membranes	Wear protective gloves; wash spills with soap and water immediately; irrigate eyes with water
Carboplatin (Paraplatin)	IV	Suspected teratogen and carcinogen; skin reaction in sensitive patients	Wear protective gloves; rinse spills thoroughly with water

When AGC is <1000 cells/mm³, patient is at risk of infection; opportunistic endogenous organisms can cause systemic and severe infections; severe neutropenia is often defined as <500 neutrophils/mm³

Assessment

Subjective data

Dyspnea on exertion
Sore throat
Perineal discomfort, pain
Rectal tenderness
Dysuria, urgency

Objective data

Elevated temperature if not masked by corticosteroids or antiinflammatory drugs
Any sudden rise or fall of temperature of even 1°F
Elevated temperature of 100.4°F (38.3°C) lasting 24 hr or longer, not associated with blood products or drugs
Elevated temperature may be caused by other factors such as atelectasis, tumor, or response of disease process
Sudden rise and fall in neutrophils may be indicative of infection
In neutropenic patients, inflammatory response (redness, heat, edema, pus formation, pain) may be diminished or absent
Respiratory
  Cough, sputum production
  Changes in breath sounds (wheezes, rales, rhonchi)
  Colds and flu
Skin and mucous membranes
  Skin breaks, puncture sites
  Redness
  Swelling
  Drainage
  Ulceration
Oral cavity
  Fissures
  Redness
  Swelling
  Ulceration
Perineum
  Excoriation
Rectum
  Fissures
  Abscess
Genitourinary system
  Frequency
  Neurologic deficit: monitor residual urine; check urine for clarity and odor
Vaginal discharge
Assess vaginal hygiene and contraceptive techniques
Prostate enlargement
Eye or ear drainage

Diagnostic tests

WBC
Differential values
  Granulocytes
    Comprise 56% to 75% of total WBC
    Responsible for fighting bacterial and fungal infection
    Life of 6 to 7 hr
    Type: neutrophils, eosinophils, basophils
  Lymphocytes
    Comprise 20% to 40% of total WBC
    Responsible for immune defenses
    B lymphocytes: humoral immunity
    T lymphocytes: cell-mediated immunity
  Monocytes
    Comprise 2% to 8% of total WBC
    Defense against bacteria and fungi
Cultures: urine, sputum, blood
Urinalysis
Chest x-ray
Pulmonary function studies

Potential complications

Septicemia

Collaborative management

Therapeutic management

Treatment based on results of cultures
  Antibiotics
  Antifungals
IV gamma globulin
Antiviral therapy
Granulocyte colony-stimulating factors (G-CSF)

Nursing management

PATIENT PROBLEM/NURSING DIAGNOSIS

● **NDX:** Risk for infection, related to depressed immune system

Check results of WBC and differential *to ensure that they are within acceptable limits;* calculate ACG
Assess patient for increasing myelosuppression; nursing management will depend on severity of condition

Assess skin and mucous membranes for signs and symptoms of infection; give special attention to skin folds and body cavities

Assess respiratory and genitourinary tract for evidence of infection

Document findings and interventions

Instruct patient and/or significant other(s) that WBC count may decrease following most chemotherapy; WBC count usually recovers before next dose; however, recovery may be delayed, and an occasional dose of chemotherapy may be rescheduled

Teach patient *to guard against infection* by the following:
  Maintaining meticulous total body hygiene including perineal care
  Avoiding crowds and persons with infections
  Maintaining good nutrition and fluid intake
  Practicing good oral hygiene after meals
  Getting adequate rest and exercise
  Reporting signs and symptoms of infection to health care personnel immediately

Place patient in noninfectious environment if AGC is <1000/mm³ or as ordered; use of reverse isolation or laminar flow room are controversial based on research findings

Use physical means *to reduce exposure to microbes*
  Instruct and ensure that personnel and visitors follow handwashing procedure with providone-iodine before entering room
  No one with infectious condition (e.g., cold, flu, skin rash,) may enter room
  Staff assigned to care for patient with neutropenia must not be assigned to care for patients who have infections, if possible
  Care for neutropenic patient first and take precautions to avoid transferring any infectious agents to neutropenic patient
  Keep room clean
    Avoid any trash in room and bathroom
    Remove food and examination trays immediately after use
    Maintain furniture, fixtures, floor, and equipment free of dust and spills
  Ensure that allied health personnel (e.g., laboratory technicians) do not bring into patient's room equipment that has been in other areas of hospital
  If patient requires transportation, avoid using elevator with potentially infectious passengers present; mask for patient may be required

Maintain skin integrity
  Avoid IM injections
  Observe IV or central line site q4h
  Change dressing daily if nonporous type is used, using aseptic technique
  Change IV tubing and bottles daily
  Avoid infiltrations that necessitate restarting IV; position IV site *to prevent stress and movement at site of insertion*

Consolidate laboratory work; clean skin with povidone-iodine scrub before puncture

Assess previous puncture sites q8h

Assess and record condition of oral cavity q8h
  Teach or assist with oral hygiene measures in morning, after food ingestion, at bedtime, and q2h to 4h when patient is awake at night
  Administer antifungal and antiviral medication as ordered
  Assess and record condition of perineum daily
  Initiate and teach perineal care to be performed after each bowel movement
  Prevent constipation (p. 956) and diarrhea (p. 955)
    Administer medications as ordered
    Avoid use of enemas and suppositories

Monitor and record vital signs q4h; take temperature more frequently if trend is beginning; report any change in temperature immediately

Institute comfort and cooling measures as indicated by condition
  Change linen and clothing *to keep patient dry*
  Avoid chilling, *which may increase temperature elevation*
  Administer antipyretics as ordered
  Mechanical cooling blanket may be ordered

Monitor intake and output; report urinary frequency, burning, or changes in character of urine

Use voiding measures when indicated *to avoid catheterization*

If catheterization is necessary
  Use strict aseptic technique for insertion
  Perform catheter care q8h to 12h

Obtain cultures as ordered (e.g., blood, urine, sputum, skin, drainage)

Assess and record respiratory status q4h; report changes in breath sounds, cough, and sputum; increases in respiratory rate; or presence of sore throat immediately

Assist and teach patient to turn, cough, and deep breathe q2h *to remove secretions and prevent site for growth of microorganisms*

Administer oxygen if ordered

Encourage mobility q8h

Turn and position immobile patient q2h *to prevent pressure sores*

Provide mild antibacterial soaps and soft cloths and towels for skin hygiene, daily and prn

Administer IV antibiotics as ordered

Monitor laboratory data daily; report changes that indicate infection

Administer gamma globulin as ordered
  Monitor for anaphylactic reaction, phlebitis, nausea, back or abdominal pain, and chills

Minimize side effects by initiating comfort measures, use of blankets, decreasing rate of infusion and pre-medicating with acetaminophen (Tylenol) as ordered

Administer colony-stimulating factors (CSFs) as ordered; assess for headache; institute interventions

Instruct patient about low-bacteria diet

Instruct about need to remove flowers and plants from environment during neutropenic phase

EXPECTED OUTCOME

Patient exhibits no signs and symptoms of infection

Patient/family teaching

Discuss signs and symptoms of infection to report to physician or nurse

Emphasize importance of avoiding persons who may be infectious or have potentially contagious conditions

Explain need to avoid persons who have been recently vaccinated

Explain need to maintain safe sex practices

Explain need to wash hands after using bathroom, before eating, and before performing any procedures

Emphasize importance of preventing injury to skin
Use electric razors
Handle knives and sharp objects carefully
Wear protective gloves when gardening and when using strong household cleaning solutions
Wear broad-brimmed hat and sunscreen when in sun
Avoid going barefoot
Wear warm clothing and boots in cold weather
Avoid cutting cuticles, corns, or calluses
Wear padded gloves when using oven

Explain need to perform oral hygiene periodically throughout the day

Emphasize importance of daily hygiene including perineal and rectal care

Emphasize importance of fluid intake of 3000 ml/day unless contraindicated; explain need to avoid using common drinking fountain

Explain need to maintain clean home environment and handle food properly

Caution patient to avoid contact with pets or other animals during neutropenic phase

Teach name of medication, dosage, time of administration, purpose, and side effects

Explain need to tell all health care personnel, especially dentists, about need *to prevent infections*

Emphasize importance of follow-up outpatient care

Ensure that patient and significant other(s) demonstrate the following:
Method for taking and recording temperature
Procedure for caring for very small cuts or breaks in skin

Home care considerations

Assess patient's ability to obtain needed protective gear such as gloves, hats, sunglasses, electric razor, dental care items; assist in procurement as needed

Assess patient's ability to provide for own physical care needs and daily living needs: cooking, housekeeping, shopping, laundry; arrange home health providers as needed

Thrombocytopenia

Reduction in the number of circulating platelets caused by destruction of bone marrow during chemotherapy; platelets circulate for about 10 days before removal from circulation

Assessment

Subjective data

Abdominal pain
Blurred vision
Headache

Objective data

Disorientation
Petechiae, easy bruising
Bleeding gums, nose
  Purpura
  Hypermenorrhea
  Blood in emesis, urine, stool; tarry stools
  Prolonged bleeding from invasive procedures
  Vaginal, rectal bleeding

Diagnostic tests

CBC
Platelet count
ABO, Rh, HLA compatibility

Collaborative management

Therapeutic management

Bleeding precautions
Stool softeners
Blood product transfusion
Safety measures

Nursing management

POTENTIAL PATIENT PROBLEM

Bleeding related to thrombocytopenia
  Monitor platelet count and coagulation studies

Anticipate time of nadir after chemotherapy (time that patient is most vulnerable to bleed)

Identify drugs and/or other factors to avoid that may lower platelet count and predispose patient to bleeding

Assess and report any signs and symptoms of bleeding

Inspect gums and oral cavity for bleeding q8h

Inspect skin q8h for increased bruising, petechiae, ecchymosis, and swelling

Inspect and palpate joints q8h for increased size and decreased mobility

Assess sensorium and neurologic status q8h

Inspect nasal cavity at least once q8h

If epistaxis occurs
  Have patient sit at 90-degree angle
  Apply pressure to nose
  Place ice pack at back of neck
  If nasal bleeding is not controlled in 10 to 15 min
    Notify physician
    Administer platelet transfusion immediately when ordered by physician

Institute safety measures as platelet count decreases below 50,000/mm³
  Avoid needle sticks when possible
  Consolidate laboratory work; apply pressure to site for 5 min and observe site q15 min for at least 1 hr
  Avoid IM injections, aspirin, aspirin-containing products, and nonsteroidal antiinflammatory drugs
  Do not take rectal T or administer medications rectally; avoid enemas
  Avoid bladder catheterization when possible
  Take BP only when necessary and pump cuff only as high as necessary
  Avoid use of the following:
    Rough towels and washcloths
    Razors
    Restraints
    Tight clothing
  Maintain clutter-free environment
Provide night-light *to prevent bumping into objects or falling*

Administer careful oral hygiene *to prevent mucosal breaks*
  Use toothettes or gauze pads
  Avoid use of dental floss or toothpicks
  Encourage use of mouth rinse q2h to 4h
    Half saline and half water
    Half saline and half hydrogen peroxide followed by saline rinse

Inspect IV or central line site q20 min to 30 min for hematoma or oozing
  Maintain pressure at site for 5 min when IV is discontinued
  Inspect q15 min for four times

Administer antacids as ordered

Test stool for blood after each bowel movement

Test urine for blood each time patient voids

Administer stool softeners as ordered *to prevent bleeding from constipation*

Avoid vaginal douches

Use lubricant during intercourse to avoid trauma

EXPECTED OUTCOMES

Patient has no bleeding due to preventable causes

Patient/family teaching

Explain relationship between platelets and bleeding risk

Teach patient signs and symptoms of bleeding to be reported to physician in any of the following areas
  Skin
  Oral
  Nasal
  Rectal
  GI tract
  Vagina
  Cerebral
  Urinary tract

Discuss emergency plan to follow if spontaneous hemorrhage occurs at home
  Have emergency numbers available
  Call paramedics
  Go to nearest emergency area

Emphasize importance of telling dentist and other medical personnel about chemotherapy and low platelet count

Emphasize importance of maintaining safe, clutter-free environment

Explain need to apply pressure at blood withdrawal site after laboratory work is completed

Emphasize importance of avoiding over-the-counter medications, especially those containing acetylsalicylic acid (i.e., aspirin), without consulting physician

Caution patient to avoid use of sharp objects when possible
  Use electric razor
  Use caution when handling knives or other equipment

Explain need to avoid harsh coughing, blowing of nose, straining, and strenuous exercise
  If cough persists, notify physician
  Take cough medication as ordered

Emphasize importance of follow-up outpatient care
  Routine laboratory appointments
  Return physician and nurse appointments

Ensure that patient and significant other(s) demonstrate the following:
  Method for applying pressure to bleeding site
    Apply dressing or clean material directly over site
    Apply pressure for 5 min

Apply ice in covered plastic bag over site once bleeding stops

Check site for further bleeding q15 min for 1 hr

Method for testing stool and urine for occult blood

Home care considerations

Discuss importance of having emergency telephone numbers immediately accessible; know nearest emergency care facility

Assist patient in obtaining medical alert identification: bracelet, necklace

Assess patient's ability to safely provide for own physical care and daily living needs; arrange home health providers as needed

Plan for sufficient, clean storage space for medical supplies: occult blood testing products, emergency dressing supplies

Anemia

Temporary reduction in the number of circulating RBCs and the level of Hgb caused by destruction of cells during chemotherapy, leading to tissue hypoxia from impaired oxygen-carrying capacity

Assessment

Subjective data

Headache, dizziness
Fatigue, irritability
Difficulty concentrating
Dyspnea
Palpitations
Feeling cold

Objective data

Syncope
Loss of color in nails and palms of hands

Diagnostic tests

Decreased Hgb and Hct (dehydration may raise Hgb/Hct); if precipitous drop in Hgb, may be caused by hemorrhaging
CBC and platelet count
Reticulocyte count
ABO, Rh compatibility
Mean cell volume (MCV)
Mean cell hemoglobin (MCH)
Mean cell hemoglobin concentration (MCHC)
Bone marrow aspirate
Total iron-binding capacity (TIBC)

Collaborative management

Therapeutic management

IV fluid therapy
Serial ECG or telemetry monitoring
Blood product transfusion
Erythropoetin administration

Nursing management

PATIENT PROBLEM/NURSING DIAGNOSIS

● **NDX:**   Fatigue related to anemia

Note signs and symptoms of fatigue, SOB, tachycardia on exertion, and/or dizziness
Adjust ADLs *to match energy level*
Monitor laboratory data
  Hgb, Hct
  MCV, MCH, MCHC, reticulocyte count
Anticipate time of nadir after chemotherapy (see Table 15-7)
Provide adequate periods of rest and sleep *to improve energy level*
  Plan nursing activities *to avoid interrupting sleep*
  Provide activity-free periods throughout the day for rest
  Schedule examinations and tests carefully
Conserve patient's energy for desired activities
  Assist with meal preparation
  Keep needed items within reach
  Assist with hygiene measures
  Plan activities after rest periods
Gradually increase activity under supervision as problem resolves
Keep patient warm *to avoid expending energy to create body warmth*
  Encourage use of warm robes, socks, and clothing
  Provide extra blankets; cotton sheets are often more comfortable
Assess systems for signs indicating anemia
  CNS: irritability, headache, dizziness
  Skin: pallor, petechiae, purpura, jaundice
  Nailbeds: pallor, blanching
  Mucous membranes: pallor, petechiae
  Bones: tenderness over ribs and sternum
  Take and record vital signs q8h
  Assess respiratory and cardiac status q8h; report tachycardia, irregular cardiac sounds, and presence of wheezes or rales
Place patient at 60-degree angle *to facilitate breathing;* position with pillows if indicated
Administer oxygen therapy as ordered
Assess extremities, abdomen, and sacrum for presence of edema; report positive findings

Observe safety precautions: instruct patient to sit at side of bed before getting up; change position slowly *to avoid positional hypotension*

Provide nutritious diet high in iron

Administer blood products when ordered (p. 258); one unit of blood will usually raise Hgb 1 g/dl

Patient/family teaching

Teach patient about the relationship between Hgb and availability of oxygen as required for normal tissue function

Teach signs and symptoms of anemia to report to physician

Emphasize importance of eating foods high in protein, vitamins, and minerals, which are necessary for RBC production

Explain need to include foods high in iron, vitamin B_{12}, and folic acid

Arrange for dietitian to teach patient and significant other foods to include in diet

Discuss methods to conserve energy
    Planned rest periods
    Adequate rest
    Activities planned after rest periods
    Assisting with ADLs
    Keeping needed items within reach

Explain need to change position slowly; use appliances (e.g., walker bars) for movement if indicated

Emphasize importance of continuing to perform ADLs and other desired activities to tolerance

Emphasize importance of follow-up care

Emphasize importance of preventing secondary problems related to tissue hypoxia: infection, tissue breakdown, and/or blood loss

Home care considerations

Assess patient's ability to provide for nutritious diet; arrange for home health provider, Meals-on-Wheels prn

Assess patient's ability to provide for own physical and daily living needs; arrange for home health provider prn

Assess patient's need for assistive devices; arrange for durable medical equipment prn

● Gastrointestinal

Nausea, vomiting, and anorexia

Caused by physiologic changes resulting from cancer, the toxicities of radiation therapy or chemotherapy, and/or psychological expectation

Assessment

Subjective data

Nausea
Anorexia

Objective data

Time of onset of nausea and vomiting before or after chemotherapy administration or radiation therapy
    Duration
    Severity
    Possible cause
        Anticipation
        Foods
        Bowel obstruction
        Other medications
        Brain metastasis
Vomitus: amount, frequency, character, color
Nutritional status (p. 23): weight loss, decreased food/fluid intake
Dehydration
    Dry mucous membranes and skin
    Poor skin turgor
    Sunken, soft eyeballs
    Concentrated urine; decreased output
Antiemetics: type, frequency, and method of administration

Diagnostic tests

Electrolytes
CBC

Potential complications

Severe dehydration
Electrolyte imbalance
Malnutrition

Collaborative management

Therapeutic management

Parenteral fluids/nutrition
Antiemetics
Sedatives/hypnotics
Relaxation/hypnosis therapy

Nursing management

PATIENT PROBLEM/NURSING DIAGNOSIS

● **NDX:** Altered nutrition: less than body requirements related to nausea/vomiting, anorexia, decreased food intake

General

Remove food trays as soon as patient has eaten *to reduce negative stimuli*

Be aware that flowers and scents may be noxious

Instruct personnel and visitors to avoid wearing colognes and perfumes or smoking, which may be noxious to patient

Provide oral hygiene materials *to enhance appetite*

Keep dentifrice and mouth rinse pleasing to patient within reach

Encourage and assist with dental and oral care before and after meals and especially after vomiting

Nausea and vomiting

Instruct patient and/or significant other about drugs that are known to cause severe emetic action such as cisplatin and nitrogen mustard

Instruct patient and/or significant other about measures used to minimize side effects

Assess history of nausea and vomiting

Assess for known or probable preexisting disease states such as diabetes or hypercalcemia

Administer antiemetics before administration of agents and q4h to 6h for 24 hr rather than prn *to maintain good control of nausea*

Administer antihistamines or barbiturates combined with an antiemetic as ordered *to decrease stimulation of the vomiting center in the brain*

If metoclopramide (Reglan) is given, assess for extrapyramidal side effects; keep diphenhydramine (Benadryl) available *to counteract side effects*

If dexamethasone (Decadron) is given, administer slowly *to prevent sensations of hot flushes and burning in perineal area*

Lorazepam (Ativan) may be given as an amnesic during chemotherapy administration *to help control nausea and vomiting*

Provide safety measures when administering these medications *to prevent physical injury*

Give chemotherapy in late afternoon or at night when possible *so a nutritious meal can be taken without anticipating nausea*

Continually evaluate effectiveness of antiemetics *to help patient find the most effective combinations of drugs*

Teach patient and/or significant other methods *to prevent nausea and vomiting*

Small, frequent meals

Small dietary intake before treatment

Avoidance of greasy or spicy foods

Rest periods before and after meals

~~iet, restful environment~~

~~itor laboratory values, CBC, electrolytes~~

~~tor vital signs~~

Maintain chart of onset of symptoms, reaction to varying dosage of medication, and frequency of administration *to determine best interventions*

Marijuana may be prescribed

Monitor intake and output *to assure adequate hydration*

Administer IV replacement fluids as ordered

Weigh patient daily: same time, clothing, and scale

Experiment with several methods *to reduce or alleviate nausea and/or vomiting before or after chemotherapy*

Withhold food and fluids for 4 to 6 hr

Eat a light, bland meal

Eat a normal meal

Take only fluids for 4 to 6 hr

Eat dry foods only

Assist patient with belching air swallowed during feeding

Avoid motions conducive to nausea (rapid or frequent change of position)

After chemotherapy

Take liquids only

Eat dry foods only

Use methods of diversion *to distract patient*

Animated conversation

Absorbing projects or activities

Use other methods *to prevent onset or reduce severity of symptoms*

Relaxation methods

Rhythmic breathing exercises

Imagery experiences

Self-hypnosis

Behavior modification techniques

Place patient in well-ventilated room *to control odors*

Room should be away from food preparation area and soiled linen and waste product storage

Remove trash frequently

Empty and remove emesis basin, bedpans, and urinals after use

Anorexia

Plan appetizing meals based on patient's preference *to enhance nutrition*

Serve food attractively arranged and at proper temperature

Avoid liquids with meals

Provide foods high in carbohydrates to promote earlier emptying of stomach

Cool foods that are bland, soft, and odorless may be tolerated more easily

Sweet foods are often preferred

Add calories and nutrients by adding supplements to food (e.g., high-protein supplements, dry milk products)

Encourage patient to chew food well to ensure easier digestion

Serve main meal when patient can best tolerate food

EXPECTED OUTCOME
Patient maintains stable weight or increases weight and improves caloric and nutritional value of food ingested

Patient/family teaching

Teach method and rationale of all aspects of ongoing care to be implemented at home

Emphasize importance of maintaining adequate food and fluid intake

Emphasize importance of reporting the following to physician or nurse

Continuous vomiting for 24 hr without food or fluid intake

Signs and symptoms of dehydration

Feeling of extreme stomach fullness and/or abdominal pain relieved by vomiting

Teach name of medication, dosage, frequency of administration, purpose, and toxic or side effects; if medication causes drowsiness, caution patient to avoid driving and participating in activities that require mental alertness for safety

Emphasize importance of follow-up outpatient care

Home care considerations

Assess patient's ability to obtain, store, and prepare nutritious meals; arrange for home health provider or have foods brought to patient as needed

Assist patient to develop relationships with community support groups for continuing nutritional and psychological counseling and support

Stomatitis/Mucositis

stomatitis: *Temporary inflammatory response of the oral mucosa to the cytotoxic effects of chemotherapy and/or radiation; may progress to ulcerative bleeding and secondary infection*

mucositis: *Temporary inflammatory response of mucous membrane*

Assessment

Subjective data

Buccal mucosa pain
Change in taste and sensation
Inability to take food and/or fluids

Objective data

Buccal mucosa
General erythema

Swelling
Bleeding
Ulceration
Infected lesions
Candida albicans: soft whitish patches; may be localized or extensive
Herpes simplex: painful clusters of vesicles or ulceration
Gram positive: dry, brownish yellow, circular, raised eruptions
Gram negative: creamy white, raised, moist, non-purulent painful ulcer
Lips
Red fissures at corners of mouth
Edema
Surface abnormalities on palpation
Ability to chew and swallow
Hydration status

Diagnostic tests

CBC, platelet count
Cultures of oral cavity

Potential complications

Infection
Malnutrition
Dehydration
Electrolyte imbalance

Collaborative management

Therapeutic management

Consult with clinical dietitian to plan diet with needed calories and nutrients that patient is able to chew and swallow
Antibacterial agents
Antifungal agents
Antiviral agents
Analgesics; topical and systemic

Nursing management

PATIENT PROBLEMS/NURSING DIAGNOSES

● **NDX:** Altered oral mucous membranes, related to effects of chemotherapy

Establish oral hygiene regimen at initiation of chemotherapy, especially if patient is receiving 5-fluouracil (5-FU), methotrexate, or bleomycin *to decrease onset of mucositis*

Assess oral cavity daily with tongue blade and light, noting color, moisture, and presence of lesions

Note color, amount, and consistency of saliva

Institute prophylactic oral hygiene regimen before, within 30 min after each meal, and q2h to 4h during waking hours *to reduce foreign flora*

Brush teeth with soft-bristled toothbrush and non-abrasive toothpaste

Use foam stick moistened with mouthwash to remove debris from mucosa if unable to tolerate brush or if platelet count is greatly decreased

Use mouthwashes with no alcohol content

Remove dentures and bridges and cleanse following oral hygiene regimen

Keep mucosa moist by frequent fluid intake and eating soft, moist food; suggest saliva substitute *to maintain moisture*

Obtain order for mild analgesia if pain is present

Assess history of alcohol use, smoking, radiation therapy, and previous and current treatment with chemotherapy

Teach patient about oral complications of chemotherapy, how to examine mouth, and complete oral care

EXPECTED OUTCOME

Oral mucosa remains clean and intact or lesions heal progressively

● **NDX:** Impaired tissue integrity related to stomatitis, pharyngitis/esophagitis, and/or rectal or vaginal mucositis related to effects of chemotherapy

Stomatitis

NOTE: Stomatitis generally occurs 5 to 7 days after chemotherapy and persists for up to 10 days

If mild stomatitis occurs

Culture oral cavity

Assess oral cavity q8h

Encourage oral hygiene regimen q2h during waking hours and q6h during the night *to reduce microorganism count*

Brush teeth with soft-bristled toothbrush and nonabrasive toothpaste q4h

Use dilute nonalcohol mouthwash or normal saline: swish, gargle, and expectorate

Baking soda (1 tsp in 8 oz of water): swish, gargle, and expectorate

Use toothette or cotton-tipped applicator to remove mucus and debris

Apply lip lubricant q2h during waking hours

Assess need for use of antifungal or antibacterial agents

Topical anesthetics such as viscous lidocaine (Xylocaine) or Orabase may be used before meals for discomfort

Use mild analgesic q3h to 4h

Encourage bland diet high in protein *to promote healing*

Encourage fluid to 2000 ml/day; avoid citrus juices

If severe stomatitis occurs

Request order for culture for oral cavity *to determine causative organism*

Assess oral cavity q8h

Practice oral hygiene q1h to 2h, including the following:

Cleaning of teeth with soft-bristled toothbrush, toothette, or gauze soaked in mouthwash–normal saline mixture

Use of antifungal and/or antibacterial agents

Use of topical anesthetics such as equal parts diphenhydramine (Benadryl) elixir (25 mg), Maalox, and viscous lidocaine (Xylocaine)

Use of moderate to strong analgesic q3h to 4h

Encourage diet (puréed) and liquids high in protein *to maintain nutrition*

If patient has difficulty in eating and maintaining fluid intake, parenteral nutrition may be necessary

If oral hygiene is difficult because of pain in oral cavity, encourage patient to rinse with 1 tsp viscous lidocaine 15 min before oral hygiene

If patient is unable to brush or rinse, irrigate mouth with syringe or soft rubber catheter using saline and water q3h to 4h

Gently clean lips with saline solution

If oral candidiasis is present, instruct patient to swish and swallow an oral suspension of nystatin (Mycostatin)

Teach patient how to examine mouth and perform oral care

Pharyngitis/esophagitis

Assess for difficulty in swallowing and for infection

Antacids may be helpful

Obtain physician's order for Sucralfate

Rectal or vaginal mucositis

Instruct female patients to report any pain, ulceration, or bleeding of mucous membrane lining perineum or vagina

Instruct patient to include frequent perineal washing after voiding; pat dry

Instruct patient to use sitz baths *to increase comfort*

Caution patient to avoid douches *to avoid further irritation*

Discuss need to avoid sexual activity while symptomatic

Instruct male patient to report signs and symptoms involving perineum

EXPECTED OUTCOME

Affected tissues heal progressively

Diarrhea

Passage of frequent stools of a soft or liquid consistency with or without discomfort caused by effects of chemotherapy on epithelium

Subjective data

Abdominal cramping

Objective data

Frequent stools
 Watery
 Bloody
 Containing mucus
 Tarry
Dehydration
 Dry mucous membranes
 Poor skin turgor
 Decreased urine output

Diagnostic tests

CBC
Electrolytes
Stool cultures

Potential complications

Electrolyte imbalance
Dehydration
Malnutrition
GI bleeding

Collaborative management

Therapeutic management

Parenteral fluids/nutrition
Antidiarrheals
Antispasmodics
Collaborate with clinical dietitian to plan meals with sufficient caloric and nutritional values that assist in controlling or do not promote diarrhea

Nursing management

PATIENT PROBLEM/NURSING DIAGNOSIS

● **NDX:** Diarrhea related to chemotherapy effects on GI mucosa

Assess usual pattern of elimination including use of laxatives
Determine other probable causes of diarrhea such as inappropriate diet, treatment side effects, infection, stress, or disease progression
Evaluate hydration and electrolyte status
 Monitor intake and output, weight, and electrolytes
 Assess frequency, character, and volume of stool
 Assess abdomen, including bowel sounds; note distention, cramping, or flatus
 Assess perineal/perianal region for skin status
Adjust diet as appropriate; include bananas and cheese; avoid hot liquids, coffee, fresh fruits, and prune juice
Include foods high in potassium to prevent weakness when laboratory values indicate a low potassium level
Encourage increased fluid intake of 3000 ml/day if not contraindicated; suggest liquids, such as Gatorade, grape juice, and fruit drinks, that contain electrolytes
Administer medications, such as Kaopectate or Lomotil as ordered, *to control diarrhea*
Observe and report early signs of constipation
Establish protocol for care of perineal area
 Gently clean area with water and mild soap after each stool; dry thoroughly and inspect for breakdown
 Apply ointments as indicated
 Use sitz baths as indicated *to increase comfort*
 Use skin barrier as needed *to promote healing*
Check and record all stools for the following:
 Frequency
 Amount
 Consistency
 Presence of blood, overt or occult
Perform perineal care if patient is unable
Apply medication to perineum as ordered *to promote healing*
Assess and record status of perineal area at least q8h; q4h if frequency of stools increases
Weigh patient daily: same time, clothing, and scale
Consult with physician *to determine possibility of interrupting treatment until diarrhea is controlled*
Assess for edema; third spacing of fluids may occur from protein deficiency and electrolyte imbalances

EXPECTED OUTCOME
Normal bowel elimination pattern is achieved

Patient/family teaching

Teach patient to perform perineal care after each defecation
 Use povidone-iodine wash or mild soap and water
 Wash with soft cloths, front to back for women
 Dry by gentle patting with soft toweling
 Wash and dry hands well
Teach patient to test stool for blood after each bowel movement
Discuss signs and symptoms of diarrhea that must be reported to physician

Emphasize importance of maintaining oral fluid intake of 3000 ml/day unless contraindicated

Explain need to avoid diet high in fiber and roughage

Explain need to take prescribed medication during episodes of diarrhea

Explain need to avoid over-the-counter medications without physician or nurse approval

Home care considerations

Assess patient's ability to obtain and store occult blood testing supplies

Assess patient's ability to provide foods for and prepare therapeutic diet; arrange for home health provider or have foods brought to patient as needed

Constipation

Passage of irregular, infrequent, hard feces; may be caused by disease process, chemotherapy, or other factors

Subjective data

Difficult, painful stool evacuation

Objective data

Absence of stool for more than 3 days
Stool
  Hard, dry
  Red-streaked
Absence of bowel sounds

Diagnostic tests

Depend on suspected cause

Potential complication

Ileus

Collaborative management

Therapeutic management

Stool softeners
Hydration: oral or parenteral
Laxatives or enemas if not contraindicated by the condition of the rectal mucosa
Collaborate with clinical dietitian to develop therapeutic meal plans that do not promote constipation

Nursing management

PATIENT PROBLEM/NURSING DIAGNOSIS

● **NDX:** Constipation related to effects of chemotherapy on the GI tract

Assess usual pattern of elimination, including use of laxatives *to establish baseline*

Identify factors that could alter usual pattern of elimination, such as immobility, chemotherapeutic drugs (vincristine, vinblastine), opiate/narcotic analgesics, low-fiber diet, or inadequate fluid intake

Assess for presence of associated signs and symptoms such as flatus, distention, or discomfort

Assess for fecal impaction

Evaluate and record time and character of bowel elimination daily

Auscultate abdomen for bowel sounds q8h *to determine prescence of ileus*

Administer enema type, amount, and solution as ordered; digital removal of feces may be necessary—follow hospital policy and procedure

If no spontaneous stool occurs within 24 hr after enema, administer stool softener, laxative, or suppository as ordered

Monitor intake and output *to ensure balance*

Force fluids to 3000 ml/day unless contraindicated

Maintain diet high in fiber and bulk

Encourage ambulation and exercise to tolerance

Perform ROM exercises q4h to 8h if patient is immobile

Provide privacy when needed
  Assist with ambulation to bathroom
  Screen patient in bed
  Do not schedule appointments or examinations at time of patient's usual evacuation

Perform perineal care after bowel movement

Assess condition of perineum daily

Apply medication to rectal area as ordered

EXPECTED OUTCOME

Easily evacuates soft, formed stool

Patient/family teaching

Emphasize importance of noting daily bowel function and consistency of stool

Discuss/demonstrate methods to enhance daily bowel movements, especially when taking vinca alkaloid medication

Take stool softener and laxative prn

Maintain fluid level at 3000 ml/24 hr unless contraindicated

Eat diet high in fiber

Administer enema if no bowel movement occurs in 3
  days
Explain need to report to physician if these methods
  fail
Explain need to avoid over-the-counter medications
  without consulting physician

Home care considerations

Assess patient's ability to obtain and prepare sufficient
fluids and foods necessary for therapeutic diet; arrange home health providers or have foods/fluids
brought to patient as needed

● Integumentary

Dermatologic

*hypersensitivity reactions: Reactions to antineo-
  plastic agents; can be very serious and/or life threatening, particularly if an anaphylactic reaction occurs;
  drugs most often associated with an anaphylactoid
  reaction include asparaginase, cisplatin (infrequent),
  and bleomycin*
*hyperpyrexia: Associated with bleomycin, especially in
  patients with lymphoma*
*erythema (Adria flaré): Associated with doxoru-
  bicin; the flare usually results when the drug is too
  concentrated of if the patient has very sensitive
  skin*

Assessment

Subjective data

Abdominal cramping
Pruritus
Photosensitivity

Objective data

Urticaria
Angioedema
Bronchospasm
Hypotension
Hyperpigmentation
Maculopapular rash
Vesicle formation
Acne
Thinning of skin and striae
Petechiae
Ecchymosis
Hives

Desquamation
Jaundice
Nail changes
  Horizontal or longitudinal banding
  Thickening of nailbed
Radiation "recall" phenomena
Blue discoloration of veins
Hyperpyrexia
  High fever
Erythema (Adria flaré)
  Redness (diffuse or streak above the vein)
  Urticaria

Collaborative management

Therapeutic management

General
  Diphenhydramine (Benadryl)
  Epinephrine
  Parenteral corticosteroids
Hyperpyrexia
  Acetaminophen
  Fluid intake
Erythema (Adria flaré)
  Ice pack to affected area

Nursing management

PATIENT PROBLEM/NURSING DIAGNOSIS

● **NDX:** Risk for impaired skin integrity related to effects of chemotherapy

Review patient's allergy history
Monitor VS and mental status
Observe patient throughout administration of drug *to
  note first signs of hypersensitivity*
Ensure that appropriate drugs and equipment are im-
  mediately available for possible emergency use; in the
  event of an anaphylactoid reaction, have the following
  available
  Diphenhydramine (Benadryl)
  Epinephrine
  Oxygen
  Airway
  Suction equipment
Be fully aware of facility procedure to follow in the
  event of such a reaction
For Adria flaré
  At first signs of itching or redness, reduce the
    amount of drug given (e.g., if giving 1 ml, reduce
    to ½ ml); flush vein well and continue adminis-
    tering drug at half dosage; if erythema and urticaria
    occur, stop IV and apply ice pack; start fresh IV and

administer remainder of drug observing for re-
peated reaction
For hyperpyrexia
Give acetaminophen q4h as ordered *to reduce temper-
ature and increase comfort*
Push oral fluids *to reduce temperature*
Advise patient to report adverse reactions immediately
Assess skin condition q8h, especially axillary and
breast folds, groin, perirectal area, and dependent
extremities
Assist with daily bath prn
Use antibacterial soaps and soft cloths
Rinse and dry well
If using lotions, do not leave skin moist
Keep linens dry and wrinkle free *to prevent skin irrita-
tion*

EXPECTED OUTCOME
Skin integrity is maintained

Patient/family teaching

Teach and assist with perianal care after each
elimination
Use soft towels or cloths
Ensure that area is kept dry
Advise patient to wear cotton clothing and underwear
Teach handwashing technique to be used after elimina-
tion and prn
Caution patient to avoid bumps, bruising, cuts, and
scratches
Explain importance of skin care to patient
Caution patient to avoid use of sharp objects (e.g.,
razors, cuticle scissors)
Explain need to always wear slippers or shoes when
out of bed
Caution patient to avoid tight or constricting
clothing
Caution patient to avoid use of rings and watches
when possible; moisture and bacteria collect underneath, and sharp edges can cause scratches or
cuts
Avoid IM injections when possible
Central line may be ordered and inserted to avoid multiple IV injections—perform daily central line care if
inserted
Consolidate laboratory work; use fingersticks when
possible; cleanse skin with povidone-iodine before
venipuncture

Home care considerations

Ensure patient has access to and storage space for
needed skin care supplies
Assess patient's ability to provide self-care; arrange
home health provider as needed

Alopecia

*Temporary loss of body hair as a result of chemothera-
peutic agents that interact with cells that are in the
anaphase of cell cycle (85% to 90% of total scalp hair
cells at any one time); hair loss in area of radiotherapy; dose-dependent antineoplastics associated with
alopecia include cyclophosphamide, doxorubicin, and
vinblastine; antineoplastics associated with thinning
rather than total hair loss include bleomycin, vincristine, 5-FU, and etoposide*

Assessment

Subjective data

Unhappy with appearance
Refuses to see visitors

Objective data

Hair loss
Scalp especially affected early
Long-term therapy
Axilla
Extremities
Pubis
Alterations in body image

Collaborative management

Nursing management

PATIENT PROBLEM/NURSING DIAGNOSIS

● **NDX:** Risk for impaired skin integrity, resulting
in hair loss related to effects of chemotherapy

Establish therapeutic nurse-patient relationship
Inform patient in advance about impending hair loss *so
patient can plan for measures that will enhance appearance and feelings of well-being*; hair loss varies among
individuals
Have patient obtain wigs, scarves, hats, or caps before
hair loss begins *so patient can become familiar with
use*
Explain to patient when to expect hair loss
Begins about 10 days after scalp is irradiated
Usually begins 1 to 2 wk after single dose of
chemotherapy; maximal loss will occur 1 to 2
months after beginning therapy
Stress temporary nature of hair loss *to alleviate concern*
Complete regrowth is usual after chemotherapy is
completed
Regrowth can begin during treatment

Tell patient to expect alterations in texture and color *(physiology of hair follicle is changed by drugs)*

Assess patient's perception of effect of hair loss on lifestyle

Short hairstyles may be preferred

Beginning hair loss may not be readily noticeable

Patient comfort may be increased by a short hairstyle when maximal amount of hair is falling out

Stress importance of periodic rather than continuous use of wigs *to allow scalp to "breathe"*

Assist with gentle scalp care during susceptible period

Wash hair with pH-balanced shampoo

Expose hair and scalp to air as much as possible *to maintain skin tone and integrity*

EXPECTED OUTCOME

Emotional response to hair loss is minimized

Patient/family teaching

Ensure that patient and significant other(s) know and understand the following:

Need to discuss feelings related to perceptions of hair loss

Importance of gentle hair and scalp care

Need to expose scalp to air as much as possible

Hair loss will be temporary throughout course of treatment

Avoiding use of dyes, color rinses, permanents, and bleaches until such time as indicated by condition of scalp, hair, and physician's direction

Home care considerations

Assist patient to contact community support groups for ongoing psychologic counseling and support

Assess patient's ability to provide for own hair and scalp care; arrange home health provider as needed

● Cardiotoxicity

Cardiac damage caused by toxicity of antineoplastic medications

Assessment

Observations/findings

Tachycardia

Extrasystoles

ST-T wave changes

Transient ECG changes

Thirty percent decrease in limb-lead QRS voltage

Predisposing medications

Doxorubicin (Adriamycin)

Daunorubicin (Daunomycin)

Concurrent use of cyclophosphamide

Predisposing factors

Previous radiation therapy near heart

Aortic stenosis

Uncontrolled hypertension

Distended neck veins

Gallop heart rhythm

Ankle edema

Diagnostic tests

ECG

Cardiac enzymes

Chest x-ray examination

Echocardiogram

Radionuclide angiography

Percutaneous endomyocardial biopsy

Potential complications

CHF

Cardiomyopathy

Dysrhythmia

Collaborative management

Therapeutic management

Serial ECG monitoring

Oxygen therapy

Cardiac medications

Nursing management

POTENTIAL PATIENT PROBLEM

Cardiotoxicity related to effects of chemotherapy

Monitor P rate and rhythm

Note significant variation in VS, skin color, T, sensorium, decreased urine output, and dyspnea, *which indicate toxicity*

Be aware that weekly low-dose injection of doxorubicin and continuous infusions may be associated with less cardiotoxicity

Be aware that by the time cardiac toxicity is clinically detectable, it is often irreversible and debilitating

Be aware of agents that place patient at risk for cardiotoxicity such as doxorubicin (adult total cumulative dose not to exceed 450 to 550 mg/m^2) and daunorubicin (total cumulative dose is 550 mg/m^2); see Heart failure (p. 146)

EXPECTED OUTCOME

Signs and symptoms of cardiotoxicity are recognized and treatment is initiated promptly

● Pulmonary Toxicity

Respiratory difficulties, temporary or chronic, related to chemotherapeutic toxicities; chemotherapeutic drugs typically associated with pulmonary toxicity include bleomycin, busulfan, and carmustine

Assessment

Subjective data

Headache
Malaise
SOB

Objective data

Toxicities associated with bleomycin include pneumonitis and interstitial fibrosis
Persons over 70 years of age who receive total cumulative dose >400 to 500 units are at greatest risk
Fine, crackling basilar rales
Dyspnea at rest, hypoxemia
Tachypnea, fever
Pneumonia (noninfectious)
Pulmonary edema
Pulmonary fibrosis
Predisposing factors
  Preexisting pulmonary disease
  Radiation therapy
  Pulmonary conditions: infection, edema, emboli
  Dry, hacking cough
  Adverse pulmonary changes are also associated with cyclophosphamide (Cytoxan) in combination with bleomycin, mitomycin, melphalan, and procarbarzine
  History of smoking

Diagnostic tests

Pulmonary function tests
ABGs
Chest x-ray

Collaborative management

Therapeutic management

Steroids
Antimicrobials
Bronchodilators
Oxygen therapy

Nursing management

POTENTIAL PATIENT PROBLEM

Pulmonary toxicity related to the effects of chemotherapy
  Be aware that once pulmonary changes are clinically detected, the disease course is often progressive
  Observe for SOB *for possible early detection*
  Auscultate chest for breath sounds q4h during course of chemotherapy; report abnormal breath sounds immediately
  Check T, P, R, and BP q4h; report T of 100.4°F (38°C) or above
  Monitor pulmonary function tests as ordered
  Teach and assist patient to turn, cough, and deep breathe q4h *to maintain adequate respirations*
  Administer oxygen cautiously when ordered; high-dose oxygen may increase reaction, especially that caused by bleomycin
  Force fluids to 3000 ml/day unless contraindicated
  Administer IV fluid therapy as ordered
  Measure intake and output q8h *to monitor for balance*
  Administer medications as ordered: corticosteroids, bronchodilators, antimicrobials
  Teach necessity of raising secretions and expectorating versus swallowing
  Assist with nebulizer treatments and respiratory physiotherapy
  See Adult respiratory distress syndrome (ARDS) (p. 311)

EXPECTED OUTCOME

Pulmonary toxicity is minimized, or signs and symptoms of pulmonary toxicity are recognized and treated promptly

● Renal

Nephrotoxicity

Dysfunction in any part of the renal system in the presence of chemotherapeutic agents that are excreted through the kidneys or act on the lining of the renal system; antineoplastic agents associated with renal dysfunction include cisplatin, methotrexate, mitomycin, 5-azatadine, nitrosoureas, and high-dose cyclophosphamide

Assessment

Subjective data

Muscle weakness
Nausea

Headache
Dysuria, frequency, urgency

Objective data

Hematuria (mild to severe), proteinuria
Oliguria, anuria
Neuromuscular irritability
Tremors, personality change
Elevated uric acid
Hyperkalemia, hyperphosphatemia
Hypocalcemia, hypomagnesemia
Hyponatremia
Elevated BUN, serum creatinine, and creatinine
  clearance
Hypertension, vomiting

DIAGNOSTIC TESTS

Electrolytes
BUN, uric acid, calcium, magnesium
Serum creatinine
Creatinine clearance
Cystoscopy

Collaborative management

Therapeutic management

IV fluid (titrate according to output)
Measure intake and output
Medications
  Bicarbonate
  Allopurinol
  Antihypertensives
  Osmotic diuretics
  Antiemetics

Nursing management

POTENTIAL PATIENT PROBLEM

Nephrotoxicity related to effects of chemotherapy
  Ensure adequate hydration and diuresis 24 hr before,
    during, and 24 to 48 hr after medication adminis-
    tration *to enhance kidney function*
  Force fluids to 3000 to 4000 ml/day unless
    contraindicated
  Enlist patient's assistance *to maintain hydration*
    Provide fluids of choice and temperature
    Dietary restrictions of protein, potassium, and
      sodium may be necessary
    Offering small amounts frequently makes taking flu-
      ids less of a chore
    Serve attractively
  Use antacids *to alleviate gastric distress*
  Use antiemetics *for control of nausea*

Administer IV fluids as ordered: usually dextrose in
  saline with electrolytes; often ordered at 200 mg/hr
  for 5 to 6 hr before, during, and after chemotherapy
  infusion
Measure intake and output; report discrepancies and
  output of less than 120 ml/hr
Test urine for occult bleeding q8h during chemotherapy infusion; slow infusion and report overt
  hemorrhaging to physician
Monitor vital signs *so early changes can be noted and
  therapy started*
Administer antihypertensive drugs as ordered *to control elevated BP*
Test urine pH as ordered
Administer sodium bicarbonate as ordered *to maintain urine pH of 7*

EXPECTED OUTCOME

Nephrotoxic effects of chemotherapy are minimized;
  signs and symptoms of nephrotoxicity are recognized
  and treated promptly

Patient/family teaching

Explain need to measure intake and output
Emphasize importance of maintaining fluid intake to
  3000 to 4000 ml/day
Discuss signs and symptoms of nephrotoxicity to report to physician
Teach name of medication, dosage, frequency,
  and toxic or side effects to report to physician
Emphasize importance of follow-up outpatient
  care
Emphasize importance of taking antihypertensive
  drugs when ordered

Hemorrhagic Cystitis

*Dose-related chemical cystitis caused by toxic effects of
  cyclophosphamide's or ifosfamide's metabolite on
  bladder mucosa*

Assessment

Observations/findings

Urinary frequency
Loss of bladder tone
Occult or gross hematuria

Diagnostic tests

Urinalysis
CBC

Collaborative management

Therapeutic management

Parenteral fluids
Bladder irrigation
Antiemetics
Sedatives

Nursing management

POTENTIAL PATIENT PROBLEM

Hemorrhagic cystitis related to effects of chemotherapy
  Encourage high fluid intake to 3000 ml/day (if not contraindicated) before and 48 hr following drug administration *to maintain kidney function*
  Encourage frequent voiding q3h to 4h; bladder should be emptied before bedtime and when patient is awake at night *to decrease irritation of bladder by stasis of high concentrations of drug in urine*
  Observe and report signs and symptoms of cystitis
    Test urine for hematuria (dipstick)
    Monitor output closely; report decrease in urine *(may be indicative of SIADH secondary to drug)*
  Administer cyclophosphamide early in the day *to prevent urine from pooling in bladder overnight*
  Indwelling catheter may be ordered
  Through-and-through bladder irrigation may be ordered *to remove drug concentrations in urine*
  Administer antiemetics and sedatives as needed
  Teach exercises to regain bladder tone

EXPECTED OUTCOME

Hemorrhagic cystitis does not occur or signs and symptoms of hemorrhagic cystitis are recognized and treated promptly

● Neurotoxicity

Damage to myelin sheath, paralysis of autonomic nerves, or CNS damage caused by effects of chemotherapeutic medications; antineoplastic agents typically associated with neurotoxicity are the Vinca (plant) alkaloids: vincristine, vinblastine, and vindesine

Assessment

Subjective data

Fatigue
Tingling, paresthesia
Muscle aches/pains
Jaw pain

Arachnoiditis (in relation to intrathecal administration)
  Back pain
  Dizziness, headache

Objective data

Tremors
Muscle weakness
  Difficulty in heel walking
  Inability to get out of chair
Foot-drop
Ptosis
Hyporeflexia to loss of deep tendon reflexes
Ataxia
Hemiplegia
Slurred speech
Hoarseness
Irritability
Seizures
Somnolence
Personality change
Coma
Arachnoiditis (in relation to intrathecal administration)
  Fever
  Stiff neck
  Vomiting
Ototoxicity
Constipation and colicky pain
Ileus
Urinary retention

Diagnostic tests

Neurologic examination
Neuroradiology studies

Collaborative management

Therapeutic management

Medications specific to symptoms
Stool softeners, laxatives
Physical therapy

Nursing management

POTENTIAL PATIENT PROBLEM

Neurotoxicity related to effects of chemotherapy
Assess for weakness/numbness of arms, hands, legs, and feet *(early signs of toxicity)*
Assess for hoarseness and jaw pain
Assess for abdominal cramping, constipation, and paralytic ileus
Perform neurologic assessment before administration of medication *for baseline information* then q4h to 8h

after infusion is completed; report changes to physician immediately

Assess ability to perform ADLs

Evaluate for discomfort or pain associated with movement

Assess pain, cardiac, respiratory, and elimination status

Provide safe, uncluttered environment *to prevent falls*

Instruct patient to sit on side of bed, stand, and then begin to walk *to prevent postural hypotension;* provide walking aids as indicated

Instruct patient to report numbness and tingling or other signs of toxicity immediately

Assure patient and significant other that changes are usually reversible when medication is stopped; discuss specifics with physician—motor weakness may take many months to resolve

Provide environment and time conducive to discussing concerns and fears

Assess color and temperature of extremities, especially hands

Assess for CNS toxicity if methotrexate or cytarabine is given intrathecally; have patient lie flat for at least 1 hr following instillation of drug

EXPECTED OUTCOME

Neurotoxicity effects are minimized

PATIENT PROBLEM/NURSING DIAGNOSIS

● **NDX:** Constipation related to neurotoxic effects of chemotherapy

Auscultate abdomen for bowel sounds q4h to 8h

Check and record daily bowel elimination *(constipation and colicky pain that develop within 2 days of drug administration are early manifestations of toxicity)*

Administer stool softeners and laxatives prophylactically

Encourage fluid to 3000 ml/day unless contraindicated *to enhance motility*

Encourage diet high in fiber *to stimulate peristalsis*

Measure intake and output

Administer enemas as ordered

Encourage mobility as tolerated

EXPECTED OUTCOME

Normal bowel motility is achieved and maintained

● Hepatotoxicity

Dysfunction of the liver induced by chemotherapeutic medications, other hepatotoxic drugs, or preexisting hepatic conditions; because the hepatocytes are not rapidly dividing cells, they are less affected by many drugs; antineoplastic agents associated with hepatic toxicity include nitrosoureas, methotrexate, 6-mercaptopurine (6-MP), cytosine arabinoside, mithramycin, asparaginase, and interferon

Assessment

Subjective data

Lethargy, weakness

Abdominal tenderness

Right upper quadrant pain

Anorexia

Digestive discomfort

Objective data

Pruritus

Jaundice

Dark urine

Sweet or sour odor of urine and breath

Clay-colored stools

Bleeding tendency
  Purpura
  Epistaxis
  Melena

Ascites

Generalized edema

Palmar erythema

Spider angiomas

Irritability

Apathy

Memory defects

Asterixis

Coma

Associated factors, preexisting or concurrent
  Viral hepatitis
  Abdominal radiotherapy
  Hepatic metastasis
  Hepatotoxic drugs
  Transfusion of blood products
  Graft vs. host disease (GVHD) (p. 836)

Diagnostic tests

Elevated
  Serum transaminase
  Bilirubin
  Alkaline phosphatase
  Cholesterol
  Fibrinogen
Decreased
  Hepatic clotting factors
  Albumin
Liver function tests

Blood clotting test, CBC
Liver biopsy
Radiologic examinations

Potential complications

Cirrhosis
Ascites
Hepatomegaly

Collaborative management

Therapeutic management

Parenteral fluids/nutrition
Blood product transfusion
Nasogastric tube

Nursing management

PATIENT PROBLEMS/NURSING DIAGNOSES

● **NDX:** Risk for impaired skin integrity related to
pruritus

Assess skin condition q8h
Bathe patient daily; use soothing baths (e.g., use cornstarch or oil) *to relieve itching*
Maintain skin hydration by application of lotion after
bath and bid, adding bath oil to water
Teach distraction, relaxation, and imagery *to prevent
scratching*
Administer skin care as needed *to decrease itching;* antihistamine drugs may be ordered
Keep nails short *to prevent scratching skin*
Encourage fluids to 3000 to 4000 ml/24 hr unless
contraindicated; fluids may be limited in presence
of edema

EXPECTED OUTCOMES

Patient states pruritus is diminished
Skin remains intact

● **NDX:** Potential for bleeding related to altered clotting mechanisms*

Assess sensorium q2h to 4h
Report changes of increased lethargy; *sign of poten-
tial bleeding*
Avoid use of drugs such as narcotics and barbitu-
rates that cause CNS depression
Observe for signs of bleeding: hematemesis, me-
lena, petechiae
Assess for abdominal distention; measure abdom-

*Not a NANDA-approved diagnosis.

inal girth; *increasing girth may indicate abdominal
bleeding*
Assess bowel sounds
Monitor vital signs and laboratory studies
If nasogastric tube is being used, maintain patency
Provide oral care; keep nostrils clean and lubricated
Maintain proper position of tube *to prevent irrita-
tion*
Place in semi-Fowler's position unless contra-
indicated
Report changes in color, bleeding, and edema to
physician *for changes in treatment plan*
Report changes in color of urine and stool that indi-
cate bleeding
Institute safety measures *to decrease bleeding tendency*
Avoid IM injections
Consolidate laboratory work
Use fingersticks when possible
Apply pressure at puncture or IV site for 5 min after
procedure has been completed; check site q15
min for four times
Carefully place furniture, equipment, and personal
items *to prevent injuries from falls or bumping into
objects*
Administer gentle oral hygiene using toothettes or
swabs
Avoid use of harsh soaps and rough towels and
cloths
Test urine and stool for occult bleeding

EXPECTED OUTCOMES

Preventable bleeding episodes are avoided
Signs and symptoms of bleeding are recognized and
treated immediately

● Gonadal Dysfunction

*Testicular or ovarian dysfunction caused by adverse
effects of chemotherapeutic drugs (e.g., nitrogen
mustard, cyclophosphamide, chlorambucil)*

Assessment

Observations/findings

Reduction of spermatocytes
Irregular menses
Amenorrhea
Menopausal symptoms: hot flushes, insomnia, irritabil-
ity, dyspareunia, vaginal dryness

Diagnostic tests

Serum follicle-stimulating hormone (FSH) level
Sperm count

Potential complication

Permanent sterility

Collaborative management

Therapeutic management

Estrogens (menopausal symptoms) (not in breast cancer)

Nursing management

PATIENT PROBLEM/NURSING DIAGNOSIS

● **NDX:** Altered sexuality patterns, related to effects of chemotherapy on the reproductive system

Obtain brief sexual history including sexual practices, sex education and attitude, and effects of disease and treatment on sexual function

Advise male patients regarding sperm banking before chemotherapy administration if appropriate

Provide contraceptive information to patients before they initiate chemotherapy if appropriate

Initiate discussion related to infertility

Encourage ventilation of feelings

Evaluate patient's and/or partner's coping skills and response to infertility

Instruct patient that infertility may be temporary or permanent (dose related)

Inform patient that sexual drive and capability usually are not physically impaired as a result of chemotherapy

Advise that antifertility effects may be reversible in some cases after therapy is terminated

Refer patient for counseling if appropriate

EXPECTED OUTCOME

Patient achieves satisfying sexual role functioning

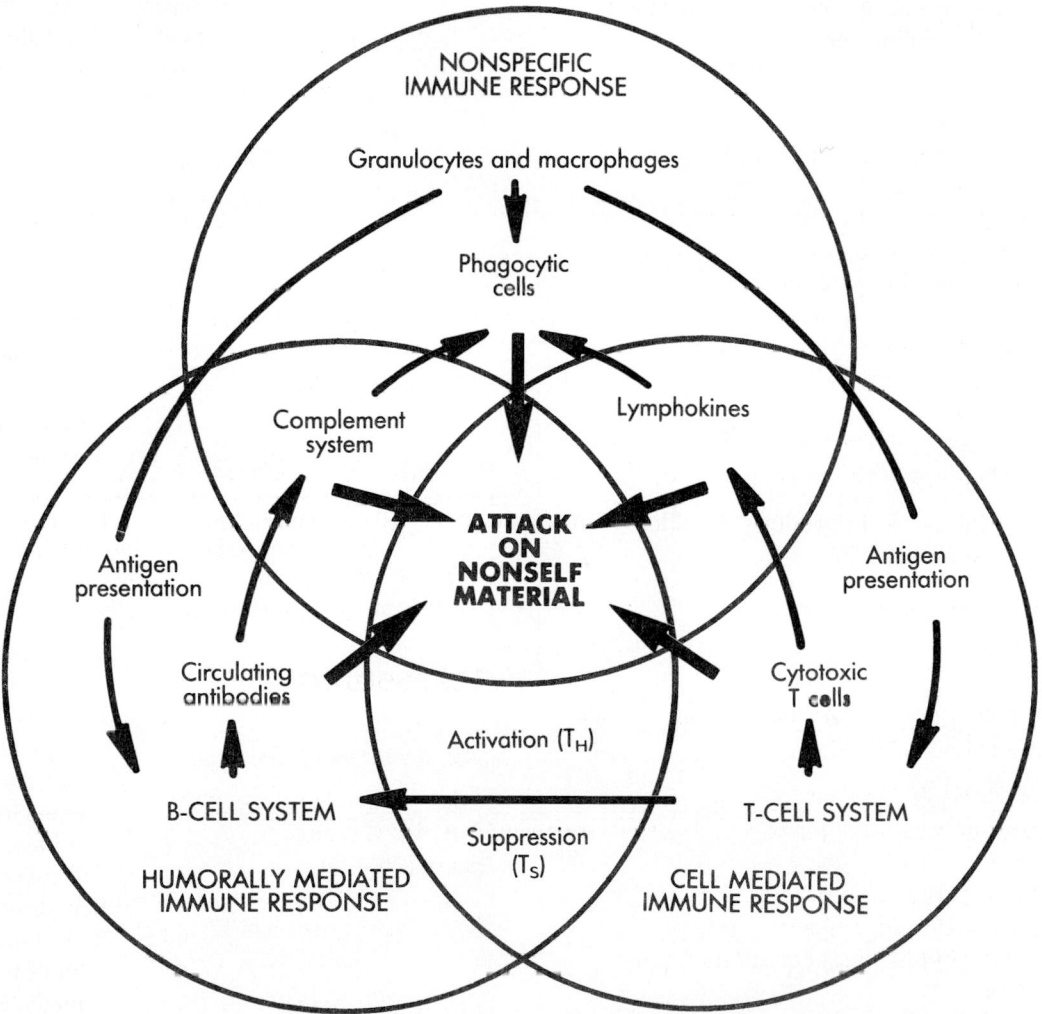

Figure 15-10   Interrelationship of nonspecific, humorally mediated, and cell mediated immune response systems. (From Phipps WJ et al: *Medical-surgical nursing: concepts and clinical practice,* ed 5, St Louis, 1995, Mosby.)

Biologic Response Modifiers

This cancer therapy is based on the theory that if the immune system recognizes tumor cells as foreign, it will mobilize and destroy them. Through research, biologic and chemical agents produced by the body, biologic response modifiers (BRMs) have been discovered. A BRM is any soluble substance capable of altering (or modulating) the immune system with either a stimula-tory or a suppressive effect (Figure 15-10). BRMs can affect the host-tumor response in three ways: (1) by modulating the individual's immune response to the tumor; (2) by direct antitumor activity, killing or suppressing growth; (3) by altering other biologic activities that indirectly affect the tumor, such as interfering with tumor cell's ability to survive or metastasize, promoting cell maturation, or interfering with transformation of normal cells into cancer cells (Table 15-9).

Table 15-9 Biologic Response Modifiers (Under Investigation)

Agent	Route of Administration	Indications Under Investigation	Side/Toxic Effects	Administration and Nursing Indications
Calmette-Guérin bacillus (BCG)	Scarification, intra-dermal by Tine technique or Heaf gun	Superficial or subcutaneous melanoma	Local, inflammatory response that increases with treatment to ulceration with eschar formation Pruritus Enlarged painful nodes, malaise, mild fever	Anesthesize area Clean skin with acetone and allow to dry Choose site that is flat and near major lymph nodes to increase absorption and that is covered by clothing that does not bind Keep areas clean and dry Apply nonmedicated, hypoallergenic cream to previous sites when needed
	Intravesical (bladder) Retain for 2 hr	Bladder (FDA approved)	Bladder irritation, infection, chills, fever, cough	Before treatment Bladder culture Have patient limit fluids for 12 hr Void before administration With first and each subsequent voiding for 6 hr add bleach equal to amount voided, close cover of toilet and flush Rehydrate patient Report fever, cough, chills to physician immediately for antibiotic therapy

Table 15-9 Biologic Response Modifiers *(Under Investigation)*—cont'd

Agent	Route of Administration	Indications Under Investigation	Side/Toxic Effects	Administration and Nursing Indications
	Intralesional	Cutaneous melanoma	Inflammatory reaction in 4 hr; fever, myalgia, nausea, vomiting for 2-3 days	
			Hypersensitivity reaction can occur: fever, chills, intravascular coagulation abnormalities, hypotension, and oliguria	Have antihistamines, corticosteroids, and emergency equipment available
			Disseminated BCG infection: persistent fever, weight loss, malaise, nausea, and vomiting	Patients with strongly positive tuberculin reaction may need diphenhydramine (Benadryl) before and after intratumor therapy
			Temporary, reversible hepatic dysfunction	Antipyretics usually control symptoms; isoniazid may be ordered
Interferons exhibit broad antiviral, antiproliferative, and immunodulatory activity	IM, IV (bolus, short-term infusion, a continuous infusion), subcutaneous, intravesical, intrathecal, or intralesional	Hairy cell leukemia (FDA approved), non–Hodgkin's lymphoma, Kaposi's sarcoma, renal cell carcinoma, malignant melanoma, multiple myeloma untreated, chronic granulocytic leukemia, mycosis furgoids, superficial bladder (intravesical), ovarian (intraperitoneal). Clinical trials for AIDS and rhino virus.	Flulike symptoms; fever (38°-40°C) 2-4 hr after injection; malaise, chills, headache, and low-grade fever may last to 20 hr after first dose	Reconstitute according to manufacturer's directions
			Chronic fatigue, irritability, impatience, low motivation, depression; sense of doom, and paranoia with high doses	Premedicate with acetominophen, then q3-4h after
				Avoid aspirin, nonsteroid antiinflammatory agents, and steroids (may hinder effectiveness)
			Nausea, altered taste, early satiety, anorexia, arthostatic hypertension; cardiovascular symptoms with history of problems	Morphine may be ordered for severe chilling (rigor) lasting more than 10 min
				Instruct patient to plan rest periods; may need to alter work habits
			Transient pancytopenia	Provide nutritional counseling
			Proteinuria with preexisting renal disease	Encourage fluid intake
				Avoid sudden position changes
				Evening administration may diminish side effects

Continued.

Table 15-9 Biologic Response Modifiers (Under Investigation)—cont'd

Agent	Route of Administration	Indications Under Investigation	Side/Toxic Effects	Administration and Nursing Indications
Thymosin fraction V	IM, subcutaneous	Small cell lung cancer, squamous cell carcinoma of head and neck	Allergic reaction, systemic itching	Antipruritics may be administered to relieve itching
Aldesleutin Interleukin-2 (IL-2) Adoptive immunotherapy	IV bolus, continuous IV infusion, intrahepatic infusion, peritoneal infusion	Advanced cancer in which standard therapy is ineffective (renal cell melanoma, colon, etc.) FDA approved for kidney and renal cancer	Symptoms are usually dose related and usually reverse in 8-21 days after IL-2	Assess baseline status of affected systems
			Disorientation, combativeness, psychosis, anxiety	Provide safety measures, explanations and reorient
			Oliguria, proteinuria, elevated creatinine and BUN	Monitor intake and output; test urine for protein; monitor laboratory values
			Anemia, thrombocytopenia	Monitor for bleeding; evaluate daily laboratory values; test stool, urine, and vomitus for blood; avoid rectal manipulation and IM injections
			Elevated bilirubin, SGOT, SGPT, LDH	Monitor laboratory values
			Erythematous rash, pruritus, desquamation	Benadryl may be given prophylactically; assess skin daily; use water-based lotion; avoid harsh products; pat skin dry
			Nausea, vomiting, mucositis, decreased appetite, diarrhea	Monitor dietary intake; prophylactic antiemetic usually given; antidiarrheal given as necessary; see Mucositis (p. 953), and Nausea and vomiting (p. 951)
			Hypotension	Monitor VS qh during infusion then q4h; albumin, dopamine, or phenylephrine may be ordered

Table 15-9 Biologic Response Modifiers *(Under Investigation)*—cont'd

Agent	Route of Administration	Indications Under Investigation	Side/Toxic Effects	Administration and Nursing Indications
			Weight gain, peripheral edema, ascites, dysrhythmias, dyspnea, pulmonary edema	Monitor intake and output; weigh daily; measure abdominal girth with ascites; elevate extremities with edema; monitor O_2 saturation
			Fever	Acetominophen given prophylactically Monitor T qh during infusion and for 24 hr Provide cooling measures prn
			Chills	Meperidine may be ordered for chills or rigor
			Flulike symptoms	Rest; acetaminophen q4h
IL-2 and LAK Adoptive immunotherapy	IL-2 given for 3 days; collect leukocytes through lymphopheresis (for 4 to 5 days); separated lymphocytes incubated with IL-2; prepared LAK cells are infused after test dose for 3 days; IL-2 infused also and for several days after LAK infusion	Melanoma, nodular lymphomas, renal cell cancer, colorectal cancer	Fever Headache Chills Nausea	Acetaminophen usually given Meperidine administered for chills or rigor Antiemetics manage nausea
			High dosages: peripheral edema, ascites, or interstitial infiltrates	Vasopressors, diuretics, and careful fluid replacement may be required
			Thrombocytopenia	May require RBC transfusion Monitor for bleeding
			Mental status changes: confusion, paranoia, hallucinations, severe disorientation	Provide safety measures, reorient continuously; haloperidol may be required
Lymphotoxin effects delayed hypersensitivity; allow higher doses of chemotherapy and radiotherapy	Intralesional injection in accessible tumors	Melanoma, bladder, and prostate cancer	—	—

Continued.

Table 15-9 Biologic Response Modifiers *(Under Investigation)*—cont'd

Agent	Route of Administration	Indications Under Investigation	Side/Toxic Effects	Administration and Nursing Indications
Monoclonal antibodies Biologic tracers that react with one specific part of the antigen's surface (an epitome) Serve as carriers of antitoxin drugs, toxins, radioisotopes, or other BRMs to tumor cells	IV by infusion pump	Lymphoma, lymphocytic leukemia, T-cell leukemia, cutaneous T-cell lymphoma, gastric and colon cancer and melanoma	Fever, chills, headache, flushing, urticaria, rash Bronchospasm, dyspnea, hypotension, tachycardia, anaphylactic reaction	Diphenhydramine usually controls mild allergic response Assess patient q15min first hr; then q30min Infusion stopped; saline; epinephrine, hydrocortisone, and diphenhydramine may be ordered; monitor VS; keep resuscitation equipment nearby
Tumor cell vaccines Provide active, specific immune stimulation	Intradermal	—	Fever, chills, headache, malaise Hepatitis	Acetominophen usually relieves symptoms
Colony-Stimulating Factors (CSF): G-CSF (granulocyte CSF) and	IV, short or continuous infusion; subcutaneously	Bone marrow destruction: iatrogenically induced: antiviral therapy in AIDS, cancer	Fever, myalgias, bone pain, fatigue	Acetaminophen usually controls symptoms
GM-CSF (granulocyte-macrophage CSF)		Chemotherapy and bone marrow transplant	Anorexia Pericardial, pleural effusions	Monitor VS, intake, output and assess heart and breath sounds; report negative findings
Increase the production of granulocytes and monocytes by stimulating stem cell and precursor cell replication and maturation		Intrinsic states: myelodysplasia, congenital cyclic neutropenia, aplastic anemia, hairy cell leukemia		

Table 15-9 Biologic Response Modifiers *(Under Investigation)*—cont'd

Agent	Route of Administration	Indications Under Investigation	Side/Toxic Effects	Administration and Nursing Indications
Erythropoietin Increases the production of RBC	Subcutaneously	Anemias: End-stage renal disease Associated with antineoplastic chemotherapy and A2T	Fever, fatigue rare	Follow manufacturer's directions Rotate sites of injection Acetaminophen usually controls symptoms
Tumor necrosis factor (TNF) has the capability of destroying malignant cells but not normal cells; activation of cells of the immune system has also been reported	IM, IV, bolus, short-term infusion	Metastatic melanoma, advanced renal cancer, others being studied		Agitation of the biologic or rapid expulsion from a syringe may result in denaturing the molecules
			Pain, erythema at injection site	Rotate IM injection sites to reduce irritation; apply cold or warm compresses; acetaminophen may increase comfort
			Fever, chills, fatigue, headache	Premedicate with acetaminophen, then continue q4h as needed Encourage and monitor fluid intake during febrile episodes
			Hypotension	Monitor VS with BP lying and standing Report negative findings

BIBLIOGRAPHY

Ackley BJ, Ladwig GB: *Nursing diagnosis handbook: a guide to planning care,* St Louis, 1993, Mosby.

Badger JM: Calming the anxious patient, *Am J Nurs* 94(5): 46, 1994.

Baker C: Factors associated with rehabilitation in head and neck cancer, *Cancer Nurs* 15(6):395, 1992.

Beare PG, Myers JL: *Principles and practice of adult health nursing,* ed 2, St Louis, 1994, Mosby.

Belcher AE: *Blood disorders,* St Louis, 1992, Mosby.

Belcher AE: *Cancer nursing,* St Louis, 1992, Mosby.

Berman A et al: Cancer chemotherapy: intravenous administration, *Cancer Nurs* 16(2):145, 1993.

Bohony J: Common IV complications and what to do about them, *Am J Nurs* 93(10) 1993.

Brock D et al: Testicular cancer, *Semin Oncol Nurs* 9(4):224, 1993.

Brown KK: Septic shock: how to stop the deadly cascade, *Am J Nurs* 94(9) 20, 1994.

Brown KK: Critical interventions in septic shock, *Am J Nurs* 94(10) 20, 1994.

Carpenito JC: *Nursing diagnosis application to clinical practice,* ed 5, Philadelphia, 1993, JB Lippincott.

Chisholm LC et al: Cancer chemotherapy: alternative administration routes, *Cancer Nurs* 16(3):237, 1993.

Davis M: Renal cell carcinoma, *Semin Oncol Nurs* 9(4):267, 1993.

Furlong TG: Neurologic complications of immunosuppressive cancer therapy, *Oncol Nurs Forum* 20(9):1337, 1993.

Helberg JL: Patients' status at home care discharge, *IMAGE J Nurs Sch* 25(2):93, 1993.

Hennessey B, Fitzgerald A, Graham D: Venous air embolism: keeping your patient out of danger, *Am J Nurs* 93(11): 54, 1993.

Johnson JR: Caring for the woman who's had a mastectomy, *Am J Nurs* 94(5): 25, 1994.

Jones DA et al: *Medical surgical nursing, a conceptual approach,* New York, 1982, McGraw-Hill.

Kelly WN et al: *Textbook of internal medicine,* Philadelphia, 1989, JB Lippincott.

Kim MJ et al: *Pocket guide to nursing diagnoses,* ed 6, St Louis, 1995, Mosby.

Hoebler L, Irwin M: Gastrointestinal tract cancer: current knowledge, medical treatment and nursing management, *Oncol Nurs Forum* 19(9):1403, 1992.

Hossan E, Stregal A: Carcinoma of the bladder, *Semin Oncol Nurs* 9(4):252, 1993.

Lam S et al: Detection and localization of early lung cancer by imaging techniques, *Chest* 103(1):12S, 1993.

LeMone P: Analysis of a human phenomenon: self-concept, *Nurs Diagn* 2(3):126, 1991.

Levy W: Chemotherapy agents: part I, *Cancer Nurs* 16(4):321, 1993.

Lynes AC: Percutaneous hepatic arterial chemotherapy and chemoembolization, *Cancer Nurs* 16(4):283, 1993.

Maxwell E: Carcinoma of the prostate, *Semin Oncol Nurs* 9(4):237, 1993.

McCance KL, Huether SE: *Pathophysiology: the biological basis for disease in adults and children,* ed 2, St Louis, 1994, Mosby.

McClosky JC: *Nursing interventions classification,* St Louis, 1992, Mosby.

McFarland GK, McFarlane EA: *Nursing diagnosis and intervention planning for patient care,* ed 2, St Louis, 1993, Mosby.

Mehmert PPA, Delaney CW: Validating impaired physical mobility, *Nurs Diagn* 2(4):143, 1991.

Micromedex On-Line Drug Evaluation Monographs: Volume 81, Micromedex, Inc: August, 1994.

Niehoff ML: Epidemiology and early detection of prostate cancer in the primary setting, *J Am Acad Physician Assist* 7(3):147, 1994.

Nieweg R et al: Nursing care for oral complications associated with chemotherapy, *Cancer Nurs* 15(5):313, 1992.

Norris J: Nursing intervention for self-esteem disturbances, *Nurs Diagn* 3(2):48, 1992.

Ouellet LL, Rush KL: A synthesis of selected literature on mobility: a basis for studying impaired mobility, *Nurs Diagn* 3(2):72, 1992.

Pack R: Descriptive epidemiology of genitourinary cancers, *Semin Oncol Nurs* 9(4):218, 1993.

Pickett M: Determinants of anticipatory nausea and anticipatory vomiting in adults receiving cancer chemotherapy, *Cancer Nurs* 14(6):334, 1991.

Quint-Kasner S: Chemotherapy agents: part II, *Cancer Nurs* 16(5):398, 1993.

Radziewicz RM, Schneider SM: Using diversional activity to enhance coping, *Cancer Nurs* 15(4):293, 1992.

Rose PG: Cervical cancer, *Emerg Med* 25(4):133, 1993.

Samet JM: The epidemiology of lung cancer, *Chest* 103(1):20S, 1993.

Skalla KA, Lacosse C: Patient education for fatigue, *Oncol Nurs Forum* 19(10):1537, 1992.

Small EJ: Prostate cancer: who to screen and what the results mean, *Geriatrics* 48(12):28, 1993.

Smith DB, Babaian RJ: The effects of treatment for cancer on male fertility and sexuality, *Cancer Nurs* 15(4):271, 1992.

Sparks SM: Exploring electronic support groups, *Am J Nurs* 92(12):62, 1992.

Stomper PC: Breast cancer, *Emerg Med* 25(4):113, 1993.

Veridiano NP: Vaginal and vulvar cancer, *Emerg Med* 25(4):149, 1993.

Watson PG: The optimal functioning plan: a key element in cancer rehabilitation, *Cancer Nurs* 15(40):254, 1992.

Woodtli MA, Van Ort S: Nursing diagnoses and functional health patterns in patients receiving radiation therapy: cancer of the head and neck, *Nurs Diagn* 2(4):171, 1991.

Yeaw EMJ: How position affects oxygenation: good lung down? *Am J Nurs* 92(3): 27, 1992.

Youngblood M et al: A comparison of two methods of assessing cancer therapy related symptoms, *Cancer Nurs* 17(1):37, 1994.

BARNES

CARE PATH® 540
TOTAL MASTECTOMY WITH
MALIGNANCY WITHOUT CC

SERVICE		PHYSICIAN		
PRIMARY NURSE		PRIMARY NURSE		
DC DATE	ADM DATE	DATE OF SURGERY	**A-8**	

Problem Number	PATIENT PROBLEMS/NURSING DIAGNOSES
#1	ALTERATION IN COMFORT
#2	ALTERATION IN COPING
#3	ALTERATION IN SELF-CONCEPT
#4	LACK OF KNOWLEDGE

#	1, 2	2, 3	1	1, 3	1
	ASSESSMENT/MONITORING	**CONSULTS**	**PROCEDURES/TEST**	**TREATMENT**	**ACTIVITY**
DAY 1 DOS	VS q 4 hrs. x1 x2 x3 x4 x5 x6 I & O Pain Control Dressing/JP patency and drainage Ability to void Circulation Emotional response/ family coping	Social Work		JP to bulb suction Incentive Spirometer/TCDB Avoid trauma to extremity	Up with assist to bathroom in PM
DAY 2 POD 1	VS q 8 hrs. if stable x1 x2 x3 I & O Pain Control Dressing/JP patency and drainage **Voiding without difficulty** Circulation Emotional response/ family coping	Social Work visit Reach to Recovery		JP to bulb suction **Uses Incentive Spirometer independently** Avoid trauma to extremity	Up as tolerated with assist if needed

SIGNATURE	INIT.	SIGNATURE	INIT.	SIGNATURE	INIT.

540

BARNES

CARE PATH® 540
TOTAL MASTECTOMY WITH
MALIGNANCY WITHOUT CC

CNS	DIETARY	RT
HOME HEALTH	OT	OTHER
PT	SW	OTHER

A-8

Problem Number	PATIENT PROBLEMS/NURSING DIAGNOSES

	1	3, 4	2, 3, 4	2, 3	INITIALS (SEE KEY AT BOTTOM)		
MEDS / IVS	NUTRITION	PATIENT/FAMILY EDUCATION	DISCHARGE PLANNING	PSYCHOSOCIAL/ EMOTIONAL/ SPIRITUAL NEEDS			
IVF IM analgesics Antibiotic if ordered	Clear liquid. Advance as tolerated to diet as prior to admission	Nursing: Pain control Positioning/mobility TCDB Incentive Spirometer Diet IV JP Primary Nursing	**Pt./family verbalizes understanding of Care Path.** **Plan of care has been mutually set with pt./family.**				
DC IVF when tolerating PO well DC IM analgesics Start oral analgesics **Pain controlled with oral analgesics**	**Tolerating diet as prior to admission**	Social Work: Assess resource needs Initiate education re: dx, prosthesis, support groups Nursing: Arm protection S/S infection BSE	Social Work: Complete high risk screening	Social Work: Assess counseling needs Initiate support Nursing: Therapeutic emotional care			
SIGNATURE	INIT.	SIGNATURE	INIT.	SIGNATURE		INIT.	

#	1, 2	2, 3	1	1, 3	1
	ASSESSMENT / MONITORING	**CONSULTS**	**PROCEDURES / TEST**	**TREATMENT**	**ACTIVITY**
DAY 3 POD 2	VS q 8 hrs. if stable x1 x2 x3 D/C I & O Except JP(s) Incision/JP patency and drainage Circulation Lab results Emotional response/ family coping	Social Work visit if needed Reach to Recovery visit	CBC **Hematocrit not decreased more than 25% from pre-op value.**	JP to bulb suction JP dressing change/ site care daily Avoid trauma to extremity	**Up ad lib**
DAY 4 POD 3	VS prior to discharge			DC Incentive Spirometer	
DISCHARGE	**No wound complications. Afebrile / VSS** **Circulation adequate.**	**Seen by Social Work** **Seen by Reach to Recovery**	**CBC stable**	**No pulmonary complications.** **JP sites clean**	**As prior to admission except restrictions to affected extremity**
	SIGNATURE	**INIT.**	**SIGNATURE**	**INIT.**	**SIGNATURE**	**INIT.**

MEDS/IVS	1 NUTRITION	3, 4 PATIENT/FAMILY EDUCATION	2, 3, 4 DISCHARGE PLANNING	2, 3 PSYCHOSOCIAL/ EMOTIONAL/ SPIRTUAL NEEDS	INITALS (SEE KEY AT BOTTOM)		
		Reach to Recovery: Peer counseling MD: Arm mobility Showering Follow-up Activity Nursing: JP care, emptying, measuring	Social Work Home care support referral if needed				
		MD: Reinforce instruction Nursing: Validate learning Review DC summary with pt. Review DC meds with pt. if prescribed					
IV site without signs of phlebitis		**Identifies support systems and resources.** **Able to verbalize/demonstrate:** **JP care/emptying and measuring** **Arm protection** **Activity/exercise** **S/Sx infection** **Importance of BSE** **MD follow-up**	**Home with appropriate level of care.**	**Verbalizes feelings R / T dx and surgery.**			

SIGNATURE	INIT.	SIGNATURE	INIT.	SIGNATURE	INIT.

Medical-Surgical Care

Metric Conversions*

LENGTH

1 in (in)	= 2.5 centimeters (cm)
1 foot (ft)	= 30 cm
1 yard (yd)	= 0.9 meters (m)
1 mile	= 1.6 kilometers (km)

MASS (WEIGHT)

1 ounce (oz)	= 28 grams (g)
1 pound (lb)	= 0.45 kilogram (kg)
1 short ton (2000 lb)	= 0.9 tonne

VOLUME

1 teaspoon (tsp)	= 5 milliliters (ml)
1 tablespoon (tbsp)	= 15 ml
1 fluid ounce (fl oz)	= 30 ml
1 cup	= 0.24 liters (L)
1 pint (pt)	= 0.47 L
1 quart (qt)	= 0.95 L
1 gallon (gal)	= 3.8 L

*Appropriate conversions to metric measures.

Mass Equivalents for Medications (Metric and Apothecary System)

Apothecary (grains)	Metric (mg)	Metric (g)
1/200	0.3	0.0003
1/150	0.4	0.0004
1/100	0.6	0.0006
1/60	1	0.001
1/30	2	0.002
1/20	3	0.003
1/15	4	0.004
1/10	6	0.006
1/8	8	0.008
1/6	10	0.010
1/4	15	0.015
1/3	20	0.020
1/2*	30	0.030
3/4	50	0.050
1	60	0.060
1½	100	0.100
2	120	0.12
2½	150	0.15
3	200	0.2
4	250	0.25
5	300	0.3
7½	500	0.5
10	600	0.6
15	1000	1.0
30	2000	2.0

*From ½ to 5 grains; the following more accurate "approximate equivalents" are also acceptable.

¼ grain = 16 mg	2½ grains = 160 mg
½ grain = 32 mg	3 grains = 200 mg
1 grain = 65 mg	4 grains = 260 mg
1½ grains = 100 mg	5 grains = 325 mg
2 grains = 130 mg	

Liquid Equivalent for Medication

Apothecary and Customary*	Metric (ml)
1 minim	0.06
5 minims	0.3
10 minims	0.6
15 minims	1
60 minims (1 fluid dram or ⅛ fl oz)	4
75 minims (1¼ fluid drams)	5.0
240 minims (4 fluid drams or ½ fl oz)	15
1 fl oz	30
2 fl oz	60
3 fl oz	90
4 fl oz	120
6 fl oz	180
8 fl oz	240
12 fl oz	360
16 fl oz (1 pt)	480
32 fl oz (1 qt)	960
35 fl oz	1000 (1 L)
64 fl oz	1825
128 fl oz (1 gal)	3650

*Minims, fluid drams, or fl oz.

24 Hr Clock System

Conventional 12 hr Time	24 hr Clock Time
12:01 AM	0001
1:00 AM	0100
1:30 AM	0130
2:00 AM	0200
3:00 AM	0300
4:00 AM	0400
5:00 AM	0500
6:00 AM	0600
7:00 AM	0700
8:00 AM	0800
9:00 AM	0900
10:00 AM	1000
11:00 AM	1100
12 noon	1200
1:00 PM	1300
2:00 PM	1400
3:00 PM	1500
4:00 PM	1600
5:00 PM	1700
6:00 PM	1800
7:00 PM	1900
8:00 PM	2000
9:00 PM	2100
10:00 PM	2200
11:00 PM	2300
12 midnight	2400

Linear Equivalents

Inches	Centimeters (cm)	Meters (m)
0.5	1.25	0.0125
1	2.5	0.025
2	5.1	0.051
3	7.6	0.076
4	10.2	0.10
5	12.7	0.13
6	15.2	0.15
7	17.8	0.18
8	20.8	0.20
9	23.0	0.23
10	25.4	0.25
12	30.5	0.30
18	45.7	0.46
24	61.0	0.61
30	76.2	0.76
36	91.4	0.91
42	106.7	1.07
48	121.9	1.22
54	137.2	1.37
60	152.4	1.52
66	167.6	1.63
72	182.9	1.83

Centigrade-Fahrenheit Equivalents*

Centigrade (C)	Fahrenheit (F)
36.0	96.8
36.5	97.7
37.0	98.6
37.5	99.5
38.0	100.4
38.5	101.3
39.0	102.2
39.5	103.2
40.0	104.0
40.5	104.9
41.0	105.8
41.5	106.7
42.0	107.6

*CONVERSION
F to C: subtract 32, then multiply by $\frac{5}{9}$.
C to F: multiply by $\frac{9}{5}$, then add 32.

Combined Care Paths and Documentation Forms

With the increased use of flow charts, 24-hour documentation forms, preprinted care plans, and timeline-based plans of care or care paths, there have been some very successful attempts at avoiding duplication of documentation. This has been achieved by combining these formats to provide one chart form. These types of combination forms save time and money and serve to streamline documentation as well as provide a single guide for all nursing staff and other multidisciplinary healthcare providers to track and monitor the patient's progress.

The Total Hip Care Path: Inpatient Phase represents a combination of a care path and a multiple day documentation tool. The Care Path for the Vaginal Delivery delineates the Standard of Care, The Standard of Practice, and the Physician's role and provides a documentation tool for the patient during the expected length of the patient's stay. In the Family Centered Maternity Unit, the Newborn documentation tools are included as part of the maternal packet since mother and baby are not separated during the hospital stay. These forms provide a comprehensive but efficient documentation system for the staff who can then focus more time on direct patient care and teaching and less time on indirect care activities, namely inefficient documentation tools.

Panorama City Medical Center

TOTAL HIP CARE PATH: In-Patient Phase
☛ *This Care Path will be INDIVIDUALIZED for each patient.*

Instructions: Initial box when intervention is implemented. Mark box with × if findings Not Within Normal Limits or intervention Not Implemented (then write documentation of the situation in the progress notes), or when Goal is Not Met. Mark box with ∅ if intervention is Not Applicable.

CARE PATH DAY	DAY 1				DAY 2				DAY 3			
PAGE 1	SURGERY DAY-ROOM #				ROOM #				ROOM #			
Write date →	DATE	N	D	E	DATE	N	D	E	DATE	N	D	E
● TESTS	X-ray _____ hip											
H/H post-op, then CBC Q AM ×3	H&H				CBC: H/H / Platelet				CBC: H/H / Platelet			
● ASSESSMENT:	*Write time done →*				*Write time done →*				*Write time done →*			
NEURO: •alert, awake •oriented ×3 •PERLA •no numbness	Assessed WNL				Assessed WNL				Assessed WNL			
CARDIO: •regular HR •peripheral pulses + •extremities warm •capillary refill 3-5 sec. •No calf tenderness •sensation intact •no edema	Assessed WNL				Assessed WNL				Assessed WNL			
RESP: •RR >10/regular •adequate depth •clear breath sounds •nailbeds pink	Assessed WNL				Assessed WNL				Assessed WNL			
GI: •bowel sounds + •no nausea/vomiting •no abd. distention •stool *(character & #)*	Assessed WNL				Assessed WNL				Assessed WNL			
GU: •clear urine •can empty bladder •no bladder distention	Assessed WNL				Assessed WNL				Assessed WNL			
SKIN: •warm, dry, intact •skin color good •no pressure ulcers to bony areas- esp. heels •IV site clear *(write type, insertion date and site)* •incision appearance - •surgical dressing - •drainage character -	Assessed WNL				Assessed WNL				Assessed WNL			
MUSCULOSKELETAL: •CSM intact____ leg •proper alignment •no int./ext. hip rotation •able to do ROM	Assessed WNL				Assessed WNL				Assessed WNL			
PAIN: location and description *(intensity in pain graph)*	No Pain: WNL				No Pain: WNL				No Pain: WNL			
BEHAVIOR: •coping effectively •no multiple requests	Assessed WNL				Assessed WNL				Assessed WNL			
** RN Teamleader concurs with above assessments		11-7 7-3 3-11				11-7 7-3 3-11				11-7 7-3 3-11		
● TREATMENTS												
VS-Duramorph x24h	see pain graph/TPR				VS q4, then QID-see TPR				VS QID-see TPR			
SCD												
TEDS with heel cut off taken off/on BID												
Heel protectors												
Abduction pillow												
ROM to extremities												
Check drainage, I&O												
I/O cath or Foley									★			
Elevated toilet seat	Start with Stage III				★				★			
Fall protocol/Trapeze												
Drains	Autovac / Hemovac				Hemovac				DC Hemovac			
Therapeutic *(write time)* Positioning (L) (R) (S)												

CARE PATH DAY PAGE 2	DAY 1 SURGERY: ROOM #		N	D	E	DAY 2 ROOM #		N	D	E	DAY 3 ROOM #		N	D	E
Write date →	DATE		N	D	E	DATE		N	D	E	DATE		N	D	E
Transfuse ___/___ units if Hct < ____/____ %															
● HYGIENE: Bath	☐ Full ☐ Partial					☐ Full ☐ Partial					☐ Full ☐ Partial				
How accomplished?	☐ Self ☐ Assist					☐ Self ☐ Assist					☐ Self ☐ Assist				
● SAFETY															
Siderails ↑															
Bed Position - low															
Call light w/in reach															
ID band correct															
● MEDICATIONS															
IV therapy	see MAR					Heplock, if no PCA ... see MAR					Heplock, if no PCA ... see MAR				
Pain Medications	see MAR & pain graph					see MAR & pain graph					see MAR & pain graph				
Antibiotic IVPB	see					see MAR					see MAR				
Iron Meds	Medication					see MAR					see MAR				
Stool Softener	Administration					see MAR					see MAR				
Antiemetic Meds	Record					see MAR					see MAR				
Antipyretic Meds	(MAR)					see MAR					see MAR				
Anticoagulant Meds	*** start Enoxaparin day after surgery					see MAR					see MAR				
Restart Home Meds	Orders made					Continue home meds		see MAR			Continue home meds		see MAR		
● DIET: As ordered		B	L	D			B	L	D			B	L	D	
Consumption *(write %)*															
Food taken per -	☐ Self ☐ Assist					☐ Self ☐ Assist					☐ Self ☐ Assist				
● PHYSICAL ACTIVITY	Bedrest					Stage 1 protocol--isometric exercises, dangling at bedside					Stage II (if drain out) -exercises, dangling tranfers to chair				
Stage Protocol															
Weight bearing						WB _____					WB _____				

● TEACHING Patient Outcomes: 1=Needs reinforcement 2=Partial understanding 3=Complete understanding/skill. *Write rating in box.*

Orient to unit routine											★				
Daily Plan of care	Review patient copy					Review patient copy									
Activity restriction															
Therapeutic position: hip flexion not > 75°															
Use of triflow, CDBE															
Use of SCD & TEDS															
Use of CPM, Trapeze															
Pain Mgt Meds/Rx															
Duramorph side effects											★				
● DISCHARGE PLANNING	Provide patient copy of care path					Order DME Refer to SNF Make HH referral									
● DAILY PATIENT GOALS	Normal vital signs					Proper position for bedside dangling					Safe transfer to chair				
	No resp. depression										Hip flexion not > 75°				
	Good pain control					Good pain control					Good pain control				
	No s/s of complications					No s/s of complications					No s/s of complications				
● InterDisciplinary Signatures. Review of Care Path done q shift by nursing						PT					PT				
	CM					CM					CM				
	11-7					11-7					11-7				
	7-3					7-3					7-3				
	3-11					3-11					3-11				

PAIN GRAPH. Patient's desired goal is _____ on 0-10 pain scale. Obtain pain rating before & after each intervention.

DATE		24	01	02	03	04	05	06	07	08	09	10	11	12	13	14	15	16	17	18	19	20	21	22	23
PAIN RATINGS Draw a dot inside the box or on the line for each pain rating.	10																								
	8																								
	6																								
	4																								
	2																								
	0																								
Respiratory Rate																									
Depth of Respiration ♣																									
Level of Arousal ♥																									
O₂ Saturation																									

See page 5 for Code Depth of Respiration and Level of Arousal

Panorama City Medical Center

Provider Initial & Date	STANDARDS OF CARE Outcomes	Target Date	STANDARDS OF PRACTICE Interventions
	Patient will be monitored for any side effects of intrathecal or epidural narcotics for early intervention; e.g. respiratory depression, itchiness, nausea or vomiting, urinary retention.	Care Path Day 1-2	**Anesthesia:** Initiate pre-printed MD order sheet & manage patient's pain × 24 hours. **Nursing:** Monitor RR, depth, level of arousal, O_2 Sat q 1 hr × 16 hrs, q 2 hrs ×2. Initiate Regional Narcotic protocol. Assess for any side effect & manage per MD orders. Notify Anesthesiologist as needed for pain mgt. × 24 hrs.
	Patient will verbalize relief or control of pain symptoms per patient's desired rating of _____ on 0-10 scale with the use of oral analgesics.	Care Path Day 3-4	**Ortho MD:** Initiate pre-printed post-op order sheet, PCA order sheet & other follow-up orders. Evaluate pain control daily. **Nursing:** Assess pain level using 0-10 scale before and after each intervention. Document on pain flow sheet. Use parenteral narcotics & offer regularly first 48 hours. Inform patient of need to report pain & rating. Change position q 2 hours; use pillows for support; relieve any pressure. Use distraction/diversional techniques. Notify surgeon for modifications in treatment plan, as needed.
	Patient will experience an absence of complication, e.g. a. hemorrhage	Care Path Day 1-5	**Nursing:** Monitor VS, note amount of bloody drainage from operative site q shift. Autotransfuse as indicated. Check H/H & platelet values daily. **Ortho MD:** Evaluate drainage output q shift and H/H & platelet values daily × 3.
	b. dislocation of prosthesis	Care Path Day 1-5	**Nursing:** Maintain therapeutic positioning q shift, to include use abduction pillow between legs at all times; maintain proper alignment; turn to unaffected side; avoid hip flexion greater than 75°. Activity restriction: avoid crossing legs; use raised toilet seat. Assess for s/s: extremity shortened, internal or external rotation, severe hip pain, unable to move leg. Notify MD. **Ortho MD:** Evaluate alignment daily & determine for any s/s.
	c. neurovascular compromise	Care Path Day 1-5	**Nursing:** Assess CSM (circulation, sensation, movement) q shift. Observe for edema or swelling. Encourage patient to do ROM q shift. **Ortho MD:** Determine neurovascular status of limb daily.
	d. deep vein thrombosis (DVT)	Care Path Day 1-5	**Nursing:** Use TEDS & SCD. Remove & reapply TEDS 2x/day- AM bath & HS. Assess pulses q shift, avoid pressure beneath knee. Assess lung status q shift. Administer anticoagulant Rx. **Ortho MD:** Order prophylactic anticoagulant medications. Check platelet status if on Enoxaparin (Lovenox) Rx. daily × 3.
	e. wound infeciton	Care Path Day 1-5	**Nursing:** Monitor VS q shift/ BID. Assess wound appearance & drainage q shift. Administer Antibiotic meds as ordered. **Ortho MD:** Check on wound appearance & other s/s daily.
	Patient will verbalize under-standing of care & demonstrate patient care skills. Any Barriers to Learning? ☐ None ☐ Language ☐ Cultural/Religious Practices ☐ Emotional ☐ Desire/Motivation ☐ Limited Learning Ability ☐ Physical Limitation	Care Path Day 4	**Nursing:** Instruct patient on daily plan. Give patient copy of Care Path. Inform on need/purpose for triflow, SCD, TEDS, abduction pillow, pain meds, ROM exercises, activity restriction & therapeutic positioning. Reinforce PT instructions on exercises. Review "After Total Hip" booklet information prior to DC. If on Enoxaparin (Lovenox) Rx, start patient teaching on self-injection of anticoagulant on post-op day 3 in preparation for DC. Provide booklet. **PT:** Provide instrucitonsd on safe transfers and use of assistive device.
	Patient will ambulate and perform transfers safely with use of assistive device.	Care Path Day 4	**Nursing:** Use trapeze when in bed. Reinforce activities upon release by PT to Nursing. Encourage exercises while in bed. **PT:** Activity per stage protocol. Instruct and supervise patient on proper use of walker or crutches, and on safe transfers. Communicate with nursing on pre-medication of patient for pain prior to activity. Communicate daily with nursing on progress with patient activity.
	Patient will be discharged home safely with family and home health follow-up. Patient & care provider knowledgeable of care after DC.	Care Path Day 4-5	**Case Manager:** Assess DC needs preop & postop - DME, Home Health follow-up. Arrange for SNF transfer, if indicated. **Nursing:** Reinforce MD/PT instructions on activity, restrictions, medications, return appt., s/s to report to MD before DC. Ensure DC orders to include prophylactic anticoagulant Rx, if indicated.

NOTE: If patient develops any other problems, nursing or the department will initiate a plan of care for that specific problem and address the interventions and outcomes in the Progress Notes for Care Path Variances.

THR care Path 7/95

PAGE 4 *PAIN GRAPH: Patient's desired goal is _____ on 0-10 scale. Obtain pain rating before and after each intervention.*

DATE		24	01	02	03	04	05	06	07	08	09	10	11	12	13	14	15	16	17	18	19	20	21	22	23
PAIN RATINGS Draw a dot inside the box or on the line for each pain rating.	10																								
	8																								
	6																								
	4																								
	2																								
	0																								
Respiratory Rate																									
Depth of Respiration ♣																									
Level of Arousal ♥																									
O₂ Saturation																									

♣ Depth of Respiration: A=Adequate and Normal N=Not Adequate and Shallow

♥ Level of Arousal: 2=Patient awake 1=Patient frequently drowsy but easily aroused O-Patient somnolent & difficult to arouse S=Normal sleep, patient easily aroused.

DATE		24	01	02	03	04	05	06	07	08	09	10	11	12	13	14	15	16	17	18	19	20	21	22	23
PAIN RATINGS Draw a dot inside the box or on the line for each pain rating.	10																								
	8																								
	6																								
	4																								
	2																								
	0																								
Respiratory Rate																									
Level of Arousal ♥																									

DATE		24	01	02	03	04	05	06	07	08	09	10	11	12	13	14	15	16	17	18	19	20	21	22	23
PAIN RATINGS Draw a dot inside the box or on the line for each pain rating.	10																								
	8																								
	6																								
	4																								
	2																								
	0																								
Respiratory Rate																									
Level of Arousal ♥																									

DATE		24	01	02	03	04	05	06	07	08	09	10	11	12	13	14	15	16	17	18	19	20	21	22	23
PAIN RATINGS Draw a dot inside the box or on the line for each pain rating.	10																								
	8																								
	6																								
	4																								
	2																								
	0																								
Respiratory Rate																									
Level of Arousal ♥																									

DATE		24	01	02	03	04	05	06	07	08	09	10	11	12	13	14	15	16	17	18	19	20	21	22	23
PAIN RATINGS Draw a dot inside the box or on the line for each pain rating.	10																								
	8																								
	6																								
	4																								
	2																								
	0																								
Respiratory Rate																									
Level of Arousal ♥																									

CARE PATH DAY	DAY 4				DAY 5				DAY 6			
PAGE 5	ROOM #				ROOM #				DISCHARGE - ROOM #			
Write date →	DATE	N	D	E	DATE	N	D	E	DATE	N	D	E
● TESTS	CBC: H/H				★				★			
CBC q AM ×3	Platelet				★				★			
● ASSESSMENT:	Write time done →				Write time done →				Write time done →			
NEURO: •alert, awake •oriented ×3 •PERLA •no numbness	Assessed WNL				Assessed WNL				Assessed WNL			
CARDIO: •regular HR •peripheral pulses + •extremities warm •capillary refill 3-5 sec. •no calf tenderness •sensation intact •no edema	Assessed WNL				Assessed WNL				Assessed WNL			
RESP: RR•>10/regular •adequate depth •clear breath sounds •nailbeds pink	Assessed WNL				Assessed WNL				Assessed WNL			
GI: •bowel sounds + •no nausea/vomiting •no abd. distention •stool (character & #)	Assessed WNL				Assessed WNL				Assessed WNL			
GU: •clear urine •can empty bladder •no bladder distention	Assessed WNL				Assessed WNL				Assessed WNL			
SKIN: •warm, dry, intact •skin color good •no pressure ulcers to bony areas- esp. heels •IV site clear (write type, insertion date and site) •incision appearance - •surgical dressing - •drain site appearance -	Assessed WNL				Assessed WNL				Assessed WNL			
MUSCULOSKELETAL •CSM intact____ leg •proper alignment •no int./ext. hip rotation •able to do ROM	Assessed WNL				Assessed WNL				Assessed WNL			
PAIN: location and description (intensity in pain graph)	No Pain: WNL				No Pain: WNL				No Pain: WNL			
BEHAVIOR: •coping effectively •no multiple requests	Assessed WNL				Assessed WNL				Assessed WNL			
** RN Teamleader concurs with above assessments				11-7 7-3 3-11				11-7 7-3 3-11				11-7 7-3 3-11
● TREATMENTS												
Vital signs BID	see TPR				see TPR				see TPR			
SCD												
TEDS with heel cut off taken off/on BID												
Heel protectors												
Abduction pillow												
ROM to extremities												
Check dressing												
I/O cath or Foley	★				★				★			
Elevated toilet seat												
Fall protocol/Trapeze												
Activity												
Therapeutic (write time) Positioning (L) (R) (S)												
● HYGIENE												
Bath	☐ Full ☐ Partial				☐ Full ☐ Partial				☐ Full ☐ Partial			
How accomplished?	☐ Self ☐ Assist				☐ Self ☐ Assist				☐ Self ☐ Assist			
● SAFETY												
Side rails↑												
Bed position - low												

CARE PATH DAY PAGE 6 Write date →	DAY 4 ROOM # DATE	N	D	E	DAY 5 ROOM # DATE	N	D	E	DAY 6 DISCHARGE - ROOM # DATE	N	D	E
Call light w/in reach												
ID band correct												
● MEDICATIONS												
Pain Meds	IM or PO: see MAR & Pain Graph				PO meds: see MAR and graph				PO meds: see MAR and graph			
Iron Meds	see MAR				see MAR				see MAR			
Stool Softener	see MAR				see MAR				see MAR			
Antiemetic Meds	see MAR				see MAR				see MAR			
Anticoagulant Meds	see MAR				see MAR				see MAR			
Continue Home Med	see MAR				see MAR				see MAR			

● DIET: As ordered		B	L	D		B	L	D		B	L	D
Consumption (write %)												
Food taken per -	☐ Self ☐ Assist				☐ Self ☐ Assist				☐ Self ☐ Assist			

● PHYSICAL ACTIVITY												
Stage Protocol	Stage III: exercises, toilet transfers gait trng walker/crutches				Continue Stage III: -toilet transfers gait trng walker/crutches				Continue Stage III: -transfer skills and gait trng & exercises			
Weight bearing	WB				WB				WB			
Occupational therapy	OT to assess ADLs				★				★			

● TEACHING Patient Outcomes: 1=Needs reinforcement 2=Partial understanding 3=Complete understanding/skill. *Write rating in box.*

Daily Plan of care												
Exercises												
Activity restriction: use abduction pillow												
Therapeutic position: hip flexion not > 75°												
Anticoagulant Rx: self-injection and s/s to report to MD	Use booklet and video											
DC instructions on meds, return appt., s/s to report to MD												
Review "After Total Hip" booklet info	"Recovering in the Hospital"				"Mastering Daily Activities & Going Home"				"Recovering At Home"			

● DISCHARGE PLANNING												
					Give info. for Home Heath follow-up				Provide equipment for home care			
					Review home care plans							

● DAILY PATIENT GOALS												
	Ambulates with walker or crutches				Ambulates with walker or crutches				Ambulates safely with device, stairs PRN			
	Safe transfers				Safe transfers				Safe transfers			
	WB as instructed				WB as instructed				WB as instructed			
	No s/s of complications				No s/s: DVT, infection				No s/s: DVT, infection			
	Good pain control				Good pain control				Good pain control			
									Know self-care for DC			

● InterDisciplinary Signatures.	PT				PT				PT			
	CM				CM				CM			
	OT											
Review of Care Path done q shift by nursing	11-7				.11-7				11-7			
	7-3				7-3				7-3			
	3-11				3-11				3-11			

ACUITY LEVEL: Patient acuity level on Care Path Day 1 (Surgery Day) and Care Path Days 2-5 is classified as 3. Acuity level on Day of Discharge is 2. Any variance from these acuity levels will be documented in the Progress Notes for Care Path Variances.

DOCUMENTATION GUIDELINES: Initialing box indicates that intervention was implemented and patient outcomes are within standards. If patient goes beyond (positive variance) or falls below (negative variance) expected daily outcomes or assessment findings are Not Within Normal Limits, or any item with a (★) symbol, nursing will document in the Progress Notes for Care Path Variances.

☞ All assigned nurses are responsible for updating, reviewing the care path, and evaluating the daily goals. Affix signature for each shift and use the end-of-shift reporting.

KAISER PERMANENTE PANORAMA CITY
Vaginal Delivery

RN Initial	Standard of Care Outcomes	Zones	Standards of Practice Interventions	Physicians
	Patient will not have excessive Bleeding during hospitalization (no more than 2 pads/hour) (see discharge info sheet).	1,2 3	Check flow and fundus at least once per shift	MD/CNM initiate preprinted orders (Zone 1)
	Patient will void at least once during the first eight hours following delivery.	1	Measure output of first voiding and record. Encourage fluid intake between meals (Zones 1, 2, 3)	Initiate follow-up orders as needed (Zone 1, 2, 3).
	Patient will not develop redness and swelling or infection in perineal area during hospitalization.	1,2,3	Continuous use of ice or iced pad to perineum per MD order. Check perineal area to determine signs of infection on admission and discharge. Check temperature and lacertation repair on admission and at discharge.	Orders patient discharge and provides instructions (Zone 3).
	Patient will report minimal discomfort from pain on oral medication.	1,2,3	Instruct patient to report onset of pain ASAP. Assess pain and record. Give MD ordered pain medication PRN. Assess effectiveness of pain medication within 1 hour and record.	
	Patient will be able to demonstrate or verbalize knowledge and skill in self care and baby care by the time of discharge. Barriers to Learning (Check those that apply) ____None ____Culture ____Religious/Spiritual Practices ____Emotional Barriers ____Desire/Motivation ____Physical Limitation ____Limited Learning Ability	1,2,3	See Postpartum Patient/ Significant Other Education and Discharge Record.	
	Patient needs will be met despite inability to speak English.	1,2,3	Use Spanish speaking nurse or interpreter for communication. Utilize Guide for Parents (20 languages) as necessary. Encourage listening and viewing of Spanish tapes and CCTV. Utilize AT&T Language line as necessary.	

Catagories	Zone 1 (0-8hours)	Zone 2 (8-16 hours)	Zone 3 (16-24 hours)

Consults:
Social Service
 	
Home Heath
 	
Lactation
  Consultant
 	
Other:
	See Education and
	  Discharge Record
	
	See Progress Notes
	
	_____
		See Education and
		  Discharge Record
		
		See Progress Notes
		
		_____
			See Education and
			  Discharge Record
			See Education and
			  Discharge Record
			See Progress Notes
			
			_____

Teaching and Discharge Planning:	See Education and
	  Discharge Record
		See Education and
		  Discharge Record
			See Education and
			  Discharge Record

Bonding:
Enfold-Enface
Actively Care
  For Infant
Encourage
  Talking to
  Infant
	_____
	
	_____
	
	_____
		_____
		
		_____
		
		_____
			_____
			
			_____
			
			_____

Safety:
  Siderails
  Bed Position
  Call Bell
	Up Down
	Up Down
	Within Reach Yes No
		Up Down
		Up Down
		Within Reach Yes No
			Up Down
			Up Down
			Within Reach Yes No

Transfer Assessment

SKIN:
- Warm/Dry _____
- Pink _____
- Pale/Cool _____
- *Other: _____

_____ _____

BREASTS:
- Soft _____

NIPPLES:
- Inverted/Flat _____
- *Other: _____

_____ _____

LOCHIA:
- Light _____
- Moderate _____
- Heavy _____

Edema Location Code
F=Feet L=Legs H=Hands
E=Eyelids G=Generalized

EPISIOTOMY/LACERATION:
- Intact _____
- Swelling _____
- *Other: _____

_____ _____

CARDIOVASCULAR:
- Heart Sounds:
- Regular/*Irregular _____
- Edema _____
- Dizziness _____
- *Other: _____

_____ _____

NEUROLOGICAL:
- Alert/Oriented _____
- *Other: _____

_____

Edema Code
4=large,pitting 3=mod. large
2=moderate 1=minimal
TR=trace

ELIMINATION:
- Distended Bladder _____
- *Other: _____

_____ _____

PSYCHOSOCIAL:
- Appropriate Affect _____
- *Depressed _____
- Infant in NICU _____
- *Other: _____

_____

IV SITE:
- Location _____
- Condition _____
- Discontinued _____

IV Condition Code
P=Patent R=Reddened
E=Edematous

IV Location Code
R=Right L=Left
A=Arm H=Hand

Transfer Assessment: Time_____   _____ **RN/LVN**

*DOCUMENT STARRED ITEMS AND/OR VARIANCES

SHIFT	INITIAL	SIGNATURE	INITIAL	SIGNATURE
☽ ☽ ☽ NOCS				
☼☼☼ DAYS				
★ ★ ★ EVES				

KASIER PERMANENTE PANORAMA CITY
Date of Birth _____

Care Path: **Newborn Record**
Catagories   **Zone 1 (0-8 hours)**   **Zone 2 (8-16 hours)**   **Zone 3 (16-24 hours)**
       Time:

Categories	Zone 1 (0-8 hours)	Zone 2 (8-16 hours)	Zone 3 (16-24 hours)

Assessment:
 	
a. Vital Signs
    Time:
 	
 Temp
 Apical Pulse
 Respiratory Rate
b. Activity
  Sleeping
  Awake
  Alert
 *Irritable
 *Lethargic
 *Jittery
  Mother/Inf.
  Interaction
	Admission Assessment
	See Back
	
	Time _____
	_____
	_____
	_____
	_____
	_____
	_____
	_____
	
	Refer to Newborn
	Discharge Instructions
		See Progress Notes
		
		Time _____
		_____
		_____
		_____
		_____
		_____
		_____
		_____
			See Newborn Discharge
			Instructions
			
			See Newborn Discharge
			Instructions
			
			See Newborn Discharge
			Instructions

Treatments:	Bath: Time _____
	Circ. Time _____
	   Vaseline _____
	   *Bleeding _____
	Gomco Mogen Sheldon
	Warming Measures:
	 Hat Warmed Blanket
	 Heat Lamp
		Circ. Time _____
		   Vaseline _____
		   *Bleeding _____
		Gomco Mogen Sheldon
		
		 *Heat Warmed Blanklet
		 Heat Lamp
			Circ. Time _____
			   Vaseline _____
			   *Bleeding
			Gomco Mogen Sheldon

Medications: Time/Init. _____ Time/Init. _____	0.5cc HBV IM RAT LAT Lot # _____ Other _____ _____	0.5cc HBV IM RAT LAT Lot # _____	HBV Recorded in KIT Date _____ Initials _____
Tests: MD Exam Urine Tox Hct. Chemstrip Newborn Screen *Other:	Time_____ Time Sent: _____ Result:_____ Time:_____ Result:_____ Time:_____ Result:_____ Time:_____ Result:_____ Time:_____ _____	*Result:_____ Time:_____ _____	*Result:_____ Time:_____ See Discharge Instructions _____

Diet:
    Time:
Breast min.   R
          L
Bottle cc.
 Other:
Suck/Swallow
*Emesis
	Observed: Yes ____ No____	Observed: Yes ____ No____	Observed: Yes ____ No____

Elimination: Time: Urine Stool: M/T			

RN Initial	Standards of Care Outcomes	Zones	Standards of Practice Interventions	Physicians
	Infant will successfully adapt to extrauterine life.	1	Observe and record skin color, activity, temperature, feeding and elimination at least once per shift.	Performs PE exam and verbalizes results to parent(s) Initiates pre-printed orders. (Zone 1) Initiates follow-up orders as needed. (Zone 1,2,3)
	Infant will be in stable condition at time of discharge.	3	See above. Observe and record.	
	Hypoglycemia will not occur during the transition period.	1	Obtain Chemstrips per MD order and document results. Notify MD if chemstrip less than 40 mg/dl and order stat blood sugar. Observe for signs of jitteriness and irritability.	
	Excessive circ bleeding will not occur during hospital stay.	1,2,3	Observe for bleeding from circ site. Apply pressure and notify OB MD for reasessment PRN.	
	Acceptance into the family unit with reciprocal interaction.	1,2,3	Observe and record parent/infant interaction.	

SKIN:		HEAD:		HEART:		EYES:	
Warm	___	Rounded	___	Regular Rhythm	___	Sclera Clear	___
Pink	___	Cephalhematoma	___	*Irreg. Rhythm	___	Discharge	___
*Pale	___	Molding	___	*Murmur	___	Edema	___
*Acrocyanosis	___	Caput	___	**ABDOMEN:**		Hemorrhage	___
*Dusky	___	Overriding		Soft/No Disten.	___	**CHEST/LUNGS:**	
*Plethoric	___	Sutures	___	*Distended	___	Breath Sounds	
*Jaundice	___	Fonts Flat/Soft	___	Bowel Sounds	___	Clear Bilat.	___
Good Turgor	___	*Fonts Bulging	___	**EXTREMITIES:**		*Abnormal	
Dry/Peeling	___	**NEUROLOGICAL**		Symet. Moves	___	BS	___
*Ecchymosis	___	**REFLEXES:**		Spontan. Moves	___	*Nasal Flaring	___
*Abrasions	___	Nml suck, root, cry	___	**ANUS:**		*Retractions	___
		Nml grasp & moro	___	Patent	___	*Grunting	___

Physical Assessment: Time _____ _____ **RN/LVN**

SECURITY: ID BAND # _____
ID Check/Shift: Days _____ **PM's** _____ **Nocs** _____
After Circ _____ **After PKU** _____ **Other** _____

*DOCUMENT STARRED ITEMS AND/OR VARIANCES

SHIFT		INITIAL	SIGNATURE	INITIAL	SIGNATURE
☽ ☽ ☽	NOCS				
☼☼☼	DAYS				
★ ★ ★	EVES				

Date of Delivery: _____ **Gravida** _____ **Para** _____

Catagories Time:	Zone 1 (0-8 hours)	Zone 2 (8-16 hours)	Zone 3 (16-24 hours)
Assessment:	Transfer Assessment	See Progress Notes	See Education and Discharge Record
a. V S : Time			
Temp.			
Pulse			
Resp. Rate			
BP			
b. Activity	Ambulate with assistance	Up ad lib	Discharge
Treatments:			
Peri Care:			
a. peri bottle	_____	Self Care	Self Care
b. ice	_____	_____	_____
c. spray	_____	Self Care	Self Care
d. tucks / oint.	_____	Self Care	Self Care
Sitz Bath	_____	_____	_____
Catherize prn	_____	* _____	* _____
	cc. _____	cc. _____	cc. _____
Fundus Check Location	_____	_____	_____
Firm	_____	_____	_____
Boggy / Massaged	_____	_____	* _____
Medications:	See MAR	See MAR	See MAR
Pain	See PRN Medication Form	See PRN Medication Form	See PRN Medication Form
Management			
Tests:			
MD / CNM Visit	Time _____	Time _____	Time _____
H&H Drawn	Time _____	Time _____	Time _____
Type / RH	Time _____	Time _____	Time _____
Other: _____	Time _____	Time _____	Time _____
Diet:	Regular	Regular	Regular
Other: _____	_____	_____	_____
Elimination:	First Voiding Measured	*First Voiding Measured	
Voiding	_____ cc Time: _____	_____ cc Time: _____	
Encourage Fluid Intake Bowel Movement	_____	_____	See Eduacation and Discharge Record

Transfer Notes: Date_____ Time _____
    Transfer from Labor and Delivery via _____

    Patient oriented to: Room _____ Visiting Policy _____ Smoking _____

                        Infant Security System _____ Blue Badge _____

                        Patient understands: Yes_____ No_____

Medical History (Include Medications other than prenatal vitamins): _____
_____
_____

Discharge Planning Needs: (See Labor and Delivery Perinatal Record 2)
    Other: _____

Educational Needs: Knowledge related to self aand baby care.
    Other: _____

TIME	NURSING OBSERVATIONS

Index